Oxford Textbook of Med

Cardiovascular Disorders

Oxford Textbook of Medicine:
Cardiovascular Disorders

Selected and updated chapters from the Oxford Textbook of Medicine, Fifth Edition

Edited by

David A. Warrell

Emeritus Professor of Tropical Medicine, Centre for Tropical Diseases, Nuffield Department of Medicine, John Radcliffe Hospital, Oxford University Hospitals NHS Foundation Trust, Oxford, UK

Timothy M. Cox

Professor of Medicine, University of Cambridge, School of Clinical Medicine, Department of Medicine, Addenbrooke's Hospital, Cambridge, UK

John D. Firth

Consultant Physician and Nephrologist, Addenbrooke's Hospital, Cambridge, UK

With Guest Editor

Jeremy Dwight

Formerly Consultant Cardiologist, Department of Cardiology, John Radcliffe Hospital, Oxford University Hospitals NHS Foundation Trust, Oxford, UK

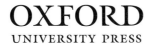

OXFORD
UNIVERSITY PRESS

OXFORD
UNIVERSITY PRESS

Great Clarendon Street, Oxford, ox2 6DP,
United Kingdom

Oxford University Press is a department of the University of Oxford.
It furthers the University's objective of excellence in research, scholarship,
and education by publishing worldwide. Oxford is a registered trade mark of
Oxford University Press in the UK and in certain other countries

Published in the United States of America by Oxford University Press
198 Madison Avenue, New York, NY 10016, United States of America

British Library Cataloguing in Publication Data
Data available

Library of Congress Control Number: 2015947233

ISBN 978–0–19–871702–7

Printed and bound in Great Britain by
Bell & Bain Ltd., Glasgow

Preface

A blizzard of medical information

Our understanding of the science of medicine continues to advance rapidly, and health and disease are always in fashion. A new outbreak of some particular infection attracts saturating media coverage, demanding instant containment, prevention, cure, and (usually) blame. A single medical paper, often without great merit, catches the eye of a news editor, and the urgent question at breakfast is 'should we all stop eating X?'. Treatment possibilities are more and more 'high tech' for those who can afford them. The findings of a preliminary clinical trial of a new biologic engineered by molecular medicine, or deployment of a complex endovascular device, are published in a carefully managed way. The new must be better than the old, and surely all (in the developed world) should have immediate access. Within a few hours commentators, some well-informed but many not so, appear out of the woodwork to expound their views.

Pretty well everyone is bombarded with medical matters by the media and has ready access to the cornucopia of medical information and misinformation that is 'Dr Google', but most patients have very limited capacity to sift the wheat from the chaff, and doctors don't have the time. The dramatic growth in the number of publications and journals in all areas of clinical medicine mean that it is now impossible for the general physician to keep track of the core literature in each specialty.

Sifting the wheat from the chaff

Doctors have always wanted ready access to reliable information, and never has the need been greater. Patients are more informed (and misinformed) about the conditions that they might or might not have. They increasingly expect to enter into a dialogue with their doctor about management options, and rightly resent the physician who routinely behaves in a paternalistic manner, although they may on occasion be very grateful when a wise doctor judges it a proper moment to say 'it's difficult, there isn't a clear right and wrong here, would you like me to tell you what I think would probably be best?'.

The fundamentals of medical practice remain as they always have been in living memory: the doctor talking with a patient, conducting a physical examination, making a diagnosis or differential diagnosis, requesting some investigations, recommending a management plan. Aside from the ability to communicate well, the key requirement is for good understanding of the basic biological and clinical aspects of diseases and their treatments, but how is this best achieved?

'The report of my death was an exaggeration'

This was the title of a statement published by Mark Twain in the New York Journal (2 June, 1897), the misunderstanding having arisen because his cousin was seriously ill in London at the time. We think that reports of the death of medical textbooks are similarly exaggerated. Never has there been greater need for doctors to have access to reliable and balanced accounts of diseases and their treatments.

Comprehensive guidelines published by specialist societies and other bodies now summarize the evidence base for many aspects of clinical practice, and (if well written) provide clear summaries of treatment and management recommendations for individual conditions. However, access to vast quantities of information does not help to put it in clinical context or organize it in terms of importance, and guidelines almost invariably assume the approach to diagnosis, the diagnosis itself, and consider the diagnosis in isolation. This is becoming more and more inappropriate. The population is aging, and with it the spectrum and complexity of disease is changing. It is increasingly irrelevant to consider one disease in isolation: many patients will have multiple co-morbidities. Diagnosis may have become easier with the advent of new and sophisticated imaging, although this has brought with it the challenge of the incidental finding, but the relative importance of each diagnosis and the way in which each affects the patient in generating the clinical presentation is becoming a greater and greater challenge.

Experienced clinicians recognize that there are many aspects of the practice of medicine that cannot be investigated by clinical trials or summarized in guidelines. This is often termed the 'art of medicine'; the method by which clinicians fuse knowledge of basic science and medical literature with accumulated experience to diagnose and treat patients. The medical textbook can describe this fusion better than any other means. Its accounts must, of course, include information from randomized controlled trials and meta-analyses of such, but must not shirk from giving a considered opinion even when the quality of evidence is poor or the situation complex. After all, the doctor may be faced with a patient unwise enough to have a disease that does not fit neatly into any category, or on which no trials of any real worth have been done, or to have many co-morbidities and be on an alarming number of medications.

The *Oxford Textbook of Medicine*

Since it first published in 1983, the *Oxford Textbook of Medicine* has sought out and obtained the best contributors to write authoritative accounts. Its approach has always been flexible. Authors have been encouraged to present information in a practical and usable format, encompassing both evidence based guidelines and their clinical experience derived from treating thousands of patients. It is of great benefit to its readers and testimony to the high quality of the book that few decline an invitation to write. The fifth edition (2010) brought the added advantage of online updates, allowing important new discoveries to be incorporated and placed within a proper context in a matter of months.

The *Oxford Textbook of Medicine: Cardiovascular Disorders*

Cardiovascular disease remains one of the main causes of morbidity and mortality, and increasingly so in the developing world. This revised and thoroughly updated edition of the cardiovascular disorders section of the *Oxford Textbook of Medicine, Fifth edition*, contains much that is new, ranging from advances in cardiac imaging to expanded coverage of heart failure and cardiac arrhythmias, recent argument that small adrenal tumours may cause hypertension, discussion of new oral anticoagulants, and recent updates of guidelines on rheumatic fever and infective endocarditis.

We hope that this new book, with its digital counterpart in the *Oxford Textbook of Medicine* online, will be a useful guide for physicians caring for patients with cardiovascular disorders, and help its many readers to sort the wheat from the chaff.

Contents

Contributors

Adrian P. Banning Professor of Interventional Cardiology, Consultant Cardiologist, Oxford University Hospitals NHS Foundation Trust, UK

Chapter 3.2, Chapter 14.1

D. Gareth Beevers Professor Emeritus, University of Birmingham Institute of Cardiovascular Sciences, City Hospital, Birmingham, UK

Chapter 17.5

Morris J. Brown Professor of Clinical Pharmacology, University of Cambridge, Addenbrookes Centre for Clinical Investigation (ACCI), Addenbrookes Hospital, Cambridge, UK

Chapter 17.3

Jonathan R. Carapetis Director, Telethon Kids Institute, University of Western Australia; Consultant, Princess Margaret Hospital for Children, Perth, Australia

Chapter 9.1

Joshua T. Chai MRC Clinical Research Training Fellow and Specialist Registrar in Cardiology, Department of Cardiovascular Medicine, University of Oxford, John Radcliffe Hospital, Oxford, UK

Chapter 13.1

Keith Channon Professor of Cardiovascular Medicine and Honorary Consultant Cardiologist at the John Radcliffe Hospital, UK

Chapter 1.1

Robin P. Choudhury Professor of Cardiovascular Medicine, University of Oxford, UK

Chapter 13.1

Andrew L. Clark Professor of Clinical Cardiology, Academic Cardiology, Hull and East Yorkshire Hospitals NHS Trust, UK

Chapter 5.2, Chapter 5.3

John G. F. Cleland Professor of Clinical Cardiology, National Heart & Lung Institute, Royal Brompton & Harefield Hospitals Trust London, UK; Honorary Professor of Cardiology, Hull York Medical School, University of Hull, UK

Chapter 5.2, Chapter 5.3

S. M. Cobbe Professor of Medical Cardiology, University of Glasgow, Glasgow, UK

Chapter 2.2, Chapter 4.2

Peter F. Currie Consultant Cardiologist & Clinical Director, Perth Royal Infirmary, Perth, and Ninewells Hospital, Dundee, UK

Chapter 9.3

Goodarz Danaei Assistant Professor of Global Health, Department of Global Health and Population; Department of Epidemiology, Harvard TH Chan School of Public Health, USA

Chapter 13.2

Alun Davies Professor of Vascular Surgery, Imperial College School of Medicine, London, UK

Chapter 14.2

Christopher Dudley Consultant Renal Physician, The Richard Bright Renal Unit, Southmead Hospital, North Bristol NHS Trust, Bristol, UK

Chapter 14.3

Jeremy Dwight Formerly Consultant Cardiologist, John Radcliffe Hospital, Oxford, UK

Chapter 2.1

Perry Elliott Director/Honorary Consultant, Inherited Heart Diseases Programme, The Heart Hospital, University College London, UK

Chapter 7.2, Chapter 7.3

Rhys D. Evans Reader, Department of Physiology, Anatomy and Genetics, University of Oxford, UK

Chapter 1.2

John D. Firth Consultant Physician and Nephrologist, Cambridge University Hospitals NHS Foundation Trust, Cambridge, UK

Chapter 16.1, Chapter 17.2, Chapter 20.1

Edward A. Fisher Leon H. Charney Professor of Cardiovascular Medicine; Director, Marc and Ruti Bell Program in Vascular Biology, and The Center for the Prevention of Cardiovascular Disease, NYU School of Medicine, USA; Visiting Professor of Cardiovascular Medicine, University of Oxford, UK

Chapter 13.1

Edward D. Folland Professor of Medicine Emeritus at University of Massachusetts Medical School, USA

Chapter 3.4, Chapter 13.5

Keith A. A. Fox Professor of Cardiology, University of Edinburgh

Chapter 13.4

David A. Gabbott Consultant Anaesthetist, Gloucestershire Hospitals NHS Foundation Trust UK; Chairman, Research Subcommittee, Resuscitation Council (UK) Executive Committee Resuscitation Council (UK)

Chapter 4.1

M. Ginks Oxford Heart Centre, Oxford University Hospitals NHS Foundation Trust, Oxford, UK

Chapter 4.2

David Gray Reader in Medicine & Honorary Consultant Physician (Retired), Department of Cardiovascular Medicine, Nottingham University Hospitals NHS Trust, Nottingham, UK

Chapter 3.1

Darren Green Clinical Lecturer in Nephrology, University of Manchester, UK

Chapter 5.4

Kaushik Guha Clinical Cardiology fellow, Royal Brompton Hospital, London, UK

Chapter 5.1

Oliver Guttmann Cardiology ST at Barts Heart Centre, London, UK

Chapter 7.2, Chapter 7.3

James L. Harrison Clinical Lecturer in Cardiology, King's College London, UK

Chapter 9.2

Catherine E. G. Head Consultant Cardiologist, Guy's and St Thomas' NHS Foundation Trust, London, UK

Chapter 18.1

Michael Henein Professor of Cardiology, Umea University, Sweden; Canterbury Christ Church University, UK

Chapter 6.1, Chapter 8.1

Andrew R. Houghton Consultant Cardiologist & Deputy Director of Medical Education, Grantham & District Hospital, Grantham, UK, and Visiting Fellow, University of Lincoln, Lincoln, UK

Chapter 3.1

Philip A. Kalra Consultant Nephrologist, Salford Royal NHS Foundation Trust, Salford, and Honorary Professor, University of Manchester, UK

Chapter 5.4

Theodoros Karamitsos Honorary Consultant Cardiologist, Oxford University Research Lecturer, Division of Cardiovascular Medicine, Radcliffe Department of Medicine, University of Oxford, John Radcliffe Hospital, Oxford University Hospitals NHS Foundation Trust, Oxford, UK

Chapter 3.3

David Keeling Oxford Haemophilia & Thrombosis Centre, Churchill Hospital, Oxford University Hospitals NHS Foundation Trust, Oxford, UK

Chapter 16.2

Andrew Kelion Consultant Cardiologist, Cardiology Department, John Radcliffe Hospital, Oxford University Hospitals NHS Foundation Trust, Oxford, UK

Chapter 3.3

Rajesh K. Kharbanda Consultant Cardiologist, John Radcliffe Hospital, Oxford University Hospitals NHS Foundation Trust, Oxford, UK

Chapter 13.4

Yasushi Kobayashi Department of Immunobiology, Yale University School of Medicine, New Haven, Connecticut, USA

Chapter 14.4

D. A. Lane Senior Lecturer in Cardiovascular Health, University of Birmingham Institute of Cardiovascular Sciences, City Hospital, Birmingham, UK

Chapter 4.2

Gregory Y.H. Lip Professor of Cardiovascular Medicine, University of Birmingham Institute of Cardiovascular Sciences, City Hospital, Birmingham, UK

Chapter 4.2, Chapter 17.5

William A. Littler Emeritus Professor of Clinical Cardiology, University of Birmingham, UK

Chapter 9.2

Kenneth T. MacLeod Reader in Cardiac Physiology, Faculty of Medicine, National Heart & Lung Institute, UK

Chapter 1.2

Steven B. Marston Professor of Cardiovascular Biochemistry, Faculty of Medicine, National Heart & Lung Institute, Imperial College, London, UK

Chapter 1.2

Jay W. Mason Professor of Medicine, Cardiology Division, University of Utah School of Medicine, Salt Lake City, Utah, USA

Chapter 7.1

Fadi Matta Staff Investigator, St. Mary Mercy Hospital, Graduate Medical Education, Research Department; Associate Professor, Department of Osteopathic Medical Specialties, College of Osteopathic Medicine, Michigan State University, Lansing, Michigan, USA

Chapter 16.1

Theresa A. McDonagh Consultant Cardiologist, King's College Hospital, Denmark Hill, London, UK

Chapter 5.1

A. D. McGavigan Professor of Cardiology, Heart and Vascular Institute, Flinders Medical Centre, Adelaide, Australia

Chapter 2.2, Chapter 4.2

William J. McKenna Professor of Cardiology, The Heart Hospital, University College London, UK

Chapter 7.2, Chapter 7.3

Fraz A. Mir Consultant Physician, Associate Lecturer, Department of Medicine, Cambridge University Hospitals NHS Foundation Trust, Addenbrooke's Hospital, Cambridge, UK

Chapter 17.3

Andrew R. J. Mitchell Consultant Cardiologist, Jersey General Hospital, Jersey, UK

Chapter 3.2, Chapter 14.1

Nicholas W. Morrell British Heart Foundation Professor of Cardiopulmonary Medicine, University of Cambridge School of Clinical Medicine, Addenbrooke's and Papworth Hospitals, Cambridge, UK

Chapter 15.1, Chapter 15.2

Peter S. Mortimer Professor of Dermatological Medicine to the University of London, Consultant Skin Physician to St George's Hospital, London and the Royal Marsden Hospital, London, UK

Chapter 19.1

Stefan Neubauer Professor of Cardiovascular Medicine, Clinical Director, Oxford Centre for Clinical Magnetic Resonance Research (OCMR), Division of Cardiovascular Medicine, Radcliffe Department of Medicine, University of Oxford, John Radcliffe Hospital, Oxford University Hospitals NHS Foundation Trust, Oxford, UK

Chapter 3.3

James D. Newton Consultant Cardiologist, Oxford University Hospitals NHS Trust, Oxford, UK

Chapter 3.2, Chapter 14.1

Jerry P. Nolan Consultant in Anaesthesia and Intensive Care Medicine, Royal United Hospital Bath, UK; Co-Chair International Liaison Committee on Resuscitation

Chapter 4.1

Jayan Parameshwar Consultant Cardiologist, Transplant Unit, Papworth Hospital, Cambridge, UK

Chapter 5.5

Janet Powell Department of Surgery & Cancer, Imperial College, London, UK

Chapter 14.2

Bernard D. Prendergast Consultant Cardiologist, Guy's and St Thomas' NHS Foundation Trust, London, UK

Chapter 9.2

Kazem Rahimi Associate Professor, Deputy Director, The George Institute for Global Health, Oxford Martin School, University of Oxford, Oxford, UK

Chapter 13.2

K. Rajappan Consultant Cardiologist, Oxford Heart Centre, Oxford University Hospitals NHS Foundation Trust, Oxford, UK

Chapter 2.2

A. C. Rankin Professor of Cardiology, University of Glasgow Medical School, Glasgow, UK

Chapter 2.2, Chapter 4.2

Nikant Sabharwal Consultant Cardiologist, Department of Cardiology, John Radcliffe Hospital, Oxford University Hospitals NHS Foundation Trust, Oxford, UK

Chapter 3.3

Nilesh J. Samani British Heart Foundation Professor of Cardiology, Department of Cardiovascular Sciences, University of Leicester, Leicester, UK

Chapter 17.4

Rana Sayeed Consultant Cardiothoracic Surgeon, Oxford Heart Centre, John Radcliffe Hospital, Oxford University Hospitals NHS Trust, Oxford, UK

Chapter 13.6

Nicholas J. Severs Professor of Cardiology, National Lung and Heart Hospital, Faculty of Medicine, Imperial College, Royal Brompton Hospital, London, UK

Chapter 1.2

Jasmeet Soar Consultant in Anaesthesia and Intensive Care Medicine, Southmead Hospital Bristol, UK; Chair, Resuscitation Council (UK)

Chapter 4.1

Krishna Somers Consultant Physician in Cardiovascular Medicine, Royal Perth Hospital, Perth, Australia

Chapter 9.4

Paul D. Stein Professor, Department of Medicine, College of Osteopathic Medicine, Michigan State University, USA
Chapter 16.1

Peter H. Sugden Professor in Biomedical Sciences, Institute for Cardiovascular and Metabolic Research, University of Reading, UK

Chapter 1.2

David Taggart Professor of Cardiovascular Surgery, University of Oxford, UK

Chapter 13.6

S. A. Thorne Consultant Cardiologist, University Hospital Birmingham, Birmingham, UK

Chapter 12.1

Adam D. Timmis Professor of Clinical Cardiology, NIHR Cardiovascular Biomedical Research Unit, Barts Heart Centre, London, UK

Chapter 13.3

Maciej Tomaszewski Professor of Cardiovascular Medicine, Institute of Cardiovascular Sciences, University of Manchester, Manchester, UK

Chapter 17.4

Thomas A. Traill Adult Cardiology Faculty, Johns Hopkins, Hospital, Baltimore, Maryland, USA

Chapter 10.1, Chapter 11.1

Steven Tsui Consultant Cardiothoracic Surgeon, Director of Transplantation, Papworth Hospital, Cambridge, UK

Chapter 5.5

Patrick Vallance President, Pharmaceuticals Research & Development, GSK

Chapter 1.1

Bryan Williams Chair of Medicine, University College London, UK

Chapter 17.1, Chapter 17.2

Abbreviations

ABPI	ankle brachial pressure index		COP	colloid osmotic pressure
ABPM	ambulatory blood pressure measurement		COPD	chronic obstructive pulmonary disease
ACE	angiotensin converting enzyme		CPFE	combined pulmonary fibrosis and emphysema
ACR	albumin/creatinine ratio		CRF	corticotrophin releasing factor
ACS	acute coronary syndrome		CRP	C-reactive protein
ACTH	adrenocorticotropic hormone		CRT	cardiac resynchronization therapy
ADH	antidiuretic hormone		CSF	colony stimulating factors
AF	atrial fibrillation		CSM	carotid sinus massage
AGE	advanced glycation end products		CT	computed tomography
AHA	American Heart Association		CTEPH	chronic thromboembolic pulmonary hypertension
AKI	acute kidney injury		CVD	cardiovascular disease
AME	apparent mineralocorticoid excess		CZT	cadmium zinc telluride
ANCA	antineutrophil cytoplasmic antibody		DAMP	damage-associated molecular pattern
ANP	atrial natriuretic peptide		DAPT	dual antiplatelet therapy
APTT	activated partial thromboplastin time		DASH	dietary approaches to stop hypertension
ARB	angiotensin receptor blocker		DBP	diastolic blood pressure
ASD	atrial septal defect		DCA	directional coronary atherectomy
AT	atrial tachycardia		DILV	double-inlet left ventricle
ATG	antithymocyte globulin		DLCO	diffusing capacity of the lung for carbon monoxide
AVN	arteriovenous nipping		DOPA	levodopa
AVNRT	atrioventricular nodal re-entrant tachycardia		DORV	double-outlet right ventricle
AVRT	atrioventricular re-entry tachycardia		DT	destination therapy
AVSD	atrioventricular septal defect		DVLA	Driver and Vehicle Licensing Agency (UK)
BCRL	breast-cancer-related lymphoedema		DVT	deep vein thrombosis
BHS	British Hypertension Society		EACTS	European Association for Cardio-Thoracic Surgery
BMI	body mass index		ECE	endothelin converting enzyme
BMP	bone morphogenetic proteins		ECG	electrocardiograph
BNP	brain natriuretic peptide		ECMO	extracorporeal membrane oxygenation
BRAO	branch artery occlusion		ECV	extracellular volume
BRVO	branch retinal vein occlusion		EHR	electronic health records
BSA	body surface area		ELCA	excimer laser coronary atherectomy
CABG	coronary artery bypass grafting		ELISA	enzyme-linked immunosorbent assay
CAD	coronary artery disease		EPBF	effective pulmonary blood flow
CCB	calcium channel blocker		EPC	endothelial progenitor cells
CETP	cholesteryl ester transfer protein		ERNV	equilibrium radionuclide ventriculography
CFA	common femoral artery		ESC	European Society of Cardiology
CHD	coronary heart disease		ESCMID	European Society of Clinical Microbiology and Infectious Diseases
CHF	congestive heart failure			
CK	creatine kinase		ESH	European Society of Hypertension
CKD	chronic kidney disease		ESR	erythrocyte sedimentation rate
CMR	cardiac magnetic resonance		FAD	flavin adenine dinucleotide
CNP	C-type natriuretic peptide		FDA	food and drug authority
CO	cardiac output		FDG	fluorodeoxyglucose

FFR	fractional flow reserve	MDCT	multidetector computed tomography
FGF	fibroblast growth factor	MEN	multiple endocrine neoplasia
FH	flame-shaped retinal haemorrhage	MERFF	myoclonic epilepsy and ragged red fibres
FISH	fluorescence in situ hybridization	MET	metabolic equivalent
GCMS	gas chromatography–mass spectrometry	MI	myocardial infarction
GDF	growth differentiation factors	MIBI	methoxyisobutylisonitrile (ligand)
GFR	glomerular filtration rate	MIC	minimum inhibitory concentration
GH	growth hormone	MLD	manual lymphatic drainage
GRA	glucocorticoid-remediable aldosteronism	MPS	myocardial perfusion scintigraphy
GRACE	global registry of acute coronary events	MPS	mucopolysaccharidosis
GTN	glyceryl trinitrate (nitroglycerine)	MR	magnetic resonance
GWAS	genome-wide association studies	MRA	magnetic resonance angiography
HAART	highly active antiretroviral therapy	MRA	mineralocorticoid antagonists
HBPM	home blood pressure measurement	MRSA	meticillin-resistant Staphylococcus aureus
HCN	hyperpolarization-activated cyclic nucleotide-gated	MUGA	multi-gated acquisition (scan)
HDL	high-density lipoprotein	MV	mitral valve
HFnEF	heart failure with a normal ejection fraction	MVP	mitral valve prolapse
HLA	human leucocyte antigen	NCCT	sodium–chloride cotransporter
HLHS	hypoplastic left heart syndrome	NICE	National Institute for Health and Care Excellence (UK)
HPLC	high-performance liquid chromatography		
HPV	hypoxic pulmonary vasoconstriction	NNH	number needed to harm
HR	heart rate	NNT	number needed to treat
HRT	hormone replacement therapy	NO	nitric oxide
IABP	intra-aortic balloon counter-pulsation	NOAC	novel oral anticoagulant
ICD	implantable cardioverter-defibrillator	NOS	nitric oxide synthase
IDH	isolated diastolic hypertension	NSAID	nonsteroidal anti-inflammatory drug
Ig	immunoglobulin	NSTEMI	non-ST-elevation myocardial infarction
IHD	ischaemic heart disease	NTS	nucleus tractus solitarius
IMA	internal mammary artery	NYHA	New York Heart Association
INR	international normalized ratio	OCT	optical coherence tomography
IRIS	immune reconstitution inflammatory syndrome	ODI	oral direct inhibitors
ISC	international society of chemotherapy	OMIM	Online Mendelian Inheritance in Man (database)
ISH	international society of hypertension	OMT	optimal medical therapy
ISH	isolated systolic hypertension	PA	pulmonary artery
IUS	intrauterine system (contraceptive)	PAH	pulmonary arterial hypertension
IVC	inferior vena cava	PAI	plasminogen activator inhibitor
IVIG	intravenous immunoglobulin	PAN	polyarteritis nodosa
IVUS	intravascular ultrasound	PANDAS	paediatric autoimmune neuropsychiatric disorders associated with streptococcal infections
JNC	Joint National Committee		
LAA	left atrial appendage	PASP	pulmonary artery systolic pressure
LAD	left anterior descending (artery)	PCC	prothrombin complex concentrate
LBBB	left bundle branch block	PCH	pulmonary capillary haemangiomatosis
LDH	lactate dehydrogenase	PCI	percutaneous coronary intervention
LDL	low-density lipoprotein	PCR	polymerase chain reaction
LGE	late gadolinium enhancement	PCWP	pulmonary capillary wedge pressure
LMWH	low molecular weight heparin	PDA	patent ductus arteriosus
LPO	left posterior oblique	PDGF	platelet-derived growth factor
LQTS	long QT syndromes	PE	pulmonary embolism
LV	left ventricle/ventricular	PET	positron emission tomography
LVAD	left ventricular assist device	PFA	profunda femoris artery
LVDD	left ventricular diastolic dysfunction	PFO	patent foramen ovale
LVEDP	left ventricular end-diastolic pressure	PISA	proximal isovelocity surface area
LVEF	left ventricular ejection fraction	PJRT	permanent junctional reciprocating tachycardia
LVH	left ventricular hypertrophy	PKA	protein kinase A
LVMI	left ventricular mass index	PKC	protein kinase C
LVOT	left ventricular outflow tract	PPCI	primary percutaneous coronary intervention
LVSD	left ventricular systolic dysfunction	PR	peripheral resistance
MAO	monoamine oxidase	PT	prothrombin time
MAPCA	major aortopulmonary collateral arteries	PTCA	percutaneous transluminal coronary angioplasty

PTH	parathyroid hormone	TAVI	transcatheter aortic valve implantation
PVA	pulmonary vein ablation	TCPC	total cavopulmonary connection
PVAD	paracorporeal ventricular assist device	TEC	transcutaneous excision catheter
PVAT	perivascular adipose tissue	TF	tissue factor
PVE	prosthetic valve endocarditis	TFPI	tissue factor pathway inhibitor
PVOD	pulmonary veno-occlusive disease	TGA	transposition of the great arteries
PVR	pulmonary vascular resistance	TGF	transforming Growth Factor
PWV	pulse wave velocity	TIA	transient ischaemic attack
RA	right atrium	TIBC	total iron binding capacity
RAAS	renin–angiotensin–aldosterone system	TLR	toll-like receptors
RAGE	receptor for advanced glycation endproducts	TNF	tumour necrosis factor
RAO	right anterior oblique (artery)	TNK	tenecteplase
RAP	right atrial pressure	TOD	target organ damage
RAVV	right atrioventricular valve	TOE	transoesophageal echocardiography
RBBB	right bundle branch block	TOR	target of rapamycin
RCA	right coronary artery	tPA	tissue plasminogen activator (alteplase)
RF	radiofrequency	TPHA	T. pallidum haemagglutination
RHD	rheumatic heart disease	TRA	thrombin receptor antagonists
RIPV	right inferior pulmonary vein	TRF	transient risk factor
ROMK	renal outer medullary potassium channel	TRP	transient receptor potential
ROS	reactive oxygen species	TTD	thiazide-type diuretic
RPR	rapid plasma reagin	TV	tricuspid valve
RV	right ventricle/ventricular	TVA	tricuspid valve annulus
RVAD	right ventricular assist device	UFH	unfractionated heparin
RVOT	right ventricular outflow tract	UIP	usual interstitial pneumonia
RVOTO	right ventricular outflow tract obstruction	UKPDS	United Kingdom Prospective Diabetes Study
SA	short-axis	URTI	upper respiratory tract infection
SADS	sudden adult death syndrome	US	ultrasound
SAECG	signal-averaged electrocardiography	VAD	ventricular assist device
SAM	systolic anterior motion of the mitral valve	VAT	ventricular activation time
SAP	serum amyloid protein	VC	vena cava
SBF	systemic blood flow	VC	vital capacity
SBP	systolic blood pressure	VEGF	vascular endothelial growth factor
SCD	sudden cardiac death	VF	ventricular fibrillation
SDH	succinate dehydrogenase	VHL	Von Hippel–Lindau (syndrome)
SFA	superficial femoral artery	VIP	vasoactive intestinal polypeptide
SIGN	Scottish Intercollegiate Guidelines Network	VLA	vertical long axis
SLE	systemic lupus erythematosus	VMA	vanillylmandelic acid
SMC	smooth muscle cell	VP	ventricular pacing
SMR	standardized mortality ratio	VSD	ventricular septal defect
SNP	single nucleotide polymorphisms	VSMC	vascular smooth muscle cells
SPECT	single photon emission computed tomography	VT	ventricular tachycardia
SR	sarcoplasmic reticulum	VTE	venous thromboembolism
SSFP	steady-state free precession (imaging)	WHO	World Health Organization
STEMI	ST-elevation myocardial infarction	WPW	Wolff–Parkinson White (syndrome)
SVC	superior vena cava	ZASP	Z-line associated protein
SVT	supraventricular tachycardia		

SECTION 1

Structure and function

CHAPTER 1.1

Blood vessels and the endothelium

Keith Channon and Patrick Vallance

Essentials

Anatomy of blood vessels

The blood vessel wall consists of the intima, the media, and the adventitia. Not all vessels have each layer, and the layers vary in size and structure between vessels. (1) The intima is made up of a single layer of endothelial cells on a basement membrane, beneath which—depending on vessel size—there may be a layer of fibroelastic connective tissue and an internal elastic lamina that provides both structure and flexibility. Embedded in the intima are pericytes. (2) The media is made up of smooth muscle cells, elastic laminae and extracellular matrix. (3) The adventitia is the outermost part of the vessel, composed mainly of fibroelastic tissue but also containing nerves, small feeding blood vessels (the vasa vasorum), and lymph vessels. The adventitia is directly related to the surrounding perivascular adipose tissue.

Function of particular constituents of blood vessels

Endothelial cells are metabolically very active and exert a profound influence on vascular reactivity, thrombogenesis and coagulation, and the behaviour of circulating cells. They produce key vasodilator mediators: nitric oxide (NO), prostanoids, and hyperpolarizing factor. Although the predominant influence of the healthy endothelium is as dilator, it also produces important vasoconstrictor factors, including endothelin, angiotensin converting enzyme (ACE), certain prostanoids, and reactive oxygen species (ROS) such as superoxide anion.

The endothelium synthesizes and releases prothrombotic and antithrombotic factors, with antithrombotic factors predominating under basal conditions. It also prevents cells from adhering fully to the vessel wall, but allows leucocytes to roll along its surface.

Vascular smooth muscle cells are remarkably plastic and may adopt a range of phenotypes: they can leave the quiescent, contractile state and enter a replicative state, undergo cell death through apoptosis, migrate into the intima, adopt a secretory phenotype that results in matrix deposition (including developing bone-like features and calcification), and can contribute to inflammation within the vessel wall.

The vessel is surrounded by adventitia and perivascular adipose tissue (PVAT), which contain adipocytes, inflammatory cells, and fibroblasts. Evidence suggests that there is continuous cross-talk between the vascular wall and perivascular tissues. PVAT secretes a wide range of adipocytokines, that have paracrine effects on the vessel wall. The vessel and its PVAT are now considered to be closely interrelated, with PVAT playing important roles in vascular homeostasis and pathophysiology.

Integrated responses of blood vessels

Blood flow elicits an endothelium-dependent dilator tone due to the production of NO, which provides a physiological counterbalance to the constrictor tone of the sympathetic nervous system. Veins differ from arteries and arterioles, and do not seem to be actively dilated by continuous release of NO.

Flow-mediated dilatation is an autoregulatory property of blood vessels that tends to oppose classical myogenic autoregulation—the process by which a blood vessel constricts in response to an increase in intraluminal pressure. There is a fourth-power relationship between resistance to flow and the radius of a blood vessel, which means that relatively small changes in the thickness or contractile state of smooth muscle in small arteries and arterioles have big effects on systemic vascular resistance.

There are important interactions between the sympathetic nervous, renin–angiotensin, and endothelin systems, with these acting in concert to control constrictor tone, and with the endothelin system providing a slowly modulating background constrictor tone. Additional endocrine signals that modulate vascular tone and function include circulating cortisol and oestrogens.

Pathophysiology

Several clinical conditions—including atherosclerosis, hypertension, hypercholesterolaemia, and diabetes—are associated with reduced NO-mediated effects. Overproduction of NO may also contribute to disease, with induction of inducible NO synthase, e.g. in sepsis leading to production of large amounts of NO and resulting in vascular paresis. Expression of adhesion molecules by the vascular endothelium is an important mechanism of cellular adhesion during inflammation and is also important in recruitment of T cells and monocytes in atherosclerosis. Impaired production and/or function of endothelial progenitor cells, particularly with ageing, may contribute to the pathogenesis of endothelial dysfunction in disease, particularly in atherosclerosis.

Introduction

Blood vessels range in size from microscopic capillaries to large vessels such as the aorta and vena cava, and vary in specialized function from tissue to tissue. They deliver oxygen and nutrients, remove waste, control the passage of cells and macromolecules from the blood into the tissues, and are equipped to sense and respond to physical and chemical signals. There are three basic layers to blood vessels—the intima, the media, and the adventitia (Fig. 1.1.1).

The intima comprises a single layer of endothelial cells on a basement membrane, beneath which—depending on vessel size—there may be a layer of fibroelastic connective tissue and an internal elastic lamina that provides both structure and flexibility. Embedded in the intima are pericytes—intriguing cells of smooth muscle cell lineage that make contact with multiple endothelial cells. The media is made up predominantly of smooth muscle cells and concentric elastic fibres making up the elastic laminae. The outermost part of the vessel is the adventitia, a less well-defined layer composed mainly of fibroelastic tissue that provides structural integrity to the vessel, but also contains nerves, small feeding blood vessels (the vasa vasorum), and lymph vessels. However, the adventitia is also in continuity with perivascular adipose tissue (PVAT) that has paracrine relationships with the vascular wall. In simple terms, the intima may be considered as the layer that transduces signals from the lumen of the vessel to the rest of the vessel wall and controls the interface with the blood; the media is the mechanical workhorse of the vessel, and the adventitia houses links to the wider environment beyond the circulation. Not all vessels have each layer, and the layers vary in size and structure between vessels. For example, capillaries are essentially endothelial cell tubes surrounded by pericytes, resistance vessels have a relatively thick media, and the large conduit arteries have a high proportion of elastic tissue and a rich vasa vasorum. In disease states, particularly atherosclerosis (see Chapter 13.1), the vessel wall may have a high content of inflammatory cells in the intima, media, and adventitia. All three layers coordinate to regulate the function of the blood vessel, and all three are involved in the pathogenesis of vascular disease.

Large arteries perform the function of mass transport; smaller arteries and arterioles provide the predominate resistance to flow, and are therefore key determinants of blood pressure; capillaries are thin-walled and contribute most to passage of nutrients, gases, and cells through to tissues; venules provide postcapillary resistance and help determine capillary pressure; and larger venules and veins dynamically regulate the total capacitance of the circulatory system.

Cellular constituents of blood vessels

Endothelium

A monolayer of endothelial cells lines the intimal surface of the entire vascular tree (Fig. 1.1.2) to form the largest endocrine/paracrine organ in the body. Endothelial cells are metabolically very active and exert a profound influence on vascular reactivity, thrombogenesis and coagulation, and the behaviour of circulating cells. Abnormalities of endothelial function have been implicated in a wide variety of diseases ranging from atheroma and hypertension to acute inflammation and septic shock.

During early development, the endothelium forms the first layer of the circulatory system and extends to produce a network of interconnecting tubes. This ability of endothelial cells to form tube-like structures is retained even when they are grown *in vitro*. *In vivo* the endothelial tubes differentiate into arteries, arterioles, capillaries, veins, and lymph vessels, and regional differences in function and structure evolve such that the properties of endothelial cells vary between arterial and venous beds, between micro- and macrovasculature, between organs, and between different parts of individual organs—perhaps the most striking example being the specialized layer of endothelial cells and pericytes that forms the blood–brain barrier. Although heterogeneity of vascular endothelium has long been recognized at the histological and immunocytochemical level, recent studies using microarray analysis of global gene expression have begun to define these differences at the molecular level and promise to have important implications for understanding physiology, pathophysiology, and therapeutics. Heterogeneity of endothelial cell function undoubtedly has such implications. For example,

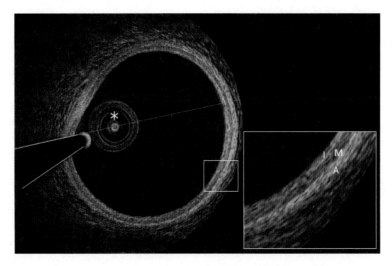

Fig. 1.1.1 Image of a human coronary artery, imaged *in vivo* using optical coherence tomography (OCT) during coronary angiography. The asterisk denotes the circular cross-section of the imaging catheter, and the dotted lines show the optical shadow cast by the coronary guidewire, adjacent to the imaging catheter. The vessel lumen appears black, with the vessel wall highlighted in yellow pseudocolour. The layers of the vessel wall—intima (I), media (M), and adventitia (A)—are shown in the magnified inset box.

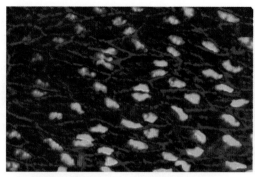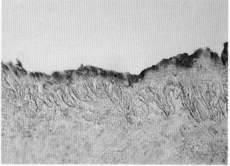

Fig. 1.1.2 Left panel: Immunostaining of an en face preparation of artery with CD31 (cell bodies red, nuclei blue), showing endothelial cells. Note that the endothelial cells are aligned in the direction of blood flow. Right panel shows a section of human internal mammary artery immunostained for endothelial nitric oxide synthase (red staining), demonstrating the endothelial cell layer on the luminal surface.

an active area of investigation involves strategies to target therapeutic agents or imaging markers to specific organs by coupling them with antibodies to proteins expressed on the endothelium of specific vascular beds. However, endothelial cells from different vessels also have many features in common and a number of pathologies, including those causing premature vascular disease, are associated with widespread changes in the behaviour of endothelial cells.

Anatomy of the endothelium

Each endothelial cell is between 25 and 50 μm long, 10 to 15 μm wide, and up to 5 μm deep, and lies with its long axis aligned in the direction of the blood flow (Fig. 1.1.2). The underlying smooth muscle cells lie radially, are about 5 to 10 μm wide, and taper at either end so that a single endothelial cell can communicate with many smooth muscle cells, and vice versa. The endothelium also comes into intimate contact with circulating cells, and the total area of the luminal surface of the endothelium is in excess of 500 m². This thin layer of cells is particularly susceptible to injury, and changes in endothelial cell morphology and turnover occur in experimental hypertension, diabetes, and atheroma.

Signal detection by endothelial cells

The endothelial cell membrane expresses a large number of receptors for circulating hormones, local mediators, and vasoactive factors released from blood cells. It can also sense changes in pressure and flow. Although the precise nature of endothelial flow, stretch, and pressure sensors is not clear, stretch of the cell membrane leads directly to the opening of a cation channel that is permeable to calcium, and flow across the cell surface leads to the opening of a potassium channel, which hyperpolarizes the cell. Recent studies suggest that members of the transient receptor potential (TRP) ion channel family may play an important role integrating stretch and other extracellular signals at the endothelial cell membrane. The intracellular signalling mechanisms linking agonist occupation of receptors or physical activation of the cell surface to mediator release is outside the scope of this chapter, but changes in the concentration of intracellular free calcium, and the temporal and spatial profile of calcium change, influence which endothelial functions are activated and therefore which message is produced by the cell. The endothelial cell also adjusts the expression and localization of certain key enzymes in response to physical or chemical stimuli. For example, changes in flow or shear stress across the endothelial cell surface lead to alterations in gene activation and can produce longer-term phenotypic alterations in the cell. One such pathway is mediated by the transcription factor KLF2, which has recently been identified as a key regulator of flow-induced vasodilatation. More recently, microRNAs (e.g. miR-126), which are endogenously expressed small non-coding RNAs that regulate gene expression at the post-transcriptional level, have been implicated in regulating endothelial cell function and angiogenesis. Translocation of enzymes from cytosol to the cell surface or to specialized invaginations in the cell surface (caveolae) in response to stimuli can also greatly alter the signalling capacity of the endothelial cell.

The endothelial cells in vascular damage and repair

Vascular endothelial cells move in response to specific chemical signals and can migrate to recover areas of endothelial damage or denudation (Fig. 1.1.3). The basic mechanisms of movement are probably the same as those required to form vessels during development or during the process of formation of new vessels in adults, e.g. in tumour angiogenesis.

Circulating endothelial cells have been identified and are increased in a variety of conditions associated with vascular damage. They are formed of two populations. The first consists of cells that have become damaged and detached and are undergoing a terminal process. The second is a population of endothelial progenitor cells (EPCs) that arise largely from the bone marrow and are instrumental in the process of vascular repair. These progenitor cells are characterized by the expression of specific cell surface markers (CD34 and CD133) and can form colonies when cultured *in vitro*. There is also increasing evidence that resident stem cells located in the vessel wall with properties of clonality, self-renewal, and multipotentiality can replace local damaged or denuded endothelial cells.

Vascular repair therefore involves three groups of endothelial cells: a mature population which migrate to areas of vascular damage, circulating EPCs, and resident stem cells.

The relationship between the number of circulating endothelial cells and cardiovascular disease is complex. On one hand, there is an increase in the number of circulating mature (dying?) endothelial cells in the presence of a wide variety of vascular diseases, and there is a positive relationship between the number of these circulating cells and the degree of impairment of endothelial function measured *in vivo*. On the other hand, the number of circulating EPCs is thought to represent the restorative capacity of the vessel wall, with low numbers being indicative of disease progression and increased cardiovascular risk. Importantly, the number of circulating EPCs appears to decrease with age, and it is likely that the ability to increase EPCs in response to vascular damage is a key feature of a healthy cardiovascular system able to repair itself.

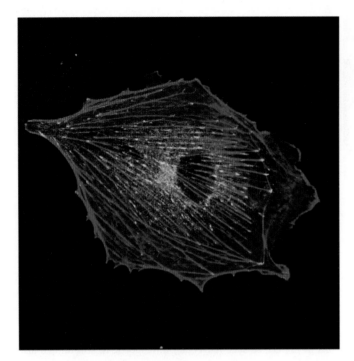

Fig. 1.1.3 An endothelial cell moving. The front end of the cell with leading lamella is on the right, stress fibres of contractile elements are seen in the centre and these end in focal adhesions. The retracting rear end of the cell is on the left.
Courtesy of Dr B. Wojciak-Stothard.

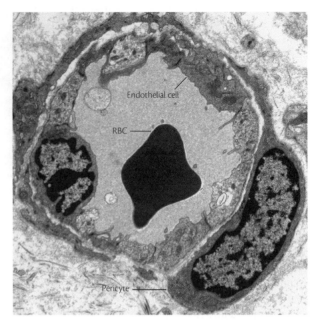

Fig. 1.1.4 Pericytes are observed outside small blood vessels in close association with endothelial cells.
Reproduced with kind permission from the Department of Pathology and Laboratory Medicine, University of Pennsylvania.

There is growing interest in the potential therapeutic delivery of EPCs—or bone marrow-derived cells capable of differentiating into EPCs and/or endothelial cells—for the treatment of cardiovascular disorders. For example, clinical studies have already been initiated in which autologous bone-marrow-derived cells have been administered to patients for the treatment of acute myocardial infarction and peripheral vascular disease. In general, the results of these early clinical experiments have been mixed, and there remain important unanswered questions regarding the optimum cell type, the timing and route of delivery (e.g. intracoronary vs intravenous), and the precise mechanism of potential beneficial effects.

In addition to EPCs, endothelium-derived microparticles have recently identified as a potential biomarker of endothelial function and cardiovascular disease. Microparticles are submicron-sized particles shed from the plasma membrane of endothelial cells in response to cell activation, cell damage, or apoptosis. The number of circulating microparticles appears to be increased in patients with cardiovascular disease, and it is possible that they play a role in the pathogenesis of disease. Microparticles have been proposed as a surrogate marker of endothelial function and vascular health; however their prognostic value remains to be determined.

Pericytes

Pericytes are about 70 μm in length and extend long cytoplasmic processes over endothelial cells in order to make multiple contacts (Fig. 1.1.4). In small capillaries, it also seems that pericytes may extend connections to more than one vessel, possibly exerting some sort of coordinating influence. The overall coverage of the endothelium by pericytes varies between vascular beds, from 10% to 50%. The junctions between pericytes and endothelial cells appear to be rich in growth factors (particularly epidermal growth factor) that are important in regulating endothelial cell growth and may

be vital for angiogenesis. Of particular importance in this interaction may be a signalling molecule known as angiopoietin and its receptor Tie2.

The nature of the junction between pericytes and endothelial cells may be important for regulating permeability at specialized sites such as the blood–brain barrier. In other areas, the contractile function of pericytes may predominate. In the retina, where pericytes are particularly prevalent, their loss is associated with impaired hierarchical organization of vessels or even vessel regression, and this might contribute to diabetic retinopathy. The only genetic disease to date in which pericyte loss has been implicated is Adams–Oliver syndrome, a rare developmental disorder characterized by scalp and limb malformations, telangiectasia, and vascular problems.

The potential roles of pericytes are listed in Box 1.1.1. These rather under-investigated cells seem to retain a plasticity that enables them to differentiate into smooth muscle cells.

Vascular smooth muscle cells

Smooth muscle cells largely lie radially around the vessel to provide contractile function. Their state of contractility is influenced by hormonal, endothelial, neuronal, and intrinsic influences, and

---

Box 1.1.1 Roles of pericytes

- Contractility
- Barrier function and regulation of permeability
- Signalling to control endothelial growth and angiogenesis
- Vascular stabilization
- Sensors of hypoxia and hypoglycaemia
- Transdifferentiation into fibroblasts for wound healing

contraction is triggered by a wave of calcium release. In some vessels, smooth muscle cells show rhythmic contraction and it may be that this, rather than a static degree of contraction, is a ubiquitous feature. The complex determinants of vascular smooth muscle cell contraction, the signalling pathways and ion channels that determine smooth muscle cell membrane potential and calcium entry, are outside the scope of this chapter, but there are many good review articles that cover this topic.

It is worth considering briefly the relationship between smooth muscle contraction and resistance to flow. There is a fourth-power relationship between resistance to flow and the radius of the vessel, which means that relatively small changes in the contractile state of smooth muscle can produce large changes in the resistance offered by the vessel. This is particularly important for small arteries and arterioles, which are the major determinants of systemic vascular resistance. The relative thickness of the vessel wall compared to the size of the lumen is also an important determinant of resistance. As the wall:lumen ratio increases, there is a comparatively larger reduction in lumen size for every incremental shortening of the smooth muscle. In this way, smooth muscle hypertrophy or hyperplasia can lead to a functional hyperreactivity of the vessel wall, exemplifying the intimate connection between structure and function.

Vascular smooth muscle cells are remarkably plastic and may adopt a range of phenotypes in response to local environmental changes. They may leave the quiescent contractile state and enter a replicative state, migrate into the intima, adopt a secretory phenotype that results in matrix deposition (including the development of bone-like features and calcification), and may, under certain conditions, contribute to inflammation within the vessel wall. Smooth muscle cells that replicate and secrete matrix contribute to the process of thickening of the vessel wall in vasculoproliferative syndromes including atherosclerosis, transplant vasculopathy, and the neointimal hyperplasia that characterizes vascular restenosis following arterial stent implantation.

Phenotypic modulation of vascular smooth muscle cells is under coordinated transcriptional regulation. In the normal vessel wall, the contractile smooth muscle phenotype is maintained by a transcriptional pathway involving signalling from the actin cytoskeleton to SRF, a ubiquitous transcription factor that functions in a smooth muscle cell-specific fashion by interacting with smooth muscle cell-restricted cofactors of the myocardin family. This actin–SRF–myocardin pathway directly regulates genes encoding contractile proteins such as smooth muscle myosin and SM22. However, in response to inflammatory and other pathological stimuli, the contractile transcriptional pathway is repressed, and alternate transcriptional pathways are activated that promote proliferation, production of inflammatory mediators, and synthesis of matrix proteins. Key mediators of the synthetic smooth muscle cell phenotype include the platelet-derived growth factor-BB (PDGF-BB) and Notch signalling pathways. Recent evidence suggests that these transcriptional pathways are also regulated in an epigenetic fashion by smooth muscle cell-specific programs for modification of histones within the chromatin structure of smooth muscle restricted genes.

As in the case of endothelial cells, there is clear heterogeneity in vascular smooth muscle cell phenotype in various vascular beds. Indeed, subsets of vascular smooth muscle cells are derived from distinct embryological precursors; vascular smooth muscle cells of the proximal aortic arch and great vessels are derived from neural crest (i.e. ectoderm), whereas vascular smooth muscle cells in the rest of the circulation are derived from somatic mesoderm. In the adult, an important example of functional heterogeneity is that the pulmonary and systemic vasculature differ markedly in their response to hypoxia. Hypoxia produces modest vasodilatation in the systemic vasculature, but marked vasoconstriction in the pulmonary circulation. This is likely an adaptive mechanism to prevent ventilation–perfusion mismatch in the presence of alveolar disease (e.g. pneumonia). However, chronic hypoxia (e.g. in the presence of chronic respiratory disease) can result in pulmonary hypertension and lead to right heart hypertrophy and failure. The precise molecular mechanisms regulating hypoxic pulmonary vasoconstriction are incompletely understood, but oxygen sensing mechanisms in the mitochondria and voltage-gated potassium channels on the plasma membrane of pulmonary vascular smooth muscle cells appear to play important roles.

Control of vascular tone

Endothelium extracts and inactivates circulating hormones, converts inactive precursors to active products, and synthesizes and releases a variety of vasoactive mediators (Fig. 1.1.5). Vasoconstrictor and vasodilator mediators allow the vessel to respond to changes in the local milieu, but the predominant background influence of the endothelium is dilator, with the removal of the endothelium leading to vasoconstriction. A basal endothelium-dependent dilator tone seems to provide a physiological counterbalance to the continuous constrictor tone of the sympathetic nervous system.

Vasodilators

The endothelium produces at least three key vasodilation mediators (Fig. 1.1.5): nitric oxide (NO), prostanoids, and hyperpolarizing factors.

Nitric oxide
Physiology
The production of NO is responsible for endothelium-dependent dilator tone that is generated by blood flow. NO is synthesized from the amino acid L-arginine by the nitric oxide synthase (NOS) enzymes (Fig. 1.1.6; see also Fig 1.1.8). The vasodilator actions of NO are mediated through the second messenger cGMP, generated when NO activates soluble guanylate cyclase (sGC) by binding to the haem group in the enzyme. A similar mechanism mediates NO signalling by inhibition of cytochrome *c* oxidase, initially in a reversible manner, but irreversibly under certain conditions. Inhibition of this enzyme decreases oxygen utilization, and the release of NO by endothelial cells appears to be an important determinant of oxygen consumption in the vasculature. However, the signalling actions of NO are much broader than modification of enzyme function by haem binding. NO modifies protein functions through numerous chemical reactions involving nitrosylation of cysteine residues and nitration of tyrosines, including ion channels, enzymes, and transcription factors, leading to change such as reduced adhesiveness of the endothelial cell for circulating white cells. A key role for endothelium-derived NO is the nitrosylation of haemoglobin, leading to changes in oxygen affinity, which appear to play a fundamental role in oxygen delivery in the microvasculature.

The arterial circulation of animals and humans is vasodilated continuously and actively by endothelium-derived NO, and inhibition of the synthesis of NO with certain guanidino-substituted

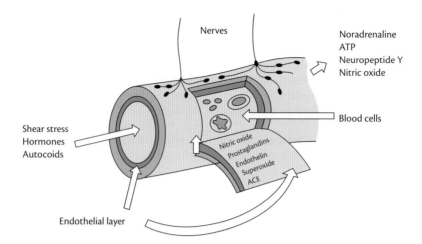

Fig. 1.1.5 Vascular endothelial cells lie at the interface between blood and the smooth muscle cells. They detect chemical and physical signals in the lumen of the blood vessel and adjust their output of biologically active mediators accordingly. This provides a mechanism of local regulation of vascular function. Rapid adjustment of vascular tone is probably achieved through a balance of endothelium-derived nitric oxide and neuronally derived noradrenaline. Endothelin provides a slowly modulating constrictor tone and angiotensin II has the capacity to fine-tune neuronal, endothelial, and smooth muscle function. ACE, angiotensin converting enzyme.

analogues of L-arginine, including N-G-monomethyl-L-arginine, leads to vasoconstriction, hypertension, and sodium retention. Shear stress—the force caused by the viscous drag of flowing blood—is an important physiological stimulus for the continuous production of NO. Shear stress increases NO production so the blood vessel relaxes, reducing the shear stress. This process of flow-mediated dilatation appears is a homeostatic mechanism to regulate blood flow and coordinate tissue perfusion. The autoregulatory action of flow-mediated dilatation opposes classical myogenic autoregulation—the process by which a blood vessel constricts in response to an increase in intraluminal pressure.

Synthesis of NO is stimulated by acetylcholine, bradykinin, and substance P, and in many vessels the release of NO accounts for the vasodilator actions of these mediators, which are known as 'endothelium-dependent vasodilators'. Circulating hormones, including insulin and oestrogens, may also act on receptors on or within the endothelial cell to stimulate the release of NO acutely

or to alter the expression of endothelial NO synthase chronically. Endothelial NO synthase (NOS) is activated either by increases in intracellular calcium, which causes binding of calmodulin, or by phosphorylation of specific serine or threonine residues in the protein, for example by the kinases Akt or PKC (Figure 1.1.8). Phosphorylation can either activate or inhibit the enzyme, for example at serine 1179 or threonine 495 respectively. Phosphorylation mediates the physiological effects of shear stress, and hormones such as insulin, oestrogen, and vascular endothelial growth factor (VEGF).

Veins differ from arteries and arterioles in that they do not seem to be actively dilated by the continuous release of NO. The venous endothelium releases NO when it is stimulated by acetylcholine or bradykinin, but not under basal conditions. Furthermore, human veins do not release much NO in response to platelet-derived mediators. Indeed, aggregating platelets constrict veins, due to the unopposed action of vasoconstricting platelet-derived mediators

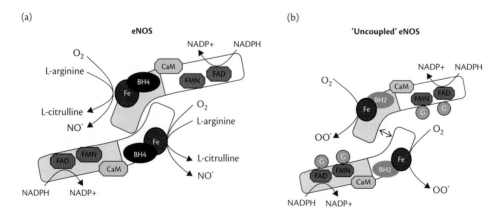

Fig. 1.1.6 (a) Nitric oxide synthases (NOS) catalyse the conversion of L-arginine and molecular oxygen to citrulline and NO. NOS enzymes are catalytically active as homodimers and require the binding of cofactors (flavin adenine dinucleotide (FAD), flavin mononucleotide (FMN), haem (Fe), and tetrahydrobiopterin (BH$_4$)) and calmodulin (CaM) for optimal activity. Each NOS dimer coordinates a single atom of zinc. (b) Under conditions where NOS are 'uncoupled', the enzyme does not catalyse the conversion of L-arginine to citrulline and NO, but instead generates superoxide or other reactive oxygen species (ROS) by reduction of molecular oxygen, driven by electron flow from NADPH via the flavin domain. Factors that cause NOS uncoupling include low levels of the cofactor tetrahydrobiopterin (BH$_4$), inadequate levels of the substrate L-arginine, or oxidative modification of the eNOS protein by glutathionylation (G) of specific cysteine residues.

on the vascular smooth muscle. The reasons for the arteriovenous difference in NO production are not fully understood, but one consequence is that the guanylyl cyclase in venous smooth muscle is relatively up-regulated and veins respond to smaller amounts of NO than do arteries or arterioles. This is of therapeutic relevance; NO is the active moiety of glyceryl trinitrate and other nitrovasodilators, and the low basal synthesis of endogenous NO by venous endothelium accounts, in part, for the venoselective action of these drugs.

Pathophysiology

Loss of NO leads to arterial vasoconstriction, has the potential to enhance platelet and white cell adhesion, and, in experimental models, may enhance atherogenesis. Several clinical conditions—including atherosclerosis, hypertension, hypercholesterolaemia, and diabetes—are associated with a functional loss of NO-mediated effects.

In the coronary vasculature, loss of NO predisposes to vasospasm and may contribute to the onset of anginal symptoms. Atherosclerotic coronary arteries constrict in response to the platelet-derived mediator serotonin (5-hydroxytryptamine), whereas healthy vessels are stimulated to produce more NO and dilate. Flow-dependent dilatation is also lost in such vessels, and the response to sympathetic stimulation is converted from dilatation to unopposed constriction. Endothelial dysfunction precedes the development of overt atheroma, and there is a relationship between risk factors for ischaemic heart disease and impaired responsiveness of coronary arteries to endothelium-dependent vasodilators. Furthermore, hypercholesterolaemia, even in the absence of angiographic evidence of atheroma in large vessels, is associated with abnormal endothelium-dependent vasodilatation in coronary and peripheral arterioles. Modified low-density lipoproteins appear to inhibit NO synthesis or accelerate its destruction, possibly by enhancing production of the superoxide anion.

Basal endothelium-dependent dilatation is also impaired in patients with essential hypertension and the degree of impairment increases with increasing blood pressure. It is not known whether the defect is a consequence or a cause of the raised pressure, but the fact that endothelial function appears to be restored by antihypertensive therapy argues in favour of such dysfunction being a response to raised pressure. Patients with diabetes show diminished endothelium-dependent dilatation, and this defect does not reverse with treatment. Thus, patients with uncontrolled hypertension, diabetes, and hypercholesterolaemia all display defects of NO-mediated vasodilatation and this could provide a common mechanism of vascular dysfunction in these diseases.

Overproduction of NO may also contribute to disease. Bacterial endotoxin and some cytokines, including interleukin (IL)-1 and interferon-γ, induce expression of a second NO synthesizing enzyme that appears in the endothelium, vascular smooth muscle, and inflammatory cells invading the vessel wall. Unlike the constitutive enzyme present in healthy endothelium (endothelial NOS, eNOS), this inducible isoform of NOS is not regulated by calcium and produces large amounts of NO. In these quantities NO, either alone or in combination with superoxide, may contribute to tissue damage in addition to causing profound vasodilatation and hypotension such as that seen in septic shock.

The NO pathway has been the basis for several important therapeutic approaches. Administration of glyceryl trinitrate, a NO donor, has been a longstanding therapy for heart failure and for

coronary ischaemia because of its ability to produce systemic venous and coronary arterial vasodilatation, respectively. Inhibitors of phosphodiesterase-5 (e.g. sildenafil, vardenafil, and tadalafil), the enzyme that inactivates cGMP, which is the key downstream signalling molecule for NO, were initially developed for hypertension, but have been much more widely used for erectile dysfunction because of their effects on augmenting blood flow into the corpous cavernosum. PDE-5 inhibitors are also used for the treatment of pulmonary hypertension, and ongoing studies are exploring their efficacy in patients with heart failure related to primarily systolic or primarily diastolic dysfunction. Activators of soluble guanylate cyclase, the enzyme that produces cGMP, have also been developed as potential therapies for systemic hypertension, pulmonary hypertension, and peripheral vascular disease (see Box 1.1.2). Other commonly used drugs, such as statins, may also exert some of their beneficial effects through 'pleiotropic' mechanisms that are not primarily dependent upon cholesterol lowering but act to increase NO bioactivity.

Prostanoids

NO appears to be the dominant vasoactive factor released from endothelial cells under basal conditions, but it is by no means the only mediator produced. The endothelium is a rich source of prostanoids, including the vasodilators prostacyclin and prostaglandins E_2 and D_2 (PGE_2 and PGD_2). However, whereas inhibition of NO leads to profound and widespread changes in vascular tone, inhibition of prostanoid synthesis with aspirin (or other nonsteroidal anti-inflammatory drugs, NSAIDs) does not, excepting in the renal vasculature where dilator prostanoids do appear to be important in the regulation of basal renal blood flow: aspirin and other NSAIDs lead to vasoconstriction in the kidney, indicating tonic release of vasodilator prostanoids in this vascular bed. Furthermore, in the fetus and newborn, indometacin leads to the closure of the ductus arteriosus and a fall in cerebral blood flow suggesting a significant contribution of endothelium-derived prostanoids to tonic vasodilatation in these beds, at least during development. The cerebral blood flow in adults also falls in response to indometacin, but not to aspirin and other cyclooxygenase (COX) inhibitors, and so the role of prostanoids is unclear. Vasodilator prostanoids are important in the vascular changes of inflammation, although whether these prostanoids derive exclusively from the endothelium is not known. The finding that the inhibition of COX-II appears to be associated with increased cardiovascular risk is important and suggests that the balance of prostanoids in the vessel wall, and between endothelium and platelets, is a key determinant of the 'stickiness' of the endothelium to platelets and other circulating cells.

Hyperpolarizing factors

An endothelium-derived hyperpolarizing factor has been identified in some animal and human blood vessels. Hyperpolarization of vascular smooth muscle cells leads to a fall in calcium entry and vascular relaxation. Increasing evidence suggests that endothelium-dependent hyperpolarization may be particularly important in small arteries and arterioles. The chemical identity of endothelium-derived hyperpolarizing factor has not been clearly established, but products of activity of cytochrome P450, the cannabinoid anandamide, and the potassium ion have all been suggested as possible candidates. Recent data also suggests that the C-type natriuretic peptide accounts for this activity in some vessels. A picture is emerging that endothelium-derived hyperpolarizing factor is not a single entity, but rather that hyperpolarization is a mechanism utilized by different mediators that vary between vessels. In addition, direct contact through gap junctions also provides a means for endothelial cells to hyperpolarize smooth muscle cells. Without specific inhibitors, it is not yet clear what role the variations in endothelial cell hyperpolarization of smooth muscle cells plays in human disease.

Vasoconstrictors

Although the predominant background influence of the endothelium is dilator, important vasoconstrictor factors are also synthesized and released.

Endothelin

The endothelins are a family of potent vasoconstrictor peptides of 21 amino acids, which are closely related to the snake-venom toxin of the Israeli burrowing asp (*Atractaspis engaddensis*). Three types of endothelin have been described—endothelin 1, 2, and 3—and there are at least two endothelin receptors in human blood vessels, the endothelin A and endothelin B receptors. Endothelins vasoconstrict and can promote the growth of vascular smooth muscle cells. Effects are mediated in part through the stimulation of increases in calcium and in part through calcium-independent mechanisms, including activation of protein kinases.

Endothelin 1 is synthesized from 'big endothelin' within human endothelial cells (Fig. 1.1.7). It is a potent and long-lasting constrictor of human blood vessels, and causes widespread vasoconstriction, hypertension, and sodium retention when infused into healthy volunteers. Antagonists of the endothelin A receptor cause vasodilatation and can lower blood pressure, indicating that there is a tonic synthesis and release of endothelin A. A number of studies suggest that there may be important interactions between the sympathetic nervous system, the renin–angiotensin system, and the endothelin system, and that these may act in concert to control constrictor tone, with the endothelin system providing a slowly modulating background constrictor tone. Endothelins also exert an important influence on sodium reabsorption in the kidney.

Although activation of endothelin B receptors on vascular smooth muscle causes constriction, activation of endothelial endothelin B receptors leads to the generation of vasodilator prostanoids and/or NO, hence endothelin can also produce transient vasodilatation in some circumstances. Binding of endothelin to endothelin B receptors also seems to be important to clear the peptide from the circulation. Stimuli for endothelin production include thrombin,

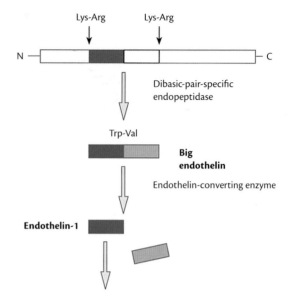

Activation of endothelin A and endothelin B receptors

Fig. 1.1.7 Endothelin-1 (ET-1), a cyclic (Cys^1–Cys^{15} and Cys^3–Cys^{11}) 21-amino acid peptide, is synthesized within the vascular endothelium as the product of an 'inactive' 39-amino acid precursor known as 'big ET-1', a conversion catalysed by a specific membrane-bound zinc metalloproteinase endothelin converting enzyme (ECE). Big ET-1, in turn, is the catalytic product of a larger (203 amino acids) precursor polypeptide termed 'preproET-1' (a conversion that is believed to be mediated by a 'furin-like' protease). The ECE-mediated conversion of big ET-1 to mature ET-1 is an essential step in the expression of full biological activity. Upon release from the vascular endothelium, ET-1 interacts with the underlying smooth muscle cells resulting in vasoconstriction. This action is mediated by two distinct G-protein-coupled receptors, ET$_A$ and ET$_B$. Although the predominant action of ET-1 is that of a vasoconstrictor, this effect is regulated by the concomitant release of vasodilatory factors (e.g. PGI$_2$, NO) by the action of ET-1 on endothelial ET$_B$-receptors. Although such an action tempers the contractile actions of ET-1, it is postulated that endothelial dysfunction (e.g. diminished ability to synthesize and/or release NO such as is seen in hypertension, atherosclerosis) results in aberrant ET-mediated vasoconstrictor tone due to a loss in concomitant endothelial regulation.

insulin, ciclosporin, adrenaline, angiotensin II, cortisol, various proinflammatory cytokines, hypoxia, and shear stress.

The concentrations of endothelins circulating in plasma are low and may not reflect local concentrations achieved within the vessel wall, making it difficult to interpret the elevated values reported in many conditions. Nonetheless, activation of the endothelin system has been implicated in the pathogenesis of a number of cardiovascular conditions. For example, a role for endothelin in the pathogenesis of vasospasm associated with subarachnoid haemorrhage and some types of renal ischaemia is suggested by experiments in animals. In addition, the increased production of endothelin has also been clearly implicated in the pathogenesis of a very rare form of secondary systemic hypertension caused by malignant haemangioendothelioma, a vascular tumour characterized by intravascular proliferation of atypical endothelial cells. In this condition, the degree of hypertension correlates with plasma levels of endothelin, and when the tumour is removed blood pressure and plasma endothelin levels fall.

The role of endothelin in the pathogenesis of pulmonary hypertension and congestive heart failure has been studied most intensely.

Box 1.1.2 Sildenafil and ADMA

The pulmonary vasculature seems to be particularly sensitive to NO and the inhibition of NO synthesis causes pulmonary hypertension. These observations have been utilized therapeutically in the form of inhaled NO treatment, and amplification of NO signalling by inhibition of cGMP phosphodiesterase with sildenafil (see Chapter 15.2). Recently, it has become clear that a naturally occurring amino acid, asymmetric dimethylarginine (ADMA), acts as an important endogenous inhibitor of NO synthesis and that the concentration of ADMA in blood is a predictor of cardiovascular risk. Accumulation of ADMA may be important in renal failure, providing a possible mechanism to link failing renal function with increased risk of atherothrombotic complications.

In pulmonary hypertension, selective ETA antagonists lower pulmonary vascular pressure in patients with advanced disease and have been approved for clinical use. However, the role of endothelin receptor antagonists in treating congestive heart failure is less clear. A substantial body of preclinical evidence indicates that selective ETA or non-selective ET_A/ET_B antagonists prevent ventricular remodelling and prolong survival in models of myocardial injury. However, although short-term studies with endothelin antagonists produced beneficial hemodynamic effects in heart failure patients, long-term studies failed to show significant effects on morbidity or mortality, and endothelin antagonists are not presently approved for heart failure.

Angiotensin converting enzyme (ACE)

ACE is located primarily on the luminal surface of the endothelium (see Fig. 1.1.5). This enzyme converts angiotensin I to angiotensin II and also metabolizes bradykinin to inactive products. The pulmonary vasculature provides the largest area of endothelium and is important in the regulation of circulating levels of angiotensin II, but the activity of endothelial ACE in systemic vessels may be more important in determining the final concentrations of angiotensin II and bradykinin that reach the blood vessel wall. Furthermore, endothelial cells also have the ability to synthesize renin and its substrate. It seems, therefore, as though the enzymatic machinery for a complete renin–angiotensin system is present within the vessel wall.

The activity of the renin–angiotensin system is clearly important in cardiovascular diseases including hypertension and heart failure, but the relative importance of local, compared with systemic, regulation of angiotensin II production is not yet clear. Furthermore, the full clinical significance of bradykinin metabolism by endothelial ACE has yet to be determined. It has been demonstrated that at least part of the vasodilator action of ACE inhibitors in certain isolated blood vessels is due to accumulation of bradykinin, which stimulates NO synthesis.

Prostanoids

The endothelium synthesizes thromboxane and the unstable prostaglandin endoperoxides PGG_2 and PGH_2. Overproduction of constrictor prostanoids by the endothelium has been implicated in animal models of diabetes and hypertension, but the significance of these findings for human disease remains uncertain.

Reactive oxygen species (ROS)

ROS can greatly influence the overall behaviour of the wall of the blood vessel and lead to an apparent defect in endothelial function even when the output of endothelial mediators is normal. ROS such as the superoxide anion (O_2^-) are synthesized within the vascular wall by multiple enzyme systems within endothelial, vascular smooth muscle ,and inflammatory cells (e.g. macrophages and neutrophils). They arise primarily from the activity of NADPH oxidases. The different forms of this enzyme can be defined by five classes of a catalytic subunit termed Nox1–5. The Nox2 enzyme typified by the neutrophil NADPH oxidase (but also expressed in endothelial cells and other inflammatory cells) is a major source of vascular superoxide. Vascular smooth muscle cells, where Nox1 and Nox4 predominate, also contribute. Stimulation by angiotensin II increases superoxide generation by Nox2 NADPH oxidases, and is a key feature of vascular pathophysiology. Other important sources of ROS are mitochondria, xanthine oxidoreductase, and NOS.

In addition to its important vasodilator properties, NO acts as a free radical scavenger. As is characteristic for such agents NO itself is also a free radical (it has an unpaired electron in its outer orbit), and as such, reacts readily with other free radicals and ROS, resulting in the formation of the reactive nitrogen species peroxynitrite (ONOO$^-$), and with other ROS to generate inorganic nitrite and nitrate (NO_3^-) in biological systems. Under certain physiological conditions (e.g hypoxia), NO can be regenerated from nitrite by nitrite reductases such as xanthine oxodoreducatse, or haemoglobin. eNOS can also generate ROS (see Fig. 1.1.6B). This aspect of eNOS function, termed 'eNOS uncoupling', occurs when levels of the cofactor for NOS, tetrahydrobiopterin (BH_4), are lowered due to oxidation or reduced biosynthesis. Uncoupling is also caused by conformational changes in eNOS due to oxidative modification of cysteine residues on the enzyme by glutathionylation. The positive feedback loop created for generation of ROS is an important pathway resulting in endothelial dysfunction and other alterations in vascular redox signalling.

Regulation of platelet function and haemostasis

The endothelium synthesizes and releases prothrombotic and antithrombotic factors. However, healthy endothelium presents a thromboresistant surface, indicating that the antithrombotic factors predominate under basal conditions.

Platelets

Endothelial cells inhibit the aggregation and adhesion of platelets, and disaggregate aggregating platelets. Two mediators are of particular importance: NO and prostacyclin (or PGE_2 in the microvascular endothelium), which act synergistically through different second messenger systems: cGMP for NO and cAMP for prostacyclin.

Thiols and sulphydryl-containing molecules react with NO to produce more stable adducts, including nitrosocysteine, nitrosoglutathione, nitrosoalbumin, and even nitrosohaemoglobin. Some of these compounds are formed in vivo and may enhance the antiplatelet effects of endothelium-derived NO. Furthermore, interaction between NO and tissue plasminogen activator leads to the formation of nitroso-tissue plasminogen activator, a molecule with fibrinolytic, antiplatelet, and vasorelaxant properties. It is not yet clear how important these NO adducts are in human physiology or pathophysiology.

Deficient production of NO has been implicated in a wide variety of cardiovascular diseases (see 'Nitric oxide' section earlier), and abnormalities of prostanoid synthesis occur in experimental models of atherosclerosis and diabetes. In the presence of a quiescent healthy endothelium, loss of basal NO alone does not lead to significant systemic platelet activation. However, loss of NO and prostacyclin at sites of endothelial damage, dysfunction, or activation promotes the formation of platelet aggregates and may contribute to thrombosis and vessel occlusion. In animals, stenosed endothelium-denuded vessels lead to cyclical variations in flow as platelets stick to the vessel wall and release vasoactive and proaggregant mediators. If this also occurs in human vessels in vivo, it might be an important mechanism of vasospasm and thrombosis.

Under basal conditions the endothelium inhibits platelet activation, but in response to certain stimuli, proaggregant, proadhesive mediators may be synthesized and released. Unstable prostaglandin endoperoxides activate platelets, platelet activating factor may be produced, and von Willebrand factor—which is synthesized and stored within endothelial cells—increases platelet adhesion. These changes occur in response to inflammatory mediators and may also result from endothelial 'injury', such as occurs during coronary artery angioplasty or stent implantation.

Coagulation

Heparan sulphate is a glycosaminoglycan closely related to heparin, but less potent, which is found on the surface of endothelial cells. Antithrombin III is also expressed on the endothelial cell surface and, together with heparan sulphate, provides a mechanism for binding and inactivating thrombin. In addition, endothelial cells participate in the activation of the anticoagulant protein C, and secretion of protein S and thrombomodulin that is found on the cell surface.

In the quiescent state, expression of anticoagulant factors predominates, but when activated the endothelium may promote coagulation. Receptors for clotting factors appear on the endothelial surface, von Willebrand factor is secreted, and tissue factor—the principal cellular initiator of coagulation—is expressed. Bacterial endotoxin, inflammatory cytokines, and glycosylated proteins activate the endothelium and shift the balance in favour of coagulation. This may occur in response to infection, inflammation, or endothelial injury. Circulating levels of von Willebrand factor are increased in some patients with diabetes or hypertension.

Fibrinolysis

The endothelial cell surface has a fibrinolytic pathway. Urokinase and tissue plasminogen activator are secreted and there are specific binding sites for plasminogen activators and plasminogen. Thrombin, adrenaline, vasopressin, and stasis of blood may be physiological stimuli for the release of tissue plasminogen activator from human endothelium.

Plasminogen activator inhibitor 1 is also synthesized and bound by endothelium, providing a pathway for local inhibition of the fibrinolytic system. Under basal conditions fibrinolysis is dominant, but the balance may be altered by a variety of local and circulating factors, including inflammatory cytokines and the atherogenic particle lipoprotein(a), which inhibits plasminogen binding and hence plasmin generation. In the presence of atherosclerosis, the fibrinolytic properties of the endothelium are diminished.

Other important aspects of vascular and endothelial biology

Cellular adhesion

The resting endothelium prevents cells from adhering fully to the vessel wall, but allows leucocytes to 'roll' along its surface. The regulation of rolling, adhesion, and migration is governed largely by specialized glycoproteins known as cell adhesion molecules, which are expressed in varying amounts on the endothelial cell surface and interact with complementary adhesion molecules on circulating cells. Endothelial-leucocyte adhesion molecule 1 (ELAM-1, also known as E-selectin), vascular adhesion molecule 1 (VCAM-1), intercellular adhesion molecule 1 (ICAM-1), and P-selectin (also known as GMP-140) are all expressed on cytokine-activated endothelium. The degree of expression and the type of adhesion molecules expressed determines the 'stickiness' of the endothelium for different cell types.

Expression of adhesion molecules is an important mechanism of cellular adhesion during inflammation and is also important in recruitment of T cells and monocytes in atherosclerosis. Increased expression of E-selectin is seen in the coronary arteries of transplanted hearts, and has been implicated in the rapid development of atherosclerosis in these vessels. NO and prostacyclin inhibit the adhesion of white cells to the endothelium and this effect may be mediated by changes in the expression or configuration of adhesion molecules. Certain endothelial cell adhesion molecules are shed into the plasma: changes in their concentration have been detected in a variety of cardiovascular diseases, but the significance of this is uncertain.

Proinflammatory cytokines

Cytokines are released from activated leucocytes in response to infection and immunological stimulation and are also produced by the vessel wall itself; IL-1, IL-6, and IL-8, and colony stimulating factors (CSF) are synthesized by endotoxin-stimulated endothelial cells, and tumour necrosis factor (TNF) by human smooth muscle cells. A large number of cytokines and chemokines alter endothelial functions, upsetting the balance of vasoactive mediators, altering thrombotic activity and the expression of adhesion molecules, or initiating apoptosis (programmed cell death). IL-1 and some other proinflammatory cytokines alter the synthesis of NO (see 'Nitric oxide' section earlier) and a variety of prostaglandins; enhance the generation of thrombin, platelet activating factor, von Willebrand factor, and plasminogen activator inhibitor; alter endothelial permeability; increase expression of ICAM-1 and VCAM-1; and may also cause endothelial cell damage and death. These findings are of direct relevance to the vascular changes occurring in inflammation and sepsis, and might also provide a link between acute or chronic immunological stimulation (e.g. infection) and the development of cardiovascular disease, including atherosclerosis or acute cardiovascular events. More recently it has been recognized that components of the innate immune pathway, such as Toll-like receptors (TLRs), are expressed by cells in the vascular wall and play a role in the pathogenesis of cardiovascular disease. These receptors recognize specific, highly conserved structural motifs in non-host pathogens, resulting in rapid activation of a coordinated innate immune response. However, TLRs may also be activated by damage-associated molecular pattern molecules (DAMPs) such as proteins released by injured or necrotic cells (e.g. heat shock proteins, HMBG1), and/or modified by oxidation (e.g. oxidized LDL), by DNA released from the nucleus, or proteins that have been glycated in diabetes (advanced glycation end products, AGE), that are recognized by RAGE, the specific receptor for AGE. These innate immune mechanisms are important in the vascular wall in atherosclerotic plaques or in the myocardium following ischaemic injury, by initiation and amplifying the pathologic inflammatory response.

Cell growth and angiogenesis

The endothelium of healthy differentiated vessels inhibits proliferation of the underlying smooth muscle. Endothelium-derived vasodilator, antiplatelet, and antithrombotic mediators (e.g. NO, prostacyclin) tend to inhibit the growth of vascular smooth muscle cells, whereas vasoconstrictor and prothrombotic mediators (e.g. endothelin, angiotensin) tend to promote it. Thus the basal state of the endothelium, in which dilatation and thromboresistance predominates, also prevents the growth of smooth muscle. The heparin-like molecules prevent cell growth and molecules similar or identical to platelet-derived growth factor (PDGF) and fibroblast growth factor (FGF) are endothelium-derived growth promoters. Others such as transforming growth factor β (TGFβ), produced by endothelial cells, may either inhibit or promote cell growth, and the precise role of this molecule *in vivo* is unclear. The basal antiproliferative effects of the endothelium may retard the development of atherosclerosis and intimal proliferation.

In addition to affecting the growth of underlying smooth muscle, endothelial cells are essential for the formation of new blood vessels. The ability of endothelial cells to initiate the formation of new vessels (angiogenesis and vasculogenesis; Fig. 1.1.8) is retained in adults, but the only place this occurs physiologically to any great extent is in the female reproductive tract. However, angiogenesis occurs in a wide range of disease states including atherosclerosis, rheumatoid arthritis, and tumour growth, and during wound healing or in response to ischaemia. Positive and negative regulators of angiogenesis have been identified and a wide variety of cytokines, growth factors, and local autacoids can act alone or in concert to promote endothelial cell growth, migration, and tube formation. Of particular interest is VEGF, a growth factor produced by smooth muscle cells in response to hypoxia, inflammatory cytokines, and certain other growth factors. There is good evidence that VEGF can promote angiogenesis in a variety of animal models and in humans. Therapeutics that inhibit angiogenesis by targeting the VEGF pathway have shown clinical benefit in diabetic retinopathy and certain cancers. Intriguingly, it appears as though VEGF can increase the production of NO by endothelial cells, and this may be one of the effector molecules mediating some of the actions of this growth factor. In order to form endothelial tubes through tissues (i.e. angiogenesis), endothelial cells must degrade matrix and they are capable of synthesizing and releasing a variety of matrix metalloproteinases. Some of these matrix metalloproteinases may, in turn, affect endothelial function by regulating cell attachment, proliferation, and migration. Failure of endothelial cells to initiate appropriate angiogenesis in response to ischaemia may lead to tissue hypoxia, while excessive or inappropriate angiogenesis may contribute to a sustained inflammatory response in the vessel wall, disrupt vessel wall architecture, or lead to haemorrhage into atherosclerotic plaques.

Transport and metabolism

The endothelium presents a permeability barrier for molecules in the bloodstream. Transfer of molecules from the bloodstream into the vessel wall across the endothelium can occur by transport through the endothelial cells or between them. The junctions between endothelial cells are maintained by specialized molecules, including cadherins, and are actively regulated. Transport between cells occurs when endothelial cells contract to leave intercellular gaps. This is an important mechanism for formation of localized oedema. Transport through cells occurs by transcytosis and is an important mechanism for the passage of some macromolecules, including insulin. In addition, specialized channels for transport of water have been identified—the aquaporins.

The endothelium is intimately involved in lipid metabolism. Lipoprotein lipase is bound to proteoglycans on the endothelial cell surface, and receptors for low-density lipoproteins are present in varying amounts. In quiescent endothelium, lipoprotein lipase is active, but there are few low-density lipoprotein receptors, indicating that healthy endothelium provides a barrier for the entry of low-density lipoproteins into the vessel wall. However, under conditions in which a low-density lipoprotein is taken into the endothelium, modification by oxidation occurs and this step may stimulate atherogenesis.

The adventitia and perivascular adipose tissue

Nerves supplying the vessel wall enter through the adventitia into the media to provide a key influence on the contraction of vascular smooth muscle cells. The sympathetic nervous system is, of course, of prime importance in determining the contractile state of the vessel. In addition, cholinergic innervation influences some vascular beds, as do purinergic nerves. Pharmacological observation suggests that not all vessels are equally affected by denervation or interruption of specific neuronal influences. Resistance vessels and capacitance veins seem to be particularly regulated by sympathetic tone, and blockade of the sympathetic system causes not only a fall in arterial pressure but also major venous dilatation that leads to postural hypotension. In the brain, local neuronal projections have been implicated in providing a link between cerebral activation and the consequent increase in blood flow.

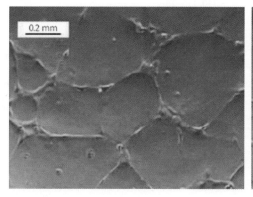 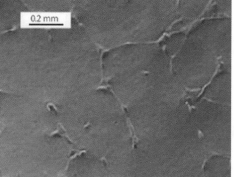

Fig. 1.1.8 Formation of new blood vessels. Endothelial cells grown in a matrix (Matrigel) form tube-like structures. The right-hand panel shows the effect of inhibiting angiogenic signals such as vascular endothelial growth factor (VEGF).

Reprinted from *Biochemical and Biophysical Research Communications*, Vol 308, Issue 4, Smith, C L *et al.*, Dimethylarginine dimethylaminohydrolase activity modulates ADMA levels, VEGF expression, and cell phenotype, pp. 984–89. Copyright (2003), with permission from Elsevier.

Lymph vessels also permeate the adventitia of large vessels and are important to remove fluid. A network of small blood vessels, the vasa vasorum, is found in the adventitia of larger blood vessels. Vasa vasorum are found mainly in vessels that have relatively thick walls with many layers of vascular smooth muscle cells. An increase in vasa vasorum may be taken as an indication of vessel wall hypoxia. Stripping the vasa vasorum in large veins may contribute to both smooth muscle and endothelial dysfunction and damage, and, in the arterial system, can stimulate smooth muscle cell replication and promote an atherogenic type of lesion. The vasa vasorum responds to vasoactive agents, but the pharmacology of these vessels is relatively poorly understood. Infiltration of the adventitia with inflammatory cells may be an important feature of atherogenesis (see Chapter 13.1), and perivascular fat may interfere with vascular function through the generation of adipokines and inflammatory cytokines; this process has been implicated in the pathogenesis of cardiovascular disease in obese individuals.

The adventitia surrounding the vascular wall also contains large numbers of adipocytes, forming the perivascular adipose tissue (PVAT). Although PVAT is typically in continuity with other surrounding adipose tissue, PVAT has particular cellular composition and pathophysiological roles that are distinct from other adipose tissue depots such as subcutaneous and visceral adipose tissue mediated by adipocytokines.

PVAT has anticontractile properties on small vessels due to a variety of vasoactive molecules produced in this tissue, such as H_2S, H_2O_2, and adipocytokines. Other infiltrating inflammatory cell types including T cells and macrophages have an equally important contribution. Most adipocytokines produced by the cells in PVAT have distinct paracrine effects on the vasculature. These can be proinflammatory/pro-atherogenic (e.g. resistin, IL-6, TNFα, MCP-1) or anti-inflammatory/anti-atherogenic (e.g. adiponectin, omentin). The balance between pro- and anti-atherogenic adipokines is influenced by conditions such as obesity and diabetes. In human PVAT, PPAR-γ signalling is a major regulator of adipocytokine production, and its dysregulation in diabetes, obesity and insulin resistance shifts the balance towards the production of proinflammatory mediators. Until recently, PVAT was considered to have mainly detrimental effects on vascular homeostasis. However, recent evidence suggests that it 'senses' proatherogenic changes in the underlying vascular wall (e.g. changes in ROS production), and can modify its biosynthetic profile by activating PPAR-γ signalling, leading to increased production of 'antioxidant' adipokines such as adiponectin and reduced production of 'pro-oxidant' adipokines such as IL-6. Therefore, increasing evidence suggests that healthy PVAT may provide local defence mechanisms against vascular injury, and its biosynthetic profile is regulated by complex interactions between PVAT, the underlying vascular wall, and systemic factors.

Further reading

Allt G, Lawrenson JG (2001). Pericytes: Cell biology and pathology. *Cells Tissues Organs*, **69**, 1–11.

Armulik A, *et al.* (2005). Endothelial/pericyte interactions. *Circ Res*, **97**, 512–23.

Asahara T, *et al.* (1997). Isolation of putative progenitor endothelial cells for angiogenesis. *Science*, **275**, 964–6.

Atkins GB, Jain MK (2007). Role of Krüppel-like transcription factors in endothelial biology. *Circ Res*, **100**, 1686–95.

Bonauer A, *et al.* (2010). Vascular microRNAs. *Curr Drug Targets*, **11**, 943–9.

Boos CJ, *et al.* (2006). Circulating endothelial cells in cardiovascular disease. *J Amer Coll Cardiol*, **8**, 1538–47.

Channon KM, Guzik TJ (2002). Mechanisms of superoxide production in human blood vessels: relationship to endothelial dysfunction, clinical and genetic risk factors. *J Physiol Pharmacol*. **53**:515-24.

Crabtree MJ, Channon KM (2011). Synthesis and recycling of tetrahydrobiopterin in endothelial function and vascular disease. *Nitric Oxide*, **25**, 81–8.

Chironi GN, *et al.* (2009). Endothelial microparticles in diseases. *Cell Tissue Res*, **335**, 143–51.

Dhaun N, *et al.* (2006). The endothelin system and its antagonism in chronic kidney disease. *J Am Soc Nephrol*, **17**, 943–55.

Earley S, Brayden JE (2010). Transient receptor potential channels and vascular function. *Clin Sci (Lond)*, **119**, 19–36.

Folkman J. (2003). Fundamental concepts of the angiogenic process. *Curr Mol Med*, **3**, 643–51.

Frantz S, *et al.* (2007). Mechanisms of disease: Toll-like receptors in cardiovascular disease. *Nat Clin Pract Cardiovasc Med*, **4**, 444–54.

Furchgott RF, Zawadzki JV (1980). The obligatory role of endothelial cells in the relaxation of arterial smooth muscle. *Nature*, **288**, 373–6.

Isner JM, Asahara T (1999). Angiogenesis and vasculogenesis as therapeutic strategies for postnatal neovascularization. *J Clin Invest*, **103**, 1232–6.

Kinlay S, *et al.* (2001). Endothelial function and coronary artery disease. *Curr Opin Lipid*, **12**, 383–9.

Margaritis M, *et al.* (2013). Interactions between vascular wall and perivascular adipose tissue reveal novel roles for adiponectin in the regulation of endothelial nitric oxide synthase function in human vessels. *Circulation*, **127**, 2209–21.

Mason JC, Haskard DO (1994). The clinical importance of leucocyte and endothelial cell adhesion molecules in inflammation. *Vasc Med Rev*, **5**, 249–75.

McDonald OG, Owens GK (2007). Programming smooth muscle plasticity with chromatin dynamics. *Circ Res*, **100**, 1428–41.

Pasqualini R, *et al.* (2010). Leveraging molecular heterogeneity of the vascular endothelium for targeted drug delivery and imaging. *Semin Thromb Hemost*, **36**, 343–51.

Rao RM, *et al.* (2007). Endothelial-dependent mechanisms of leukocyte recruitment to the vascular wall. *Circ Res*, **101**, 234–47.

Ross R (1999). Atherosclerosis—an inflammatory disease. *N Engl J Med*, **340**, 115–26.

Tse D, Stan RV (2010). Morphological heterogeneity of endothelium. *Semin Thromb Hemost*, **36**, 236–45.

Vallance P, *et al.* (1997). Infection, inflammation and infarction: does acute endothelial dysfunction provide a link? *Lancet*, **349**, 1391–2.

Vallance P, Leiper J (2004). Cardiovascular biology of the asymmetric dimethylarginine:dimethylarginine dimethylaminohydrolase pathway. *Arterioscler Thromb Vasc Biol*, **24**, 1023–30.

Vane JR, *et al.* (1998). Cyclooxygenases 1 and 2. *Annu Rev Pharmacol Toxicol*, **38**, 97–120.

CHAPTER 1.2

Cardiac physiology

Rhys D. Evans, Kenneth T. MacLeod, Steven B. Marston, Nicholas J. Severs, and Peter H. Sugden

Essentials

The function of the heart is to provide the tissues of the body with sufficient oxygenated blood and metabolites to meet the moment-to-moment needs as dictated by physical activity and postural and emotional changes.

Functional anatomy of the cardiac myocyte

Cardiac myocytes are the contractile cells of the heart and constitute the bulk of heart mass. There are differences between the myocytes of the ventricles, the atria, and the conduction system: ventricular myocytes are elongated cells, packed with myofibrils (the contractile apparatus) and mitochondria (for ATP production). Myofibrils are repeating units (sarcomeres) made up of thin actin filaments anchored at the Z-discs at either end of the sarcomere, and thick myosin filaments which interdigitate and interact with the thin filaments. Contraction results from sarcomere shortening produced by the ATP-dependent movement of the thin and thick filaments relative to one another. Transverse (T-) tubules facilitate extracellular Ca^{2+} entry into the cytoplasm (sarcoplasm) for signalling and contraction. Atrial myocytes differ from ventricular myocytes, having few T-tubules but more abundant caveolae. Myocytes of the conduction system are small and possess only a rudimentary myofibrillar structure.

Myocytes are attached to their neighbours and to the extracellular matrix to allow transmission of force. At some regions of contact (the intercalated discs), specialized structures (the gap junctions) contain channels which form contiguous electrical connections between a myocyte and its neighbours, and allow passage of ions and small molecules.

Cardiac action potential

A potential difference (the membrane potential) is maintained across the plasma membrane (sarcolemma) such that the inside of the cell is negative compared to the outside by about 90 mV. This is caused largely by the efflux of K^+ from the cell through K^+ channels and down its concentration gradient until the electronegative force retaining K^+ in the cell balances the tendency for efflux.

The sarcoplasmic reticulum (SR) surrounds the myofibrils and is a reservoir of the Ca^{2+} which participates in myofibrillar contraction. T-tubules are deep, finger-like indentations of the sarcolemma that abut the SR at junctional regions in register with the Z-discs of the superficial sarcomeres.

When a myocyte is electrically excited, Na^+ channels open and Na^+ enters the cell down its own concentration gradient, producing a rapid inward current and depolarizing the cell towards its equilibrium potential: the initial phase (phase 0) of the action potential. As the myocyte depolarizes, L-type Ca^{2+} channels in the sarcolemma and T-tubules open and Ca^{2+} enters the cell down its concentration gradient. The Na^+ channels close rapidly, but the L-type Ca^{2+} channels remain open for longer, maintaining depolarization: phases 1 and 2 of the action potential, where the tendency to depolarize is balanced by repolarizing outward current flow carried by a variety of K^+ channels. The membrane potential in phase 2 is relatively stable and hence this phase is also known as the plateau phase.

Ca^{2+} entry in close apposition to the junctional SR causes SR Ca^{2+}-release channels to open, discharging about half of the SR Ca^{2+} reservoir into the cytoplasm (Ca^{2+}-induced Ca^{2+}-release). This increase in Ca^{2+} concentration (the Ca^{2+} transient) is sensed by a Ca^{2+}-binding protein (troponin C) that is a component of the thin filament regulatory complex (the troponin–tropomyosin complex). This initiates myofibrillar contraction, which starts about halfway through phase 2.

As the L-type Ca^{2+} channels close, outward current flow through K^+ channels predominates and the myocyte repolarizes towards the K^+ equilibrium potential (phase 3). Ca^{2+} is removed from the cytoplasm and returned to the SR in an ATP-requiring process mediated by the sarcoplasmic/endoplasmic Ca^{2+}-ATPase (SERCA2). Ca^{2+} is also expelled from the cell by the plasma membrane Na^+,Ca^{2+} exchanger, which is electrogenic (three Na^+ exchanged for one Ca^{2+}) and tends to prolong the plateau phase. The behaviour of the Na^+,Ca^{2+} exchanger is complex because—depending on the Na^+ and Ca^{2+} concentrations and the membrane potential—it can reverse, thus mediating Ca^{2+} entry and repolarization. This occurs at depolarized potentials, and more so when intracellular Na^+ is increased. In phase 4, repolarization is complete and the myocyte is electrically quiescent until the next depolarization.

Cardiac pacemaker and regulation of contractility

The sinoatrial node ('pacemaker') contains modified myocytes that exhibit a different form of action potential from ventricular myocytes because of differences in the expression of ion channels. The cell depolarizes spontaneously and gradually during phase 4 until an action potential is produced. This partly results from the presence of hyperpolarization-activated cyclic nucleotide-gated (HCN) channels which are absent from ventricular myocytes and which carry an inward-depolarizing Na^+ current. Depolarization is then mediated by Ca^{2+} channel opening. The stimulus is transmitted in a controlled manner via the conduction system to all regions of the heart.

Whole organ physiology

Cardiac contractility is controlled largely by the sympathoadrenal system and the parasympathetic nervous system. β-Adrenergic stimulation increases the tendency of the L-type Ca^{2+} channel to open (positive inotropism). β-Stimulation also increases relaxation (positive lusitropism) by stimulation of SERCA2 and an increased rate of release of Ca^{2+} from the troponin complex. The positive chronotropic effects of β-stimulation result from increased HCN channel opening, causing an increased frequency of pacemaker depolarization. These effects are all opposed by the (cholinergic) muscarinic receptors of the parasympathetic nervous system.

The energy requirements of the heart during rest and exertion are influenced by ventricular volume, outflow resistance (blood pressure), venous return, and the activity of the autonomic nervous system. An increase in ventricular volume increases wall tension during contraction, and an augmented myocardial oxygen supply is then required to maintain the same systemic blood pressure and stroke volume.

The normal integration of the venous return, heart rate, stroke volume, and arterial blood pressure ensures that there is an adequate supply of oxygen and nutrients to the tissues. The activities of the sympathetic and parasympathetic nervous systems contribute to the adjustment of cardiac performance to immediate needs—the former by increasing heart rate and myocardial contractility during exertion and emotion, the latter by maintaining a relatively slow heart rate at rest. Vagal fibres in the heart are distributed mainly to the sinoatrial node and the atria; sympathetic innervation is to both the atria and the ventricles. There is a normal diurnal variation in autonomic function, with an increased sympathetic outflow in the mornings, soon after wakening.

Coronary flow occurs largely in diastole. It is finely adjusted to meet metabolic requirements and may increase five- or sixfold during strenuous exercise. The inner layers of the ventricular muscle normally receive a slightly greater blood flow than the outer layers. Haemodynamic and ventilatory responses during exercise take 2 to 3 min to equilibrate and adjust to an increased workload and reach a new steady state. Regular exercise to least 60% of maximal heart rate about three times a week improves effort tolerance. Measurement of the cardiovascular response to exercise provides an objective assessment of cardiac function.

Introduction

The function of the heart is to pump sufficient oxygenated blood containing nutrients, metabolites, and hormones to meet moment-to-moment metabolic needs and preserve a constant internal environment. The heart has two essential characteristics—contractility and rhythmicity. The nervous system and neurohumoral agents modulate relationships between the venous return to the heart, the outflow resistance against which it contracts, the frequency of contraction, and its inotropic state; there are also intrinsic cardiac autoregulatory mechanisms. An understanding of the molecular mechanisms governing cardiac cell behaviour and the mechanical, electrical, and hormonal control of the heart at a whole organ level is essential for the understanding of cardiac pathophysiology.

Cardiac myocytes

Cardiac myocytes are the contractile cells of the heart, and include ventricular and atrial myocytes, as well as cells specialized to provide the electrical impulse and conduction system. Myocytes constitute the bulk of the cellular volume, but because they are large cells they are fewer in number, being outnumbered by endothelial cells, smooth muscle cells of the vasculature, and fibroblasts. Ventricular myocytes are believed to be terminally differentiated cells in mammals, incapable of replication; this is less clear for the atrial myocyte. Terminal differentiation has important consequences for the heart in terms of its limited ability to survive haemodynamic insults or stresses, but also means that the myocardium is essentially resistant to malignant transformation.

Morphology of the ventricular myocyte and its contractile machinery

The ventricular myocyte is an elongated cell (100–150 μm long and 20–35 μm wide) and is packed with striated myofibrils (the contractile elements) that alternate with rows of mitochondria (Fig. 1.2.1). Each myofibril is roughly cylindrical (2–3 μm in diameter), stretches the length of the cell, and is anchored at each end in a fascia adherens junction. The myofibril comprises sarcomeres arranged in series. Sarcomeres consist of two arrays of filaments: thin filaments, comprised predominantly of the protein actin, interdigitated with thick filaments of myosin. The characteristic striated appearance arises from the organization of these filaments within the myofibril (Fig. 1.2.1). The thick filaments are confined to the A-band at the

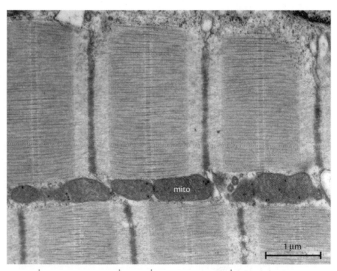

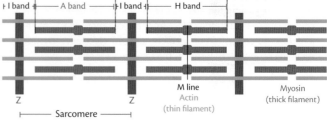

Fig. 1.2.1 Upper panel: Electron micrograph of ventricular myocyte showing the structure of the myofibrils. Portions of two myofibrils are shown in the field, with a row of mitochondria (mito) between. Lower panel: Diagrammatic representation of the arrangement of the thick and thin filaments in relation to the striated pattern seen in microscopy.

centre of the sarcomere. The thin filaments extend out from either side of the Z-disc (Z-line), crossing the I-band, and penetrate partially into the A-band, where they overlap and interact with the thick filaments. Each Z- to Z-disc repeat constitutes a sarcomere, and the distance between consecutive Z-discs (the sarcomere length) is a measure of the contractile state of the myofibril. At the centre of the sarcomere lies the M-line. Each myofibril contains 70–80 sarcomeres. Myocytes have an irregular 'branched' morphology; through these branches, each ventricular myocyte typically connects to 10 or more of its neighbours to form the three-dimensional branching, syncytium-like structure of the myofibre.

Structure of the contractile apparatus

Thick filaments

The myosin molecule comprises two heavy chains (molecular mass ~200 kDa) and two pairs of light chains (mass 18–28 kDa). The myosin heavy chains are arranged as dimers, with a tail and two heads (Fig. 1.2.2). The tails are packed together to form the shaft of the thick filament, while the heads protrude from the filament and lie close to the thin actin filaments. The myosin heads are the motor units of muscle: they bind and hydrolyse ATP to ADP and convert the free energy of hydrolysis into mechanical work through their interaction with actin in the thin filaments (for details see 'The mechanism of myocyte contraction').

Thin filaments

Each thin filament comprises about 300 globular actin subunits (mass 42 kDa). The actin monomers have sites for interaction with the myosin heads and with a regulatory protein complex that confers Ca^{2+} sensitivity. The latter consists of the troponin complex and the elongated protein α-tropomyosin (Fig. 1.2.2). Troponin complexes are located at intervals along the actin filament. Tropomyosin forms two continuous strands along the thin filament and is responsible for cooperative propagation of regulatory signals.

Other structural components of the sarcomere

The thin filaments are attached to the Z-discs in a regular array with filaments on each side in opposite orientation (Fig. 1.2.1). The main structural component of the Z-disc is the actin cross-linking protein α-actinin. Z-discs are also associated with the T-tubules and costameres (see below), and contain a number of additional proteins believed to be associated with cell signalling. The M-line (Fig. 1.2.1) contains the protein myomesin that cross-links the thick filaments to maintain their orientation. In addition, the giant protein titin (connectin) extends from the M-line to the Z-disc. Titin contains multiple binding sites for multiple sarcomeric proteins, including myosin-binding protein-C (MyBP-C; Fig. 1.2.2). It contributes to elasticity, passive tension, and thick filament positioning in the sarcomere.

Intermediate filaments, costameres, and the plasma membrane skeleton

The myofibrils are held in position by scaffold-like webs of intermediate filaments made from a (non-contractile) protein, desmin. Desmin filaments are anchored to costameres, which circumscribe the lateral plasma membrane. Apart from maintaining the spatial organization of the contractile apparatus, the costameres mechanically couple the cells laterally to the extracellular matrix. Associated with the costameres, but closely applied to the entire cytoplasmic aspect of the lateral plasma membrane, is the membrane skeleton, a peripheral membrane protein network of dystrophin and spectrin. The costameres, membrane skeleton, and intermediate filaments are linked to the glycocalyx and extracellular matrix by sets of integral plasma membrane proteins, notably the integrins and the components of the dystrophin–glycoprotein complex.

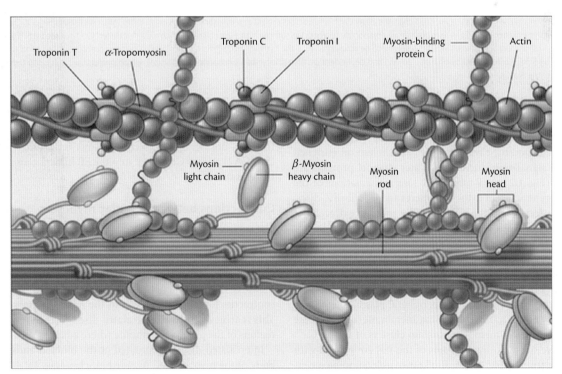

Fig. 1.2.2 Structural arrangement of contractile proteins in the filament overlap zone of the sarcomere.

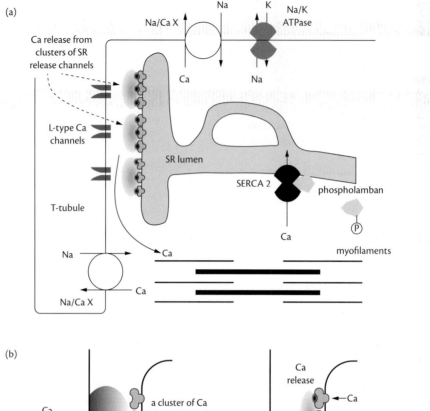

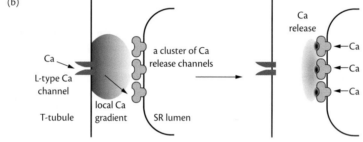

Fig. 1.2.3 EC coupling in the heart. (a) L-type Ca^{2+} channels allow Ca^{2+} influx across the plasma membrane, creating I_{Ca}. This influx increases the local Ca^{2+} concentration around a cluster of SR Ca^{2+}-release channels (ryanodine receptor) in sufficient amounts to open them (Ca^{2+}-induced Ca^{2+}-release). (b) The opening of clusters of SR Ca^{2+}-release channels allows SR Ca^{2+} reservoir to be discharged into the cytoplasm. Ca^{2+} fluxes combine to initiate contraction. The contraction process is terminated (1) by SERCA2 (regulated by phospholamban and dependent on phospholamban phosphorylation state), which pumps Ca^{2+} back into the SR, and (2) by the plasma membrane Na/CaX which expels Ca^{2+} from the cell.

Coupling of the plasma membrane to the SR

The plasma membrane (sarcolemma) contains openings of transverse (T)-tubules and the caveolae, which are cholesterol-enriched pits in which signal-transducing and water-channel proteins are concentrated (Fig. 1.2.3a). T-tubules are long invaginations of the plasma membrane adjacent to the costameres and myofibril Z-discs, and penetrate deeply into the cell. T-tubules mediate extracellular Ca^{2+} (Ca^{2+}_o) entry into the cell through the L-type Ca^{2+} channels. Each myofibril is surrounded by a network of interconnecting membranous tubules and cisternae known as the sarcoplasmic reticulum (SR) (Fig. 1.2.3a). At multiple sites within this network, the membranes form flattened sacs, the junctional SR (JSR) cisternae, which press tightly against the peripheral plasma membrane and T-tubules (Fig. 1.2.3b). The plasma membrane and T-tubule domains facing the JSR membrane contain clusters of L-type Ca^{2+} channels, while the apposing domains of the JSR are packed with Ca^{2+}-release channels (Fig. 1.2.3), also known as 'ryanodine receptors' because of their sensitivity to interference by the plant alkaloid ryanodine. The JSR is the major reservoir of cytoplasmic Ca^{2+}.

This close spatial arrangement is important in control of the Ca^{2+} transient required for myofibrillar contraction. Following contraction, the sarcoplasmic/endoplasmic reticulum Ca^{2+}ATPase 2 (SERCA2) pumps Ca^{2+} back into the SR lumen, causing myofibrillar relaxation.

Connections between cardiac myocytes

The myocyte can function as an autonomous contractile unit. To produce a heartbeat, the contractile capabilities of the ~3 billion myocytes that constitute the human heart have to be electromechanically synchronized. This requires both an orderly spread of the wave of electrical activation and the effective transmission of contractile force from one cell to the next, throughout the heart. This is achieved by the intercalated discs, formed from specialized regions of the plasma membrane where adjacent cells interact.

Intercalated discs are situated at the blunted ends of the main body of the myocyte and its side branches (Fig. 1.2.4). Three types of cell junction—the gap junction, the fascia adherens, and the desmosome—connect the adjacent membranes at the disc. The

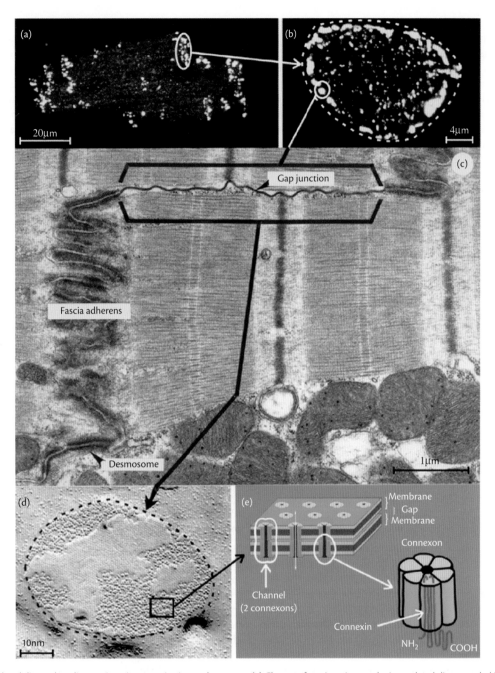

Fig. 1.2.4 The intercalated disc and cardiac gap junction organization and structure. (a) Clusters of gap junctions at the intercalated discs revealed in a single ventricular cardiac myocyte by immunoconfocal microscopy. (b) One disc-cluster of gap junctions viewed *en face* (reconstruction from a stack of serial optical sections). One of these immunolabelled spots corresponds to a single gap junction. (c) Electron micrograph illustrating the three types of cell junction of the intercalated disc. Gap junctions occur where the adjacent plasma membrane profiles run in close contact. The fascia adherens and the desmosome are characterized by a much wider intermembrane space (*c*.25 nm). (d) Viewing the membrane *en face* by freeze-fracture reveals the gap junction as a cluster of particles (connexons). (e) The gap junction channel consists of a pair of connexons (hemichannels), one contributed by each of the adjacent plasma membranes. Each connexon is itself formed from six connexin molecules. The specific connexin type or types within the connexon is a major determinant of the functional properties of the gap junction channel.
Reprinted from Severs NJ (2000). The cardiac muscle cell. *BioEssays*, **22**, 188–99 (Fig. 5). With permission from Wiley-Blackwell.

fascia adherens and desmosome are forms of anchoring junction; gap junctions contain clusters of connexons (Fig. 1.2.4). These junctions are clusters of intercellular channels which span two closely apposed plasma membranes and directly link adjacent cytoplasmic compartments of neighbouring cells. They form the sites of electrical coupling between individual cardiac myocytes and permit direct cell-to-cell transmission of chemical signals (ions and small molecules of <1 kDa). The combination of connexin isoforms constituting a gap junction channel is a major determinant of its functional properties, and varies in different cardiomyocyte subsets. This arrangement renders the myocardium into a functional syncytium.

Cardiac myocyte subtypes

Atrial myocytes are significantly different to the ventricular myocytes described above; they are long and slender, with few or no

T-tubules but more abundant caveolae. By producing the peptide hormone atrial natriuretic peptide (ANP; atrial natriuretic factor), they also function as secretory cells. Natriuretic peptides participate in the control of sodium and water balance and hence of blood pressure.

A third, heterogeneous, group of modified and morphologically distinct myocytes makes up the pacemaker and conduction system. These cells show some resemblance to ventricular and atrial cells, but their primary function is impulse generation and its timed distribution to the contractile myocytes at the appropriate point in the cardiac cycle.

Myocytes of the sinoatrial and atrioventricular nodes are typically small (c.5 μm diameter), containing just a few rudimentary myofibrils, and small, sparse, gap junctions. These features contribute to poor coupling, which in the atrioventricular node is essential to slowing of conduction to ensure time for atrial ejection. The cell population is morphologically heterogeneous: cells of the compact atrioventricular node, and those of the surrounding areas (the transitional cells and posterior nodal extension), are distinctive, and myocytes of the His–Purkinje system show a range of morphologies according to their location, progressively increasing in size and myofibril content, and with more developed intercalated discs distally, towards the ventricular myocardium.

The cardiac action potential

The membrane potential

Electrical activity of the heart (membrane potential; action potential) is based on differential distribution of ions across the cellular membranes. This distribution is achieved by the action of ion-transport proteins, including ion pumps and channels.

Ion channels

Electrical excitation of myocytes involves the movement of ions through specific channels. These are 'excitable' proteins embedded in membranes that contain pores capable of opening or closing in response to a stimulus, which could be a change in membrane potential, a neurotransmitter or hormone, an intracellular second messenger or ion, or mechanical stretch of the membrane. On opening, a channel becomes selectively permeable to a restricted series of ions. There are many different types of channel, often named after the most permeant ion they pass, e.g. Na^+, Ca^{2+}, and K^+ channels. Ions move down their electrochemical gradients through the channel at high rates (>10^6 ions/s), distinguishing them from other ion-transport proteins (e.g. the Na^+,K^+-ATPase or pump, and the Na^+,Ca^{2+} exchanger (Na/CaX); see below 'The Na^+,Ca^{2+} exchanger (Na/CaX) and the Na^+,K^+-ATPase') which move ions across plasma membranes several orders of magnitude more slowly. Hence cardiac excitation provides a means of coordinating the contractile activities of the four chambers and is the basis for the electrocardiograph (ECG) (see Chapter 3.1).

Origin of the membrane potential

Cardiac membrane potential is determined by three factors: (1) ionic concentrations across the sarcolemma; (2) the permeability (conductance) of the sarcolemma to specific ions; and (3) the activity of electrogenic pumps that maintain the ionic concentration gradients. When a ventricular myocyte is at rest (diastole), there is a potential difference of about −90 mV across the plasma membrane, the inside of the cell being negative with respect to the outside. This is principally caused by plasma membrane permeability to K^+. The extracellular concentration of K^+ (K^+_o) is about 4 mmol/litre, and the intracellular (cytoplasmic) concentration (K^+_i) is about 140 mmol/litre, so K^+ tends to diffuse out of the cell down its concentration gradient, resulting in the interior becoming negatively charged. An equilibrium is thus established where the electronegative force retaining K^+ inside the cell (mostly derived from negatively charged proteins) balances its tendency to diffuse out of the cell down its concentration gradient. This is termed the equilibrium potential (E) and can be calculated from the Nernst equation (see Table 1.2.1 for E values of relevant ions). At this potential, there will be no net flux of K^+ ions through K^+ channels and, if the membrane is only permeable to K^+, then the membrane potential will be equal to E_K.

The membrane potential at any moment is dependent upon the equilibrium potentials for all permeant species and their relative permeabilities. The actual transmembrane potential difference at rest and the calculated E_K are rarely the same owing to a small leakage, mainly of Na^+ into the cell down its concentration gradient (Na^+_o = 140 mmol/litre, Na^+_i = 7–10 mmol/litre). To counteract this leak and to maintain the concentration gradients of Na^+ and K^+ upon which the generation of the membrane potential depends, the plasma membrane Na^+,K^+-ATPase uses free energy derived from the hydrolysis of ATP to pump these ions against their concentration gradients. This process is electrogenic (three Na^+ extruded for two K^+ entering) and generates 3 to 10 mV of the membrane potential.

The action potential

The action potential is divided into five phases (Fig. 1.2.5). The currents that flow are described in Table 1.2.1, Table 1.2.2, and Fig. 1.2.5. Depolarization from the resting potential is mediated by inward current flow.

Phase 0 of the action potential

When a myocyte is electrically stimulated, Na^+ channels open and allow Na^+ ions to enter the cell. The channels open by sensing potential difference more positive than about −65 mV across the cell membrane (Fig. 1.2.5). Excitation depolarizes the cell membrane slightly and this increases the probability of Na^+ channel opening. A cardiac myocyte contains many thousands of Na^+ channels, hence the current (I) generated by the movement of Na^+ ions into the cell (I_{Na}) is the sum of the small currents that flow though each individual channel. Positive charge is taken into the cell, the membrane potential increases towards the equilibrium potential for Na^+ (E_{Na} = +70 mV, Table 1.2.1), and the cell depolarizes (Fig. 1.2.5). The Na^+ current causes the rapid upstroke (phase 0) of the action potential. The propagation velocity of the action potential across the whole heart is related to the rate of the rapid upstroke. Following activation and opening, the channels close very rapidly, even though the myocyte remains depolarized, a process termed 'inactivation'. Inactivated channels cannot open again until the cell repolarizes, causing the refractory period during which a further stimulus cannot evoke another action potential (Fig. 1.2.5).

The inactivation of each channel decreases the total number of Na^+ channels that are conducting such that I_{Na} almost entirely inactivates within the first 5 ms of the action potential (the overall action potential in humans at rest lasts c.350 ms). Some Na^+ channels do not inactivate so rapidly, allowing a small inward current

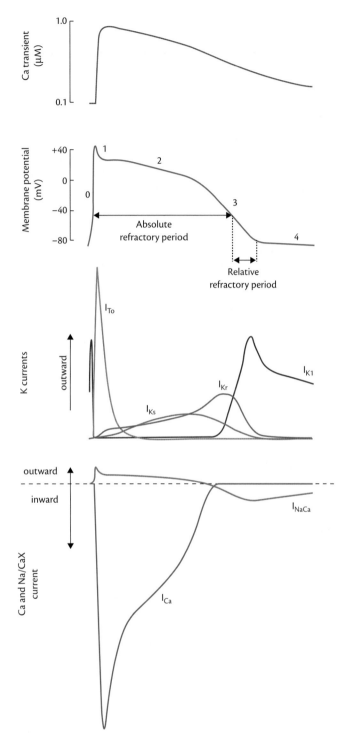

Fig. 1.2.5 Ca^{2+} transient, membrane potential, K^+ currents, and Ca^{2+}-related currents during a ventricular myocyte action potential. The inward Na^+ current that produces the rapid upstroke of the action potential is not shown Top panel: Changes in cytoplasmic Ca^{2+} concentration during the action potential (Ca^{2+} transient). Upper middle panel: Phases of the ventricular myocyte action potential. For a period between phase 0 and about midway through phase 3, cardiac muscle cannot be excited with another stimulus: the absolute refractory period. From about halfway through phase 3 until just before the end of phase 3, cardiac muscle is in its relative refractory period, when a stronger stimulus than normal is required to initiate an action potential. The states of refractoriness are related to the ability of ion channels to recover from a stimulus. This recovery is both voltage- and time-dependent. Lower middle panel: K^+ currents during one action potential. All K^+ currents (I_{TO}, I_{Ks}, I_{Kr}, and I_{K1}) repolarize the myocyte because of outward K^+ movement. Bottom panel: Ca^{2+}-related currents during one action potential. Because of the inward movement of Ca^{2+}, Ca^{2+} current (I_{Ca}) is depolarizing. The Na/CaX produces both outward and inward current ($I_{Na,Ca}$) depending on the phase of the action potential. The inward Na^+ current is roughly 8 to 10 times the size of the Ca^{2+} current and has largely inactivated by the time of the peak Ca^{2+} current.

Table 1.2.1 Ion concentrations in the quiescent myocyte, and their calculated equilibrium potentials (E). E is calculated from the Nernst equation, $E = (RT/zF)\ln(a_o/a_i)$, where E is in volts, T is the absolute temperature, R is the gas constant, F is the Faraday constant, z is the valency, and a_o and a_i are the extracellular and intracellular activities of the ion in question

Ion	Intracellular concentration (mmol/litre)	Plasma concentration (mmol/litre)	Calculated E (mV)
Na^+	10	140	+70
K^+	140	4.5	−91
Ca^{2+}	0.0001	2.3	+131
Cl^-	20	110	+45

to persist during the plateau phase of the action potential (phase 2, see below).

Phase 1 of the action potential

The characteristic notch observed in phase 1 of the action potential in ventricular myocytes (Fig. 1.2.5) is caused by a transient outward current (I_{TO}), carried mainly by K^+ ions flowing out of the cell (I_{TO1}), but also by some Cl^- current (I_{TO2}), that partially repolarizes the membrane. The current inactivates within 30–40 ms but is important in determining action potential duration. A component of I_{TO} appears to be dependent upon intracellular Ca^{2+} concentration (raised Ca^{2+}_o increases I_{TO}): this is the probable mechanism underlying action potential shortening during tachycardia.

Phase 2 of the action potential

Several currents flow during phase 2 (the action potential plateau), including I_{Ca} (Fig. 1.2.5). L-type ('long lasting') Ca^{2+} channels, which take longer to activate and inactivate than Na^+ channels, open within 3–5 ms of the start of the upstroke and allow Ca^{2+} to flow into the cell (I_{Ca}). L-type Ca^{2+} channels activate at more positive voltages than Na^+ channels (around −35 mV). The influx of Ca^{2+} maintains depolarization (Fig. 1.2.5, Tables 1.2.1 and 1.2.2), and initiates Ca^{2+}-induced Ca^{2+}-release (CICR) from the SR through the SR Ca^{2+}-release channels, causing the myocyte to contract (see below). Hence, Ca^{2+} has a role in both membrane potential and signal transduction/inotropy. In addition, a slow delayed rectifier K^+ current (I_{KS}) exports K^+ in phase 2.

The plateau phase (phase 2) of the action potential (Fig. 1.2.5) is prolonged in ventricular myocytes because of the properties of several types of K^+ channel that give rise to several different K^+ currents. The main repolarizing current, I_K, is composed of two distinct currents, one activating more rapidly (I_{Kr}) than the other (I_{Ks}) (see Table 1.2.2). Both channels open at positive membrane potentials and close (deactivate) at negative potentials. The plateau of the action potential is the result of a balance of inward (Ca^{2+}) and outward (K^+) current flow.

Phase 3 of the action potential

The final phase of repolarization begins with the termination of I_{Ca} and progressively increasing K^+ current (I_{Kr} and I_{Ks}) (Fig. 1.2.5). As repolarization proceeds, the Na/CaX responds to the increase in cytoplasmic Ca^{2+} concentration and produces an inward current ($I_{Na,Ca}$) through the exchange of three Na^+ entering the cell for one Ca^{2+} expelled; by producing an inward current, the Na/CaX slows

repolarization and prolongs the plateau. In ventricular myocytes, complete repolarization and a return to a negative resting membrane potential is eventually achieved by (the large) I_{K1} (the 'inward rectifier'; Fig. 1.2.5; Table 1.2.2). The channel through which this current flows possesses peculiar characteristics. Normally, because of the relative concentrations of K^+ inside and outside the cell, there is outward movement of K^+ ions that becomes larger the more positive the displacement from E_K. However, the I_{K1} current flows through a channel that first increases its conductance but then decreases it as the cell depolarizes away from E_K (anomalous rectification). Thus, there is outward flow of repolarizing current only over a narrow voltage range (around −30 to −80 mV)—another reason for the prolonged cardiac action potential because a large, rapid, outward K^+ current does not flow despite the membrane potential approaching 0 mV during the plateau phase.

I_{K1} underlies the main flow of K^+ giving rise to the membrane potential. The channels through which I_{K1} flows are numerous in ventricular cells, fewer in atrial cells, and absent in pacemaker cells. The current is therefore large in ventricular cells and this is the reason that the resting membrane potential of ventricular myocytes lies near E_K, whereas atrial cells have a more positive resting membrane potential, and SA nodal cells do not have a stable resting potential.

Phase 4 of the action potential

This phase relates to the membrane potential during the electrically silent period between excitatory events in ventricular myocytes (Fig. 1.2.5); phase 4 is stable in these cells.

Regional variations in action potential

The configuration of the cardiac action potential differs regionally within the heart (Fig. 1.2.6) because ion-channel expression varies between cells. In the sinoatrial node, I_{Na} is very small and the main current responsible for the depolarizing upstroke is I_{Ca}, carried mainly by L-type Ca^{2+} channels. The only repolarizing current is I_K. I_{K1} is absent and, as mentioned above, this partially explains why sinoatrial node cells have a more depolarized 'diastolic' potential than ventricular myocytes. Sinoatrial node cells depolarize spontaneously during phase 4 (Fig. 1.2.6), owing to the absence of I_{K1} and the presence of a current activated on hyperpolarization called the 'funny' current (I_f), carried mainly by Na^+ through hyperpolarization-activated cyclic nucleotide-gated (HCN) channels, and current ($I_{Ca,T}$) resulting from an influx of Ca^{2+} through voltage-dependent T-type ('transient') Ca^{2+} channels (abundant in these cells) (Table 1.2.2). Phase 4 is often termed the 'pre- or pacemaker potential' in nodal cells and is caused by the gradual decrease in I_K and increase in I_f and $I_{Ca,T}$ (Fig. 1.2.6). Once the cell has depolarized to a voltage at which L-type Ca^{2+} channels open (the threshold), a more rapid depolarization (caused by $I_{Ca,L}$) occurs, forming the upstroke (phase 0) of the sinoatrial node action potential. Acetylcholine (ACh) activates $I_{K,ACh}$, which helps drive the membrane potential towards E_K and slows the rate of depolarization, while β-adrenergic stimulation increases the slope of the pacemaker potential and heart rate through an effect on I_f, affecting heart rate (Fig. 1.2.7).

Atrial and ventricular myocytes do not have pacemaker potentials and spontaneously discharge only when injured or when there is abnormal ionic balance. The longest action potential is in Purkinje fibres (Fig. 1.2.6) and this acts as a 'gate' preventing retrograde activation by depolarization of adjacent ventricular myocytes.

Table 1.2.2 Plasma membrane currents in the cardiac myocyte

Current	Name	Activated by	Blocked by	Gene	Protein	Function
Inward currents						
I_{Na}	(Fast) Na$^+$ current	Depolarization	Tetrodotoxin, local anaesthetics	SCN5A	Nav1.5	Rapid upstroke of action potential
$I_{Ca,L}$	L-type Ca^{2+} current ('long lasting')	Depolarization	Verapamil, Cd^{2+}, dihydropyridines	CACNA1C	Cav1.2	Ca^{2+} influx that activates CICR, provides some Ca^{2+} for contraction
$I_{Ca,T}$	T-type Ca^{2+} current ("transient")	Activates on depolarization but at more negative potentials than L-type current	Ni^{2+}, mibefradil	CACNA1G CACNA1H	Cav3.1 Cav3.2	Channel density high in pacemaker and conducting tissue so may contribute to pacemaker activity. Role in ventricular cells unclear
I_f	Hyperpolarization-activated, cyclic nucleotide-gated cation channel	Hyperpolarization, noradrenaline, cAMP	Cs$^+$, ZD7288, ivabradine, zatebradine, cilobradine	HCN2 HCN4		Exists in sinoatrial node and Purkinje fibres bringing membrane potential slowly to threshold
Inward and outward (reversible) current						
$I_{Na/Ca}$	Na/CaX current	Ca$^{2+}_i$	Ni^{2+}, KB-R7943	NCX1		Expels Ca^{2+} from the cell, maintains inward current flow near end of action potential, at positive potentials may reverse and mediate Ca^{2+} influx
Outward currents						
I_{TO}	Transient outward current	Depolarization	4-Aminopyridine	KCNA4 KCND2 KCND3	Kv1.4 Kv4.2 Kv4.3	Early repolarization (notch)
I_{Cl}	Chloride current	cAMP		CFTR		Early repolarization
$I_{Cl,Ca}$	Ca^{2+}-activated chloride current	Ca^{2+}		CLCA1		Early repolarization
I_{Kur}	Ultra-rapid delayed rectifier	Depolarization	Tetraethylammonium, Cs$^+$, Ba^{2+}, 4-aminopyridine, flecainide, nifedipine, diltiazem, bupivacaine, propafenone, quinidine	KCNA5	Kv1.5	Repolarization of cell
I_{Kr}	Rapid delayed rectifier	Depolarization	Tetraethylammonium, Cs$^+$, Ba^{2+}, E-4031, dofetilide, D-sotolol, cisapride, BRL32872	KCNH2	herg, Kv11.1	Repolarization of cell
I_{Ks}	Slow delayed rectifier	Depolarization	Chromanol 293B	KCNQ1	KvLQT1	Repolarization of cell
I_{K1}	Inward (anomalous) rectifier	Depolarization from E_K Conductance of channel increases then decreases to zero at 0 mV	Cs$^+$, Rb$^+$, Ba^{2+}, intracellular Mg^{2+}, spermidine, spermine	KCNJ2 KCNJ12	Kir2.1 Kir2.2	Prolongs action potential duration, background K$^+$ conductance,
I_p	Na$^+$/K$^+$ pump current	Na^+_i, K^+_o	Cardiac glycosides			Maintains low [Na$^+$]$_i$,
$I_{K,ACh}$	Acetylcholine-activated K$^+$ current (inward rectifier)	ACh	Ba^{2+}	KCNJ3 KCNJ5	Kir3.1 Kir3.4	Muscarinic receptor-coupled. Activates additional K$^+$ channels so slowing pacemaker potential

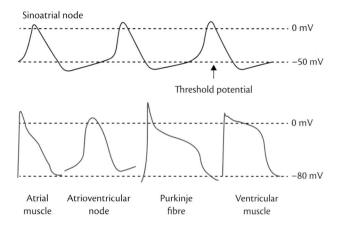

Fig. 1.2.6 Regional configurations of the action potential. In the sinoatrial (SA) and atrioventricular (AV) nodes, the cells spontaneously depolarize during diastole (phase 4 depolarization). When the membrane potential reaches a threshold, the complete action potential is initiated. Because the SA nodal cells have the fastest phase 4 depolarization, they act as the cardiac pacemaker.

The mechanism of myocyte contraction

Excitation–contraction coupling

The electrical events throughout the heart initiate and regulate contraction (Fig. 1.2.5). Coupling of the electrical excitation of the heart to contraction (termed excitation–contraction coupling

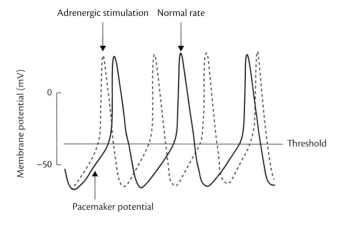

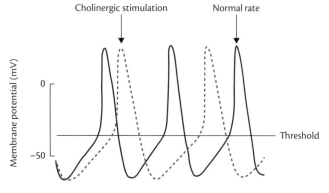

Fig. 1.2.7 Change in heart rate produced by altering the phase 4 slope of the pacemaker potential in the sinoatrial (SA) node. β-Adrenergic stimulation increases, and cholinergic stimulation decreases, the slope of the pacemaker potential, affecting the time taken to reach threshold.

or EC coupling) by Ca^{2+} ions involves the interaction of several proteins involved in Ca^{2+} homeostasis (Fig. 1.2.3). The T-tubules carry depolarization deeply into the cell. During diastole, when cytoplasmic Ca^{2+} concentrations are low ($c.0.1\,\mu mol/litre$), Ca^{2+} is sequestered by the Ca^{2+}-buffering protein calsequestrin within the JSR. Depolarization then opens the L-type Ca^{2+} channels in the T-tubule and plasma membrane allowing influx of Ca^{2+} (Figs. 1.2.3 and 1.2.5) and producing I_{Ca} (Fig. 1.2.5). Ca^{2+} influx increases the local Ca^{2+} concentration around clusters of SR Ca^{2+}-release channels sufficiently to open them (i.e. CICR), the number of channels activated in this way being mainly, though not exclusively, determined by the size of the Ca^{2+} current. CICR provides amplification as the small 'trigger' Ca^{2+} influx through the L-type Ca^{2+} channels evokes a much larger release of Ca^{2+} from the SR into the cytoplasm; also, the release of Ca^{2+} from the SR is under precise control as it is closely matched to the amount of Ca^{2+} influx. Cytoplasmic Ca^{2+} concentration rises to between 1 and $3\,\mu mol/litre$ (Fig. 1.2.5). The release of Ca^{2+} ceases because the L-type Ca channels inactivate so the trigger influx declines, leading to closure of SR Ca^{2+} release channels.

The mechanism of myofibrillar contraction

Ca^{2+} release from the SR activates the contractile apparatus of the sarcomere (Figs. 1.2.2 and 1.2.8). The temporal relationship between the action potential, the Ca^{2+} transient, and the subsequent development of tension is shown in Fig. 1.2.9. Sarcomere shortening is caused by the interaction of motor protein myosin in the thick filaments with actin in the thin filaments (Fig. 1.2.8). Myosin heads bind and hydrolyse ATP, retaining bound ADP and phosphate and trapping the free energy of hydrolysis within the myosin molecule. The myosin–ADP–phosphate complex then binds to actin, leading to the release of the stored energy by a conformational change that moves the actin filament by about 10 nm relative to the thick filament. This is known as the cross-bridge cycle (Fig. 1.2.8) and results in the sliding of the thin filament past the thick filaments, and sarcomere shortening. If the muscle is under load, the cross-bridge cycle generates force and work is done (the maximum efficiency is more than 60% in intact muscle). The mechanical characteristics of contracting muscle can be described in terms of the relationship between shortening speed and force, and between sarcomere length and force (Fig. 1.2.10a). Maximum force is produced under isometric conditions, while maximum shortening speed is observed in unloaded muscle. Power output is the product of force and velocity and is optimal at about 30% of maximum shortening speed (Fig. 1.2.10a).

The isometric force produced by a muscle depends on the sarcomere length, being optimal at 2.00–2.25 μm where the overlap of thick and thin filaments is such that all the myosin cross-bridges can interact with actin (Fig. 1.2.10b). In the heart, the sarcomere length is generally less than optimal, with 'preload' stretching the sarcomere to 2.1 μm at the end of diastole and the sarcomere shortening to 1.6 μm during systole. In this length range, stretching the cardiac muscle when it is relaxed leads to increased force in the subsequent contraction. This characteristic is responsible in part for the Frank-Starling mechanism of the heart.

Control of contraction by Ca^{2+}

Muscle contraction is initiated by an increase in cytoplasmic Ca^{2+}, which binds to the troponin complex of the thin filament. Troponin comprises three subunits. Troponin C is a Ca^{2+}-binding protein;

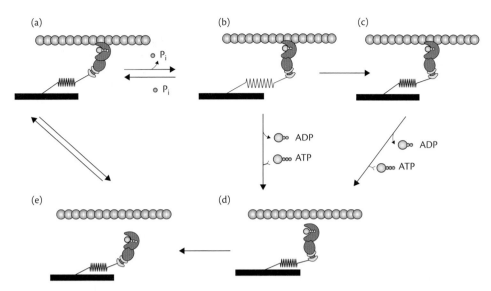

Fig. 1.2.8 The cross-bridge cycle. Exchange of ATP with ADP (a) on either a load-bearing (b) or a resting-length myosin head (c) results in a conformational change in the myosin head, causing a rapid dissociation of the myosin head from actin ((b) to (d) and (c) to (d), respectively). Following detachment from actin, the ATP is hydrolysed to ADP and Pi, both of which remain tightly bound to the myosin head (e). Hydrolysis is accompanied by a major conformational change which represents the reversal or a repriming of the power stroke. If an actin site is within reach of the myosin head, it will bind rapidly and reversibly to the actin site (a). When the myosin head binds actin, the interaction can promote a major change in conformation (the power stroke) which is accompanied by the dissociation of Pi ((a) to (b)). This step approximates to isometric contraction (no relative movement of actin and myosin) whereas the (a) to (c) steps approximate to an isotonic contraction (relative movement, with a release of the myosin 'spring'). This power stroke consists of a reorientation of part of the myosin head that results in the displacement of the tip by up to 10 nm.

Reproduced with permission from S. Weiss and M. A. Geeves.

in cardiac myocytes, the thin filament is activated when a single Ca^{2+} ion binds to troponin C. Troponin I is the inhibitory subunit. In relaxed muscle, the Ca^{2+} concentration is low and troponin I binds to a site on actin which blocks the binding of myosin cross-bridges, thus preventing cross-bridge cycling. In the presence of activating Ca^{2+} concentrations, Ca^{2+} binds to troponin C, which binds troponin I preventing its interaction with actin, permitting actin–myosin interaction. The third component, troponin T, binds to troponin C and troponin I and also to tropomyosin, independently of the Ca^{2+} concentration, thereby anchoring the regulatory complex on the thin filament (Fig. 1.2.2).

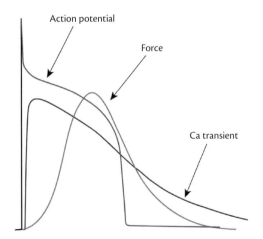

Fig. 1.2.9 The relationship between the action potential, the Ca^{2+}-transient and the generation of force. The peak of force production is not achieved until near the end of the plateau phase of the action potential and lags behind the peak of the Ca^{2+}-transient, reflecting the time required for Ca^{2+}-induced Ca^{2+}-release and cross-bridge cycling.

The Ca^{2+}-sensitivity of cardiac myocytes is increased by stretch, promoting relaxation at the start of diastole (short sarcomere lengths) and activating contraction at start of systole (long sarcomere lengths). Moreover, this 'stretch activation' is delayed so that the enhanced contractility is synchronized with systole, thus contributing to the Starling effect.

Termination of contraction

Sarcoplasmic/endoplasmic reticulum ATPase type 2 (SERCA 2)

Contraction is terminated predominantly by Ca^{2+} reuptake into the SR by activation of SERCA2, an ATP-requiring Ca^{2+} pump expressed in the network of non-junctional SR surrounding the myofibrils (Figs. 1.2.3a). SERCA2 activity is regulated by the extent of phosphorylation of the SERCA2-associated protein phospholamban.

The Na^+,Ca^{2+} exchanger (Na/CaX) and the Na^+,K^+-ATPase

The sarcolemmal Na/CaX contributes to lowering cytoplasmic Ca^{2+} during the latter part of the action potential and during diastole (Fig. 1.2.5 and Table 1.2.2). The Na/CaX utilizes the energy associated with the concentration and electrical gradients for Na^+ to expel Ca^{2+} from the cell. It is electrogenic, promoting depolarization under these conditions. The exchange is sensitive to Na^+_i concentration: when membrane potential is near its diastolic level and Na^+_i is at normal physiological concentration, the Na/CaX will eject Ca^{2+} from the cell; if Na^+_i increases by a few mmol/litre and the membrane potential becomes depolarized, the exchanger can reverse and mediate Ca^{2+} entry.

The sarcolemmal Na^+,K^+-ATPase is responsible for Na^+_i extrusion. Cardiac glycosides (e.g. digoxin) inhibit the Na^+,K^+-ATPase, preventing Na^+ extrusion, which indirectly reverses the Na/CaX into Ca^{2+}_o uptake mode. Under these conditions, Ca^{2+} uptake by

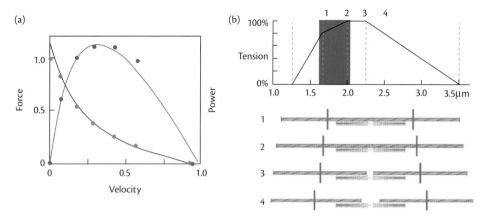

Fig. 1.2.10 Force–velocity–power relationship in cardiac muscle. (a) Force-velocity relationship (red symbols, black line). Maximum force is produced under isometric conditions (velocity $V = 0$), while maximum shortening speed is observed in unloaded muscle (force $P = 0$). The force–power relationship (blue symbols, green line) is a parabola with maximum power being produced at an intermediate force and velocity. (b) Length–tension relationship in cardiac muscle. At sarcomere length greater than $2.0\,\mu m$, isometric tension depends on the amount of overlap between myosin cross-bridges and actin filaments. At shorter sarcomere lengths (down to $1.6\,\mu m$), tension is reduced because of interference of thin filaments from opposite ends of the sarcomere. Below $1.6\,\mu m$ sarcomere length, myosin filaments interfere with the Z-line and tension falls rapidly. The range of sarcomere lengths during a normal cardiac cycle is shown in blue.

the SR may be increased, thereby augmenting the cardiac Ca^{2+} pool and facilitating CICR. The net effect of the cardiac glycosides is to increase the cytoplasmic concentration and availability of Ca^{2+} resulting in an increased force of contraction.

Ventricular myocytes possess other, minor, systems to decrease cytoplasmic Ca^{2+} concentrations, including the plasma membrane Ca^{2+} ATPase and mitochondrial Ca^{2+} uptake. SERCA2 and Na/CaX contribute about 70% and 25%, respectively, towards relaxation, though these figures vary greatly between species.

Whole organ physiology

The cardiac cycle

Electrical events initiate the cardiac cycle with depolarization of the sinoatrial (SA) node in the upper right atrium (Fig. 1.2.11). Cardiac

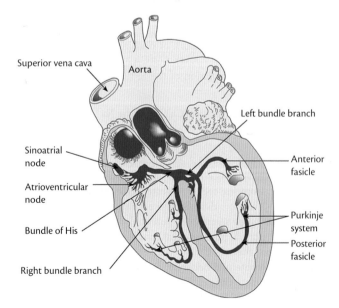

Fig. 1.2.11 Diagram of the heart showing the impulse-generating and impulse-conducting system.

From Junqueira LC, Carneiro J, (2005). *Basic histology*, 11th edn. McGraw-Hill, New York.

muscle acts as a functional syncytium. Communication between neighbouring cells is mediated by gap junctions which form arrays of cell-to-cell channels. The generated action potential spreads from the sinoatrial node across the functional syncytium at a speed of 1.0 to 1.2 m/s. The first mechanical response is atrial systole.

The cell-to-cell conduction of the electrical impulse from atrium to ventricle normally occurs only through the atrioventricular (AV) node (Fig. 1.2.11), a region of slow conductance at 0.02 to 0.1 m/s. This delays activation of the cells of the bundle of His and allows time for completion of ventricular filling. The conduction velocity in the bundle of His is from 1.2 to 2.0 m/s. The impulse passes via the right bundle branch and the two branches of the left bundle, and spreads rapidly (2.0–4.0 m/s) through the Purkinje fibres and each muscle cell to produce an orderly sequence of ventricular contraction (Fig. 1.2.11). Atrial and ventricular depolarization (P wave and QRS complex) and repolarization (T wave) can be recorded on the ECG (Fig. 1.2.12).

The specialized cells of pacemaker tissue have an inherent rhythmicity that is shared by the sinoatrial node, the atrioventricular node, and Purkinje tissue. Unlike other myocardial cells, these cells do not maintain a diastolic intracellular potential of about –90 mV, but tend to depolarize spontaneously. Because the sinoatrial node has the fastest inherent discharge (depolarization) rate, and because there is a brief period after depolarization of the whole heart during which a further stimulus is ineffective—the absolute refractory period—the sinoatrial node is normally the pacesetter for the heart. However, if this does not occur, pacemaker tissue in the atrioventricular node, the bundle of His, or the Purkinje system will assume this role, in which case the heart rate is then considerably slower.

Mechanical events

The mechanical events following depolarization of the atrial and ventricular muscle and their timing in relation to the ECG, to pressure and flow changes, and to heart sounds are shown in five phases in Fig. 1.2.13. After the P wave, and coinciding with atrial systole, 'a' waves appear in left atrial and right atrial pressure tracings due to atrial contraction, and an 'a' wave can be seen in the jugular venous pulse. Atrial contraction increases ventricular filling by about 10% (phase 1).

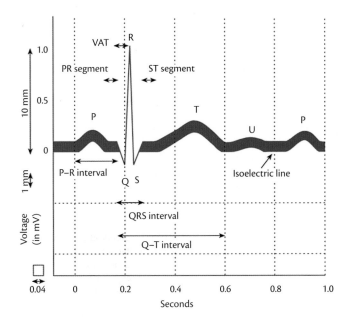

Fig. 1.2.12 Diagram of electrocardiographic complexes, intervals, and segments. VAT, ventricular activation time.

From Goldschlager N, Goldman MJ (1989). *Principles of clinical electrocardiography*, 13th edn. Appleton and Lange, East Norwalk, CT.

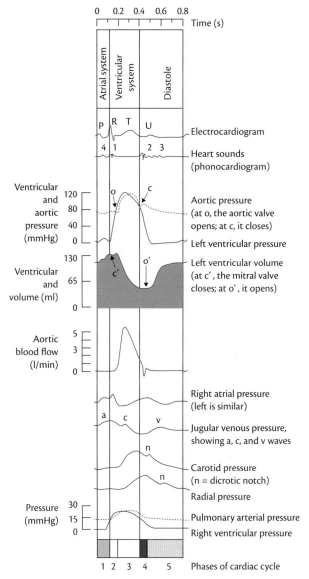

Fig. 1.2.13 Events of the cardiac cycle at a heart rate of 75 beats/min. The phases of the cardiac cycle, identified by the numbers at the bottom, are: (1) atrial systole; (2) isovolumetric ventricular contraction; (3) ventricular ejection; (4) isovolumetric ventricular relaxation; and (5) ventricular filling. Note that late in systole, aortic pressure actually exceeds left ventricular pressure. However, the momentum of the blood keeps it flowing out of the ventricle for a short time. The pressure relationships in the right ventricle and pulmonary artery are similar. The jugular venous pulse is similar in form to that seen in the right atrial pressure tracing. The 'c' wave interrupts the 'x' descent of the 'a' wave. The decline in pressure from the peak of the 'v' is the 'y' descent; the rate of decline reflects speed of ventricular filling. Atr. syst, atrial systole; ventric. syst, ventricular systole.

Modified with permission from Ganong WF (2005). *Review of medical physiology*, 22nd edn. McGraw-Hill, New York.

The onset of ventricular contraction coincides with the peak of the R wave of the ECG; a rapid rise in intraventricular pressure closes the mitral and tricuspid valves, causing the first heart sound. During this short isovolumetric period (phase 2 of Fig. 1.2.13), the pressure rises rapidly in the ventricles. When ventricular pressures exceed those in the pulmonary artery and aorta, the outflow valves open and ventricular ejection follows. The highest flow rate is in early systole, and pressures in the aorta and pulmonary artery rise. Normally, between 50 and 70% of the ventricular volume is ejected during systole, and this can be seen in the volume curve included in Fig. 1.2.13 (phase 3).

The jugular venous pulse, during ventricular contraction, has a positive deflection in early systole, the 'c' wave, due to right ventricular contraction and bulging of the tricuspid valve into the right atrium. Descent of the tricuspid ring caused by ventricular contraction then produces a negative 'x' descent, but as atrial inflow continues the pressure rises in the atria and great veins, producing the 'v' wave. This reaches its peak just before the opening of the tricuspid valve, declining during early ventricular filling as the negative 'y' descent. The changes in the pulmonary veins and left atrium are similar.

As the strength of ventricular contraction declines, coinciding with the end of the T wave, the aortic and pulmonary valves close, producing the dicrotic notch seen on both aortic and pulmonary artery pressure tracings in Fig. 1.2.13. Aortic closure slightly precedes pulmonary closure, and together these are responsible for the two components of the second heart sound. A short period of further rapid decline in ventricular pressure ensues without change in the ventricular volume (the period of isovolumetric ventricular relaxation, phase 4), and at the end of this the mitral and tricuspid valves open. There is a pressure gradient from atrium to ventricle so that a period of rapid ventricular filling follows, which coincides with the timing of the third heart sound. The rapid ventricular filling is reflected in the shape of the ventricular volume curve, and is followed by a period of slower filling (phase 5) with a final sudden small increment from the next atrial contraction as diastole ends (phase 1).

Third heart sounds are normally audible in children and young adults, but over the age of about 40 years this usually indicates elevation of ventricular end-diastolic pressure (most frequently in the left ventricle). The myocardium and valvular structures become stiffer with ageing, and large increases in ventricular end-diastolic pressure are then required to tense valvular structures and generate audible vibrations. A fourth heart sound almost always indicates abnormal ventricular function, with increased end-diastolic pressure. A fourth heart sound precedes the Q wave of the ECG, and must be distinguished from a normal splitting of the two components of the first heart sound. The latter occurs after the Q wave (Figs. 1.2.12 and 1.2.13).

Normal volumes, pressures, and flows

The blood volume in normal adults is about 5 litres (haematocrit 45%), and, of this, about 1.5 litres are in the heart and lungs—the central blood volume. The pulmonary arteries, capillaries, and veins contain about 0.9 litres, with only about 75 ml being in the pulmonary capillaries at any one instant. The volume of blood in the heart is about 0.6 litres. Left ventricular end-diastolic volume is about 140 ml, stroke volume about 90 ml, and end-systolic volume around 50 ml, reflecting an ejection fraction (stroke volume/end-diastolic volume) of between 50 and 70%. The right ventricular ejection fraction is similar.

Of the 3.5 litres in the systemic circulation, most—at least 60% of the total blood volume—is in the veins. The systemic veins containing most of the blood volume are easily distensible, and input of blood into the contracting heart is associated with only small changes in venous pressure. By contrast, ejection of blood into the much less distensible arterial tree produces large pressure changes.

The normal values for pressures generated in the heart and great vessels during the cardiac cycle are shown in Table 1.2.3. Pressures are measured with reference to a zero pressure arbitrarily set at 5 cm below the sternal angle with the patient recumbent. 'Normal' arterial blood pressure is considered later (see below 'Regulation of systemic arterial blood pressure').

Cardiac output is the product of stroke volume and heart rate. It is related to body size and is best expressed as litre/min per m² of body surface area: the 'cardiac index'. The mean cardiac index under resting and relaxed conditions is 3.5 litre/min per m², and values below 2 and above 5 are abnormal. The cardiac index declines with age. In persons of average size, resting oxygen consumption is about 240 ml/min, and the difference in oxygen content between arterial and mixed venous blood is about 40 ml/litre (arteriovenous oxygen difference), giving a basal cardiac output of 6 litre/min. In normal subjects, the arteriovenous difference in oxygen content at rest is maintained within narrow limits, from 35 to 45 ml/litre; values of 55 ml/litre and above are always abnormal.

Pulmonary or systemic vascular resistance is estimated by dividing the difference between mean inflow pressure (pulmonary artery or aortic) and mean outflow pressure (left atrial or right atrial) in mmHg by the flow in litre/min through the respective circulations.

In normal subjects and patients without intracardiac shunts, this flow is the cardiac output. Normal pulmonary vascular resistance is less than 2 mmHg/litre per min (16 MPa s m⁻³,160 dyn s cm⁻⁵). Arterial blood pressure is the product of cardiac output and total peripheral resistance.

Stroke work is the integral of instantaneous ventricular pressure with respect to stroke volume, but is usually estimated as the product of stroke volume and mean ejection pressure. The orderly sequence of contraction in the normal cardiac cycle coordinates changes in instantaneous pressure and flow, so maximizing the transfer of energy to the circulation. Normal left ventricular work output at rest is about 6 kg/m² per min.

Myocardial mechanics

When a muscle is activated to contract, it develops a potential for doing work. In isolated skeletal and heart muscle preparations, the stretching force applied to the muscle—and therefore the length of the muscle—can be varied before contraction; this is the *preload*. The activated muscle will begin to shorten when it has generated a force sufficient to overcome that exerted by the attached weight or load against which it contracts. When the force exerted by the load is so arranged that it is not applied to the relaxed muscle and is applied only after the muscle has begun to develop tension, it is termed the *afterload*. If this load is so large that the activated muscle is unable to overcome it, and so cannot shorten, the contraction produces tension only, and the contraction is isometric. When shortening does occur, external work is done. If the load is constant during the shortening, the contraction is said to be *isotonic*; if it changes, it is *auxotonic*.

The tension produced by both skeletal and cardiac muscle during contraction depends on initial fibre length; during afterloaded isotonic contractions from a particular length, the amount and the speed of fibre shortening and the tension developed all depend upon the afterload. Over a range of loads the initial velocity of muscle shortening is most rapid and the most extensive shortening occurs when the load is smallest.

The inverse relationship between initial velocity of fibre shortening and load in an isotonic contraction is a fundamental one for both skeletal and cardiac muscle. There is, however, a major difference between the two types of muscle in that the relationship at any one length is constant in a skeletal muscle, whereas in cardiac muscle there are variations in inotropic state that are accompanied by considerable changes in the relationship between force and velocity. A positive inotropic effect produces a more extensive contraction from the same initial length and afterload, and a faster maximum velocity of shortening (V_{max}). An increase in initial fibre

Table 1.2.3 Normal resting values for pressures in the heart and great vessels

Site	Systolic pressure (mmHg)	Diastolic pressure (mmHg)	Mean pressure (mmHg)
Right atrium	'a' up to 7, 'v' up to 5	'y' up to 3, 'x' up to 3	Less than 5
Right ventricle	Up to 25	End pressure before 'a' up to 3; end pressure on 'a' up to 7	Not applicable
Pulmonary artery	Up to 25	Up to 15	Up to 18
Left atrium (direct or indirect pulmonary capillary wedge)	'a' up to 12, 'v' up to 10	'x' up to 7, 'y' up to 7	Up to 10
Left ventricle	120	End pressure before 'a' up to 7; end pressure on 'a' up to 12	Not applicable

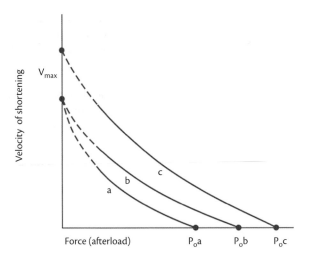

Fig. 1.2.14 Idealized relationships between velocity of fibre shortening and afterload or force developed during contraction of a strip of cardiac muscle under three different conditions. Curves a and b were obtained with the muscle in the same inotropic state but with a longer initial fibre length (greater preload) for curve b. Curves b and c were obtained with initial fibre length the same but with contractility increased in c by the addition of a drug producing a positive inotropic effect. The terms V_{max} and P_0 describe, respectively, a hypothetical maximum shortening velocity in the absence of any load (hence the broken lines), and the force developed in an isometric contraction. An increase in initial fibre length increases P_0 but not V_{max}; a positive inotropic change increases both P_0 and V_{max}.

length with no increase in inotropic state increases the force of contraction but does not, however, change the maximum velocity of shortening. This is illustrated in Fig. 1.2.14.

The contraction of the intact heart can be visualized as being similar mechanically to the afterloaded contraction of an isolated muscle strip. For the left ventricle, the preload is the distending force which stretches the muscle fibres in end-diastole, and the initial afterload is the force the ventricle must generate in order to open the aortic valve and eject blood. At the end of ejection, the ventricular muscle is isolated from the peripheral circulation, with the afterload then supported by the competent aortic valve, and the muscle relaxes against a comparatively small force. Relaxation of the heart is an active process due to withdrawal of calcium ions from the cytoplasm surrounding the myofibrils. 'Active' relaxation is still proceeding in the ventricular wall when the atrioventricular valves open, and, if it is delayed—as in the hypoxic heart—the slower relaxation increases the stiffness of the ventricular wall and reduces filling. Wall thickness is also a determinant of relaxation rate and compliance. For this reason, filling pressures are higher for the thicker and stiffer left ventricle than for the thinner and more distensible right ventricle (Table 1.2.3). When the left ventricle is hypertrophied due to chronic pressure overload, as in systemic hypertension or aortic stenosis, it becomes stiffer and filling pressures may then be abnormally high.

Regulation of cardiac function

Four essential factors determine the performance of the heart: (1) venous return, (2) outflow resistance (afterload), (3) inotropic state or contractility, and (4) heart rate. Changes in cardiac performance are accomplished by mechanisms that alter these four determinants.

Venous return, preload, and the Frank–Starling relationship

The relationship described independently by Frank and Starling between end-diastolic fibre length and force of contraction is shown in Fig. 1.2.15. When the ventricle ejects against a constant pressure, variations in venous return alter the degree of stretch of the muscle fibres in diastole, and this determines contraction strength and work output. The number of active force-generating sites in each fibre increases as it lengthens so that, within limits, the force of contraction and stroke work are positively related to end-diastolic fibre length. The relationship is curvilinear when stroke work is plotted against end-diastolic pressure as an index of preload, reflecting the exponential relationship between end-diastolic pressure and end-diastolic volume. When stroke work is plotted against end-diastolic volume, the relationship between stroke work and preload is linear.

The response of the heart at any particular time depends upon: (1) the intrinsic state of the muscle, i.e. the biochemistry and contractile machinery; (2) the prevailing neurohumoral state, e.g. increased sympathetic outflow produces a more forceful contraction at any end-diastolic fibre length; (3) extrinsic inotropic influences—drugs which have either positive or negative inotropic effects.

End-diastolic fibre length is determined by the force distending the ventricle at end-diastole, and end-diastolic pressure provides a reasonable indication of this force when the ventricle has normal distensibility or compliance; this is the preload. The systemic venous return and the elastic properties of the myocardium produce the end-diastolic distending pressure for the right ventricle, and the pulmonary venous return and myocardial elasticity that for the left ventricle. For clinical purposes, it is convenient to equate venous return with preload because, as it changes from beat to beat, it adjusts the strength of the subsequent ventricular (and atrial)

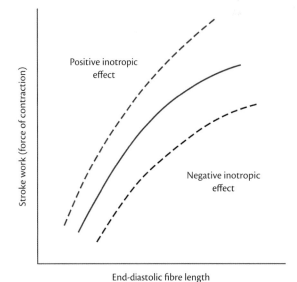

Fig. 1.2.15 The relation between left ventricular end-diastolic fibre length and left ventricular stroke work showing displacement upward and to the left with an increase in contractility and downward and to the right with a reduction in contractility. Similar but not identical curves are obtained by plotting left ventricular stroke work as one measure of the force of contraction against ventricular end-diastolic pressure or volume (see text). Similar function curves may be obtained from both ventricles and both atria.

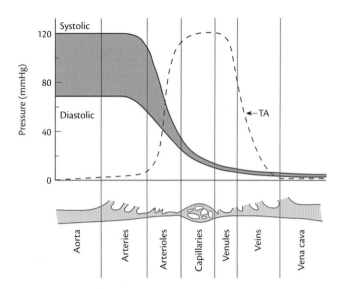

Fig. 1.2.16 Diagram of the changes in pressure as blood flows through the systemic circulation. The total cross-sectional area of the vessels (TA) increases from 4.5 cm² to 4500 cm² in the capillaries. The major resistance to flow is at the arteriolar level.

Modified and reproduced with permission from Ganong WF (2005). *Review of medical physiology*, 22nd edn. McGraw-Hill, New York.

contraction by varying the force stretching the relaxed cardiac muscle and changing end-diastolic fibre length.

Outflow resistance or afterload

Pulmonary and aortic valve opening pressures are determined largely by the pulmonary and systemic vascular resistances, as shown for the latter in Fig. 1.2.16. These resistances, together with an inertial component dependent upon the mass of blood within the vessels, the compliance (stiffness) of the vessels, and the physical characteristics of each vascular tree combined with the pulsatile nature of the flow, constitute the impedance to ventricular outflow. This is the load against which the ventricle must contract and shorten. As this load is not applied in diastole to the relaxed muscle, it then being supported by competent aortic and pulmonary valves, it is described clinically as the afterload: it becomes applied to the muscle only after the ventricle has begun to develop tension.

Regulation of systemic arterial blood pressure

The regulation of the systemic circulation is well adapted to the vital function of maintaining constant, adequate cerebral perfusion. There is a need to maintain a relatively constant arterial blood pressure when there are changes in posture and circulating blood volume. The baroreceptors mediate rapid responses to alterations in aortic pressure, while a variety of hormonal and physical factors regulate the circulating blood volume.

Baroreceptors

The baroreceptor regulatory system comprises two groups of stretch receptors: one group in the carotid sinuses near the bifurcations of the common carotid arteries in the neck and a second group in the arch of the aorta. These respond to an increase in central arterial pressure by the firing of impulses, which pass by the glossopharyngeal and vagus nerves to the solitary tract nucleus in the medulla and inhibit sympathetic outflow. Efferent impulses from these central connections pass via the right vagus nerve mainly

to the sinoatrial node, and via the left vagus mainly to the atrioventricular node. The effect is to decrease the heart rate and the force of atrial contraction. There is also attenuation of sympathetic discharge to arteriolar smooth muscle in the limbs and visceral circulation, resulting in a release of peripheral arteriolar constriction and, therefore, peripheral vasodilatation. Thus the immediate response to a rise in arterial pressure is slowing of the heart rate, reduced force of atrial contraction, and reduced vascular resistance. The net effect of this negative feedback system is to offset the elevation in blood pressure. Conversely, a lowering of blood pressure diminishes stimulation of the stretch receptors and reduces afferent traffic to the solitary tract nucleus, resulting in reduced inhibition of sympathetic outflow. There is, then, a quickening of the heart rate and peripheral vasoconstriction so that the blood pressure increases. The changes in heart rate take place within 1 to 2 s and changes in vasomotor control within 5 or 6 s.

Baroreceptor mechanisms effectively modulate the responses of blood pressure to postural change. Additionally, they adapt to maintain the normal circadian variation in blood pressure (see below 'Diurnal variation in autonomic function'). They also maintain elevated arterial blood pressure in systemic hypertension. Sensory input to the reflex is reduced in disorders of the autonomic nervous system, and in the prolonged weightlessness of space flight.

Blood volume

The circulating blood volume is relatively small, and a large proportion is contained in the veins (Fig. 1.2.16) so that any change in blood volume will affect venous return and, therefore, cardiac output and blood pressure. When blood volume is large and the veins full, there is little reduction in venous return on standing and cardiac output is maintained. However, when effective blood volume is reduced and the veins are relatively empty, on standing there is pooling of blood in the veins of the legs and a reduction in venous return and cardiac output so that arterial blood pressure falls. Baroreceptor responses become evident within a couple of beats, the heart rate increases, and cardiac output and blood pressure are restored. Circulating blood volume is kept relatively constant by a combination of mechanisms which involve the actions of natriuretic peptides, the renin–angiotensin–aldosterone system, vasopressin, and osmolality.

Natriuretic peptides

The discovery of secretory granules in the atria of the heart, and the demonstration in 1981 that they produce a natriuretic factor that inhibits the reabsorption of sodium in the distal tubule of the kidney, enhanced understanding of the regulation of blood volume and cardiac performance. Three natriuretic peptides have subsequently been identified.

- *ANP* is present in the circulation, and concentrations increase during volume expansion. The right atrium contains about 2 to 4 times as much activity as the left, and release of the hormone is mediated largely by atrial distension. The effect is to produce a diuresis and to reduce cardiac and circulating blood volume. ANP also has a vasodilator action and opposes the vasoconstricting effects of noradrenaline and angiotension II.

- The second natriuretic peptide was identified in brain tissue and is now referred to as *B-type natriuretic peptide*. Large amounts are found in the ventricles of the heart, and circulating levels are increased in ventricular hypertrophy and cardiac failure. B-type and ANP have similar actions.

◆ The third natriuretic peptide to be identified was *C-type natriuretic peptide*. It is distributed widely in tissues, circulating concentrations are low, and it appears to have actions similar to the other two peptides, but with a greater vasodilator effect on veins.

These three peptides contribute to the regulation of cardiac and circulating blood volume and of blood pressure. Both B-type natriuretic peptide and N-terminal pro-brain natriuretic peptide are useful adjuncts to the clinical evaluation of dyspnoeic patients in that levels are elevated when the dyspnoea is due to cardiac failure.

Renin–angiotensin system

This system, which is both local and systemic, is of major importance in the regulation of circulating blood volume and the maintenance of normal blood pressure. Enhanced activity of systemic renin and angiotensin increases the production of aldosterone, which promotes reabsorption of sodium by the kidney and expansion of circulating blood volume. All components of the renin–angiotensin system are distributed widely throughout tissues—including the brain and the heart—and increased activation of the system increases the risk of cardiovascular events. Angiotensin II is a potent vasoconstrictor that has a number of additional important actions on the vasculature (Fig. 1.2.17). The angiotensin converting enzyme (ACE) inhibitors in clinical use diminish angiotensin II production locally and in the circulating blood.

Both local and general effects appear important in mediating the benefits that accrue from the use of these drugs in the management of hypertension and congestive cardiac failure, and in the reduction in rates of recurrence of coronary events in ischaemic heart disease. The mechanisms mediating the latter include antioxidant effects and a reduction in the production of potentially damaging free radicals, anti-inflammatory effects, and augmentation of the profibrinolytic effects of bradykinin. The more recently developed angiotensin II receptor blocking drugs (ARBs) have now been shown to produce similar outcomes.

Regulation of nitric oxide production

A recently recognized contribution to endothelial function, which affects the afterload, is related to nitric oxide production, and its inhibition by asymmetric dimethylarginine (ADMA). Asymmetric dimethylarginine is produced by the physiological degradation of methylated proteins. ADMA inhibits the production of nitric oxide, which is derived directly from L-arginine, present in all cells. ADMA levels are regulated by the balance between its production and its metabolism. The balance may be disrupted in clinical situations, for example in renal impairment. Reduced renal function increases the level of ADMA and this reduces endothelial dilatation.

Ventricular volume and afterload

Ventricular volume also has a major effect on afterload, as pressure is equal to force per unit area. The force acting radially on the inner surface of the whole ventricle at any time during systole is the product of the intraventricular pressure and ventricular surface area at that time. If the left ventricle is assumed to be a sphere (surface area = πd^2), the force opposing ejection at any time during contraction is the product of the intracavity pressure and πd^2 at that time. Thus, a doubling in left ventricular diameter from a normal value of 5 cm to 10 cm would result in a fourfold increase in the force opposing ejection for the same intracavity systolic pressure; the ventricle would need to develop greatly increased wall tension to overcome that force. Because wall tension developed during systole is the major determinant of myocardial oxygen consumption, the contraction will clearly be much less efficient in the larger heart for the same stroke volume and ejection pressure (stroke work).

During a normal heartbeat, the afterload is greatest at the beginning of ejection (rapid rise in pressure and maximum volume; Fig.

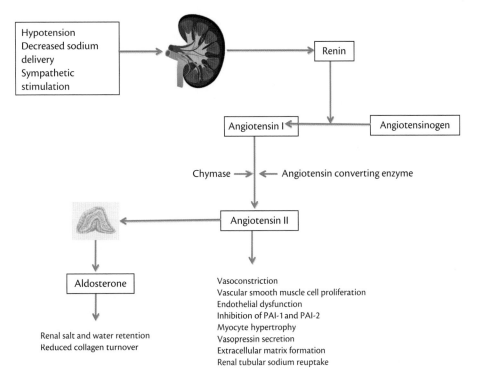

Fig. 1.2.17 The renin–angiotensin system. ACE, angiotensin converting enzyme; PAI, plasminogen activator inhibitor.

1.2.13), but decreases thereafter as the pressure reaches a plateau and then declines as the ventricle becomes smaller. There is, therefore, a matching of the afterload to the declining intensity of the contraction as it proceeds to completion, and fibres shorten at a relatively constant rate. This is less obvious in a large heart where the volume change during ejection is a smaller proportion of the total ventricular volume.

The end-diastolic volume is influenced by preload, afterload, circulating blood volume, the inotropic state of the ventricle, heart rate, and neurohumoral influences. It is smaller in the erect than in the horizontal position because of reduced venous return, and it decreases with a moderate increase in heart rate because of an associated positive inotropic effect. The proportion of end-diastolic volume ejected during systole, the ejection fraction (normal 50–70%), is a useful index of overall left ventricular function and is easily measured noninvasively by gated blood-pool scanning and two-dimensional echocardiographic techniques. The ejection fraction increases with exercise and with positive inotropic interventions. Values for right ventricular ejection fraction are of the same order as those for the left side of the heart.

Role of the sympathoadrenal system in normal and failing hearts

Catecholamines have positive inotropic, lusitropic, and chronotropic effects on the normal heart. The inotropic effect of catecholamines on the force of contraction is mediated by a PKA-mediated phosphorylation of the L-type Ca^{2+} channel, which increases the probability of channels opening when the cell is depolarized, thus increasing I_{Ca}. Positive lusitropism (myocardial relaxation) is achieved by a PKA catalytic subunit-mediated phosphorylation of phospholamban which inhibits SERCA2 in its hypophosphorylated state (Fig. 1.2.8a). Phosphorylated phospholamban does not inhibit SERCA2. The effect of phospholamban phosphorylation is thus to activate SERCA2 and stimulate Ca^{2+} reuptake into the SR. In addition, protein kinase A phosphorylates cardiac troponin I, and this increases the rate of dissociation of Ca^{2+} from troponin C, increasing the rate of dissociation of myosin cross-bridges from actin (i.e. stimulating relaxation). Positive chronotropism is achieved by increasing the frequency of depolarization in the sinoatrial node. Upon stimulation of the sympathoadrenal system, I_f (generated by HCN channels) is activated to depolarize the membrane to the threshold level more quickly and increase the rate of production of action potentials. The positive chronotropism of the sympathoadrenal system is in part mediated by the binding of cAMP to these HCN channels. This shifts their voltage dependence of activation to more depolarized potentials and increases both the rate of channel opening and the maximal current level. The net result is an increased frequency of depolarization and the heart rate increases.

In heart failure, the myocyte becomes unresponsive to β-adrenergic agonists, and consequently phosphorylation of the proteins responsible for the control of contractility is diminished. The $β_1$-adrenergic receptor abundance is decreased and the expression of proteins which antagonize $β_1$-receptor signalling is increased, thus the efficacy of β-agonism is diminished. Many drugs that mitigate heart failure are targeted at the proteins that regulate the inotropic state. There is evidence also that SERCA2 expression is decreased and this may contribute to the elevated cytoplasmic Ca^{2+} concentrations sometimes seen in diastole during heart failure and the poorer contraction of the heart in this condition.

Myocardial function is greatly altered by changes in inotropic state or contractility. Positive inotropic effects are thought to be mediated by activation of excitation–contraction coupling mechanisms and are associated with an increased influx of calcium ions into myocardial cells and a more powerful contraction. Changes in the intensity of excitation–contraction coupling are independent of the Frank–Starling mechanism. Increases in the intensity shift the curve upwards and to the left, and decreases shift it downwards and to the right (Fig. 1.2.15). With a positive inotropic effect, the force of contraction, however measured, is increased for a given end-diastolic fibre length and, if the afterload is the same, the initial velocity of fibre shortening is also increased (Fig. 1.2.14); in the intact heart, there is more complete emptying during systole. Increased sympathetic stimulation, some drugs, and an increase in heart rate itself (the staircase or Bowditch phenomenon; postectopic potentiation, see 'Heart rate', next section) have positive inotropic effects. Myocardial depressants, such as hypoxia and most anaesthetic drugs, have negative inotropic effects. Increased parasympathetic stimulation produces acetylcholine-mediated negative inotropic effects that are confined almost entirely to the atria because of the anatomical distribution of vagal endings in the myocardium.

It is difficult to measure inotropic changes accurately in the human heart because changes in the intensity of excitation–contraction coupling and changes in the Frank–Starling relationship, though separate, are nevertheless closely linked. The peak rate of change of intraventricular pressure (peak dP/dt) is a useful index of change in contractility, provided that preload, afterload, and heart rate remain constant.

Heart rate

Frequency of contraction is the fourth essential determinant of cardiac performance. Heart rate during rest and exertion may vary from 45 to 200 beats/min in the healthy young adult. As changes can occur within seconds, an increase in heart rate is the usual and most effective way of producing a rapid increase in cardiac output. It plays the major role in the response to exercise, during which stroke volume does increase (more so in athletes and when in the erect, rather than the supine, position) but the changes are less marked than those of rate. In addition, an increase in contraction frequency itself produces a positive inotropic effect, whereby the force of contraction increases and reaches a new steady state within a few beats. This is termed the 'positive staircase', Treppe, or Bowditch effect. It may be a consequence of an augmented movement of calcium ions into myocardial cells with increased frequency of action potentials, combined with diminished time for outward movement of calcium between beats. More forceful contractions also follow premature beats—the phenomenon of postextrasystolic potentiation—and the mechanism is probably the same. The extrasystole occurring prematurely is a weak contraction because of decreased filling time and an uncoordinated activation of the ventricle when the ectopic focus is within the ventricle. The next beat is delayed because of the refractory period of the extrasystolic beat, but is a more powerful contraction because of increased filling time and ventricular volume, and increased contractility. Calcium-dependent changes similar to those of the Bowditch effect are probably responsible for the latter. Recently it has become clear that intrinsic circadian clocks are involved in the control of heart rate, with time-of-day dependent oscillations in clock gene expression. The cardiomyocyte circadian clock influences many myocardial processes, including ion channels.

Coronary blood flow

Coronary blood flow accounts for about 4% of the cardiac output. The heart extracts most (70%) of the oxygen carried in the coronary circulation; the arteriovenous difference for oxygen across the heart being about 110 ml/litre, while that for the whole body is only about 40 ml/litre under resting conditions. Therefore, large increases in myocardial oxygen requirements must be met largely by increases in coronary blood flow, and this may increase five- or sixfold during strenuous exercise. The greater part of this flow is to the left ventricle, of which at least two-thirds occurs during diastole because of the throttling effect systole has on myocardial perfusion. The main coronary arteries are on the superficial surface of the heart, and because of this, and the hindrance to coronary flow during systole, the subendocardial region of the left ventricle is more vulnerable to perfusion deficits in relation to oxygen need than the outer two-thirds of the muscle wall. Despite these mechanical problems, flow is normally evenly distributed throughout the myocardium so that when regional coronary blood flow is measured using injected radioactive microspheres (in dogs), the ratio of endocardial to epicardial flow is approximately unity. In fact, the inner layers of the heart probably receive slightly more blood (up to 10%) than the outer layers. This is consistent with the subendocardium developing more tension than the subepicardium, and is evidence for a greater rate of myocardial oxygen consumption in the inner layers.

Myocardial oxygen requirements and coronary blood flow are finely adjusted.

The nervous system and the heart

The heart is richly supplied with adrenergic nerves, whose terminals reach atrial and ventricular muscle fibres and impinge upon all pacemaker tissue, including the sinoatrial and atrioventricular nodes and Purkinje fibres. Sympathetic stimulation leads to an increase in myocardial contractility and heart rate, and in the rate of spread of the activation wave through the atrioventricular node and the Purkinje system. This is mediated by local noradrenaline release, which interacts with β-adrenergic receptors. The key elements in these regulatory mechanisms are calcium ions and cAMP. The activated β-receptor increases adenylcyclase activity and the conversion of ATP to cAMP. Peptide cotransmitters, released with noradrenaline and acetylcholine, have recently been isolated and also influence autonomic function. Neuropeptide Y is a peptide of 36 amino acids that is colocated with noradrenaline in most sympathetic nerves and is released with sympathetic stimulation. It is a powerful pressor agent with direct arteriolar vasoconstrictor action and also potentiates the pressor action of noradrenaline.

The distribution of parasympathetic fibres is much more limited, being confined to the sinoatrial and atrioventricular nodes and the atria, with few, if any, fibres reaching the ventricles in humans, except perhaps in relation to coronary arteries and Purkinje tissue. The effects of parasympathetic nerve stimulation are mediated by local acetylcholine release, which slows the heart rate and speed of conduction through the atrioventricular node and Purkinje tissue, and depresses atrial contractility. The negative inotropic effects are associated with a lowering of the concentration of intracellular cAMP.

The effect of the nervous system on the heart at any one time is the sum of the activities of these two opposing control systems. They usually vary reciprocally. Under resting conditions, vagal inhibitory effects predominate, maintaining a slow heart rate, there being virtually no sympathetic outflow. With exercise, there is withdrawal of vagal activity and an increase in sympathetic outflow. Afferents from stretch receptors in the carotid sinus and aortic arch—the baroreceptors—also have a considerable effect on cardiac performance, this effect being mediated via the adrenergic nervous system and vagal withdrawal. A fall in blood pressure reduces stretching in the carotid sinus and inhibitory afferent traffic so that the sympathetic outflow increases. As a consequence of this combined vagal and adrenergic effect, there is a quickening of the heart rate within one or two beats, a positive inotropic effect, and also a constriction of veins and arterioles that increases preload and afterload. Elevation of pressure in the carotid sinus has the reverse effects. In cardiac failure, there is a reduced variability in heart rate due to these autonomic mechanisms as there is then a predominance of adrenergic activity.

There are also mechanoreceptors in all four chambers of the heart (identified in dogs) and in the coronary vessels, which give rise to depressor reflexes. Their clinical relevance is uncertain, but they may contribute, e.g. to the bradycardia and hypotension occurring in some patients with acute myocardial infarction and to the syncope that patients with critical aortic stenosis may experience with the onset of exercise when there is sudden left ventricular distension. Vagal afferents from reflexogenic areas in the infarcting left ventricle may be responsible for the bradycardia, gastric distension, nausea, and vomiting which frequently occur with the onset of inferior or posterior myocardial infarction, but not usually of anterior infarction, which is generally associated with a marked increase in sympathetic activity. The cardiac receptors connected to afferent fibres running in cardiac sympathetic nerves, however, are very important because they are responsible for the perception of cardiac pain. Receptors have also been identified (in animals) at the junction of pulmonary veins with the atrial wall. These respond to mechanical distension with increased sympathetic outflow to the sinus node and inhibition of secretion of antidiuretic hormone from the posterior lobe of the pituitary gland. The result is a quickening of the heart rate and diuresis.

Autonomic efferent activity

The autonomic outflow to the heart is controlled by multiple integrative sites within the central nervous system, with complex interactions between afferent and central inputs. Autonomic responses are mediated through the suprapontine and bulbospinal pathways—both those arising 'reflexively' and those arising from various types of volitional or central 'command'. Nevertheless, intrinsic mechanisms are sufficient for adequate cardiac function in the absence of autonomic control, as prolonged survival after cardiac transplantation has shown. But in the denervated heart, there is blunting of the normally rapid physiological adjustments mediated by the autonomic nervous system.

Diurnal variation in autonomic function

Variations in vascular tone and control of blood pressure and of hormone secretion and platelet function occur in a predictable way throughout the 24-h cycle. In normal subjects, there is a circadian rhythm of blood pressure changes that is not seen in patients, after cardiac transplantation, who have denervated hearts. There is a decline in both blood pressure and heart rate at night, and increases in both soon after wakening. This is due to a normal adrenergic surge in the early morning, which results in increased vascular tone and blood pressure. Increased forearm vascular resistance in the morning, with a reduction in the afternoon and evening, can be clearly identified in humans by assessing responses to α-adrenergic blockade. It is presumed that this occurs in coronary vessels as well. Measurable early morning increases in circulating catecholamines and in the propensity for platelets to aggregate can also be documented.

The circadian rhythm of autonomic function is correlated with a significant tendency for myocardial infarction and sudden cardiac death to occur more frequently in the morning, soon after wakening. There is also an increase in the occurrence of angina pectoris in the early morning, independent of the level of physical activity.

Exercise and the heart: cardiac reserve

The heart responds to exercise with an increase in cardiac output, and values of 30 litres/min may be achieved in a trained athlete. Exercising muscles extract more oxygen from the blood, but the response of the cardiac output is the ultimate determinant of delivery of oxygen to tissues and is the limiting factor for aerobic exercise.

The cardiac response to exercise involves all the mechanisms already discussed. Interaction within the central nervous system between higher and autonomic centres augments sympathetic discharge, and there is a withdrawal of parasympathetic outflow. The heart rate increases immediately, and redistribution of peripheral flow increases venous return and preload. There is venoconstriction, particularly in the large-volume splanchnic circulation, and vasoconstriction and increased oxygen extraction in inactive parts. In active parts, there is vasodilation. This is most evident in the vascular beds of the exercising skeletal muscles and of the heart. The overall effect is a marked lowering of total peripheral vascular resistance, which reduces afterload and encourages greater systolic emptying of the left ventricle. Stroke volume increases during exercise in the upright position. During light to moderate exercise (running or cycling), up to about 80% of maximum exercise capacity there is an almost linear relationship between work intensity and heart rate response, cardiac output, and oxygen uptake. With further exercise, the heart rate and cardiac output responses level off while additional increases in oxygen consumption ($c.500$ ml) occur by increased oxygen extraction and a greater widening of the arteriovenous difference for oxygen.

The venous return increases in relation to the elevated cardiac output. Vasodilation in the working muscles that receive the bulk of the redirected blood permits high flow rates into the capacitance vessels. Because of adrenergically mediated venoconstriction, the capacity of this system is reduced, so that blood moves rapidly into the right atrium. Venous return is also enhanced by the pumping action of the rhythmically contracting working muscles, by a decrease in intrathoracic pressure with forced inspiration, and by an increase in intra-abdominal pressure. The augmented pulmonary blood flow results in only slight increases in pulmonary artery pressure because of the distensibility of the large pulmonary arteries, an increased area of the pulmonary capillary bed due to the recruitment of more capillaries, and the low resistance offered by the normal pulmonary circulation (see Table 1.2.3).

The elevated cardiac output and larger stroke volume result in increased systolic blood pressure and pulse pressure, even though the afterload itself is reduced. Enhanced neurohumoral activity from adrenergic stimulation of the heart and the suprarenal glands (increased circulating adrenaline and noradrenaline) effect positive inotropic changes, to which tachycardia also contributes because of the Bowditch effect. There is a shift in the Frank–Starling relationship to the left, increased speed and force of cardiac contraction, and elevated ejection fraction and stroke volume. Peak dP/dt is increased, and there is a rapid rise in coronary blood flow to meet myocardial oxygen requirements that increase linearly with the product of systolic blood pressure and heart rate. During moderate exercise, these changes together result in a decreased or unaltered end-diastolic volume and decreased end-systolic volume. With severe exercise, end-diastolic dimensions and end-diastolic fibre length are slightly increased and the Frank–Starling mechanism then operates and further augments the force of contraction.

The haemodynamic and ventilatory responses evoked by an increase to a new steady workload take about 2 to 3 min to equilibrate and adjust oxygen supply to the greater demand. Protocols for exercise testing are therefore usually based on work increments at 3-min intervals to allow time for a new 'steady state' to occur, e.g. in the standard Bruce exercise protocol. A steady state becomes progressively more difficult to maintain as maximal exercise capacity is approached. Glycogen is used by the working skeletal muscles as a source of stored energy, and the anaerobic metabolism which ensues produces lactic acidosis and thereby further increases ventilation. As all cardiopulmonary transport mechanisms reach maximum levels, shortness of breath, fatigue, and muscle pain become limiting symptoms; motivation is then the final determinant of the duration of exercise. Ageing reduces the efficacy of cardiopulmonary transport mechanisms and, of course, exercise capacity. The heart rate response at peak exercise reflects this. In healthy individuals aged 20 years it is about 200 beats/min, and at 65 years about 170 beats/min.

When exercise stops, the cardiopulmonary and metabolic changes return rapidly to resting levels, the rate following an exponential pattern in the first few minutes; the excretion and metabolism of lactate and other substances, and the dissipation of heat generated take longer (time constant of about 15 min or more). Reduced circulatory function slows the recovery rate.

Training effects

Regular exercise to about 60% of maximal heart rate for 20 to 30 min three times a week is the minimum requirement for improved effort tolerance due to a training effect. The resting heart rate becomes slower, while the cardiac output is maintained by an increased end-diastolic volume and ejection fraction, and therefore stroke volume. In a 'trained' exercising individual, there is a reduced heart rate response to a standard submaximal workload, and systemic blood flow is more effectively distributed away from visceral and skin circulations to working muscles. Changes in muscle mitochondria permit increased oxygen consumption. There is suggestive animal evidence that prolonged endurance training increases the calibre of coronary arteries and enlarges capillary surface area relative to cardiac muscle mass. Myocardial protein synthesis increases. Adrenergic mechanisms appear to be involved in mediating this response. Rhythmic exercise (e.g. running) and isometric exercise (e.g. weightlifting) have different physiological effects. The blood pressure rises disproportionately during the latter. The mechanisms are partly reflex and partly mechanical from the contracting muscles. Isometric exercise training is not recommended for cardiac patients because of the increased afterload it imposes.

Regular exercise has other effects: it increases feelings of well-being and lowers blood pressure in normotensive and mildly hypertensive subjects. There are also diverse exercise-related hormonal changes, including the reduction of glucose-stimulated insulin secretion—of particular relevance to patients with type 2 diabetes. Regular exercise also improves the availability of nitric oxide, with its important vascular effects. These are considered elsewhere.

To summarize, changes in the four essential determinants of cardiac function—preload, afterload, heart rate, and contractility—combine to augment cardiac output and oxygen delivery during exercise. Measurement of the cardiovascular response to exercise is essential for the objective assessment of cardiac function.

Further reading

Bers DM (2001). *Excitation-contraction coupling and cardiac contractile force*, 2nd edition. Kluwer, Dordrecht.

Durgan DJ, Young ME (2010). The cardiomyocyte circadian clock: emerging roles in health and disease. *Circ Res*, **106**, 647–58.

Ganong WF (2005). *Review of medical physiology*, 22nd edition. McGraw Hill, New York.

Houser SR, Margulies KB (2003). Is depressed myocyte contractility centrally involved in heart failure? *Circ Res*, **92**, 350–8.

Jones NL, Killian KJ (2000). Exercise limitation in health and disease. *N Engl J Med*, **243**, 632–41.

Kaestner L (2012). *Calcium signalling: approaches and findings in the heart and blood*. Springer Science Media, Berlin.

Kardami E, *et al.* (2010). *Cardiac cell biology*. Springer Science Media, Berlin.

Katz AM (2006). *Physiology of the heart*, 4th edition. Lippincott Williams and Wilkins, Philadelphia, PA.

Ko Y-S, *et al.* (2004). Three-dimensional reconstruction of the rabbit atrioventricular conduction axis by combining histological, desmin, and connexin mapping data. *Circulation*, **109**, 1172–9.

Libby P, *et al.* (ed.) (2008). *Braunwald's heart disease: a textbook of cardiovascular medicine*, 8th edition. Saunders Elsevier, Philadelphia.

Opie LH (2013). *Stunning, hibernation and calcium in myocardial ischemia and reperfusion*. Kluwer Academic Publishers, Boston, MA.

O'Rourke B (2010). Be still, my beating heart: never! *Circ Res*, **106**, 238–9.

Severs NJ (2000). *The cardiac muscle cell. BioEssays*, **22**, 188–99.

Severs NJ, *et al.* (2004). Gap junction alterations in human cardiac disease. *Cardiovasc Res*, **62**, 368–77.

Solaro RJ, Tardiff JC (2013). *Biophysics of the failing heart: physics and biology of heart muscle*. Springer Science Media, Berlin.

Willis MS, Homeister JW, Stone J (2014). *Cellular and molecular pathobiology of cardiovascular disease*. Academic Press–Elsevier, Amsterdam.

Young ME (2006). The circadian clock within the heart: potential influence on myocardial gene expression, metabolism, and function. *Am J Physiol Heart Circ Physiol*, **290**, 1–16.

Zipes DP, Jalife J (2013). *Cardiac electrophysiology*, 6th edition. Saunders-Elsevier, Philadelphia, PA.

SECTION 2

Clinical presentation
of heart disease

Chest pain, breathlessness, and fatigue

Jeremy Dwight

Essentials

Chest pain, breathlessness, and fatigue are common diagnostic challenges. They have a broad differential diagnosis that includes a number of life-threatening pathologies.

Chest pain

The most reliable discriminating feature for angina, as opposed to other causes of chest pain, is its constricting nature, a fixed and predictable relationship to exertion, and that is relieved, within a few minutes, by rest or glyceryl trinitrate.

The ECG is used to triage patients with chest pain on admission to the Emergency Department, with treatment by thrombolysis or angioplasty after a brief confirmatory history in patients with significant ST elevation. However, these represent only a small fraction of those presenting with chest pain, and patients without ST elevation present the greater diagnostic challenge. A detailed history is needed to establish whether the pain is cardiac, and to inform the risk stratification process that determines the nature and time course of subsequent therapy and investigation.

The character of pain in acute coronary syndromes is similar to exertional angina, but usually more severe. It usually reaches maximal intensity over the course of a few minutes: pain reaching its maximum intensity instantaneously suggests an alternative cause.

Aortic dissection is a rare but important cause of chest pain: its pain is very sudden in onset, usually described as tearing or ripping, and the patient may report that it migrates from the front to the back of the chest. Pain with this description, loss of peripheral pulses, blood pressure difference between the two arms (>20 mmHg), and mediastinal widening on the chest radiograph are the most helpful diagnostic indicators.

Pericarditis occurs most commonly following myocardial infarction or viral infection. The pain is usually sharp and precordial, its onset is often sudden, and it is characteristically worse on inspiration, but is relieved by sitting up and leaning forward. A pericardial friction rub heard over the sternum may be positional and can appear and disappear within hours.

Breathlessness and fatigue

Most patients find it impossible to distinguish between cardiac and pulmonary causes of dyspnoea. The New York Heart Association classification is used to classify the extent of disability.

In the diagnosis of left ventricular failure, the most helpful features in the history are exertional breathlessness, orthopnoea, paroxysmal nocturnal dyspnoea, or a history of myocardial infarction. Tachycardia, cyanosis, and an elevated jugular venous pressure are features of heart failure, but they are also features of the major differential diagnoses. A displaced apex on palpation is helpful and relatively specific. A third heart sound has a high specificity (90–97%) but low sensitivity (31–51%) for detecting left ventricular dysfunction. Basal inspiratory crackles are suggestive of pulmonary oedema but have a sensitivity and specificity as low as 13 and 35%, respectively.

Other considerations

The cardiovascular history routinely includes assessment of risk factors and those aspects of the patient's past medical history that make cardiovascular disease more likely. The presence of numerous risk factors may, on occasion, prompt the physician to proceed to further investigation even in the face of a relatively unconvincing history.

Most diagnoses are made on the basis of the history, and the physician is always compelled to return to the initial history and examination to put the findings of any investigations into context and to plan therapy appropriate for the individual patient.

Introduction

The symptoms of chest pain, breathlessness, and fatigue present a frequent diagnostic challenge in the outpatient and acute medical departments as well as the Emergency Department. They have a broad differential diagnosis that includes a number of life-threatening pathologies.

As with all clinical presentations, the initial presenting symptom will prompt a differential diagnosis that the physician must narrow down, using a thorough history, to one or two possibilities. The onset, nature, and precipitating causes of symptoms need to be accurately defined, with carefully directed questions used to assess their relevance. The process involves a partnership between the patient and their doctor, and is enhanced by explaining the reasoning behind the questions asked and their relevance to making a diagnosis. In this way history-taking is a useful opportunity to assist the patient to a better understanding of their symptoms and to improve their compliance with any management plan.

The cardiovascular history routinely includes assessment of risk factors such as age, occupation, diabetes, hypertension, smoking, hypercholesterolaemia, drugs (both therapeutic and recreational), and a family history. It should also record those aspects of the patient's past medical history that make cardiovascular disease more likely, such as stroke, transient ischaemic attack, claudication, vascular surgery, renal disease, or connective tissue disease. The presence of numerous risk factors may, on occasion, prompt the physician to proceed to further investigation even in the face of a relatively unconvincing history.

Armed with a differential diagnosis obtained from the history, the physical examination is directed to identifying further supporting evidence. In isolation, however, there are surprisingly few examination findings that will provide a definitive diagnosis.

The cardiologist has a large armamentarium of diagnostic tools available to assist in making a diagnosis—ECG, echocardiography, coronary angiography, MRI, etc. These may appear to threaten to displace history-taking with the allure of high-definition images and impressive software. However, most diagnoses are made on the basis of the history, and the physician is always compelled to return to the initial history and examination to put the findings of any investigations into context and to plan therapy appropriate for the individual patient.

Chest pain

Chest pain accounts for up to 20% of all medical consultations and is one of the commonest presentations to the Emergency Department. In the community setting musculoskeletal or gastrointestinal causes are most common, whereas cardiac causes are more frequent in the Emergency Department (Table 2.1.1).

The circumstances of chest pain

Chest pain on exertion: angina pectoris

They who are afflicted with it are seized while they are walking (more especially if it be uphill and soon after eating) with a painful and most disagreeable sensation of the breast, which seems as if it would

Table 2.1.1 Cardiovascular causes of chest pain and differential diagnoses

Frequency as cause of chest pain	Cardiovascular	Noncardiovascular
Common	Angina	Oesophageal reflux
	Acute coronary syndromes	Pleurisy
	Pericarditis	Spinal root compression
	Pulmonary embolism	Costochondritis
	Syndrome X	Muscular/ arthropathies
	Tachyarrhythmias	
Uncommon	Valvular heart disease	Pneumothorax
	Pulmonary hypertension	Herpes zoster
	Aortic dissection	Peptic ulcer disease
	Myocarditis	Pulmonary or mediastinal tumours
	Takotsubo cardiomyopathy	Mediastinitis

extinguish life, if it were to increase or continue, but the moment they stand still, all this uneasiness vanishes. (Heberden 1768)

Unfortunately for the physician, the descriptors used by patients with angina are highly variable and include burning, heaviness, tightness, pressure, squeezing, aching, and strangling. Patients may not describe pain and it is preferable to ask for symptoms of discomfort in the chest. Most patients with angina recognize the pain as being worrying or serious. The location of the discomfort is usually retrosternal and may radiate to the arms, neck, and jaw (Fig. 2.1.1). Less commonly the pain may be felt in the back and upper abdomen.

The most reliable discriminating feature for angina as opposed to other causes of chest pain is a fixed and predictable relationship to exertion that is relieved within a few minutes by rest or glyceryl trinitrate (nitroglycerine). The discomfort characteristically occurs when walking on an incline and compels the patient to stop. In some cases the characteristic symptoms occur at the start of exertion and then ease, which is termed 'walk-through angina'. Surprisingly, patients may still be able to perform substantial anaerobic exercise without limitation. Angina is often worse in cold weather, in a cold wind, or after eating. Occasionally the pain is only present at the start of the day, when the patient is shaving or brushing their teeth. Symptoms of chest discomfort occurring after rather than during exertion, or which are present continuously throughout the day, are not due to angina.

Taking a careful history of the time course of relief with rest and glyceryl trinitrate is important. Many patients mistakenly report a response to glyceryl trinitrate when their pain has taken more than 15 min to resolve, but a response to glyceryl trinitrate is only helpful diagnostically when it occurs within a few minutes. Oesophageal spasm also responds to glyceryl trinitrate and may produce similar discomfort, but the pain is not related to exertion and is nearly always associated with symptoms of reflux. The three key clinical features of anginal pain are that it is (1) a constricting discomfort in the front of the chest, neck, shoulders, jaw, or arms; (2) precipitated by exertion; (3) relieved by rest or GTN within about 5 min. These features are used to identify patients with typical angina (all three features), atypical angina (two features), or noncardiac pain (one or none of these features). In the United Kingdom this classification has been incorporated into recent National Institute for Health and Care Excellence (NICE) guidelines for management of chest pain of recent onset.

Chest pain at rest

Chest pain due to ischaemia that occurs at rest has a broader differential diagnosis. The important life-threatening differential diagnoses are myocardial infarction, aortic dissection, and pulmonary embolism. Rest pain due to angina without infarction is usually accompanied by a history of exertional angina, but there are a few exceptions. Arrhythmias, e.g. paroxysmal atrial fibrillation, may precipitate angina at rest and a history of palpitations should be sought in those with unpredictable symptoms. Emotional stress may also precipitate an attack. An important example of this is Takotsubo cardiomyopathy where chest pain is accompanied by a characteristic pattern of left ventricular damage in the absence of significant coronary disease. Nocturnal angina may be precipitated by nightmares or the onset of pulmonary oedema, but a history of exertional angina is nearly always present. Where nocturnal chest pain is present in the absence of exertional symptoms a history of

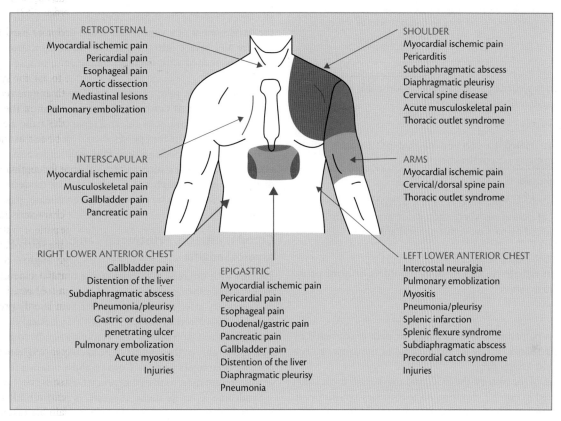

RETROSTERNAL
Myocardial ischemic pain
Pericardial pain
Esophageal pain
Aortic dissection
Mediastinal lesions
Pulmonary embolization

SHOULDER
Myocardial ischemic pain
Pericarditis
Subdiaphragmatic abscess
Diaphragmatic pleurisy
Cervical spine disease
Acute musculoskeletal pain
Thoracic outlet syndrome

INTERSCAPULAR
Myocardial ischemic pain
Musculoskeletal pain
Gallbladder pain
Pancreatic pain

ARMS
Myocardial ischemic pain
Cervical/dorsal spine pain
Thoracic outlet syndrome

RIGHT LOWER ANTERIOR CHEST
Gallbladder pain
Distention of the liver
Subdiaphragmatic abscess
Pneumonia/pleurisy
Gastric or duodenal
penetrating ulcer
Pulmonary embolization
Acute myositis
Injuries

EPIGASTRIC
Myocardial ischemic pain
Pericardial pain
Esophageal pain
Duodenal/gastric pain
Pancreatic pain
Gallbladder pain
Distention of the liver
Diaphragmatic pleurisy
Pneumonia

LEFT LOWER ANTERIOR CHEST
Intercostal neuralgia
Pulmonary emoblization
Myositis
Pneumonia/pleurisy
Splenic infarction
Splenic flexure syndrome
Subdiaphragmatic abscess
Precordial catch syndrome
Injuries

Fig. 2.1.1 Differential diagnosis of chest pain according to location and radiation. Serious intrathoracic or sub diaphragmatic diseases are usually associated with pains that begin in the left anterior chest, left shoulder, or upper arm, the interscapular region, or the epigastrium. The scheme is not all inclusive (e.g. intercostal neuralgia occurs in locations other than the left, lower anterior chest area).
From Miller AJ: *Diagnosis of chest pain.* New York, Raven Press (LWW), 1988, p. 175.

acid reflux (relief on sitting up or with antacids, and discomfort on drinking hot fluids) should be sought. Reflux symptoms are common and may coexist with angina, and the patient may find it impossible to differentiate between the two.

Particular causes of chest pain

Acute coronary syndromes

The term 'acute coronary syndrome' encompasses myocardial infarction and unstable angina, conditions which are usually caused by a common pathology—the rupture or erosion of an atheromatous plaque. Because of the need for rapid assessment and treatment, the ECG is often used to triage patients with chest pain on admission to the Emergency Department. Where there are classic features of ST elevation infarction, treatment is commenced with thrombolysis or angioplasty after a brief confirmatory history (see Chapter 13.4). However, patients with ST elevation represent only a small fraction of those presenting with chest pain, and those without ST elevation present the greater diagnostic challenge. Some will simply have dyspepsia or musculolskeletal pain, whereas those at the other end of the spectrum will be at imminent risk of myocardial infarction. The history has two important roles: first to establish whether the pain is cardiac, and secondly to contribute to the risk stratification process that determines the nature and time course subsequent therapy and investigation.

The character of pain in acute coronary syndromes is similar to exertional angina, but usually more severe. It usually reaches maximal intensity over the course of a few minutes. Pain reaching its maximum intensity instantaneously suggests an alternative cause, in particular, aortic dissection. The patient should be asked to describe exactly what they were doing at the onset of the pain: sudden onset during a specific movement will suggest a musculoskeletal origin.

The classical description of the pain of myocardial infarction is of a heavy, crushing or constricting pain. In comparison to angina the duration of pain in myocardial infarction is longer (>15 min), and with increasing duration myocardial infarction is more likely, but the pain rarely lasts more than a few hours. Infarction is more likely to be associated with systemic symptoms (breathlessness, sweating, nausea and vomiting) and does not respond to glyceryl trinitrate. About one-half of patients will have a history suggestive of worsening exertional angina, or short-lived episodes of chest pain at rest before presentation. The pain of an acute coronary syndrome usually discourages the patient from attempting any exertion and does not improve with exercise. Although the history alone cannot definitively rule out myocardial infarction, it can be used to assess the probability of this condition (Box 2.1.1).

During the examination the patient should be asked to map out the distribution of the pain. Highly localized pain of less than a few centimetres in distribution is unlikely to ischaemic in origin.

> **Box 2.1.1** Risk stratification for acute myocardial infarction and acute coronary syndrome according to components of the chest pain history
>
> Low risk:
>
> - Pain that is pleuritic, positional, or reproducible with palpation, or is described as stabbing
>
> Probably low risk:
>
> - Pain not related to exertion or that occurs in a small inframammary area of the chest
>
> Probably high risk:
>
> - Pain described as pressure, is similar to that of a prior myocardial infarction or worse than prior anginal pain, or is accompanied by nausea, vomiting, or diaphoresis
>
> High risk:
>
> - Pain that radiates to one or both shoulders or arms or is related to exertion

Tenderness on palpation of the chest wall or pain exacerbated by rotation of the thorax or passive movements of the arms or neck suggest musculoskeletal pain.

Components of the history, the ECG, and markers of myocardial damage are used in non-ST elevation acute coronary syndromes to determine the risk of subsequent events in the TIMI (Thrombolysis in Myocardial Infarction) risk score (Table 2.1.2) and a scoring system based on the GRACE (Global Registry of Acute Coronary Events) registry. Great emphasis has been placed on the use of troponin estimation in determining the risk of subsequent events in these patients and this is undoubtedly a useful tool. However, in the absence of definitive ECG changes or troponin rise, the patient may still score 5 on the TIMI risk score from the history alone, giving a risk of 25% of major cardiovascular adverse events in the next 14 days. For further discussion see Chapter 13.4.

There are no specific findings on cardiovascular examination in acute coronary syndromes. In the context of severe coronary disease the patient may present with the clinical features of left ventricular failure (see 'Particular causes of breathlessness') or cardiogenic shock. Features of increased sympathetic tone, pallor, tachycardia,

Table 2.1.2 TIMI risk score for non-ST elevation acute coronary syndromes

Clinical feature	Points
Age ≥65 years	1
At least three risk factors for coronary disease[a]	1
Prior demonstration of significant coronary artery stenosis	1
ST deviation on ECG	1
Severe anginal symptoms (e.g. ≥2 anginal events in the last 24 h)	1
Use of aspirin in previous 7 days	1
Elevated cardiac markers (e.g. troponin)	1

[a] Family history, hypertension, hypercholesterolaemia, diabetes, current smoking.

From Antman et al. JAMA 2000; 284:835–842.

and sweating are often present in infarction, but are also features of all causes of severe chest pain. A pansystolic murmur may indicate the development of a ventricular septal defect or papillary muscle rupture and severe mitral regurgitation, complications which are usually associated with haemodynamic compromise and left ventricular failure.

The presence or peripheral vascular disease increases the probability of coexistent coronary disease and the patient should be examined for carotid, femoral, and renal bruits and an abdominal aortic aneurysm. The foot pulses should also be assessed.

The presence of neck and/or chest wall tenderness will point to alternative diagnoses such as cervical spondylopathy, costochondritis, or nerve entrapment. Hypochondrial tenderness suggests a gastrointestinal cause, e.g. peptic ulcer disease, pancreatitis, or gallstones.

Coronary spasm, Prinzmetal's angina, syndrome X, atypical angina

Patients with unpredictable angina due to the occurrence of coronary spasm, either in the context of coronary disease or with normal coronary arteries, have been described. The diagnosis should only be considered in the patient with a classical description of ischaemic chest pain that usually responds rapidly to glyceryl trinitrate, preferably in the context of ECG changes (ST elevation in the case of Prinzmetal's angina). Cocaine abuse is now a frequent cause of this presentation to the Emergency Department.

Syndrome X, as its name suggests, is poorly understood. This label (whether it can properly be called a diagnosis is debatable) is often attached to patients with cardiac-sounding chest pain and a normal angiogram. This finding is more common in women. The pain often has features atypical of angina. It is often of submammary location or radiation, and precipitating factors are highly variable. This diagnosis should only be considered after other causes of chest pain have been carefully excluded, since it may expose the patient to a lifetime of inappropriate treatment and anxiety.

The term 'atypical chest pain' is meaningless (especially for the patient) and is best avoided. There are, however, many patients for whom a confident diagnosis cannot be made. Serious pathology can be excluded and the patient can be reassured that they have an excellent prognosis. It is better to leave the diagnosis at 'chest pain,? cause' than to inappropriately label the patient as having 'atypical angina' or syndrome X.

Aortic dissection

Aortic dissection is a rare but important cause of chest pain: up to one-half of all patients with an untreated proximal aortic dissection die within 48 h. The pain of aortic dissection is very sudden in onset, is usually described as tearing or ripping, and the patient may report that it migrates from the front to the back of the chest. There should be a particularly high index of suspicion when chest pain is associated with neurological features such as hemiplegia or paraplegia due to involvement of the carotid vessels and spinal arteries, but these are present in less than 20% of cases. Risk factors in the history include hypertension, Marfan's syndrome, a bicuspid aortic valve, previous aortic valve replacement, cocaine usage, and the third trimester of pregnancy. Of the clinical features (see Box 2.1.2) aortic pain (as described above), loss of peripheral pulses, blood pressure difference between the two arms (>20 mmHg), and mediastinal widening on the chest radiograph are the most helpful. In

Box 2.1.2 Clinical features associated with aortic dissection

- Sudden onset tearing, ripping chest pain that migrates to the back
- Loss of peripheral pulses
- Blood pressure difference >20 mmHg between arms
- Hemiparesis
- Paraparesis
- Diastolic murmur
- Pleural effusion (usually left sided)
- Hoarseness
- Horner's syndrome
- Bilateral testicular tenderness
- Pulsatile stenoclavicular joint
- Superior vena cava obstruction
- Pulsus paradoxus (with pericardial tamponade)

the absence of these features the incidence of aortic dissection is less than 5%. The absolute level of blood pressure in unhelpful in discriminating aortic dissection from other causes of chest pain.

Pericarditis

Pericarditis occurs most commonly following a myocardial infarction or viral infection. The patient may describe a preceding viral illness with fever and cough. The pain is usually sharp and precordial. The onset is often sudden. It is characteristically worse on inspiration and relieved by sitting up and leaning forward, and it can be accompanied by classic pleuritic pain. A less typical description occurs when a pericardial effusion has developed and the pain arises from pericardial distension, when the pain may be a dull restrosternal ache or pressure. Radiation of pericarditic pain occurs to all those areas associated with myocardial infarction, but radiation to the trapezius ridges is pathognomic of the diagnosis.

The patient is usually well and not compromised haemodynamically (except where there is pericardial tamponade). Clinical examination may initially be normal. A pericardial friction rub heard over the sternum may be positional and appear and disappear within hours. Repeated examination may be helpful, including auscultation of the patient lying flat in expiration. The ECG finding of concave ST elevation in multiple lead is helpful, but ECG findings are equivocal or normal in 40 to 50% of cases.

Breathlessness and fatigue

Breathlessness (or dyspnoea, derived from Greek words meaning painful or difficult breathing) is the endpoint of a variety of pathologies and is mediated by a series of neural pathways, the sensory inputs of which originate in the lungs, chest wall, and peripheral and sensory chemoreceptors (see Fig. 2.1.2). Patients may describe the sensation of breathlessness as tightness, wheeze, 'inability to get enough air', sighing, choking, or suffocating. Heart failure, asthma, and chronic obstructive airways disease account for about three-quarters of hospital admissions with breathlessness in industrialized nations. Symptom clusters have been described for these pathologies, but most patients find it impossible to distinguish between cardiac and pulmonary causes of dyspnoea.

The time course of the illness is an important aid to the diagnosis in patients with dyspnoea but must be interpreted in the context

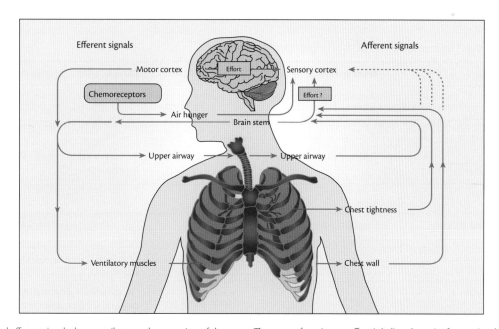

Fig. 2.1.2 Efferent and afferent signals that contribute to the sensation of dyspnoea. The sense of respiratory effort is believed to arise from a signal transmitted from the motor cortex to the sensory cortex coincidently with the outgoing motor command to the ventilatory muscles. The arrow from the brainstem to the sensory cortex indicates that the motor output of the brainstem may also contribute to the sense of effort The sense of air hunger is believed to arise, in part, from increased respiratory activity within the brainstem, and the sensation of chest tightness probably results from stimulation of vagal-irritant receptors. Although afferent information from airway, lung, and chest wall receptors most likely passes through the brainstem before reaching the sensory cortex, the dashed lines indicate uncertainty about whether some afferents bypass the brainstem and project directly to the sensory cortex.

From Manning HL, Schwartzstein RM *New England Journal of Medicine* 333. 1547–1553. http://content.nejm.org/cgi/content/extract/333/23/1547.

Table 2.1.3 New York Heart Association classification of breathlessness according to severity

Class I	No limitation—ordinary physical activity does not cause undue fatigue, dyspnoea, or palpitation
Class II	Slight limitation of physical activity—comfortable at rest, but ordinary physical activity results in fatigue, dyspnoea, or palpitation
Class III	Marked limitation of physical activity—comfortable at rest, but less than normal activity produces symptoms
Class IV	Inability to carry out any physical activity without discomfort

of the patient's day-to-day activities. Even when the disease progresses gradually the patient may report a recent onset of symptoms because they have (often subconsciously) adapted their lifestyle over the course of many months. This is particularly true of patients with chronic heart failure.

Until relatively recently, symptoms of fatigue and breathlessness in heart failure have been assumed to be due purely to a combination of poor cardiac output and pulmonary congestion. However, in patients with heart failure the correlation between symptoms and left ventricular ejection fraction is very poor. Changes in skeletal and respiratory muscle function appear to contribute significantly to symptoms, a hypothesis that is supported by the response observed to exercise training programmes in patients with chronic heart failure, and which may account for part of the considerable variability in disability in patients with similar haemodynamic and echocardiographic findings. Because of the contribution of fatigue it is more helpful to ask about a change in exercise tolerance in patients with suspected heart failure, since this may correlate more closely with the underlying pathology. The New York Heart

Association (NYHA) classification is used to classify the extent of disability (Table 2.1.3).

The time course of onset of breathlessness can be particularly useful in determining the underlying pathology (Table 2.1.4). Breathlessness of dramatic onset (over minutes) is suggestive of pulmonary embolism, pulmonary oedema, upper airway obstruction, or a pneumothorax. Chronic dyspnoea presents in the context of worsening breathlessness over a period of months or years is typical of chronic obstructive airways disease, interstitial lung disease, or anaemia, but may also be a feature of heart failure. Acute on chronic dyspnoea indicates an exacerbation of breathlessness in a patient with established disease.

Chronic obstructive airways disease, asthma, and heart failure are common in the population of industrialized countries and most elderly patients presenting to the Emergency Department with breathing difficulties will have a prior history of pulmonary or cardiac disease. However, it is important not to automatically attribute any deterioration in symptoms as being due to progression of their underlying disease process. Alternative causes should be considered, and this situation is often a major diagnostic challenge. A common example is a sudden deterioration in the patient with long-standing well-controlled heart failure, which should prompt consideration of further pathology such as a silent myocardial infarction, pulmonary embolism, or arrhythmia.

Breathlessness at rest occurs in pulmonary embolism or pulmonary oedema, and with a pneumothorax. Exertional dyspnoea occurs in left ventricular failure and chronic obstructive airways disease. Psychogenic breathlessness is frequently present at rest and is associated with sighing, features of hyperventilation such as perioral or peripheral paraesthesiae, and chest tightness. The presence of breathlessness at rest but not on exertion strongly suggests a functional origin.

Table 2.1.4 Conditions causing breathlessness classified by the rate of onset

Acute	Acute on chronic	Chronic
Asthma	Infective exacerbation of COPD	COPD
Myocardial infarction	Decompensated chronic heart failure	Cardiac failure
PE	PE complicating congestive cardiac failure or COPD	Anaemia
Cardiogenic pulmonary oedema (secondary to ischaemia, valvular disease, arrhythmias)	Pneumothorax complicating COPD or asthma	Pulmonary vascular disease (PE, pulmonary hypertension)
Pneumonia	Atrial fibrillation/flutter complicating COPD or cardiac failure	Parenchymal lung disease, e.g. UIP, sarcoid
Noncardiogenic pulmonary oedema	Chordal rupture in chronic nonrheumatic mitral regurgitation	Pleural disease, e.g. effusion, asbestosis
Pulmonary haemorrhage		Chest wall disease e.g. kyphosis, ankylosing spondylitis
Spontaneous pneumothorax		Neuromuscular disorders, e.g. muscular dystrophy, polio, myasthenia gravis
Chest trauma		Malignancy
Upper airway obstruction		Obesity/deconditioning
Hyperventilation syndrome		Sleep apnoea
		Silent myocardial ischaemia

COPD, chronic obstructive pulmonary disease; PE, pulmonary embolism; UIP, usual interstitial pneumonia.

Particular causes of breathlessness

Left ventricular failure

The incidence of left ventricular failure in the community is 1 to 2%. It is important to attempt to identify the cause during the initial assessment. A history of ischaemic or valvular heart disease, alcohol abuse, smoking, diabetes, hypertension, and a family history are important.

Patients with left ventricular failure commonly present to the outpatient clinic, but may present for the first time to the Emergency Department. An acute presentation is more likely when there has been a rapid rise in the left atrial pressure generating pulmonary oedema. In severe cases this is associated with haemoptysis in the form of frothy pink sputum. This type of presentation occurs with myocardial infarction, mitral valve papillary muscle or chordal rupture, malignant hypertension, tachyarrhythmias, and endocarditis with major valve destruction. Where a rise in left atrial pressure occurs over a longer time course, sustained elevated left atrial pressures are compensated for by increased lymphatic drainage and structural changes in the pulmonary capillary and alveolar basement membrane and patients more commonly present with fatigue, exertional breathlessness, and orthopnoea. Prolonged increases in left atrial pressure are associated with pulmonary hypertension and the associated clinical features of right ventricular enlargement, tricuspid regurgitation, and a loud pulmonary second sound. This type of presentation is more frequently a feature of patients with an idiopathic, ischaemic, hypertensive, or alcoholic cardiomyopathy.

Clinical findings that help in assessing impaired left ventricular function or elevated left atrial filling pressures are shown in Table 2.1.5.

The most helpful features in the history are exertional breathlessness, orthopnoea, paroxysmal nocturnal dyspnoea, or a history of myocardial infarction. Breathlessness that is worse on lying flat and relieved promptly on sitting up is characteristic for orthopnoea. Patients with chronic obstructive airways disease may also describe orthopnoea, but this is usually present only in the setting of severe disease and chronic breathlessness at rest. Paroxysmal nocturnal dyspnoea is due to the development of interstitial oedema and typically occurs 2 to 4 h after the onset of sleep. The patient usually stands up or sits on the side of the bed and symptoms resolve over the course of 10 to 15 min. This is usually a frightening and memorable experience for the patient, and to avoid these symptoms they will sleep propped up on pillows or, in severe cases, in a chair. However, a history of paroxysmal nocturnal dyspnoea or orthopnoea is only present in 20% of patients with heart failure and its absence does not exclude the diagnosis. Ankle oedema is supportive of a diagnosis of heart failure, but dependent oedema is often present in older people and in patients with chronic obstructive airways disease, and the astute physician should avoid the common mistake of assuming that 'ankle oedema means cardiac failure means diuretic prescription'.

The clinical examination findings are used to support a suspected diagnosis of heart failure, but they are not always helpful. Tachycardia, cyanosis, and an elevated jugular venous pressure are features of heart failure, but they are also features of the major differential diagnoses, pulmonary embolism, and chronic obstructive airways disease. Although jugular venous pressure correlates with left atrial pressure it may be misleading in the presence of isolated right ventricular dysfunction, tricuspid regurgitation, and pulmonary hypertension. A displaced apex on palpation is helpful and relatively specific. Basal inspiratory crackles (rales) are suggestive of pulmonary oedema but can be present in fibrotic lung disease infection and chronic airways disease and have a sensitivity and specificity as low as 13% and 35% respectively. The third sound is a low-pitched sound heard in mid-diastole, best with the bell of the stethoscope placed lightly over the apex. It can be confused with a split second sound, but is later in diastole and has a much longer duration. It has a high specificity (90–97%) but low sensitivity (31–51%) for detecting left ventricular dysfunction.

Fever and purulent sputum usually point to a diagnosis of an infective exacerbation of chronic bronchitis or chest infection. In older people, however, a chest infection may precipitate decompensation of heart failure.

Left ventricular failure is highly unlikely in the presence of a genuinely normal ECG. Evidence of a previous myocardial infarction on the ECG, in particular the presence of Q waves in the anterior chest leads is highly predictive of left ventricular dysfunction.

The most useful finding on chest radiography is cardiomegaly, but heart size may be normal, particularly in diastolic heart failure. Changes of pulmonary venous distension, pulmonary oedema, and pleural effusion are more common in acute presentations, but are frequently absent in patients presenting with chronic breathlessness.

Following clinical assessment, including ECG and chest radiography, there may still be considerable uncertainty about the diagnosis of the cause of breathlessness, particularly in patients presenting to the Emergency Department. Measurement of blood brain natriuretic peptide (BNP) may assist in a more rapid and accurate diagnosis in this circumstance, a level below 100 pg/ml (>300 pg/ml for NT-proBNP) making the diagnosis of left ventricular failure highly unlikely and alternative diagnoses should be considered. High levels (>500 pg/ml) are strongly suggestive of heart failure. Intermediate levels are more difficult to interpret as there are a number of confounding factors for BNP measurement (Table 2.1.6)

As with troponin (see Chapter 13.4), BNP levels must be interpreted in the context of the history, clinical findings and other investigations. Scoring systems have been devised using BNP and other clinical and investigation findings in acute dyspnoea (Fig. 2.1.3).

Given the relatively poor predictive value of the clinical history and physical signs in the diagnosis of left ventricular failure, open access to echocardiography may appear superior to clinical

Table 2.1.5 Helpful and relatively specific clinical findings for predicting heart failure in patients presenting with dyspnoea

History	Examination
Orthopnoea	Elevated jugular venous pressure
Paroxysmal nocturnal dyspnoea	Cardiomegaly
Recent onset peripheral oedema	Third or fourth heart sound
Prior history of heart failure	Basal crepitations
Previous myocardial infarction	Positive hepatojugular reflux
	Peripheral oedema beyond mid-calf

Adapted from Badgett RG. Lucey C.T., Mulrow C.D, Can the clinical examination diagnose left-sided heart failure in adults? JAMA 1997; 277: 1712–1719.

Table 2.1.6 Confounding factors in the interpretation of BNP measurements

Increased BNP	Decreased BNP
Increasing age	Obesity
Female sex	Cardioactive drugs
Pulmonary disease	ACE inhibitors
Systemic hypertension	Spironolactone
Hyperthryoidism	β-Blockers (long term)
Cushing's syndrome	Diuretics
Glucocorticoid usage	
Conn's syndrome	
Hepatic cirrhosis with ascites	
Renal failure	
Paraneoplastic syndrome	
Subarachnoid haemorrhage	

assessment. However, there are important arguments for careful clinical assessment. Firstly, echocardiography is not always available in the emergency setting. Secondly, cardiac and noncardiac causes of dyspnoea, particularly chronic obstructive pulmonary disease (COPD), often coexist, and where there is dual pathology, deciding which treatment to escalate is more dependent on the appropriate interpretation of the symptoms, clinical signs, and chest radiographic findings than echocardiographic parameters. Thirdly, heart failure is frequently present in the presence of apparently preserved systolic function on echocardiography.

Airways disease

The clinical features of heart failure and airways disease are often difficult to distinguish. Patients with lung disease tend to use the terms 'chest tightness' or 'restriction', whereas the patient with heart

Clinical and investigation findings	Points
Elevated NT-proBNP	4
Interstitial oedema on chest radiograph	2
Orthopnoea	2
Absence of fever	2
Current loop diuretics	1
Age >75	1
Crepitations (rales) on lung examination	1
Absence of cough	1

Fig. 2.1.3 Scoring system to predict whether a patient presenting to the Emergency Department has congestive heart failure (CHF). The patient's total score (maximum 14) is obtained by adding the points that they score for each clinical or investigation feature

Reprinted from *Am J Heart*, Vol 151 (1), Baggish A.L et al, A validated clinical and biochemical score for the diagnosis of acute heart failure: the Pro-BNP Investigation of Dyspnoea in the Emergency Department (PRIDE) acute heart failure score, pp48–54. Copyright (2006), with permission from Elsevier.

failure is more inclined to describe the sensation of 'not being able to get enough air'. Patients are more likely to have COPD if they have a self-reported history of COPD, wheezing on examination (although this can be a feature of heart failure), a forced expiratory time of 9 s or more, and laryngeal descent. Clearly COPD is very unlikely in the absence of a smoking history and in patients under 45 years of age. Patients with COPD and left ventricular failure may suffer from a chronic cough, although in the case of heart failure this is usually a dry cough and more prominent at night.

Fluid retention giving rise to an elevated jugular venous pressure and ankle oedema can occur in association with hypoxia, but only if saturations are persistently less than 93%. Ankle oedema may also be a feature of chronic CO_2 retention. Although often cited as a cause of the clinical features of right heart failure in COPD, true right ventricular failure is relatively uncommon and the mechanism of fluid retention is complex. COPD and heart failure often coexist.

The chest radiograph may be unhelpful and patients with emphysema and left ventricular failure may not have any radiological features of pulmonary congestion or oedema. In these situations systolic heart failure can only be ruled out by echocardiography.

Pulmonary embolism

Pulmonary embolism is a common differential diagnosis in patients with breathlessness and should be considered in any presenting with breathlessness without clinical signs of left ventricular failure. The acute presenting symptoms are of breathlessness (usually of sudden onset), chest pain (classically pleuritic, but central with large pulmonary emboli), and less commonly haemoptysis, cough, and syncope. The differential diagnosis depends on the predominant presenting feature, i.e. pleuritic pain (chest infection with pleurisy, pericarditis), central chest pain (myocardial infarction), dyspnoea (COPD or heart failure). Chronic pulmonary embolic disease and pulmonary hypertension present with exertional breathlessness, and patients may complain of central chest pain that is due to right ventricular subendocardial ischaemia. The diagnosis of pulmonary embolism cannot easily be excluded without investigation and the exclusion of an alternative, more likely, cause of breathlessness is crucial to the initial assessment.

Most patients with acute pulmonary embolism are breathless or tachypnoeic (respiratory rate >20/min) and in the absence of these findings haemoptysis and pleuritic chest pain are usually due to another cause. See Chapter 16.1 for further discussion of examination findings and diagnostic strategy in patients with suspected pulmonary embolism.

Dyspnoea with preserved left ventricular function

Where breathlessness is present in the context of preserved left ventricular function, diastolic heart failure should be considered. This diagnosis can only be made in the context of an appropriate history and examination findings. Echocardiographic parameters of diastolic dysfunction (see Chapter 3.2) are common in the community setting, but more than 50% of individuals with such an echocardiographic diagnosis are asymptomatic and the presence of diastolic dysfunction in a patient with breathlessness should not automatically lead to a diagnosis of the clinical syndrome of diastolic heart failure. COPD, ischaemic heart disease, and obesity are common in individuals with diastolic dysfunction, and diastolic heart failure can be overdiagnosed. Hypertension, coronary disease, and left ventricular hypertrophy are important causes of diastolic dysfunction and in their absence diastolic heart failure is rare. Alternative causes for dyspnoea should be always be excluded, in particular, chronic thromboembolic disease, airways disease, sleep apnoea, and silent ischaemia.

Further reading

Badgett RG, Lucey CR, Mulrow CD (1997). Can the clinical examination diagnose left-sided heart failure in adults? *JAMA*, **277**, 1712–19.

Bugiardini R, Merz CNB (2005). Angina with normal coronary arteries. A changing philosophy. *JAMA*, **293**, 477–84.

Cayley WE (2005). Diagnosing the cause of chest pain. *Am Fam Physician*, **72**, 2012–21.

Chunilal SD, *et al.* (2003). Does this patient have pulmonary embolism? *JAMA*, **290**, 2849–58.

Cooper A, Timmis A, Skinner J; Guideline Development Group (2010). Assessment of recent onset chest pain or discomfort of suspected cardiac origin: summary of NICE guidance. http://guidance.nice.org.uk/CG95/Guidance/pdf/English

Davie AP, *et al.* (1997). Assessing diagnosis in heart failure: which features are any use? *Q J Med*, **90**, 335–9.

Gehlbach BK, Geppert E (2004). The pulmonary manifestations of left heart failure. *Chest*, **125**, 669–82.

Global Registry of Acute Coronary Events (GRACE). Center for Outcomes Research, University of Massachusetts Medical School. http://www.outcomes-umassmed.org/grace/

Hurst JW, Morris DC (2001). *Chest pain*. Futura, Armonk, NY.

Klompas, M (2002). Does this patient have acute thoracic aortic dissection? *JAMA*, **287**, 2262–72.

Mahler, DA (1990). *Dyspnoea*. Futura, Armonk, NY.

Manning HL, Schwartzstein RM (1995). Pathophysiology of dyspnea. *N Engl J Med*, **333**, 1547–53.

Marcus GM, *et al.* (2005). Association between phonocardiographic third and fourth heart sounds and objective measures of left ventricular function. *JAMA*, **293**, 2238–44.

Miller AJ (1988). *Diagnosis of chest pain*. Raven Press, New York.

Scano G, Stenardi L, Grazzini M (2005). Understanding dyspnoea by its language. *Eur Resp J*, **25**, 380–5.

Straus SE, *et al.* (2000). The accuracy of patient history, wheezing, and laryngeal measurements in diagnosing obstructive airway disease. CARE-COAD1 Group. Clinical assessment of the reliability of the examination-chronic obstructive airways disease. *JAMA*, **283**, 1853–7.

Swap CJ, Nagurney JT (2005). Value and limitations of chest pain history in the evaluation of patients with suspected acute coronary syndromes. *JAMA*, **294**, 2623–9.

Wang CS, *et al.* (2005). Does this dyspneic patient in the emergency department have congestive heart failure? *JAMA*, **294**, 1944–56.

CHAPTER 2.2

Syncope and palpitation

K. Rajappan, A. C. Rankin,
A. D. McGavigan, and S. M. Cobbe

Essentials

Syncope

Syncope is a transient episode of loss of consciousness (T-LOC) due to cerebral hypoperfusion. Its causes can be subdivided on the basis of pathophysiology, including (1) neurally mediated—or reflex—syncope; (2) orthostatic hypotension; (3) cardiac causes; and (4) cerebrovascular or psychogenic causes.

Neurocardiogenic syncope, or simple faint, is the commonest cause and is benign, but it is always important to exclude or establish the diagnosis of cardiac syncope, because this has an adverse prognosis that may be improved with appropriate treatment. Cardiac arrhythmia should be considered in all patients who have syncope associated with any of the following: (1) exertion, chest pain, or palpitations; (2) a past medical history of heart disease; (3) abnormal cardiovascular findings on examination; (4) an abnormal ECG; and (5) a family history of sudden cardiac death in people younger than 40 years old or with an inherited cardiac condition.

Initial assessment of the patient with syncope by clinical history, examination, and 12-lead ECG will indicate a probable diagnosis in most patients and guide further investigation (if required). Documentation of cardiac rhythm during syncope is extremely useful, especially if it is associated with palpitations, but this is usually difficult to obtain because of the intermittent and typically infrequent nature of the symptom. External or implanted loop recorders, which can store the rhythm before, during, and after an episode, are increasingly used when the diagnosis remains unclear. In patients with structural heart disease in whom arrhythmia is suspected, programmed electrical stimulation of the ventricles may induce sustained monomorphic ventricular tachycardia: this is a relatively specific response, shows that the patient is at risk of recurrent ventricular arrhythmia, and makes an arrhythmic origin of syncope likely, but the diagnostic yield of electrophysiological testing is low in patients with a structurally normal heart.

Palpitation

Palpitation is the awareness of one's heart beating—it may be due to an awareness of an abnormal cardiac rhythm, or an abnormal awareness of normal rhythm. It is most commonly due to premature beats (ectopics) and is benign. Correlation between symptoms and cardiac rhythm is the initial aim of investigations in patients presenting with palpitations.

Syncope

Definition

Syncope is defined as a transient loss of consciousness, with loss of postural tone, usually resulting in falling. It is often of sudden onset, with prompt spontaneous recovery. The underlying mechanism is reduced cerebral perfusion, which may be due to a variety of cardiovascular—or less commonly cerebrovascular—causes. It is a common presentation, producing 1 to 3% of Emergency Department visits and up to 6% of hospital admissions. The cause is often initially uncertain and assessment must first differentiate syncope from other causes of loss of consciousness, such as epileptic seizures.

Prognosis

The prognosis depends on the aetiology, with most patients having a benign condition, although recurrent syncope can produce anxiety and reduction in quality of life regardless of the underlying cause. The exceptions are cardiac causes of syncope, which have been reported to have 1-year mortality rates as high as 18 to 33%. An important aim in the evaluation of syncope is to identify this subgroup of patients: clues may come from the history, examination, and the 12-lead ECG (Box 2.2.1).

Differential diagnosis

The initial evaluation of the patient with possible transient loss of consciousness should include history, examination, supine and upright blood pressure, and 12-lead ECG (Fig. 2.2.1). It is important to establish that loss of consciousness (syncope) occurred to enable differentiation from nonsyncopal causes such as falls, drop attacks, and transient ischaemic attacks. In the absence of 'red flag' features of cardiac syncope (Box 2.2.1) and with a normal 12-lead ECG, a single episode of syncope requires no further investigation or treatment, other than reassurance. In patients with recurrent syncope, or a single episode in a high-risk individual, further investigation and treatment will depend on the suspected diagnosis.

The causes of syncope can be subdivided on the basis of pathophysiology, namely (1) neurally mediated—or reflex—syncope, (2) orthostatic hypotension, (3) cardiac causes, and (4) cerebrovascular or psychogenic causes (Table 2.2.1). The history is most important. For example, it may strongly suggest a vasovagal origin, or an epileptic seizure. However, the diagnosis may be complicated by an overlap in features, such as convulsive movements during a vasovagal episode due to anoxic convulsive seizures. It is

---

Box 2.2.1 Features associated with cardiac syncope

History of syncopal episode

- Occurs during exertion*
- Occurs when supine*
- Associated palpitations
- Associated chest pain

Past medical history

- Known structural heart disease*
- Previous myocardial infarction*
- History of heart failure*
- Valvular heart disease*

Family history

- Family history of sudden death*

Examination

- Presence of murmur*
- Signs of heart failure*
- Carotid bruit

12-lead ECG

- Evidence of atrioventricular block
- Bundle branch block
- Evidence of previous infarction
- Left ventricular hypertrophy
- Long QTc interval
- Features of Brugada syndrome

* Denotes a 'red flag' feature of the history or examination that suggests urgent assessment is required and a high chance of recurrent syncope exists.

---

increased sympathetic activity and catecholamine levels. The vigorous contraction of relatively empty ventricles results in the activation of mechanoreceptors that would normally respond to stretch in the left ventricular wall. Afferent nerve fibres conduct to the cerebral medulla and activate the reflex withdrawal of peripheral sympathetic tone and activation of vagal parasympathetic activity. The resultant vasodilatation and bradycardia cause reduced cerebral perfusion and loss of consciousness. However, there is debate about these mechanisms and other factors may be involved in the aetiology of syncope, as illustrated by the documentation of neurocardiogenic syncope—despite cardiac denervation—in orthotopic heart transplant recipients. Certainly, it is well recognized that vasovagal syncope can result from other stimuli, such as pain, emotional shock, or the sight of blood: in these instances the reflex activation is central in origin.

The development of tilt testing has allowed the study of the pathophysiology of neurocardiogenic syncope. The patient is strapped to a tilt table and is tilted, head upright, usually at 70° for up to 45 min. Protocols that use additional provocation with isoprenaline or nitrates are commonly used. Blood pressure and cardiac rhythm are monitored throughout the tilt test. In neurocardiogenic syncope, the patient classically maintains normal blood pressure initially, until the sudden onset of syncope is associated with severe hypotension and bradycardia, often preceded by tachycardia. These features resolve with return to the supine posture. Some patients have a mainly vasodepressor response, with hypotension and little change in heart rate, while others have a marked cardioinhibitory response, with severe bradycardia or asystole of several seconds duration (Fig. 2.2.2). Most have a mixed response of hypotension and bradycardia.

Carotid sinus hypersensitivity

An abnormal sensitivity of a normal reflex is responsible for syncope. Activation of the carotid sinus baroreceptors (e.g. by physical pressure, such as carotid sinus massage) results in sympathetic withdrawal and parasympathetic activation. Bradycardia is usually a prominent feature.

Situational reflex-mediated syncope

In susceptible individuals, similar abnormal reflex sensitivity can result in syncope in response to afferent activity from other mechanoreceptor activation. Syncopal responses to cough, micturition, defecation, or swallowing have been reported.

Orthostatic hypotension

Hypotension may occur in patients in whom there are abnormalities in the autonomic control of cardiovascular function. Abnormalities of afferent or efferent pathways, or of peripheral vascular control, can result in low blood pressure in the upright posture, i.e. orthostatic hypotension. The clinical presentation can be divided into four subgroups:

- *Initial orthostatic hypotension*—symptoms occurring within 30 s of standing diagnosed with active standing blood pressure measurement (syncope is rare).
- *Classical orthostatic hypotension*—symptoms occur between 30 s and 3 min diagnosed with active standing blood pressure measurement. It is usually due to classical autonomic failure or drug therapy (syncope is rare).

increasingly recognized that many patients who attend clinics for epilepsy have been misdiagnosed and are suffering from recurrent syncope: some of these patients have potentially lethal ventricular arrhythmias for which they should be receiving treatment.

Neurally mediated syncope

There are many disorders of autonomic control that can cause syncope. The most common is neurocardiogenic syncope, or simple faint, which is due to an increased sensitivity of normal reflex responses. By contrast, autonomic dysfunction may produce abnormal neurovascular control that results in orthostatic hypotension.

Vasovagal syncope

Vasovagal syncope is the most common cause of syncope. It can affect all age groups and varies from infrequent episodes associated with obvious triggering factors to frequent unprovoked collapses, which may be debilitating. The pathophysiology most commonly involves venous pooling of blood and reduced venous return to the heart in response to upright posture. Reduced cardiac output and blood pressure stimulate arterial baroreceptors with resultant

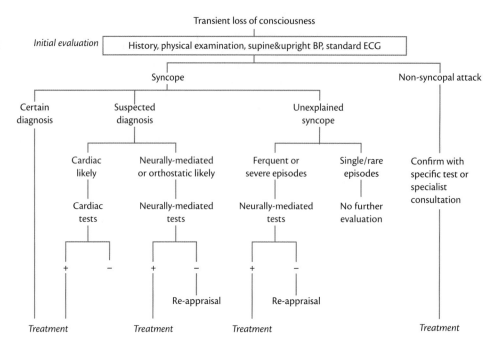

Fig. 2.2.1 A flow diagram showing the evaluation of loss of consciousness, proposed by the Task Force on Syncope of the European Society of Cardiology. The most useful cardiac tests are echocardiography, prolonged ECG monitoring, stress test, electrophysiological study and implantable loop recorder. Neurally mediated tests include tilt test, carotid sinus massage and implantable loop recorder. BP, blood pressure; ECG electrocardiogram.

Reproduced with permission from Brignole M, *et al.* (2004) Guidelines on management (diagnosis and treatment) of syncope—update 2004. *Europace*, **6**, 467–537.

- *Delayed*—symptoms occur between 3 and 45 min of standing and there is a more prolonged prodrome with a gradual fall in blood pressure resulting in syncope with or without a reflex (abrupt blood pressure fall) component, usually diagnosed with tilt table testing.

- *Reflex syncope*—typically occurring in young healthy females, onset between 3 and 45 min; blood pressure is usually maintained until syncope and diagnosed by tilt table testing.

Postural orthostatic tachycardia syndrome is not classically associated with syncope.

Orthostatic hypotension is more common in elderly patients, where it may be multifactorial, often exacerbated by drugs (Box 2.2.2). Nocturnal symptoms may occur, with a fall in blood pressure exacerbated by sudden rising from a warm bed.

Autonomic failure is an uncommon cause of syncope and patients may present with other features, including disturbances of bowel, bladder, or sexual function. Pure autonomic failure can be acute or chronic, primary (of unknown origin) or secondary to systemic disease. Multiple system atrophy is characterized by autonomic dysfunction, parkinsonism, and ataxia. Orthostatic hypotension may be a marked feature (the Shy–Drager syndrome), with additional parkinsonian features or cerebellar symptoms. Secondary autonomic failure can result from the central or peripheral involvement of certain diseases, including multiple sclerosis, cerebral tumour, diabetes, and amyloidosis.

Cardiac syncope

Loss of consciousness of cardiac origin may result from some substantial disturbance of cardiovascular function or from abnormalities of heart rhythm, with resultant reduced cerebral perfusion. The importance in establishing the diagnosis of cardiac syncope is the associated adverse prognosis, which may be improved with appropriate treatment. The probability of cardiac syncope is increased in the presence of structural cardiovascular disease identified from the history, clinical examination, or the ECG (Box 2.2.1).

Tachycardia

Syncope may be caused by tachycardia, most commonly ventricular, but supraventricular tachycardia can also be associated with loss of consciousness if it is very fast or in patients with structural heart disease. Syncope, rather than cardiac arrest, may result from self-terminating ventricular tachycardia or from sustained tachycardia with hypotension at the onset, but with a subsequent recovery of blood pressure. Whether or not a tachycardia causes syncope is related to its rate, underlying left ventricular function, and the patient's baroreceptor sensitivity.

Cardiac arrhythmia should be considered in all patients with structural heart disease presenting with syncope. Ventricular tachycardia most commonly occurs in patients with structural heart disease (e.g. prior myocardial infarction), but may also occur in patients with structurally normal hearts. For example, torsades de pointes in a patient with the long-QT syndrome is an important diagnosis to consider in young people with a history of loss of consciousness and possible epilepsy, in whom the episodes of collapse may be due to syncope caused by ventricular arrhythmia.

Bradycardia

A sudden decrease in heart rate, onset of ventricular standstill, or asystole may be a cause of syncope. When due to sinoatrial dysfunction (sick sinus syndrome) this is not associated with a poor prognosis, but syncope due to intermittent complete atrioventricular block is. Syncope in a patient with a permanent pacemaker may indicate pacemaker malfunction.

Table 2.2.1 Causes of syncope

Neurally mediated	Vasovagal or neurocardiogenic syncope
	Carotid sinus hypersensitivity
	Situational (micturition, defecation, cough, swallow)
Orthostatic hypotension	Primary autonomic failure
	Pure autonomic failure
	Multiple system atrophy (parkinsonian, cerebellar)
	Secondary autonomic failure (diabetic, amyloid neuropathy)
	Postural orthostatic tachycardia syndrome
	Drugs and alcohol
	Volume depletion (haemorrhage, diarrhoea)
Cardiac syncope	
Bradycardia	Atrioventricular block
	Sinoatrial disease
Tachycardia	Ventricular arrhythmia
	Structural heart disease
	Previous myocardial infarction
	Cardiomyopathy
	Structurally normal heart
	Long-QT or Brugada syndrome
	Supraventricular arrhythmia
Structural cardiovascular disease	Aortic stenosis
	Hypertrophic cardiomyopathy
	Atrial myxoma or thrombus
	Pulmonary embolism
Cerebrovascular or psychogenic	
Neurological	Migraine
	Subclavian steal
	Vertebrobasilar disease
Psychogenic	Anxiety, depression, and hyperventilation

Structural cardiovascular disease

Aortic stenosis may be associated with syncope, particularly during sudden exertion when the demand for increased cardiac output cannot be met because of the mechanical obstruction. Hypertrophic cardiomyopathy may also be associated with syncope, either because of outflow obstruction or ventricular arrhythmia. Obstruction of blood flow through the mitral valve by an atrial myxoma or thrombus is an uncommon cause of syncope. A number of other cardiac diseases may be associated with loss of consciousness by a variety of mechanisms (arrhythmia, reflex-mediated, or haemodynamic), including myocardial infarction, pulmonary embolism, congenital heart disease, or cardiac tamponade. Vascular diseases may also be involved, such as aortic dissection and extracranial vascular disease.

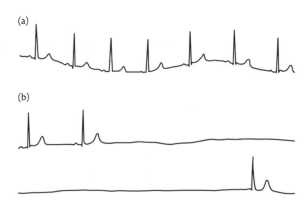

Fig. 2.2.2 Cardioinhibitory response to tilt testing. (a) After 6 min of head-up tilting at 70° the patient complained of presyncope. Heart rate was 60/min but blood pressure was 70 mmHg. (b) By 7 min the patient had lost consciousness, associated with an asystolic pause of 10 s duration and an unrecordable blood pressure. Recovery was rapid following the patient's return to the supine position.

Cerebrovascular or psychogenic causes of syncope

When epilepsy is excluded, neurological conditions are rare causes of loss of consciousness, but possible diagnoses include migraine, vertebrobasilar vascular disease, and subclavian steal syndrome. However, in most cases these will not result in true syncope.

A psychogenic origin of loss of consciousness implies the absence of neurally mediated, neurological, or cardiac abnormalities, and may occur in association with anxiety, depression, and conversion disorders. For instance, apparent syncope may occur during tilt testing but with normal pulse and blood pressure. Hyperventilation may be an associated mechanistic factor in psychogenic syncope.

Assessment of the patient with syncope

Careful assessment of the patient's history, a full physical examination and the 12-lead ECG will indicate a likely diagnosis in over 50% of patients with a history of syncope. Further investigations will be prompted by the initial evaluation (Fig. 2.2.1).

History

The importance of the clinical history in assessing a patient with syncope cannot be overemphasized. If possible, an eyewitness description of the patient during the syncopal event should be obtained. Features associated with increased risk of cardiac syncope should be sought (Box 2.2.1).

Provocative factors

Vasovagal syncope is classically associated with upright posture, often with aggravating circumstances such as prolonged standing, a hot environment, or hunger. However, episodes may also occur when seated, including while driving. Specific stimuli may be responsible for neurocardiogenic syncope in susceptible individuals. Ventricular arrhythmia, in particular torsades de pointes in the long-QT syndrome, may be provoked by sudden stimuli such as a noise, such as an alarm clock, or exercise, in particular swimming. Exertional syncope is a feature of aortic stenosis or hypertrophic cardiomyopathy. Syncope may also be triggered by coughing, micturition, and more rarely swallowing or laughing.

Preceding symptoms

Sweating and feeling hot or nauseated may precede vasovagal syncope. Cardiac arrhythmia may be associated with palpitation, chest pain, or breathlessness. Bradycardia, such as intermittent complete

Box 2.2.2 Common drugs that may cause postural hypotension

- Diuretics
- α-Adrenergic receptor blockers
- β-Adrenergic receptor blockers
- ACE inhibitors
- Angiotensin II receptor antagonists
- Calcium channel blockers
- Nitrates
- Opiates
- Ethanol
- Tricyclic antidepressants
- Bromocriptine
- Phenothiazines
- Levodopa

heart block, may produce no preceding symptoms and may cause loss of consciousness without warning. Sinoatrial dysfunction is a cause of symptoms of dizziness and light-headedness in addition to syncope. A psychogenic origin may be suggested by multiple associated symptoms including hyperventilation, paraesthesiae in fingers and lips, palpitation, and chest pain, which may precede syncope. Epilepsy may be preceded by a characteristic aura, which would strongly point away from cardiac syncope as the diagnosis.

The syncopal episode

In syncope the duration of loss of consciousness is usually short, with recovery after a few minutes. A longer duration of loss of consciousness suggests an alternative diagnosis. An exception to this is when the patient has remained upright during the attack, possibly aided by well-meaning but misguided helpers. Incontinence is a feature of epileptic seizure but may also occur (uncommonly) with syncope. Description of the patient during the episode is of great value. The classic description of an episode of syncope due to cardiac arrhythmia—in particular sudden-onset severe bradycardia—is of a sudden loss of colour, becoming deathly pale, with flushing on recovery (Stokes–Adams attack). Cyanosis may be a feature of an arrhythmic origin of syncope. Convulsive movements during the episode would raise the possibility of epilepsy, but they also occur with cardiac syncope. Although any cause of syncope can be associated with injury, its absence may point to a nonsyncopal or psychogenic origin.

The recovery period

By contrast to the postictal phase following epilepsy, there is commonly a rapid recovery of cerebral function following syncope. Vasovagal syncope may be followed by persisting nausea or vomiting and general malaise; in older people this phase may be prolonged.

Family history

There are a few specific causes of syncope in which a family history of syncope or sudden death may have prognostic significance. Long-QT syndrome is hereditary and may be associated with sudden death. A family history of syncope is of adverse prognostic significance in hypertrophic cardiomyopathy.

Investigation

The investigation of cardiac disease and arrhythmia are dealt with in the appropriate chapters, but the approach to the patient with syncope is described briefly here. Dependent on the history, further investigations may not be necessary with the exception of a 12-lead ECG. For example, the diagnosis of vasovagal syncope is a clinical one and other investigations are likely to have a low diagnostic yield. By contrast, if the history or examination points to a clear cause of syncope, investigations appropriate to the underlying cause should be performed.

Electrocardiogram

An ECG should be performed on all patients with syncope. This may provide evidence of aetiology of syncope, such as the long-QT syndrome, or of structural heart disease, such as prior myocardial infarction or left ventricular hypertrophy. An arrhythmia may be documented if it is sustained, and there may be evidence of sinoatrial disease or conduction system disease, such as 'trifasicular' block, bundle branch block, or first- or second-degree block. In those over the age of 40 carotid sinus massage (CSM) with digital pressure to the carotid artery for up to 5 s may cause marked bradycardia in carotid sinus hypersensitivity, with pauses of more than 3 s duration. Although it is recommended that CSM is avoided in patients with carotid bruits or a stroke or TIA within past 3 months, the incidence of adverse events is extremely rare.

Active standing

Measurement of lying and standing blood pressure is made using a sphygmomanometer (not an automated blood pressure cuff, as is commonly done) for a period of 3 min or until diagnostic criteria are reached. The test is diagnostic when there is a symptomatic fall in systolic blood pressure from baseline of 20 mmHg or more or diastolic blood pressure of 10 mmHg or more, or a decrease in systolic blood pressure to less than 90 mmHg. An asymptomatic fall, although suggestive, is not diagnostic when taken in context of the background incidence of postural hypotension which is up to 30% in the unselected elderly population and up to 60% in the hospitalized population.

Ambulatory monitoring

Documentation of cardiac rhythm during syncope is extremely useful, especially if it was associated with palpitations, but is difficult to obtain because of the intermittent and usually infrequent nature of the symptom. In patients admitted with high-risk syncope, in-hospital monitoring is recommended. Holter monitoring is usually only useful in individuals with recurrent syncope occurring more than once a week or in those where there are underlying ECG abnormalities (in particular conduction abnormalities which do not automatically meet the criteria for bradycardiac pacing). Real-time event recorders are of limited value in the investigation of syncope because they require a conscious patient to make the recording. Loop recorders, which have automatic rhythm detection algorithms and which can also be activated by the patient facilitating retrospective rhythm analysis, can be used for periods of 1 to 4 weeks and are useful for investigating syncope with an intermediate frequency. Implantable loop recorders have a greater diagnostic yield than conventional monitoring and can now be implanted in an outpatient setting. They are indicated in the evaluation and treatment of infrequent (>4-week interval), high risk, and recurrent syncope.

Tilt testing

When the history is suggestive of vasovagal syncope, the tilt test may be of value in confirming the diagnosis, but a negative test does not exclude the diagnosis. Adjuvant provocation (isoprenaline or nitrate) may increase the sensitivity, but the incidence of false positive tests with tilt testing has been reported as 5 to 20%. As such, its use is probably best limited to investigation of recurrent symptoms with an atypical history in patients in whom there are no features to suggest cardiac syncope.

Electrophysiological testing

Abnormal sinus node function or evidence of atrioventricular conduction disease may be elicited by electrophysiological testing, but demonstrating bradycardia during ambulatory monitoring more reliably makes both of these diagnoses. In patients with structural heart disease in whom arrhythmia is suspected, programmed electrical stimulation of the ventricles can induce sustained monomorphic ventricular tachycardia. This is a relatively specific response, shows that the patient is at risk of recurrent ventricular arrhythmia, and makes an arrhythmic origin of syncope likely. The diagnostic yield of electrophysiological testing is low in patients with a structurally normal heart.

Other investigations

Assessment for structural heart disease is important. Physical examination will detect most significant valve disease, but other diagnoses, such as hypertrophic cardiomyopathy or atrial myxoma, may produce little in the way of clinical signs. An echocardiogram is therefore worthwhile in cases where the diagnosis remains unclear. Exercise testing is useful in patients with a history of syncope during or immediately after exercise. Exercise testing is diagnostic if Mobitz II second-degree or third-degree atrioventricular block develop during exercise even without syncope.

Troponin measurement is not indicated in patients with syncope in the absence of features suggestive of an acute coronary syndrome. Approximately 10% of patients over the age of 60 presenting to the Emergency Department with syncope will have an elevated troponin, and although this is an independent risk factor for subsequent serious events, the finding rarely changes management appropriately or contributes to the final diagnosis.

A strong suspicion of diagnoses other than syncope should lead to other investigations, including electroencephalography and brain imaging, but these have a low diagnostic yield in patients with syncope and should not be routine.

Treatment

Neurocardiogenic syncope may require no treatment other than reassurance and avoidance of provocative factors. Management of vasovagal syncope, bradycardia, and cardiac arrhythmia are discussed in Chapter 4.1 of this book and Chapter 24.5.4 of the *Oxford Textbook of Medicine*. In up to one-third of patients the aetiology of syncope may not be found: these patients have a good outcome unless they have underlying heart disease.

Palpitation

The symptom of palpitation is defined as an awareness of one's heart beating. This may be due to an awareness of an abnormal heart rhythm but it may also be due to an abnormal awareness of normal rhythm. A careful and detailed history can provide a likely diagnosis. The most important aim in investigation is to correlate symptoms with cardiac rhythm.

History

A description of the symptom should include an estimate of heart rate, duration of symptom, regularity of rhythm, suddenness of onset and offset. It may be helpful to ask the patient to tap with their finger to describe their palpitation. Trigger factors, including exercise, and aggravating factors such as alcohol and caffeine should be detailed. The length of history may be of interest.

Sinus tachycardia

An awareness of a rapid heart rate of gradual onset and offset is often associated with feelings of alarm and panic in patients with anxiety.

Premature/ectopic beats

Symptomatic atrial and ventricular premature or ectopic beats commonly occur in normal individuals, and often generate considerable anxiety resulting in consultation.

In the absence of coronary disease, premature ventricular ectopic beats (PVCs) at a frequency of 1 per hour or more were recorded during Holter monitoring in the Framingham study in 33% of men and 32% of women. PVCs have also been recorded in 0.8% of a healthy military population during a standard 12-lead ECG. These are important factors to remember when discussing their significance with the patient. The patient may describe 'missed beats' or forceful beats. These symptoms relate to the pause that follows a premature beat. The premature beat produces a short diastolic filling interval and the low ventricular volume results in reduced ventricular contraction with a small stroke volume. However, the subsequent pause provides a long diastolic filling period and the resultant stretching of the ventricular walls is associated with an increased and forceful systolic contraction. The combination of the diminished premature beat and the enhanced postextrasystolic beat is responsible for the symptoms. Benign ectopy is indicated by the absence of a history of other cardiovascular symptoms or family history of sudden death, their occurrence at rest and resolution with exercise, and a normal clinical cardiovascular examination and resting ECG. Multifocal ventricular ectopy, and PVCs at a frequency of more than 20 000 in 24 h, are more indicative of potentially significant cardiac pathology and require further investigation.

Atrial fibrillation

This common arrhythmia may produce a variety of symptoms depending on ventricular rate, irregularity, and persistence. Paroxysmal atrial fibrillation is characterized by self-terminating episodes of atrial fibrillation, when there may be a rapid and irregular ventricular response. The patient is aware of an increased heart rate and often describes the irregular nature of the symptom. The variations in diastolic interval produce symptoms by similar mechanisms to that described above for premature beats, with 'missed' and 'forceful' beats. Patients with sinoatrial dysfunction may be most symptomatic on termination of the atrial fibrillation, which can be followed by sinus bradycardia or prolonged sinus pauses. Atrial fibrillation may be persistent or permanent, and the severity of symptoms will be related to the ventricular rate and irregularity.

Paroxysmal supraventricular tachycardia

A history of sudden-onset, rapid, regular palpitation in a healthy patient with no underlying structural heart disease is suggestive of paroxysmal supraventricular tachycardia. It may stop spontaneously or with vagotonic manoeuvres, or the patient may have had to attend hospital for intravenous therapy. In addition to palpitation, patients commonly report fatigue, malaise, light-headedness, or dyspnoea, but because they have normal hearts such episodes of tachycardia are usually well tolerated. Polyuria is a common associated symptom, which results from the release of atrial natriuretic peptide secondary to atrial stretch.

Ventricular tachycardia

Ventricular arrhythmias can present with the symptom of palpitation, but more severe symptoms such as syncope or cardiac arrest also occur. Characteristically the symptom of palpitation would be the sudden onset and offset of a rapid regular heart rhythm. A history of structural heart disease should be sought.

Investigation

Electrocardiogram

The first aim is to document cardiac rhythm during symptoms. This may be possible with a standard ECG if the arrhythmia is sustained or persistent. Atrial or ventricular premature beats, or evidence of structural heart disease, e.g. myocardial infarction, may be documented. The presence of pre-excitation indicates the diagnosis of Wolff–Parkinson–White syndrome and suggests symptoms due to episodes of atrioventricular re-entry tachycardia. Other ECG signs indicative of primary electrical heart disease are: a corrected QT interval greater than 460 ms or less than 320 ms (long or short QT syndrome); right bundle branch block with 'coved' ST elevation (Brugada syndrome); epsilon waves and/or T wave inversion with QRS duration greater than 100 ms in the right precordial ECG leads (arrhythmogenic right ventricular cardiomyopathy); and high voltages in the precordial leads with Q wave formation and ST changes (hypertrophic cardiomyopathy).

Ambulatory monitoring

The success of ambulatory monitoring in documenting the rhythm during symptoms will be dependent on the frequency of symptoms. If they occur daily then a 24 or 48 h Holter recording should suffice. However, palpitation is often infrequent and other patient-activated devices can be of more value. These include hand-held, patient-activated event recorders that allow the telephonic transmission of recordings. These devices do not allow retrospective recording and require symptoms of sufficient duration to allow their use. Shorter episodes may be captured using loop recorders. Implantable loop recorders may be helpful where symptoms are infrequent and may also be effective in monitoring therapy once implanted for diagnostic purposes.

Other investigations

Thyroid function and a full blood count are of particular importance in patients with atrial arrhythmias or sinus tachycardia respectively. Electrolytes are routinely analysed. In patients with paroxysmal symptoms, a history of hypertension, sweating, and anxiety during attacks, urinary metanephrines for the investigation of phaeochromocytoma are indicated. Echocardiography is performed in most patients with palpitations and documented arrhythmias: in patients with ventricular ectopy, however, it is usually indicated only in those with suspected structural heart disease or those at a high risk of development of serious ventricular arrhythmias or sudden cardiac death.

Electrophysiological studies

Invasive studies are of most value in determining the mechanism of a previously documented tachyarrhythmia, particularly with a view to treatments such as radiofrequency catheter ablation.

Management

Documentation of the cardiac rhythm during palpitation allows appropriate management, with reassurance as the only treatment in those with sinus tachycardia or premature beats. The treatment of other cardiac arrhythmias is discussed in Chapter 4.1.

Lifestyle advice

Advice regarding lifestyle with palpitations revolves around reassurance where it is felt to be benign, and avoiding precipitants where these can be identified. Although caffeine, other stimulants, alcohol, and stress are often quoted as potential triggers (and this may be true of ectopy, for example), it is much more common for many arrhythmias to occur without any avoidable trigger. Exercise as a trigger for palpitations is unusual and may signify adrenaline-dependent arrhythmias such as some forms of ventricular tachycardia (see Chapter 4.1). Syncope has a number of effects on lifestyle. Simple lifestyle measures may be employed to improve symptoms in specific situations: for example, increased fluid and salt intake. Where there is warning before syncope occurs this may be used to prevent injury or complete syncope by adopting a position lying down or with feet elevated. It is crucial for those who suffer syncope to avoid situations that might put them at harm, such as swimming alone or bathing (showering is preferred). Driving restrictions may apply for both palpitations and syncope. In the United Kingdom clear guidance is provided by the Driver and Vehicle Licensing Agency (DVLA) as to who can and cannot drive with these symptoms, investigations that are required, and the duration of driving bans for both a normal driving licence and heavy goods/passenger vehicle licences.

Further reading

Benditt DG, Sutton R (2005). Tilt-table testing in the evaluation of syncope. *J Cardiovasc Electrophysiol*, **16**, 356–8.

Brignole M. (2007). Diagnosis and treatment of syncope. *Heart*, **93**, 130–6.

Brignole M, *et al.* (2004). Guidelines on management (diagnosis and treatment) of syncope—update 2004. *Europace*, **6**, 467–537.

Grubb BP (2005). Neurocardiogenic syncope and related disorders of orthostatic intolerance. *Circulation*, **111**, 2997–3006.

Moya A, *et al.* (2009). Guidelines for the diagnosis and management of syncope (version 2009): the Task Force for the Diagnosis and Management of Syncope of the European Society of Cardiology (ESC). *Eur Heart J*, **30**, 2631–71.

NICE (2010). *Transient loss of consciousness*. Clinical Guideline 109.

Raviele A, *et al.* (2011). Management of palpitations: a position paper from the European Heart Rhythm Association. *Europace*, **13**, 920–34.

Strickberger SA, *et al.* (2006). AHA/ACCF Scientific Statement on the evaluation of syncope: from the American Heart Association Councils on Clinical Cardiology, Cardiovascular Nursing, Cardiovascular Disease in the Young, and Stroke, and the Quality of Care and Outcomes Research Interdisciplinary Working Group; and the American College of Cardiology Foundation: in collaboration with the Heart Rhythm Society: endorsed by the American Autonomic Society. *Circulation*, **113**, 316–27.

SECTION 3

Clinical investigation of cardiac disorders

CHAPTER 3.1

Electrocardiography

Andrew R. Houghton and David Gray

Essentials

The resting 12-lead ECG

The ECG has been recognized as a valuable diagnostic tool since the end of the 19th century. The normal ECG waveform consists of P, QRS, and T waves (and sometimes U waves)—P waves result from atrial depolarization, QRS complexes from ventricular depolarization, and T waves from ventricular repolarization. The standard 12-lead ECG utilizes 4 limb electrodes and 6 precordial electrodes to generate 12 leads or 'views' of the heart's electrical activity. There are six limb leads (termed I, II, III, aVR, aVL, and aVF) and six precordial leads (termed V1, V2, V3, V4, V5, and V6). Supplementary 'views' can be obtained by using additional leads, such as V7, V8, and V9 to assess the posterior aspect of the heart and right-sided chest leads to look for a right ventricular myocardial infarction.

Assessment of the 12-lead ECG—this should be done in a methodical manner, working through each aspect in turn. Conventionally, the heart rate, rhythm and axis are assessed before inspection of each component of the waveform—the P wave, PR interval, QRS complex, ST segment, T wave, QT interval, and U wave, with each component having its own range of normal attributes.

Myocardial hypertrophy—the ECG can be a specific but generally insensitive tool for detecting myocardial hypertrophy: (1) left ventricular hypertrophy can be assessed using a number of diagnostic criteria, including the Cornell criteria and the Romhilt–Estes scoring system; (2) right ventricular hypertrophy is indicated by a dominant R wave in lead V1 with right axis deviation; (3) left atrial hypertrophy is indicated by broad, bifid P waves; and (4) right atrial hypertrophy by tall P waves.

Conduction blocks—(1) left anterior hemiblock results from a block of conduction in the anterosuperior fascicle and is a cause of left axis deviation; (2) left posterior hemiblock results from a block of conduction in the posteroinferior fascicle and is a cause of right axis deviation; (3) left and right bundle branch blocks both cause broadening of the QRS complexes by prolonging ventricular depolarization, and both exhibit characteristic diagnostic features.

Ventricular pre-excitation—causes shortening of the PR interval and can result from Wolff–Parkinson–White-type pre-excitation, short PR-type pre-excitation, or Mahaim-type pre-excitation (for discussion of the 12-lead ECG in arrhythmia, see Chapter 4.1).

Acute coronary syndromes

The ECG is the most useful bedside triage tool in acute coronary syndromes, with utility in diagnosis, in location of the site of ischaemia/infarction, and as a prognostic indicator.

ST elevation myocardial infarction (STEMI)—the first indication of infarction on the ECG is usually ST segment elevation, which occurs within a few hours. The J point (the origin of the ST segment at its junction with the QRS complex) is elevated by 1 mm or more in two or more limb leads, or by 2 mm in two or more precordial leads. The ST segment returns to the baseline over the next 48 to 72 h, during which Q waves and symmetrically inverted T waves appear. Some patients develop left bundle branch block, either transiently or permanently. The ECG of a completed infarct shows new Q waves greater than 2 mm, R waves reduced in size or absent, and inverted T waves.

Non-ST-elevation myocardial infarction (NSTEMI)—ECG changes are more variable than in STEMI. The ECG may be normal on first presentation and remain unchanged throughout the acute admission; there may be transient ST segment depression indicative of myocardial ischaemia; in 20 to 30% the only change will be T wave inversion.

Difficulties in interpretation of the ECG in acute coronary syndromes—the ECG diagnosis of acute myocardial infarction can pose challenges in the setting of right ventricular infarction, atrial infarction, coronary artery spasm, reciprocal changes, 'stuttering' infarction, noninfarct ST-segment elevation, late presentation, left bundle branch block, prior infarction, pre-excitation, and T wave inversion.

Clinical decision-making—incorrect interpretation of an ECG can lead to inappropriate patient triage, either missing the opportunity to provide appropriate reperfusion therapy, or leading to inappropriate treatment with attendant risk. Up to 12% of those with a high-risk ECG are missed on admission to the Emergency Department, yet pressure to provide treatment promptly to fulfil audit 'targets', e.g. door-to-balloon time for primary percutaneous coronary intervention (PCI), should not replace accuracy in diagnosis. It is sometimes better to repeat the ECG than to make an incorrect diagnosis. It is easy to place too much reliance on minor changes on the ECG; it is gross changes of ST elevation or depression within the parameters above that should determine treatment.

Exercise ECG testing

Exercise ECG testing is better as an indicator of prognosis than as a diagnostic tool. The sensitivity of exercise ECG testing, the proportion with coronary disease correctly identified by the test, is 68% (range 23–100) and specificity, the proportion free of disease correctly identified by the test, is 77% (range 17–100). In multivessel disease, these figures are 81% (range 40–100) and 66% (range 17–100), respectively. This means that exercise testing frequently yields both false-positive results—incorrectly diagnosing disease when coronary arteries are normal or minimally diseased—and false-negative results—missing coronary disease when a flow-limiting, even critical left main stem, coronary stenosis is present.

Appearance of symptoms or ECG changes early in an exercise test is generally associated with more severe and extensive coronary disease and a poor prognosis. Changes within the first 3 min usually indicate severe coronary disease affecting the left main stem or the proximal segments of at least one major coronary artery. Multivessel coronary disease is more likely with ST segment down-sloping, delayed ST normalization after exercise, increased number of leads affected, and lower workload at which ECG changes appear.

The resting 12-lead ECG

History

The first electrocardiogram (ECG), of an exposed frog's heart, was performed by Marey in 1876 using the mercury capillary electrometer that had recently been invented by Gabriel Lippmann. Two years later the British physiologists John Burdon Sanderson and Fredrick Page demonstrated that recordings of the frog heart's electrical activity consisted of two phases (which were subsequently to become known as the QRS complex and T wave). The first human ECG was published in 1887 by Augustus D Waller, who had worked under Sanderson in the Department of Physiology at the University College of London. While working at St Mary's Hospital, London, Waller used a capillary electrometer to record the ECG of a laboratory technician, Thomas Goswell.

Electrocardiography was developed further by the Dutch physiologist Willem Einthoven, who witnessed a demonstration by Waller at the First International Congress of Physiology in Basle, Switzerland, in 1889. Although Einthoven made considerable improvements to the technique of recording ECGs with the capillary electrometer, it was only with his invention of the string galvanometer at the turn of the century that high-quality ECG recording became possible. Within a decade of Einthoven's publication of the first string galvanometer ECG recordings in 1902, a commercial ECG machine became available. Manufactured by the Cambridge Scientific Instrument Company, the first machine was delivered to Sir Thomas Lewis, who would play a major role in developing the clinical application of electrocardiography. Einthoven's invention led to him being awarded the Nobel Prize in 1924.

Einthoven was also the first to use the PQRST notation to describe the ECG waveforms. In the early ECG recordings, the waveforms were named ABCD (four deflections were recognized).

Mathematical correction, using differential equations, was used to correct and improve ECG recordings, and it was traditional that mathematical notation used letters from the latter half of the alphabet. The letters N and O were already used elsewhere, so it was decided to begin the notation at P.

Over the following years further refinements were undertaken, most notably in the 1930s when the use of the chest leads was first described. At around the same time Frank Wilson invented the 'indifferent electrode' (also known as the 'Wilson central terminal'). This led to the development of the 'unipolar' limb leads VR, VL, and VF ('V' stands for 'voltage'). In 1942 the American cardiologist Emanual Goldberger increased the voltage of these leads by 50%, leading to the term 'augmented' leads (aVR, aVL, and aVF), and the 12-lead ECG which remains familiar today finally took shape.

Although the format of the 12-lead ECG has remained essentially unchanged since that time, there have nevertheless been other significant developments in electrocardiography over more recent years. Ambulatory ECG recorders and implantable cardiac monitors have gained a central role in the investigation of patients with suspected arrhythmias, and the use of intracardiac ECG recording has enable the rapid development and widespread use of electrophysiological studies.

Normal ECG appearances

The ECG waveform

The three fundamental deflections on the normal ECG are termed the P wave, the QRS complex, and the T wave (Fig. 3.1.1). The origins of each deflection are as follows.

P wave

The P wave results from depolarization of the atrial myocardium. Depolarization of the sinoatrial node itself, which triggers normal atrial depolarization, cannot be seen on the surface ECG (although it can be identified in intracardiac recordings). However, the presence of a P wave with normal morphology and orientation is generally taken to infer normal sinoatrial node depolarization.

Repolarization of the atrial myocardium is represented on the ECG by the Ta wave (the atrial equivalent of the ventricular T wave). The Ta wave is seen as a small asymmetrical deflection after the P wave, with an opposite polarity to the preceding P wave. The Ta wave is often hidden within the QRS complex and is therefore not easily seen—in fact, it is unusual to be able to appreciate the Ta wave at all. However, it can extend right through to the following ST segment, where it can be mistaken for the ST-segment depression of myocardial ischaemia (particularly because the Ta wave is most likely to be seen extending into the ST-segment during

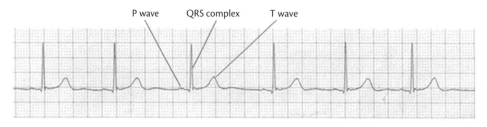

Fig. 3.1.1 Basic ECG waveform.

exercise-induced sinus tachycardia). There is one case report of a positive Ta wave (after an inverted P wave) giving the erroneous impression of an acute ST segment elevation myocardial infarction.

QRS complex

The QRS complex represents depolarization of the ventricular myocardium. Of all the deflections, the QRS complex can exhibit the greatest variability in appearance. As a result, the individual components of the QRS complex can be labelled in upper case (Q, R, or S) or lower case (q, r, or s) to represent the relative size of the component. For example, QRS complexes with a small Q wave deflection can be termed qRS complexes, and those QRS complexes with no Q wave component and a small R wave component can be termed rS complexes.

T wave

The T wave (together with the preceding ST segment) represents repolarization of the ventricular myocardium.

The 12 conventional ECG leads

Lead nomenclature

It is important to emphasize that the term 'lead' does not refer to the electrode connecting the ECG machine to the patient. For a standard 12-lead ECG recording, 10 electrodes are used to generate the 12 conventional ECG leads. The 12 leads can be categorized as limb (or frontal plane) leads (I, II, III, aVR, aVL, aVF) and chest (or precordial) leads (V1, V2, V3, V4, V5, V6). The 12 leads can also be categorized as bipolar (I, II, III) or unipolar (aVR, aVL, aVF, V1, V2, V3, V4, V5, V6). The leads aVR, aVL, and aVF can be further described as 'augmented' leads, as they are modified versions of the original VR, VL, and VF leads, having a voltage amplification of 50%.

The bipolar leads are generated by measuring the potential (voltage) between two electrodes. One electrode acts as a positive terminal and the other as a negative terminal. For instance, lead I measures the potential between the left arm electrode (positive) and right arm electrode (negative). Lead I is obtained by subtracting the right arm vector from the left arm vector. Similarly, lead II measures the potential between the left leg electrode and the right arm electrode, and lead III measures the potential between the left leg electrode and the left arm electrode.

The augmented unipolar leads measure the voltage between a single positive electrode and a 'central' point of reference generated from the other limb electrodes. Thus aVR uses the right arm electrode as the positive terminal, aVL uses the left arm electrode, and aVF uses the left leg electrode. The three bipolar leads and the three augmented unipolar leads together comprise the six limb leads that view the heart in the frontal plane.

The unipolar chest leads measure the voltage between six electrodes placed across the surface of the chest and a central point of reference, providing a view of the heart that is perpendicular to the frontal plane leads. For all 12 ECG leads, it is conventional that a wave of depolarization moving towards a lead generates a positive (upward) deflection on the ECG recording and vice versa.

The six limb leads (frontal plane leads)

Because the limbs act as linear conductors, it does not matter whereabouts the limb electrodes are attached on each limb. The six limb leads provide general spatial information (being less localized

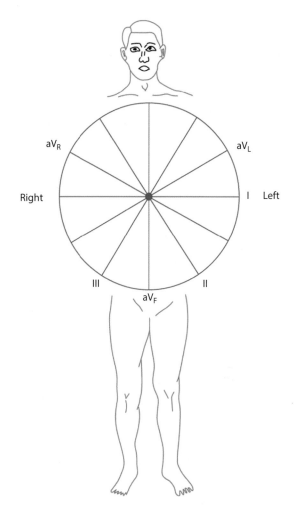

Fig. 3.1.2 The six limb leads and their 'view' of the heart. Note that leads II, III, and aVF are inferior to the heart, I and aVL are anterolateral to the heart, and aVR looks into the cavity of the heart.

than the six chest leads). Figure 3.1.2 shows the orientation of the six limb leads in relation to the heart. In simple terms one can visualize lead aVR as 'looking' at the heart from the right shoulder, lead aVL from the left shoulder and lead aVF from the feet. Lead I 'looks' at the heart from the left horizontal position. Similarly, the 'views' of leads II and III are shown in Fig. 3.1.2.

The six chest leads (precordial leads)

For the chest (precordial) leads, each of the six electrodes is attached to a particular site on the chest wall. The chest electrodes act as positive terminals, and the indifferent terminal is formed from a combination of leads R, L and F. The location of each electrode is important, in contrast to the limb leads. The surface positions of the chest electrodes is shown in Fig. 3.1.3, and the relation between the chest leads and the heart in Fig. 3.1.4. The electrodes are placed as follows:

- The V_1 electrode is placed at the right sternal edge in the fourth intercostal space

- The V_2 electrode is placed at the left sternal edge in the fourth intercostal space

- The V_3 electrode is placed midway between the V_2 and V_4 electrodes

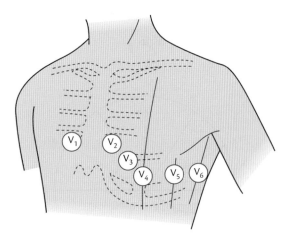

Fig. 3.1.3 Surface positions of the chest electrodes.

- The V_4 electrode is placed at the left midclavicular line in the fifth intercostal space

- The V_5 electrode is placed at the left anterior axillary line in a horizontal line with V_4

- The V_6 electrode is placed at the left midaxillary line in a horizontal line with V_4 and V_5

Reading a normal 12-lead ECG

Figure 3.1.5 shows a normal 12-lead ECG. As is conventional, this shows the leads arranged in four columns, each column containing three leads. In addition, a rhythm strip runs along the bottom of the ECG across its whole width. This is conventionally lead II, but any one of the 12 leads can be used for the rhythm strip as required. The ECG is recorded at a paper speed of 25 mm/s, and at a sensitivity of 10 mm/mV. The speed and sensitivity settings can also be adjusted on most ECG machines, if required, and so it is important that the actual recording speed and sensitivity are always noted on the ECG for future reference.

In the following paragraphs we will describe the appearances of the normal ECG, looking at each wave, interval and segment in turn. We will assume that the patient is in normal sinus rhythm, and that a standard paper speed (25 mm/s) and calibration (10 mm/

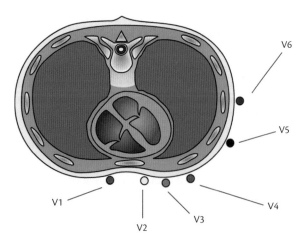

Fig. 3.1.4 The chest leads and their anatomical relationship to the heart.
Return to the top

mV) have been used—this should always be checked before reading any ECG.

Identification details

Before reading the ECG, check the patient's details (the patient's name and at least one other form of identification, such as date of birth or identification number, should be recorded on the ECG) and the date and time on which the ECG was recorded. It is good practice to note on the ECG any relevant clinical features. For instance, a note that the patient was experiencing chest pain or palpitations at the time the ECG was recorded can prove invaluable later on. Indeed, ECG interpretation should always take into account the appropriate clinical context. For instance, the ECG shown in Fig. 3.1.5 can be interpreted as showing normal sinus rhythm in a patient who is well. However, in a patient who is unconscious and pulseless, the same ECG would be interpreted as showing pulseless electrical activity, a cardiac arrest rhythm. Before interpreting any ECG it is therefore appropriate (and important) to ask, 'How is the patient?'

Rate

A normal heart rate is between 60 and 100 beats/min. A rate below 60 beats/min is termed bradycardia; a rate greater than 100 beats/min is termed tachycardia. Heart rate normally applies to the ventricular rate, as shown on the ECG by the rate of QRS complexes. However, the atria have their own rate, as shown by the P wave rate. The atrial and ventricular rates are usually the same, and there is a 1:1 ratio between P waves and QRS complexes. However, the rates can differ; for instance, in complete heart block (Figure 3.1.6), the atrial rate is usually greater than the ventricular rate, and both rates should therefore be quoted.

Ventricular rate can be calculated in two different ways. One method necessitates counting the number of large (5 mm) squares between two adjacent QRS complexes. This figure is then divided into 300 to give the ventricular rate per minute. For instance, if there are 5 large squares between QRS complexes, the ventricular rate is 300/5 = 60 beats/min. The same method can be used to calculate atrial rate, counting the large squares between two consecutive P waves.

If the heart rhythm is irregular, the square-counting method is not so useful. An alternative method is to count the number of QRS complexes in a certain time period, and then multiply the number up to obtain a rate per minute. Traditionally one counts the number of QRS complexes in a period of 30 large squares, which equates to 6 s of recording (a paper speed of 25 mm/s covers 5 large squares per second, or 300 large squares per minute). One then multiplies the result by 10 to obtain the rate per minute. Thus if there are 8 QRS complexes within 30 large squares, then the ventricular rate is 8 × 10 = 80 beats/min. Once again, the same method can be used to calculate atrial rate.

Rhythm

A detailed description of arrhythmias can be found in Chapter 4.1. In general terms, the assessment of rhythm on the ECG requires careful attention to the following:

- Whether there is ventricular activity (QRS complexes) and what is the ventricular rate

- Whether there is atrial activity (P waves) and what is the atrial rate

- Whether the heart rhythm is regular or irregular

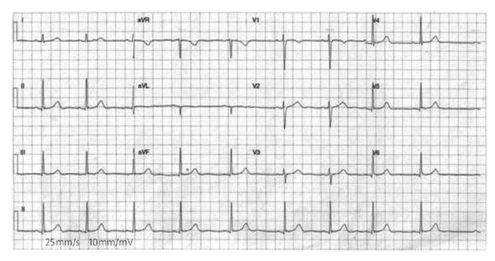

Fig. 3.1.5 A normal 12-lead ECG.

• Whether the QRS complexes are normal or broad (broad complexes indicating either a ventricular origin to the rhythm or aberrant conduction of a supraventricular rhythm)

• Whether there is a relationship between P waves and QRS complexes.

Assessing the ECG along these lines will provide a basis upon which to describe the rhythm and begin to identify the nature of the arrhythmia.

Axis

The concept of axis is often regarded as one of the hardest principles to grasp when learning ECG interpretation. The concept is, nonetheless, straightforward: axis refers to the overall direction in which the wave of depolarization travels. There is a QRS (ventricular) axis, which is what most people refer to when discussing cardiac axis, but the P wave has its own axis too, representing the overall direction of depolarization in the atria. The T wave also has an axis, in this case referring to the overall direction of the wave of repolarization. In this section the discussion is confined to the QRS (ventricular) axis, but the same principles apply to P wave and T wave axes too.

As the ventricles depolarize, the wave of depolarization travels through the atrioventricular node, into the bundle of His, and then to the ventricular myocardium via the Purkinje fibres. The overall direction of this depolarization wavefront is usually towards the apex of the heart. If, by convention, we regard the 'view' that lead I has of the heart (a horizontal line to the left of the heart) as 0°, and any angle clockwise from that line is positive (and any angle anticlockwise from that line is negative), then the normal ventricular depolarization wavefront travels through the ventricles at an angle of approximately +60° (Fig. 3.1.7).

As Fig. 3.1.7 illustrates, the six limb leads 'view' the heart from different angles. Lead I is taken as the horizontal reference point, 0°.

Moving in a clockwise (positive) direction, lead II views the heart from an angle of +60°, lead aVF from an angle of +90°, and lead III from an angle of +120°. Moving anticlockwise from lead I, lead aVL views the heart from an angle of −30°, and lead aVR from an angle of −150°. This system of looking at axis, using the six limb leads, is known as the hexaxial reference system.

The shaded area in Fig. 3.1.7 shows the normal range for the QRS axis, which lies between −30° and +90°. This does vary with body morphology—tall, slim individuals tend to have axes towards the rightward (+90°) end of the normal range; short, overweight individuals have axes towards the leftward (−30°) end of the normal range. An axis more negative (anticlockwise) than −30° is abnormal and termed left axis deviation. Similarly, an axis more positive (clockwise) than +90° is abnormal and termed right axis deviation. Left axis deviation is seen in left anterior hemiblock (see below), inferior myocardial infarction and also in ostium primum atrial septal defect. Right axis deviation is seen in left posterior hemiblock, right ventricular hypertrophy, lateral myocardial infarction, ostium secundum atrial septal defect, and Wolff–Parkinson–White (WPW) syndrome.

There are a number of ways to calculate the QRS axis. One method is to look for which of the six limb leads has a QRS complex in which the R wave and S wave are closest to being equal (i.e. in which the positive and negative deflections cancel each other out). The QRS axis will be at right angles to this 'equipolar' lead, but could be pointing in either direction. For instance, if the equipolar lead is lead III (which looks at the heart from +120°), then the QRS axis will be at right angles to this, namely either +30° or −150° (refer back to Fig. 3.1.7). Next, find which lead is at right angles to the equipolar lead—in this example, the answer would be lead aVR. Now, if the QRS axis is −150°, then you would expect a positive QRS complex in lead aVR (because the wave of depolarization would be travelling directly towards it). If, however, the QRS

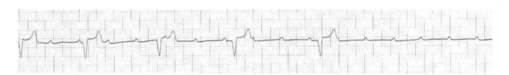

Figure 3.1.6 Complete heart block: complete dissociation of atrial (P waves) and ventricular (QRS complexes) rate.

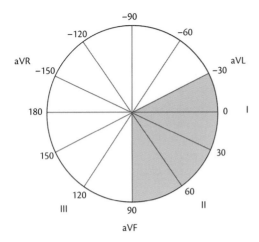

Fig. 3.1.7 The standard convention for describing the orientation of cardiac axis, and the corresponding 'views' of each of the six limb leads. The shaded area represents the normal range for the QRS axis.

complex in lead aVR is negative, the depolarization must be moving away from it and the QRS axis must be therefore be +30°. This method works whichever limb lead is equipolar, as every limb lead has another lead at right angles to it.

An alternative and quick method of checking whether the QRS axis is within the normal range is simply to look at leads I and II. If the QRS complex in lead I is positive (or at least equipolar), then the QRS axis must lie somewhere in the range of –90° to +90°. Similarly, if the QRS complex in lead II is positive, then the QRS axis must lie somewhere in the range -30° to +150°. Therefore we can say that if the QRS complexes in leads I and II are both positive then the QRS axis must lie somewhere in the range –30° to +90°. Thus a positive QRS complex in leads I and II means the QRS axis is within the normal range; a positive QRS complex in lead I and a negative QRS complex in lead II indicate left axis deviation; a negative QRS complex in lead I and a positive QRS complex in lead II indicate right axis deviation.

More precise calculations of the QRS axis can be made by measuring the individual R and S waves in each of the limb leads and using vector analysis to plot out the overall direction of depolarization, but this degree of precision is usually unnecessary.

P wave

The P wave represents atrial depolarization. P waves are usually upright except in leads aVR and V1 (and sometimes V2), where they can be inverted (or biphasic). P waves are seen most clearly in lead II and this is usually the lead of choice for the rhythm strip so that atrial activity can be assessed clearly.

P waves can be inverted in other leads, indicating that atrial depolarization has been initiated somewhere other than the sinoatrial node. For instance, an ectopic focus of depolarization near the

atrioventricular node will give rise to inverted P waves in the inferior leads (II, III, and aVF) as the wave of atrial depolarization will spread upwards rather than downwards.

P waves are normally no broader than three small squares (0.12 s) and no taller than 2.5 mm. The features of atrial hypertrophy are discussed later.

PR interval

The PR interval is measured from the beginning of the P wave to the beginning of the QRS complex. A normal PR interval is between 0.12 s and 0.20 s in adults.

A long fixed PR interval is termed first-degree atrioventricular block and results from a delay in conduction between the atria and ventricles (Fig. 3.1.8). In second-degree atrioventricular block the PR interval may gradually increase with each beat before a P wave is not conducted (Mobitz type I or Wenckebach phenomenon), or may be fixed and long (or normal) with intermittent nonconduction of P waves (Mobitz type II). In third-degree atrioventricular block and also in atrioventricular dissociation the PR interval will vary because of the absence of any association between atrial and ventricular activity. See Chapter 4.1 for further discussion.

A short PR interval is seen in ventricular pre-excitation (see below) or when the focus of atrial depolarization arises not from the sinoatrial node but from the vicinity of the atrioventricular node.

QRS complex

The QRS complex represents ventricular depolarization. The first negative deflection of the complex is termed the Q wave and the first positive deflection the R wave (whether or not it follows a Q wave). A negative deflection after an R wave is termed an S wave. If the deflections are small, lower-case letters (q, r, and s) are used. Thus it is possible to have QRS complexes, qRS complexes, rS complexes, and so on.

Normal 'physiological' q waves are usually narrow (no more than 0.04 s in duration) and small (less than 25% the amplitude of the following R wave) and result from the left to right depolarization of the interventricular septum ('septal q waves'). Larger Q waves may be pathological, although can be normal in leads III and aVR, and may also been seen in lead aVL if the QRS axis is greater than +60°.

The normal QRS complex duration is less than 0.12 s. The amplitude of the QRS complex varies normally from lead to lead and, in the precordial leads, normally increases progressively from lead V1 to V6. At least one R wave in the precordial leads must be at least 8 mm in height, and the tallest R wave should be no more than 27 mm (and the deepest S wave no more than 30 mm), and the sum of the tallest R wave and the deepest S wave should be no more than 40 mm. In the limb leads, the R wave height should be no more than 13 mm in lead aVL and 20 mm in lead aVF.

ST segment

The ST segment should be horizontal and should not normally deviate by more than 1 mm above or below the isoelectric line

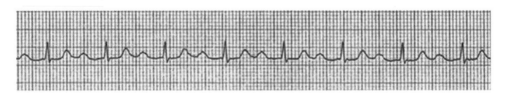

Fig. 3.1.8 First-degree atrioventricular block (long PR interval).

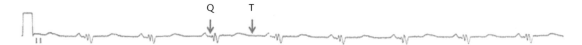

Fig. 3.1.9 A prolonged QT interval. Measurement can be difficult since the precise beginning and end of the interval may not be easy to determine, particularly if the end of the T wave is obscured by a superimposed U wave or the following P wave.

(which is the line between end of the T wave and the start of the subsequent P wave).

T wave

T waves in the limb leads are normally concordant—if the QRS complex is positive, the subsequent T wave is upright, and vice versa. The T wave is normally inverted in lead aVR and upright in leads I and II.

With regard to the precordial leads, normal T waves are always upright in leads V4 to V6. A flat or inverted T wave is found in lead V1 in 20% of adults, and in lead V2 in 5% of adults (in which case, the T wave should be inverted in lead V1 as well). An inverted T wave in lead V3 can, rarely, be found in normal young adults. T waves should not change their orientation—an inverted T wave is not normal if previous ECGs show that it was previously upright.

There are no strict criteria for normal T wave size, so 'tall' and 'small' T waves are not well defined and deciding on their presence tends to be a subjective judgement. 'Tall' T waves can occur in early acute myocardial infarction ('hyperacute' T waves) and in hyperkalaemia ('tented' T waves). Small T waves can be seen in hypokalaemia.

QT interval

The QT interval is measured between the start of the QRS complex and the end of the T wave. The normal range for the QT interval varies according to heart rate. It is therefore convenient to correct the measured QT interval to what it would be if the heart rate were 60 beats/min. This is done most commonly using Bazett's formula, in which the measured QT interval (in seconds) is divided by the square root of the RR interval (in seconds), to give the corrected QT interval (QTc). The normal range for the QT interval at a heart rate of 60 beats/min, and thus for the QTc, is between 0.35 s and 0.45 s (men) or 0.46 s (women) (Figure 3.1.9).

U wave

The T wave is occasionally followed by a U wave, most clearly seen in the right precordial leads, which has the same orientation as the T wave and is usually no more than one-third of its size. The physiological origin of the U wave is still debated, but is often said to relate to afterdepolarizations in the ventricles.

Myocardial hypertrophy

Left ventricular hypertrophy

Evidence of left ventricular hypertrophy on the ECG is a significant risk factor for cardiovascular morbidity and mortality. A number of diagnostic ECG criteria for left ventricular hypertrophy have been developed which, in general, are relatively specific (>90%) but not very sensitive (20–60%). The diagnostic criteria shown in Box 3.1.1 are commonly used.

The Cornell criteria involve measuring the S wave in lead V3 and the R wave in lead aVL. Left ventricular hypertrophy is indicated by a sum of more than 28 mm in men and more than 20 mm in women.

The Romhilt–Estes scoring system allocates points for the presence of certain criteria, with a score of 5 indicating left ventricular hypertrophy and a score of 4 indicating probable left ventricular hypertrophy. Points are allocated as follows:

- 3 points for (a) R or S wave in limb leads of 20 mm or more, (b) S wave in right precordial leads of 25 mm or more, or (c) R wave in left precordial leads of 25 mm or more
- 3 points for ST segment and T wave changes ('typical strain') in a patient not taking digitalis (1 point with digitalis)
- 3 points for P-terminal force in V1 greater than 1 mm deep with a duration greater than 0.04 s
- 2 points for left axis deviation (beyond –15°)
- 1 point for QRS complex duration greater than 0.09 s
- 1 point for intrinsoid deflection (the interval from the start of the QRS complex to the peak of the R wave) in V5 or V6 greater than 0.05 s.

A left ventricular 'strain' pattern (ST-T wave abnormalities) is associated with around double the risk of myocardial infarction and stroke as left ventricular hypertrophy in the absence of strain.

Left ventricular hypertrophy cannot be assessed reliably using the ECG in patients with bundle branch block, previous myocardial infarction or WPW syndrome; visualization via echocardiography or cardiac MRI is required.

An example of left ventricular hypertrophy is shown in Fig. 3.1.10.

Right ventricular hypertrophy

As with left ventricular hypertrophy, the ECG criteria for right ventricular hypertrophy tend to be relatively specific but not very

---

Box 3.1.1 Diagnostic criteria for left ventricular hypertrophy

Limb leads

- R wave >11 mm in lead aVL
- R wave >20 mm in lead aVF
- S wave >14 mm in lead aVR
- Sum of R wave in lead I and S wave in lead III >25 mm

Precordial leads

- R wave of ≥25 mm in the left precordial leads
- S wave of ≥25 mm in the right precordial leads
- Sum of S wave in lead V1 and R wave in lead V5 or V6 >35 mm (Sokolow–Lyon criteria)
- Sum of tallest R wave and deepest S wave in the precordial leads >45 mm

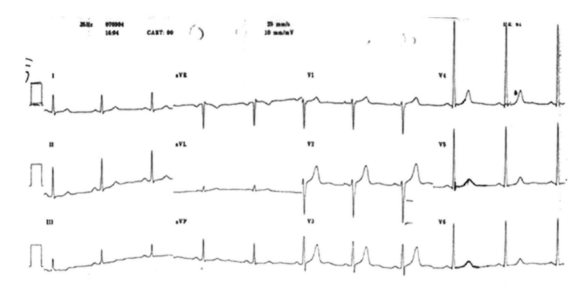

Fig. 3.1.10 Left ventricular hypertrophy.

sensitive. Right ventricular hypertrophy shifts the QRS complex axis rightwards as well as producing higher-voltage QRS complexes in the right precordial leads. ECG criteria include:

- a dominant R wave (R wave ≥ S wave) in lead V1, in the presence of a normal QRS duration
- a QRS complex axis of greater than +90°.

These criteria are supported by:

- ST segment depression and T wave inversion in the right precordial leads
- deep S waves in the lateral precordial and limb leads.

It is not essential for all these criteria to be present, but the greater the number of features present, the greater the likelihood of right ventricular hypertrophy. It is prudent to remember that a dominant R wave in lead V1 can also be seen in right bundle branch block, WPW syndrome, and a posterior wall myocardial infarction.

Atrial hypertrophy

Left atrial hypertropy

Left atrial depolarization is responsible for the terminal portion of the normal P wave. Left atrial hypertrophy increases the voltage and duration of this depolarization, and thus usually evidences itself by abnormalities of the terminal portion of the P wave. The P wave duration is prolonged, and it becomes bifid in lead II and biphasic, with a predominant negative component, in lead V1. So-called 'P mitrale' can be seen in the left atrial enlargement that results from mitral valve stenosis (hence the term) and also in association with conditions that cause left ventricular hypertrophy, such as hypertension (most commonly) and aortic stenosis (Fig. 3.1.11).

Right atrial hypertrophy

Right atrial hypertrophy increases the voltage, but not the duration, of the P wave, and this is usually best seen in the inferior and right precordial leads. A P wave height greater than 2.5mm is regarded as abnormal. So-called 'P pulmonale' can result from right ventricular hypertrophy or from tricuspid valve stenosis (Fig. 3.1.12).

The hemiblocks

The left bundle branch divides into anterosuperior and posteroinferior fascicles. A block of either fascicle (hemiblock) causes a deviation of the QRS axis.

Left anterior hemiblock

Block of the anterosuperior fascicle leads to left anterior hemiblock. This causes a leftward shift in the QRS axis, as the right/inferior region of the left ventricle depolarizes first (via the posteroinferior fascicle) and then the wave of depolarization spreads to the left/superior region. Although this hemiblock introduces a minor delay in ventricular depolarization, the QRS duration remains within the normal range (up to 120 ms). The QRS axis shifts to the left (beyond −30°). As a similar axis shift can result from an inferior myocardial infarction, the diagnosis of left anterior hemiblock requires the presence of left axis deviation in the absence of an abnormal q wave in lead aVF.

Left posterior hemiblock

Block of the posteroinferior fascicle leads to left posterior hemiblock. This causes a rightward shift in the QRS axis, as the left/superior region of the left ventricle depolarizes first (via the anterosuperior fascicle) and then the wave of depolarization spreads to the right/inferior region. As with left anterior hemiblock, the QRS duration remains within the normal range (up to 120 ms). The QRS axis shifts to the right (beyond +90°). However, right axis deviation can occur in several conditions (most commonly right ventricular hypertrophy, but also in lateral myocardial infarction and WPW syndrome). It is therefore not possible to diagnose left posterior hemiblock with certainty from the 12-lead ECG alone.

Bundle branch block

Left bundle branch block

Left bundle branch block (LBBB) leads to a delay in left ventricular depolarization, as the left ventricle is depolarized via the right-sided

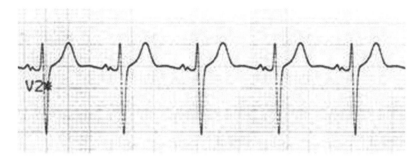

Fig. 3.1.11 Left atrial hypertrophy ('P mitrale').

Purkinje system. In addition, the interventricular septum depolarizes from right to left instead of the usual left to right. Thus, in LBBB:

- The QRS duration is prolonged (≥120 ms)

- The normal 'septal' q waves usually seen in the lateral leads are absent

- A secondary r wave is not seen in lead V1 (this distinguishes LBBB from right bundle branch block (RBBB) with clockwise cardiac rotation).

These findings may be accompanied by ST segment depression and T wave inversion in the lateral precordial and limb leads, broad QS waves in the right precordial leads and broad R waves in the lateral leads, and R wave notching ('M-shaped' QRS complexes).

An example of LBBB is shown in Fig. 3.1.13. The extensive nature of the ECG changes means that further interpretation of the QRS complexes, ST segments or T waves cannot be made. The difficulties of diagnosing myocardial infarction in the setting of LBBB are discussed later.

Right bundle branch block

RBBB leads to a delay in right ventricular depolarization, as the right ventricle is depolarized via the left-sided Purkinje system. However, the normal left to right activation of the interventricular septum is preserved. The ECG changes seen in RBBB are therefore not as extensive as in LBBB. The QRS duration is prolonged (≥120 ms) and the right ventricular leads contain a second positive wave (and, conversely, the left ventricular leads contain a second negative wave). Thus, in RBBB:

- the QRS duration is prolonged (≥120 ms)

- lead V1 contains a second positive wave (rsR′)

- lead V6 contains a second negative wave (qRs).

These findings may be accompanied by deep slurred S waves in the lateral precordial and limb leads, and abnormal ST-T wave changes in the right precordial leads.

An example of RBBB is shown in Fig. 3.1.14.

Ventricular pre-excitation

The normal progression of a wave of depolarization is from the sinoatrial node through the atria to the atrioventricular node, and then through the bundle of His and the Purkinje fibres to the ventricular myocardium. However approximately 1 in 1000 of the population has an accessory pathway—an alternative pathway from atria to ventricles that bypasses part of this normal route. Such a pathway initiates depolarization of the ventricles at a slightly earlier stage in the cardiac cycle than would otherwise be the case, hence the term 'ventricular pre-excitation'. This is because the accessory pathway lacks the inherent delay to conduction that is normally found in the atrioventricular node, thus allowing faster conduction of the wave of depolarization from atria to ventricles.

There are several types of pathway that can give rise to ventricular pre-excitation.

WPW-type pre-excitation

WPW-type pre-excitation is exemplified by WPW syndrome. In WPW syndrome an accessory pathway, the bundle of Kent, connects the atria to the ventricles and bypasses the atrioventricular node altogether. This shortens the time between the onset of atrial depolarization and the onset of ventricular depolarization, and hence one of the ECG features of WPW syndrome is a short PR interval (<0.12 s). Because the accessory pathway leads directly to the ventricular myocardium, and not into the His–Purkinje system, the subsequent initial ventricular depolarization progresses slowly, as conduction of the wave of depolarization cannot take advantage of the rapidly-conducting Purkinje fibres. This gives rise to a delta wave—a slurred initial upstroke of the QRS complex. These features can be seen in the ECG from a patient with WPW syndrome in Fig. 3.1.15.

Conduction between atria and ventricles can be via the accessory pathway, or via the atrioventricular node, or via both routes, or

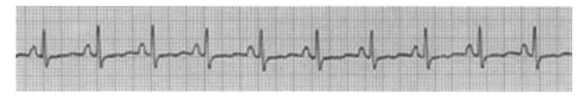

Fig. 3.1.12 Right atrial hypertrophy ('P pulmonale').

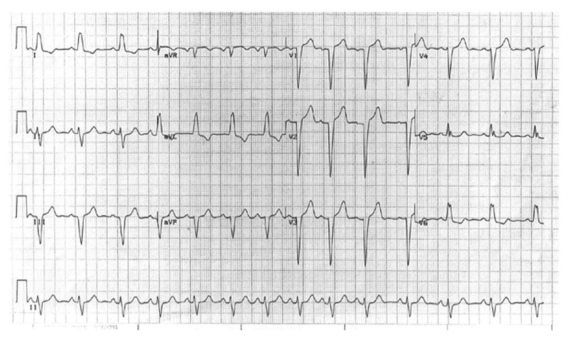

Fig. 3.1.13 Left bundle branch block.

can vary from one to another. If conduction does not occur via the accessory pathway, the ECG will appear normal and the pathway is said to be 'concealed'.

The appearances of the delta wave can vary from patient to patient. Indeed, the ECG appearances of the QRS complex can be used, to a limited extent, to predict the likely location of the accessory pathway. However, the exact location can only be found with electrophysiological studies. The QRS complex morphology in WPW syndrome can mimic LBBB, RBBB, or acute myocardial infarction. WPW syndrome can also lead to repolarization (and therefore T wave) abnormalities. Great care must be thus taken in diagnosing these conditions in the presence of WPW syndrome.

The existence of two atrioventricular pathways (the normal atrioventricular node and the abnormal bundle of Kent) provides a substrate for atrioventricular re-entry tachycardia, which is discussed in more detail in Chapter 4.1.

Short PR-type pre-excitation

A short PR interval in the absence of a delta wave/abnormal QRS complex is often referred to as Lown–Ganong–Levine syndrome, in which an atrio-His accessory pathway bypasses the slow-conducting part of the atrioventricular node. Identical appearances can also be seen with a fast-conducting atrioventricular node. The presence of an atrio-His accessory pathway is a substrate for atrioventricular nodal re-entry tachycardia. For further discussion see Chapter 4.1.

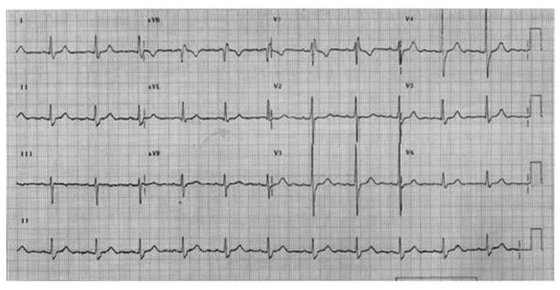

Fig. 3.1.14 Right bundle branch block.

Mahaim-type pre-excitation

Mahaim fibres, first described in the 1930s, are atriofascicular or atrioventricular accessory pathways that connect the atrioventricular node to the right bundle or the right ventricle. Patients with Mahaim-type pre-excitation have a normal PR interval with a LBBB QRS complex morphology and are prone to re-entry tachycardia. For further discussion see Chapter 4.1.

Acute coronary syndromes

Sudden disruption of existing coronary plaque may partially or totally occlude a coronary artery, causing myocyte necrosis. Symptoms of severe, centrally located chest pain develop suddenly, usually accompanied by breathlessness due to left ventricular dysfunction and tachycardia, pallor, sweating, nausea and extreme anxiety due to sympathetic drive. The American College of Cardiology and the European Society of Cardiology classification of myocardial ischaemia and infarction recognizes that acute changes in coronary atheroma produce a spectrum of disease, the acute coronary syndromes (ACS):

◆ *Unstable angina*, where coronary plaque has ruptured but stabilizes without major change in the lumen of the coronary artery: the ECG may be normal, or indicate a previous myocardial infarction, or dynamic ST depression and/or T wave inversion may appear. Serum troponin level, a marker of myocyte necrosis, is within normal limits.

◆ *Non-ST elevation myocardial infarction (NSTEMI)*, where plaque is ruptured with partial occlusion of a major coronary artery: ECG signs are variable—the ECG may be normal, or indicate a previous myocardial infarction, or ST depression may appear transiently or symmetrically inverted T waves may appear. Troponin levels are elevated.

◆ *ST elevation myocardial infarction (STEMI)* where thrombosis from a ruptured plaque completely occludes a coronary artery: the ECG shows ST segment elevation initially, then resolves within a day or two, with new Q waves and inverted T waves appearing in the leads subtending the infarcted area. Troponin levels are elevated.

For discussion of the clinical features and management of ACS, see Chapters 2.1, 13.5, and 13.6.

Role of the ECG in acute coronary syndromes

The ECG remains the most useful bedside triage tool in the emergency setting, whether in the community, en route to hospital, or in the Emergency Department. Accurate interpretation is essential—misinterpretation of the ECG can be as high as 12% and lead to inappropriate management. The ECG is used to diagnose ACS, to locate the site of ischaemia and infarction (see Table 3.1.1) and to identify areas of impaired perfusion (see 'Reciprocal changes').

Of those who suffer a STEMI, the initial ECG is diagnostic in 50%, abnormal but not diagnostic in 40%, and normal in the remainder. Repeat ECGs may be necessary to confidently diagnose or exclude an acute coronary syndrome, as diagnostic changes may not appear for several hours. Serial recordings increase the sensitivity to 95%.

The presenting ECG and prognosis in acute coronary syndrome

About 22% of all patients with acute chest pain will present with T wave inversion, 28% with ST segment elevation, 35% with ST segment depression, and 15% with a combination of ST segment elevation and depression. T wave inversion is most likely to be associated with angiographically normal coronary arteries. Those with ST segment depression are more likely to have three-vessel disease. Mortality at 1 month is 1.7% in those with T wave changes, 5.1% with ST segment elevation or depression, and 6.6% with both depression and elevation. Severe ST segment depression (>2 mm in two contiguous leads) is associated with an increased risk of death at 1 year.

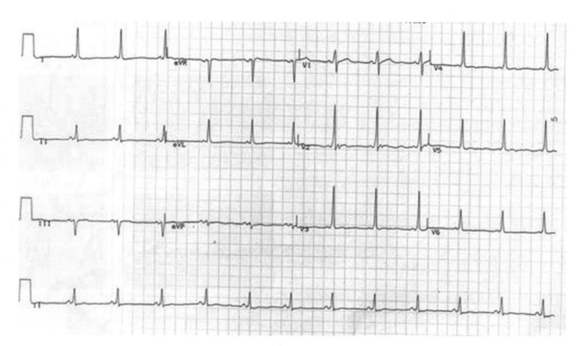

Fig. 3.1.15 WPW syndrome, showing the short PR interval and delta wave.

The presenting ECG and probability of acute coronary syndrome

New, or presumed new, ST segment deviation greater than 0.1 mV, however transiently, or T wave inversion in multiple precordial leads, is highly indicative of ACS. Q waves, ST segment depression of 0.05–0.1 mV or T wave inversion greater than 0.1 mV have an intermediate probability of ACS. T wave flattening or inversion less than 0.1 mV (in leads with dominant R waves) or a normal ECG has a low probability of ACS. The likelihood of NSTEMI is increased threefold in chest pain with ST segment depression in three leads or >0.2 mV.

The presenting ECG and triage

The presenting ECG can be used to triage patients with acute cardiac-sounding chest pain:

- ST elevation present—immediate reperfusion should be considered, by primary percutaneous coronary intervention (PCI) (or by intravenous thrombolysis if primary PCI unavailable).

- ST elevation not evident—immediate treatment with anti-platelet drugs and anti-ischaemic drugs, with consideration of coronary angiography where appropriate. Risk stratification using tools such as GRACE or TIMI scoring, can help identify those most likely to benefit from early coronary angiography and revascularization.

- Elevation is present—consider PCI or intravenous thrombolysis.

ST segment elevation myocardial infarction

The ECG changes of myocardial infarction, first described in 1920, reflect myocardial ischaemia, injury, and myocyte necrosis. Within an hour or so of occlusion of a coronary artery, the T wave becomes more prominent, exceeding one-half the height of the preceding R wave in the ECG leads subtending the infarcted area (see Fig. 3.1.16). Many patients present later than this, so these changes may pass unnoticed. In up to 50%, the presenting ECG is normal. The first documented indication of infarction is usually ST segment elevation which occurs within a few hours. The J point (the origin of the ST segment at its junction with the QRS complex) is elevated by 1 mm or more in two or more limb leads, or by 2 mm in two or more precordial leads.

The ST segment returns to the baseline over the next 48 to 72 h, during which Q waves and symmetrically inverted T waves appear. Some patients develop LBBB, either transiently or permanently. The ECG of a completed infarct shows new Q waves greater than 2 mm, R waves reduced in size or absent, and inverted T waves. This classical evolution of STEMI is seen in about 50 to 66% of patients.

Reperfusion therapy, by primary PCI (or thrombolysis where primary PCI is unavailable) may alter this natural sequence of changes in the ECG. If treatment is given with thrombolysis, then an ECG performed 90 min after initiation should show that ST elevation has been reduced by at least 50% from pretreatment levels (Fig. 3.1.17). If chest pain persists and the ST segments remain elevated, coronary angiography and rescue PCI should be considered. Where available, primary PCI should be offered in preference to thrombolysis.

Resolution of ST segment elevation predicts 30-day mortality. With greater than 70% ST segment resolution, mortality is 2.1%; with 30–70% ST segment resolution 5.2%; with no ST segment resolution 5.5%; and with worsening ST segment elevation 8.1%.

Non-ST elevation myocardial infarction

ECG changes in NSTEMI are more variable than in STEMI. The ECG may be normal on first presentation and remain unchanged throughout the acute admission. There may be transient ST segment depression indicative of myocardial ischaemia. In 20 to 30%, the only change will be T wave inversion. Risk-scoring systems have been developed, e.g. by the Trials In Myocardial Infarction group (www.timi.org), for use in patients with ACS. These are described in Chapter 13.5: with regard to NSTEMI, ST segment deviation greater than 0.5 mm is one of the recorded parameters.

Table 3.1.1 Location of infarction and affected coronary artery

ECG leads affected	Site of infarction	Most likely artery occluded (positive predictive value)
V3 and V4	Anterior	Left anterior descending (96%)
I, aVL and V1 to V6 (in extensive infarction)		
V1 and V2	Septal	
V1 to V4	Anteroseptal	
I, aVL and V3 to V6	Anterolateral	
II, III and aVF	Inferior	Right coronary (80%)
		Right or circumflex (94%)
I, aVL and V6	Lateral	Circumflex (75%)
I and aVL (high lateral)		
ST depression in V1 and V2 followed by development of prominent R waves in lead V1 or V2	Posterior	Circumflex (75%)
	Lateral or posterior	Right or circumflex (94%)
II, III and aVF with aVL, V5 and V6	Inferolateral	Right coronary (93%)

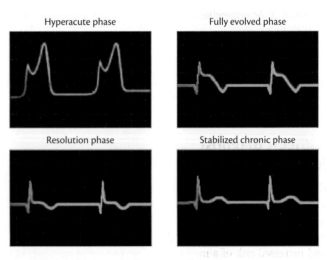

Hyperacute phase   Fully evolved phase

Resolution phase   Stabilized chronic phase

The evolving infarction: ST elevation, followed by development of new Q waves and inverted T waves

Fig. 3.1.16 Evolution of STEMI over several days.

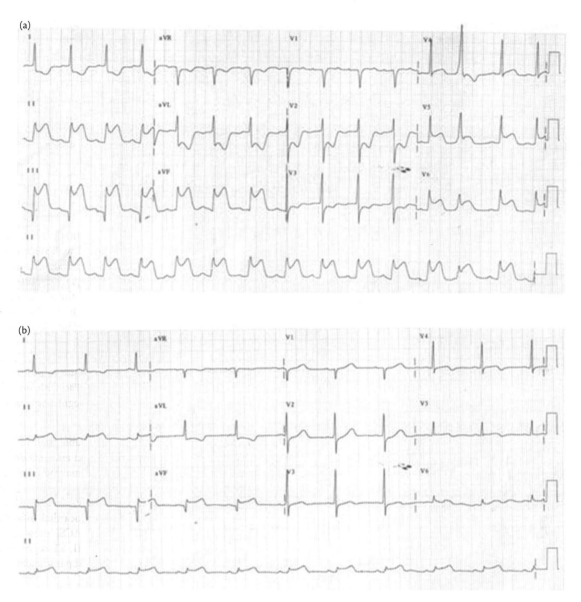

Fig. 3.1.17 (a) Acute inferolateral ST segment elevation myocardial infarction. (b) Substantial (but not complete) resolution of ST segment elevation 90 min after the initiation of thrombolysis.

The extent of ST depression identifies those who are most likely to benefit from early revascularization (FRISC II trial). Mortality with early invasive therapy is 4% with ST segment depression, 2% with no ECG changes, and 0.2% with T wave inversion.

Difficult diagnoses in acute myocardial infarction

Right ventricular infarction

The ECG provides prognostic as well as diagnostic information. An inferior infarction generally carries a good prognosis unless it is associated with a right ventricular infarction, when there is a six-fold increased risk of a major in-hospital complication, including ventricular fibrillation, reinfarction, and death. The right ventricle is involved in about 50% of those with an inferior infarction, occurring with occlusion of the right coronary artery, causing a transmural infarct of the inferoposterior wall and the posterior septum.

To determine whether the right ventricle is involved in an inferior infarction, an ECG should be recorded with the anterior chest leads placed on the right side of the chest, in equivalent (but mirrored) positions to a standard 12-lead ECG. The right ventricle is involved if there is greater than 1 mm ST segment elevation in chest lead 'right V4' (RV4); this has a sensitivity of 100%, specificity of 87%, and positive predictive value of 92% for occlusion of the right coronary artery proximal to the right ventricular branch. If these changes are absent, the right ventricle has been spared (Fig. 3.1.18).

Atrial infarction

This occurs in up to 10% of myocardial infarcts in conjunction with ventricular infarction. A clue to its presence is PR segment displacement but there may also be an abnormal P wave. It can cause rupture of the atrial wall and is frequently associated with atrial arrhythmias including atrial fibrillation, atrial flutter, and atrioventricular nodal rhythm.

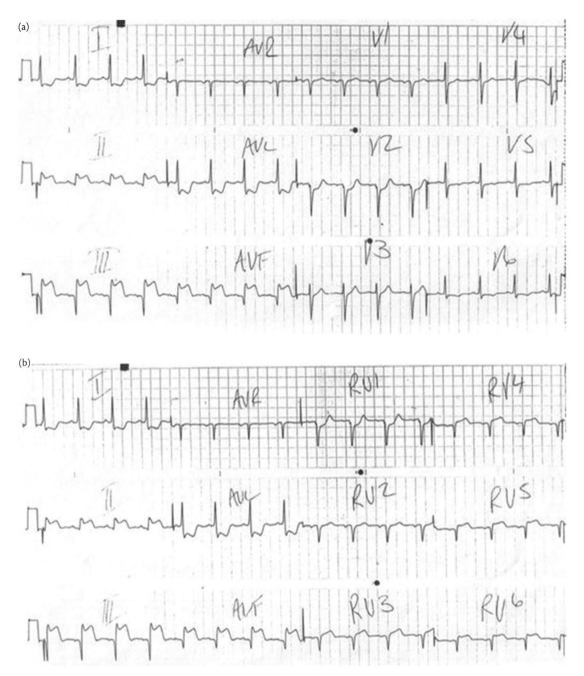

Fig. 3.1.18 (a) Inferior ST segment elevation myocardial infarction. (b) Inferior ST segment elevation myocardial infarction with right ventricular involvement (note the right ventricular chest leads, with ST segment elevation in lead RV4).

Coronary artery spasm

The pain of Prinzmetal's or variant angina is not usually triggered by exercise, emotion, cold, or a meal but tends to occur at rest, accompanied by transient, marked ST segment elevation. This rapidly reverts to normal when the pain resolves spontaneously or with glyceryl trinitrate. Atrioventricular block or ventricular arrhythmia may accompany spasm-induced myocardial ischaemia. Spasm sufficient to cause myocardial ischaemia, myocardial infarction, and sudden death can follow cocaine use.

Reciprocal changes—septal ischaemia or posterior infarction?

ST or 'reciprocal' depression may be seen in leads remote from the site of a STEMI. For example, ST depression may be seen in leads V1 to V4 in an inferior STEMI. There are two explanations. First, in a right-dominant system (70% of the population), the right coronary artery supplies the posterior interventricular septum, which becomes ischaemic with an inferior STEMI; the ischaemia resolves within a few days as septal perforating arteries from the left anterior descending artery dilate in response to ischaemic stress. Second, in a left-dominant system, the circumflex supplies the posterior interventricular septum; if this occludes, a 'true posterior infarction' follows.

Difficulties in diagnosing STEMI

'Stuttering' infarction

Symptoms of myocardial infarction are usually severe and of sudden onset. Occasionally, the onset of symptoms is not so clear cut and

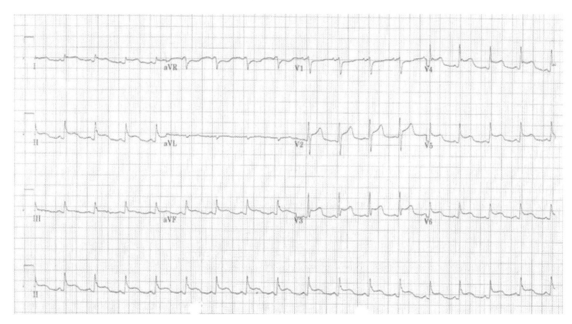

Fig. 3.1.19 Widespread elevation of the ST segments (concave upwards) in a case of pericarditis.

chest pain may resolve but recur at intervals over several hours. The time of arterial occlusion is at best a guess but for practical purposes is taken as the time that symptoms increase or are at their worst.

Noninfarct causes of ST segment elevation

Pericarditis may mimic the pain of myocardial infarction but is usually relieved by sitting forward and is accompanied by a pericardial rub. The ST segments are elevated diffusely, do not fit the usual lead pattern for an inferior or anterior infarction, and, unlike the convexity of STEMI, are concave upwards (Figure 3.1.19). Prinzmetal's angina, caused by coronary artery spasm, can also mimic myocardial infarction. This usually occurs at rest, with marked ST elevation during pain and a brisk response to glyceryl trinitrate. The ST segment can be elevated chronically in left ventricular aneurysm, left ventricular hypertrophy, LBBB, hypertrophic cardiomyopathy, acute cor pulmonale, hypothermia, and cocaine abuse. A normal variant is so-called 'high take-off' where serial ECGs show consistent ST elevation across most ECG leads; patients should be given a copy of the ECG to show to medical personnel to avoid unnecessary investigations and treatment.

Late presentation

Patients who present to hospital outside the 12-h time limit for reperfusion are sometimes diagnosed as 'missed infarction'. The ECG may show signs characteristically seen later in the infarction process, with ST segments only slightly elevated, with established Q waves and inverted T waves. Over the next few days, the ST segment fully returns to baseline and Q waves and T waves deepen.

LBBB

Recognition of acute STEMI in pre-existing LBBB is challenging, but the Sgarbossa criteria help. Five points are scored for ST elevation ≥1 mm in at least one lead with a positive QRS complex, 3 points for ST depression ≥1mm in leads V1-V3, and 2 points for ≥5 mm ST elevation in leads with a negative QRS complex. A score ≥3 points has a 90% specificity (but a poor sensitivity) for acute myocardial infarction.

ECG changes of 'old' infarction

Q waves, once formed, usually persist indefinitely and so are a reliable indicator of a previous myocardial infarction (Fig. 3.1.20). However there are several other causes of a Q wave that may cause confusion, the most common being hypertrophic cardiomyopathy and idiopathic cardiomyopathy. Rarer causes include myocarditis, cardiac amyloid, neuromuscular disorders (e.g. muscular dystrophy, myotonic dystrophy, Friedreich's ataxia), scleroderma, sarcoidosis and an anomalous coronary artery.

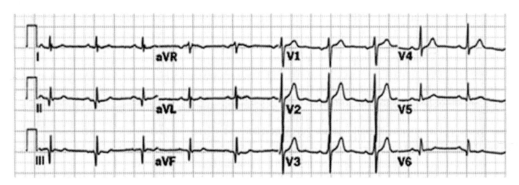

Fig. 3.1.20 'Old' inferior myocardial infarction: pathological Q waves in leads II, III, and aVF.

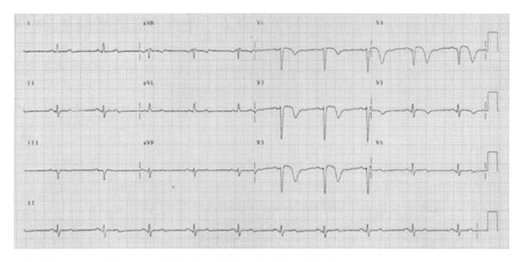

Fig. 3.1.21 Recent anterior ST segment elevation myocardial infarction with 'arrowhead' T wave inversion.

Pre-excitation

WPW syndrome makes interpretation of the ECG more complicated. It may mask a myocardial infarction if conduction via the bypass tract is towards the left ventricle, as a Q wave will not be apparent. WPW may also simulate an infarction due to a negative delta wave in the inferior leads producing Q waves. Serial or previous ECGs will reveal the true diagnosis. Patients with WPW syndrome should be given a copy of their ECG to avoid confusion and unnecessary future investigations.

T wave inversion

Atypical ECG features are seen in up to half of all infarctions in the early stages. Alone, these changes are not diagnostic. They can occur in ventricular aneurysm, electrolyte abnormalities, myocarditis, and subarachnoid haemorrhage, and with some drugs. Serial ECGs are necessary to establish a firm diagnosis.

Deep, symmetrical 'arrowhead' T waves developing during an infarction are most often due to proximal occlusion of the left anterior descending coronary artery (Fig. 3.1.21).

Where errors occur

Incorrect interpretation of an ECG leads to inappropriate patient triage and misses the opportunity to provide reperfusion therapy, whether by angioplasty or thrombolysis. In the worst case scenario, inappropriate thrombolysis might lead to a haemorrhagic stroke or ruptured aneurysm. Up to 12% of those with a high-risk ECG, i.e. ST segment elevation of at least 0.1 mV, ST segment depression of at least 0.05 mV, or T wave inversion of at least 0.2 mV in two or more contiguous leads, are missed on admission to the Emergency Department.

The ECG provides a 'snapshot' of electrical events within the heart, when the clinician really needs a 'movie' to monitor the dynamic changes of an acute coronary syndrome. If a diagnosis cannot be made on the presenting ECG but the history suggests an acute coronary syndrome, the patient should be admitted to a monitored area, a review by a specialist should be arranged, and the ECG should be repeated if symptoms get worse or if ST segment changes are seen on the monitor. This will ensure prompt and appropriate treatment.

While it may be important to provide treatment promptly to fulfil audit targets, e.g. door-to-balloon time for primary PCI, speed should not replace accuracy in diagnosis. It is sometimes better to repeat the

ECG than to make an incorrect diagnosis. It is easy to place too much reliance on minor changes on the ECG; it is clear changes of ST elevation or depression within the parameters above, that should determine treatment.

Exercise ECG testing

ECG changes on exercise were first reported in patients with chronic stable angina in the early 1900s. Exercise testing was adopted into routine clinical practice soon after a standardized exercise protocol was developed.

Cardiovascular responses to exercise in normal subjects and in coronary disease

Normally on treadmill exercise, heart rate increases as a result of diminished vagal and increased sympathetic outflow. Heart rate increases on commencing exercise and reaches a plateau during each stage of the exercise test. A rapid increase may be due to lack of fitness, prolonged bed rest, anaemia, or dehydration. Systolic blood pressure increases in line with increased cardiac output, while diastolic pressure is near constant or falls slightly due to vasodilatation. On stopping the test, heart rate slows within a few minutes to pretest levels and both systolic and diastolic blood pressure falls, often to below pretest levels, as a result of vasodilatation.

With cardiac disease, the maximum cardiac rate may be attenuated (even in the absence of a β-blocker) due to sinus node disease, coronary heart disease, or postinfarction (with or without β-blockade). Failure to achieve the maximum predicted heart rate, calculated as 220 minus age, is suggestive of cardiac disease. Brady- and tachyarrhythmias including atrial fibrillation may occur. Exercise-induced hypotension, even a transient fall in blood pressure at (near-)maximum heart rate, is indicative of severe heart disease and increases the risk of ventricular fibrillation. On stopping exercise, systolic pressure falls to resting levels (or lower) within minutes, where it may remain for several hours. In some, venous pooling may cause a precipitous drop in systolic pressure.

ECG changes with exercise in normal subjects and in coronary disease

In normal subjects, exercise-induced tachycardia causes shortened PR, QRS, and QT intervals, increased P wave amplitude, and

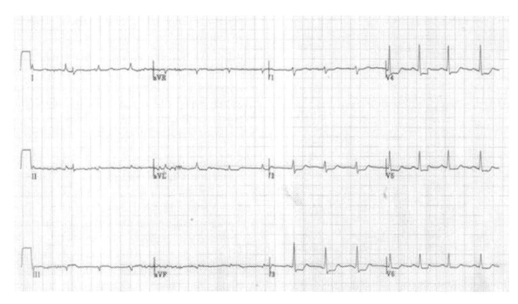

Fig. 3.1.22 ECG recorded during an exercise treadmill test, showing anterolateral ST segment depression after 3 min of exercise using the Bruce protocol.

down-sloping of the PR segment. R waves and T waves may diminish and S waves increase at maximum exercise. The J point (the isoelectric point where the S wave reaches the baseline) may become depressed in all leads and the ST segment may become up-sloping.

The most helpful ECG marker of exercise-induced myocardial ischaemia is the ST segment which becomes depressed with increasing heart rate. This is due to shortening of the action potential due to ischaemia, setting up electrical gradients between endocardium and epicardium. Horizontal or down-sloping ST depression, measured 60 to 80 ms after the J point, of 1 mm (0.10 mV) or more for 80 ms in at least three complexes is considered significant (Fig. 3.1.22), but the leads in which ST depression appear do not reliably localize the site of myocardial ischaemia.

Other indicators of myocardial ischaemia include:

- ST segment elevation—this indicates severe ischaemia due to proximal disease or coronary spasm, or an aneurysmal or dyskinetic left ventricle. Unlike exercise-induced ST segment depression, the ECG site of ST segment elevation is relatively specific for the coronary artery involved

- T wave inversion—this may occur with exercise-induced hyperventilation

- Normalization of an inverted T wave—this alone is not indicative of coronary disease

- U wave inversion—this is relatively specific for coronary artery disease but is relatively insensitive; in precordial leads, it usually indicates left anterior descending coronary artery disease

Exercise protocols

Various protocols have been developed but the most widely used are the following.

Bruce protocol

This is a multistage test with 3-min walking periods during which a steady state is reached before the workload is increased by increasing the speed and slope of the treadmill. It is clearly only suitable for those whose walking is not limited by other considerations, e.g. musculoskeletal or neurological. For older patients or those with limited exercise capacity, the test can be modified to include two stages with lower workload demands.

Bicycle ergometry

This is often combined with radionuclide imaging (see Chapter 3.3), which increases the sensitivity and specificity of the test. Cycling avoids motion artefact, and so ECG recordings are clearer. The patient pedals at a comfortable speed of between 60 and 80 revolutions/min; the test is terminated if speed cannot be maintained above 40 revolutions/min. Exercise workload begins at 25 W and resistance is increased every 2 min in 25-W increments by applying either an electronic or mechanical brake.

The workload achieved during exercise is measured in metabolic equivalents or METs. This allows comparison of different protocols. A MET is 3.5 ml/min per kg, the resting Vo_2 for a 40-year-old 70-kg male. METs equivalent to normal daily activities have been estimated (Table 3.1.2).

Conducting the exercise test

Who should have an exercise test?

Deciding who should and who should not undergo an exercise test requires clinical judgement and the test should not be organized as a routine. Exercise testing is used to:

- assess functional capacity and estimate prognosis in the evaluation of chest pain

- assess patients with known coronary artery disease

- establish prognosis after myocardial infarction either pre-discharge (submaximal test) or 4–6 weeks postdischarge (symptom-limited)

- assess the effectiveness of coronary revascularization

- assess patients with symptoms of exercise-induced cardiac arrhythmia

- risk-stratify before noncardiac surgery in patients with or at high risk of coronary disease

Table 3.1.2 Table of MET equivalents

Occupation	METs	Activity	METs
Receptionist	1–2	Carrying a suitcase	7
Professional (active)	1.5–2.5	Cleaning floor	4
Homemaker	1.5–4	Washing clothes	5
Farm worker	3.5–7.5	Cooking	3
Construction worker	4–8.5	Gardening	4
Miner	4–9	Push mower	5
Postal carrier	2.5–5	Sex	5
		Bed-making	5–6

♦ determine the efficacy of rate-responsive pacemakers.

Exercise testing may also be indicated in selected asymptomatic individuals:

♦ in specific occupations for licensing purposes (e.g. airline pilots, bus or heavy goods vehicle drivers; see Chapter 13.8)

♦ with more than two cardiovascular risk factors for risk stratification

♦ wishing to commence a strenuous exercise programme

♦ to assess cardiovascular risk due to prior to major surgery.

Who should not have an exercise test?

In its 2010 guideline on assessing chest pain of recent onset, the National Institute for Health and Care Excellence (NICE) recommended that exercise testing should no longer be used to diagnose or exclude stable angina in those without known coronary artery disease. Some conditions are considered to be absolute contraindications to exercise testing but even in these patients a submaximal test may be informative.

Exercise testing is inappropriate:

♦ in healthy individuals with a low risk factor profile—the false-positive rate is increased (see below)

♦ with unstable medical conditions such as unstable angina; severe congestive cardiac failure; uncontrolled ventricular or supraventricular arrhythmia; myocarditis; severe pulmonary hypertension; drug toxicity; haemodynamic instability; symptomatic aortic stenosis; active thromboembolic disease; hypertension with systolic blood pressure >200 mmHg or diastolic blood pressure >110 mmHg

♦ in extreme obesity

♦ when taking specific medication—digoxin depresses the ST segment (Figure 3.1.23); type 1 antiarrhythmics and tricyclic antidepressants may be proarrhythmic

♦ in vasoregulatory disorders—pulse and blood pressure changes are unpredictable.

Patients with aortic stenosis may fail to report symptoms of angina, breathlessness, and syncope. Although severe symptomatic aortic stenosis is considered an absolute contraindication to exercise testing, a medically supervised symptom-limited test in those who appear to be asymptomatic during their everyday activities may identify those who warrant cardiac catheterization and valve replacement.

Who should supervise an exercise test—cardiac technician, specialist nurse, or physician?

Patients with new- or recent-onset chest pain thought to be angina are often referred to a rapid-access chest pain clinic for assessment, where a specialist nurse carries out an initial assessment and then an exercise test. Experience shows that this approach is safe, provided a physician is available for consultation and advice. There are some high-risk situations where the test, if it must be carried out, should be supervised by a physician. These include patients whose symptoms are unstable, aortic stenosis, known severe coronary disease, severe or moderate systemic or pulmonary hypertension, severe left ventricular dysfunction, congestive or hypertrophic cardiomyopathy, or a history of ventricular tachycardia or second or third-degree atrioventricular block.

Risks of exercise testing

Exercise testing is generally considered a safe procedure but full resuscitation facilities, including defibrillator, emergency drug kit, airways management equipment, and oxygen are essential. Serious complications are rare. The risk of myocardial infarction and sudden death is less than 1 in 1000, more when testing patients after myocardial infarction or with malignant ventricular arrhythmia.

When to stop an exercise test

Reasons for stopping a test include:

♦ achieving 90% of the maximum predicted heart rate

♦ symptoms—establish if these are typical symptoms of chest pain or breathlessness; exercise may continue provided that symptoms are not distressing or severe

♦ systolic blood pressure—if systolic blood pressure falls below baseline levels or if systolic increases to greater 250 mmHg or diastolic to greater than 115 mmHg

♦ change in ECG—if more than 2 mm ST segment depression or more than 1 mm ST segment elevation; or if LBBB (this may look remarkably like ventricular tachycardia at fast heart rate) or arrhythmia develops

♦ clinical signs—if signs of poor peripheral perfusion such as cyanosis appear

♦ symptoms of central nervous system dysfunction—dizziness, near syncope, or ataxia

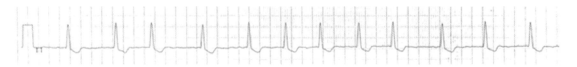

Fig. 3.1.23 Depression of the ST segments caused by digoxin.

* serious arrhythmia—ventricular tachycardia, multifocal ectopics, ventricular couplets

* technical difficulties—failure of blood pressure recording or poor ECG trace

* patient request—distressing symptoms of fatigue, breathlessness, wheeze or claudication; maximal patient effort; or inability to maintain speed of treadmill.

Recovery period

It is important to observe the patient into the recovery period until the pretest heart rate and blood pressure have been restored. Minor ECG abnormalities early in recovery are common but late changes usually indicate myocardial ischaemia.

Interpreting the results of an exercise test

Like all medical tests, the exercise test is not a perfect indicator of the presence or absence of disease. Nevertheless, a test is often described as:

* positive—chest pain develops with or without ST displacement; blood pressure falls; arrhythmia occurs; the patient fails to complete the first two stages of the Bruce protocol or reach 90% of predicted maximum heart rate

* negative—the patient completes uneventfully three stages of the Bruce protocol or reaches 90% of predicted maximum heart rate

* indeterminate—90% predicted heart rate is not reached; symptoms occur which are not typical of cardiac pain with a normal ECG throughout.

A positive test does not necessarily mean that the patient has coronary disease, nor does a negative test mean the patient has some other, noncardiac, cause for chest pain. The exercise test has limited use as a diagnostic test for coronary disease.

Limitations and strengths of the exercise test

The exercise test as a diagnostic tool

The sensitivity of the exercise test, the proportion with coronary disease correctly identified by the test, is 68% (range 23–100) and specificity, the proportion free of disease correctly identified by the test, is 77% (range 17–100). In multivessel disease, these figures are 81% (range 40–100) and 66% (range 17–100) respectively.

This means that exercise testing frequently yields false-positive results, incorrectly diagnosing disease when coronary arteries are normal or minimally diseased; and false-negative results, missing coronary disease when a flow-limiting, even critical left main stem, coronary stenosis is present.

Selection of patients for exercise testing is important as a false-positive result is more likely when an individual has few predisposing risk factors for coronary disease or the prevalence of coronary disease prevalence in the population is low.

Example 1

A positive test in a middle-aged man with multiple coronary risk factors (smoking, dyslipidaemia, hypertension, diabetes mellitus, and family history) and typical chest pain on exertion (who is highly likely to have coronary disease) is most likely to be correct.

Example 2

A positive test in a young woman with atypical chest pain and few or no cardiovascular risk factors is likely to be incorrect and may lead to other, more invasive tests including coronary angiography. The prevalence of coronary disease is lower in women than men and the specificity of exercise testing is lower in women, which means that the test is more likely to be positive in the absence of coronary disease, possibly due to increased catecholamine secretion during exercise contributing to coronary vasoconstriction.

The exercise test as an indicator of prognosis

Although the exercise test is of limited value as an aid to diagnosis, it is more reliable as a marker of prognosis.

Generally, appearance of symptoms or ECG changes early in the test is associated with more severe and extensive coronary disease and a poor prognosis (Table 3.1.3). Changes within the first 3 min usually indicate severe coronary disease affecting the left main stem or the proximal segments of at least one major coronary artery.

Multivessel coronary disease is more likely with ST segment down-sloping, delayed ST normalization after exercise, increased number of leads affected, and lower workload at which ECG changes appear.

Difficulties with exercise testing

Baseline ECGs that make interpretation of the exercise test difficult

ECG patterns that may make exercise-induced changes hard to recognize include:

* ST depression or elevation at rest

* ventricular strain patterns—left and right ventricular hypertrophy

Table 3.1.3 Prognostic indicators on treadmill testing

	Indicators of a good prognosis	Indicators of a poor prognosis
ST segment	No displacement or up-sloping	2 mm or more depression in stage 1 Bruce- within 3 minutes Down-sloping or horizontal
Duration of exercise	9 minutes (>9 METs)	Unable to complete stage 2 Bruce or equivalent (<6.5 METs)
Heart rate at onset of limiting symptoms	Reaches maximum predicted heart rate (220 – age)	Unable to attain >120/min off β-blocker
Systolic BP response	Maintained or increased	Sustained decrease >10 mmHg or failure to rise with exercise
Changes on exercise	No changes	Ventricular tachycardia U wave inversion T wave normalization
Recovery	Recovers normal heart rate <10 min	Delayed recovery >10 min
Symptoms	None or atypical	Test terminated due to increasing angina on exercise

- ◆ T wave changes—inversion secondary to previous infarction or 'strain'
- ◆ conduction abnormalities—LBBB affects ST segment and T wave; RBBB affects ST segment and T wave changes in V1, V2, and V3
- ◆ prolonged QT interval.

Alternative tests that do not rely on the ECG to identify myocardial ischaemia are dobutamine stress echocardiography, radionuclide thallium or MIBI stress test, or cardiac MRI (see Chapters 3.2 and 3.3).

Medication and exercise testing

β-Blockers and rate-modifying calcium antagonists may mask myocardial ischaemia by limiting exercise-induced tachycardia and so delay the appearance of ST depression. Blood pressure lowering medication may blunt the normal exercise-induced rise in pressure. Digoxin may induce or accentuate ST depression on the resting ECG.

Medication may be continued if the indication for exercise testing is to assess the efficacy of treatment but should be temporarily stopped in all other circumstances. Specific rules apply if assessing for driving licensing purposes—always check local rules, but generally, antianginal drugs must be stopped at least 48 h prior to the assessment.

ST segment depression in the absence of symptoms

Asymptomatic, exercise-induced ST segment depression, or 'silent ischaemia', is seen in 60% of patients with coronary disease but does not increase the risk of cardiac death compared with those who report angina.

Technical issues

Current ECG machines filter out motion and muscle artefact to facilitate measurement of the ST segment. Because leads placed on the limbs produce motion artefact, moving these to the torso exaggerates the degree of change and increases the amplitude of the R wave, potentiating exercise-induced ST segment changes. It can be difficult to identify ST segment depression during exercise. If there is any doubt about the extent of ST segment depression on the running ECG, most automated machines will provide a filtered 12-lead ECG for comparison with baseline.

Exercise testing in special groups

Peri- and postmyocardial infarction

Exercise testing after myocardial infarction may be performed for risk stratification and selection for revascularization. A submaximal predischarge test to identify residual ischaemia appears to be safe, with 0.05% morbidity and 0.02% mortality. An abnormal blood pressure response or low exercise capacity predicts a poor outcome and is an indication for urgent revascularization. Evidence of myocardial ischaemia, especially at low workload, is an indication for referral for coronary angiography.

Elderly patients

Advanced age alone is not a contraindication to exercise testing, provided that the individual can walk at a reasonable speed. If mobility is limited, dobutamine stress echocardiography, radionuclide

thallium or MIBI stress test, or cardiac MRI are alternative means of identifying ischaemia (see Chapters 3.2 and 3.3).

Asymptomatic individuals

Testing may be undertaken in asymptomatic individuals, generally a low-risk population, as part of health screening, for insurance purposes, or for risk stratification. Up to 12% of middle-aged men and up to 30% of women will have an abnormal exercise test in the absence of symptoms; the risk of a cardiac event is low unless the test result indicates a poor prognosis. The presence of cardiovascular risk factors increases the likelihood of coronary disease.

Cardiac arrhythmia

Exercise testing can be useful in evaluating cardiac arrhythmia, supplementary to ambulatory monitoring and electrophysiological studies. In about 10%, it may provoke an arrhythmia.

Further reading

Bruce, RA, Fisher LD (1987). Exercise-enhanced assessment of risk factors for coronary heart disease in healthy men. *J Electrocardiol*, **20** (Suppl. October), 162.

Corrado D, *et al.* (2010). Recommendations for interpretation of 12-lead electrocardiogram in the athlete. *Eur Heart J*, **31**, 243–59.

Cura FA, *et al.* (2004). ST segment resolution 60 minutes after combination treatment of abciximab with reteplase or reteplase alone for acute myocardial infarction (30-day mortality results from the resolution of ST segment after reperfusion therapy substudy). *Am J Cardiol*, **94**, 859–63.

Einthoven W (1912). The different forms of the human electrocardiogram and their signification. *Lancet*, **1**, 853–61.

Gianrossi R, *et al.* (1989). Exercise-induced ST segment depression in the diagnosis of coronary artery disease: a meta-analysis. *Circulation*, **80**, 87–98.

Hancock EW, *et al.* (2009). AHA/ACCF/HRS recommendations for the standardization and interpretation of the electrocardiogram: Part V: Electrocardiogram changes associated with cardiac chamber hypertrophy. *J Am Coll Cardiol*, **53**, 992–1002.

Houghton AR, Gray D (2014). *Making sense of the ECG*, 4th edition. Hodder Arnold, London.

Joint European Society of Cardiology/American College of Cardiology Committee (2000). Myocardial infarction redefined—a consensus document of the joint European Society of Cardiology/American College of Cardiology Committee for the Redefinition of Myocardial Infarction. *Eur Heart J*, **21**, 1502–13.

Kligfield P, *et al.* (2007). Recommendations for the standardization and interpretation of the electrocardiogram: Part I: The electrocardiogram and its technology. *J Am Coll Cardiol*, **49**, 1109–27.

Knaapen P, van Loon RB, Visser FC (2005). A rare cause of ST segment elevation. *Heart*, **91**, 188.

Levy D, *et al.* (1990). Determinants of sensitivity and specificity of electrocardiographic criteria for left ventricular hypertrophy. *Circulation*, **81**, 815–20.

Lloyd Jones DM, *et al.* (1998). Electrocardiographic and clinical predictors of acute myocardial infarction in patients with unstable angina pectoris. *Am J Cardiol*, **81**, 1182–6.

Marey EJ (1876). Des variations électriques des muscles et du coeur en particulier étudiés au moyen de l'électromètre de M Lippman. *C R Acad Sci (Paris)*, **82**, 975–7.

Mason JW, *et al.* (2007). Recommendations for the standardization and interpretation of the electrocardiogram: Part II: Electrocardiography diagnostic statement list. *J Am Coll Cardiol*, **49**, 1128–35.

Mueller C, *et al.* (2004). Prognostic value of the admission electrocardiograph in patients with unstable angina/ST segment elevation myocardial infarction treated with very early revascularisation. *Am J Med*, **117**, 145–50.

National Institute of Health Care Excellence (2010). *Chest pain of recent onset*. NICE clinical guideline 95: Available at https://www.nice.org.uk/guidance/cg95 (accessed 25 November 2015).

Rautaharju PM, *et al.* (2009). AHA/ACCF/HRS recommendations for the standardization and interpretation of the electrocardiogram: Part IV: The ST segment, T and U waves, and the QT interval. *J Am Coll Cardiol*, **53**, 982–91.

Savonitto S, *et al.* (1999). Prognostic value of the admission electrocardiogram in acute coronary syndromes. *JAMA*, **281**, 707–13.

Surawicz B, *et al.* (2009). AHA/ACCF/HRS recommendations for the standardization and interpretation of the electrocardiogram: Part III: Intraventricular conduction disturbances. *J Am Coll Cardiol*, **53**, 976–81.

Wagner GS, *et al.* (2009). AHA/ACCF/HRS recommendations for the standardization and interpretation of the electrocardiogram: Part VI: Acute ischemia/infarction. *J Am Coll Cardiol*, **53**, 1003–11.

Waller AD (1887). A demonstration on man of electromotive changes accompanying the heart's beat. *J Physiol (Lond)*, **8**, 229–34.

CHAPTER 3.2

Echocardiography

Adrian P. Banning, Andrew R. J. Mitchell, and James D. Newton

Essentials

Ease of use, rapid data provision, portability, and safety mean that echocardiography has become the principal investigation for almost all cardiac conditions. A modern transthoracic echocardiography examination combines real-time two-dimensional (2D) imaging of the myocardium and valves with information about velocity and direction of blood flow obtained by Doppler and colour-flow mapping. A complete examination can be performed in most patients in less than 30 min.

Valvular heart disease—echocardiography has revolutionized the diagnosis and follow-up of patients with these conditions. Serial cardiac catheterization to assess severity and progress of valvular stenosis has been almost completely superseded by Doppler echocardiography, and the role of invasive investigation is increasingly limited to the assessment of the coronary arteries prior to revascularization.

Transoesophageal echocardiography—this is now a routine investigation in many centres. Under sedation, an ultrasound probe is passed into the oesophagus to a position behind the heart, producing excellent resolution of cardiac structures. It is used diagnostically in many emergency situations, including aortic dissection and suspected prosthetic mechanical valve dysfunction, and as an additional method of monitoring cardiac performance during cardiac and noncardiac surgery.

Other technological developments—these include (1) stress echocardiography—used to detect occult coronary disease and predict cardiac risk; (2) use of contrast agents—these improve visualization of the endocardium in patients with poor acoustic windows and allow some estimation of myocardial perfusion; and (3) real-time three-dimensional imaging—this is available on modern platforms and allows detailed assessment of myocardial and valve function.

History of echocardiography

- 1842—Christian Doppler observed that the pitch of a sound varies if the source is moving
- 1880—first piezoelectric crystals developed
- 1912—Richardson develops sonar technique using sound waves to detect underwater objects

- 1929—Sokolov uses ultrasound to identify flaws in metal components
- 1954—heart visualized with ultrasound by Carl Herz and Inge Edler
- 1960s—multielement scanners lead to development of two-dimensional (2D) echocardiography
- 1970s—Doppler colour-flow mapping used to evaluate valve disease
- 1970s—transoesophageal and stress echocardiography developed
- 1980s—ultrasound contrast agents developed
- 1990s—intracardiac and intracoronary ultrasound in wider use
- 2000s—development and refinement of three-dimensional (3D) echocardiography and advances in myocardial deformation imaging.

Principles of echocardiography

The transducer used for most echocardiographic examinations contains piezoelectric crystals that emit ultrasound frequencies of 2.5 to 5 MHz. Most of the sound energy is scattered or absorbed, but reflection occurs at interfaces between tissues of different acoustic impedance (e.g. between blood and muscle). The transducer collects these reflections and the time delay between emission and reception is calculated. This allows the depth of the reflection to be derived and its position to be displayed on a screen as a dot (pixel). The brightness of the dot is related to the magnitude of the reflected signal. In general, higher-frequency transducers allow better discrimination between structures, but the increased attenuation leads to reduced penetration.

There are three main echocardiographic techniques: two-dimensional (2D; cross-sectional), M-mode, and Doppler.

Two-dimensional echocardiography (cross-sectional)

Cross-sectional images are constructed as the ultrasound beam sweeps across the heart in a sector (Fig. 3.2.1). Between 50 and 100 cross-sections are presented each second, giving the impression of a moving picture. These images are readily interpretable by an observer with knowledge of cardiac anatomy, and this technique is the cornerstone of modern echocardiography.

M-mode echocardiography

M-mode echocardiography preceded modern 2D imaging. Unlike 2D imaging, which uses a series of sweeps across the heart, M-mode uses a single static beam of ultrasound pulses at a very high frequency. The narrow beam is analogous to a vertical mineshaft

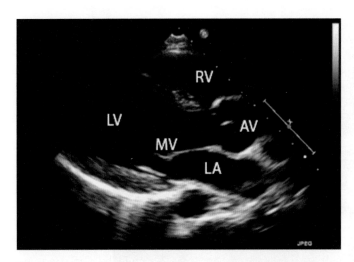

Fig. 3.2.1 Parasternal long-axis view of the heart using 2D echocardiography. The sector images through the right ventricle (RV) to the left ventricle (LV). In this view, 2D echocardiography provides useful data on the structure and function of the aortic valve (AV) and mitral valve (MV).

passing through various layers of rock. Displayed in real time, this results in reflections from cardiac structures being displayed as horizontal lines, with superficial structures at the top of the screen and the deeper structures at the bottom (Fig. 3.2.2). These data are interpretable when one knows which structure each line represents. The technique has excellent spatial resolution; hence, with the advent of 2D echocardiography and Doppler, M-mode is now principally used for measurement of cardiac chamber dimensions and observation of the relative movement of cardiac structures to each other; for example, the relationship of the anterior leaflet of the mitral valve to the septum in hypertrophic cardiomyopathy.

Doppler echocardiography

The Doppler principle allows the velocity and direction of movement of an object (blood or myocardium in the case of cardiac ultrasonography) to be calculated from the shift in the frequency of a reflected waveform relative to the observer. Cardiac imaging

employs pulsed-wave, continuous-wave, and colour Doppler techniques. Pulsed-wave Doppler allows information about flow to be obtained from a particular point within the heart. The range of detectable velocities is limited, and the technique is used for sampling normal and low velocities (e.g. mitral valve flow). Continuous-wave Doppler identifies the peak velocity encountered along the whole of the ultrasound beam and is particularly valuable for measuring high-velocity jets, as seen in aortic valve disease (Fig. 3.2.3), for example. It is important to remember that failure to align the transducer exactly parallel to flow results in measurement of artefactually low velocities and potentially an underestimation of valvular stenosis.

Colour Doppler allows a dynamic representation of the direction and velocity of flow to be superimposed on to a 2D image of the heart. Velocities towards the transducer are usually coded in red and velocities away in blue (Fig. 3.2.4). Turbulent and high-velocity flow produces variable velocities and results in a mosaic pattern that is ideal for characterization of regurgitant lesions. This technique is now so sensitive that it can detect trivial regurgitation during the closure of many normal heart valves.

Tissue Doppler echocardiography uses the same principles but by changing the settings the direction and velocity of the myocardium is encoded rather than the blood pool. Pulse-wave Doppler can then be used to interrogate a specific part of the myocardium and provide detailed information on myocardial mechanics in both systole and diastole (Fig 3.2.5).

Transthoracic echocardiography

Imaging is performed using dedicated echocardiography equipment with the patient lying on their left hip in the left lateral position and with their left arm behind their head to open the rib spaces. Ultrasound cannot travel through bone and thus cardiac imaging is performed via intercostal spaces to the left of the sternum and at the apex of the heart in the axillary line. These 'echo windows' provide standard views described as the parasternal short and long axis and apical two-, four-, and five-chamber views. Useful additional views can also be obtained from the subcostal

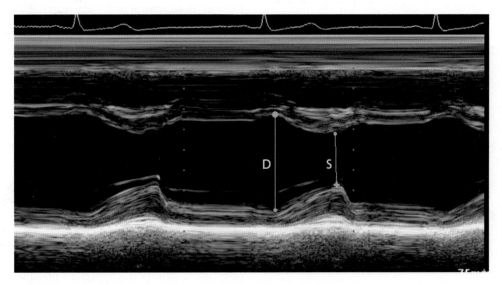

Fig. 3.2.2 M-Mode view of the left ventricle. The high imaging frequency of M-mode allows accurate measurements of structures to be made, in this case the diastolic (D) and systolic (S) cavity size.

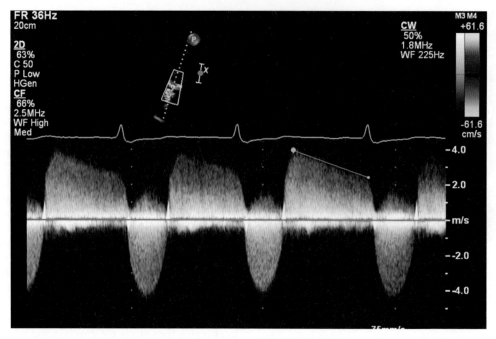

Fig. 3.2.3 Continuous-wave Doppler of the aortic valve showing aortic regurgitation (flow towards the probe above the line). Calculations can be performed using on-machine software to instantly provide useful haemodynamic data.

and suprasternal approach in some patients. A standard echocardiography examination involves 2D imaging from the parasternal, apical, and subcostal approaches supported by M-mode measurements, continuous, pulsed, and colour Doppler and tissue Doppler imaging.

Valvular heart disease

Transthoracic echocardiography is the investigation of choice for patients with suspected valvular heart disease. All four cardiac valves can be visualized and interrogated by Doppler and 2D echocardiography. Concomitant abnormalities in ventricular performance can be assessed simultaneously.

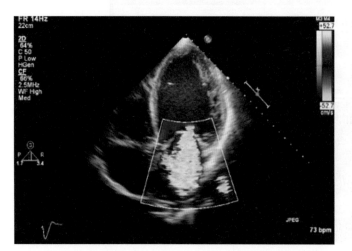

Fig. 3.2.4 Colour-flow mapping of mitral regurgitation. There is high-velocity flow in systole from the left ventricle into the left atrium through the mitral valve

Aortic stenosis

2D echocardiography can usually image the aortic valve cusps; if they are thin and freely mobile, it is unlikely that there is significant aortic stenosis. However, if the valve cusps are thickened and calcified, interrogation by continuous-wave Doppler is mandatory. The severity of aortic stenosis is usually expressed as the peak pressure difference (or gradient) across the valve, and is calculated from the maximum flow velocity (V) using the modified Bernoulli equation (pressure gradient $= 4\,V^2$). In patients with normal left ventricular systolic function, a peak gradient measured by Doppler of over 65 mmHg or a mean gradient of over 40 mmHg suggests significant aortic stenosis. The aortic valve area can be estimated using the continuity equation which requires measurement of the left ventricular outflow tract diameter on 2D echo and the pulse-wave velocity at this point using Doppler (Fig. 3.2.6). Severe stenosis usually equates to a valve area of less than 1.0 cm^2 but should be indexed to the patient's body surface area.

When chronic critical outflow obstruction results in declining left ventricular function and reduced cardiac output, the gradient produced by any degree of valve obstruction also falls. Doubt about the severity of the stenosis can usually be resolved by enhancing left ventricular function by administering intravenous dobutamine and evaluating the gradient during increased flow.

Aortic regurgitation

Assessment of the mechanism and severity of aortic regurgitation requires a combination of all three echocardiography modalities. M-mode may demonstrate fluttering of the anterior leaflet of the mitral valve and, in the setting of acute severe aortic regurgitation, may reveal premature closure of the mitral valve. 2D echocardiography will occasionally demonstrate prolapse of one more of the aortic cusps, but even severe aortic regurgitation can occur through an aortic valve that appears to be structurally normal.

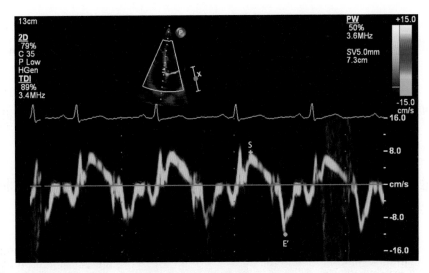

Fig. 3.2.5 Tissue Doppler of the basal interventricular septum allowing measurement of the systolic contraction (S) and early passive relaxation (E') phase.

The severity of aortic regurgitation can be estimated using continuous-wave and colour Doppler (see Chapter 14.1, Figs. 14.1.3 and 14.1.4), although assessment can be difficult as it is influenced by left ventricular function and blood pressure. Doppler-derived pressure half-time and measurement of regurgitant fraction and/or flow convergence zone are valuable when there is uncertainty over lesion severity. M-mode and colour Doppler can be combined and, when the regurgitant jet fills more than 50% of the left ventricular outflow tract, the regurgitation is classified as severe. Flow within the descending thoracic aorta can be measured using pulse-wave Doppler and in severe aortic regurgitation there is typically holodiastolic flow reversal—analogous to the collapsing pulse.

In patients with severe asymptomatic aortic regurgitation, serial increase in left ventricular dimensions or a progressive fall in ejection fraction are indications for surgery. However, any increase in ventricular dimension should be at least 0.5 cm before it is regarded as significant, given the limited reproducibility of echocardiographic parameters.

Mitral stenosis

Mitral valve stenosis is well visualized using either M-mode or cross-sectional echocardiography. Its severity can be determined by estimating the area of the valve orifice either by direct planimetry of the 2D short-axis image or from the Doppler pressure half-time (mitral valve area = 220/pressure half-time). A valve area of less than 1.0 cm² usually indicates severe mitral stenosis (Fig. 3.2.7). The mean gradient across the valve can also be measured by Doppler and is in excess of 10 mmHg in severe stenosis. Transthoracic echocardiography is also used to assess the suitability of the mitral valve for balloon dilation, although transoesophageal imaging is necessary to exclude left atrial thrombus.

Mitral regurgitation

Transthoracic echocardiography will usually demonstrate the mechanism and severity of mitral regurgitation. 2D imaging identifies abnormalities of the valve leaflets and colour-flow shows jet direction and area (Fig. 3.2.8). Severe mitral regurgitation is suggested by increased left ventricular end-diastolic dimension and

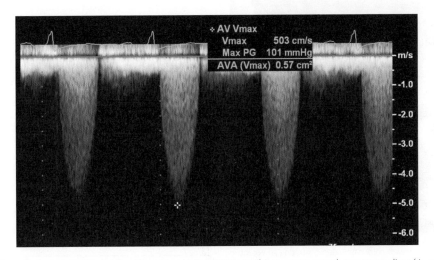

Fig. 3.2.6 Continuous-wave Doppler through the aortic valve. The peak velocity is 503 cm/s. This equates to a peak pressure gradient (A_0 max PG) of 101 mmHg. Previous measurements of the left ventricular outflow tract diameter and velocity allow a calculated aortic valve area to be derived, in this case 0.57 cm².

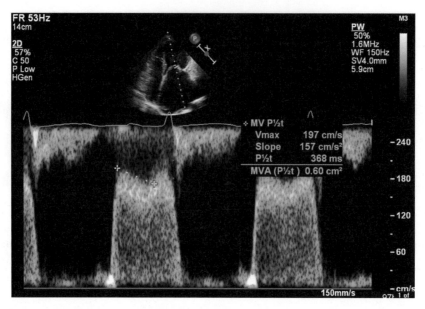

Fig. 3.2.7 Pulse-wave Doppler at the mitral valve leaflet tips in a patient with severe mitral valve stenosis. The pressure half-time is calculated as 368 ms giving an estimated valve area of 0.6 cm².

hyperdynamic function due to volume overload. Precise quantification of the amount of regurgitation is demanding as it is influenced by left ventricular function, the direction of the jet, and left atrial size. Various algorithms have been devised to improve quantification of mitral regurgitation, including measurement of the flow convergence zone and the proximal isovelocity surface area (PISA) method, but most centres simply classify the extent of regurgitation as mild, moderate, or severe (Table 3.2.1).

Pulmonary and tricuspid valve disease

In adults, 2D imaging of the pulmonary valve may be difficult, particularly if there is lung disease. Despite this, accurate Doppler information is usually obtainable. Tricuspid stenosis is very uncommon, but some degree of tricuspid regurgitation is detectable even in healthy individuals. Measurement of the peak velocity of tricuspid regurgitation (V) is valuable as, in the absence of pulmonary

valve disease, it can be used to estimate pulmonary artery (PA) systolic pressure:

PA systolic pressure (mmHg) = $4V^2$ + right atrial pressure (usually 5–10 mmHg)

Prosthetic valves

Transthoracic echocardiography is commonly performed as part of the routine follow-up of prosthetic valves. It is usually able to

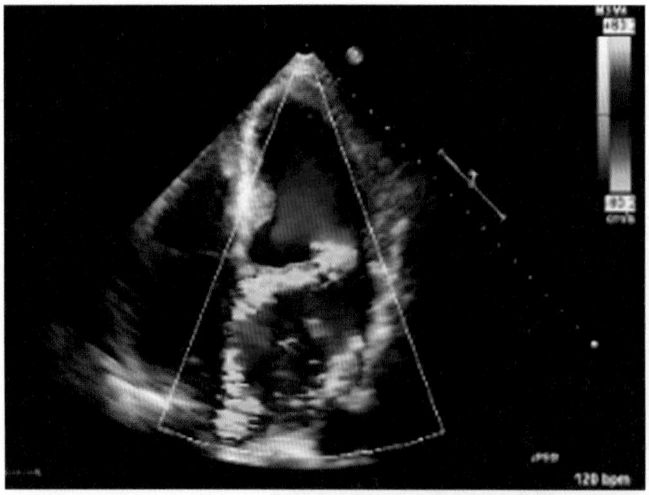

Table 3.2.1 Classification of mitral regurgitation

	Mild	Severe
Specific signs of severity		
Vena contracta	<0.3 cm	>0.7 cm
Jet size	<4 cm² or <20% left atrium	>40% left atrium
	Small and central	Large and central or wall-impinging and swirling
PISA radius	None/minimal (<0.4 cm)	Large (>1 cm)
Pulmonary vein flow		Systolic reversal
Valve structure		Flail or rupture
Supportive signs of severity		
Pulmonary vein flow	Systolic dominant	
Mitral inflow	A-wave dominant	E-wave dominant (>1.2 m/s)
CW trace	Soft and parabolic	Dense and triangular
LV and LA	Normal size LV if chronic MR	Enlarged LV and LA if no other cause

CW, continuous wave; LA, left atrium; LV, left ventricle; PISA, proximal isovelocity surface area.

Fig. 3.2.8 Apical four-chamber view with colour-flow demonstrating an eccentric jet of mitral regurgitation from the left ventricle (LV) to the left atrium (LA). In this case the leak is due to prolapse of the posterior mitral valve leaflet.

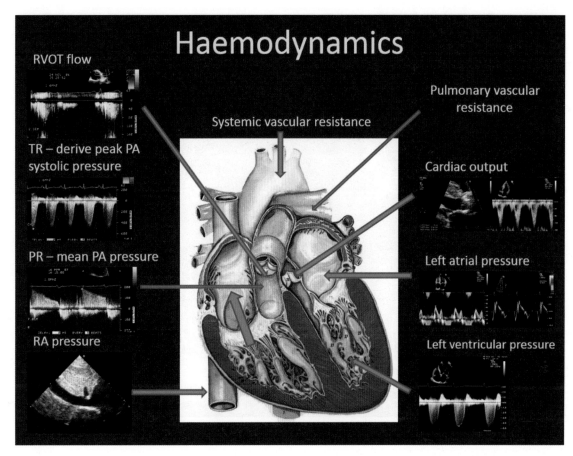

Fig. 3.2.9 An example of the haemodynamic parameters that can be estimated with a standard transthoracic echocardiography data set.

assess biological valves accurately, but for mechanical mitral valve prostheses in particular, attenuation artefact produced by the metal may be problematic. Transoesophageal imaging is recommended when transthoracic imaging is suboptimal or if improved resolution is required, for example, in patients with suspected prosthetic valve endocarditis.

Haemodynamic assessment

Using Doppler to evaluate flow across all four cardiac valves and with the great vessels the pressure within each cardiac chamber can be estimated and a comprehensive description of the current haemodynamic status provided (Fig. 3.2.9). This can be extremely helpful in the setting of intensive cardiorespiratory support although obtaining clear and accurate imaged in critically ill patients can be very challenging.

Abnormal left ventricular function

In most patients, a full transthoracic echocardiography study will confirm or refute a clinical suspicion of left ventricular dysfunction and identify the likely aetiology of any abnormality. Systolic and diastolic left ventricular function can be assessed and a variety of methods can be used to derive an estimate of left ventricular ejection fraction. The most accurate methods use imaging in two orthogonal planes or a 3D technique to model the whole left ventricle (Fig. 3.2.10).

The normal ejection fraction (calculated from the end-diastolic and end-systolic volumes) is greater than 55%. An ejection fraction of 45 to 54% equates to mild left ventricular dysfunction, 30 to 44% to moderate dysfunction, and less than 30% to severe dysfunction.

In patients with ischaemic heart disease, assessment of regional wall motion is valuable. Segments may be described as normokinetic, hypokinetic, akinetic, dyskinetic, or aneurysmal. Detection of a regional wall motion abnormality in patients presenting with left ventricular systolic dysfunction supports an ischaemic aetiology.

The echocardiographic assessment of diastolic dysfunction is complex, but increasingly important in the assessment of patients with heart failure presenting with a normal ejection fraction. Impaired diastolic filling is indicated by a combination of echocardiographic findings routinely measured. Measurements of early diastolic filling E (the peak early diastolic flow velocity) compared to that associated with atrial filling (A) giving an E/A ratio greater than 1.0 are often used as an indicator of diastolic dysfunction but rely on the patient being in sinus rhythm and can be misleading in severe diastolic dysfunction where pseudo normalization may occur. The ratio of tissue Doppler measurement of peak early diastolic mitral annular tissue velocities (e') in combination with peak early diastolic filling (E) providing a ratio (E/e') is also used as an indicator of diastolic dysfunction. A ratio greater than 15 is strongly supportive of diastolic dysfunction. The presence of an enlarged left atrium is an important discriminator as left atrial size is rarely normal in the presence of significant diastolic dysfunction. These parameters are commonly abnormal in the elderly population and only support a diagnosis of diastolic heart failure in conjunction with appropriate clinical features.

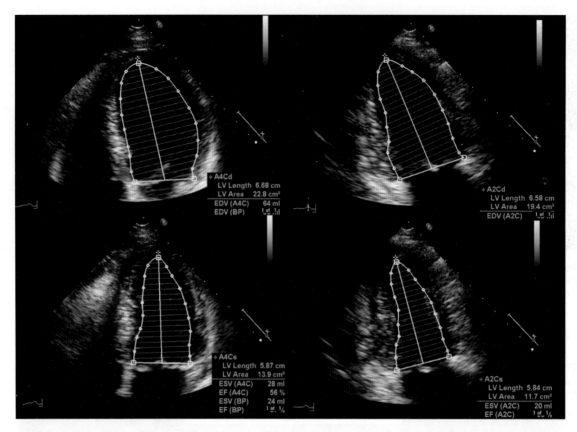

Fig. 3.2.10 Apical four-chamber and two-chamber views in end diastole and end systole with an overall ejection fraction derived from the change in volume.

Pulmonary artery pressure

Estimation of pulmonary artery pressure from a tricuspid regurgitant jet is possible from the majority of echocardiographic examinations (see above). Causes of an elevated pulmonary artery systolic pressure (>35 mmHg) include left heart failure, valvular disease (particularly mitral valve disease), pulmonary embolic disease, chronic obstructive airways disease, and pulmonary vascular disease.

Left ventricular hypertrophy

Left ventricular hypertrophy is detected by echocardiography and a measurement of left ventricular mass can also be derived. Transthoracic echocardiography may also detect intracardiac thrombus, particularly in patients with impaired systolic ventricular function (Fig. 3.2.11).

Minor concentric left ventricular hypertrophy is common in patients with hypertension. In hypertrophic cardiomyopathy, 2D imaging may demonstrate asymmetrical septal hypertrophy with disproportionate thickening of the interventricular septum compared with the left ventricular free wall, or dramatic concentric hypertrophy with left ventricular cavity obliteration. Other characteristic features of hypertrophic cardiomyopathy include systolic anterior motion of the mitral valve and partial midsystolic closure of the aortic valve, which usually correlates with the presence of outflow tract obstruction. In the absence of conditions that may induce ventricular hypertrophy (e.g. aortic stenosis), these findings are diagnostic of hypertrophic cardiomyopathy. Colour Doppler can demonstrate turbulence in the outflow tract and continuous-wave Doppler may detect characteristic 'dynamic' gradients that

increase in severity as systole progresses. Other associated echocardiographic abnormalities in hypertrophic cardiomyopathy include mitral regurgitation and severe diastolic dysfunction.

Atrial fibrillation

Most patients with atrial fibrillation should undergo echocardiography as it excludes a structural cause for atrial fibrillation (e.g. mitral stenosis) and facilitates thromboembolic risk stratification. It also allows measurement of left atrial dimensions, which

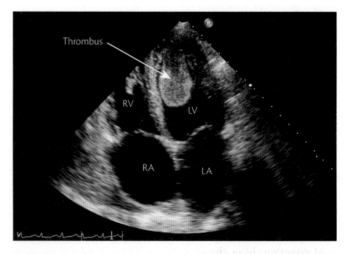

Fig. 3.2.11 Apical four-chamber view showing the left ventricle (LV), left atrium (LA), right ventricle (RV), and right atrium (RA). There is a large thrombus attached to the left ventricular apical septum.

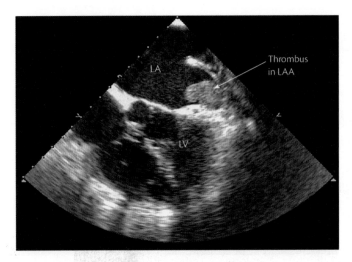

Fig. 3.2.12 Transoesophageal echocardiography of a patient with atrial fibrillation. There is a large thrombus filling (and extending from) the left atrial appendage (LAA). LA, left atrium; LV, left ventricle.

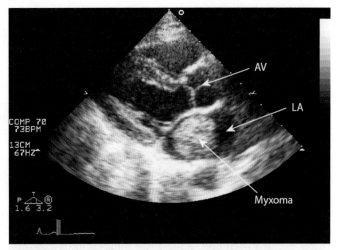

Fig. 3.2.13 Transoesophageal echocardiography revealing a large myxoma in the left atrium (LA) and close to the mitral valve.

is valuable as cardioversion is less likely to be successful when this is large. Identification of left ventricular hypertrophy can guide the choice of antiarrhythmic drug therapy. Transoesophageal echocardiography can be useful to facilitate cardioversion in patients with atrial fibrillation of unknown duration by excluding intracardiac thrombus, particularly in the left atrial appendage (Fig. 3.2.12).

Following an embolic event or stroke

Echocardiography is the investigation of choice when a cardiac source of an embolus is suspected. It should be considered in all patients presenting with embolic occlusion of a peripheral artery, or thromboembolic episodes in more than one vascular territory. Echocardiography should not, however, be performed in circumstances when the result is unlikely to influence patient management. In patients with ischaemic stroke and a low likelihood of atheromatous arterial disease, an echocardiogram can be considered as, occasionally, it will detect occult abnormalities such as a cardiac thrombus or atrial myxoma (Fig. 3.2.13). Contrast studies with Valsalva manoeuvre should be considered to exclude paradoxical embolism through a cardiac shunt from the right heart. In patients with a high clinical suspicion of a cardiac source of embolus, in whom transthoracic echocardiography is normal, transoesophageal echocardiography is recommended.

Pericardial disease

Echocardiography is not routinely indicated in patients with uncomplicated pericarditis. It can, however, diagnose the presence of pericardial fluid and is useful when a pericardial effusion is suspected and percutaneous drainage is being considered. Echocardiographic signs of pericardial tamponade include exaggerated respiratory variation in the mitral valve Doppler, presystolic closure of the aortic valve, and (particularly) right atrial and right ventricular diastolic collapse (Fig. 3.2.14). Constrictive pericarditis is a difficult diagnosis to make using standard echocardiographic techniques. Patients may complain of episodic breathlessness and fluid retention, have characteristic abnormalities of the venous pressure, and have subtle abnormalities on mitral and tricuspid valve inflow Doppler patterns.

Pulmonary embolism

Echocardiography can be useful in patients with pulmonary embolism as it can demonstrate right ventricular dilation and/or impaired right ventricular systolic function. Tricuspid regurgitant velocity can be used to estimate pulmonary artery systolic pressure, although it is unusual for this to be more than 70 mmHg acutely. Exceptionally, 2D imaging may show a thrombus within the right heart or the proximal pulmonary arteries. Although echocardiography is diagnostically useful when it demonstrates features consistent with pulmonary embolism, it cannot exclude the diagnosis.

Infective endocarditis

Echocardiography cannot be used to exclude endocarditis but is valuable when endocarditis is suspected clinically while there is insufficient data to make a formal diagnosis. Under these circumstances, a typical vegetation (Fig. 3.2.15) detected by an experienced observer is regarded as a major criterion in the Duke diagnostic classification, and this may facilitate appropriate management.

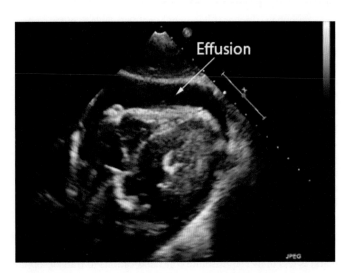

Fig. 3.2.14 Apical four-chamber view demonstrating a large pericardial effusion. There is collapse of the right ventricle suggesting cardiac tamponade.

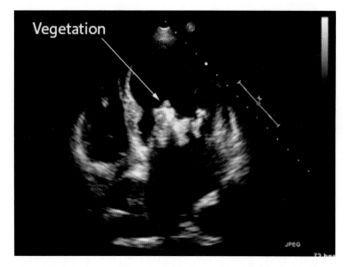

Fig. 3.2.15 Apical four-chamber view demonstrating a large vegetation involving the mitral valve.

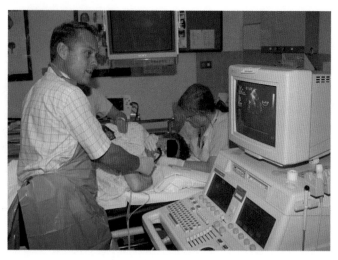

Fig. 3.2.16 Transoesophageal echocardiography.

Transoesophageal echocardiography should be performed when there is a suspicion of aortic root abscess, if prosthetic endocarditis is suspected, or occasionally, in cases where there is persistent diagnostic doubt and the additional sensitivity and spatial resolution of echocardiography might be valuable.

Congenital heart disease

Echocardiography is the diagnostic modality of choice for patients with suspected congenital heart disease. Detailed transthoracic cardiac imaging is possible in cooperative infants and children, but occasionally sedation or a short anaesthetic may be required. Rates of cardiac catheterization have been reduced by miniaturization of transoesophageal probes that facilitate diagnosis and follow-up of complex congenital heart disease.

Fetal echocardiography is performed when surveillance obstetric ultrasound is abnormal or in cases where previous history suggests a possible cardiac problem.

Transoesophageal echocardiography

Transoesophageal echocardiography is now available in many centres (Fig. 3.2.16). The ultrasound probe is similar to the endoscope used for upper gastrointestinal investigation, except that there are no optical fibres. Transoesophageal echocardiography is an invasive procedure for which the patient's written consent is (usually) required. After fasting for a minimum of 4h, a local anaesthetic spray (10% lidocaine) is applied to the upper pharynx and the patient is usually sedated, typically with a short-acting intravenous benzodiazepine (e.g. midazolam 2mg). The probe is manipulated into the oesophagus where its position behind the heart produces excellent resolution, particularly of posterior cardiac structures. Blood pressure and oxygen saturation are monitored throughout, and both resuscitation equipment and the benzodiazepine antagonist flumazenil should be readily available.

Even though transoesophageal echocardiography is commonly performed in high-risk, haemodynamically unstable patients, the rate of serious complications (aspiration and oesophageal rupture/tears) is less than 1%. Absolute contraindications to transoesophageal echocardiography include oesophageal tumours, strictures, diverticulae, and varices.

Who should have a transoesophageal echocardiogram?

The principal indications for transoesophageal echocardiography are listed in Box 3.2.1. The principal advantages over transthoracic imaging are improved spatial resolution and the ability to image posterior structures such as the left atrium and descending aorta. It is valuable in a number of emergency situations, including suspected aortic dissection, prosthetic mechanical valve failure, and possible endocarditis. Transoesophageal echocardiography may be used to image the heart in patients in whom data from transthoracic imaging is unsatisfactory due to obesity, lung disease, or chest deformity. Other indications include screening for left atrial thrombus before cardioversion of atrial fibrillation, and monitoring cardiac performance during cardiac and some noncardiac surgery.

Valve disease

Patients with mitral stenosis are at particular risk of thromboembolism, and transthoracic echocardiography has limited sensitivity for the detection of left atrial thrombus. Transoesophageal echocardiography is recommended in those patients with mitral stenosis if embolic events occur despite therapeutic anticoagulation, and may demonstrate spontaneous echocardiography contrast (smoke-like echoes produced by the interaction of erythrocytes and plasma proteins under conditions of stasis). This is an independent predictor of left atrial thrombus and cardiac thromboembolic events. Transoesophageal echocardiography is also used to assess anatomy and exclude left atrial thrombus before balloon valvuloplasty in patients with mitral stenosis and to assess anatomy, severity, and suitability for surgical repair in patients with mitral regurgitation. In patients with mitral prostheses, reverberation artefact overlying the left atrium limits the ability of transthoracic imaging to detect paraprosthetic regurgitation. Transoesophageal imaging provides excellent visualization of the left atrium and is particularly recommended under these circumstances.

Endocarditis

Characteristic vegetations or evidence of abscess formation identified by echocardiography are increasingly used as diagnostic criteria in patients with possible endocarditis. The excellent spatial resolution (<1 mm) of transoesophageal echocardiography makes it

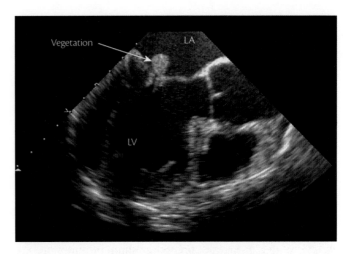

Fig. 3.2.17 Transoesophageal echocardiography demonstrating a large vegetation attached to the mitral valve. LA, left atrium; LV, left ventricle.

superior to transthoracic imaging for the detection of vegetations and its sensitivity may exceed 90% (Fig. 3.2.17). Transoesophageal echocardiography should be considered when there is a high clinical suspicion of endocarditis but blood cultures are sterile and transthoracic imaging is not diagnostic, or under circumstances when the sensitivity of transthoracic imaging is particularly poor, for example prosthetic valves or calcific valvular disease. Transoesophageal echocardiography is also recommended if there is a possibility of aortic root abscess formation as this complication is not easily identified using transthoracic imaging and surgery may be required.

Aortic disease

Transthoracic imaging of the aorta is limited to the proximal aortic root and the arch in most patients. Using transoesophageal imaging,

most of the ascending and the entire descending thoracic aorta can be visualized and image quality is improved. This is particularly useful in patients with suspected acute aortic dissection and, in many cases, it is the only imaging necessary before emergency surgery (see Chapter 14.1, Figs. 14.1.8 and 14.1.9). Large, mobile, or pedunculated aortic atheromas in the descending aorta which can be associated with ischaemic stroke may be detected by transoesophageal echocardiography (Fig. 3.2.18). Transoesophageal imaging of the aorta has also been recommended in suspected cases of cholesterol embolization and to assess thromboembolic risk prior to cardiac intervention or surgery.

Thromboembolism

In patients with thromboembolism, there has been extensive debate over the value of imaging with transoesophageal echocardiography. Clinical examination, electrocardiography, and transthoracic echocardiography provide sufficient information to determine optimal management in the majority. However, transoesophageal echocardiography is indicated when embolic events occur in anticoagulated patients with native or prosthetic valvular

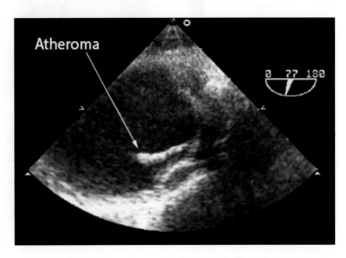

Fig. 3.2.18 Transoesophageal echocardiography of the descending aorta (AO). There is a prominent, eccentric and mobile atherosclerotic plaque.

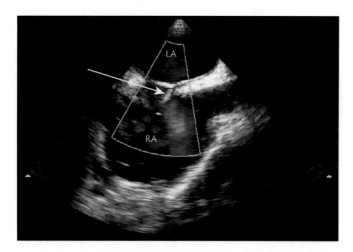

Fig. 3.2.19 Transoesophageal echocardiography of the interatrial septum. The flap of the patent foramen ovale can be seen where the septum primum is overlapped by the septum secundum. There is colour flow through it (arrowed) from the left atrium (LA) to the right atrium (RA).

heart disease, especially if endocarditis is suspected, or when transthoracic images are inconclusive. In patients with unexplained or cryptogenic ischaemic stroke, wider use of transoesophageal echocardiography has been advocated. Transthoracic echocardiography and exclusion of alternative pathologies such as thrombophilia and carotid stenoses should precede the transoesophageal examination, but under these circumstances minor cardiac structural abnormalities are more likely to be clinically relevant.

Transoesophageal echocardiography is superior to the transthoracic approach for imaging the interatrial septum for atrial septal aneurysm (a redundant bulge in the area of the fossa ovale, with respiratory movement >10 mm) and assessing patency of the foramen ovale (Fig. 3.2.19). However, the clinical relevance of such atrial septal abnormalities can be questionable as the relationship

to the thromboembolic event is commonly speculative. Currently, anticoagulation is the usual management following an otherwise unexplained, single, embolic event, but occasionally a percutaneous or surgical correction of the defect is recommended.

Stress echocardiography

Diagnosis of reversible ischaemic myocardial dysfunction is now possible using echocardiography. Imaging can be performed either during or immediately after exercise, but more commonly an intravenous infusion of dobutamine is used to mimic the cardiac response to exercise. Development of reversible systolic regional wall motion abnormalities suggests coronary artery disease. Stress echocardiography also has an increasing role in risk stratification before general surgical procedures and in assessing myocardial viability before revascularization. The use of transpulmonary contrast agents to opacify the left ventricle and enhance endocardial definition greatly reduces the number of inconclusive scans, allows more accurate assessment of left ventricular function, and allows some measure of myocardial perfusion to be made (Fig. 3.2.20).

Intracardiac echocardiography

Miniaturization of echocardiography probes has led to the development of echocardiography from within the heart. Small, flexible catheters with ultrasound transducers (Fig. 3.2.21) can be manoeuvred within the heart to provide very high resolution images of intracardiac structures. This has been particularly useful during percutaneous closure of atrial septal defects and during radiofrequency ablation procedures (Fig. 3.2.22).

Three-dimensional echocardiography

Real-time, 3D image acquisitions with both transthoracic and transoesophageal echocardiography are now available on most

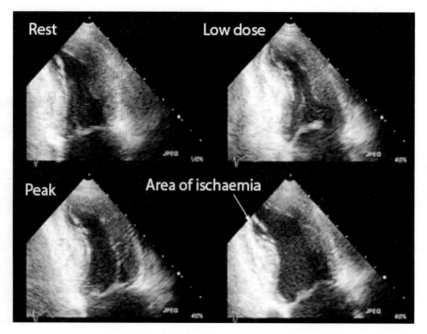

Fig. 3.2.20 A sequence of apical two-chamber images during a stress echo. At peak stress a wall motion abnormality in the inferior apex is evidence which persists into the recovery phase.

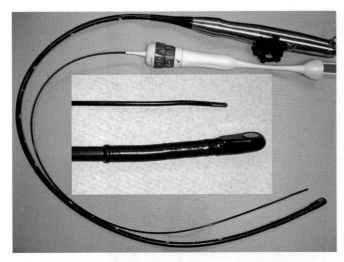

Fig. 3.2.21 Comparison of an intracardiac echocardiography probe with a standard transoeophogeal echocardiography probe with a close-up view of the tip of the probes. The intracardiac probes are for single use only; the transoeophogeal probes are sterilized after each procedure.

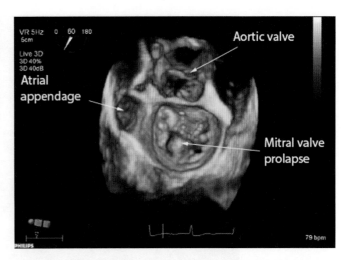

Fig. 3.2.23 3D transoesophageal echocardiography of the mitral valve. The images show prolapse of the central portion of the posterior leaflet with three ruptured chordae. The whole of the mitral valve is in view and oriented to mimic the view of the cardiac surgeon at the time of mitral valve repair.

high-end echocardiography machines. Some systems acquire a series of gated images to reconstruct the entire heart during a cardiac cycle. This image can then be manoeuvred and slices cut away to visualize the area of interest (Fig. 3.2.23). Regional wall tracking can also allow a 3D model of left ventricular function to be acquired and provides an accurate assessment of left ventricular function (Fig. 3.2.24) as well as identifying areas of left ventricular dysynchrony. Transthoracic 3D acquisition is limited by frame rate and image quality in the same way as 2D echocardiography. Transoesophageal 3D echocardiography usually produces clear 3D images particularly of the mitral valve and is excellent for examination of prosthetic mitral valves (Fig 3.2.25). It is particularly helpful in displaying and communicating pathology, as views familiar to cardiac surgeons can be recreated and displayed.

Echocardiography in the emergency setting

Echocardiography equipment increases in sophistication but also continues to miniaturize, and now several small portable ultrasound

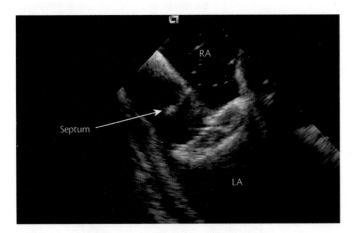

Fig. 3.2.22 Intracardiac echocardiography from the right atrium (RA). An atrial septal defect is being closed using a percutaneous approach. The disk in the left atrium (LA) has been deployed and is about to be pulled tight to the interatrial septum.

devices are available (Fig. 3.2.26). These are increasingly available in emergency and intensive care departments. A hand-held 'screening ultrasound' can be performed in a matter of seconds to exclude pericardial effusion, recognize left ventricular dysfunction or pulmonary embolism and to diagnose most valvular abnormalities. This is proving extremely useful in the management of critically ill patients.

It is important to recognize that these devices cannot perform a full echocardiogram and a more detailed study is needed if the screening scan is abnormal or inconclusive. In critically ill patients with sepsis or severe metabolic derangement left ventricular function is often abnormal; however, this is not always imply that left ventricular dysfunction is the cause of the presentation. Repeat examination following treatment of the underlying illness often reveals that this finding is transient and is not always an indication of primary cardiac disease.

The advent of portable ultrasound has prompted the development of several types of emergency ultrasound including:

◆ FAST scan—focused assessment with sonography for trauma

◆ FEEL scan—focused echocardiography in emergency life support

◆ FICE scan—focused intensive care echocardiography

◆ FATE scan—focused transthoracic echocardiography

Each of these require specific training, mentoring, and accreditation to become proficient. Full training in transthoracic echocardiography typically requires 2 years and over 500 scans performed and reported.

Limitations of echocardiography

Despite the rapid and major advances in ultrasound technology and the widespread use of echocardiography it is important to recognize and understand the limitations of the technique. These include:

◆ Reliance on acoustic windows—clear images are impossible in some patients.

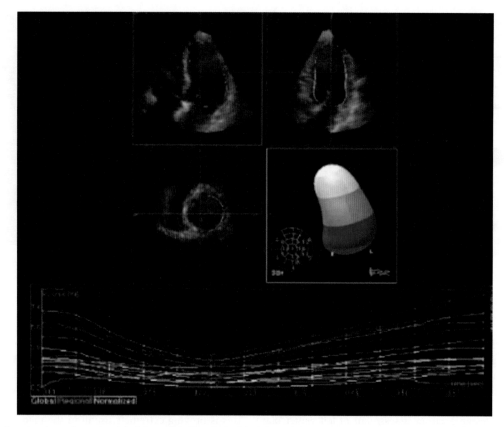

Fig. 3.2.24 3D transthoracic echocardiography of the left ventricle. The whole of the left ventricle is captured over four cardiac cycles and stitched together to create a single volume of data. Corrections for foreshortening can be made, the volume traced over time, and a 3D 'model' of the left ventricle created with each segment shaded a different colour.

◆ Evaluation at rest—the vast majority of echo is performed with the patient resting so dynamic lesions such as outflow tract gradients of mitral regurgitation can be underestimated.

◆ Subjective assessments—precise quantification of cardiac function and valve disease can be challenging and often a more subjective opinion is required, which depends critically on the operator's experience and training.

◆ Evaluation of complex structures such as the right ventricle remains a major challenge—3D techniques are showing promise but are not in mainstream use.

◆ The scope of an 'echo' is broad indeed and to measure every parameter possible would take more than 60 min. Like any other test, it is most powerful when the pre-test probability has been

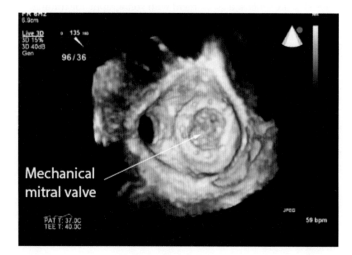

Fig. 3.2.25 3D transthoracic echocardiography of a mechanical prosthetic mitral valve. The sutures placed by the surgeon are visible as a row of dots around the sewing ring.

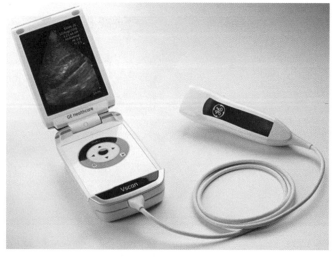

Fig. 3.2.26 Hand-carried ultrasound allows rapid assessment of cardiac function and can exclude a pericardial effusion.

considered and a specific question asked: for example, 'Is there important aortic stenosis to explain symptoms and signs?'

Further reading

Cheitlin MD, *et al.* (2003). ACC/AHA/ASE guideline update for the clinical application of echocardiography: summary article. *Circulation*, **108**, 1146.

Douglas PS, *et al.*(2011) ACCF/ASE/AHA/ASNC/HFSA/HRS/SCAI/ SCCM/SCCT/SCMR 2011 appropriate use criteria for echocardiography. *J Am Soc Echo*, **24**, 229.

Feigenbaum H (2004). *Feigenbaum's echocardiography*. Lea & Febiger, Philadelphia, PA.

Flachskampf FA, *et al.* (2001). Recommendations for performing transesophageal echocardiography. *Euro J Echocardiol*, **2**, 8.

Leeson P, Becher H, Mitchell ARJ (2007). *Echocardiography*. Oxford University Press, Oxford.

Rimington H, Chambers J (1998). *Echocardiography: a practical guide for reporting*. Parthenon, London.

Zoghbi WA, *et al.* (2003). Recommendations for evaluation of the severity of native valvular regurgitation with two-dimensional and Doppler echocardiography. *J Am Soc Echo*, **16**, 777.

CHAPTER 3.3

Cardiac investigations: nuclear and other imaging techniques

Nikant Sabharwal, Andrew Kelion, Theodoros Karamitsos, and Stefan Neubauer

Essentials

Myocardial perfusion scintigraphy

Myocardial perfusion scintigraphy (MPS) provides physiological information about the coronary circulation, in contrast to the anatomical information provided by angiography.

Three radionuclide-labelled perfusion tracers are routinely used in single photon emission computed tomography (SPECT) imaging: thallium-201 and the technetium-99 m-labelled complexes sestamibi and tetrofosmin. Imaging is performed following tracer injection during stress (exercise or pharmacological) and at rest; comparison allows determination of whether regional perfusion is normal, or if there is inducible hypoperfusion or infarction/scar.

Myocardial perfusion imaging is minimally invasive, and—in contrast to other methods of investigation—can be performed regardless of overall exercise capacity, abnormalities of the resting electrocardiogram (ECG), pacemakers, obesity, claustrophobia, renal dysfunction, iodine allergy, or acoustic windows.

In the investigation of a patient with possible coronary artery disease, a normal SPECT study is very reassuring, predicting a very low chance of cardiac death or nonfatal myocardial infarction over the following few years (<1% per year). High-risk markers on SPECT provide additional prognostic value to clinical, exercise test, and even angiographic variables, and decisions about revascularization can be usefully informed by SPECT imaging.

ECG-gated SPECT allows images to be taken throughout the cardiac cycle, when comparison of end-systolic and end-diastolic images then allows volumetric analysis and calculation of left ventricular ejection fraction.

Positron emission tomography (PET)

Using PET, myocardial perfusion imaging can be performed with nitrogen-13 ammonia or rubidium-82, and metabolic imaging with fluorine-18 fluorodeoxyglucose (FDG). Cardiac PET is expensive, but image quality is superior to SPECT and absolute flow quantification is possible. PET is gaining a significant foothold in the developed world, largely driven by the roll-out of scanners for oncological imaging and the availability of generator-supplied rubidium-82 as a perfusion tracer. Imaging using oxygen-15-water is considered the gold standard for absolute quantification of myocardial perfusion (though static perfusion images cannot be obtained), and metabolic imaging with FDG occupies the same position in the assessment of myocardial viability.

Cardiac MRI

MRI uses the magnetic properties of the hydrogen nucleus, radio waves, and powerful magnets, to provide high-quality still and cine images of the cardiovascular system with and without the use of exogenous contrast (gadolinium). Cardiovascular MRI (CMR) is the gold standard method for the three-dimensional analysis of cardiothoracic anatomy, the assessment of global and regional myocardial function, and viability imaging (late gadolinium enhancement technique). Using first-pass perfusion imaging under vasodilator stress, CMR has high diagnostic accuracy for the identification of myocardial ischaemia. Oedema imaging using T2-weighted techniques is useful for the identification of acute coronary syndromes and myocardial inflammation. Coronary MRI is feasible, and particularly indicated for anomalous coronaries. Its spatial and temporal resolution is inferior to CT or conventional angiography, and the identification and grading of stenoses remains challenging. Molecular imaging may in future allow visualization of unstable plaque. Novel techniques such as T1 and T2 mapping have been recently developed and offer a quantitative measure of tissue characteristics. CMR also provides important prognostic data for many cardiovascular diseases. CMR is now an essential component of an advanced cardiovascular imaging service, and it is anticipated that its role will continue to grow.

Cardiac CT

Multidetector computed tomography (MDCT) is a fast and noninvasive method for the visualization of the coronary arteries. In comparison to CT imaging of other organs, it requires a scanner with at least 64 detectors and ECG gating. CT can be used to assess the overall burden of coronary atheroma in terms of calcification, and angiographic images can be obtained following power injection of iodinated X-ray contrast.

The spatial and temporal resolution of cardiac CT remains inferior to invasive angiography. Its positive predictive value is limited by artefacts, particularly in relation to calcified plaques, though in experienced hands this may be less of a problem than the literature suggests. However, the great strength of the technique lies in its extremely high negative predictive value, which exceeds 99% in most studies. Hence cardiac CT is an excellent test to rule out coronary stenoses in patients with low to intermediate likelihood of disease. With further technical developments it is likely that coronary CT will replace invasive coronary angiography for many diagnostic purposes.

Nuclear imaging

Introduction to myocardial perfusion scintigraphy

Myocardial perfusion scintigraphy (MPS) can provide information on (1) viable vs infarcted myocardium on the resting scan; (2) inducible hypoperfusion on the stress scan (in comparison with rest); and (3) regional and global left ventricular function, both at rest and post-stress.

The procedure is versatile and minimally invasive, and is not limited by overall exercise capacity, abnormalities of the resting ECG, pacemakers, obesity, claustrophobia, renal dysfunction, iodine allergy, or acoustic windows. Indeed, it is very difficult to identify any patient who is not suitable for nuclear perfusion imaging, and as a result the technique has matured into a first-line procedure for the assessment of coronary artery disease in many countries. Over 5 million nuclear cardiology procedures were undertaken in the United States of America in 2001.

Basic principles of MPS

An intravenous injection of a radiopharmaceutical tracer is administered, which enters intact myocardial cells and is retained within them to allow time for subsequent imaging.

Usually, the comparison of stress and rest images determines whether regional myocardial perfusion is uniform, or if there are inducible or reversible perfusion defects (corresponding to inducible ischaemia) or fixed perfusion defects (corresponding to infarction) (Fig. 3.3.1).

There are currently three radiopharmaceutical perfusion tracers used in single photon emission computed tomography (SPECT) imaging: thallium-201, and two technetium-99 m-labelled agents, sestamibi and tetrofosmin. All are monovalent cations, roughly the same size as a hydrated potassium ion. Following injection, they are delivered to the myocardium in proportion to blood supply, and enter the cells down the electrochemical gradient.

Thallous-201 chloride has been in use since the mid-1970s. It is produced in a commercial cyclotron, and has a half-life of 73 h. It emits photons of varying energies (predominantly 68–80 keV). Following myocardial uptake, thallium-201 gradually re-equilibrates with the extracellular space (redistribution). Therefore, following injection of 80 MBq during stress (exercise or pharmacological), imaging must be performed immediately (within 10 min). A redistribution scan 3–4 h later reflects resting viability/perfusion without the need for a second injection. Nevertheless, a second injection of thallium (40 MBq) may be administered at rest to optimize the assessment of myocardial viability.

Sestamibi and tetrofosmin are organic complexes with technetium-99 m. Technetium-99 m is widely available in nuclear medicine departments from a generator, and is used to label a freeze-dried product in a vial. Technetium-99 m emits γ-rays at 140 keV and has a half-life of 6 h. Sestamibi and tetrofosmin bind to intracellular components, and hence their distribution at the time of imaging (typically 30–60 min after injection) reflects myocardial perfusion at the time of injection. Separate injections are required for stress and rest imaging, either on separate days (typically 400 MBq on each day) or on the same day (with a larger second dose—750 MBq after 250 MBq—to swamp residual activity). Sublingual glyceryl trinitrate (GTN) can be given before the resting injection of sestamibi or tetrofosmin to maximize the detection of myocardial viability.

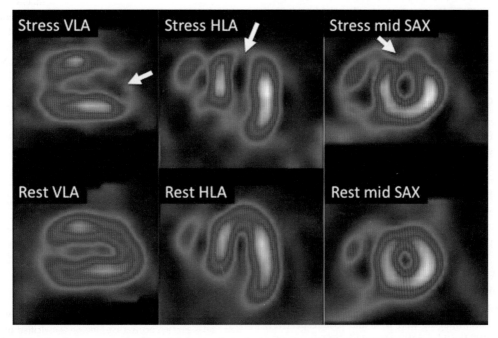

Fig. 3.3.1 Myocardial perfusion imaging—an example of inducible hypoperfusion in the anterior wall and apex. Panels from left to right show representative vertical long axis (VLA), horizontal long axis (HLA), and mid short-axis (SAX) slices, with stress above rest. The white arrows show a perfusion defect on the stress slices which resolves at rest.

Photons emitted from the patient are imaged by a gamma camera, the head of which is essentially a large crystal of sodium iodide. Absorption of a gamma photon produces a burst of photons within the visible range (scintillation), which is detected by underlying photomultiplier tubes. The gamma camera rotates around the patient over a 180° arc from right anterior oblique (RAO) to left posterior oblique (LPO). A planar image is acquired at each of a series of 32–64 steps, and these can be gated to the patient's ECG to provide functional information on the processed scan. Acquisition usually takes 15–20 min. The planar projections are reconstructed to give sets of vertical long-axis, horizontal long-axis, and short-axis slices. Stress and rest slices are viewed side by side to facilitate comparison.

A new generation of gamma cameras is becoming available, which use cadmium zinc telluride (CZT) as solid-state detectors, rather than sodium iodide. These cameras have far higher sensitivity and spatial resolution, offering the potential for substantially reduced acquisition times (2–5 min) and/or tracer dose reductions.

Principles of stress testing for MPS

The wide range of stress modalities available to nuclear cardiology is one of its major advantages. Exercise (or physiological) stress can be achieved with a treadmill or bicycle following a specified protocol, such as the Bruce protocol. This is the preferred method, mimicking 'real world' stress and providing valuable physiological data. The increase in myocardial oxygen demand provokes secondary coronary arteriolar dilatation. The radiopharmaceutical is injected at peak stress, and the patient maintains exercise for a further 1–2 min while it is being taken up by the myocardium.

Patients unable to exercise can undergo pharmacological stress. Vasodilators such as adenosine or dipyridamole can be injected or infused intravenously to induce maximal coronary arteriolar dilatation, provoking flow heterogeneity between coronary vascular beds. These two vasodilators are contraindicated in patients with significant airways disease and unpaced second- or third-degree atrioventricular block. Regadenoson is a recently introduced selective adenosine A_{2A} receptor agonist which can safely be used in asthmatics. For patients unable to exercise where there is a contraindication to a vasodilator drug, inotropic stress with escalating doses of dobutamine (± atropine) can be used.

Some practical considerations for MPS

The overall radiation exposure of a patient undergoing a stress-rest technetium study is 8–10 mSv, which is greater than for a diagnostic coronary angiogram, but without the invasive and vascular complications.

Cost-effectiveness studies have been performed with SPECT in both Europe and the United States of America. In general, diagnostic strategies that utilize MPS are more cost-effective than those that do not. This has helped to drive a significant increase in the number of SPECT procedures performed worldwide.

Clinical value of MPS in the investigation of known or suspected coronary artery disease

In a large meta-analysis of 33 studies the sensitivity and specificity of myocardial perfusion imaging were 87% and 73% respectively. The normalcy rate, which removes the referral bias of false-positive

patients being referred on for coronary angiography, was 91%. Similar results are available for vasodilator and dobutamine stress. More importantly, a wealth of prognostic data is available. The value of a normal SPECT study is beyond doubt, with a meta-analysis including just under 21 000 patients followed up for 2.3 years demonstrating a risk of cardiac death or nonfatal myocardial infarction of 0.7% per year. Follow-up studies extending up to 7 years have demonstrated similar low event rates.

High-risk markers on SPECT have incremental prognostic value over electrocardiographic and clinical variables. They include multivessel disease patterns, a large burden of ischaemia (>10% of myocardium), transient ischaemic left ventricular dilatation, left ventricular ejection fraction (LVEF) <0.4 (see 'Assessment of left ventricular volume and function'), and lung uptake (only with thallium-201).

SPECT is also able to add prognostic data when risk scores such as the Duke treadmill score are applied to exercise ECG variables (Fig. 3.3.2), and can stratify risk in specific populations such as patients after myocardial infarction or with diabetes mellitus, women, and patients with an abnormal ECG (e.g. left bundle branch block).

More recent data have emphasized the value of MPS even in patients with proven coronary artery disease. In a large retrospective study from Cedars-Sinai Hospital (Los Angeles, California), patients managed conservatively had higher event rates than those managed with revascularization if they had inducible hypoperfusion that was more extensive than 10% of the left ventricular myocardium (see Fig. 3.3.3). The COURAGE trial failed to show any prognostic benefit of percutaneous coronary intervention (PCI) plus optimal medical therapy (OMT) over OMT alone. However, a nuclear substudy suggested that PCI was better at reducing inducible hypoperfusion than OMT alone, and that event rates were lower for patients with greater decreases in inducible hypoperfusion. The implication, which requires further research, is that MPS could be used to identify a subgroup of patients in whom, despite OMT, the prognosis could be improved by PCI.

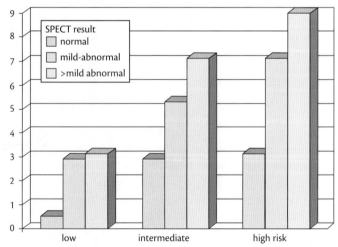

hard events/year (%)

SPECT result
- normal
- mild-abnormal
- >mild abnormal

Result of exercise ECG (Duke treadmill score)

Fig. 3.3.2 Incremental value of myocardial perfusion imaging over exercise ECG: hard event rates per year as a function of exercise SPECT in patients initially stratified by low, intermediate, and high Duke treadmill scores.

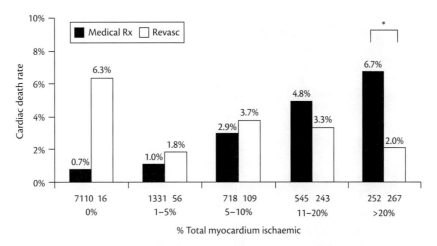

Fig. 3.3.3 Annualized cardiac death rate according to ischaemic burden and treatment strategy. Increasing ischaemia appears to be better treated with revascularization in this retrospective study.
From Hachamovitch, R. et al, 'Comparison of the Short-Term Survival Benefit Associated With Revascularization Compared With Medical Therapy in Patients With No Prior Coronary Artery Disease Undergoing Stress Myocardial Perfusion Single Photon Emission Computed Tomography', *Circulation*. 2003; 107: 2900–2907.

Nuclear techniques are well suited to the identification of myocardial viability, which predicts functional recovery (identified by echocardiography) in approximately 80% of dysfunctional segments after revascularization. Comparative studies with low-dose dobutamine echocardiography (see Chapter 3.2), positron emission tomography (PET), and cardiovascular magnetic resonance (CMR) have been performed. Each test is broadly similar in its ability to predict functional recovery. SPECT has also been used to assess success of revascularization procedures.

In the acute setting, resting SPECT may be performed in patients attending the Emergency Department with chest pain and a nondiagnostic initial ECG. A normal perfusion scan is associated with a low risk of future events, lower likelihood of requiring cardiac catheterization, and lower costs owing to the shorter hospital stay and fewer subsequent investigations.

Assessment of left ventricular volume and function using nuclear techniques

Nuclear cardiology techniques have been used for the noninvasive assessment of left ventricular function since the early 1970s. Three radionuclide techniques are available for assessing left ventricular function: first-pass radionuclide ventriculography, equilibrium radionuclide ventriculography, and gated myocardial perfusion SPECT. The first is rarely performed nowadays and will not be considered further.

Equilibrium radionuclide ventriculography (ERNV)

This investigation, also affectionately (but inaccurately) known as multigated acquisition (MUGA), is performed following labelling of red blood cells with technetium-99 m-pertechnetate. This is usually performed *in vivo* following a preceding injection of stannous pyrophosphate. For a simple assessment of LVEF, gated planar imaging of the blood pool is performed in a LAO 45° projection to optimize separation of the left and right ventricular cavities. This method is independent of left ventricular geometry, and hence very accurate and reproducible.

The wide availability of echo (with its lack of radiation exposure) has led to a substantial decrease in the number of ERNV studies performed. However the radionuclide method can still be valuable when a quick and reproducible assessment of LVEF is required, for example in the monitoring of patients undergoing chemotherapy with anthracyclines or trastuzumab.

ECG-gated myocardial perfusion SPECT

SPECT acquisition during MPS can be gated at no extra inconvenience, cost, or risk to the patient. Tomographic slices are reconstructed for each of 8 or 16 frames, and can be played as a cine for visual assessment. Left ventricular volumes and LVEF can be derived following endomyocardial border definition. Gated SPECT (Fig. 3.3.4) can be very useful in identifying attenuation artefacts (which appear as fixed perfusion defects but demonstrate normal wall motion). Indices of left ventricular function (ejection fraction and end-systolic volume) provide independent prognostic information, and in particular are powerful predictors of cardiac death. Importantly, changes in regional and global function from post-stress to rest imaging can help unmask multivessel ischaemia which has been underestimated by the visible regional perfusion defects.

Positron emission tomography (PET)

PET scanners employ coincidence detection of 511-keV photons travelling 180° apart following annihilation of a positron with an electron. Perfusion can be assessed with nitrogen-13-ammonia (requiring an on-site cyclotron) or rubidium-82 (from a generator). Metabolism is assessed with fluorine-18 fluorodeoxyglucose (FDG), which has become widely commercially available with the growth of oncological PET. Absolute myocardial perfusion can be derived using both nitrogen-13-ammonia and rubidium-82, but is best done with oxygen-15-water (though this tracer requires a cyclotron and does not permit myocardial imaging). Cardiac PET studies are no longer confined to research centres, mainly due to the rapid increase in oncological studies requiring combined PET/ CT scanners.

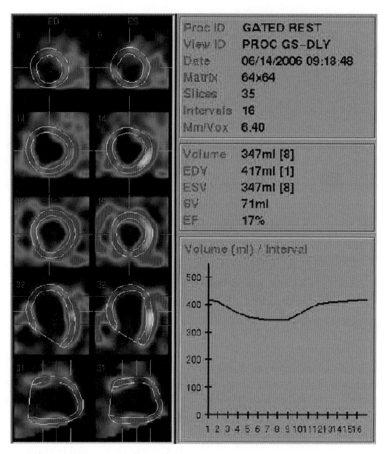

Fig. 3.3.4 Gated SPECT to assess left ventricular systolic function at rest in a patient with an extensive anteroapical and septal infarct and poor left ventricular systolic function. Left column: end-diastolic frame showing (from top to bottom) apical, mid, and basal short-axis slices, horizontal and vertical long-axis slices. Right column: end-systolic frame showing corresponding slices. Right column: calculated volumes and ejection fraction (middle panel), with time-volume curve (bottom panel).

Comparison of nuclear techniques with other imaging modalities

For physiological assessment of known or suspected coronary artery disease, the alternatives to SPECT and PET are exercise electrocardiography, stress (exercise or dobutamine) echocardiography, and stress CMR (with vasodilator stress for perfusion or dobutamine for wall motion). The exercise ECG is inferior, mainly due to its dependence on exercise ability and the poor sensitivity and specificity of ECG changes.

Stress echocardiography is a good alternative technique, with a slightly lower sensitivity but higher specificity in comparative studies. It is physician-intensive and operator-dependent, but harmonic imaging and microbubble contrast agents have greatly improved image quality. An important advantage over the radionuclide techniques is the avoidance of ionizing radiation, which makes it particularly attractive for younger patients.

Cardiac MRI can assess regional and global left ventricular systolic function during a dobutamine infusion, similar to stress echocardiography. Alternatively, gadolinium can be used as a first-pass myocardial perfusion tracer during vasodilator stress, with late-enhancement used to identify infarction. Two recent comparative studies have suggested that CMR is a good alternative to SPECT, though whether it is better remains a matter of controversy.

In practice, the different modalities should be regarded as largely interchangeable, with local clinical expertise being more important than any marginal differences in technical performance between them. Functional imaging, however performed, is recommended in the latest National Institute for Health and Care Excellence (NICE) guidelines for the assessment of patients with chest pain of recent onset.

Cardiac MRI

Introduction

Cardiovascular MRI (CMR) has undergone significant advancement in terms of imaging capabilities, ease of use, and speed of acquisition over the past 15 years. A study of cardiovascular anatomy, left and right ventricular function, and viability/fibrosis (late gadolinium enhancement) with a modern CMR scanner can be performed in less than 30 min by an experienced operator. These improvements have led to the widespread adoption of CMR in clinical practice.

How CMR works

MRI is typically based on the magnetic properties of the hydrogen nucleus, though other nuclei can also be used. Hydrogen nuclei (protons), which are abundant in the human body, behave like small spinning magnets that have an alignment (magnetic moment) parallel to the direction of the external magnetic field and a rotation (*precession*) frequency proportional to the strength of the field. Radio waves in the form of a radiofrequency pulse transmitted into the patient cause the alignment of the protons to change (i.e. the magnetic moments in that region are flipped out at an angle (flip angle) to the magnetic field (*excitation*). When this radiofrequency pulse is turned off, the protons in the patient's body return to their neutral position (*relaxation*), emitting their own weak radio-wave signals, which are detected by receiver coils and used to produce an image. The contrast between tissues (e.g. heart muscle and fat) depends on the tissue density of hydrogen atoms (proton density), and on two distinct MR relaxation processes that affect the net magnetization: the longitudinal relaxation time (T1), and transverse relaxation time (T2). The differences in these parameters in distinct tissues are used to generate contrast in MR images. Image contrast can also be modified by modulating the way the radiofrequency pulses are played out (the MR sequence): For example, in so-called T1-weighted images, myocardial tissue is dark whereas fat is bright. On the other hand, T2-weighted images highlight unbound water in the myocardium and are used to demonstrate myocardial oedema due to inflammation or acute ischaemia.

CMR requires advanced technology, including a high-field superconducting magnet which produces a homogeneous and stable magnetic field (typically 1.5 Tesla, although 3.0-T systems are increasingly being used), gradient coils within the bore of the magnet which generate the gradient fields, a radiofrequency amplifier to excite the spins with radiofrequency pulses, and a radiofrequency antenna (coil), which receives the radio signals coming from the patient. A computer and specific software are also needed to control the scanner and generate (reconstruct) the images. To prevent artefacts from cardiac motion, most CMR images are generated with ultrafast sequences gated to the R wave of the ECG. Respiratory motion, which is another factor that can produce artefacts, is eliminated by acquiring most CMR images in end-expiratory breathhold. When acquisition is long and cannot be completed within one breath-hold, special free-breathing sequences that track the diaphragm's position (navigators) are used.

CMR safety

MRI scan subjects and operators are not exposed to ionizing radiation and there are no known detrimental biological side effects of MRI, if safety guidelines are followed. Ferromagnetic objects can be attracted by the scanner becoming projectiles that could lead to significant patient or operator injury and also damage the scanner. The presence of certain medical implants and devices (e.g. most pacemakers and defibrillators, cochlear implants, cerebrovascular clips) is a contraindication for routine MR scanning, but nearly all prosthetic cardiac valves, coronary and vascular stents, and orthopaedic implants are safe in a 3-T (or less) MR environment. There are now MRI conditional pacemakers (generator and leads) available. Whenever there is uncertainty regarding a particular device or implant, the CMR operator should consult a more detailed source of information, such as reference manuals, dedicated web sites (e.g. <http://www.mrisafety.com>), or the manufacturer's product information when available. Claustrophobia may be a problem in a small minority of patients, and mild sedation usually helps to overcome this. In the vast majority of patients, gadolinium contrast agents are safe—safer than iodine-based contrast. Recently, gadolinium-containing contrast agents have been linked with the development of a rare systemic disorder called nephrogenic systemic fibrosis. The patients at risk for developing this disease are those with acute or chronic severe renal insufficiency (glomerular filtration rate <30 mL/min/1.73 m^2); or acute renal dysfunction of any severity due to the hepatorenal syndrome or in the perioperative liver transplantation period. To date, there is no evidence that other patient groups are at risk. Many MR centres use gadolinium agents that are tightly bound to a cyclic chelate, for which the incidence of nephrogenic systemic fibrosis is near zero. Moreover, it is unknown whether immediate haemodialysis protects against nephrogenic systemic fibrosis. Therefore, gadolinium-based contrast media should be avoided in high-risk patients unless the diagnostic information is essential and not available with noncontrast enhanced CMR or other imaging modalities.

Applications of CMR

Normal and pathological anatomy

Historically, the first widespread application of CMR was the three-dimensional analysis of cardiovascular anatomy. By providing excellent soft tissue contrast, cardiovascular anatomy can be assessed in virtually any imaging plane (coronal, transverse, sagittal), or individualized double-angulated planes. The latter is particularly valuable in complex congenital heart disease.

Myocardial function and mass

CMR is now the accepted gold standard for quantification of left and right ventricular function. Using steady-state free precession techniques that provide excellent delineation of the blood-myocardium interface, long-axis and short-axis cine views (Fig. 3.3.5) can be obtained during all phases of the cardiac cycle (cine-CMR). Planimetry of each short-axis slice and summation of slice volumes allow precise determination of systolic and diastolic left and right ventricular volumes, stroke volumes, and ejection fraction with high reproducibility. Ventricular mass can also be determined by multiplication of the myocardial volume by its specific weight of 1.05 g/cm^3. The excellent inter-study reproducibility of volume and mass measurements by CMR has allowed reductions of sample sizes of 80–97% to achieve the same statistical power for demonstrating a given change in left ventricular volumes, ejection fraction, or cardiac mass.

Analysis of regional myocardial function is feasible both at rest and during pharmacological stress, typically using dobutamine. Dobutamine stress CMR has high sensitivity and specificity for detecting ischaemic heart disease and is particularly useful in patients with difficult acoustic windows.

Blood flow

Phase contrast mapping of velocities through planes transecting blood flow in the main pulmonary artery and the ascending aorta can provide accurate measurements of cardiac output, shunt flow, aortic or pulmonary regurgitation and, indirectly, of mitral and tricuspid regurgitation. For stenotic jets, the peak velocity can be measured on through-plane velocity-encoded images. Peak pressure gradients can be estimated according to the modified Bernoulli equation. Valve morphology can be assessed with the use of SSFP cine images and valve area can be assessed with accuracy by direct planimetry using cross-sectional cine images, although valve structure is generally better assessed by echocardiography. Bicuspid aortic valves or fused valve leaflets can be readily identified. CMR is an excellent technique for the quantitative assessment of regurgitation. If a single valve is affected, the regurgitant volume can be measured from the difference in left and right ventricular stroke volumes. If both the mitral and tricuspid valves are affected, the regurgitant

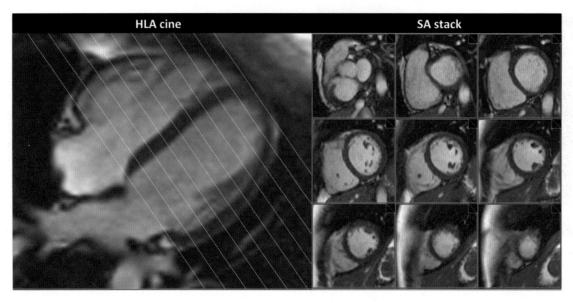

Fig. 3.3.5 End-diastolic still images from multiple contiguous short-axis SSFP cines that encompass the left ventricle, from base to apex. Note the position of the short-axis (SA) slices marked on the still frames of end-diastolic horizontal long axis (HLA) cine image and the excellent delineation of the myocardium from the blood and the surrounding tissue.

volumes can be calculated by subtracting the flow in main pulmonary artery and the ascending aorta, measured by CMR velocity mapping, from the left and right stroke volumes (measured by the volumetric method), respectively. This technique compares favourably with measurements from catheterization and Doppler echocardiography techniques. For pulmonary and aortic regurgitation, direct measurement of regurgitant volume is also possible using CMR velocity mapping. These CMR techniques have high interstudy reproducibility and can be used for the longitudinal follow-up of patients with valve disease over time.

Apart from the evaluation of patients with valve pathologies, flow imaging by CMR is regularly used in assessing patients with congenital heart disease. By measuring flow in the ascending aorta and main pulmonary artery with velocity encoding CMR, the pulmonary-to-systemic flow ratio (Q_p/Q_s) can be determined. These CMR measurements show excellent correlation with calculations obtained from oximetry during haemodynamic catheterization.

Myocardial viability

The assessment of myocardial viability using gadolinium-based contrast agents (late gadonium enhancement—LGE technique) has revolutionized the use of CMR in cardiology. Gadolinium chelates are extracellular tracers that cannot cross cell membranes. In normal myocardium the myocytes are densely packed and the extracellular space and vascular volume represents less than 15% of the myocardial volume, hence after injection of gadolinium there are only few gadolinium molecules in a myocardial sample volume. By contrast, when the membranes of myocytes rupture, gadolinium molecules can penetrate into the myocytes and stay there, even late after gadolinium injection, such that in scar tissue the interstitial space is expanded and increased gadolinium concentration is found (Fig. 3.3.6). In practice, on inversion-recovery T1-weighted sequences obtained 5–10 min after gadolinium administration, nonviable myocardium (scarred or irreversibly injured) shows high signal intensity, whereas normal and viable (stunned, hibernating) myocardium shows low signal intensity.

Myocardial infarction (acute or chronic) has a characteristic LGE pattern due to the wavefront of myocardial necrosis that always involves the subendocardium at the core of the infarct (Fig. 3.3.7). The LGE technique has undergone extensive histopathological validation. The superb spatial resolution of LGE-CMR allows the detection of even small subendocardial infarcts that might otherwise be missed by lower spatial resolution techniques such as SPECT. Several studies have demonstrated an inverse relationship between the transmural extent of myocardial infarction and segmental functional recovery after revascularization. In practice, segments which show more than 50% scarring are considered nonviable, whereas segments with only subendocardial enhancement (<50%)

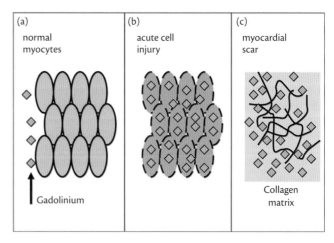

Fig. 3.3.6 Mechanism for late gadolinium enhancement (LGE) in acute and chronic myocardial damage: (a) Densely packed myocytes with intact cell membrane—gadolinium chelates only in the vessels and extracellular space. (b) Acute myocardial damage with ruptured cell membranes of myocytes—intracellular accumulation of gadolinium chelates. (c) Chronic myocardial damage with loss of myoctes and replacement by scar tissue—mostly collagen fibres that are filled with gadolinium chelates.

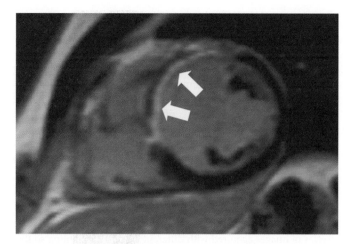

Fig. 3.3.7 Short-axis late gadolinium enhancement (LGE) image at the midventricular level in a patient with near transmural antero-septal myocardial infarction (white arrows).

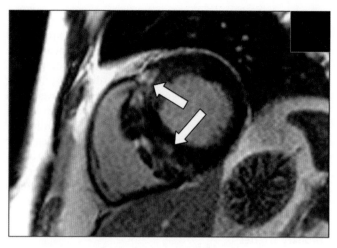

Fig. 3.3.8 Short-axis late gadolinium enhancement (LGE) image at the midventricular level in a patient with hypertrophic cardiomyopathy. Note the patchy LGE due to fibrosis in the hypertrophied septum (white arrows), including both left-right ventricular junctions.

have a high likelihood of functional recovery. CMR can also assess myocardial viability using a low-dose dobutamine protocol in a way analogous to echocardiography, but in practice, this is rarely required. Several CMR techniques, including LGE, can also identify areas of microvascular obstruction (no-reflow phenomenon) after revascularization in patients with acute myocardial infarction.

LGE-CMR in nonischaemic cardiomyopathies

Specific patterns of regional fibrosis and scarring have also been described for many nonischaemic cardiomyopathic processes (Fig. 3.3.8). For example, the majority of patients with hypertrophic cardiomyopathy show patchy fibrosis in the hypertrophied septum involving left/right ventricular junctions, whereas about a third of patients with dilated cardiomyopathy show a midwall band of septal fibrosis. Furthermore, most patients with myocarditis have subepicardial LGE in the lateral left ventricular wall. Several other patterns of LGE exist for other rarer cardiomyopathies such as cardiac amyloidosis or sarcoidosis. The LGE technique is a major part of nearly every scanning protocol and provides valuable diagnostic and pathophysiological insights in both ischaemic and nonischaemic cardiomyopathies.

Myocardial perfusion

Regional myocardial perfusion can be measured during the first pass of a gadolinium-based contrast agent. Using sequential multi-slice fast gradient-echo CMR, passage of the contrast agent through the heart chambers and the myocardial tissue can be followed. From a series of such images, regional time–signal intensity curves can be derived. Pharmacological vasodilatation (with adenosine, dipyridamole, or reganedoson) induces a three- to fivefold increase of blood flow in myocardial areas subtended by normal coronary arteries, whereas no (or only minimal) change is found in areas subtended by stenotic coronary arteries. Thus, contrast arrival in these areas is delayed, and they therefore appear hypointense (dark) compared to adjacent normal myocardium (Fig. 3.3.9). A large number of clinical trials have assessed the feasibility, safety and diagnostic accuracy of stress perfusion CMR. A recent meta-analysis (2,125 patients) showed that first-pass perfusion CMR under vasodilator stress has excellent sensitivity (89%) and very good specificity (80%) to diagnose coronary artery disease with quantitative coronary

angiography as the gold standard. The CE-MARC study compared the diagnostic accuracy of stress perfusion CMR with single photon emission computed tomography (SPECT) and showed that both techniques have similar specificity but CMR is more sensitive to detect ischaemia compared to scintigraphy. It should be noted that CMR perfusion techniques have higher spatial resolution than nuclear techniques (by at least an order of magnitude) and can be used to study the transmural aspect of myocardial perfusion. The clinical implications of this higher resolution (that allows, for example, demonstrating very small perfusion defects not seen on nuclear imaging) remain to be established.

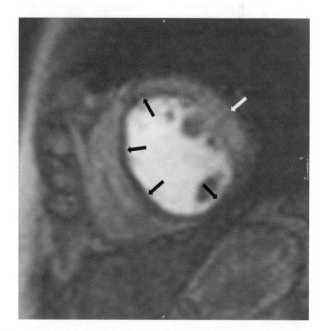

Fig. 3.3.9 Example of a stress perfusion scan. Short-axis stress perfusion at the midventricular level showing an extensive perfusion defect (black arrows) in the anterior wall, septum and the inferior wall. The lateral wall (white arrow) has relatively normal perfusion.

Myocardial oedema

Various technical improvements have enabled the wide clinical use of T2-weighted CMR for the qualitative or semi-quantitative detection of myocardial oedema and inflammation, primarily in acute coronary syndromes and myocarditis. Despite these improvements, a few well-recognized limitations of conventional T2-weighted techniques remain including the need for a 'normal' reference region of interest, in either remote myocardium or skeletal muscle. This can lead to false-negative results when these reference areas are also affected in systemic processes. Novel quantitative T2 and T1 mapping techniques have been developed to overcome these limitations. Myocardial haemorrhage in patients with acute myocardial infarction can also be assessed using T2-weighted CMR.

Coronary arteries

CMR of the coronary arteries remains a technical challenge because of their small size (up to 4 mm) and continuous, complex movement. Fast, flow-sensitive gradient-echo sequences allow imaging of proximal coronary arteries using breath-hold or navigator techniques, with a maximum in-plane resolution of about 700 μm². However, the sensitivity for coronary stenosis is only 60–90% because of the inferior spatial resolution compared to CT or invasive coronary angiography. Further developments (parallel acquisition, gradient performance, intravascular contrast agents, higher-field magnets) might in the future allow the development of high-resolution MR coronary angiography with CT-like quality. At present, MR coronary angiography can be used for diagnosis of anomalous coronary arteries or coronary aneurysms.

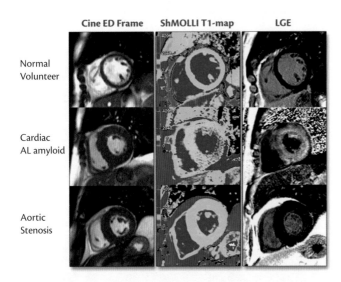

| | Cine ED Frame | ShMOLLI T1-map | LGE |

Normal Volunteer

Cardiac AL amyloid

Aortic Stenosis

Fig. 3.3.10 Cardiac magnetic resonance (CMR) end-diastolic frame from cine (left panel), ShMOLLI noncontrast T1 map (middle panel), and late gadolinium enhancement (LGE) images (right panel) in normal volunteer, aortic stenosis patient, and cardiac amyloid patient. Note the markedly elevated myocardial T1 time in the cardiac amyloid patient (1170 ms, into the red range of the colour scale) compared to the normal control (955 ms) and the patient with aortic stenosis and left ventricular hypertrophy (998 ms). ED, end-diastolic.

Reprinted from the *Journal of the American College of Cardiology*, Vol 6, Issue 4, Karamitsos, Theodoros D, et al, Noncontrast T1 Mapping for the Diagnosis of Cardiac Amyloidosis, 488-497, Copyright (2013) with permission from Elsevier.

Iron overload

The most common cause of iron overload cardiomyopathy is repeated blood transfusions in patients with transfusion-dependent anaemias (e.g. β-thalassaemia major) and in primary hemochromatosis. The cardiomyopathy is reversible if chelation is commenced early, but diagnosis is often delayed because of the late onset of symptoms and patients often die from heart failure. T2* MRI allows the accurate quantification of cardiac and liver iron levels. This allows identification of patients who are at risk of developing heart failure (i.e. those with myocardial T2* <10 ms), allowing more aggressive iron chelation therapy to be administered.

Novel CMR techniques: T1 and T2 mapping

T1 and T2 mapping refers to parametric maps that are generated from a series of images acquired with different T1 or T2 weighting so that each pixel can be assigned a T1 or T2 value. These maps are usually displayed using colour or thresholded scales to enable quantitative visual interpretation. Each tissue type exhibits a characteristic range of normal T1 and T2 relaxation times at a particular field strength, deviation from which may be indicative of disease. Myocardial T1-mapping methods are used for native (i.e. without the use of gadolinium-based contrast agents) and also for post-contrast T1 measurements. In combination with haematocrit, these T1 measurements enable the quantification of extracellular volume fraction (ECV).

Elevated native T1 times and ECV in the myocardium have been reported in several commonly encountered cardiac conditions including myocardial infarction, myocarditis, hypertrophic and dilated cardiomyopathy, cardiac amyloidosis (Fig. 3.3.10), cardiac involvement in systemic diseases and diffuse fibrosis in patients with aortic stenosis. Native myocardial T1 values may be lowered by water–protein interactions, fat, or iron content and thus can also serve as a diagnostic tool in characterizing Anderson–Fabry disease, fat in cardiac masses, and myocardial siderosis.

T2 mapping can detect oedematous myocardial territories in a variety of cardiac pathologies, including acute myocardial infarction, myocarditis, takotsubo cardiomyopathy, and heart transplant rejection.

CMR and prognosis

The evolving prognostic evidence base of is rapidly expanding for both ischaemic and nonischaemic cardiomyopathies. The

---

Box 3.3.1 Limitations of coronary CT

- Radiation exposure, which is highly dependent on the scanner being used and the mode of gating: Calcium scoring alone delivers approximately 1 mSv. Angiography with retrospective gating on a 64-slice scanner could deliver as much as 15 mSv, while prospective gating on a 320-slice scanner may routinely deliver <1 mSv.

- Iodinated X-ray contrast required. This can problematic for patients with renal dysfunction or hypersensitivity.

- Beta-blockade required to achieve low heart rate (preferably <60 bpm) to minimize motion artefacts in angiography.

- Calcium and stents can cause blooming and beam-hardening artefacts, obscuring the lumen.

Table 3.3.1 Assessment of patients with stable chest pain (according to NICE Clinical Guideline 95)

Estimated likelihood of CAD[a]	
<10%	Consider noncardiac causes of chest pain
10–29%	Offer CT calcium score:
	1–400 offer CT angiography
	>400 follow pathway for >60% probability of CAD
30–60%	Offer noninvasive functional imaging (MPS with SPECT or stress echocardiography or first-pass contrast-enhanced magnetic resonance perfusion or magnetic resonance imaging for stress-induced wall motion abnormalities)
	If positive offer invasive coronary angiography
>60%	Invasive coronary angiography

[a] According to type of chest pain, age, sex, and risk factor profile (see NICE Clinical Guideline 95)

CAD, coronary artery disease; MPS, myocardial perfusion scintigraphy

completion of ongoing multicentre trials and registries is expected to provide more outcome and cost-effectiveness data which will further strengthen the clinical role of CMR.

Cardiac CT

Multidetector computed tomography (MDCT) can be used to produce high-quality anatomical images in a variety of cardiac pathologies (e.g. complex congenital heart disease). However, its most widespread use is in the noninvasive anatomical assessment of the coronary arteries. The entire coronary tree is imaged during a single breath-hold over a few cardiac cycles (or even a single cycle if the scanner has sufficient detectors).

A stack of transaxial slices is acquired, covering the thorax between the carina and the diaphragmatic border of the heart. This is achieved over a few cardiac cycles, depending on the number of detectors. Coronary calcification is assessed from a noncontrasted scan. For angiographic imaging (to assess for luminal stenoses), an

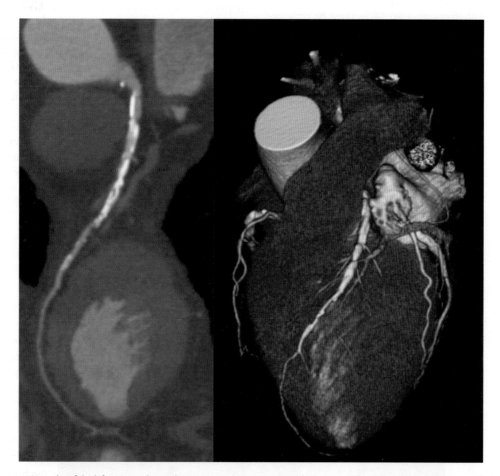

Fig. 3.3.11 CT coronary angiography of the left anterior descending coronary artery. Note how the heavy calcification makes it difficult to exclude or confirm significant luminal stenosis at several locations.

Image courtesy of Dr N. Sabharwal, Oxford Heart Centre.

intravenous power injection of an iodinated X-ray contrast agent is given, typically 60–80 ml at 5–6 ml/s, followed by a saline flush. Following a breath-hold, the scan is triggered once the left side of the circulation is sufficiently opacified. The timing can be judged either by using an initial test bolus, or by a bolus tracking method where a test slice is monitored until the Hounsfield value in the ascending or descending aorta exceeds a certain threshold.

In order to image the coronary arteries free of motion, ECG gating is required. Prospective gating is now the preferred method, with the patient being imaged (and irradiated) for only a brief period of the cardiac cycle, typically at 75% of the R-R interval. This usually represents end-diastole, when the coronary arteries (particularly the right coronary) are at their stillest. Retrospective gating offers imaging throughout the cardiac cycle, which can be valuable when heart-rate control is poor or information about cardiac function is required. However, radiation exposure is relatively high, and the prospective method is routinely preferred.

High-quality angiographic images also depend on the patient having a relatively slow heart rate (<65 and preferably <60 bpm), which is achieved by giving a β-blocker, either orally or intravenously. Many centres also give sublingual GTN prior to the study to achieve coronary vasodilatation.

Once the scan has been acquired and reconstructed, it must be carefully examined. The thin transaxial slices must be reviewed, and a number of tools are available to help reorientate the images to display the coronary arteries and other cardiac structures.

Some of the technical limitations of cardiac CT are shown in Box 3.3.1.

Clinical uses of cardiac CT

CT coronary calcium scoring

The ability of CT to detect and quantify calcified structures is unrivalled by other imaging techniques. Pathological studies indicate that coronary calcification is an integral part of the atherosclerotic process, and unique to it (with the possible exception of patients with renal failure). Specifically, the square root of the extent of calcification is directly proportional to the square root of the overall extent of atheromatous plaque. On a non-contrast-enhanced CT scan, the Agatston score is used to quantify the total amount of coronary calcium, and assesses the area and density of plaques in all arteries.

The coronary calcium score is a good measure of the overall coronary atheroma burden, and predicts the likelihood of luminal coronary stenoses, as well as the risk of cardiac events over at least 10 years of follow-up. In particular, a score of zero predicts an extremely low risk.

Stand-alone coronary calcium scoring may be valuable in the risk stratification of asymptomatic patients or those with atypical chest pain. However, its value in patients with possible angina is less straightforward: up to 10% of patients with no coronary calcification will nevertheless have a significant coronary stenosis due to soft plaque. Moreover, the location of calcification is a poor guide to the exact location of luminal stenoses, which are typically caused by noncalcified soft plaques. Therefore, in patients with possible angina, most authorities would regard coronary calcium scoring as complementary to angiography rather than an alternative, though this is at variance with the NICE guidance (see Table 3.3.1).

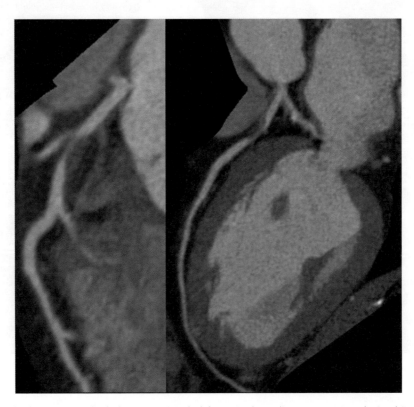

Fig. 3.3.12 CT coronary angiography showing a critical soft plaque stenosis in the left anterior descending coronary artery also involving the first diagonal. No calcification is present.

CT coronary angiography

Multidetector CT is unique among the noninvasive imaging modalities in providing anatomical (rather than physiological) information about the coronary arteries. Invasive coronary angiography remains the gold standard, as CT does not yet approach its spatial or temporal resolution. However, for the exclusion of coronary stenoses CT appears extremely reliable, with a negative predictive value that approaches 99% in the literature. Positive predictive values are less robust, largely due to artefacts, particularly in relation to calcified plaques (Fig. 3.3.11). These observations make CT coronary angiography particularly suitable for the diagnostic investigation of patients with low to intermediate probability of obstructive coronary disease (Fig. 3.3.12).

As well as its role in patients with stable chest pain, cardiac CT is increasingly used in low-risk patients admitted with acute chest pain, where it is cost-effective compared with alternative strategies.

CT can also be useful in certain groups of patients with established coronary disease. It offers a very straightforward way of assessing graft patency after coronary artery bypass surgery, and can also be valuable in the exclusion of stent obstruction (though artefact can make this difficult for smaller stents).

Acknowledgements

The authors of the CMR section acknowledge support from the National Institute for Health Research Oxford Biomedical Research Centre Programme. Professor Stefan Neubauer also acknowledges support from the Oxford British Heart Foundation Centre of Research Excellence.

Further reading

Nuclear imaging

Anagnostopoulos D, *et al.* (2012). Myocardial perfusion scintigraphy: technical innovations and evolving clinical applications. *Heart*, **98**, 353–9.

Berman DS, *et al.* (2006). Roles of nuclear cardiology, cardiac computed tomography, and cardiac magnetic resonance: noninvasive risk stratification and a conceptual framework for the selection of noninvasive imaging tests in patients with known or suspected coronary artery disease. *J Nuclear Med*, **47**, 1107–18.

Cardiac Radionuclide Imaging Writing Group (2009). ACCF/ASNC/ACR/AHA/ASE/SCCT/SCMR/SNM 2009 appropriate use criteria for cardiac radionuclide imaging: a report of the American College of Cardiology Foundation Appropriate Use Criteria Task Force, the American Society of Nuclear Cardiology, the American College of Radiology, the American Heart Association, the American Society of Echocardiography, the Society of Cardiovascular Computed Tomography, the Society for Cardiovascular Magnetic Resonance, and the Society of Nuclear Medicine. *Circulation*, **119**, e561–87.

Dilsizian V, Narula J (2013). *Atlas of nuclear cardiology*, 4th edition. Springer, New York.

NICE (2010). *Assessment and diagnosis of recent onset chest pain or discomfort of suspected cardiac origin.* Clinical guideline 95. www.nice.org.uk/guidance/CG95

Sabharwal NK, Loong C, Kelion A (2008). *Oxford handbook of nuclear cardiology.* Oxford University Press, Oxford.

Zaret B, Beller GA (2010). *Clinical nuclear cardiology: state of the art and future directions*, 4th edition. Mosby, London.

Computed tomography

Taylor AJ, *et al.* (2010). ACCF/SCCT/ACR/AHA/ASE/ASNC/NASCI/SCAI/SCMR 2010 Appropriate use criteria for cardiac computed tomography. *J Cardiovasc Comput Tomogr*, **4**, 407.e1–407

Williams MC, *et al.* (2011). Cardiac and coronary CT comprehensive imaging approach in the assessment of coronary heart disease. *Heart*, **97**, 1198–205.

MRI

American College of Cardiology Foundation Task Force on Expert Consensus D, Hundley WG, Bluemke DA et al. (2010). ACCF/ACR/AHA/NASCI/SCMR 2010 expert consensus document on cardiovascular magnetic resonance: a report of the American College of Cardiology Foundation Task Force on Expert Consensus Documents. *J Am Coll Cardiol*, **55**, 2614–62.

Bluemke DA, *et al.* (2008). Noninvasive coronary artery imaging: magnetic resonance angiography and multidetector computed tomography angiography: a scientific statement from the American Heart Association Committee on Cardiovascular Imaging and Intervention of the Council on Cardiovascular Radiology and Intervention, and the Councils on Clinical Cardiology and Cardiovascular Disease in the Young. *Circulation*, **118**, 586–606.

Eitel I, Friedrich MG. (2011). T2-weighted cardiovascular magnetic resonance in acute cardiac disease. *J Cardiovasc Magn Reson*, **13**, 13.

Greenwood JP, *et al.* (2012). Cardiovascular magnetic resonance and single-photon emission computed tomography for diagnosis of coronary heart disease (CE-MARC): a prospective trial. *Lancet*, **379**, 453–60.

Hamon M, *et al.* Meta-analysis of the diagnostic performance of stress perfusion cardiovascular magnetic resonance for detection of coronary artery disease. *J Cardiovasc Magn Reson*, **12**, 29.

Karamitsos TD, *et al.* (2009). The role of cardiovascular magnetic resonance imaging in heart failure. *J Am Coll Cardiol*, **54**, 1407–24.

Kim RJ, *et al.* (2000). The use of contrast-enhanced magnetic resonance imaging to identify reversible myocardial dysfunction. *N Engl J Med*, **343**, 1445–53.

Moon JC, *et al.* (2013). Myocardial T1 mapping and extracellular volume quantification: a Society for Cardiovascular Magnetic Resonance (SCMR) and CMR Working Group of the European Society of Cardiology consensus statement. *J Cardiovasc Magn Reson*, **15**, 92.

Salerno M, Kramer CM. (2013). Advances in parametric mapping with CMR imaging. *JACC Cardiovasc Imaging*, **6**, 806–22.

Cardiac catheterization and angiography

Edward D. Folland

Essentials

Cardiac catheterization/angiography is indicated for evaluation of patients with coronary, valvular, and congenital heart disease in whom diagnostic or therapeutic decisions cannot be made on the basis of noninvasive tests. Most patients presenting for cardiac catheterization have coronary artery disease: catheterization and coronary angiography are integral parts of interventional treatments for patients experiencing ischaemic coronary syndromes.

Technique and diagnostic utility—vascular access is usually obtained percutaneously from the femoral, radial, or brachial artery (for the left heart), or the femoral, internal jugular, or brachial/antecubital vein (for the right heart). Key information that can be obtained by cardiac catheterization/angiography include (1) pressures within cardiac chambers; (2) cardiac output; (3) quantitative estimation of left ventricular function; (4) diagnosis and quantitation of intracardiac shunts; (5) calculation of systemic and pulmonary vascular resistances; (6) assessment of cardiac valves; and (7) details of coronary arterial anatomy and function.

Therapeutic utility—cardiac catheterization/angiography permits interventions, particularly coronary angioplasty/stenting (see Chapters 13.5 and 13.6), that are of great and increasing therapeutic importance.

Introduction

Invasive cardiac diagnosis by means of catheterization and angiography developed hand in hand with cardiac surgery throughout the 20th century. It answered the need for precise information about cardiac physiology and anatomy, which arose in the 1940s when surgical techniques for the treatment of congenital and rheumatic heart disease first became available. A few years earlier, in 1929, Werner Forsman of Germany successfully and safely passed a filiform urinary catheter from a median basilic vein into the right atrium of his own heart and documented it on X-ray film. Although this feat cost him his own job, it enabled Andre Cournand and Dickenson Richards a decade later to use catheters for sampling blood, measuring pressure and flow, and injecting radio-opaque contrast medium (angiography) into the intact, beating human heart, ushering in the era of invasive cardiac diagnosis. Cournand, Richards, and Forsman later won the Nobel Prize for their important work. This chapter reviews the diagnostic applications of cardiac catheterization and angiography.

Indications for cardiac catheterization and angiography

Catheterization entails some degree of risk and discomfort, and is expensive, hence patients should be carefully selected. In broadest terms, it is indicated for detailed evaluation of those with coronary, valvular, and congenital heart disease, once they have been identified as candidates for surgery or other forms of intervention. It may also be indicated for patients whose diagnosis is uncertain from noninvasive evaluation.

Coronary artery disease

Most patients presenting for cardiac catheterization have coronary artery disease. Angiography of the coronary arteries performed during cardiac catheterization is essential for patients in whom revascularization is indicated. In spite of the limitations discussed later in this chapter, no other imaging modality, including MRI and CT (see Chapter 3.3), can as yet provide the detailed anatomy of the entire coronary circulation that is needed for planning revascularization procedures such as coronary artery bypass surgery and percutaneous intervention.

Coronary angiography is indicated for patients with chronic stable angina that persists in spite of reasonable efforts at pharmacological therapy. It is also indicated for patients whose survival would be improved by revascularization, regardless of symptoms. Such patients are those with severe stenosis of the main left coronary artery and those with severe two- and three-vessel coronary artery disease in combination with impaired left ventricular function. These patients may be identified by the following features of stress testing: ischaemia at low workload (especially in stage 1 of the Bruce protocol), marked depression of the electrocardiographic ST segment (>2 mm), failure to augment systolic blood pressure during exercise, and large exercise-induced defects or increased lung uptake during radionuclide perfusion imaging (see Chapters 3.1 and 3.3). In addition, patients with high-risk clinical presentations such as acute myocardial infarction, unstable angina, and post-myocardial infarction ischaemia are candidates for angiography. Patients having acute myocardial infarction are best served by immediate percutaneous coronary intervention if this is available in a timely manner (see Chapters 13.5 and 13.6). Finally, catheterization is sometimes indicated to obtain a definitive diagnosis when noninvasive testing has yielded equivocal or inconsistent results.

Valvular disease

Catheterization was once considered essential prior to the surgical treatment of valvular heart disease. This is no longer the case because of advances in noninvasive testing using ultrasound and Doppler techniques. Nevertheless, catheterization is frequently helpful for gathering the information needed to properly select patients for surgical therapy, and to guide the surgeon in providing optimum treatment, the most common issue being to assess the need for coronary artery revascularization, particularly among those with aortic stenosis, who commonly have coronary artery disease. Haemodynamic studies may also be necessary in cases where noninvasive diagnostic data are limited or equivocal. By contrast, it is often possible to avoid catheterization in young patients in whom noninvasive studies yield unequivocal conclusions and there is no evidence of coronary artery disease.

Congenital disease

Most patients with congenital heart defects can be definitively diagnosed by transthoracic or transoesophageal ultrasound, CT, or MRI (see Chapters 3.2 and 3.3). As in valvular disease, catheterization is most useful in cases where the abnormality is unusually complex, the noninvasive data are incomplete, or the patient is suspected of having coronary artery disease. Catheterization is particularly useful in quantifying shunt flow and pulmonary vascular resistance, both of which are important considerations in the treatment of intracardiac defects. The physical passage of a systemic venous catheter across the atrial septum into a pulmonary vein or the left ventricle is diagnostic of an atrial septal defect.

Pericardial disease

Pericardial tamponade and constriction lend themselves particularly well to diagnosis by catheterization. Although ultrasonography has superseded catheterization as a rapidly available method of confirming the clinical diagnosis of tamponade, it is usually inconclusive for patients with pericardial constriction. At catheterization, patients with both conditions usually demonstrate equalization of all intracardiac diastolic pressures, with unique pressure waveforms exhibited in the right atrium and right ventricle usually distinguishing the two diagnoses (Fig. 3.4.1).

Congestive heart failure

The aetiology and pathophysiology of congestive heart failure are readily elucidated by catheterization. States of pressure and volume overload as well as systolic and diastolic dysfunction of the ventricles can be easily identified, as explained in detail later in this chapter. Furthermore, catheterization is uniquely suited for identifying transient or reversible causes of left ventricular dysfunction caused by ischaemia or myocardial hibernation due to underlying coronary artery disease. Sometimes exercise or other interventions are performed during a catheter study to elicit transient abnormal haemodynamic function. Myocardial biopsy performed during catheterization can sometimes identify the aetiology of primary myocardial dysfunction.

Pulmonary vascular disease

Patients with primary pulmonary hypertension (see Chapter 15.2) should undergo catheterization to measure pulmonary vascular pressure and resistance. Certain vasodilating drugs may or may not benefit the patient, depending upon their effect on pressure and resistance during acute administration. Pulmonary angiography performed during right heart catheterization is traditionally

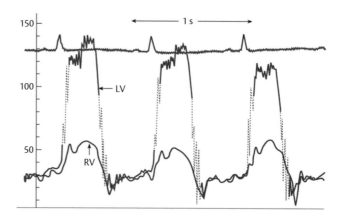

Fig. 3.4.1 Pericardial constriction. This is a tracing of simultaneous left ventricular (LV) and right ventricular (RV) pressure in a patient with pericardial constriction. Generally, the diastolic pressure of the left ventricle is higher than that of the right ventricle. For patients with a constriction, the pericardium determines the diastolic compliance of both chambers, causing the diastolic pressures to be equal. Note also the typical 'dip–plateau' pattern or 'square-root sign' of both chambers in diastole. Although diastolic ventricular pressures are also equal for patients having tamponade, the dip–plateau pattern is usually absent.

regarded as the most definitive test for pulmonary embolism, although in most cases the diagnosis can be secured by CT angiography or radioisotope lung scanning.

Practicalities of cardiac catheterization

Preparing the patient

Precatheterization evaluation should consist of a careful history and examination, particularly aimed at eliciting details of prior cardiac procedures, reactions to contrast medium, renal function, peripheral vascular status, and haemostatic function. The patient should be carefully advised of the indications, alternatives, risks, discomforts, and expected benefits of the procedure. The skilled clinician does this while building the patient's confidence and avoids creating undue alarm. Following an uncomplicated diagnostic catheterization the patient should usually expect to go home the same day and to resume customary physical activities within a day or two.

Vascular access

The traditional approach to vascular access is via a cut-down near the antecubital fossa, with isolation and mobilization of the brachial or antecubital vein and the brachial artery for right and left heart catheterization thereby allowing arterial and venous access. After the procedure the arterial entry site is repaired by suture and the vein is usually tied off. However, although this approach has the advantage of enabling early postprocedure ambulation and the security of direct arterial closure in anticoagulated patients, it has the disadvantage of being time-consuming for most physicians and less cosmetic for the patient. Hence the cut-down approach is now seldom used, with percutaneous arterial catheterization becoming increasingly popular.

Percutaneous vascular access is achieved by direct puncture with a needle through which a flexible spring guide wire is passed into the vessel. Catheters may then be passed into the vessel over the guide wire. Following the procedure haemostasis is achieved by applying pressure over the puncture site until bleeding stops.

Percutaneous access is frequently employed at the femoral site, although it may also be used at brachial, axillary, internal jugular, and radial locations. It has the advantage of speed, simplicity, and—when performed from the femoral vessels—frees the upper body and arms during angiographic filming. However, it has the disadvantage of sometimes requiring several hours' immobilization of the catheterization site following the procedure. Nevertheless, the femoral approach remains popular, especially when smaller catheters (4 and 5 French) and arterial closure devices enable earlier ambulation. In recent years the percutaneous approach to the radial artery has become the preferred choice of many physicians because it is associated with fewer bleeding complications and shortens hospital time.

Right heart catheterization

Right heart catheterization can be performed from any of the approaches described above. Although traditionally performed with a stiff, woven Dacron, end-hole catheter, it is often done with a flexible, balloon-tip, flow-directed catheter (Swan–Ganz) because this is safer and enables the measurement of cardiac output by thermodilution.

Catheterization of the right heart is indicated by itself for the study of pulmonary vascular disease and haemodynamic response to exercise or drug administration. It is indicated in combination with left heart catheterization for patients requiring haemodynamic study of valvular, congenital, or myocardial disease, and for patients being studied primarily for coronary artery disease who also have heart failure, valvular, or pulmonary disease.

Left atrial pressure can be measured indirectly via right heart catheterization by wedging the tip of the catheter in a pulmonary arteriole, or by occluding a pulmonary artery branch with the inflated balloon at the tip of a Swan–Ganz catheter. In either case, this creates a static column of blood from the tip of the catheter, through the pulmonary capillary bed, to the left atrium. This static column of blood has the effect of extending the tip of the catheter to the left atrium for pressure-measuring purposes. The resulting pressure is identical to the directly measured left atrial pressure, except that it is delayed temporally by approximately 80 ms. This pressure, commonly known as the pulmonary (artery) capillary wedge (PCW) pressure, is very useful in the management of left heart failure and shock, and for estimating the diastolic gradient across the mitral valve in patients with mitral stenosis.

Left heart catheterization

Left heart catheterization is generally performed in conjunction with coronary angiography, but is specifically required for the assessment of left ventricular function and assessment of stenosis or regurgitation of the left-sided valves (mitral and aortic). It is most often accomplished by femoral, radial, or brachial arterial access, and by retrograde crossing of the aortic valve to enter the left ventricle. Left heart catheterization may also be achieved by controlled puncture of the interatrial septum with a catheter originating from the right femoral vein (trans-septal left heart catheterization): this can then be used to measure left atrial pressure directly, and be passed antegradely through the mitral valve to measure pressure and perform angiography of the left ventricle. Retrograde access of the left atrium from the left ventricle is technically difficult and seldom done.

The left ventricle may also be entered via transthoracic needle puncture. This approach, known as direct left ventricular puncture, is occasionally necessary for studying patients who have both mitral and aortic mechanical prosthetic valves. The passage of the needle into the left ventricle from the cardiac apex is facilitated by echocardiographic guidance.

Information obtained from cardiac catheterization and angiography

Intracardiac pressures

Methodology

Pressure at the tip of the catheter is transmitted through the fluid inside the catheter (usually saline) to a transducer, which converts the pressure signal to an electrical signal that can then be amplified, displayed on a screen, and stored as a digital time recording. Once calibrated, the pressure at the tip of the catheter can be read graphically from the recording screen and analysed electronically. The fidelity of recording depends upon the physical characteristics of the fluid-filled catheter, stopcocks, connecting tubing, and the pressure transducer itself. A fluid-filled system is usually capable of responding to transient pressure changes up to 20 or occasionally 30 Hz, which is of sufficient fidelity to reproduce diagnostically useful pressure waveforms from the heart. However, it is not responsive enough to accurately reproduce the rate of rise of left ventricular pressure during the isovolumic phase of systole (dP/dt). This requires responsiveness to transient pressure changes of at least 60 Hz, of which fluid-filled catheter systems are not capable. For such applications catheter-tip manometers are available (Millar catheters) in which the transducer is placed at the catheter tip, eliminating the need for an intervening column of fluid. These devices are expensive and are used only when such fidelity is required, usually in research applications.

Normal intracardiac pressures

The upper limits of all normal intracardiac pressures measurable from a right heart catheter are approximate multiples of six, hence they are easily remembered by the 'rule of sixes' (Table 3.4.1). For example, the mean right atrial pressure is 6 mmHg or less, mean left atrial pressure is 12 mmHg or less. A further aid to remembering normal pressures is the 'corollary of continuity', which means that contiguous chambers have a common pressure when the intervening valve is open. For example, the right ventricle and right atrium are essentially a common chamber when the tricuspid valve is open in diastole, therefore the upper limit of right ventricular end-diastolic pressure is the same as the upper limit of the normal right atrial pressure, or 6 mmHg. This assumes there is no significant stenosis or regurgitation across the tricuspid valve, and that the right ventricle has normal compliance. The same condition applies to the mitral valve in diastole and the pulmonic and aortic valves in systole. Another practical rule is that the pulmonary artery diastolic and pulmonary artery capillary pressures approximate each other in the absence of severe pulmonary vascular disease. Once this has been established for any given patient, the pulmonary artery diastolic pressure can be followed as a surrogate for pulmonary capillary wedge pressure in situations where a pulmonary artery catheter is used for intensive-care monitoring.

All intracardiac pressures rise and fall phasically with breathing due to transmission of shifting intrapleural pressure during

Table 3.4.1 Normal intracardiac pressures[a]

Location	Phasic pressure (mmHg)	Mean pressure (mmHg)
Right atrium		3 ± 2
Right ventricle		
Systole	24 ± 4	
Diastole	5 ± 3	
Pulmonary artery		13 ± 5
Systole	24 ± 6	
Diastole	13 ± 5	
Pulmonary capillary		
Wedge		9 ± 3
Left atrium		9 ± 3
Left ventricle		
Systole	120 ± 18	
Diastole	10 ± 5	

[a] These values are derived from 100 consecutive catheterization studies of patients proven to have no evidence of heart disease at the West Roxbury Veterans Administration Hospital from 1955 to 1980. An easy way to remember the upper limits of normal values (≤2 standard deviations above mean) is that they are generally multiples of the number 6.

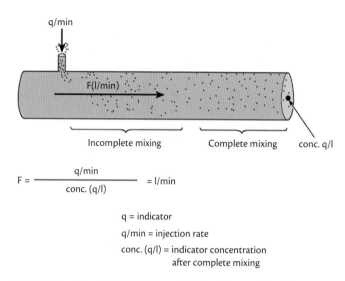

$$F = \frac{q/min}{conc.\ (q/l)} = l/min$$

q = indicator
q/min = injection rate
conc. (q/l) = indicator concentration
after complete mixing

Fig. 3.4.2 The Fick principle. The flow rate (F) through a vessel (cardiac output, in this case) can be measured if an indicator is added to the flowing liquid at a known rate (q/min) and the concentration (q/litre) of the indicator is measured after complete mixing has occurred.

respiratory effort. Usually this variation is no more than a few mmHg from inspiration to expiration, but it can be quite marked in patients with obstructive lung disease. Standards of normal pressure are based upon measurements taken during resting respiration, averaging several respiratory cycles. Pressures in the catheterization laboratory should be similarly measured: asking a patient to hold their breath may generate misleading data.

Waveforms

The shape of intracardiac pressure waveforms carries useful diagnostic information. Atria and ventricles have characteristic waveforms, the left-sided chambers normally demonstrating similar patterns at relatively higher pressures than right-sided chambers. The state of volume loading and the relative compliance or 'stiffness' of the respective ventricles during diastolic filling determines pressures in the right and left atria. The left ventricle is generally thicker, stiffer, and less compliant to the stretch of increasing volume than the right ventricle; hence the left atrial and left ventricular diastolic pressures are higher than the respective pressures in the right heart. Conditions such as pericardial constriction and tamponade alter this normal relationship (see Fig. 3.4.1).

Cardiac flow and output

Measurement of cardiac output was one of the earliest applications of catheterization. Most methods entail application of the indicator dilution theory (the Fick principle), summarized graphically in Fig. 3.4.2, which can be stated simply as follows: the rate of flow can be measured if an indicator substance is added to the moving vehicle (e.g. blood) at a known rate, and the concentration of the indicator is also known proximal and distal to the point where the indicator is added. The indicator can be any readily measured substance such as oxygen, indocyanine green dye, or saline, the temperature of which is known and different from that of the bloodstream.

Cardiac output by oximetry

In this method, commonly called the Fick method, the indicator is oxygen that is carried physiologically by the blood. The method requires that the subject be in a metabolic steady state where the use of oxygen is constant. Such a steady state exists at rest and also during exercise, provided that the workload is constant for at least 3 min. As seen in Fig. 3.4.3, the pulmonary blood flow can be calculated when the oxygen consumption rate is known and the oxygen contents of blood in systemic and pulmonary arteries are known. In the absence of intracardiac shunts the pulmonary blood flow equals the systemic blood flow, or cardiac output.

Dye dilution

This method entails the rapid injection of a known quantity of indocyanine dye into the pulmonary artery. Blood is then sampled by withdrawal at a constant rate from a systemic artery. The sampled blood passes through a spectrophotometer, which is calibrated to measure the concentration of dye. A concentration curve is inscribed when the injected bolus of dye passes the sampling point (Fig. 3.4.4). Dividing the quantity of dye injected by the area of the time–concentration curve (corrected for recirculation as indicated by the dashed line in Fig. 3.4.4) yields the cardiac output. This method is now seldom used.

Thermodilution

Measurement of cardiac output by thermodilution uses the same principle as dye dilution, with the indicator being 'negative calories' (the difference between the caloric content of the injected bolus of cool saline and the caloric content of the same quantity of the subject's blood). The downstream 'concentration' of injected negative calories is measured as a transient drop in temperature by a thermistor at the tip of the injection catheter several centimetres from the point of injection. Dividing the negative calories injected by the area of the distal time–temperature curve yields cardiac output. The advantages of speed, automaticity, and repeatability of this method make it particularly suitable for serial measurements during different haemodynamic states.

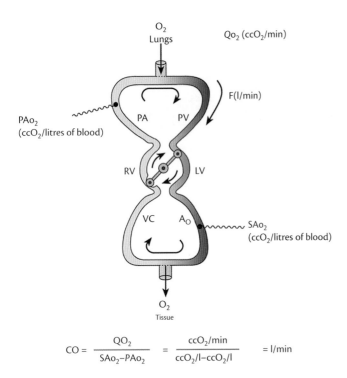

$$CO = \frac{Q_{O_2}}{SA_{O_2} - PA_{O_2}} = \frac{ccO_2/min}{ccO_2/l - ccO_2/l} = l/min$$

Fig. 3.4.3 Cardiac output measured by oximetry. This is an application of the Fick principle in which oxygen is the indicator carried by flowing blood. The patient's metabolism must be at steady state, a condition where oxygen consumption and utilization are matched. It requires three measurements: oxygen consumption rate (Q_{O_2}), systemic arterial oxygen content (SA_{O_2}), and pulmonary arterial oxygen content (PA_{O_2}). Ao, aorta; cc, volume in ml; CO, cardiac output; LV, left ventricle; PV, pulmonary vein; RV, right ventricle; VC, vena cava.

Angiographic output

This is the only commonly used method that does not employ the indicator dilution or Fick principle. The left ventricular stroke volume calculated from quantitative angiography is multiplied by the heart rate to yield the left ventricular output. In the absence of valvular regurgitation this is the same as cardiac output. As explained in greater detail later in the chapter, this method is particularly useful in assessing mitral and aortic valvular regurgitation.

Quantitative angiography

Quantitative left ventricular angiography enables the measurement of left ventricular volume at instants throughout the cardiac cycle. Radiographic contrast medium is injected rapidly into the left ventricle and the shadow image of the opacified ventricle captured electronically at a particular frame rate in any chosen projection. The most common projection is $30°$ right anterior oblique at a framing rate of 30 images/s. In this view the image of the left ventricle is parallel to its long axis, resembling an ellipse. Arvidsson and Greene first suggested that the volume of the left ventricle could be calculated from the volume formula for an ellipsoid, the three-dimensional structure created by rotating an ellipse on its long axis. Dodge and Sandler improved upon this concept by deriving the minor hemi-axes from an idealized ellipse of the same length and area as the projected image of the ventricle. This method is still commonly used and is often referred to as the area–length method. Images captured at end diastole and end systole are analysed and corrected for magnification to yield end-diastolic and end-systolic

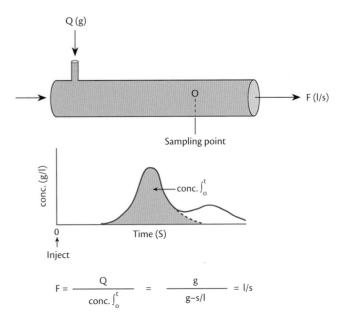

$$F = \frac{Q}{conc. \int_o^t} = \frac{g}{g\text{-}s/l} = l/s$$

Fig. 3.4.4 Cardiac output measured by dye curve. The concentration curve of indocyanine green dye generated by sampling distal to an injection point can be analysed to yield cardiac output. See text for more details. Thermodilution cardiac output employs the same principle, except that temperature is the measured indicator. F, flow or cardiac output; Q, quantity of indicator injected.

volumes, the difference between these volumes being the stroke volume and the product of the stroke volume and heart rate, the angiographic left ventricular output. These indices are useful in the assessment of left ventricular function and valvular regurgitation as discussed later in this chapter.

Intracardiac shunts

The same methods of oximetry and indicator dilution used in measuring cardiac output can be employed for the detection and quantitation of intracardiac shunts. Under normal resting conditions, blood is approximately 75% saturated as it returns from the body to the right heart and pulmonary artery. As it leaves the lungs in the pulmonary veins blood is 99% saturated. Intracardiac shunts can be detected, localized, and quantified by measuring the oxygen saturation in various locations. Left-to-right shunts will cause a step-up in the saturation of the blood at the location of the shunt; for example, in a patient with an atrial septal defect the saturation will rise in the right atrium, whereas with a ventricular septal defect the saturation will rise in the right ventricle. A patient with Eisenmenger's syndrome (pulmonary hypertension and right-to-left shunting) will exhibit a drop in saturation at the location of the shunt, namely at the left atrium or ventricle in the case of atrial and ventricular septal defects, respectively. The degree of the change in saturation is proportional to the size of the shunt, and enables calculation of the shunt flow in either direction in litres/min. Figure 3.4.5 presents a scheme and formulae for calculating shunt volume.

Vascular resistance

Blood flow through the pulmonary and systemic circulations can be compared to the flow of an electric current through a circuit. Pressure is the driving force analogous to voltage, flow rate is analogous to current, and the impediment to flow through the vascular bed is resistance. Pressure, flow, and resistance relate to each other in a fashion analogous to Ohm's law:

resistance = pressure / flow

In the above formula 'pressure' is the difference in mean pressure across the systemic vascular bed (systemic arterial pressure − right atrial pressure) or the pulmonary vascular bed (pulmonary artery pressure − left atrial pressure). In the absence of intracardiac shunts 'flow' is the same for both circulations and is measured as cardiac output by methods already described. In cases of intracardiac shunting the systemic and pulmonary flows will differ according to the degree of shunting, and can be calculated as described under the section on cardiac shunts and in Fig. 3.4.5. Normal values for pulmonary vascular and systemic vascular resistance are expressed either in dynes cm^{-5} or Wood units and are shown in Table 3.4.2. Total pulmonary resistance is a useful concept for expressing the total resistance against which the right ventricle must work, and includes not only the pulmonary vascular resistance but also the resistance engendered by the static pressure in the left atrium.

Table 3.4.2 Normal vascular resistance[a]

Location	Resistance (dynes s cm^{-5})[b]
Total systemic resistance	1276 ± 371
Total pulmonary resistance	185 ± 57
Pulmonary vascular resistance	55 ± 18

[a] The values are derived from 100 consecutive catheterization studies of patients proven to have no evidence of cardiac disease at the West Roxbury Veterans Administration Hospital during the years 1955–1980.

[b] Divide these values by 10 to obtain values in MPa s m^{-3}.

Hence, pulmonary vascular disease, left heart failure, or both, can increase the total pulmonary resistance.

Measurement of resistance is useful for assessing the state of the pulmonary circulation in congenital heart disease with intracardiac shunting: high pulmonary vascular resistance may preclude the safe correction of an intracardiac shunt, particularly if the shunt is from right to left. It is also useful in diagnosing the relative contribution of left heart failure and pulmonary vascular disease in patients with pulmonary hypertension, and is the best indicator of the effectiveness of vasodilating drugs for patients with pulmonary hypertension.

Valvular stenosis

Valvular stenosis is assessed by measuring the transvalvular pressure gradient and by calculating the valvular orifice area using a formula introduced in the late 1940s by cardiologist Richard Gorlin and his father, an engineer. The Gorlin formula for valve area was initially developed for patients with rheumatic mitral stenosis. It is based upon a study which utilized data from right heart catheterization alone, validated by relatively crude intraoperative estimates of valve area using the index finger of surgeon Dwight Harken during closed mitral commissurotomy operations at the Peter Bent Brigham Hospital in Boston, Massachusetts. Although its validation was relatively crude, the formula has stood the test of time and remains the standard for the haemodynamic assessment of valvular stenosis. In its generalized form it is expressed as follows:

$$\text{valve area} = \text{TFR} / \left(K \sqrt{m} \right)$$

where K is a constant unique to mitral or aortic valve analysis (38 and 44.5, respectively), TFR is the transvalvular flow rate, and m is the mean pressure gradient in mmHg during the time when the valve is open.

In aortic valve applications TFR (i.e. cardiac output normalized for the time that the valve is actually open) is the cardiac output divided by the product of heart rate and systolic ejection period. In mitral valve applications it is the cardiac output divided by the product of heart rate and diastolic filling period. Cardiac output is the effective systemic blood flow as determined by Fick, thermodilution, or dye dilution methods, unless there is associated valvular regurgitation, in which case it is the total left ventricular output as determined by quantitative left ventricular angiography.

Figure 3.4.6 shows tracings that demonstrate typical gradients from patients with aortic and mitral stenosis. The ranges of calculated valve area associated with various levels of stenosis for both aortic and mitral valves are displayed in Table 3.4.3. In general,

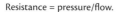

Resistance = pressure/flow.

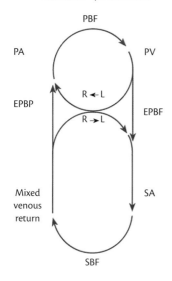

$$SBF\,(\text{l/min}) = \frac{O_2\ \text{consumption (ml/min)}}{SAo_2 - \text{mixed } Vo_2) \times 10}$$

$$PBF\,(\text{l/min}) = \frac{O_2\ \text{consumption (ml/min)}}{(PVo_2 - PAo_2) \times 10}$$

$$EPBF\,(\text{l/min}) = \frac{O_2\ \text{consumption (ml/min)}}{(PVo_2 - \text{mixed } Vo_2) \times 10}$$

Shunt flow (l/min):

$$L \rightarrow R = PBF - EPBF$$
$$R \rightarrow L = SBF - EPBF$$

Fig. 3.4.5 Quantitation of intracardiac shunts. Shunts between the left and right sides of the heart due to septal defects can be quantified by oximetry using this scheme. Oxygen content is measured in units of cc oxygen per decilitre of blood. EPBF, effective pulmonary blood flow, i.e. that part of the systemic venous return that actually passes through the lungs and is oxygenated; PBF, pulmonary blood flow; mixed Vo_2, mixed systemic venous oxygen content; PAo_2, pulmonary artery oxygen content; PVo_2, pulmonary vein oxygen content; SAo_2, systemic artery oxygen content; SBF, systemic blood flow.

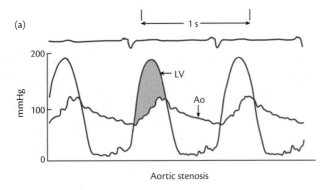

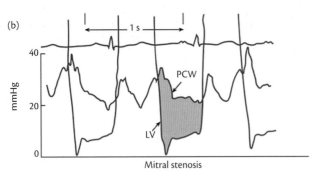

Fig. 3.4.6 Pressure gradients associated with valvular stenosis. The upper panel shows simultaneous tracings of left ventricular (LV) and ascending aortic (Ao) pressure in a patient with severe aortic stenosis. The mean systolic gradient across the aortic valve is 60 mmHg. The lower panel shows simultaneous tracings of left ventricular (LV) and pulmonary capillary wedge (PCW) pressure in a patient with severe mitral stenosis. The mean diastolic pressure gradient across the valve is 16 mmHg. The respective valvular gradients are cross-hatched.

procedures performed for the relief of anatomical stenosis are expected to be beneficial in symptomatic patients with severe valvular obstruction. However, many factors enter into such a decision and individual clinical judgement is required. Although patients with large transvalvular gradients generally experience the best result from intervention, the gradient by itself can be misleading due to its exponential relationship to cardiac output.

Valvular regurgitation

Qualitative assessment

Regurgitation of all four cardiac valves can be qualitatively assessed by angiography. The downstream side of the valve in question is opacified by a rapid injection of radiographic contrast medium. Regurgitation is visualized as upstream leakage of contrast across

Table 3.4.3 Calculated valve areas associated with various degrees of mitral and aortic stenosis

Severity	Valve area (cm²)	
	Aortic	Mitral
Mild	>1.2	>2.0
Moderate	0.8–1.2	1.1–2.0
Severe[a]	<0.8	≤1.0

[a] 'Severe' stenosis is generally considered to be sufficient to warrant surgical correction.

the closed valve. In the case of mitral regurgitation systolic opacification of the left atrium occurs during injection of the left ventricle. In aortic regurgitation diastolic opacification of the left ventricle occurs during supravalvular injection of the aorta. The degree of regurgitation is graded on an arbitrary scale from mild (1+) to severe (4+).

Quantitative assessment

Aortic and mitral regurgitation can be quantified in terms of regurgitant flow in litres/min or regurgitant fraction as a percentage of left ventricular output. Regurgitant flow is the difference obtained by subtracting the effective forward flow (Fick method described earlier) from the total left ventricular output (angiographically derived). It is the best method for measuring the severity of regurgitation, provided that the left ventricular angiogram, which itself may change cardiac output, is performed soon after the Fick measurement. Furthermore, both measurements must be made with considerable care to ensure accuracy. Regurgitation is considered clinically severe when 50% or more of the total left ventricular output is simply shuttling or regurgitating across the defective valve. The ability to quantify regurgitation across either valve is lost when both mitral and aortic valves are leaky.

Left ventricular function

Global function

Global function of the left ventricle is broadly described by its ability to generate pressure and flow under particular conditions of preload and afterload. Plotting the pressure and volume of the left ventricle at instants in time for a single cardiac cycle generates a pressure–volume loop displayed in Fig. 3.4.7. Most of the commonly used indices of left ventricular function can be derived from such a loop, including end-diastolic volume, end-systolic volume, stroke volume, ejection fraction, end-diastolic pressure, and dP/dt. Of these, the ejection fraction is most useful because it correlates with prognosis in a variety of cardiac diseases.

Grading angiographic wall motion in various segments of the left ventricle as normal, hypokinetic, akinetic, or dyskinetic assesses the regional function of the left ventricle. Regions of abnormal function generally correspond to locations of infarcted or ischaemic myocardium.

Contractility

This parameter is difficult to assess in the intact heart because all pressure and volume indices are dependent upon preload and afterload. Although ejection fraction is clinically useful it can be misleading in situations of high afterload (e.g. severe aortic stenosis) and low afterload (e.g. severe mitral regurgitation). The concept of 'elastance' has gained favour as a useful index of intrinsic contractility because it is relatively independent of loading conditions. Elastance is the slope of the line generated by plotting the end-systolic left ventricular pressure from a series of pressure–volume loops generated at differing afterloads created by the infusion of pressor or vasodilator drugs. The method is laborious and generally reserved for research applications.

Diastolic function

Diastolic function of the left ventricle is best appreciated from the slope of the pressure–volume loop during the period from mitral valve opening to its closure at the onset of systole. The curve becomes steeper as the left ventricle becomes less compliant due

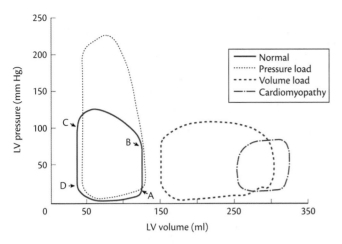

Fig. 3.4.7 Pressure–volume loops. Simultaneously plotting the instantaneous pressure and volume of the left ventricle throughout a single cardiac cycle produces these loops. The loop is a synthesis of most information relevant to left ventricular function. In this figure a loop from a normal patient is contrasted with those from patients with pressure load (hypertension or aortic stenosis), volume load (aortic or mitral regurgitation), and cardiomyopathy. Point A represents mitral valve closure; segment A–B, isovolumic contraction; point B, aortic valve opening; segment B–C, systolic ejection; point C, aortic valve closure; segment C–D, isovolumic relaxation; point D, mitral valve opening; and segment D–A, diastolic filling.

to the effects of hypertrophy, ischaemia, or infiltrative disease. In general, left ventricular end-diastolic pressure (LVEDP) rises as diastolic compliance falls, accounting for the high left atrial pressure and heart failure seen in diastolic left ventricular dysfunction.

Assessment of coronary arterial anatomy and function

Disease of the coronary arteries can be characterized at catheterization by both anatomical and functional assessment. Coronary angiography images the lumen of the vessel, which has been rendered radio-opaque by injection of radiographic contrast medium. It is a shadowing technique that displays the impact of the lesion on the arterial lumen but does not image the plaque *per se*. Intracoronary ultrasonography provides a tomographic image of the vessel wall and is capable of demonstrating the thickness and sonic density of the vessel wall and any associated plaque, hence angiography and intravascular ultrasonography are complementary methods of assessing vascular anatomy. To learn the haemodynamic importance of a coronary lesion it may be necessary to analyse its effect on function by measuring pressure and flow in the affected vessel. All these anatomical and functional modalities may be accomplished by catheterization.

Coronary arteriography or angiography

Coronary arteriography or angiography is presently the single most essential application of cardiac catheterization. The anatomy of coronary arteries in living, conscious humans was first demonstrated by nonselective injection of the aortic root. In the early 1960s David Littmann developed a loop catheter that enabled the injection of contrast medium preferentially in the outer circumference of the aortic root, opacifying the left and right coronary arteries simultaneously. At the time it was commonly believed that selective injection of contrast material into a coronary artery would have fatal consequences. This changed when Mason Sones accidentally performed

the first selective coronary angiogram without harm. He was intending to inject the left ventricle, but the catheter recoiled across the aortic valve and into the right coronary artery. Sones, a cardiologist by training, went on to develop a safe method of selective coronary angiography from the brachial artery cut-down approach using the flexible-tip catheter bearing his name. At the same time Melvin Judkins, a radiologist by training, was perfecting his own method of selective coronary angiography, using preshaped catheters, from a percutaneous femoral artery approach. Both methods have continued to be practised, although the percutaneous femoral, or Judkins' approach, has become most popular because of its speed and simplicity. However—as stated previously—in recent years there has been a return to the arm approach using percutaneous catheterization of the radial artery, which enables more rapid patient ambulation, and the radial artery approach is also associated with fewer serious access site complications.

Normal coronary anatomy is demonstrated in Fig. 3.4.8. A patient's anatomy is considered to be right (80%)- or left (20%)-dominant, depending upon whether the posterior descending artery arises from the right or left coronary artery, respectively.

Atherosclerotic disease is manifest by lesions that encroach upon the opacified lumen of the coronary artery (Fig. 3.4.9). Various approaches are used to grade the severity of these lesions. Most commonly a visual estimate of the percentage of the stenotic reduction in luminal diameter is given to each lesion, with severity quantified by comparing the minimal lumen diameter within a lesion to the diameter of the nearest normal segment of artery. This can be done manually using callipers or automatically using computer-based systems for edge detection and contrast densitometry. Quantitative coronary angiography is a complex subject because it requires attention to many variables, such as selection of view and frame, and choice made from among several analytical techniques.

Early work by Lance Gould determined that a lesion must impair coronary blood flow to be clinically important. Although flow at rest is not usually reduced until stenosis reduces vessel diameter by 90%, flow under stress may be impaired when the diameter is reduced by 70%. The clinical impact of a stenosis of any given severity is also dependent upon the degree of collateral flow into the vascular bed distal to the stenosis.

Coronary physiological measurements (pressure and flow)

Flow and pressure may be directly measured in the coronary artery by means of special guide wires that have pressure transducers or Doppler flow transducers mounted near their tips. As mentioned above, the flow at rest may be normal across a particular coronary artery stenosis. Coronary flow normally increases after maximal vasodilatation induced by local vasodilators. The quotient of the vasodilated flow divided by the resting flow, which is called the coronary flow reserve, is normally greater than 2. If not, the lesion in question is considered to be haemodynamically important. Pressure can be measured in the coronary artery at a location distal to a lesion using a guide wire with a transducer at its tip. The quotient of pressure distal to a lesion compared to the proximal pressure during maximal vasodilatation is called the fractional flow reserve. A quotient less than 0.75 is considered to be clinically important. The measurement of fractional flow reserve has proven useful in selecting vessels in need of revascularization.

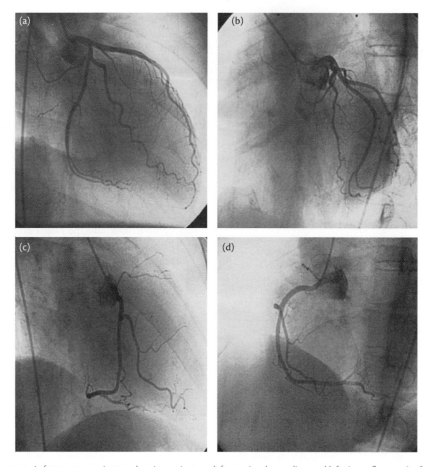

Fig. 3.4.8 Normal coronary anatomy. Left coronary angiogram showing main stem, left anterior descending, and left circumflex arteries from right anterior oblique view (a) and left anterior oblique view (b). Right coronary angiogram showing right coronary and posterior descending arteries from right anterior oblique view (c) and left anterior oblique view (d).

Intravascular ultrasonography (IVUS)

IVUS is accomplished by advancing a catheter over a guide wire previously placed into a coronary artery. The catheter has a miniature ultrasound transducer near its tip, which enables rotational Doppler imaging of the vessel wall in a plane perpendicular to its axis. IVUS is particularly useful for assessing the nature of angiographically questionable lesions, determining the true size of the vessel prior to stent deployment, and assessing the completeness of stent deployment. It is also probably the best method for serial studies of coronary anatomy during drug treatment trials, because it is able to image the plaque itself and is therefore a more sensitive method than angiography.

Complications of cardiac catheterization

Although cardiac catheterization is a relatively safe procedure, it is nevertheless important for both the patient and the referring physician to recognize the nature and likelihood of potential complications. Table 3.4.4 lists the complications of bilateral heart catheterization, including coronary, left ventricular, and aortic angiography, in a prospective study of valvular heart disease from the United States Veterans Administration. Even though these data were collected over 30 years ago from a particularly high-risk group of patients, the frequency of complication is a realistic estimate of what should currently be expected. The rate of each particular complication will vary with the age and general health of the patient. For

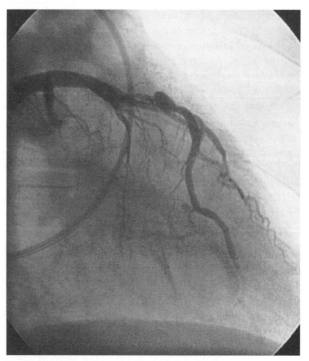

Fig. 3.4.9 Atherosclerotic coronary artery disease. The constrictions and blunt terminations seen in this patient's coronary angiogram represent atherosclerotic lesions.

Table 3.4.4 Complications of cardiac catheterization from a prospective study of 1559 procedures performed on 1483 United States veterans having valvular heart disease during the years 1977–1982[a]

Type of complication	Frequency (%)
Death within 24 h	0.1
Death between 24 h and 30 days	0.1
Stroke	0.3
Transient cerebral ischaemia	0.1
Myocardial infarction	0.2
Peripheral arterial embolism	0.1
Access site complications	1.7
Cardiac tamponade	0.3
Ventricular fibrillation	0.5
Arrhythmia other than ventricular fibrillation	1.5
Primary hypotension	0.5
Reaction to contrast medium (allergic and renal)	1.8
Arterial perforation or dissection	0.3
Miscellaneous complications	1.4
Patients having one or more of the above complications	6.9

[a] Although this is a high-risk group of patients undergoing extensive study, the rates are very comparable to what should be expected today. In fact, some complications, especially bleeding, are now more frequent because of aggressive anticoagulation and antiplatelet treatments given to many patients before and during catheterization.

example, the risk of vascular complication is considerably increased by the presence of vascular disease, and the risk of renal failure due to contrast medium is particularly high in diabetic patients with pre-existing renal dysfunction. Access site complications (bleeding, haematoma, arteriovenous fistula, pseudoaneurysm, and occlusion) have received particular attention in recent years because of the use of aggressive anticoagulation and antiplatelet treatments during percutaneous coronary intervention. Use of smaller gauge catheters and careful location of arterial puncture site is important. Vascular closure devices enable earlier ambulation of patients having femoral procedures.

In counselling the patient regarding the likelihood of untoward events it is important to give individualized advice based on the patient's particular circumstances. The decision to recommend catheterization must be based on the anticipation that its benefits justify its risk and cost.

Further reading

De Bruyne B, *et al.* (2012). Fractional flow reserve guided-PCI versus medical therapy in stable coronary disease. *N Engl J Med*, **367**, 991–1001.

Kern M (2011). *The cardiac catheterization handbook*, 5th edition. Elsevier, Philadelphia, PA.

Moscucci M (2013). *Grossman and Baim's cardiac catheterization, angiography and intervention*, 8th edition. Lippincott Williams and Wilkins, Baltimore, MD.

Tonino PA, *et al.* (2009). Fractional flow reserve versus angiography for guiding percutaneous coronary intervention. *N Engl J Med*, **360**, 213–24.

Cardiac arrhythmias

CHAPTER 4.1

Cardiac arrest

Jasmeet Soar, Jerry P. Nolan, and David A. Gabbott

Essentials

Cardiovascular disease is the most common cause of sudden cardiac arrest, which causes over 60% of adult coronary heart disease deaths. In Europe, the annual incidence of out-of-hospital cardiopulmonary arrests treated by emergency medical systems is 38 per 100 000.

Survival from cardiac arrest depends on a sequence of interventions—the Chain of Survival—comprising (1) early recognition and call for help, (2) early cardiopulmonary resuscitation (CPR), (3) early defibrillation, and (4) postresuscitation care. The division between basic life support and advanced life support (ALS) is arbitrary—the resuscitation process is a continuum.

Starting CPR

1. Check the patient for a response—and if they do not respond:

2. Turn the patient on their back, open the airway, and check for breathing and circulation—and if the patient has no signs of life, no pulse, or if there is any doubt.

3. Start CPR immediately.

Initial resuscitation

1. The compression to ventilation ratio is 30:2, with a chest compression rate of 100 to 120/min and depth for compression of 5 to 6 cm.

2. Use whatever equipment is available immediately for airway and ventilation.

3. Do continuous chest compressions with no pause for ventilations once the trachea is intubated—good quality chest compressions with minimal interruption for other procedures improves outcome.

4. When the defibrillator arrives, apply the electrodes to the patient and analyse the rhythm.

Advanced life support

Continue CPR and proceed to:

1. Treat shockable cardiac arrest rhythms (ventricular fibrillation/pulseless ventricular tachycardia—VF/VT) with attempted defibrillation.

2. Treat nonshockable rhythms (asystole and pulseless electrical activity, PEA) by treating the underlying cause.

3. Identify and treat reversible causes—hypoxia, hypovolaemia, electrolyte (hyperkalaemia, hypokalaemia, hypocalcaemia) or metabolic disorders (acidaemia), hypothermia, tension pneumothorax, tamponade, toxic substances, thromboembolism (pulmonary embolism or coronary thrombosis).

4. Minimizing interruptions to chest compressions will improve patient survival.

Postresuscitation care

The quality of postresuscitation care determines the patient's final outcome if resuscitation is successful. Consider therapeutic hypothermia and early percutaneous coronary intervention (PCI) in comatose survivors of cardiac arrest to improve neurological outcome and survival.

Do not attempt resuscitation (DNAR)

Decisions about CPR should be considered at the request of any person with capacity, as part of end-of-life care for a person with terminal illness, and as part of the care of patients with acute severe illness who might die.

Some patients will have made a clear statement of their wish not to receive CPR (e.g. 'living will'), and such a decision should be respected.

The decision-making process must comply with all relevant legislation, including that related to capacity, discrimination, and human rights. Discussions, decisions, and reasons for decisions should be recorded clearly in the patient's notes.

Introduction

Survival from cardiac arrest depends on a sequence of interventions—the 'chain of survival' (Fig. 4.1.1)—all four links in the chain must be strong:

- Early recognition and call for help
- Early cardiopulmonary resuscitation (CPR)
- Early defibrillation
- Postresuscitation care

Historical perspective

Current CPR techniques were first described relatively recently: the first report of external defibrillation was in 1956, mouth-to-mouth ventilation in 1958, and chest compressions in 1960.

Epidemiology

Sudden cardiac arrest causes over 60% of adult coronary heart disease deaths. In Europe, the annual incidence of out-of-hospital

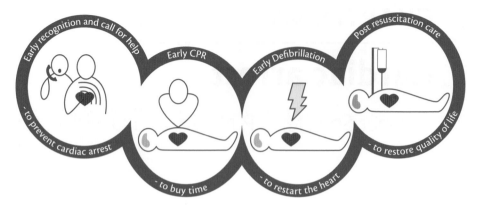

Fig. 4.1.1 The chain of survival.

cardiopulmonary arrests treated by emergency medical services is 38 per 100 000, with the annual incidence of VF/VT arrest being 17 per 100 000. Survival to hospital discharge is 10.7% for all-rhythm and 21.2% for VF cardiac arrest.

One-third of those developing a myocardial infarction die before reaching hospital. Usually the presenting rhythm is VF/VT in 25% of cases. The initial treatment for VF/VT is attempted defibrillation—with each minute's delay without CPR the chances of a successful outcome decrease by 7 to 10%.

Factors influencing the incidence of in-hospital cardiac arrest include the criteria for hospital admission and use of do not attempt (cardiopulmonary) resuscitation (DNAR) orders. The incidence of primary cardiac arrest in hospital is 1.5 to 3.0/1000 admissions, with 15 to 20% survival to hospital discharge. In two-thirds of in-hospital cardiac arrests the first monitored rhythm is asystole or pulseless electrical activity (PEA).

Prevention

Out-of-hospital, recognition of the importance of chest pain enables victims or bystanders to call the emergency medical service who can initiate treatment that can prevent cardiac arrest. In-hospital cardiac arrests are usually not sudden or unpredictable: in about 80% there is deterioration in clinical signs during the preceding few hours. Hypoxia and hypotension are often unnoticed, or are recognized but not acted upon or treated poorly. The cardiac arrest rhythm is usually PEA or asystole and prognosis is poor. Earlier recognition and treatment can prevent some cardiac arrests, deaths, and unanticipated intensive care unit (ICU) admissions. Recognition of this underlies the increasing usage of early warning scores to identify sick patients, which also enables decision making about DNAR orders.

Cardiopulmonary resuscitation

The division between basic life support and advanced life support (ALS) is arbitrary—the resuscitation process is a continuum. The keys steps are:

- Cardiorespiratory arrest is recognized immediately.
- Help is summoned.
- CPR (chest compressions and ventilations) is started immediately and, if indicated, defibrillation attempted as soon as possible (ideally, within 3 min of collapse).

The sequence of actions and outcome depends on:

- Location—out-of-hospital/in-hospital? Witnessed/unwitnessed? Monitored/unmonitored?

- Skills of the responders—in some public places (e.g. airports, railway stations) staff may be trained in CPR and defibrillation. Automated external defibrillator (AED) programmes with rapid response times in airports, on aircrafts, or in casinos, and studies using police officers have achieved survival rates as high as 49 to 74%. General practitioners and dental practitioners should have an AED on their premises.

- Number of responders—single responders must ensure that help is coming. If others are nearby, several actions can be undertaken simultaneously.

- Equipment available—AEDs are available in some public places. Staff working in hospitals usually have immediate access to resuscitation equipment and drugs.

- Response system to cardiac arrest and medical emergencies—outside hospital the emergency medical service should be summoned. In hospital, the resuscitation team can be a traditional cardiac arrest team (called when cardiac arrest is recognized). Alternatively, hospitals can have strategies to recognize patients at risk of cardiac arrest and summon a team (e.g. medical emergency team, rapid response team, or critical care outreach team) before cardiac arrest occurs.

Risks to the rescuer

There are few reports of harm to rescuers from doing CPR. Gloves should be worn: eye protection, aprons, and face masks may be necessary. A pocket mask with filter, or a barrier device with one-way valve, should be used to minimize risk during rescue breathing. However, the risk of infection is lower than perceived: there are reports of transmission of tuberculosis and severe acute respiratory syndrome (SARS), but HIV transmission has never been reported. It is sensible to wear full personal protective equipment when the victim has a serious infection (e.g. tuberculosis or SARS). Mouth-to-mouth ventilation should be avoided in hydrogen cyanide or hydrogen sulphide poisoning, as should contact with corrosive chemicals (e.g. strong acids, alkalis, paraquat) or substances (e.g. organophosphates) that are absorbed through the skin or respiratory tract.

Starting CPR

CPR should be started as shown in Box 4.1.1.

Box 4.1.1 Starting CPR

1. Check the patient for a response
   - If you see a patient collapse or apparently unconscious:
     - shout for help
     - assess responsiveness (shake their shoulders) and seek a verbal response

2. If the patient does not respond
   - Agonal breathing (occasional gasps, slow, laboured, or noisy breathing) is common immediately after cardiac arrest—do not mistake this for a sign of life.
   - Turn patient on to their back and open the airway.

3. Open airway, check breathing, and check for circulation
   - Open the airway using a head tilt chin lift.
   - Look in the mouth and remove any visible foreign body or debris.
   - A patent airway takes priority over concerns about a potential cervical spine injury, but minimize neck movement if cervical spine injury is suspected.
   - Keeping the airway open, look, listen, and feel (for up to 10 s) to determine if the patient is breathing normally (an occasional gasp, slow, laboured, or noisy breathing is not normal) and simultaneously feel for a carotid pulse.

4. If the patient has no signs of life, no pulse, or if there is any doubt, start CPR immediately
   - Ensure help is coming.
   - If alone, leave the patient to get help.
   - Give 30 chest compressions (depth 5–6 cm, rate 100–120 compressions/min, allowing complete chest recoil at end of each compression) followed by two ventilations (compression–ventilation ratio=30:2).
   - The hand position for chest compression is the middle of the lower half of the sternum.
   - Allow the chest to recoil completely after each compression.
   - Take the same amount of time for compression and relaxation.
   - Use whatever equipment is available immediately for airway and ventilation. Use a pocket mask (which can be supplemented with an oral airway), a supraglottic airway (e.g. laryngeal mask airway (LMA)) and self-inflating bag, or bag mask. Attempt tracheal intubation only if trained and competent to do so.
   - Use an inspiratory time of 1 s and enough volume to produce a normal chest rise. Add supplemental oxygen as soon as possible.
   - Avoid rapid or forceful breaths to prevent gastric distension.
   - Once the patient's trachea has been intubated, continue chest compressions uninterrupted at a rate of 100 to 120/min, and ventilate the lungs at approximately 10 breaths/min.

   - If airway and ventilation equipment are unavailable, give mouth-to-mouth ventilation. If there are clinical reasons to avoid mouth-to-mouth contact, or you are unwilling or unable to do this, do chest compressions until help or airway equipment arrives.
   - When the defibrillator arrives, apply the electrodes to the patient and analyse the rhythm. See ALS for further steps.
   - Providing CPR is tiring—change the individual undertaking compressions every 2 min to ensure high-quality chest compressions with minimal interruption.

5. If the patient is not breathing and has a pulse (respiratory arrest)
   - Ventilate the patient's lungs (as described above) and check for a circulation every 10 breaths (about every minute).
   - If there are any doubts about the presence of a pulse, start chest compressions.

Cardiopulmonary resuscitation—mechanism of action

Chest compressions create blood flow by increasing intrathoracic pressure and compressing the heart directly. However, perfusion of the brain and myocardium is (at best) 25% of normal. The coronary perfusion pressure achieved during CPR correlates with return of spontaneous circulation (ROSC). In the presence of VF, chest compressions increase the likelihood that attempted defibrillation will be successful, and pauses in chest compressions of just 5 s before shock delivery almost halves the chances of successful defibrillation. Frequent interruptions in chest compressions reduce survival from cardiac arrest. Each time chest compressions are stopped the coronary perfusion pressure decreases rapidly, and on resuming chest compressions it takes time to build up to the coronary perfusion pressure present just before compressions were interrupted (Fig. 4.1.2).

Advanced life support (ALS)

The ALS algorithm enables a standardized approach to cardiac arrest management (Fig. 4.1.3). Once CPR has started, assess the patient's rhythm as soon as possible. Heart rhythms associated with cardiac arrest comprise:

- Shockable rhythms—VF/VT. In adults, the most common rhythm at the time of cardiac arrest is VF, which may be preceded by a period of VT, by a bradyarrhythmia, or less commonly by supraventricular tachycardia (SVT).
- Nonshockable rhythms—asystole and pulseless electrical activity (PEA). PEA is cardiac electrical activity in the absence of any palpable pulses.

Treatment of shockable rhythms (VF/VT)

Shockable rhythms should be treated as shown in Box 4.1.2.

During CPR

Resume chest compressions immediately after a shock. Even if a defibrillation attempt is successful in restoring a perfusing rhythm, it is rare for a pulse to be palpable immediately after defibrillation,

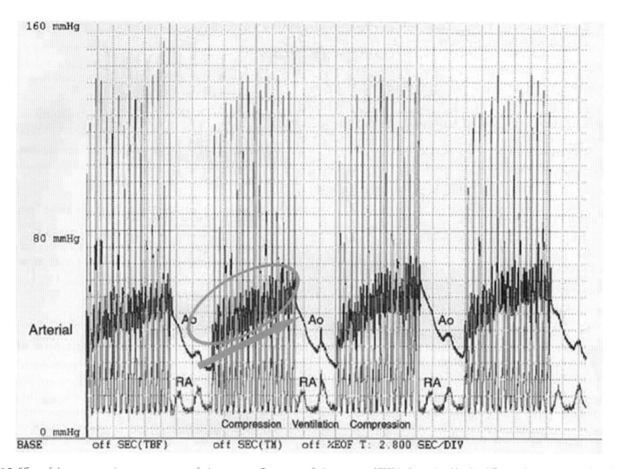

Fig. 4.1.2 Effect of chest compressions on coronary perfusion pressure. Coronary perfusion pressure (CPP) is determined by the difference between aortic diastolic pressure and right atrial pressure. The lower border of the dark band (marked by the orange ellipse) depicts the aortic diastolic pressure and thus CPP. This increases progressively as chest compressions are continued but decreases to base levels each time compressions are stopped. Note also that CPP continues to increase and does not plateau after 15 compressions. Uninterrupted chest compressions will generate a higher CPP.
Reproduced from Resuscitation, 39;3;10, Efficacy of chest compression-only BLS CPR in the presence of an occluded airway, Kern, Hilwig, Berg & Ewy, © 1998 with permission from BMJ Publishing Group Ltd.

and delay in trying to palpate a pulse will further compromise the myocardium if a perfusing rhythm has not been restored. If a perfusing rhythm has been restored, giving chest compressions does not increase the chance of VF recurring.

The vasopressor adrenaline is given to increase coronary perfusion pressure during CPR. A recent meta-analysis showed no statistically significant difference between vasopressin and adrenaline for ROSC, death within 24 h, or death before hospital discharge.

There is no evidence that giving any antiarrhythmic drug routinely during human cardiac arrest increases survival to hospital discharge. In the prehospital setting, the use of amiodarone (300 mg intravenously) in VF refractory to shock (three failed defibrillation attempts) improves the short-term outcome of survival to hospital admission in comparison with placebo and lidocaine.

Monitored and witnessed cardiac arrest

If a patient has a monitored and witnessed VF/VT cardiac arrest in the cardiac catheter laboratory or immediately after cardiac surgery give up to three successive defibrillatory shocks before starting chest compressions. There is a good chance of successful defibrillation in these settings.

The precordial thump

The mechanical energy of a precordial thump is converted to electrical energy, which may be sufficient to achieve cardioversion. The

electrical threshold of successful defibrillation increases rapidly after the onset of arrhythmia, and the amount of electrical energy generated falls below this threshold within seconds. A precordial thump (delivered using the ulnar edge of a tightly clenched fist to deliver a sharp impact to the lower half of the sternum) is most likely to be successful in converting VT to sinus rhythm, and successful treatment of VF by precordial thump is much less likely. Recent evidence suggests that the precordial thump rarely works in clinical practice and its use has been de-emphasized in recent guidelines.

Nonshockable rhythms (PEA and asystole)

Nonshockable rhythms should be treated as shown in Boxes 4.1.3 and 4.1.4 , with care taken to identify and treat reversible causes of PEA and asystole during CPR, as described below.

Airway and ventilation

Tracheal intubation provides the most reliable airway during CPR, but should be attempted only by trained rescuers. Acceptable alternatives include the laryngeal mask airway (LMA), i-gel airway, ProSeal LMA, or Laryngeal Tube, which are supraglottic devices that can be inserted without the need for laryngoscopy. Compared with bag mask ventilation, early ventilation with a supraglottic device reduces the incidence of gastric distension and subsequent

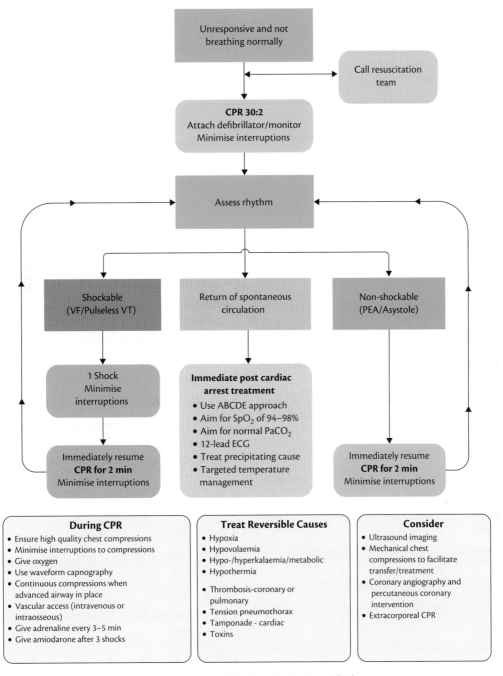

Fig. 4.1.3 The advanced life support algorithm. Reproduced with permission of the Resuscitation Council (UK).

regurgitation, and enables more effective ventilation of the lungs of an unconscious patient. Continuous chest compressions should be performed without stopping for ventilations if such an alternative airway has been inserted, but if excessive gas leakage results in inadequate ventilation of the patient's lungs, then chest compressions should be interrupted to enable ventilation. Waveform capnography should be used to confirm correct placement of a tracheal tube; it also provides an indication of the quality of CPR (higher values indicate better pulmonary blood flow). A sudden increase in end-tidal carbon dioxide values suggests return of spontaneous circulation.

Drug delivery

Peak drug concentrations are higher and circulation times are shorter when drugs are injected into a central vein compared with a peripheral vein. However, insertion of a central venous catheter requires interruption of CPR and is associated with several potential complications: peripheral venous cannulation is quicker, easier, and safer. Flush drugs injected peripherally with at least 20 ml of fluid and elevate the extremity for 10 to 20 s to facilitate drug delivery to the central circulation. Use the intraosseous route in adults when the intravenous route is impossible. The tracheal route is no longer recommended for drug delivery during adult CPR.

Box 4.1.2 Treatment of shockable rhythms (VF/VT)

- Start CPR and assess rhythm to diagnose VF/VT: resume chest compressions while charging the defibrillator to 150 to 200 J biphasic (or 360 J monophasic).
- Once defibrillator charged, stop chest compressions and give shock.
- Immediately resume chest compressions (30:2) without reassessing the rhythm or feeling for a pulse.
- Continue CPR for 2 min, then pause briefly to check the monitor.
- If VF/VT persists resume chest compressions while charging the defibrillator to 150 to 360 J biphasic (360 J monophasic):
  - Once defibrillator charged, stop chest compressions and give a further (2nd) shock.
  - Resume CPR immediately and continue for 2 min.
  - Pause briefly to check the monitor.
- If VF/VT persists resume chest compressions while charging the defibrillator to 150 to 360 J biphasic (360 J monophasic):
  - Once defibrillator charged, stop chest compressions and give a further (3rd) shock.
  - Resume CPR immediately and continue for 2 min. During CPR give adrenaline 1 mg intravenously and amiodarone 300 mg intravenously.
  - Pause briefly to check the monitor.
- Give further shocks after each 2-min period of CPR and after confirming that VF/VT persists.
- Give further adrenaline 1 mg intravenously every 3 to 5 min (alternate loops).

  If organized electrical activity compatible with a cardiac output is seen, check for a pulse.
- If a pulse is present, start postresuscitation care.
- If no pulse is present, continue CPR and switch to the nonshockable algorithm (Boxes 4.1.3 and 4.1.4).
  - If asystole is seen, continue CPR and switch to the nonshockable algorithm (Boxes 4.1.3 and 4.1.4).

  There is no strong outcome data, but the balance of evidence favours the use of anti-arrhythmics in cardiac arrest.

* Give amiodarone after 3 shocks (300 mg IV push + 150 mg IV push if no cardioversion + continued infusion if cardioversion achieved).

Box 4.1.3 Treatment for PEA

- Start CPR 30:2.
- Give adrenaline 1 mg intravenously as soon as intravascular access is achieved.
- Continue CPR 30:2 until the airway is secured—then continue chest compressions without pausing during ventilation.
- Recheck the rhythm after 2 min:
  - If organized electrical activity is seen, check for a pulse and/or signs of life.
- If pulse and/or signs of life are present, start postresuscitation care.
- If no pulse and/or signs of life are present (PEA):
- Continue CPR.
- Recheck the rhythm after 2 min and proceed accordingly.
- Give further adrenaline 1 mg intravenously every 3 to 5 min (alternate loops).
  - If VF/VT at rhythm check, change to the shockable side of algorithm (Box 4.1.2).
  - If asystole or an agonal rhythm seen at rhythm check:
- Continue CPR.
- Recheck the rhythm after 2 min and proceed accordingly.
- Give further adrenaline 1 mg intravenously every 3 to 5 min (alternate loops).

- Hyperkalaemia, hypokalaemia, hypocalcaemia (acidaemia and other metabolic disorders)
- Hypothermia
- Tension pneumothorax
- Tamponade
- Toxic substances
- Thromboembolism (pulmonary embolism or coronary thrombosis)

Use of ultrasound imaging during advanced life support

The use of ultrasound during advanced life support requires considerable expertise. Interruptions to chest compressions must be minimized. There are no studies demonstrating that outcome is improved, but no doubt that potentially reversible causes of cardiac arrest can be detected, e.g. cardiac tamponade.

Waveform capnography during ALS

Recent guidelines recommend the use of waveform capnography whenever endotracheal intubation is performed to ensure the tube is placed in the trachea, monitor the quality of chest compression during CPR, identify return of spontaneous circulation, and provide prognostic information (low end-tidal CO_2 is associated with poor outcome).

Reversible causes

Reversible causes should be identified and treated during CPR in all cardiac arrests. These can be divided into two groups of four, based upon their initial letter—either H or T:

- Hypoxia
- Hypovolaemia

Box 4.1.4 Treatment for asystole

◆ Start CPR 30:2.

◆ Check that the leads are attached correctly without stopping CPR.

◆ Give adrenaline 1 mg intravenously as soon as intravascular access is achieved.

◆ Continue CPR 30:2 until the airway is secured, then continue chest compressions without pausing during ventilation.

◆ Recheck the rhythm after 2 min and proceed accordingly.

◆ If VF/VT occurs, change to the shockable rhythm algorithm (Box 4.1.2).

◆ Give adrenaline 1 mg intravenously every 3 to 5 min (alternate loops).

Mechanical chest compression

Automated mechanical chest compression devices can be used by appropriately trained staff, but randomized controlled trials have not demonstrated benefit.

Defibrillation

Defibrillation is the passage of sufficient current across the myocardium to depolarize a critical mass of the cardiac muscle simultaneously, which enables the natural pacemaker tissue to resume control. Success is defined as termination of fibrillation or—more precisely—the absence of VF/VT at 5 s after shock delivery, although the ultimate goal is ROSC.

Factors affecting defibrillation success

Transthoracic impedance

In adults, impedance is normally 70 to 80 Ω, but in the presence of poor technique it may rise to 150 Ω, halving the current delivered and thereby reducing the chance of successful defibrillation. The factors influencing transthoracic impedance are listed in Table 4.1.1.

Table 4.1.1 Factors influencing transthoracic impedance

Chest hair	Hair increases impedance and can cause burns to the patient's chest
Electrode size	The total electrode area should be a minimum of 150 cm². Larger electrodes have lower impedance, but excessively large electrodes may result in less transmyocardial current flow
Coupling agents	If using manual paddles, gel pads are preferable to electrode pastes and gels because the latter can spread between the two paddles, creating the potential for a spark
Paddle force	Apply paddles firmly to the chest wall to reduce transthoracic impedance by improving electrical contact at the electrode–skin interface and reducing thoracic volume. The optimal force of application is 8 kg in an adult

Electrode position

During defibrillation, transmyocardial current is likely to be maximal when electrodes are placed so that the part of the heart that is fibrillating lies directly between them (i.e. ventricles in VF/VT, atria in AF). This means that the optimal electrode position may not be the same for ventricular and atrial arrhythmias.

Pads versus paddles

Self-adhesive defibrillation pads are safe, effective, and preferable to defibrillation paddles. When used for initial monitoring of a rhythm and shock delivery, both pads and paddles enable quicker delivery of the first shock compared with attaching standard ECG electrodes. Pads make it easier to minimize interruption to chest compressions and to charge the defibrillator during chest compressions.

Shock energy and waveforms

There are currently two main types of waveforms used for defibrillation (Fig. 4.1.4): monophasic and biphasic (e.g. truncated exponential, rectilinear). The optimal defibrillation energy dose should achieve defibrillation and ROSC and minimize myocardial injury, and also reduce the need for repetitive shocks (which also limits myocardial injury). Although energy levels are selected for defibrillation, it is the transmyocardial current flow that actually achieves defibrillation, the optimal current for defibrillation using a monophasic waveform being in the range of 30 to 40 A, with indirect evidence suggesting 15 to 20 A using biphasic waveforms. Because they require less energy, biphasic devices have smaller capacitors and need less battery power, hence they are smaller, lighter, and more easily portable.

First-shock efficacy for long duration VF/VT is greater with biphasic (86–98%) than monophasic waveforms (54–91%), although a survival advantage has yet to be demonstrated. Some defibrillator manufacturers recommend escalating energy doses with successive shocks, while others favour fixed-energy dose shocks. There is currently no evidence supporting one strategy over the other.

Defibrillator safety

The operator must ensure that everyone is clear of the patient before delivering a shock, also that no oxygen is flowing across the chest. Oxygen masks should be moved to a distance greater than 1 m away, with tracheal tubes or supraglottic devices left connected to a breathing circuit or bag device. New guidelines in 2010 recommend that chest compressions continue while the defibrillator is charging. Once the defibrillator is charged, all rescuers should stand clear for shock delivery. Chest compressions should continue immediately after the shock. Safety issues should be addressed whilst chest compressions are ongoing in order to minimize interruptions to chest compressions.

Postresuscitation care

The quality of postresuscitation care significantly influences the patient's ultimate outcome. The airway, breathing, circulation, disability, and exposure (ABCDE) system approach should be applied.

Airway and breathing

Consider tracheal intubation, sedation and controlled ventilation in patients with obtunded cerebral function after ROSC. Both hypoxaemia and hyperoxaemia may be harmful to the reperfused brain. Adjust the inspired oxygen to maintain an oxygen

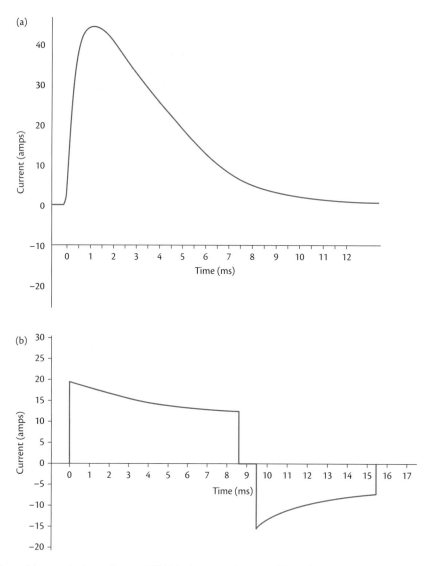

Fig. 4.1.4 Defibrillation waveforms: (a) monophasic waveform and (b) biphasic truncated exponential waveform.

saturation of 94 to 98%. Hypocapnia induced by hyperventilation causes cerebral ischaemia after cardiac arrest. There are no data to support the targeting of a specific $Paco_2$ after resuscitation in this situation, but it is reasonable to adjust ventilation to achieve normocapnia.

Circulation

Haemodynamic instability is common after cardiac arrest and manifests as hypotension, low cardiac output, and arrhythmia. This is partly caused by reperfusion injury and is usually transient, often reversing within 24 to 48 h. The postresuscitation period is associated with marked elevation in plasma cytokine concentrations and with a sepsis-like syndrome and multiple organ dysfunction.

A 12-lead ECG should be recorded as soon as possible. Acute S-T segment elevation or new left bundle branch block in a patient with a typical history of acute myocardial infarction is an indication for reperfusion therapy by emergency percutaneous coronary intervention.

Disability and exposure

Cerebral perfusion

Immediately after ROSC there is a period of cerebral hyperaemia, but global cerebral blood flow decreases after 15 to 30 min of reperfusion and there is generalized hypoperfusion. Normal cerebral autoregulation is lost, leaving cerebral perfusion dependent on mean arterial pressure. Under these circumstances, hypotension will compromise cerebral blood flow severely and will compound any neurological injury, hence after ROSC the aim should be to maintain mean arterial pressure at the patient's usual level.

Control of seizures

Seizures and/or myoclonus occur in 5 to 15% of patients who achieve ROSC and in about 40% of those who remain comatose. Per se, they are not related significantly to outcome, but status epilepticus—and in particular status myoclonus—is a poor prognostic sign. Prolonged seizures can cause cerebral injury and should be controlled with benzodiazepines, phenytoin, propofol, or a barbiturate.

Temperature control

Treatment of hyperthermia

Hyperthermia is common in the first 48 h after cardiac arrest, and the risk of a poor neurological outcome increases for each degree of body temperature over 37°C. Any hyperthermia occurring in the first 72 h after cardiac arrest should be treated with antipyretics or active cooling.

Therapeutic hypothermia

Mild hypothermia suppresses many of the chemical reactions associated with reperfusion injury, including free radical production, excitatory amino acid release, and calcium shifts, which can in turn lead to mitochondrial damage and apoptosis (programmed cell death).

Unconscious adult patients with spontaneous circulation after out-of-hospital VF cardiac arrest should be cooled to a temperature of 32 to 34°C as soon as possible and maintained at this level for at least 12 to 24 h. Induced hypothermia might also benefit unconscious adult patients with spontaneous circulation after out-of-hospital cardiac arrest from a nonshockable rhythm, or cardiac arrest in hospital. The patient should be rewarmed slowly (0.25°C/h), with avoidance of hyperthermia, but the optimum target temperature, rate of cooling, duration of hypothermia, and rate of rewarming have yet to be determined.

Prediction of prognosis after cardiac arrest

Of 24 132 patients admitted to ICUs in the United Kingdom after cardiac arrest, 42.9% survived to leave intensive care and 28.6% survived to hospital discharge. Of those discharged from hospital, 80% return immediately to their normal residence.

Two-thirds of those dying after admission to ICU following out-of-hospital cardiac arrest do so from neurological injury, as do a quarter of those admitted following in-hospital cardiac arrest. A means of predicting neurological outcome that can be applied to individual patients immediately after ROSC would be extremely useful, but none is available.

Clinical tests

There are no neurological signs that can predict outcome in the first few hours after ROSC. By 3 days after the onset of coma relating to cardiac arrest, 50% of patients with no chance of ultimate recovery have died. The absence of pupillary light reflexes or an absent motor response to pain on day 3 are independently predictive of a poor outcome (death or vegetative state) with very high specificity. The use of therapeutic hypothermia influences the reliability of these clinical predictors and may mean that prognostication has to be delayed until 3 days after the return to normothermia.

Electrophysiological tests

Median nerve somatosensory evoked potentials in normothermic patients, comatose for at least 72 h after cardiac arrest, predict poor outcome with 100% specificity. Bilateral absence of the N20 component of the evoked potentials in comatose patients with coma of hypoxic-anoxic origin is uniformly fatal. A normal or a grossly abnormal EEG both predict outcome reliably, but an EEG between these extremes does not.

Other issues

Cardiac electrophysiological assessment

The possible requirement for an implantable cardioverter defibrillator (ICD) should be considered in any patient who has been resuscitated from cardiac arrest in a shockable rhythm outside the context of proven acute ST segment elevation myocardial infarction. All such patients should be referred before discharge from hospital for assessment by a cardiologist with expertise in heart rhythm disorders.

Audit and research

All CPR attempts should be audited to ensure that practice complies with published standards. Lack of uniformity in cardiac arrest reporting makes it difficult to evaluate the impact on survival of individual factors, such as new drugs or techniques. New interventions that improve survival rate only slightly are highly significant because cardiac arrest is common and kills thousands of people every year. However, individual hospitals or health care systems are unlikely to have sufficient patients to identify subtle effects or eliminate confounders, but by adopting uniform definitions and collecting standardized data on the process and outcome of CPR in many patients and systems it may be possible to identify relatively small but important changes in outcome. Changes in the resuscitation process could then be introduced and evaluated more widely.

The Utstein style template was established by consensus among a group of resuscitation experts and this standardized format should be followed when collecting data for audit or research.

Many countries are now establishing national cardiac arrest registries that collate data from individual hospitals, e.g. National CPR registry in the USA and National Cardiac Arrest Audit in the UK.

Decisions relating to cardiopulmonary resuscitation

Decisions about CPR should be considered:

- at the request of any person with capacity.

- as an essential part of end-of-life care for a person with terminal illness.

- as an essential part of the care of a patient with acute severe illness who has suffered an event from which no recovery can reasonably be expected, or who is deteriorating despite treatment.

Some patients will have made a clear statement of their wish not to receive CPR (e.g. 'living will'), but in other cases discussions about CPR can be difficult. They are best approached on an individualized basis that puts the decision within the context of the patient's prognosis, care, and treatment. Some will want to discuss and engage in decisions about their end-of-life care, and others will not. Their views should be respected and explored sensitively, and discussions, decisions, and reasons for decisions should be recorded clearly in the patient's notes.

Decisions about CPR should be made by the most senior doctor available and all members of the health care team looking after the patient should be informed. Any decision should be reviewed at the patient's request, if those close to the patient request a review, and if there is a significant change in the patient's clinical condition.

The decision-making process must comply with all relevant legislation, including that related to capacity, discrimination, and human rights. The courts in England have stated that there is a presumption that the patient will be involved in decisions about CPR unless such discussions would cause them harm, and when a decision not to attempt CPR (DNACPR) is made because CPR would not be successful, it is expected that the decision and the reasons for it would be explained to them. A patient, or their relative, does not have a right to demand CPR, but the physician must proceed very carefully if their decision that CPR should not be attempted is at variance with the patient's view or that of their family. They would be well advised to obtain advice from senior clinical colleagues and other appropriate sources (e.g. legal, medical defence union) in this circumstance.

Likely developments over the next few years

International CPR guidelines are updated every 5 years. Defibrillator technology is evolving rapidly, and many have several other functions as well as defibrillation. New defibrillators already have the ability to provide real-time feedback on depth and rate of chest compression, and on ventilation rate and volumes. In the near future, AEDs will be able to analyse the rhythm without interruption of chest compressions, which will enable continuous CPR with just a short pause for shock delivery. Analysis of VF waveforms will indicate when a shock is likely to achieve ROSC and will reduce the incidence of postshock asystole or PEA, thus minimizing the number of ineffective and potentially harmful shocks given to the patient.

Several mechanical chest compressing devices are available, but as yet none has been shown to improve long-term survival after cardiac arrest. It is likely that the efficiency of these devices will be improved.

The use of transthoracic echocardiography in the peri-arrest period to identify reversible causes of cardiac arrest will become more popular. This will require increased training in echocardiography and wider availability of echocardiography machines.

Hypothermia provides significant protection from ischaemia and hypoxia. The possibility of cooling patients rapidly just before cardiac arrest, e.g. during exsanguinating haemorrhage in the military setting, may enable the patient to be transported for definitive surgery in a state of 'suspended animation'. This technology has been applied successfully in animal models.

Further reading

Abella BS, *et al.* (2005). Quality of cardiopulmonary resuscitation during in-hospital cardiac arrest. *JAMA*, **293**, 305–310.

Atwood C, *et al.* (2005). Incidence of EMS-treated out-of hospital cardiac arrest in Europe. *Resuscitation*, **67**, 75–80.

Bernard SA, *et al.* (2002). Treatment of comatose survivors of out-of-hospital cardiac arrest with induced hypothermia. *N Engl J Med*, **346**, 557–563.

Cretikos M, *et al.* (2006). Guidelines for the uniform reporting of data for Medical Emergency Teams. *Resuscitation*, **68**, 11–25.

Cullinane M, *et al.* (2005). *An acute problem? National Confidential Enquiry into Patient Outcome and Death 2005 report.* http://www.ncepod.org.uk/2005report/.

Deakin CD, Nolan JP, European Resuscitation Council (2010). European Resuscitation Council Guidelines for Resuscitation 2010. Section 3: Electrical therapies: automated external defibrillators, defibrillation, cardioversion and pacing. *Resuscitation*, **81**, 1293–304.

Deakin CD, *et al.* (2010). European Resuscitation Council guidelines for resuscitation 2010. Section 4. Adult advanced life support. *Resuscitation*, **81**, 305–52.

Decisions relating to cardiopulmonary resuscitation. Joint statement from the BMA, the Resuscitation Council (UK) and RCN (October 2007) www.resus.org.uk.

Edelson DP, *et al.* (2006). Effects of compression depth and pre-shock pauses predict defibrillation failure during cardiac arrest. *Resuscitation*, **71**(2), 137–45.

Gabbott D, *et al.* (2005). Cardiopulmonary resuscitation standards for clinical practice and training in the UK. *Resuscitation*, **64**, 13–19.

Hypothermia after Cardiac Arrest Study Group (2002). Mild therapeutic hypothermia to improve the neurological outcome after cardiac arrest. *N Engl J Med*, **346**, 549–56.

Koster RW (2009). Precordial thump: Friend or enemy? *Resuscitation*, **80**(1), 2–3.

Langhelle A, *et al.* (2005). Recommended guidelines for reviewing, reporting, and conducting research on post-resuscitation care: the Utstein style. *Resuscitation*, **66**, 271–83.

Lloyd MS, *et al.* (2008). Hands-on defibrillation: an analysis of electrical current flow through rescuers in direct contact with patients during biphasic external defibrillation. *Circulation*, **117**, 2510–2514.Nolan J, *et al.* (eds) (2011). *Advanced life support*, 6th edition. Resuscitation Council UK, London.

Nolan JP, *et al.* (2015). Part 1; Executive summary: 2015 International Consensus on Cardiopulmonary Resuscitation and Emergency Cardiovascular Care Science with Treatment Recommendations. *Resuscitation*, **95**, Suppl 1, e1–32.

Nolan JP, *et al.* (2008). Post-cardiac arrest syndrome: epidemiology, pathophysiology, treatment, and prognostication. A Scientific Statement from the International Liaison Committee on Resuscitation; the American Heart Association Emergency Cardiovascular Care Committee; the Council on Cardiovascular Surgery and Anesthesia; the Council on Cardiopulmonary, Perioperative, and Critical Care; the Council on Clinical Cardiology; the Council on Stroke. *Resuscitation*, **79**(3), 350–79.

Nolan JP, Soar J (2008). Airway and ventilation techniques. *Curr Opin Crit Care*, **14**, 279–86.

Nolan JP, Soar J (2009). Defibrillation in clinical practice. *Curr Opin Crit Care*, **15**, 209–15.

Oddo M, Rossetti AO (2011). Predicting neurological outcome after cardiac arrest. *Curr Opin Crit Care*, **17**, 254–9.

Sandroni C, *et al.* (2007). In-hospital cardiac arrest: incidence, prognosis and possible measures to improve survival. *Intensive Care Med*, **33**, 237–245.

Soar J, *et al.* (2015). Part 4: Advanced life support: 2015 International Consensus on Cardiopulmonary Resuscitation and Emergency Cardiovascular Care Science with Treatment Recommendations. *Resuscitation*, **95**, e71–122.

Soar J, Nolan JP (2008). Cardiopulmonary resuscitation for out of hospital cardiac arrest, Editorial. *BMJ*, **336**, 782–3.

CHAPTER 4.2

Cardiac arrhythmias

M. Ginks, Gregory Y. H. Lip, D. A. Lane, S. M. Cobbe, A. D. McGavigan, and A. C. Rankin

Essentials

The term cardiac arrhythmia (or dysrhythmia) is used to describe any abnormality of cardiac rhythm. The spectrum of cardiac arrhythmias ranges from innocent extrasystoles to immediately life-threatening conditions such as asystole or ventricular fibrillation.

The key to the successful diagnosis of cardiac arrhythmias is the systematic analysis of an ECG (see Chapter 3.1) of optimal quality obtained during the arrhythmia.

Continuous monitoring is necessary for identification when arrhythmias are intermittent. Ambulatory ECG recordings are of most value when they provide correlation between the patient's symptoms and the cardiac rhythm at that moment. Alternative strategies for the detection of infrequent arrhythmias include the use of a patient-activated recorder, which is applied and activated during symptoms, or an external or implanted loop recorder.

More detailed investigation of cardiac arrhythmias is undertaken by invasive cardiac electrophysiological testing. Multipolar electrodes are inserted transvenously to record electrograms from the atrium, ventricle, His bundle, and coronary sinus. Electrophysiological mapping is an essential part of radiofrequency ablation.

Bradycardias

Bradycardia is defined as a ventricular rate of less than 60 beats/min. The principal indications for active intervention in bradycardia are symptomatic (disturbances of consciousness, fatigue, lethargy, dyspnoea, or bradycardia-induced tachyarrhythmias) or prognostic (prevention of sudden cardiac death).

In the presence of haemodynamic compromise, immediate attempts to increase heart rate should be employed, using atropine, isoproterenol (isoprenaline), and/or temporary cardiac pacing (transvenous or transcutaneous). Following stabilization, factors causing or contributing to the presentation should be sought and corrected—especially, acute ischaemia and infarction, concomitant drug therapy, hypothermia, or electrolyte disorders.

Specific disorders causing bradycardia include (1) sinoatrial disease ('sick sinus syndrome'); (2) neurocardiogenic syncope (e.g. carotid sinus hypersensitivity); and (3) atrioventricular (AV) conduction disorders ('heart block').

AV block—the commonest cause of AV block is idiopathic fibrosis of the His–Purkinje system, and the severity (degree) of block can be classified as (1) first-degree—defined as a PR interval greater than 0.2 s, which produces no symptoms and does not require treatment; (2) second-degree—when there is intermittent failure of conduction from atrium to ventricle, either with a characteristic pattern of increasing PR-interval duration preceding the nonconducted P-wave (Mobitz type I, Wenckebach) or without (Mobitz type II). Pacemaker implantation is not necessary for Mobitz type I in most cases, but is usually required for Mobitz type II; (3) third-degree (complete) AV block—when there is complete dissociation between atrial and ventricular activity, which is an indication for permanent pacemaker implantation, except in the context of an acutely reversible condition.

Tachycardias

The principal mechanisms responsible for tachyarrhythmias are (1) abnormal automaticity; (2) triggered activity; or (3) re-entry. Most clinically important sustained tachycardias appear to arise on the basis of re-entry, which requires the presence of a potential circuit comprising two limbs with different refractoriness and conduction properties.

The first and most important step in the diagnosis and management of tachycardias is to determine whether the arrhythmia arises within the atria and/or AV junction, or from the ventricles, which can often be achieved by careful analysis of a 12-lead ECG.

Diagnosis—it is safe to assume that virtually all narrow-complex tachycardias have a supraventricular origin, but wide-complex tachycardias (QRS duration ≥0.12 s) may arise either from the ventricle or from supraventricular mechanisms, and few areas in cardiology cause more difficulty—or result in more mismanagement—than the diagnosis of wide-complex tachycardias. Careful scrutiny of the 12-lead ECG may reveal diagnostic features, but the commonest reason for error is that the clinical context is not considered, or erroneous conclusions are drawn from it: key issues to recognize are (1) elderly patients or those with a history of ischaemic heart disease are most likely to have ventricular arrhythmia; (2) the patient's haemodynamic status is a poor predictor of the type of tachycardia; (3) ventricular tachycardia can present with a history of paroxysmal self-terminating episodes.

Treatment—R-wave synchronized, direct current (DC) cardioversion under general anaesthesia or deep sedation is the most effective and immediate means of terminating sustained tachycardias, and should be employed when tachycardia is associated with haemodynamic compromise. In patients with tachycardia who are haemodynamically stable, manoeuvres that produce transient vagal stimulation, such as the Valsalva manoeuvre or carotid sinus massage, may be employed. The response to intravenous adenosine, which will often terminate arrhythmias dependent on the AV node, may be of therapeutic or diagnostic value, and should be considered in all patients with tolerated regular tachycardia. In the long term, tachycardias can be treated with antiarrhythmic drugs (usefully categorized by the Vaughan Williams classification), implantable cardioverter–defibrillators (ICDs), radiofrequency catheter ablation, or arrhythmia surgery. In all cases an assessment of the underlying precipitating cause (i.e. ischaemic heart disease, electrolyte disturbance, structural heart disease, genetic predisposition, or drug therapy) is required before planning subsequent long-term therapy.

Atrial fibrillation

Rhythm management—if it is clinically appropriate to attempt chemical cardioversion, the drugs of choice are the class Ic agents (e.g. flecainide) for patients without significant underlying heart disease; class III drugs (e.g. sotalol or amiodarone) are somewhat less effective but are safer in the presence of left ventricular dysfunction or ischaemic heart disease. Normally, only one drug should be tried in any individual patient: if drug therapy fails, DC cardioversion is commonly effective.

Unless the patient has been therapeutically anticoagulated for several weeks, cardioversion (by chemical or electrical means) should not be attempted without transoesophageal echocardiography if the arrhythmia has been present for longer than 48 h because of the risk of thromboembolism. Anticoagulation plus rate control with a β-blocker, calcium channel blocker, or digoxin should be considered in these circumstances. Prophylaxis against thromboembolism should be considered in all patients with atrial fibrillation.

Paroxysmal atrial fibrillation—drug therapy may not be necessary for patients with infrequent paroxysms, or a 'pill in the pocket' approach can be used in those without structural heart disease, whereby they take a dose of an antiarrhythmic drug after the onset of arrhythmia. No drug is entirely satisfactory for recurrent paroxysmal atrial fibrillation: a β-blocker is often prescribed as first-line therapy.

Persistent atrial fibrillation—usually requires electrical cardioversion to achieve sinus rhythm and has a high recurrence rate even after successful cardioversion. The key decision is whether to employ a rhythm or rate-control strategy. In general, a rate-control strategy (AV nodal blocking drug, e.g. β-blocker, calcium channel blocker, or digoxin) should be employed in patients with few or minor symptoms, elderly patients, and those with contraindications to antiarrhythmic therapy or cardioversion. A rhythm-control strategy (elective cardioversion) may be best in more severely symptomatic or younger patients, or in those with atrial fibrillation due to a treated precipitant. If symptoms are clearly attributable to atrial fibrillation and are refractory to antiarrhythmic drugs then catheter ablation can be considered.

Prevention of stroke—this is the key priority among patients with atrial fibrillation, and requires individual assessment of a patient's stroke risk, using the CHA_2DS_2-VASc score. Patients with one or more stroke risk factors should be considered for oral anticoagulation. Formal assessment of a patient's risk of bleeding with treatment should also be undertaken using the HAS-BLED score and both the

HAS-BLED and SAMe-TT_2R_2 scores can help inform management decisions. Discussion and incorporation of patient preferences for treatment is advocated and regular review of the treatment strategy over time is essential.

Atrial flutter

It is important to attempt to terminate atrial flutter since the ventricular rate is often poorly controlled by AV nodal blocking drugs: this may be achieved by chemical or electrical cardioversion, or by catheter ablation. Prophylaxis against thromboembolism should be given as for atrial fibrillation.

Supraventricular tachycardias

The term supraventricular tachycardia encompasses three types of arrhythmia: AV nodal re-entrant tachycardia (AVNRT), AV re-entry tachycardia (AVRT), and atrial tachycardia (AT) in order of reducing frequency.

Termination of an attack of AVNRT is achieved by producing transient AV nodal block by vagotonic manoeuvres, adenosine, or verapamil. Drug prophylaxis is undertaken with β-blockers, a combined β-blocker/class III agent such as sotalol, or with AV nodal blocking drugs such as verapamil or digoxin. Curative treatment is by radiofrequency ablation.

Attacks of AVRT are treated in the same way as AVNRT. Antiarrhythmic prophylaxis may be effective, but radiofrequency ablation offers high success rates with low incidence of complications and should be considered early.

Pre-excitation syndromes

The term 'pre-excitation' (seen as a delta wave on the ECG) refers to the premature activation of the ventricle via one or more accessory pathways that bypass the normal AV node and His–Purkinje system. When seen in conjunction with palpitations this is Wolff–Parkinson–White syndrome. The main prognostic concern is pre-excited atrial fibrillation, which can be very rapid and degenerate into ventricular fibrillation. Patients with pre-excitation should be offered a cardiac electrophysiological study as first-line therapy, with a view to radiofrequency ablation.

Ventricular tachycardia

Ventricular tachycardia (VT) normally occurs in individuals with overt heart disease, but is also seen in young and apparently healthy subjects, when occult cardiac disease or cardiac genetic syndromes should be considered.

Sustained VT is a medical emergency. Immediate DC cardioversion is necessary if the patient is hypotensive; haemodynamically tolerated VT may be terminated pharmacologically, with intravenous β-blocker or amiodarone being the usual first-choice options. Unless there is a clear precipitating factor, the risk of sudden death is high and patients should be considered for an implantable cardioverter–defibrillator.

Polymorphic VT, of which torsades de pointes is a well-recognized type associated with acquired or congenital prolongation of the QT interval, is an unstable rhythm with varying QRS morphology that undergoes spontaneous termination or degenerates into ventricular fibrillation. In patients with this condition, it is essential to discontinue predisposing drugs or other agents and to avoid empirical antiarrhythmic drug therapy. Intravenous magnesium sulfate is a safe and effective emergency measure. Intravenous isoprenaline or temporary pacing may also be required.

Ventricular fibrillation

The management of cardiac arrest due to ventricular fibrillation is discussed in this chapter. Patients who survive an episode should be assessed carefully to determine the risk of recurrence and may require an implantable cardioverter–defibrillator or antiarrhythmic therapy as for patients with ventricular tachycardia.

Genetic syndromes

These are inheritable causes of cardiac arrhythmia, and can be divided into ion channel diseases ('channelopathies') and heart muscle diseases. Ion channel diseases include the congenital long-QT syndromes, short-QT syndrome, Brugada syndrome, and catecholaminergic polymorphic VT. Heart muscle diseases include hypertrophic cardiomyopathy and arrhythmogenic right ventricular cardiomyopathy.

General principles

Definition

The term cardiac arrhythmia (or dysrhythmia) is used to describe an abnormality of cardiac rhythm of any type. Normal cardiac electrophysiology is discussed in Chapter 3.1. The spectrum of cardiac arrhythmias ranges from innocent extrasystoles to immediately life-threatening conditions such as asystole or ventricular fibrillation. Arrhythmias may occur in the absence of cardiac disease, but are more commonly associated with structural heart disease or external provocative factors.

Symptoms of cardiac arrhythmias

The symptoms produced by bradyarrhythmias depend on the extent of cardiac slowing. They may include sudden death, syncope (Stokes–Adams attacks), or dizziness/presyncope. Continuous bradycardia without asystolic pauses may produce symptoms of fatigue, lethargy, dyspnoea, or cognitive impairment.

The symptoms caused by tachyarrhythmias depend on a variety of factors including the heart rate, the difference between the rate during the arrhythmia and the preceding heart rate, the degree of irregularity of the rhythm, and the presence or absence of underlying cardiac disease. Symptoms of tachycardia include a feeling of rapid palpitation, chest discomfort or dyspnoea, syncope or sudden death. The differential diagnosis of palpitation and syncope is discussed in Chapter 2.2.

Investigation of arrhythmias

History-taking must include a detailed description of the symptoms associated with the arrhythmia. Evidence should be sought for factors that may precipitate the arrhythmia (e.g. exercise, alcohol, or drug therapy) and for the presence of underlying cardiac disease, in particular valvular heart disease, myocardial ischaemia/infarction, or congestive heart failure. Examination of the pulse may be unremarkable if the arrhythmia is intermittent. Physical examination for evidence of structural heart disease is essential. A 12-lead ECG

should be performed both during the arrhythmia and once it has resolved (if possible, when the patient presents acutely).

A full blood count (in cases of sinus tachycardia), thyroid function (sinus tachycardia and atrial arrhythmias), and electrolyte testing (potassium for both atrial and ventricular arrhythmias and calcium and magnesium for sustained ventricular arrhythmias) are routinely performed. Although troponin is often measured routinely in the patients presenting to the Emergency Department, a minor rise in troponin should not be regarded as diagnostic of an acute coronary syndrome as the precipitating cause. Further investigations to establish the presence of structural heart disease and to determine ventricular function may include chest radiography, echocardiography, exercise stress testing, coronary angiography, or MRI.

Electrocardiography

The key to the successful diagnosis of cardiac arrhythmias is the systematic analysis of ECG (see Chapter 3.1) of optimal quality obtained during the arrhythmia (Table 4.2.1). Ideally, this should be a 12-lead ECG and may be compared to the ECG in intrinsic rhythm.

Ambulatory electrocardiography

Continuous monitoring is necessary for identification when arrhythmias are intermittent. Ambulatory (Holter) ECG is normally performed for periods of 24 to 48 h using a portable recorder. High-speed or automatic replay facilities enable the identification of intermittent arrhythmias, as well as the quantification of extrasystoles and assessment of parameters of heart rate variability. Interpretation of recordings requires knowledge of possible artefacts, such as those caused by movement or loss of electrode contact. It is important to allow for physiological variability in the sinus rate, also appreciating that minor abnormalities such as extrasystoles or brief (3–4 beat) runs of supraventricular arrhythmias are usually of no significance. Ambulatory ECG recordings are of most value when they provide correlation between the patient's symptoms and the cardiac rhythm at that moment. Patients should be

Table 4.2.1 Principles of ECG diagnosis of arrhythmias

Obtain 12-lead or multichannel recordings if possible	
Atrial activity	P-waves visible?
	Normal P-wave morphology and axis?
	Flutter/fibrillation waves?
	Atrial rate?
Ventricular activity	Ventricular rate?
	Regular or irregular?
	Normal QRS morphology and duration?
	Bundle branch block or bizarre QRS morphology?
	Variation in QRS morphology/axis?
Atrioventricular relationship	PR interval—fixed or varied?
	Retrograde P-waves?
	Atrial versus ventricular rate?

issued with a diary card and asked to note any symptoms suggestive of arrhythmia during the recording.

Alternative strategies for the detection of infrequent arrhythmias include the use of a patient-activated recorder, which is applied and activated during symptoms, or an external or implanted loop recorder. Loop recorders continually record the ECG signal, but only have sufficient memory to retain a few minutes of data. In the event of symptoms, the patient activates the device, thus 'fixing' the previous few minutes of recording for subsequent analysis. External loop recorders are usually used for up to 7 days, while an implanted event recorder can last for up to 3 years.

Cardiac electrophysiological study

More detailed investigation of cardiac arrhythmias is undertaken by invasive cardiac electrophysiological testing. Multipolar electrodes are inserted transvenously to record electrograms from the atrium, ventricle, His bundle, and commonly from the coronary sinus (Fig. 4.2.1). The site of conduction delays within the heart may be identified, or accessory pathways localized. Sustained arrhythmias may be initiated and their pattern of activation in the heart studied in detail; if necessary the mechanism of the arrhythmia can be clarified using pacing manoeuvres (Fig. 4.2.2). Electrophysiological mapping is an essential part of radiofrequency ablation (see below), and modern three-dimensional mapping systems have facilitated ablation of complex arrhythmias.

Bradycardias

Aetiology and mechanisms

Bradycardia is defined as a ventricular rate of less than 60/min, and results from a reduction in the rate of normal sinus pacemaker activity, or from disturbances of atrioventricular (AV) conduction. Sinus bradycardia may be physiological, for example during sleep and in athletes. Pathological bradyarrhythmias can result from intrinsic degenerative disease of the sinus or AV node, or the conducting system. Bradycardia may also be due to extraneous factors such as sympathetic withdrawal, vagal stimulation, drug effects, myocardial ischaemia/infarction, infiltration, or surgical trauma and also miscellaneous conditions such as hypothyroidism, hypothermia, jaundice, or raised intracranial pressure.

General principles of management

The principal indications for active intervention in bradycardia are symptomatic (disturbances of consciousness, fatigue, lethargy,

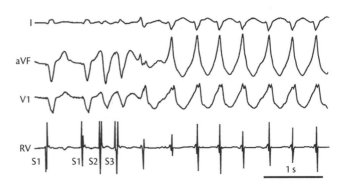

Fig. 4.2.2 Induction of ventricular tachycardia by programmed stimulation. Ventricular pacing stimuli (S1) at 100 beats/min are followed by two extrastimuli (S2 and S3). Sustained monomorphic ventricular tachycardia is induced. Surface leads I, aVF, V$_1$, and the intracardiac electrogram from right ventricular apex (RV) are shown.

dyspnoea, or bradycardia-induced tachyarrhythmias) or prognostic (prevention of sudden cardiac death). Particular attention should be given to the history and ECG documentation of the rhythm disturbance. Drugs interfering with sinoatrial or AV nodal function should be withdrawn if possible, although under certain circumstances (e.g. tachycardia–bradycardia syndrome) it may be necessary to combine pacemaker implantation with continued drug therapy.

Acute management of bradycardia

General principles can be applied to patients presenting with overt bradycardia, regardless of aetiology (Table 4.2.2). In the presence of haemodynamic compromise, immediate attempts should be made to increase heart rate. Transient increases in sinus rate or the ventricular escape rate in complete AV block may be achieved with atropine or isoproterenol (isoprenaline). However, drug treatment is only of temporary value, and temporary or permanent cardiac pacing

Table 4.2.2 General principles of acute management of the patient with bradycardia

Assess the patient	Respiratory status
	Blood pressure
	Symptoms
Examine the ECG	Sinus rate
	Ventricular rate
	AV relationship
	QRS morphology and duration
If haemodynamic compromise	Atropine
	Isoproterenol
	Temporary pacing
Look for precipitants	Ischaemia/infarction
	Vasovagal episode
	Thyroid status
	Electrolyte imbalance
	Hypothermia
	Drug therapy

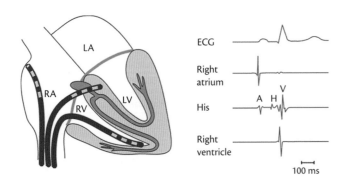

Fig. 4.2.1 Electrophysiological study. Illustration of lead placement (left). Quadripolar leads have been inserted from the femoral vein and the tips are shown positioned to allow recording and pacing from the high right atrium, His bundle, and the right ventricular apex. Intracardiac electrograms (right) show recordings from atrium (A), His bundle (H), and right ventricle (V).

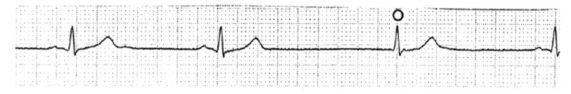

Fig. 4.2.3 Sinus bradycardia. The heart rate is less than 40 beats/min, and the sinus rate is so slow that an escape junctional beat is seen (open circle), preceding the P-wave.

is indicated for persistent bradycardia (see 'Pacemaker therapy', below). Temporary pacing is also indicated where frequent Stokes–Adams attacks are occurring. Pacing can be performed transcutaneously using an external pacing system in the emergency situation if facilities for transvenous pacing are not immediately available.

Following stabilization, factors causing or contributing to the presentation should be sought and corrected, especially acute ischaemia and infarction, concomitant drug therapy, or electrolyte disorders. Analysis of the ECG will allow identification of the conduction disorder and plans for long-term management can be instituted.

Specific causes of brachycardia

Sinoatrial disease

Sinoatrial disease, often referred to as 'sick sinus syndrome', results in inappropriate sinus bradycardia, sinus pauses, or junctional rhythm (Fig. 4.2.3) in the absence of extrinsic factors. The condition is most commonly caused by idiopathic degeneration of the sinus nodal cells, particularly in older people, and is associated in about 20% of cases with idiopathic bundle branch fibrosis (see 'Aetiology of atrioventricular block'). Occasionally, sinoatrial disease is caused by ischaemia due to obstruction of the right coronary artery. Conduction block may occur between the sinus node and the atrium (sinoatrial exit block), resulting in 'dropped' P-waves (Fig. 4.2.4). More prolonged suppression of sinus node activity results in periods of sinus arrest, which are terminated by an escape beat from the sinus node, AV node, or ventricle (Fig. 4.2.5a). Where the sinus rate is permanently slower than the junctional rate, continuous AV junctional rhythm will be present. Patients with sinoatrial disease have an increased predisposition to atrial tachyarrhythmias (tachycardia–bradycardia syndrome), and prolonged pauses may follow termination of tachycardia (Fig. 4.2.5b).

Sinoatrial disease can cause symptomatic bradycardia, dizziness, or syncope, but may be asymptomatic. The diagnosis is normally made from 12-lead or ambulatory ECG recording. Investigation should focus on excluding extrinsic causes of bradycardia, and on demonstrating the correlation between bradycardia or pauses and symptoms. Pacemaker implantation is indicated for the relief of symptoms (see below). Prognosis is not improved by pacemaker implantation in sinus nodal disease and thus pacemaker implantation in asymptomatic patients is not indicated.

Neurocardiogenic syncope

Conditions where patients suffer reflex-induced attacks of bradycardia or hypotension are described in Chapter 2.2.

Patients with carotid sinus hypersensitivity and reproducible symptoms of presyncope or syncope on carotid sinus massage should undergo permanent pacemaker implantation (see 'Permanent pacemaker therapy').

In patients with recurrent vasovagal syncope, it is recommended to maintain good hydration and salt intake. Isometric exercises may be helpful. Medical therapy with agents as diverse as α-agonists, β-blockers, vagolytic agents (disopyramide, hyoscine), ephedrine, mineralocorticoids, or antidepressants is often tried, but the evidence base for the efficacy of drug therapy is weak. Spontaneous resolution of symptoms occurs in many patients. There is little evidence to support pacemaker implantation even in those with predominant bradycardia as the response to tilt testing, but it may be considered in selected individuals with intractable symptoms.

Atrioventricular conduction disorders

Impairment of AV conduction may occur either within the AV node (intranodal) or within the His–Purkinje system (infranodal). Intranodal block is not associated with QRS abnormalities, while distal (infranodal) block is commonly associated with bundle branch block. Bundle branch block (particularly left bundle branch block) is a common finding in elderly patients with a history of fatigue, dizziness, and syncope. Although both left and right bundle branch block are associated with an increased risk of developing complete AV block, bundle branch block as an isolated finding is not sufficient evidence to attribute symptoms to conduction disease; fewer than one-half of patients with bundle branch block and syncope have a final diagnosis of cardiac syncope. There are two exceptions. Alternating left and right bundle branch block (although rare in the absence of higher-grade AV block) is an indication for pacemaker insertion in the absence of documented

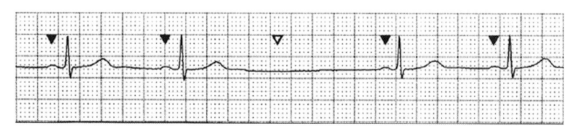

Fig. 4.2.4 Sinoatrial exit block. A pause occurred because of the absence of a P-wave (open arrow). The timing of the sinus beats, however, is not interrupted, indicating that the sinus node discharged but the impulse failed to excite the atria.

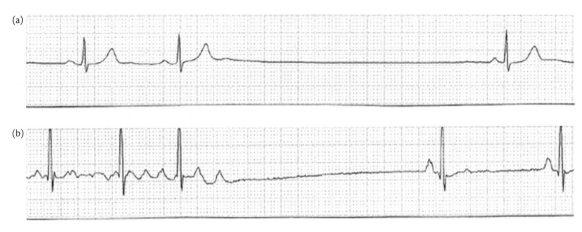

Fig. 4.2.5 Sinus arrest. (a) A pause of 4 s results from failure of the sinus node to discharge. (b) Termination of atrial fibrillation is followed by a sinus pause of 2.5 s due to sinus arrest in a patient with bradycardia/tachycardia syndrome.

symptomatic 2:1 or third-degree AV block. Trifascicular block (a triad of first-degree heart block, left-axis deviation, and right bundle branch block) may be considered sufficient evidence for symptomatic conduction disease requiring pacing where no other cause for symptoms has been identified. However, further evidence of more advanced conduction disease with prolonged ECG monitoring is usually sought.

Aetiology of atrioventricular block

The causes of AV block are shown in Box 4.2.1. The commonest is idiopathic fibrosis of the His–Purkinje system, which occurs with increasing frequency from the seventh decade of life onwards, is associated with sinoatrial disease in up to 25% of cases, and results in progressive impairment of AV conduction.

Atrioventricular block may occur acutely in myocardial infarction (Fig. 4.2.6). Inferior myocardial infarction predominantly affects AV nodal conduction by vagal overactivity, and possibly adenosine release from ischaemic myocardium. First-degree, second-degree, or third-degree AV block may occur, but are commonly transient, particularly with the advent of primary percutaneous coronary intervention (PCI). Spontaneous recovery of normal conduction generally occurs within 7 to 10 days. By contrast, AV block secondary to anterior myocardial infarction is normally due to extensive infarction of the interventricular septum involving both the left and right bundle branches. This may result in type II second-degree block or complete AV block, with a low probability of recovery of normal conduction.

Any drug slowing AV conduction may potentially produce AV block. The risk is greater when such drugs are used in combination. Intravenous verapamil in patients already receiving β-adrenoceptor blockers is particularly hazardous. Vagally mediated conduction disturbances occur as a physiological finding in highly trained athletes, and in young people during sleep, or in neurocardiogenic syncope. Atrioventricular conduction disturbances arise in structural congenital heart disease such as endocardial cushion defects, but also as an isolated congenital abnormality, commonly in association with maternal systemic lupus erythematosus.

First-degree atrioventricular block

First-degree AV block is defined as a PR interval greater than 0.20 s (Fig. 4.2.7). This produces no symptoms and does not require treatment, although the risk of progression to higher-degree AV block should be considered.

Second-degree atrioventricular block

In second-degree AV block, there is intermittent failure of conduction from atrium to ventricle. In type I (Wenckebach) second-degree block, a characteristic pattern of increasing PR interval duration followed by a nonconducted P-wave is seen (Fig. 4.2.8). The QRS morphology is commonly normal. Type I (Wenckebach) second-degree AV block usually indicates block in the AV node, and is normally associated with a reliable subsidiary pacemaker and a low risk of progression to complete heart block. In most instances pacemaker implantation is not necessary unless recurrent presyncope or syncope suggest the occurrence of an intermittent higher-degree block. By contrast, in type II second-degree AV block (commonly called Mobitz type II AV block) there is a sudden failure of conduction, without a preceding increase in the PR interval (Fig. 4.2.9). Regular nonconducted P-waves may result in high-degree block, with 2:1 or 3:1 conduction. Type II second-degree AV block is generally indicative of extensive infranodal conduction abnormality, with a high risk of progression to complete AV block. Guidelines therefore recommend permanent pacemaker implantation even in the absence of symptoms.

Box 4.2.1 Causes of atrioventricular block

- Idiopathic conducting system fibrosis
- Acute myocardial ischaemia/infarction
- Infiltration—calcific aortic stenosis, sarcoidosis, scleroderma, syphilis, tumour
- Infection—diphtheria, rheumatic fever, endocarditis, Lyme disease
- Drugs—digoxin, verapamil or diltiazem, β-blockers, antiarrhythmic drugs
- Surgical trauma, radiofrequency ablation
- Congenital heart block, congenital heart disease
- Vagal—athletic heart, carotid sinus, and vasovagal syndrome
- Myotonic dystrophy

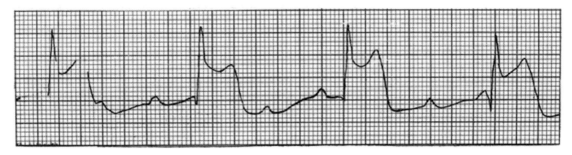

Fig. 4.2.6 Complete heart block in a patient with acute myocardial infarction. There is a narrow-QRS complex escape rhythm with ST-segment elevation, ventricular rate 45 beats/min.

Third-degree atrioventricular block

The characteristic feature of third-degree (complete) AV block is dissociation between atrial and ventricular activity (Figs. 4.2.6 and 4.2.10). The ventricular rate is regular and slower than the atrial rate. An escape rhythm arising above the bifurcation of the bundle of His will produce a narrow-QRS morphology, commonly with a relatively stable escape rhythm (50–60/min). A more distal escape rhythm results in widened bundle branch block morphology complexes with a slower escape rate (20–30/min). Complete AV block in patients with atrial fibrillation is often missed. It is recognized by the presence of a slow, regular ventricular response. High-degree AV block can be intermittent, and the resting ECG may be normal or only show evidence of mild conducting system disturbance such as first-degree AV block or bundle branch block. If there is clinical suspicion, ambulatory ECG recording is required, for prolonged periods if necessary.

The presence of complete AV block, except in the context of an acutely reversible condition, should be regarded as an indication for permanent pacemaker implantation. This is urgent in patients who are having Stokes–Adams attacks; their prognosis is poor without pacemaker implantation, and markedly improved by permanent pacing, after which outcome will depend on the presence and extent of any underlying cardiac disease. Permanent pacing also improves prognosis in asymptomatic patients with complete AV block. One exception to this general rule is congenital complete heart block, where the escape rhythm is often relatively fast (50–60/min) with a narrow-QRS morphology. Many patients remain asymptomatic well into adult life, although there is a small risk of syncope or sudden death. Pacemaker implantation should be considered if there are symptoms, if there are abrupt pauses, if the average heart rate is below 50/min, or in patients over 40 years of age.

Asystole

The term asystole is used when the ECG shows a complete cessation of both atrial and ventricular activity. This appearance may be mimicked by disconnected ECG cables or other artefacts, but since asystole causes cardiac arrest the distinction is virtually always obvious. Ventricular standstill occurs when there in ongoing 'p' wave activity without QRS complexes.

Pacemaker therapy

Basic principles

The basis of pacemaker therapy is the local depolarization of the myocardium by an electric current passed through an electrode in contact with the heart (atrium or ventricle). Activation of the remainder of the atria or ventricles occurs by direct cell-to-cell conduction. The minimum current necessary to stimulate the heart during diastole is known as the pacing threshold. Pacemaker systems consist of one or more intracardiac catheter electrodes, introduced into the heart via the venous system, and a pulse generator, which contains the circuitry for generating and timing the pacing stimulus, as well as for sensing spontaneous cardiac depolarizations. The pacing stimulus is delivered between the active pole at the tip of the electrode catheter and an indifferent electrode sited either on the same catheter 1–2 cm proximal to the tip (bipolar pacing), or utilizing the can of an implanted pulse generator (unipolar pacing). Satisfactory pacing requires stable electrode contact with the myocardium. The standard sites for endocardial atrial and ventricular pacing are the right atrial appendage and the right ventricular apex respectively (Fig. 4.2.11), although screw-in active fixation leads allow placement at other atrial and ventricular sites.

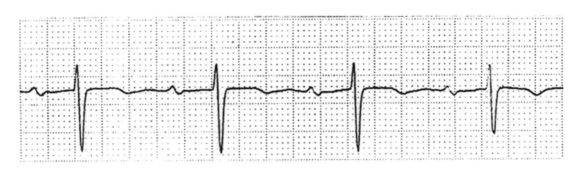

Fig. 4.2.7 First-degree heart block. The PR interval is prolonged (0.32 s).

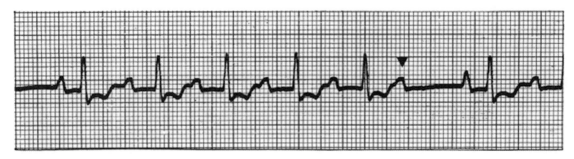

Fig. 4.2.8 Second-degree heart block, type I (Wenckebach). The PR interval progressively prolongs until there is a failure of conduction following a P-wave (arrow).

An external pulse generator is used for temporary pacing. For permanent pacing, it is usually implanted deep to the subcutaneous fat layer in the prepectoral region (Fig. 4.2.11). The generator contains a timer set to deliver pacing stimuli at a preset pulse interval (e.g. 1000 ms). Pacemakers normally operate in the demand mode, whereby if spontaneous activation of the cardiac chamber is sensed via the electrode, the delivery of a pacing stimulus is inhibited and the timer circuit of the generator is reset. Pacing in the fixed-rate mode results in the delivery of stimuli regardless of the spontaneous activity of the chamber being paced.

Temporary ventricular pacing

Temporary pacing is indicated in patients with bradycardia causing haemodynamic compromise, or as a prelude to permanent pacemaker implantation in those with significant recurring symptoms, or high-risk AV block. It is recommended that in those patients with an indication for a permanent system this should arranged urgently where possible to avoid the complications associated with temporary pacemaker insertion.

In patients undergoing anaesthesia for noncardiac surgery the standard indications for pacing apply. The role for temporary pacing in patients with first-degree heart block and left bundle branch block or with trifascicular block remains controversial. Temporary pacing is recommended by the American College of Cardiology/American Heart Association for those procedures where heart block may be promoted, but there is little evidence to support this approach and progression to haemodynamically significant AV block unresponsive to pharmacological therapy is exceedingly rare.

Facilities for radiographic screening, continuous ECG monitoring, and defibrillation are required. The pacing electrode is introduced under aseptic conditions via an intravascular sheath into the subclavian, internal jugular, or femoral vein and the tip advanced under radiographic guidance to the right ventricular apex. Nonsustained ventricular tachycardia, or occasionally ventricular fibrillation, may occur during catheter manipulation. Once the electrode is at an acceptable site, pacing is initiated, and the minimum output necessary to achieve stable ventricular capture is determined. The pacing threshold should ideally be less than 1 V, at a pulse width of between 0.5 and 2 ms. If the pacing threshold is unsatisfactory, the electrode is repositioned until an acceptable site is found. Care should be taken to determine that the electrode is stable by asking the patient to take deep breaths or to cough while pacing at threshold. The electrode is then secured at the site of insertion and the pulse generator set to an output of at least 3 V above the pacing threshold.

Permanent pacemaker therapy

Indications for permanent pacing therapy are given in Table 4.2.3. Two scenarios are quite common and can cause confusion. Elderly patients presenting with symptomatic AV block (particularly in the context of chronic atrial fibrillation) or sinus node disease are frequently on rate-slowing drugs. It is usual to withdraw these agents before assessing the need for pacing therapy. This is particularly common where multiple agents (e.g. digoxin and β-blockade) have been used. However, if patients have been on these agents for many years then the presentation with symptomatic bradycardia should be taken as an indication of progressive conduction disease and increasingly long-term pacing is required, particularly where these agents are required for control of tachyarrhythmias. The second scenario is the patient with evidence of conduction disease presenting

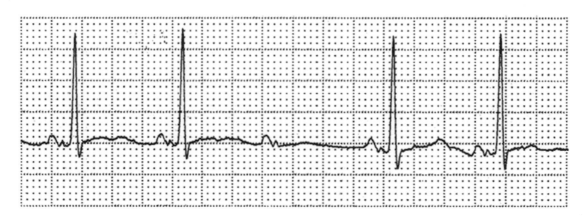

Fig. 4.2.9 Second-degree heart block, type II. A nonconducted P-wave occurs without preceding prolongation of the PR interval.

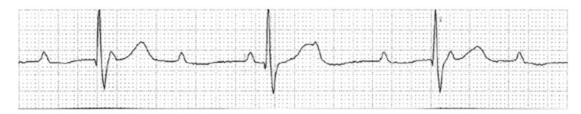

Fig. 4.2.10 Third-degree (complete) heart block. Atrial activity does not conduct to the ventricles, and there is a regular escape rhythm of 35 beats/min.

with syncope where a class I indication is not met but there is a high index of suspicion and no other cause has been identified. These are patients with sinus node disease manifesting as pauses (>3 s) on a prolonged monitoring or advanced conduction disease (trifascicular block) on a 12-lead ECG. It should be remembered that there is no prognostic benefit in permanent pacing in patients with either of these conditions. Ideally an attempt should be made to correlate pauses with symptoms or identify a more extensive conduction disease with prolonged monitoring. Nocturnal pauses are common in this population and are not an indication for pacing unless they are very prolonged, associated with symptoms, or the history is strongly suggestive of an arrhythmic cause for syncope (other causes having been excluded). Patients with sinus node disease have an increased susceptibility to neurally mediated bradycardia and hypotension, which may explain why a significant proportion continue to have symptoms after pacemaker insertion.

Pacing is not indicated in patients with unexplained falls; however, there may be an argument for pacing in the context of conduction disease and a classic history in selected cases, in an attempt to prevent further events.

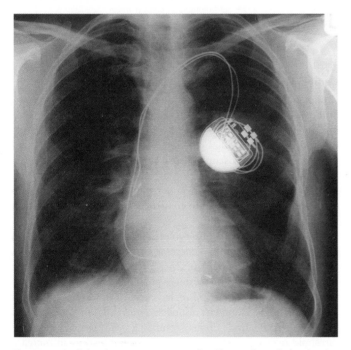

Fig. 4.2.11 Dual-chamber permanent pacemaker. Chest radiograph showing the pacemaker generator (in a subcutaneous pocket in the pectoral region), which is connected to electrodes that pass via the left subclavian vein and superior vena cava to the heart. The tips of the electrodes are in the right atrial appendage and the right ventricular apex.

Permanent pacing electrodes are normally inserted via the left or right cephalic, axillary, or subclavian vein. Once the electrode is in a satisfactory position, it is secured and connected to the implanted pulse generator. Most pulse generators are powered by lithium batteries and have a life of approximately 7 to 8 years, after which the generator is replaced. The rate, output voltage, pulse width, and other pacemaker functions can be modified noninvasively by means of telemetry via a transmitter/receiver placed on the skin over the pulse generator. The amplitude and pulse width of the pacing stimulus are usually set at nominal values (e.g. 3.5 V, 0.5 ms), but are adjustable and can be reduced to prolong the life of the battery, provided there is a sufficient safety margin between the pulse generator output and the pacing threshold.

Pacing mode selection

The nomenclature used to describe pacing mode is given in Table 4.2.4, and ECG examples of the principal pacing modes are shown in Fig. 4.2.12. Atrial demand (AAI) pacing is used for sinoatrial disease in the absence of AV block. Ventricular pacing (VVI) is the simplest and technically easiest mode of pacing, and is required for AV conduction disturbances. However, VVI pacing does not permit AV synchrony or an increase in pacing rate in response to an increase in sinus (atrial) rate. Dual-chamber (DDD) pacemakers have electrodes in both the right atrium and ventricle. If the sinus cycle length is greater than the pulse interval, atrial demand pacing occurs. Following the atrial stimulus, a programmable AV delay commences. If no spontaneous ventricular depolarization is sensed before the end of this interval, a pacing stimulus is delivered via the ventricular electrode. If the sinus cycle length is shorter than the pulse interval, no atrial stimulus is given, but the AV delay is triggered by the sensed atrial activity, followed by a paced ventricular beat, if a conducted ventricular activation does not occur. By this means, the ventricular rate tracks the atrial rate up to a programmable maximum, allowing the heart to increase its rate in a physiological manner in response to metabolic demand. An alternative, and simpler, approach to achieve a rate response is the use of an activity sensor such as an accelerometer in the pulse generator. Such devices detect bodily movement and increase the pacing rate according to a programmable algorithm. Rate response can be utilized in either single- or dual-chamber pacemakers, and is designated by the suffix 'R' (e.g. AAIR, VVIR, DDDR).

The advantage of DDD pacing over VVI pacing lies in the maintenance of AV synchrony and rate responsiveness, but this is achieved at the expense of increased complexity, complications, and cost. DDD pacing reduces the risk of atrial fibrillation by virtue of pacing the atrium and avoiding retrograde atrial activation via the AV node and has a lower incidence of the pacemaker syndrome (see below). However, large-scale randomized trials comparing DDD with VVI(R) pacing have failed to substantiate survival

Table 4.2.3 Indications for permanent pacing therapy

Indications for pacing	Conducting tissue disease	Details	Class of indication	Level of evidence
In patients with persistent bradycardia	Sinus node disease.	Pacing is indicated when symptoms can clearly be attributed to bradycardia	I	B
	Acquired AV block	Pacing is indicated in patients with third- or second-degree type 2 AV block irrespective of symptoms	I	C
	Acquired AV block	Pacing should be considered in patients with second-degree type 1 AV block which causes symptoms or is found to be located at intra- or infra-His levels at EPS	IIa	C
In patients with intermittent (documented) bradycardia	Sinus node disease (including brady-tachy form)	Pacing is indicated in patients affected by sinus node disease who have documentation of symptomatic bradycardia due to sinus arrest or sinus- atrial block	I	B
	Intermittent/ paroxysmal AV block (including AF with slow ventricular conduction)	Pacing is indicated in patients with intermittent/paroxysmal intrinsic third- or second- degree AV block	I	C
	Reflex asystolic syncope	Pacing should be considered in patients ≫40 years with recurrent, unpredictable reflex syncope and documented symptomatic pause/s due to sinus arrest or AV block or the combination of the two	IIa	B
	Asymptomatic pauses (sinus arrest or AV block)	Pacing should be considered in patients with a history of syncope and documentation of asymptomatic pauses >6 s due to sinus arrest, sinus-atrial block or AV block	IIa	C
In patients with BBB	BBB, unexplained syncope, and abnormal EPS	Pacing is indicated in patients with syncope, BBB and positive EPS defined as HV interval of >70 ms, or second- or third-degree His–Purkinje block demonstrated during incremental atrial pacing or with pharmacological challenge	I	B
	Alternating BBB	Pacing is indicated in patients with alternating BBB with or without symptoms	I	C
In patients with undocumented reflex syncope	Carotid sinus syncope	Pacing is indicated in patients with dominant cardioinhibitory carotid sinus syndrome and recurrent unpredictable syncope	I	B

AF, atrial fibrillation; AV, atrioventricular; BBB, bundle branch block; EPS, electrophysiology study.

benefits from DDD pacing, at least during follow-up periods of up to 3 years.

Cardiac resynchronization pacing in patients with reduced ejection fraction and an indication for permanent pacing is supported by evidence from a number of small randomized trials. The benefits have to be weighed against the added complexity of these devices and the complication rates. It should, however, be standard practice to perform an echocardiogram to assess left ventricular function in all patients undergoing permanent pacing, as up to 10% may have evidence of significant left ventricular dysfunction.

Table 4.2.4 Pacemaker mode nomenclature

Chamber-paced		Chamber-sensed		Mode		Additional features	
A	Atrium	A	Atrium	I	Inhibited	R	Rate responsive
V	Ventricle	V	Ventricle	T	Triggered		
D	Dual (A and V)	D	Dual (A and V)	D	Dual (I and T)		
		O	Neither	O	Fixed rate		

See text for examples.

Complications of pacemaker insertion

Complications of temporary or permanent pacemaker implantation include those of central venous cannulation (e.g. bleeding, pneumothorax), perforation of the heart by the electrode tip leading to pericardial effusion and cardiac tamponade, and macroscopic or microscopic displacement of the electrode resulting in an increase in the pacing threshold or failure to capture. A chest radiograph should be taken after pacemaker insertion to exclude pneumothorax and to confirm that the electrode position is satisfactory.

Permanent pacing may be complicated by the development of infection around the pulse generator, or by mechanical erosion of the generator through the skin. Once infection is established, or the skin is breached, it is almost never possible to eradicate infection with antibiotics: removal and replacement of the pacing system is required. The development of oedema and inflammation around the implanted electrode tip may result in a steady rise in the pacing threshold over the first few weeks, which can lead to an increase of the pacing threshold such that capture is lost (Fig. 4.2.13a), although the process is normally mild and self-limiting. Lead dislodgement occurs in up to 4.2% of patients with a dual-chamber and 1.4% with a single-chamber system.

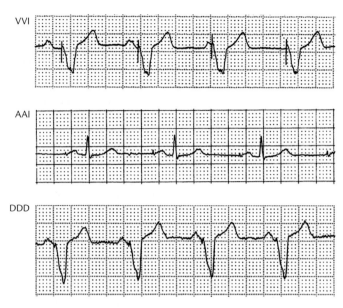

Fig. 4.2.12 Permanent pacemaker modes. Ventricular demand pacing, VVI (upper) with broad-complex ventricular complexes following the stimulus. Dissociated atrial activity can be seen. Atrial demand pacing, AAI (middle) with low amplitude bipolar pacing spike preceding the P-waves. Dual-chamber pacemaker, DDD (lower) with paced ventricular complexes following each P-wave (atrial tracking).

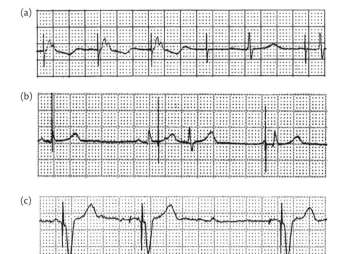

Fig. 4.2.13 Pacemaker malfunction. (a) Failure to capture. The fourth stimulus fails to capture the ventricle. (b) Undersensing. The atrial pacemaker has failed to sense the preceding atrial activity and therefore delivered the second stimulus. This has captured the atrium, with the P-wave in the ST segment, and subsequent conduction to the ventricle. (c) Oversensing. This dual-chamber pacemaker has sensed an electrical artefact through the ventricular lead and as a result has suppressed ventricular pacing, with the absence of ventricular activation following the third P-wave.

Demand pacemakers require an adequate intracardiac signal to recognize activation of the chamber in question, to inhibit output. The pacing stimulus will not be suppressed ('undersensing') if the intracardiac signal is of insufficient amplitude, resulting in inappropriate pacemaker firing (Fig. 4.2.13b). This phenomenon is commoner in atrial pacing, owing to the lower amplitude of atrial compared with ventricular electrograms. Conversely, detection of extraneous electrical activity (e.g. skeletal muscle activity) via the pacing electrode can result in inappropriate inhibition of the pacemaker output (oversensing) (Fig. 4.2.13c). Oversensing is commoner with unipolar than bipolar pacing modes because of the inclusion of the pulse generator can in the electrical circuit, and its proximity to the pectoral muscles. For the same reason, unipolar pacemaker systems are more prone to the problem of local skeletal muscle stimulation. Damage to the conductor or insulation of the pacing electrode may occur due to trauma at the site of ligation or to compression between the clavicle and first rib. This may result in oversensing, skeletal muscle stimulation, or short-circuiting leading to premature battery depletion.

Patients receiving AAI pacemakers may subsequently develop AV block, resulting in a recurrence of syncope and requiring upgrade of the pacing system to a DDD unit. Some patients with VVI pacemakers, particularly those with sinoatrial rather than AV disease, will manifest retrograde ventriculoatrial conduction during ventricular pacing. This sometimes causes symptoms of fatigue, dizziness, or hypotension ('pacemaker syndrome'), which are associated with the presence of atrial cannon waves occurring as a result of simultaneous atrial and ventricular contraction. Upgrade of the system to a dual-chamber unit is necessary if symptoms are troublesome. Newer pacing systems allow DDD pacemakers to act as single-chamber atrial pacemakers, automatically switching to dual-chamber pacing should AV conduction fail, providing the benefits of atrial pacing with a lower risk of pacemaker syndrome.

Follow-up

Many patients with long-standing heart block treated by permanent pacing have no underlying cardiac rhythm, hence failure of the pacing system for whatever reason may be fatal and patients require follow-up in a pacemaker clinic. As well as detection of the complications described above, the function of such a clinic is to assess the status of the pulse generator battery, and to maximize its life by programming the pulse generator output to the minimum consistent with a satisfactory safety margin. The design of pulse generators and the battery characteristics normally allow prediction of the expected replacement date several months if not years ahead. However, premature battery depletion or pacemaker failure does occur, and patients should therefore be assessed at least annually by the clinic.

Managing patients with permanent pacemakers

Patients with a permanent pacing system can usually lead a perfectly normal life without limitations regarding physical activity. Driving is usually allowed 1 week after implantation. Patients should avoid strong electromagnetic fields and specific risks (arc welding machines). Domestic appliances are not usually a problem unless faulty, and mobile phones are safe unless used in close proximity (<15 cm) to the device. Electronic surveillance systems and metal detectors at airports can affect pacemaker function.

A significant proportion of patients with pacemaker and CRT devices will subsequently develop an indication for investigation with MRI. This has led to the development of MRI-compatible devices which are now used routinely in younger patients or those where this form of imaging is likely to be required. Although the use of MRI in patients with pacemakers should be avoided, where the benefits of this investigation are thought to outweigh the risks, imaging can be relatively safely performed. Imaging should take place after consultation with the implanting cardiologist and a cardiac physiologist should be in attendance during the procedure.

Radiotherapy can also affect pacemaker function. Reprogramming is required before and after treatment in those patients who are pacing dependent. Where the device lies directly within the radiotherapy field the pacemaker needs to be repositioned.

In patients presenting with recurrent syncope, palpitations, or falls with a pacemaker *in situ* the cause is rarely due to pacemaker malfunction, although a pacing check is usually performed. Interrogation of modern pacing devices may also provide useful information in patients with suspected tachyarrhythmias.

Tachycardias

Mechanisms of arrhythmogenesis

The principal mechanisms responsible for tachyarrhythmias are those of abnormal automaticity, triggered activity, or re-entry (Fig. 4.2.14). There is a complex interaction between the underlying substrate, such as previous myocardial infarction, a triggering event such as an extrasystole, and modulating influences, of which sympathetic stimulation and myocardial ischaemia are the most important.

Automaticity

Abnormal automaticity is defined as an inappropriate increase in the rate of discharge of a tissue that has physiological pacemaker properties (sinus node, AV node, or Purkinje fibres) or the pathological development of automaticity in atrial or ventricular myocytes (Fig. 4.2.14a). Such abnormalities are most commonly seen in the presence of ischaemia, sympathetic stimulation, or drug toxicity, especially digoxin. Automatic tachycardias are characterized by an absence of initiation by extrasystoles, either spontaneously or during electrophysiological testing.

Triggered activity

The term 'triggered activity' is used to define an impulse initiation associated with a preceding action potential, and can be induced *in vitro* in tissues that do not demonstrate physiological automaticity. Two characteristic forms of depolarization may cause triggered activity.

Early after-depolarizations

These occur during the plateau phase of the action potential, prior to repolarization (Fig. 4.2.14b), and are more evident at slow heart rates, particularly in the presence of hypokalaemia and hypomagnesaemia. Mutations in cardiac Na^+ or K^+ channels, or drugs that prolong myocardial repolarization by inhibiting one or more components of the outward potassium current, I_K, (class IA and class III antiarrhythmics, tricyclic antidepressants, antihistamines, organophosphorus insecticides, and many others) predispose to the appearance of early after-depolarizations *in vitro*. These changes are associated with the congenital and acquired long-QT syndromes and the arrhythmia torsades de pointes (see 'Torsades de pointes and the long-QT syndromes').

Delayed after-depolarizations

These are subthreshold depolarizations occurring after full repolarization of the action potential (Fig. 4.2.14c). Their amplitude is increased by tachycardia or intracellular calcium overload, and may reach a threshold at which an action potential is generated, potentially initiating a sustained tachycardia. Delayed after-depolarizations can be induced experimentally by digitalis overload, and are the likely mechanism of digitoxic arrhythmias.

Re-entry

Most clinically important sustained tachycardias, whether of atrial, junctional, or ventricular origin, arise on the basis of re-entry. The establishment of a re-entry tachycardia requires the presence of a potential circuit comprising two limbs with different refractoriness and conduction properties (Fig. 4.2.14d). A premature beat can be conducted in one limb of the circuit, but the other limb may still be refractory, resulting in unidirectional conduction block. If conduction is sufficiently slow, the tissue distal to the site of block in the refractory limb will have regained excitability before the arrival of the depolarizing wavefront, and conducts the activity retrogradely. This results in reactivation of the initial conducting pathway and thus a circus movement tachycardia is established. Macro re-entry is defined as the occurrence of a re-entry circuit over a large area of the heart, such as in the presence of an accessory pathway (Fig. 4.2.15a). Micro re-entry occurs in a relatively small area of the heart, for example at the border zone of an old myocardial infarction, where conduction velocity is markedly slowed (Fig. 4.2.15b). The characteristic feature of a re-entrant tachycardia is that an appropriately timed extrastimulus can induce unidirectional block and initiate the arrhythmia. The tachycardia may be terminated by extrastimuli that depolarize the tissue ahead of the circulating wave front and thus interrupt the circus movement.

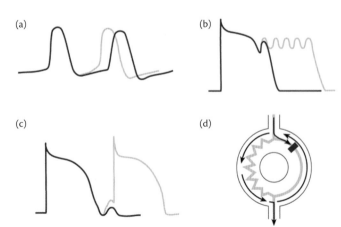

Fig. 4.2.14 Mechanisms of arrhythmia. (a) Increased automaticity. (b) Triggered activity due to early after-depolarizations. (c) Triggered activity due to delayed after-depolarizations. (d) Re-entry circuit. See text for details.

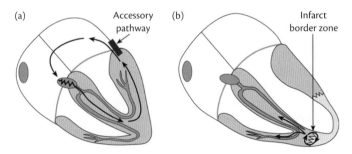

Fig. 4.2.15 Examples of re-entry tachycardias. (a) Macro re-entry circuit involving an accessory pathway, which results in atrioventricular re-entry tachycardia. (b) Micro re-entry circuit at the border zone of a myocardial infarction.

Differential diagnosis of tachycardias

General principles

The first and most important step in the diagnosis and management of tachycardias is to determine whether the arrhythmia arises within the atria and/or AV junction, or from the ventricles. An essential element in the differential diagnosis is to distinguish between tachycardias with normal QRS-complex morphology and duration ('narrow-complex tachycardias'), and those where the QRS complexes are abnormal in morphology and increased in duration ('broad-complex tachycardias'). A guide to the differential diagnosis of tachyarrhythmias is provided in Fig. 4.2.16.

Narrow-complex tachycardias

Narrow-complex tachycardias arise through mechanisms that result in ventricular activation via the AV node and His–Purkinje system and therefore show normal QRS morphology and duration (≤0.12 s) during tachycardia. Careful study of all leads of the ECG is necessary to assess regularity of QRS complexes and to identify the presence of atrial activity (P-waves) (Fig. 4.2.16). The relationship of the PR to the RP interval is helpful in determining mechanism of narrow-complex tachycardias. In supraventricular tachycardias (see 'Supraventricular tachycardia'), P-waves may not be visible, or may occur immediately following the QRS complex. A long RP interval is found in atrial tachycardia, atypical AV nodal re-entry tachycardia and AV re-entry involving a slowly conducting accessory pathway as the retrograde limb. Atrial flutter waves are most commonly evident in the inferior limb leads or in lead V1.

Broad-complex tachycardias

Few areas in cardiology cause more difficulty, or result in more mismanagement, than the diagnosis of broad-complex tachycardias. Whereas it is safe to assume that virtually all narrow-complex tachycardias have a supraventricular origin, broad-complex tachycardias (QRS duration ≥0.12 s) may arise either from the ventricle or from supraventricular mechanisms, the latter occurring if there is bundle branch block, either pre-existing or functional (aberration) as a result of the high rate (Fig. 4.2.16). An additional cause of aberrant conduction is activation of the ventricles via an accessory pathway.

If the broad QRS morphology during tachycardia is identical to that in sinus rhythm, then a supraventricular origin is likely, with fixed bundle branch block. However, no ECG in sinus rhythm may be available, and difficulties in diagnosis and management arise when ventricular tachycardia is not recognized and is misdiagnosed as 'SVT with aberration'. This usually happens as a result of a number of failings and misconceptions, the commonest being that the clinical context is not considered:

- *Age of the patient*—middle-aged or older individuals presenting with a recent history of broad-complex tachycardia, and who give a history of myocardial infarction or congestive heart failure, are more likely to have ventricular than supraventricular tachycardia. However, ventricular tachycardia can also arise in young patients.

- *Haemodynamic status of the patient*—it is often assumed that ventricular tachycardia should cause haemodynamic collapse, whereas patients may in fact be haemodynamically stable if the rate is not excessively fast or if underlying cardiac function is good. Conversely, supraventricular tachycardias may cause syncope, hypotension, or shock if sufficiently rapid, or if there is underlying heart disease.

- *Nature of the episodes of palpitation*—it is often not appreciated that ventricular tachycardia can present with a typical history of paroxysmal self-terminating episodes, just as in the case of supraventricular tachycardia.

The importance of making a correct diagnosis in broad-complex tachycardia is twofold. First, inappropriate acute therapy of the tachyarrhythmia can be avoided. In particular, the use of verapamil in ventricular tachycardia misdiagnosed as supraventricular

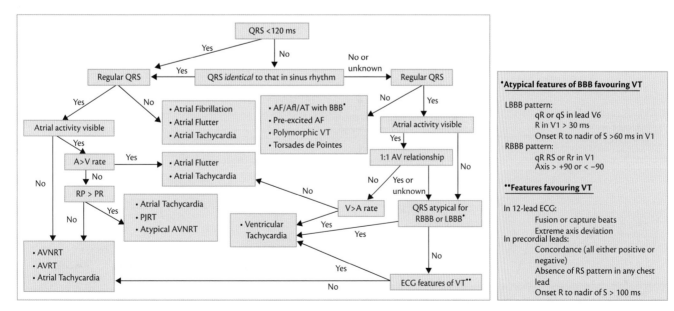

Fig. 4.2.16 Algorithm for diagnosis of tachycardia from 12-lead ECG. A, atrial rate; AF, atrial fibrillation; Afl, atrial flutter; AT, atrial tachycardia; AVNRT, atrioventricular nodal re-entrant tachycardia; AVRT, atrioventricular re-entrant tachycardia; BBB, bundle branch block; LBBB, left bundle branch block; PJRT, permanent junctional reciprocating tachycardia; PR, PR interval; RBBB, right bundle branch block; RP, RP interval; V, ventricular rate; VT, ventricular tachycardia. See text for details.

Table 4.2.5 Diagnostic use of intravenous adenosine

Arrhythmia	Response
Atrial tachycardia	Transient AV block reveals atrial arrhythmia
Atrial flutter	Rarely terminated
Atrial fibrillation	
AVNRT	Terminates tachycardia by anterograde (AV) block
AVRT	
Ventricular tachycardia	Not terminated
	1:1 VA conduction may be blocked, revealing AV dissociation

For abbreviations, see Fig. 4.2.16.

tachycardia is associated with a high risk of haemodynamic collapse as a result of its negative inotropic effect, coupled with its lack of efficacy in terminating ventricular tachycardia. Secondly, if the original arrhythmia has been misdiagnosed, then the adverse prognostic significance of ventricular tachycardia will be overlooked. Appropriate investigation and long-term management may not be instituted. It is therefore important that a diagnosis of SVT with aberration is made only if the ECG displays typical left or right bundle branch block with none of the features suggestive of VT listed in Fig. 4.2.16. In addition to attention to the history and 12-lead ECG, the response to transient AV nodal blockade with adenosine will assist diagnosis in many patients (Table 4.2.5).

General principles of management

Many cardiac arrhythmias are benign and require no intervention. The main indications for treatment are to relieve symptoms, or to prevent complications such as myocardial ischaemia, cardiac failure, embolism, or arrhythmic sudden death. Precipitating factors such as myocardial ischaemia/infarction, infection, thyrotoxicosis, alcohol, electrolyte disorders, or drug toxicity must be sought and treated if possible. The therapy indicated will commonly be influenced by the presence of underlying structural heart disease such as myocardial ischaemia/infarction or left ventricular dysfunction and can include drug therapy, device implantation, or radiofrequency ablation.

Acute management of tachycardia

An algorithm for the treatment of tachyarrhythmias is shown in Fig. 4.2.17. Assessment of the patient's cardiorespiratory status takes precedence. R-wave synchronized, direct current (DC) cardioversion under general anaesthesia or deep sedation is the most effective and immediate means of terminating sustained tachycardias, and should be employed when the tachycardia is associated with haemodynamic compromise (Fig. 4.2.18). Although atrial flutter may respond to low-energy cardioversion (50–100 J), other arrhythmias normally require energies of 100 to 360 J for termination (100–150 J for biphasic shocks). The use of DC shock in the termination of ventricular fibrillation is discussed later in this chapter.

In patients with haemodynamically stable tachycardias, manoeuvres that produce transient vagal stimulation such as the Valsalva manoeuvre or carotid sinus massage may be employed. Similarly, adenosine is used pharmacologically to produce transient slowing or block of the sinus node or AV node (see 'Adenosine'). Vagal manoeuvres or adenosine will often terminate arrhythmias dependent on the AV node, and are also useful diagnostic tools, since transient interruption of AV nodal conduction may reveal the tachycardia mechanism (Table 4.2.5). Atrial tachyarrhythmias will

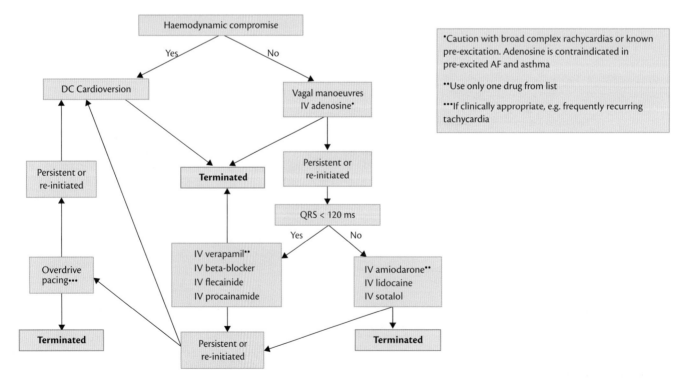

Fig. 4.2.17 Algorithm for the acute management of tachyarrhythmias.

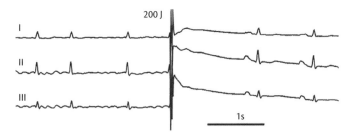

Fig. 4.2.18 Synchronized DC cardioversion of atrial fibrillation. A 200 J DC shock is delivered during atrial fibrillation to coincide with the R-wave of the QRS complex. This shock terminates the arrhythmia with restoration of normal sinus rhythm.

Table 4.2.6 Classification of antiarrhythmic drug activity

		ECG effect				Tissue effect			
		HR	PR	QRS	QT	SA node	Atrium	AV node	Ventricle
Class	Ia	0	0/−	+	++	0	++	−	++/−
	Ib	0	0	0	0/−	0	0	0	++/−
	Ic	0	+	++	+	0	++	0/+	++/−
Class	II	−	+	0	0	++	++	++	+/0
Class	III	0/−	0/+	0	++	0/+	++	0/+	++/−
Class	IV	0/−	+	0	0	0/+	+/−	++	0
Digoxin		0/−	+	0	0	0/+	0/−	++	0/−
Adenosine		−	+	0	0	++	0/−	++	0

ECG effect: +, increases; −, decreases; 0, no effect; HR, heart rate. Tissue effect: +, antiarrhythmic activity; −, potential adverse or proarrhythmic effect; 0, no effect.

not normally be terminated by vagal stimulation or adenosine, but an increase in AV block reveals the underlying atrial rhythm.

Re-entry tachycardias may be terminated by the delivery of appropriately timed extrastimuli that depolarize part of the re-entry circuit prior to the arrival of the wave front and interrupt the arrhythmia. Simple overdrive pacing can be effective in the termination of atrial flutter, AV nodal re-entry, AV (orthodromic) re-entry tachycardia, or sustained ventricular tachycardia (Fig. 4.2.19). The cardiac chamber in question is paced for brief periods, e.g. 6 to 12 beats, at a rate just above that of the tachycardia, with repeated attempts sometimes necessary at gradually increasing rates. Overdrive atrial or ventricular pacing may result in degeneration into atrial and ventricular fibrillation respectively, hence facilities for immediate defibrillation must be available. Implantable antitachycardia pacing facilities are incorporated into implantable cardioverter–defibrillators (see 'Implantable cardioverter–defibrillators').

Treatments for tachycardias

Antiarrhythmic drug therapy

The Vaughan Williams classification is based on the effects of antiarrhythmic drugs in isolated normal tissue, and although many drugs act by more than one mechanism, the classification is still in widespread use. The effects of the major classes of antiarrhythmic drug activity at the tissue level, and the associated electrocardiographic changes, are listed in Table 4.2.6. Individual drugs are described in Table 4.2.7.

Class I activity

Class I antiarrhythmic drugs act by inhibiting the rapid inward sodium current. Class Ia agents (e.g. quinidine, procainamide, and

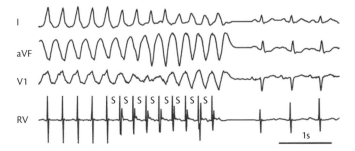

Fig. 4.2.19 Termination of ventricular tachycardia by overdrive ventricular pacing. During ventricular tachycardia a burst of eight stimuli (S) results in termination of the tachycardia and resumption of normal sinus rhythm. Surface leads I, aVF, V1, and intracardiac electrograms from the right ventricular apex (RV) are shown.

disopyramide) increase the cardiac action potential duration and have intermediate effects on the onset and recovery kinetics of the sodium channel and hence on intracardiac conduction. Class Ib agents (e.g. lidocaine and mexiletine) shorten the cardiac action potential duration and have very rapid offset kinetics that result in minimal slowing of normal intracardiac conduction. Class Ic drugs (e.g. flecainide and propafenone) have no major effect on action potential duration, but produce the most long-lasting effect on cardiac sodium channel kinetics and the most marked slowing of intracardiac conduction.

Class II activity

Class II activity is defined as antagonism of the arrhythmogenic effects of catecholamines. The commonest agents in this class are the competitive β-adrenoceptor blockers. Other agents such as propafenone have a weak β-receptor blocking activity, and amiodarone (see next paragraph) exhibits a noncompetitive sympatholytic effect.

Class III activity

The class III mode of antiarrhythmic activity comprises lengthening of the cardiac action potential duration and hence of the effective refractory period. Drugs in this class possess a broad spectrum of activity against atrial, supraventricular, and ventricular arrhythmias. Currently available class III agents act by inhibiting the rapid component of the outward potassium current I_{Kr}. Dofetilide and ibutilide are examples of drugs with 'pure' class III antiarrhythmic actions. Sotalol is a non-selective β-adrenoceptor antagonist that also possesses class III activity. Amiodarone possesses antiarrhythmic activity in all four Vaughan Williams classes.

Class IV activity

Class IV drugs (e.g. verapamil and diltiazem) reduce the inward calcium current I_{Ca} in sinoatrial and AV nodal tissues. They are used to prevent or interrupt re-entry arrhythmias involving the AV node (e.g. AV nodal re-entry tachycardia), or to slow the ventricular response in atrial fibrillation or flutter. The dihydropyridine calcium antagonists, such as amlodipine and nifedipine, have no antiarrhythmic action.

Table 4.2.7 Commonly used antiarrhythmic drugs

	Principal indication	Dose		Adverse effects
		IV	Oral	
Class Ia				
Quinidine	AF cardioversion	–	1–2 g/day	Hypersensitivity, GI symptoms, QT prolongation, hypotension
Disopyramide	AF prophylaxis VT termination	2 mg/kg	300–600 mg/day	Negative inotropy, QT prolongation, parasympathetic blockade (accelerated AV conduction, urinary retention, dry mouth, blurred vision)
Procainamide	AF cardioversion VT termination	100 mg/5 min up to 1000 mg1–6 mg/min	2–6 g/day	Hypotension, QT prolongation, GI upset, lupus syndrome
Class Ib				
Lidocaine (lignocaine)	VT termination VT/VF prophylaxis	100 mg bolus 1–4 mg/min	Ineffective	CNS—confusion, dysarthria, fits
Class Ic				
Flecainide	AF cardioversion AF prophylaxis WPW prophylaxis	2 mg/kg	100–300 mg/day	Proarrhythmia, negative inotropy, CNS disturbance
Propafenone	AF cardioversion AF prophylaxis WPW prophylaxis	–	450–900 mg/day	Proarrhythmia, negative inotropy, CNS disturbance, bronchoconstriction
Class II				
Various, e.g. bisoprolol	AF prophylaxis AF rate control SVT prophylaxis Sudden death prophylaxis	–	5–10 mg/day	Bradycardia, -ve inotropy, cold extremities, bronchoconstriction, lethargy
Class III				
Sotalol	AF termination AF prophylaxis WPW prophylaxis VT prophylaxis	2 mg/kg	160–320 mg/day	Bradycardia, negative inotropy, cold extremities, bronchoconstriction, lethargy, QT prolongation
Amiodarone	AF termination AF prophylaxis WPW prophylaxis VT prophylaxis	300 mg in 30–60 min, then 900 mg/24 h	0.6–1.2 g/day loading first 2 weeks, then 100–400 mg/day	Bradycardia, photosensitivity, skin pigmentation, hypo- or hyperthyroidism, alveolitis, hepatitis, peripheral neuropathy, epidydimitis
Class IV				
Verapamil	SVT termination SVT prophylaxis AF rate control	5–10 mg	240–480 mg/day	Negative inotropy, AV block, flushing, constipation
Other				
Digoxin	AF rate control		0.125–0.25 mg/day	Anorexia, nausea, vomiting, AV block, atrial and ventricular arrhythmias
Adenosine	SVT termination	3–12 mg by incremental bolus		Flushing, chest pain, bronchospasm, transient AV block

AF, atrial fibrillation; SVT, supraventricular tachycardia (atrioventricular nodal and atrioventricular re-entrant tachycardia); VT, ventricular tachycardia; WPW, Wolff–Parkinson–White syndrome.

Digoxin

The antiarrhythmic activity of digoxin is not explained within the Vaughan Williams classification and appears to be mediated predominantly through vagal stimulation. It is used to slow ventricular rate in atrial fibrillation.

Adenosine

Adenosine, a naturally occurring purine nucleoside, is used pharmacologically to produce transient slowing or block of the sinus node or atrioventricular node. It is of particular value in view of its extremely short plasma half-life ($c.2\,$s), which confers safety. It must be administered by rapid intravenous bolus injection, using incremental doses usually from 6 to 18 mg, to achieve the desired therapeutic effect. Adenosine is contraindicated in pre-excited atrial fibrillation or in severe asthma and cautioned in patients with known pre-excitation syndrome (see 'Pre-excitation syndromes (Wolff–Parkinson–White syndrome)').

Nonpharmacological therapy
Cardioversion

External electrical cardioversion, as described above, can be used electively to restore normal rhythm in patients with persistent arrhythmia. Failure of external cardioversion of atrial fibrillation occurs in some patients as a result of various factors, including increased transthoracic impedance due to obesity, prolonged atrial fibrillation, left ventricular dysfunction, and left atrial dilatation. Internal cardioversion can be successful in many of these patients. The procedure involves the introduction of specialized electrode catheters that permit DC shock delivery between electrodes in the right atrium and the pulmonary artery or coronary sinus, providing a current field that achieves depolarization of both atria.

Implantable cardioverter–defibrillators

Patients identified as being at high risk of sudden cardiac death, e.g. a history of spontaneous or inducible sustained ventricular arrhythmias or out-of-hospital cardiac arrest, may be treated with an implantable cardioverter–defibrillator (ICD). A transvenous rate-sensing/shocking electrode is introduced via the subclavian vein to the right ventricular apex, with the generator implanted in the pectoral region (Fig. 4.2.20). If a heart rate above the threshold programmed by the device is recognized, a shock is delivered between the intracardiac shocking electrode and the generator casing. Some devices also include a right atrial electrode to sense atrial activation. A third lead lying in a tributary of the coronary sinus can be implanted to pace the left ventricle and help restore electromechanical synchrony in those with heart failure, reduced ejection fraction, and evidence of dyssynchrony (cardiac resynchronization therapy). An ICD can be programmed to deliver initial antitachycardia ventricular pacing for tolerated tachycardias, with shock delivery available for faster rates or if pace-termination fails. ICDs are expensive, complex, and require regular specialist follow-up.

For patients without an indication for pacing, cardiac resynchronization therapy or requirement for antitachycardia pacing (i.e. sustained monomorphic ventricular tachycardia), a subcutaneous ICD (S-ICD) is an alternative treatment option for prevention of sudden cardiac death. The lead is tunnelled superficial to the sternum and connected to a generator in an axillary pocket (Fig. 4.2.21).

Radiofrequency ablation

Selective ablation of part of a re-entry circuit, an arrhythmic focus, or the AV node is used increasingly in the management of arrhythmias, and offers the opportunity of curative treatment. Radiofrequency energy is delivered between the tip of an intracardiac electrode positioned at the appropriate site and an indifferent

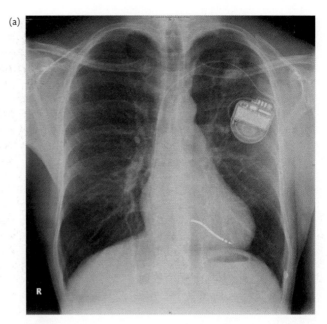

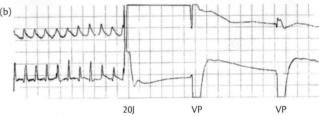

Fig. 4.2.20 Implantable cardioverter–defibrillator (ICD). (a) Chest radiograph showing the ICD generator in the left pectoral region, connected to a lead which passes via the left subclavian vein and superior vena cava to the heart. The tip of the lead is in the right ventricular apex. Cardiac rhythm is sensed from the electrodes at the tip of the lead, and shocks can be delivered between the metal casing of the generator and the right ventricular coil (thick portion of lead). (b) Discharge from an ICD. A rapid polymorphic ventricular tachycardia is terminated by a 20 J shock from the device. Electrograms shown are retrieved from the memory of the device, upper tracings from the shocking circuit (generator can to ventricular coil) and lower tracings from the sensing circuit (bipolar electrodes at the tip of the catheter in the right ventricle. The shock is followed by ventricular pacing (VP).

surface electrode placed over the scapula. The energy produces a localized necrotic lesion 2 to 3 mm in diameter, which results in local conduction block. Current indications for radiofrequency ablation are listed in Table 4.2.8, and specific issues are discussed below in relation to individual arrhythmias.

Arrhythmia surgery

The 'maze' procedure for atrial fibrillation involves creating a series of lines of conduction block in the left and right atria, either by incisions or by ablation. This prevents the development of atrial re-entry circuits while permitting AV conduction. Surgical management of recurrent ventricular tachycardia by mapping and resection of the re-entry circuit is occasionally performed, but has been largely superseded by ablation or ICD therapy.

Specific causes of arrhythmias
Extrasystoles

The term extrasystole is used to describe a premature beat arising from a focus other than the sinus node. Extrasystoles are also

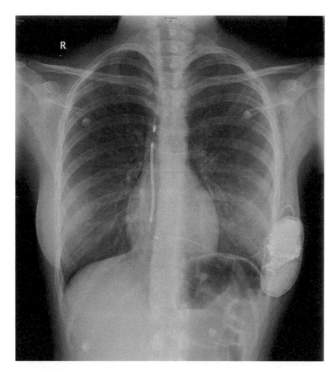

Fig. 4.2.21 CXR showing subcutaneous ICD connected to a generator in an axillary pocket.

described as premature beats, premature contractions, premature depolarizations, or ectopic beats.

Atrial extrasystoles

Atrial extrasystoles are recognized by a premature P-wave of different morphology from the sinus P-wave (Fig. 4.2.22a), which can

Table 4.2.8 Indications for radiofrequency ablation

Diagnosis	Ablation target	Success	Comments
AVRT	Accessory pathway	+++	
Pre-excited AF	Accessory pathway	+++	
AVNRT	Slow pathway	+++	0.5–1 % risk of CHB
Atrial flutter	TVA–IVC isthmus	+++	
Focal atrial tachycardia	Tachycardia focus	++	
Paroxysmal AF	Pulmonary vein isolation	++	Moderate recurrence rate
Persistent AF	Extensive LA ablation	+	Often requires >1 procedure
Permanent AF	AV node	+++	Requires permanent pacing, does not cure AF
Scar-related ventricular tachycardia	Re-entry circuit	+	High recurrence rate
Focal ventricular tachycardia	Site of origin	++	Especially RVOT focus

AVRT, atrioventricular re-entry tachycardia; AF, atrial fibrillation; AVNRT, atrioventricular nodal re-entry tachycardia; LA, left atrial; CHB, complete heart block; TVA, tricuspid valve annulus; IVC, inferior vena cava; RVOT, right ventricular outflow tract.

be hidden within the ST segment or T-wave of the preceding sinus beat. Premature atrial extrasystoles that occur before full recovery of the AV node will be followed by prolongation of the PR interval, or, if sufficiently premature, complete failure of conduction (Fig. 4.2.22b). Nonconducted atrial extrasystoles must be distinguished from sinus arrest or second-degree AV block.

An atrial extrasytole will commonly reset the sinoatrial node, such that the next sinus beat occurs earlier than expected with respect to the preceding sinus beat, and the pause is less than compensatory.

Atrial extrasystoles are a common finding in healthy people, particularly with increasing age, but are more frequent in the presence of increased atrial pressure or stretch such as in cardiac failure or chronic mitral valve disease. Patients should be reassured that the arrhythmia is benign and that drug treatment is rarely necessary. If treatment is required on symptomatic grounds, β-adrenergic blockers may be used, but class I antiarrhythmic drugs should be avoided in view of their proarrhythmic risk.

Junctional extrasystoles

Junctional extrasystoles are identified by the appearance of a premature, normal QRS complex in the absence of a preceding P-wave. The atria as well as the ventricles may be activated, resulting in an inverted P-wave simultaneous with the QRS complex, or inscribed within the ST segment. The significance and management of junctional extrasystoles are similar to those of atrial extrasystoles.

Ventricular extrasystoles

Ventricular extrasystoles are identified by the appearance of a bizarre, wide QRS complex not preceded by a P-wave (Fig. 4.2.23). There is commonly ST segment depression and T-wave inversion. Ventricular extrasystoles may be intermittent, or occur with a fixed relationship to the preceding normal beats, i.e. 1:1, 1:2 (bigeminy or trigeminy). Ventricular extrasystoles occur in otherwise normal hearts, but are found particularly in the presence of structural heart disease. Benign ventricular ectopy is common and indicated by the following: normal resting 12-lead ECG, structurally normal heart on echo, absence of other cardiac symptoms, resolution with exercise and the absence of a family history of early cardiac disease or sudden cardiac death. Ventricular ectopics occur commonly in the acute phase of myocardial infarction, but are also seen in the postinfarction phase, and in the presence of severe left ventricular hypertrophy or dysfunction of whatever cause. While the presence of frequent ectopy following myocardial infarction conveys an adverse prognosis, their suppression with class I agents (flecainide) actually increases mortality. Extrasystoles may produce symptoms that require treatment in a minority of cases. The safest option is β-blockade.

Atrial arrhythmias

Atrial fibrillation

Mechanisms

Studies of patients with paroxysmal atrial fibrillation suggest that the arrhythmia may be triggered by one or more rapidly discharging foci, which are commonly situated in the pulmonary veins.

In the presence of a heterogeneous substrate, it is thought that such a trigger gives rise to high frequency re-entry in certain areas (rotors) which perpetuate fibrillatory conduction. Rapid atrial activation induces a process of electrical remodelling, which renders cardioversion and maintenance of sinus rhythm more difficult ('atrial fibrillation begets atrial fibrillation'). The initial mechanism

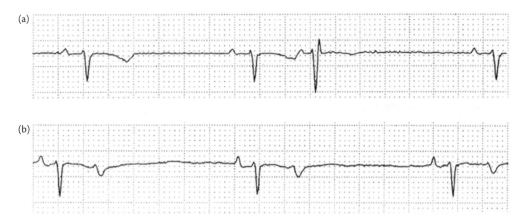

Fig. 4.2.22 Atrial extrasystoles. (a) An atrial extrasystole, with an abnormal P-wave at the end of the preceding T-wave, occurs following a sinus beat. (b) Blocked atrial extrasystoles. In the same patient, atrial extrasystoles occur following each sinus beat. They are earlier than those in (a), and the AV node is refractory because of the proximity of the atrial extrasystoles to the preceding beat, and conduction is blocked.

of remodelling is thought to be intracellular calcium overload resulting in shortening of the atrial refractory period, although more prolonged atrial tachyarrhythmias result in down-regulation of calcium entry and dedifferentiation of atrial myocytes. Structural changes, including interstitial fibrosis, also occur and further perpetuate the arrhythmia.

Classification and aetiology

Atrial fibrillation is a common arrhythmia affecting 1% of the population, the incidence increases with advancing age to 5 to 10% in very elderly individuals. It is classified as paroxysmal (self-terminating episodes <7 days duration but usually <48 h), persistent (terminates after 7 days or following intervention, e.g. electrical cardioversion), and permanent (where there is no strategy to terminate the arrhythmia).

There are numerous causes of the arrhythmia (Box 4.2.2), but in many instances no obvious aetiological factor can be identified, and the patient is described as having 'lone' atrial fibrillation. Atrial fibrillation carries adverse prognostic significance, in part through its association with organic heart disease but also as an important risk factor for the development of stroke and systemic embolism as a result of stasis and thrombus formation in the left atrium. The risk of stroke is particularly high in patients with mitral stenosis or mitral valve replacement and permanent atrial fibrillation.

Presentation

Patients with structurally normal hearts with a relatively slow ventricular rate may be asymptomatic and only picked up during routine screening. The onset of atrial fibrillation may trigger palpitations, fatigue, breathlessness, or angina in patients with underlying coronary disease. Presentation with syncope is relatively uncommon but may occur in the context of sinus node disease where spontaneous reversion to sinus rhythm is associated with prolonged sinus node recovery. Atrial fibrillation may be detected at the time of presentation or during the investigation of stroke.

Atrial fibrillation results in loss of the atrial contribution to left ventricular filling, which can result in a worsening of heart failure. Symptoms and impairment of left ventricular function ('tachycardiomyopathy') arise as a result of a rapid uncontrolled ventricular rate. In addition, uncontrolled atrial fibrillation can cause further impairment of ventricular filling in mitral stenosis and conditions associated with left ventricular diastolic dysfunction such as hypertensive left ventricular disease and aortic stenosis.

Diagnosis

The characteristic ECG findings in atrial fibrillation of recent onset are of rapid, irregular 'f' waves at a rate of 350 to 600/min. These are associated with an irregular ventricular response because of variable conduction through the AV node (Fig. 4.2.24a). With increasing duration of persistent atrial fibrillation, the amplitude of the 'f' waves diminishes until they are no longer visible. Under these circumstances, atrial fibrillation is diagnosed by the absence of P-waves and the irregular ventricular response (Fig. 4.2.24b).

Atrial fibrillation is classified into three patterns: paroxysmal, persistent, or permanent. In paroxysmal atrial fibrillation,

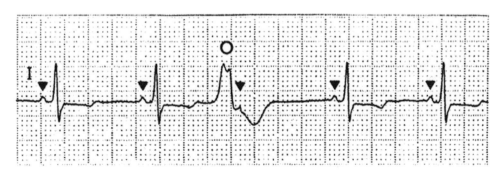

Fig. 4.2.23 Ventricular extrasystole (open circle). No retrograde atrial activation occurs, and the P-wave sequence is undisturbed (arrowed).

Box 4.2.2 Aetiology of atrial fibrillation

- Increased atrial pressure—mitral valve disease, congestive heart failure, left ventricular hypertrophy, restrictive cardiomyopathy, pulmonary embolism
- Atrial volume overload—atrial septal defect
- Myocardial ischaemia/infarction
- Thyrotoxicosis
- Alcohol
- Sinoatrial disease
- Infiltration—constrictive pericarditis, tumour
- Infection— systemic, e.g. pneumonia; cardiac: myo/pericarditis
- Cardiac or thoracic surgery
- Idiopathic—'lone' atrial fibrillation

spontaneously terminating attacks of palpitation last anything from a few seconds to a few days. The ventricular rate is often rapid and the patient may be severely symptomatic. The term 'persistent atrial fibrillation' is used to describe instances where the arrhythmia is not self-terminating, but where sinus rhythm can be restored by electrical or pharmacological cardioversion. Permanent atrial fibrillation describes the situation where both patient and physician accept the arrhythmia and rhythm control (i.e. the restoration of sinus rhythm) is not being pursued. At this stage, the ventricular rate is often slower and the patient may be unaware of the irregular pulse or of palpitations.

General principles of management

Appropriate management of atrial fibrillation depends on the presence or absence of symptoms, haemodynamic status, duration of arrhythmia and the presence of factors affecting the successful maintenance of sinus rhythm. Management is based on the prevention of thomboembolic complications and the use of a rate- or rhythm-control strategy. In asymptomatic patients trials have failed to demonstrate a mortality or morbidity benefit from restoring and maintaining sinus rhythm with antiarrhythmic therapy. There is a general consensus that in the elderly asymptomatic or mildly symptomatic patient, particularly with long-standing atrial fibrillation, a rate-control strategy is sufficient.

Emergency presentation

Atrial fibrillation of recent onset may terminate spontaneously, particularly if associated with an acute febrile illness. However, outside the context of an acute febrile illness, an attempt to restore sinus rhythm should be made unless the arrhythmia is obviously long-standing (>48 h) or is associated with advanced organic heart disease. Underlying precipitating factors such as thyrotoxicosis should be corrected before attempting cardioversion.

Chemical cardioversion may be achieved with class Ia, Ic, or III agents. Class Ia agents accelerate the ventricular rate by virtue of their anticholinergic action on the AV node and must be used in combination with AV nodal blocking agent (e.g. digoxin, β-blocker, or calcium channel blocker). For patients without significant underlying heart disease, the current drugs of choice are the class Ic agents (e.g. flecainide 2 mg/kg intravenously over 30 min). Class III drugs are somewhat less effective but are safer in the presence of left ventricular dysfunction or ischaemic heart disease. Options include sotalol (1.5 mg/kg intravenously over 30 min) or amiodarone (300 mg intravenously over 30 min followed by 900 mg/24 h until cardioversion). The class III agents ibutilide and vernakalant have approval for this indication in certain areas. Normally, only one drug should be tried in any individual patient. If drug therapy fails, DC cardioversion is commonly effective.

Given that atrial fibrillation is a risk factor for the development of intracardiac thrombus formation, cardioversion, by chemical or electrical means, should not be attempted acutely if arrhythmia has been present for longer than 48 h. Anticoagulation plus rate control with a β-blocker, calcium channel blocker, or digoxin should be considered in these circumstances. However, in the presence of haemodynamic compromise, the benefit of achieving sinus rhythm may outweigh the potential risk of embolism and attempt to restore sinus should be made. Transoesophageal echocardiography is useful in this situation to exclude left atrial thrombus.

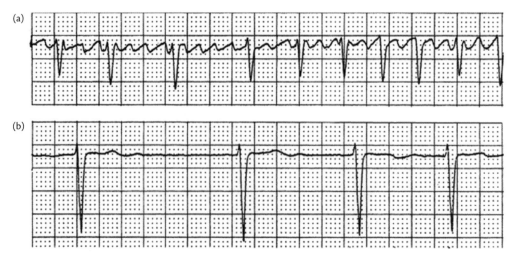

Fig. 4.2.24 Atrial fibrillation. (a) Coarse atrial fibrillation of recent onset. (b) Fine atrial fibrillation in a patient with long-standing valvular disease. Surface V1 leads are shown.

The strategy used will therefore depend upon the clinical presentation and is summarized in Box 4.2.3.

Paroxysmal atrial fibrillation

Paroxysmal atrial fibrillation is a self-terminating, recurrent arrhythmia, often associated with marked symptoms of palpitations. The goal of treatment is the maintenance of sinus rhythm and the amelioration of symptoms. In patients with infrequent paroxysms, drug therapy may not be necessary, or a 'pill in the pocket'

Box 4.2.3 Cardioversion for atrial fibrillation

1. Defined onset <48 h with minor symptoms, haemodynamic stability and no intercurrent illness

   50% or more of patients will cardiovert spontaneously particularly in the context of prior paroxysmal symptoms. Rate control with oral β-blockade (e.g. bisoprolol 5 mg) may be all that is required initially. Administration of LMWH is indicated in case cardioversion does not occur spontaneously within 24 h. Early echocardiography is required to assess for structural heart disease. In the presence of normal LV function and absence of a history of ischaemic heart disease consider oral flecainide loading (300 mg) or IV flecainide (2 mg/kg over 30 min). In the context of coronary disease or LV dysfunction consider oral sotalol 80 to 160 mg twice daily.

2. Defined onset >48 h/no defined onset, with minor symptoms, haemodynamic stability and no intercurrent illness

   Rate control with oral β-blockade or rate-limiting calcium channel blocker as first line. Oral digoxin if other agents are contraindicated. Commence warfarin. Outpatient review and decision regarding rate or rhythm control depending on symptoms.

3. Defined onset >48 h/no defined onset, with haemodynamic instability and no intercurrent illness

   Oral digoxin loading pending urgent echocardiographic assessment, then β-blockade if required (in the absence of cardiogenic shock or severe LV dysfunction or aortic stenosis on echo). Consider IV amiodarone and TOE-guided cardioversion in patients failing to respond (emergency cardioversion may be required without TOE in patients in imminent danger of cardiorespiratory arrest).

4. Rapidly conducted atrial fibrillation in conjunction with intercurrent illness

   In the context of a prior diagnosis of well-controlled permanent atrial fibrillation treatment should be directed at the underlying illness and continuing current rate control medication. Patients with new-onset atrial fibrillation should be treated with rate control (as above) and anticoagulation with LMWH. Where haemodynamic compromise is felt to be due to atrial fibrillation rather than the underlying illness, chemical or electrical cardioversion may be attempted depending on the duration of the arrhythmia (see above); however, the early recurrence rate is high.

LMWH, low molecular weight heparin; LV, left ventricular; TOE, transoesophageal echocardiography.

---

approach can be used with selected patients without structural heart disease. For this, the patient takes a dose of an antiarrhythmic drug after the onset of arrhythmia (e.g. flecainide 100 mg), if this has previously been shown to be safe and effective under hospital supervision.

In those with recurrent paroxysmal atrial fibrillation, prophylactic therapy should be considered. No drug is entirely satisfactory and a β-blocker is often prescribed as first-line therapy. If this is ineffective, other antiarrhythmic therapy should be started. Class Ic agents (flecainide or propafenone) are effective and reasonably safe in the absence of underlying ischaemia, history of coronary artery disease, or left ventricular dysfunction, and are usually co-prescribed with an AV nodal blocking drug. Sotalol (80–160 mg twice daily) is also effective and well tolerated. Amiodarone is effective but can be associated with significant adverse effects and should be reserved for when the above measures fail. In the tachycardia–bradycardia syndrome, implantation of a permanent pacemaker may be required to control bradycardia and to allow antiarrhythmic therapy for the treatment of tachycardia. Catheter ablation may be considered as first line or for those in whom pharmacological therapy has failed. The goal of catheter ablation is to achieve electrical isolation of the pulmonary veins; clinical success rates are 70 to 80% from a single procedure.

Persistent atrial fibrillation

Persistent atrial fibrillation is not self-terminating, usually requires electrical cardioversion to achieve sinus rhythm, and has a high recurrence rate even after successful cardioversion. The key decision is whether to employ a rhythm or rate control strategy. The AFFIRM trial showed no overall mortality benefit of a rhythm-control strategy in patients in whom a rhythm-control strategy in not indicated on the basis of symptoms. In general, a rate-control strategy should be employed in asymptomatic or mildly symptomatic individuals, in older people, and in those with contraindications to antiarrhythmic therapy or cardioversion. This group should be treated as having permanent atrial fibrillation. In more severely symptomatic or younger patients, or in those with atrial fibrillation due to a treated precipitant, a rhythm-control strategy may be more appropriate. However, treatment choice has to be tailored to the individual and both options should be discussed with the patient. In patients with multiple comorbidities (e.g. chronic obstructive pulmonary disease, heart failure, ischaemic heart disease), the contribution of atrial fibrillation to the patient's limitation may not be immediately clear. In such cases an attempt at restoring sinus rhythm may be worthwhile to clarify whether a rhythm-control strategy is justified. Prophylaxis of thromboembolism should be considered in both groups.

If a rhythm-control strategy is adopted, elective cardioversion should be scheduled. Given that cardioversion may be associated with embolism, patients undergoing this procedure should be treated with warfarin or a NOAC for at least 3 weeks beforehand and this should be continued long term if warranted according to risk stratification, and for at least 4 weeks in those at low risk of thromboembolism. There is a high risk of recurrent atrial fibrillation (up to 50% at 1 year) and antiarrhythmic prophylaxis should be considered. First-line therapy is often a simple β-blocker followed by a class Ic agent if there is no structural heart disease. Amiodarone may also be considered, and treatment prior to cardioversion increases the likelihood of its success. Finally, radiofrequency ablation may be employed but this requires more

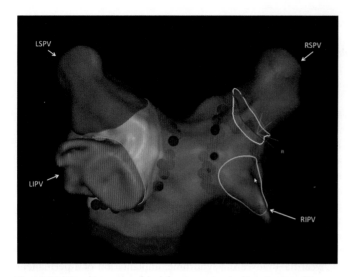

Fig. 4.2.25 Virtual geometry of the left atrium using the Carto 3 system (Biosense Webster, Diamond Bar, CA, USA). The view is a posterior view. The pulmonary veins are shown and the veins are labelled (RSPV, right superior pulmonary vein; RIPV, right inferior pulmonary vein; LSPV, left superior pulmonary vein; LIPV, left inferior pulmonary vein). Lesions produced by sequential application of radiofrequency energy are shown by the red spheres, encircling the pulmonary veins to produce electrical isolation.

extensive left atrial ablation compared to paroxysmal atrial fibrillation (Fig. 4.2.25), with a lower success rate, and often requires more than one procedure.

Permanent atrial fibrillation

In permanent atrial fibrillation, restoration of sinus rhythm is not feasible or is unsuccessful and chronic management involves control of ventricular rate. Traditionally, the mainstay of treatment has been digoxin, at a dose titrated to achieve adequate slowing in the ventricular rate at rest, with therapeutic plasma concentrations. However, despite adequate rate control at rest, patients commonly have an uncontrolled heart rate on exercise. Control of rate response with other AV nodal blocking drugs such as β-blockers or verapamil is associated with improved rate control which is especially important if the duration of diastole is critical, as in mitral stenosis or ischaemic heart disease. Often a combination of AV nodal blocking drugs is required. In cases where adequate rate control cannot be achieved despite combination therapy, radiofrequency ablation of the AV node and implantation of a permanent pacemaker (or cardiac resynchronization pacemaker) is an option, although this commits the patient to lifelong pacing therapy.

Prevention of thromboembolism

Atrial fibrillation patients have a fivefold increased risk of stroke compared to age- and sex-matched peers without atrial fibrillation. However, individual stroke risk varies and is dependent upon the presence of other stroke risk factors such as increasing age, previous stroke or transient ischaemic attack (TIA), hypertension, heart failure, diabetes mellitus, vascular disease (peripheral or coronary artery disease), and female sex; the more risk factors that are present, the greater the risk of stroke. Importantly, when stroke occurs in the presence of atrial fibrillation, the severity is greater, survival is poorer, residual

neurological deficit is greater, patients are more likely to require nursing home/residential care, and risk of recurrent stroke within 12 months is increased.

Oral anticoagulation for stroke prevention. Anticoagulant therapy significantly reduces the risk of stroke and death in atrial fibrillation patients. Accordingly current clinical guidelines (see Table 4.2.9) recommend effective stroke prevention with oral anticoagulation, either as a vitamin K antagonist (VKA, e.g. warfarin) or one of the non-VKA oral anticoagulants (NOACs), for all atrial fibrillation patients except those patients at extremely low risk of stroke (see Table 4.2.10). These low-risk patients are defined as men and women aged under 65 years with no stroke risk factors. It is important to formally assess each patient's individual risk of stroke to inform appropriate treatment decisions.

Stroke risk assessment: CHA_2DS_2-VASc. The National Institute for Health and Care Excellence (NICE), American Heart Association/American College of Cardiology/Heart Rhythm Society, and European Society of Cardiology (ESC) guidelines advocate the use of CHA_2DS_2-VASc to assess stroke risk (see Table 4.2.9). CHA_2DS_2-VASc is an acronym for the stroke risk factors which comprise it (see Table 4.2.10): congestive heart failure, hypertension, age 75 years or more, diabetes mellitus, previous stroke or TIA, vascular disease, age 65 to 74 years, and female sex. The presence of each risk factor scores 1 point, except for age 75 years or over and previous stroke/TIA, which score 2 points each; the maximum score is 9. The ACCP9 guidelines recommend assessing stroke risk using the older $CHADS_2$ score: congestive heart failure, hypertension, age 75 years or more, diabetes mellitus (1 point for each), and previous stroke or TIA (2 points); maximum score is 6. In those with a $CHADS_2$ score of 0, the ACCP guidelines recommend consideration of 'non-$CHADS_2$' risk factors, that is, age 65 to 74, female gender and vascular disease. The CHA_2DS_2-VASc score incorporates the $CHADS_2$ score but offers a more comprehensive assessment of stroke risk by including additional risk factors (vascular disease, age 65–74 years, and female sex, placing greater emphasis on age ≥75 years) and it also allows further risk stratification of patients with a $CHADS_2$ score of 0. Indeed, patients designated as 'low risk' on the basis of a $CHADS_2$ score of 0 are not truly low risk, and thus treatment decisions made on the basis of $CHADS_2$ score of 0 (i.e. no therapy or aspirin monotherapy) may result in ineffective stroke prevention.

The duration of paroxysms of atrial fibrillation required to increase the risk of thromboembolism in patients who are asymptomatic has been studied in the ASSERT trial where atrial arrhythmias were detected in patients with pacemaker implants. The annual incidence of stroke increased markedly from around 1% in those with episodes less than 17 h to approximately 5% per annum in those with episodes greater than 17 h. See Chapter 16.1 for further discussion.

Bleeding risk assessment: HAS-BLED. Decisions regarding OAC or antithrombotic therapy also require formal assessment of the patient's risk of bleeding with treatment. The NICE and ESC guidelines recommend the use of the HAS-BLED score to assess bleeding risk (see Table 4.2.9). The HAS-BLED acronym stands for uncontrolled hypertension, abnormal renal and/or hepatic function, previous stroke, prior bleed or bleeding predisposition, labile INRs

Table 4.2.9 Current guidelines for the antithrombotic management of atrial fibrillation

Guidelines	Assessment of stroke risk	Assessment of bleeding risk	Treatment recommendations	Other recommendations
NICE (2014)	CHA$_2$DS$_2$-VASc	HAS-BLED	Offer OAC[a] when CHA$_2$DS$_2$-VASc ≥2, taking into consideration bleeding risk Consider OAC[a] for men with CHA$_2$DS$_2$-VASc ≥1, taking into consideration bleeding risk Review need for OAC at least yearly Do **not** offer aspirin monotherapy for stroke prevention in AF Only consider dual antiplatelet therapy if OAC contraindicated in patients with CHA$_2$DS$_2$-VASc ≥2	OAC with VKA TTR ≥65% Assess TTR at each visit Correct modifiable reasons for poor INR control[c] Consider alternative OAC if TTR cannot be improved[d] NOACs In accordance with NICE STAs
ESC (2012)	CHA$_2$DS$_2$-VASc	HAS-BLED	Consider patients' treatment preferences No antithrombotic therapy if patient <65 years with lone AF (including females) (i.e. CHA$_2$DS$_2$-VASc = 0) OAC[a] recommended if CHA$_2$DS$_2$-VASc ≥2 Consider OAC[a] if CHA$_2$DS$_2$-VASc ≥1 Consider APT (mono- or dual therapy) only if patient refuses OAC	NOAC preferred to VKA in majority of AF patients initiating OAC NOACs Assess renal function before initiation (CrCl) Not recommended in those with severe renal impairment (CrCl<30 ml/min) In accordance with licensed indications VKAs INR 2–3; TTR control paramount
ACCP (2012)	CHADS$_2$	No formal bleeding risk assessment or tool specified	Tailor treatment decisions based on patients' treatment preferences and bleeding risk No therapy if CHADS$_2$ = 0 If patients with CHADS$_2$ = 0 choose therapy, aspirin monotherapy or dual APT is recommended; if non-CHADS$_2$ risk factors are present (age 65–74, female gender, vascular disease), OAC recommended If CHADS$_2$ = 1, OAC recommended over aspirin monotherapy or dual APT If CHADS$_2$ ≥2, OAC recommended or aspirin monotherapy or dual APT if OAC refused/contraindicated	Dabigatran[b] preferred over VKAs

ACCP, American College of Chest Physicians; APT, antiplatelet therapy; CHADS$_2$, congestive heart failure (recent), hypertension, age≥75 years, diabetes mellitus, previous stroke or transient ischaemic attack; CHA$_2$DS$_2$-VASc, congestive heart failure, hypertension, age ≥75 years, diabetes mellitus, previous stroke or TIA, vascular disease, age 65–74 years, female sex; CrCl, creatinine clearance; ESC, European Society of Cardiology; HAS-BLED, uncontrolled hypertension, abnormal renal and/or hepatic function, previous stroke, prior bleed or bleeding predisposition, labile INRs (if on VKA), elderly, concomitant interacting drugs and alcohol (drink) excess; INR, international normalized ratio; NICE, National Institute for Health and Care Excellence; NICE STA, National Institute of Clinical Excellence single technology appraisal; NOAC, non-vitamin K antagonist oral anticoagulant; OAC, oral anticoagulation; TTR, time in therapeutic range, VKA, vitamin K antagonist.

[a] Either vitamin K antagonist (most commonly warfarin) or non-vitamin K antagonist oral anticoagulant (apixaban, edoxaban, dabigatran, or rivaroxaban).

[b] At the time the ACCP guidelines were published, dabigatran was the only NOAC approved by the US FDA.

[c] Cognitive function; adherence to VKA; illness; drug interactions; lifestyle factors (diet and alcohol interactions).

[d] If reason for poor TTR is non-adherence to OAC, switching to a NOAC is not recommended.

(if on VKA), elderly, concomitant interacting drugs, and alcohol (drink) excess; with 1 point for the presence of each risk factor (see Table 4.2.10), with a maximum score of 9. Some factors within the HAS-BLED score are modifiable and a patients' HAS-BLED score can be reduced by ensuring blood pressure is well controlled (<140/90 mmHg), maintaining INR control within the therapeutic range (INR 2.0–3.0), omitting nonessential antiplatelets or NSAIDs, and minimizing alcohol intake (≤8 units/week). A high HAS-BLED score (≥3) does not indicate withholding of OAC but warrants caution and should encourage more regular review and control of modifiable bleeding risks. In addition, OAC should not be withheld exclusively because of the risk of falls.

Prediction of INR control: SAMe-TT$_2$R$_2$. Oral anticoagulation treatment options for stroke prevention in atrial fibrillation include VKAs and NOACs (see Figure 4.2.26). The SAMe-TT$_2$R$_2$ score (see Table 4.2.10), made up of routine demographic and clinical risk factors, can be used to identify upfront those newly diagnosed non-anticoagulated atrial fibrillation patients who are likely to have poor INR control on a VKA (SAMe-TT$_2$R$_2$ score >2) and who may require more frequent INR monitoring and other interventions to help them achieve adequate TTR and for whom a NOAC might be a more effective option. Use of the SAMe-TT$_2$R$_2$ score is recommended by an ESC Task Force on Anticoagulants in Heart Disease to aid decision-making, rather

Table 4.2.10 Risk stratification scores to assess stroke risk (CHA_2DS_2-VASc), bleeding risk (HAS-BLED), and predict INR control ($SAMe$-TT_2R_2)

CHA_2DS_2-VASc	Definition	Score	HAS-BLED	Definition	Score	$SAMe$-TT_2R_2	Definition	Score
Congestive heart failure	Symptoms of HF and/or objective evidence of LV systolic dysfunction (on echocardiography)	1	Hypertension	Systolic blood pressure >160 mmHg	1	Sex	Female	1
Hypertension	Elevated blood pressure (>140/90 mmHg) or receiving antihypertensive medication	1	Abnormal renal function	Chronic dialysis, renal transplantation, serum creatinine ≥200 mmol/litre	1	Age	<60 years	1
Age	≥75 years	2	Abnormal liver function	Chronic hepatic disease (e.g. cirrhosis), biochemical evidence of hepatic derangement[a]	1	Medical history	≥2 of the following: hypertension, diabetes, CAD/MI, PAD, CHF, stroke, pulmonary dx, hepatic or renal dx	1
Diabetes mellitus		1	Stroke	Ischaemic or haemorrhagic	1	Treatment	Interacting drugs (e.g. amiodarone)	1
Stroke/TIA/TE	Previous stroke, transient ischaemic attack or thromboembolism	2	Bleeding	History of bleeding or bleeding predisposition (e.g. anaemia)	2	Tobacco use	Current or ex-smoker (within 2 years)	2
Vascular disease	PAD, myocardial infarction, aortic plaque	1	Labile INR	TTR <60%	1	Race	Non-white ethnicity	2
Age	65–74 years	1	Elderly	>65 years	1			
Sex category	Female	1	Drugs or drink	Concomitant antiplatelets or NSAIDs or excessive alcohol (≥8 units/week) (1 point for each)	1 or 2			
Maximum score		9			9			8

CAD, coronary artery disease; CHF, congestive heart failure; dx, disease; HF, heart failure; INR, international normalized ratio; LV, left ventricular; NSAIDs, nonsteroidal anti-inflammatory drugs; PAD, peripheral arterial disease; TTR, time in therapeutic range.

[a] + Bilirubin >2 upper limit of normal (ULN) in association with aspartate aminotransferase/alanine aminotransferase/alkaline phosphatase>3 ULN.

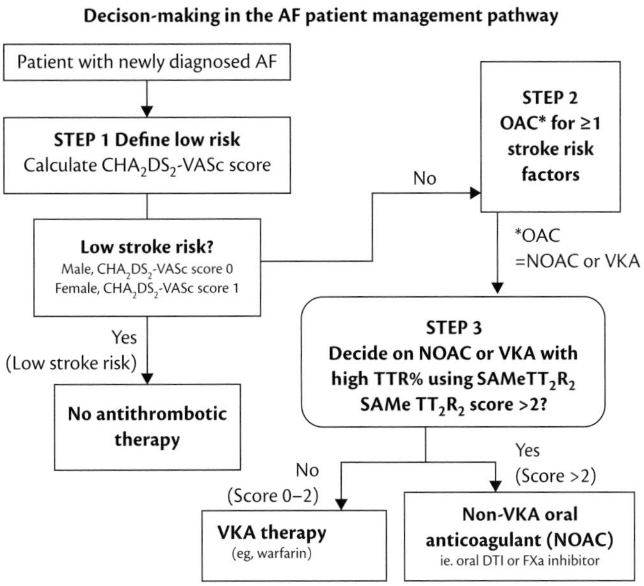

Decison-making in the AF patient management pathway

Fig. 4.2.26 The approach to decision-making in the AF patient management pathway using the CHA$_2$DS$_2$-VASc, HAS-BLED and SAMe-TT$_2$R$_2$ scores.

than subjecting atrial fibrillation patients to a 'trial of warfarin' which may put such patients at risk of stroke during the initial period of treatment.

Patient preferences for treatment. All of the most recent clinical guidelines advocate the importance of eliciting patients' preferences regarding antithrombotic therapy and incorporating them into the decision-making process. Central to informed decision-making is patient education. The clinician's role is to provide patients with information about their own risk of stroke, the benefits of OAC in reducing this risk, and their risk of bleeding with such treatment to allow them to make appropriate treatment decisions, and to respect their views and beliefs. Patients with better knowledge about atrial fibrillation, who understand the necessity of OAC for stroke prevention, despite having awareness and/or concerns about the bleeding risk associated with OAC, are more likely to adhere to treatment.

Use of oral anticoagulation in the United Kingdom and globally. Despite the overwhelming evidence of the benefit of OAC for stroke prevention in atrial fibrillation, two recent sizeable observational studies have demonstrated that large proportions of patients at risk of stroke (CHA$_2$DS$_2$-VASc score ≥2 or CHADS$_2$ score of ≥2) still do not receive OAC. In the first cohort from the Global Anticoagulant Registry in the FIELD (GARFIELD) study, of 10 614 AF patients in 19 countries, 40.7% of patients with a CHA$_2$DS$_2$-VASc score of 2 or more did not receive OAC. More than one-half of the reasons given for withholding OAC therapy for patients at risk of stroke in the GARFIELD registry were linked to physician choice (i.e. bleeding risk, concerns over patient adherence, falls risk). Perhaps a more worrying finding from the GARFIELD registry revealed that approximately one-quarter of patients with a CHA$_2$DS$_2$-VASc score of 2 or more were receiving antiplatelet monotherapy. A similar underuse of OAC in patients at high of stroke and overuse in those at low risk was seen in the Euro Heart Survey which was conducted a decade ago. The recent analysis in 1857 general practices in the United Kingdom, utilizing the GRASP-AF tool (which assessed

stroke risk on the basis of the CHADS$_2$ score and recommends treatment based on the 2006 NICE guidelines), demonstrated that 34.0% of patients with a CHADS$_2$ score of 2 or more, with no documented contraindication to OAC, were receiving OAC and the use of antiplatelet therapy rose as stroke risk increased. Use of OAC declined significantly among patients aged 80 years or over (47.4% vs 64.5%; p <0.001), while antiplatelet therapy increased in this age group. Consequently those patients at greatest risk of stroke (i.e. elderly patients and those with multiple comorbidities) are the very patients who are least likely to receive adequate preventative therapy against stroke. This is despite very clear evidence from the Birmingham Atrial Fibrillation in The Aged (BAFTA) study which demonstrated that warfarin was more effective in preventing strokes than aspirin in patients aged 75 years or over (2.5% vs 4.9% per year; RR 0.52 [95% CI 0.33–0.80]), with a similar risk of major bleeding (1.9% vs 2.0% per year; RR 0.96 [95% CI 0.53–1.75]) and from an individual patient-data meta-analysis of approximately 9000 atrial fibrillation patients which confirmed that OAC was efficacious in reducing ischaemic stroke regardless of the patient's age, whereas the protective effect of aspirin declined significantly with age. The lack of OAC prescription among atrial fibrillation patients at risk of stroke was not related to their bleeding risk or comorbidities.

Guidelines for stroke prevention in atrial fibrillation. Effective prevention of stroke for atrial fibrillation patients requires OAC, either with a VKA or one of the NOACs (see Table 4.2.9 and Figure 4.2.26). If patients are prescribed a VKA, the most important consideration is their anticoagulation control (INR 2.0–3.0), evidenced by a time in therapeutic range (TTR) of 65% or more. Patient education about factors that may affect their INR control (e.g. diet, alcohol intake, and interacting drugs) is important, and regular INR monitoring and assessment of the reasons for poor anticoagulation control is essential. Indeed, a recent trial demonstrated that a one-off intensive education session significantly improved TTR 6 months after warfarin initiation in an inception cohort compared to usual care. Consideration and correction (where possible) of the reasons for poor anticoagulation need to be addressed (see Figure 4.2.26 and Table 4.2.9). Currently four NOACs—apixaban, dabigatran, edoxaban, and rivaroxaban—are NICE approved and available for stroke prevention in atrial fibrillation (see Table 4.2.11 and Figure 4.2.26). For patients who are OAC-naive, the NOACs are broadly preferred over a VKA for the majority of patients. Strict adherence to licensed indications is essential and a recent European Heart Rhythm Association document offers excellent practical guidance on the use of NOACs in practice. Renal function must be assessed prior to initiating a NOAC and the creatinine clearance, using the Cockroft–Gault formula, must be calculated. NOACs should not be used in patients with severe renal impairment (CrCl <30 ml/min), although rivaroxaban 15 mg once daily, edoxaban 30mg once daily, and apixaban 2.5 mg twice daily can be used with caution in patients with CrCl

15 to 29 ml/min. Regular monitoring of a patients' renal function for the duration of NOAC treatment is advocated; the frequency of renal function testing is dependent of the degree of renal impairment (see Table 4.2.11). Dose reductions are required in patients with moderate renal impairment and according to other factors (see Table 4.2.11 'Dose reductions' for specific criteria for each NOAC).

Aspirin monotherapy is not an effective treatment strategy for stroke prevention in patients with atrial fibrillation and consequently the clinical guidelines actively discourage its use. Dual antiplatelet therapy, with aspirin and clopidogrel, should only be considered in patients with a CHA_2DS_2-VASc score of 2 or more in whom any OAC use is refused or contraindicated, given the increased risk of bleeding with dual antiplatelets and reduced efficacy compared to OAC. Left atrial appendage occlusion devices should only be considered if OAC is contraindicated or the patient refuses OAC; they are not a first-line

Table 4.2.11 Novel oral anticoagulants for stroke prevention in atrial fibrillation

Drug characteristics	Apixaban	Dabigatran	Edoxaban	Rivaroxaban
Mechanism	Oral direct factor Xa inhibitor	Oral direct thrombin inhibitor	Oral direct factor Xa inhibitor	Oral direct factor Xa inhibitor
Half-life (h)	9–14	12–17	10–14	5–13
Excretion	25% renal; 75% faecal	80% renal	50%	66% liver, 33% renal
Dose	5 mg twice daily	150 mg twice daily	60 mg once daily	20 mg once daily
Dose in renal impairment[b] (30–49 ml/min)	2.5 mg twice daily[a]	110 mg twice daily	30 mg once daily*	15 mg once daily
Dose reductions	If ≥2 of following: serum creatinine >133 µmol/l; age ≥80 years; body weight ≤60 kg	≥80 years; concomitant verapamil; HAS-BLED score ≥3[c]	≥1 of the following: CrCl mL/min 15–50 mL/min; body weight ≤60 kg; on ciclosporin, dronedarone, erythromycin, or ketoconazole	No dose reduction except for renal function
Drug interactions	Anticoagulants, antiplatelets, NSAIDs; ketoconazole, itracronazole, voriconazole, posaconazole, HIV protease inhibitors (ritonavir), rifampicin, St John's wort, phenobarbital, phenytoin, carbamazepine	Anticoagulants, antiplatelets, NSAIDs; systemic ketoconazole, ciclosporin, tacrolimus, itraconazole, verapamil; quinidine, dronedarone, amiodarone, clarithomycin, rifampicin, St John's wort, phenytoin, carbamazepine, SSRIs, SNRIs	Anticoagulants, antiplatelets, NSAIDs †Ciclosporin, dronedarone, erythromycin, or ketoconazole Quinidine, verapamil, amiodarone Phenytoin, carbamazepine, phenobarbital, or St. John's Wort	Anticoagulants, antiplatelets, NSAIDs; ketoconazole, fluconazole, itracronazole, voriconazole, posaconazole quinidine, HIV protease inhibitors (ritonavir), clarithomycin, erythromycin, dronedarone, rifampicin, St John's wort, phenobarbital, phenytoin, carbamazepine
Take with/after food	No	Yes	No	Yes
Check renal function	Divide CrCl by 10; e.g. CrCl 60 ml/min monitor every 6 months; if decline in renal function is suspected (e.g. hypovolaemia, dehydration) or concomitant use of certain medicinal products, check renal function			

* if CrCl 15–50mL/min

† Reduce dose to 30mg once daily if use of concomitant use of ciclosporin, dronedarone, erythromycin, or ketoconazole.

[a] Dose reduction if serum creatinine >133 µmol/litre plus age ≥80 years and/or body weight ≤60 kg.

[b] Dabigatran not to be used if CrCl <30 ml/min; edoxaban, rivaroxaban, and apixaban not be used if CrCl <15 ml/min; rivaroxaban and apixaban only to be used if CrCl 15–29 ml/min with caution and regular review (at least 3 monthly).

[c] On an individual basis based on stroke and bleeding risk.

Adapted from Camm AJ et al. (2012) ESC Committee for Practice Guidelines (CPG). 2012 focused update of the ESC Guidelines for the management of atrial fibrillation: an update of the 2010 ESC Guidelines for the management of atrial fibrillation. *Eur Heart J*, **33**, 2719–47 and Heidbuchel H et al. (2013) European Heart Rhythm Association. European Heart Rhythm Association Practical Guide on the use of new oral anticoagulants in patients with non-valvular atrial fibrillation. *Europace*, **15**, 625–51.

alternative to OAC and the risks of LAAO need to be carefully discussed with the patient. Regardless of the stroke prevention treatment strategy selected after discussion with the patient, treatment decisions and stroke and bleeding risk assessments should be reviewed at least annually as a patients' risk may change and treatment may need to be altered. One of the NICE 2014 recommendations is to offer patients with atrial fibrillation 'a personalized package of care including measures to prevent stroke' and this involves matching the right OAC drug to the patient on the basis of their stroke and bleeding risk assessment and overall clinical background/profile; ability to do this requires knowledge of the results of the individual trials.

Net clinical benefit of OAC: NOACs versus warfarin. The most appropriate stroke prevention strategy involves balancing the benefit of treatment (i.e. reduction in stroke) against the possibility of serious bleeding (i.e. intracranial haemorrhage) associated with treatment for each patient; an evaluation of the net clinical benefit. An analysis of the net clinical benefit of warfarin was undertaken in a large (>180 000) cohort of Swedish patients, with stroke and bleeding risk assessed by CHA_2DS_2-VASc and HAS-BLED respectively. This study found that OAC treatment was associated with a positive net clinical benefit for all patients, except those with a CHA_2DS_2-VASc score of 0, confirming their truly low-risk status. Those with high stroke and high bleeding risk fared best from warfarin therapy; there were 12 fewer ischaemic strokes per 100 years at risk compared to not giving warfarin. What about the net clinical benefit of the NOACs against warfarin? There will never be a direct head-to-head comparison of the NOACs, therefore the next best option is an indirect comparison of the NOACs with warfarin. A similar analysis modelled the net clinical benefit of the NOACs apixaban, dabigatran, and rivaroxaban against warfarin in a real-world cohort of Danish atrial fibrillation patients. All four NOACs offered a net clinical benefit superior to warfarin among patients with a CHA_2DS_2-VASc score of 2 or more or a $CHADS_2$ score of 1 or more, despite the risk of bleeding. Among patients with a CHA_2DS_2-VASc score of 1, both doses of dabigatran and apixaban were associated with better net clinical benefit. In patients with a $CHADS_2$ score of 0 and a high risk of bleeding, only dabigatran 110 mg twice daily and apixaban displayed a beneficial net clinical

outcome. If the risk of stroke and the risk of bleeding are high, the NOACs have a risk-benefit profile superior to that of warfarin.

Atrial flutter

Atrial flutter is caused by a macro re-entrant circuit in the right atrium (Fig. 4.2.27), which produces a typical electrocardiographic 'sawtooth' pattern of atrial activity with a rate close to 300/min (Fig. 4.2.28). In the common form of the arrhythmia, flutter waves are negative in leads II, III, and aVF and positive in lead V1. Atrial flutter may be associated with either a regular or irregular ventricular response. Flutter with 2:1 AV conduction produces a regular tachycardia of 150/min and should always be considered in the differential diagnosis of a regular, narrow-QRS tachycardia of this rate. Occasionally, flutter occurs with 1:1 AV conduction producing a ventricular rate approaching 300/min. Class I antiarrhythmic drugs may predispose to this by causing a relative slowing of the atrial rate and allowing 1:1 conduction through the AV node. The flutter waves may not be seen easily with faster ventricular rates, and transient slowing of AV conduction may be necessary to make the diagnosis (Fig. 4.2.28).

The underlying causes of atrial flutter are the same as those of atrial fibrillation (Box 4.2.2). Although atrial flutter may last for many months or occasionally years, it usually degenerates into atrial fibrillation unless cardioversion or catheter ablation is undertaken. Atrial flutter also carries a risk of thromboembolism, and anticoagulation is indicated before and after cardioversion as for atrial fibrillation. It is important to attempt to terminate atrial flutter since the ventricular rate is often poorly controlled by AV nodal blocking drugs. Termination may be achieved by chemical or electrical cardioversion as described above for atrial fibrillation. Bursts of atrial overdrive pacing at a rate approximately 10% above the atrial flutter rate are also used: this may restore sinus rhythm or precipitate atrial fibrillation. Prophylaxis against atrial flutter is undertaken using the same agents as in paroxysmal atrial fibrillation; indeed the conditions often coexist and patients may manifest either flutter or fibrillation at different times. Treatment of atrial flutter by radiofrequency ablation creates a line of conduction block between the tricuspid valve annulus and the inferior vena cava, interrupting the isthmus through which the re-entry circuit must pass (Fig. 4.2.27). This achieves cure in 90 to 95% of cases and is increasingly used as a first-line therapy.

Atrial tachycardia

Atrial tachycardia usually results in an atrial rate between 120 and 250/min. There may be a degree of AV block, although 1:1 AV conduction can occur. The ECG shows regular P-waves which do not show the same 'sawtooth' appearance as in atrial flutter (Fig. 4.2.28). Atrial tachycardia may occur as a result of sinus node re-entry, with sudden paroxysms of tachycardia with a normal P-wave morphology. Automatic atrial tachycardia manifests an abnormal P-wave morphology, commonly with a prolonged PR interval. The rate characteristically accelerates or 'warms up' before reaching a rate of 125 to 200/min. Atrial tachycardia with AV conduction block is a manifestation of digitalis toxicity. Multifocal atrial tachycardia, in which rapid, irregular P-waves of three or four different morphologies are seen, may occur in severely ill elderly patients or in association with acute exacerbation of pulmonary disease.

Management includes drug treatment or cardioversion, as for atrial fibrillation. Focal atrial tachycardia may be amenable to treatment with radiofrequency ablation with success rates approaching 75%, although recurrence rate is high.

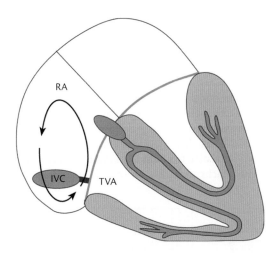

Fig. 4.2.27 Mechanism of atrial flutter. Typical atrial flutter results from a counterclockwise re-entry circuit in the right atrium. The isthmus between the tricuspid valve annulus (TVA) and inferior vena cava (IVC) forms a critical part of this circuit, and linear ablation to create block can prevent recurrent atrial flutter.

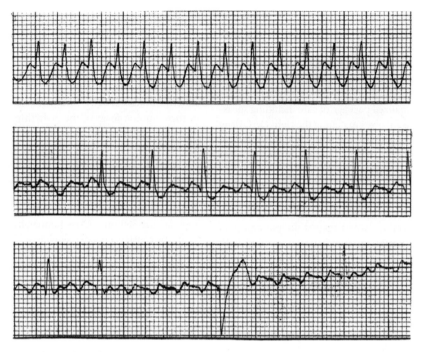

Fig. 4.2.28 Atrial flutter with 1:1 AV conduction (above), 2:1 conduction (middle), and following adenosine administration (below) (6 mg intravenous injection 10 s previously).

Supraventricular tachycardia

Although all atrial arrhythmias are by definition supraventricular in origin, the term supraventricular tachycardia is commonly reserved for those in which the AV node is an obligate part of a re-entry circuit—AV nodal re-entrant tachycardia (AVNRT) or AV re-entry tachycardia (AVRT). Correct recognition of these arrhythmias has achieved additional importance with the development of effective curative measures.

Atrioventricular nodal re-entry tachycardia

Mechanism

This is the commonest cause of paroxysmal re-entry tachycardia manifesting regular, normal QRS complexes. The basis of the arrhythmia is the presence of two functionally distinct pathways in the region of the AV node (Fig. 4.2.30). The 'fast' pathway conducts more rapidly, but has a longer refractory period. The 'slow' pathway has slower conduction properties but a shorter refractory period. During sinus rhythm, AV nodal conduction occurs via the fast pathway with a normal PR interval (Fig. 4.2.30a). If a sufficiently premature atrial extrasystole arises, conduction in the fast pathway is blocked, but slow pathway conduction may continue, resulting in an abrupt increase in the AH interval as recorded in the His bundle electrogram. This corresponds to an increased PR interval on the surface ECG (Fig. 4.2.30b). If conduction down the slow pathway is sufficiently delayed to allow the fast pathway to recover excitability

before activation reaches the distal end of the pathways, retrograde activation occurs via the fast pathway. The stage is then set for a re-entry circuit with anterograde conduction via the slow pathway and retrograde conduction via the fast pathway ('slow/fast AV nodal re-entry'; Fig. 4.2.30c). Characteristically, anterograde activation of the ventricles and retrograde activation of the atria occur virtually simultaneously, resulting in the P-wave being 'buried' within the QRS complex, or producing a very small distortion of the terminal QRS, recognition of which requires careful comparison with the ECG during sinus rhythm (Fig. 4.2.31).

A less common variant of AV nodal re-entry tachycardia may arise where anterograde conduction during tachycardia is via the fast pathway with retrograde conduction via the slow pathway ('fast/slow AV nodal re-entry', also termed 'atypical AVNRT'). Under these circumstances, the atrium is activated well after the QRS complex, characteristically producing an inverted P-wave, with the RP interval greater than the PR interval during tachycardia, termed 'long RP tachycardia' (Fig. 4.2.32).

Clinical features

Atrioventricular nodal re-entry tachycardia commonly presents in young adults, although it may appear at any age. The natural history is of episodic paroxysmal tachycardia. Attacks occur at random intervals, although clustering of attacks may occur interposed with periods of relative freedom from symptoms. Atrioventricular nodal re-entry tachycardia has no specific association with other

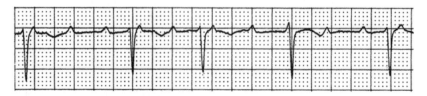

Fig. 4.2.29 Atrial tachycardia, with variable AV conduction. Lead V1.

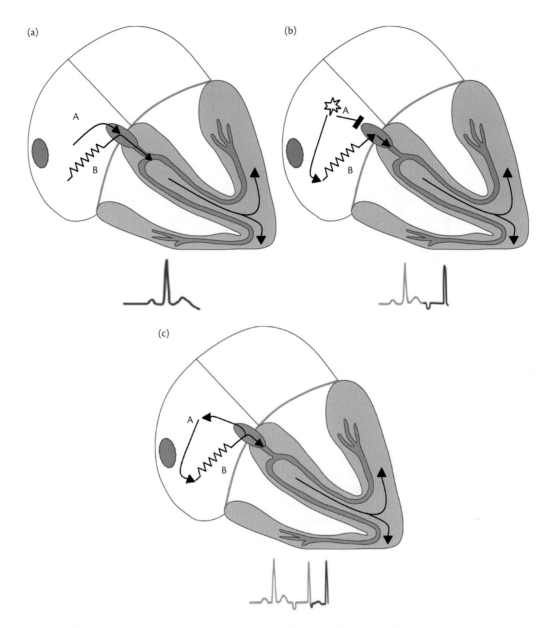

Fig. 4.2.30 Atrioventricular nodal re-entry tachycardia. Mechanism of initiation by atrial extrasystole. See text for details.

organic heart disease. Palpitations are normally well tolerated unless the tachycardia is particularly rapid, prolonged, or if the patient has other heart disease.

Management

Termination of an attack of AV nodal re-entry tachycardia is achieved by producing transient AV nodal block. This may be achieved by vagotonic manoeuvres, by intravenous adenosine (3–18 mg) (Fig. 4.2.31), or by intravenous verapamil (6–18 mg). Drug prophylaxis of AV nodal re-entry tachycardia is undertaken with β-blockers, a combined β-blocker/class III agent such as sotalol, or AV nodal blocking drugs such as verapamil or digoxin. Curative treatment of AV nodal re-entry tachycardia by radiofrequency ablation is increasingly used as a first-line therapy, and is indicated if patients are refractory to drugs, intolerant of side effects, or unwilling to take long-term medication. Radiofrequency energy is delivered to the 'slow' pathway, which lies between the compact AV node and the tricuspid annulus. Ablation at this site is normally

curative in over 90% of cases, but carries a small risk (0.5–1%) of inducing complete heart block.

Atrioventricular re-entry tachycardia

Mechanism

In contrast to AV nodal re-entry tachycardia, the substrate for AV re-entry is the presence of a second atrioventricular connection, separate from the AV node. This accessory pathway can lie anywhere along the mitral or tricuspid annuli. Anterograde pathway conduction produces ventricular pre-excitation and is discussed in the 'Pre-excitation syndromes' section below. However, some accessory pathways only conduct in the retrograde (ventriculoatrial) direction and are termed 'concealed', since there is no clue to their presence on the resting ECG. The anterograde limb of the re-entrant circuit is the AV node, with retrograde atrial activation occurring over the accessory pathway (see Fig. 4.2.33). This is termed orthodromic tachycardia and normally produces a narrow-complex QRS morphology. Retrograde atrial activation can

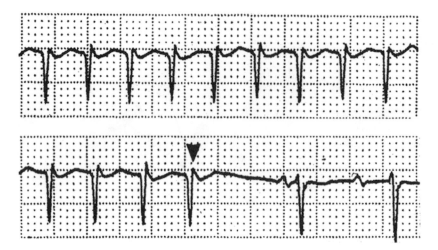

Fig. 4.2.31 Atrioventricular nodal re-entrant tachycardia. Rapid narrow-complex tachycardia with no apparent P-waves (upper) responding to 6 mg adenosine with restoration of sinus rhythm (lower). Close inspection reveals a positive deflection of the terminal QRS during tachycardia (pseudo R′, arrowed) which is absent during sinus rhythm. This is due to retrograde atrial activity coincident with ventricular activation. Lead V1.

be identified by the presence of a characteristic inverted P′-wave early in the ST segment, an important diagnostic feature of AV re-entry tachycardia (Fig. 4.2.34). Rarely, an accessory pathway with slow retrograde conduction may allow a stable, incessant re-entrant circuit with a long RP interval, referred to as permanent junctional reciprocating tachycardia.

Clinical features
Features are similar to AV nodal re-entry tachycardia, although accessory pathways are the more common tachycardia substrate in children. Patients have a similar relapsing course of symptoms interspersed with periods of relative quiescence. Multiple pathways can be present within the same patient and are more common if there is coexisting structural heart disease such as Ebstein's anomaly (see Chapter 12).

Management
As with AV nodal re-entry tachycardia, the AV node is an obligate part of the circuit and attacks may be aborted by vagotonic manoeuvres or with intravenous adenosine. Antiarrhythmic therapy may be effective, but radiofrequency ablation offers high success rates with low incidence of complications and should be considered early in a patient's treatment.

Pre-excitation syndromes (Wolff–Parkinson–White syndrome)
The term 'pre-excitation' refers to the premature activation of the ventricle via one or more accessory pathways that bypass the normal

AV node and His–Purkinje system. Accessory pathways with electrophysiological properties of normal myocardium may lie at any point in the AV ring, the commonest sites being in the left free wall or the posteroseptal region (Fig. 4.2.33). The characteristic electrocardiographic appearance is of early activation of the ventricular myocardium adjacent to the insertion of the accessory pathway. There is no AV delay via the pathway, hence the PR interval is shortened, but slow intraventricular conduction results in slurred initiation of the QRS complex (the delta wave; Fig. 4.2.35), before the remainder of the ventricle is excited via the normal His–Purkinje system. The ECG appearances of a delta wave occur in approximately 1.5 per 1000 of the population, but many individuals never experience paroxysmal tachycardias. The degree of pre-excitation during sinus rhythm is variable: it may be intermittent if the refractory period of the accessory pathway is close to the sinus cycle length (Fig. 4.2.35), or inapparent if the delta wave is obscured due to rapid AV nodal conduction. In such instances, transient slowing of AV nodal conduction (e.g. by adenosine) will enhance the proportion of the ventricle excited by the accessory pathway and reveal pre-excitation. The Wolff–Parkinson–White syndrome describes the combination of the symptoms of palpitation and the presence of pre-excitation on the ECG.

Mechanisms of orthodromic and antidromic tachycardia
The mechanism for orthodromic AV re-entry tachycardia is illustrated in Fig. 4.2.32. A premature atrial extrasystole may find the pathway refractory but be conducted through the AV node to the

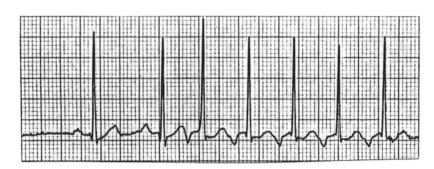

Fig. 4.2.32 Atypical atrioventricular nodal re-entry tachycardia ('long RP'). Inverted P-waves precede the QRS complex during tachycardia (compare with preceding sinus beats)

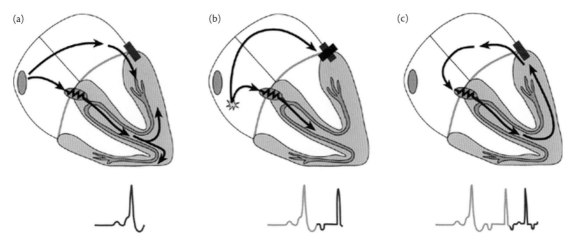

Fig. 4.2.33 Atrioventricular re-entry tachycardia. Mechanism of initiation by atrial extrasystole. See text for details: if the accessory pathway were concealed the ECG in sinus rhythm would not show the characteristic delta wave.

ventricles (Fig. 4.2.33b). If sufficient delay has occurred by the time the ventricular insertion of the accessory pathway is depolarized, the pathway may have recovered excitability and allow retrograde activation from the ventricle to atrium, with the establishment of a re-entry circuit (Fig. 4.2.33c). Since the circuit involves activation of the ventricles via the His–Purkinje system, the QRS morphology during re-entry tachycardia is normal, unless a rate-related bundle branch block develops. If bundle branch block is seen at a lower heart rate than a documented narrow-complex tachycardia, this is diagnostic of an accessory pathway ipsilateral to the bundle branch block (Coumel's sign).

A rare form of AV re-entry tachycardia has anterograde conduction via the accessory pathway and retrograde conduction via the AV node (antidromic tachycardia). The QRS morphology of this tachycardia is broad and grossly abnormal with appearances dependent upon the site of insertion of the accessory pathway.

Pre-excited atrial fibrillation

The major prognostic concern in Wolff–Parkinson–White syndrome is pre-excited atrial fibrillation. Conduction via an accessory pathway with a short refractory period, bypassing the normal AV nodal slowing, may result in very rapid conduction to the ventricle (Fig. 4.2.36) that can degenerate into ventricular fibrillation. The degree of pre-excitation during atrial fibrillation varies, giving a characteristic pattern of an irregular ventricular response with QRS morphology ranging from normal to fully pre-excited. The risk of sudden death is increased if the shortest R-R interval is less than

250 ms during pre-excited atrial fibrillation, and is an indication for urgent cardioversion and early radiofrequency ablation.

Management of the symptomatic patient with ventricular pre-excitation

The AV node is a part of the re-entry circuit in both ortho- and antidromic tachycardia, and adenosine and other AV nodal blocking drugs may be effective. However, adenosine may precipitate pre-excited atrial fibrillation and should be used with caution. In patients with known Wolff–Parkinson–White syndrome presenting with AV re-entrant tachycardia, drugs which also act on the accessory pathway such as flecainide or sotalol may be preferred. In pre-excited atrial fibrillation, AV nodal blocking drugs such as digoxin or verapamil should be avoided, because of the risk of ventricular fibrillation; treatment should be with antiarrhythmic therapy such as flecainide or by DC cardioversion. Patients with Wolff-Parkinson-White syndrome should be offered radiofrequency ablation as first-line therapy. This abolishes the risk of pre-excited atrial fibrillation as well as preventing further attacks of AV re-entry tachycardia. Careful mapping of the AV annulus using an electrode catheter is necessary to identify the site of the accessory pathway, at which the interval between the atrial and ventricular electrograms is at a minimum. Passage of the radiofrequency current causes heating of the catheter tip and results in the disappearance of accessory pathway conduction within a few seconds (Fig. 4.2.37). The success rate of ablation varies according to the location of the pathway, but is usually over 90% in experienced hands.

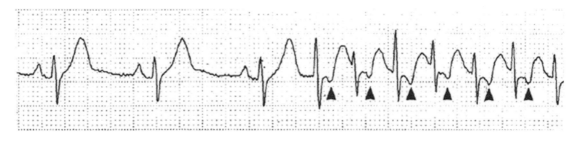

Fig. 4.2.34 Initiation of atrioventricular re-entry tachycardia. The third sinus beat is followed by the onset of narrow-complex tachycardia, initiated by an atrial extrasystole (obscured by T-wave). Retrograde atrial activation, with inverted P-waves in the ST segment (arrows), are seen during tachycardia.

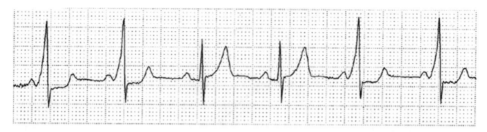

Fig. 4.2.35 Intermittent pre-excitation in Wolff–Parkinson–White syndrome. The first two beats show the characteristic short PR interval and delta wave. The middle two beats, however, show that the pre-excitation was intermittent. The pathway has become refractory, with normal PR interval and QRS morphology. Pathway conduction returns to cause pre-excitation in the final two beats.

Approach to the asymptomatic patient with ventricular pre-excitation

Patients with Wolff–Parkinson–White syndrome should be evaluated carefully for the risk of pre-excited atrial fibrillation, even in the absence of symptoms. The risk of sudden death due to rapid pre-excited atrial fibrillation is very low among adults who have not had any symptomatic tachycardias, but is higher in symptomatic patients. If pre-excitation is intermittent, this indicates a long refractory period of the pathway and a low risk of life-threatening tachycardias. Abrupt disappearance of the delta wave in response to exercise testing, or during Holter monitoring, or with the administration of a class Ia or Ic antiarrhythmic drug, also suggests a low risk. Some centres advocate diagnostic electrophysiological studies to identify a high-risk group with short pathway refractory periods and inducible tachycardia or pre-excited atrial fibrillation. The general tendency is for accessory pathway conduction to become slower with increasing age, and spontaneous disappearance of conduction is well documented.

Other pre-excitation syndromes

Other forms of pre-excitation include the Mahaim pathway, a direct AV or atriofasicular connection with decremental conduction properties similar to AV nodal tissue. Evidence for direct atrionodal pathways associated with a short PR interval but no delta wave remains controversial and has not been established histologically.

Ventricular tachycardia

Definitions

Ventricular tachycardia is defined as the presence of three or more consecutive ventricular beats at a rate of 120/min or greater. It is considered to be sustained if an individual salvo lasts for 30 s or more, and nonsustained if the duration is between 3 beats and 30 s. Monomorphic ventricular tachycardia demonstrates a consistent QRS morphology during each paroxysm. Polymorphic ventricular

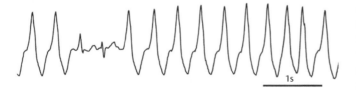

Fig. 4.2.36 Pre-excited atrial fibrillation. Conduction via an accessory pathway results in an irregular broad-complex tachycardia. The third and fourth beats show less pre-excitation, with activation mainly through the normal conducting system, with more normal QRS-complex morphology. Lead V1.

tachycardia demonstrates a constantly changing QRS morphology, often without discrete QRS complexes. Polymorphic ventricular tachycardia may degenerate into ventricular fibrillation and the ECG distinction between the two is difficult. Torsades de pointes is a polymorphic VT in association with QT interval prolongation and is discussed in more detail later in the chapter.

ECG characteristics

The presence of AV dissociation is a particularly important feature to seek in a broad-complex tachycardia as it makes the diagnosis of ventricular tachycardia virtually certain (Fig. 4.2.38a). A careful search for P-waves perturbing the QRS complex or T-waves is necessary, ideally using multi-lead recordings. Occasionally, a fortuitously timed P-wave allows the development of a capture beat of normal QRS morphology without interrupting the tachycardia. A fusion beat occurs when activation of the ventricle is partly via the normal His–Purkinje system and partly from the tachycardia focus (Fig. 4.2.38b). Fusion and capture beats are diagnostic of ventricular tachycardia, but are commonly present only if the ventricular rate is relatively slow. Although AV dissociation is diagnostic of ventricular tachycardia, it is not invariable. Retrograde ventriculoatrial conduction may occur, giving either 1:1 conduction or higher degrees of block (Fig. 4.2.38c).

The QRS duration in ventricular tachycardia is commonly greater than 0.12 s, and values greater than 0.14 s are particularly suggestive of ventricular tachycardia. Although the QRS morphology may superficially resemble left or right bundle branch block, the morphology is commonly atypical (see Fig. 4.2.16). Ventricular tachycardia arising from the right ventricular free wall has a left bundle branch block-like pattern, whereas left ventricular free wall tachycardias show right bundle branch block morphology. The presence of concordant positive or negative QRS complexes across the chest leads is suggestive of ventricular tachycardia, as is the existence of extreme axis deviation. ECG features consistent with VT are listed in Fig. 4.2.16.

Aetiology

Sustained monomorphic ventricular tachycardia commonly occurs in the presence of structural heart disease, but also arises in structurally normal hearts. It rarely occurs in the acute phase of myocardial infarction, but may be seen in the subacute phase (>48 h), or may arise many years later, particularly in association with left ventricular scar or aneurysm formation. The arrhythmia also occurs in other forms of structural heart disease associated with ventricular dilatation or fibrosis such as dilated cardiomyopathy, hypertrophic cardiomyopathy, or previous ventriculotomy (e.g. following repair

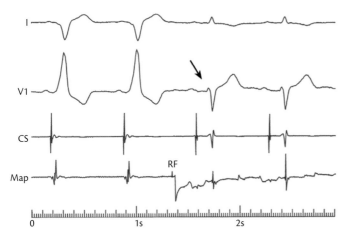

Fig. 4.2.37 Radiofrequency ablation of an accessory pathway. The patient had Wolff–Parkinson–White syndrome with evidence of ventricular pre-excitation on the surface electrogram during sinus rhythm (short PR interval, delta wave). One beat after switching on the radiofrequency (RF) current the QRS becomes normal, indicating successful ablation of the accessory pathway. This was a left-sided accessory pathway, as shown by the short interval between left atrial and left ventricular activation recorded from the coronary sinus (CS). This interval is prolonged following ablation of the pathway. Surface leads I, V1, and intracardiac electrograms from CS and mapping catheter (Map) are shown.

of Fallot's tetralogy). Ventricular tachycardia may degenerate into ventricular fibrillation. Sustained monomorphic tachycardia can occur as a proarrhythmic response to antiarrhythmic drugs, particularly class I agents.

Although ventricular tachycardia normally occurs in individuals with overt heart disease, it is also seen in young and apparently healthy subjects. In these, occult cardiac disease or cardiac genetic

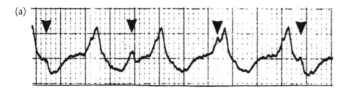

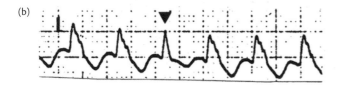

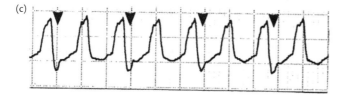

Fig. 4.2.38 Sustained monomorphic ventricular tachycardia. (a) Ventricular tachycardia with atrioventricular dissociation. P-waves (arrowed) are seen to have no relationship to the ventricular activation. Lead V1. (b) Ventricular tachycardia with fusion beat (arrow). Lead V1. (c) Ventricular tachycardia with 2:1 ventriculoatrial conduction. Lead III. P-waves (arrows) follow every second ventricular complex.

syndromes should be considered (see 'Genetic syndromes'). There remain a few patients with documented ventricular tachycardia in whom no structural heart disease is evident on clinical, ECG, or echocardiographic examination. The tachycardia may arise from the outflow tract of the right or left ventricle, or from one of the fascicles of the left bundle branch, and is amenable to radiofrequency ablation.

Acute management of ventricular tachycardia

Rapid ventricular tachycardia may present with cardiac arrest, syncope, shock, anginal chest pain, or left ventricular failure, but slower tachycardias in patients with preserved cardiac function may be well tolerated. Sustained ventricular tachycardia is a medical emergency. If the patient is pulseless or unconscious, immediate DC cardioversion is necessary. If the patient is conscious but hypotensive, urgent DC cardioversion under general anaesthesia or deep sedation is used. Haemodynamically tolerated tachycardias may be terminated by drug therapy (see Fig. 4.2.17). Adenosine may be administered in the presence of haemodynamic stability to exclude the differential diagnoses of SVT with aberrancy or antidromic AVRT, but is likely to be ineffective in terminating VT (see Table 4.2.6). Amiodarone 300 mg over 20 min (ideally via a central vein) followed by 900 mg/24 h may be effective in restoring sinus rhythm. Intravenous lidocaine (lignocaine) 100 mg, repeated if necessary after 5 min, can be used in refractory cases. Sotalol 1.5 mg/kg intravenously is more effective, but its use is restricted by its negative inotropic action. Second-line drugs for the termination of ventricular tachycardia include procainamide and disopyramide. Flecainide is contraindicated in view of the risk of developing incessant tachycardia. Verapamil should be avoided as it may cause clinical deterioration. The only exception to this is in the rare instance of patients with structurally normal hearts who have ventricular tachycardia that is known to respond to verapamil, e.g. LV fascicular tachycardia. All antiarrhythmic drugs have significant negative inotropic actions that may further impair the haemodynamic status of the patient if sinus rhythm is not restored. For this reason, no more than one antiarrhythmic drug should normally be given before recourse to alternative therapy, usually DC cardioversion. Overdrive termination of ventricular tachycardia following insertion of a temporary pacing lead may be effective, particularly if the tachycardia is relatively slow. Facilities for cardioversion must be available in view of the risk of acceleration or degeneration into ventricular fibrillation.

Secondary prevention

Ventricular tachycardia is a potentially life-threatening condition. Unless the acute episode was clearly precipitated by some transient or reversible factor, there is a high probability of recurrent attacks, which may result in sudden death. Prognosis is worse if the arrhythmia was poorly tolerated, or if there is severe left ventricular dysfunction.

Clinical evaluation of the patient after restoration of sinus rhythm should be supported by ECG, echocardiography, and/or radionuclide ventriculography. Coronary angiography should be considered to identify the presence of significant coronary artery disease, which may act as a trigger to ventricular tachycardia. Unless there is a clear precipitating factor such as drug toxicity, electrolyte abnormality, or acute ischaemia, the risk of sudden death is high and patients should be considered for a secondary prevention ICD (see

Fig. 4.2.20). A meta-analysis of three secondary prevention trials of patients resuscitated from ventricular fibrillation or ventricular tachycardia causing haemodynamic compromise showed defibrillators to be better than antiarrhythmic drug therapy in preventing death from any cause (Fig. 4.2.39a).

Primary prevention

Patients with left ventricular dysfunction of any cause are at risk of sudden death from ventricular tachycardia or fibrillation and implantable defibrillators are appropriate for a subgroup of these patients as part of a primary prevention strategy. Those with nonsustained ventricular tachycardia, in whom sustained tachycardia can be induced at electrophysiological testing, have a better survival with defibrillator implantation compared with drug therapy. The Sudden Cardiac Death in Heart Failure Trial (SCD-HeFT) expanded the indications to include patients with class II/III heart failure and an ejection fraction less than 30%, even in the absence of known arrhythmia (Fig. 4.2.39b). Patients with QRS duration greater than 120 ms appear to derive the largest benefit.

Antiarrhythmic therapy

Implantable defibrillator therapy is not affordable in all countries, and not appropriate for patients with New York Heart Association (NYHA) class IV heart failure or other conditions causing a severely limited prognosis. Medical therapy is necessary for many patients, but is limited by a relative lack of evidence from randomized controlled trials. β-Adrenoceptor blockers are comparable

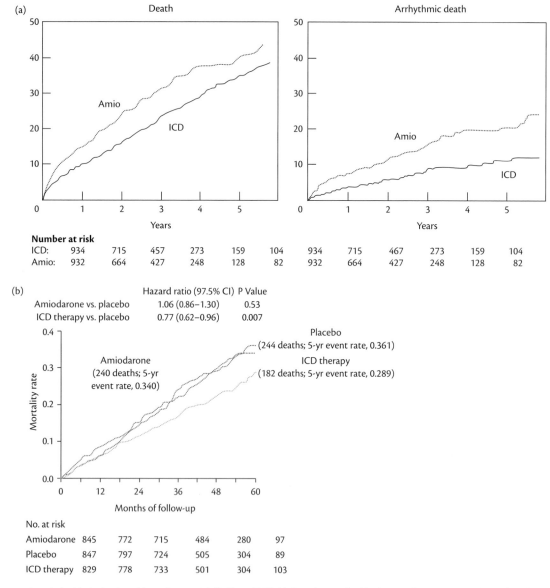

Fig. 4.2.39 Improved survival with the implantable cardioverter–defibrillator (ICD). (a) Cumulative risk of fatal events for ICD or amiodarone (amio) from a meta-analysis of trials of secondary prevention, showing reduced death with ICD (left panel), due to reduced arrhythmic death (right panel). (b) Improved survival with ICD compared to amiodarone or placebo in a study of primary prevention in patients with heart failure.

(a) Reproduced with permission from Connolly SJ, *et al.* (2007), *Eur Heart J*, **28**, 1598–660; (b) Bardy GH, *et al.* (2005), *New Engl J Med*, **352**, 230. Copyright ©2005 Massachusetts Medical Society. All rights reserved.

to conventional antiarrhythmic agents in the prevention of recurrent ventricular tachyarrhythmias. Since they have been shown to reduce the risk of sudden death in unselected survivors of myocardial infarction and in patients with chronic heart failure, they should be used routinely in the prophylaxis of ventricular tachycardia if tolerated. Amiodarone did not improve mortality compared to placebo in the SCD-HeFT trial. The class I antiarrhythmics should not be used for this indication as they were associated with a higher rate of arrhythmic deaths in the Cardiac Arrhythmia Suppression Trial.

Other therapies

Radiofrequency ablation is used in the management of ventricular tachycardia, particularly in those with no structural heart disease. Right or left ventricular outflow tract tachycardia and fascicular tachycardia are particularly amenable to ablation. Radiofrequency ablation of critical areas of slow conduction in scar-related ventricular tachycardias is now frequently undertaken but success rates are lower than for other types of ablation and this approach is often reserved for the treatment of recurrent tachycardia in patients with implantable defibrillators.

Direct surgical management of recurrent ventricular tachycardia involves aneurysmectomy, endocardial mapping, and resection of the area containing the micro re-entry circuit. The indications for surgery have been reduced considerably since the advent of the ICD and the emergence of catheter ablation, since the surgical mortality is up to 10 to 15%. Where medically intractable ventricular tachyarrhythmias are associated with very poor left ventricular function, cardiac transplantation should be considered if catheter ablation fails.

Nonsustained ventricular tachycardia

The mechanism and causes of nonsustained ventricular tachycardia (Fig. 4.2.40) are similar to those of sustained ventricular tachycardia. There is often slight variation in the R-R interval, particularly if the salvo involves only a few beats. Short salvos of nonsustained ventricular tachycardia are often asymptomatic. Apart from the instances where nonsustained ventricular tachycardia produces troublesome symptoms, the major clinical significance of the arrhythmia is as a risk marker for sustained ventricular tachycardia or sudden cardiac death in patients with left ventricular dysfunction or hypertrophy. Patients with structural heart disease, in particular those with severe left ventricular dysfunction, with QRS duration greater than 120 ms or heart muscle disease, should be considered for an implantable defibrillator as primary prevention of sudden cardiac death. If no structural heart disease or ion channel disease is present, and the patient is asymptomatic, no treatment is indicated as long-term follow-up of such patients indicates a good prognosis with no excess risk of sudden death.

Polymorphic ventricular tachycardia

Polymorphic ventricular tachycardia is an unstable rhythm with varying QRS morphology. It is most commonly seen in the acute phase of myocardial infarction. It either undergoes spontaneous termination or degenerates into ventricular fibrillation. If episodes of polymorphic ventricular tachycardia are frequent in the early hours of myocardial infarction, they can be suppressed by β-blockade.

Torsades de pointes and the long-QT syndromes

Torsades de pointes is a characteristic type of polymorphic ventricular tachycardia with a typical undulating variation in QRS morphology as a result of variation in axis. It occurs in association with a prolonged QT interval during sinus rhythm. Long-QT syndromes may be acquired or congenital; the latter are discussed later in the chapter.

Aetiology

Although class Ia and III antiarrhythmic drugs are the best-known causes of acquired long-QT syndrome, a very large number of noncardiac drugs inhibit the outward potassium current I_{Kr}, and may cause significant lengthening of the QT interval either singly or in combination (Table 4.2.12). Episodes of torsades de pointes are often multifactorial in origin, with prolongation of the QT interval by an I_{Kr} inhibitor in association with predisposing factors such as bradycardia or pauses, hypokalaemia, or hypomagnesaemia. All of these predispose to early after-depolarizations *in vitro* and this mechanism appears to be the likely cause of torsades de pointes in the acquired syndromes. The prognosis of the acquired long-QT syndromes is excellent, provided the underlying predisposing factors are identified and corrected. However, it is increasingly recognized that there is a genetic predisposition to the development of acquired long-QT syndrome in the face of predisposing factors, leading to the concept that patients developing acquired long-QT syndrome have reduced 'repolarization reserve' as a result of a *forme fruste* of the congenital syndrome.

ECG characteristics

Torsades de pointes is an atypical ventricular tachycardia characterized by a continuously varying QRS axis ('twisting of points') (Fig. 4.2.41). Episodes of torsades are commonly repetitive and normally self-terminating, although they may degenerate into ventricular fibrillation. Paroxysms of torsades de pointes are associated in the preceding beats with evidence of marked QT prolongation, and frequently with morphological abnormalities of the T-wave such as T-U fusion, gross increases in T-wave amplitude, or T-wave alternans. In the acquired long-QT syndromes a slowing of the heart rate, and in particular a postextrasystolic pause, is often

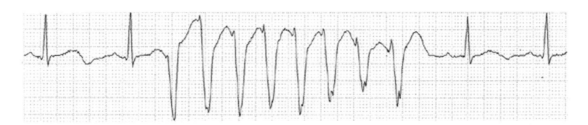

Fig. 4.2.40 Nonsustained ventricular tachycardia.

Table 4.2.12 Causes or contributory factors in acquired long-QT syndromes

Drug induced	Antiarrhythmic drugs—classes Ia, III
	Macrolide antibiotics—erythromycin
	Antifungals—ketoconazole
	Psychotropics—tricyclic/tetracyclic antidepressants, antipsychotics
	Antihistamines—terfenadine, astemizole
	Antiemetics—domperidone, ondansetron
	Synthetic opioid—methadone
Electrolyte disturbances	Hypokalaemia, hypomagnesaemia, hypocalcaemia
Metabolic	Hypothyroidism, starvation, anorexia nervosa, liquid protein diet
Bradycardia	Sinoatrial disease, AV block
Toxins	Organophosphorus insecticides, heavy metal poisoning

associated with initiation of the arrhythmia. This produces a characteristic 'short–long–short' sequence of initiation (Fig. 4.2.41).

Acute management

The common clinical presentation is of recurrent dizziness or syncope, and the condition may easily be misdiagnosed as self-terminating polymorphic ventricular tachycardia or ventricular fibrillation unless the characteristic morphology of torsades de pointes and the associated QT interval prolongation is recognized. It is essential to discontinue predisposing drugs or other agents and to avoid empirical antiarrhythmic drug therapy, which may worsen the arrhythmia. Individual paroxysms of torsades de pointes are normally self-limiting, but if they are persistent, cardiac arrest will occur and emergency defibrillation is necessary. Intravenous magnesium sulfate (8 mmol over 10–15 min, repeated if necessary) is a safe and effective emergency measure for the prevention of recurrent paroxysms of tachycardia. If torsades de pointes is associated with bradycardia and pauses, the heart rate should be increased to between 90 and 100/min by atrial or ventricular pacing or isoproterenol (isoprenaline) infusion. Hypokalaemia and hypomagnesaemia should be sought and corrected if necessary.

Accelerated idioventricular rhythm

The term 'accelerated idioventricular rhythm' is used to describe a continuous ventricular rhythm with a rate less than 120/min. Idioventricular rhythm commonly occurs in the setting of acute myocardial infarction and appears to be a marker of successful reperfusion therapy. No active treatment is necessary.

Ventricular fibrillation

Ventricular fibrillation is defined as a chaotic, disorganized arrhythmia with no identifiable QRS complexes (Fig. 4.2.42). The mechanism is of multiple, unstable re-entry circuits. The electrocardiographic pattern depends on the duration of fibrillation: recent-onset fibrillation is described as 'coarse', with a peak-to-peak amplitude of around 1 mV (1 cm). With increasing duration of cardiac arrest, the amplitude of ventricular fibrillation diminishes and such 'fine' ventricular fibrillation is less likely to be amenable to successful electrical defibrillation.

Ventricular fibrillation may occur during acute myocardial ischaemia often initiated by an R on T extrasystole, and is the principal cause of death in the first 2 h following acute myocardial infarction (Fig. 4.2.42). Ventricular fibrillation during myocardial infarction is subdivided into primary, occurring without warning in an otherwise stable patient, and secondary, where fibrillation occurs in the context of left ventricular failure or cardiogenic shock. Ventricular fibrillation occurring in chronic heart disease is most commonly a result of degeneration of rapid ventricular tachycardia,

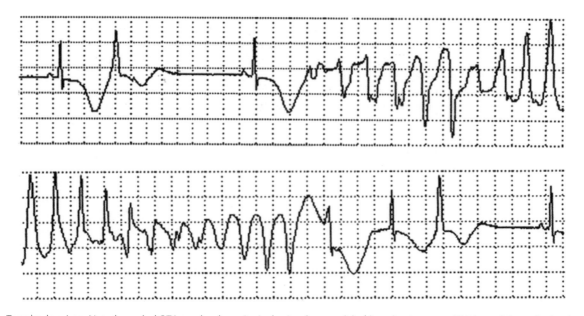

Fig. 4.2.41 Torsades de pointes. Note the marked QT interval prolongation in the sinus beats, and the 'short–long' pattern of R-R intervals immediately prior to initiation of the arrhythmia. Ambulatory monitoring recording is shown (continuous tracing).

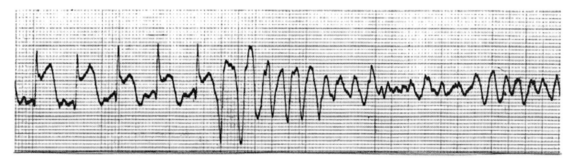

Fig. 4.2.42 Ventricular fibrillation complicating acute myocardial infarction. The arrhythmia is initiated by an 'R on T' ventricular extrasystole.

whose causes have been described above. Rarer causes of fibrillation are listed in Box 4.2.4.

Ventricular fibrillation is rarely self-terminating, and normally causes cardiac arrest with the rapid onset of pulselessness, unconsciousness, and apnoea. The management of cardiac arrest due to ventricular fibrillation is discussed in Chapter 4.2.

Patients who survive an episode of ventricular fibrillation should be assessed carefully to determine the risk of recurrence. If ventricular fibrillation has occurred in the first few hours of a typical ST-elevation myocardial infarction, the risk of recurrent cardiac arrest is low, and no specific prophylactic therapy other than assessment and treatment of residual ischaemia and conventional postinfarction β-blockade is indicated. However, in many instances ventricular fibrillation arises as a result of acute ischaemia in patients with known, extensive heart disease who have not sustained an acute infarction. These patients remain at high risk of recurrent ventricular fibrillation, and should be evaluated fully by exercise testing and coronary arteriography with a view to revascularization, and managed with an ICD or antiarrhythmic therapy as discussed in the section on ventricular tachycardia.

Genetic syndromes

Ion channel diseases

Congenital long-QT syndromes

The congenital long-QT syndromes (LQTS) are inherited conditions due to mutations in genes encoding ion channel proteins.

Box 4.2.4 Causes of ventricular fibrillation

- Acute myocardial ischaemia
- Acute myocardial infarction—primary or secondary
- Advanced organic heart disease with poor LV or RV function
- Severe LV hypertrophy
- Ventricular tachycardia/torsades de pointes
- Electrical—electrocution, lightning, unsynchronized DC shock, competitive ventricular pacing
- Pre-excited atrial fibrillation
- Profound bradycardia
- Hypoxia, acidosis
- Genetic syndromes (e.g. long-QT syndrome, Brugada syndrome)

They are mainly autosomal dominant and are subclassified according to the underlying gene defect (Table 4.2.13). Most cases are either LQT1 or LQT2, due to mutations affecting either the slow (I_{Ks}) or rapid (I_{Kr}) components of the outward potassium current. In the less common LQT3, the inward sodium current (I_{Na}) is affected. Lengthening of ventricular repolarization, and hence of the QT interval, occur as a result either of reduced outward current flow via I_{Kr} or I_{Ks} or increased duration of current flow via I_{Na}. The arrhythmia, torsades de pointes, has characteristics consistent with triggered activity.

Attacks of torsades de pointes in the congenital syndromes are commonly associated with sympathetic stimulation such as exercise, waking, or fright, and are associated with increases in sinus rate. Cardiac events are particularly associated with exercise in LQT1, with auditory stimulation in LQT2, and can occur during sleep in LQT3. Paroxysms may produce syncope, which if prolonged may be complicated by convulsion, leading to misdiagnosis as epilepsy. A family history of recurrent syncope or sudden death may be obtained. Sinus bradycardia is commonly seen in these syndromes.

The diagnosis of long-QT syndrome can be challenging and is not based on the ECG characteristics alone. The finding of a long QT interval on an ECG in patients with a history of syncope or palpitations or a routine ECG in asymptomatic patients can cause considerable anxiety among clinicians. The probability of LQTS can be assessed using the Schwartz score (Table 4.2.14).

The prognosis of untreated congenital long-QT syndrome is poor, with a high incidence of sudden death in childhood. Factors associated with high risk include personal history of aborted sudden cardiac death or syncope and corrected QT interval greater than 500 ms.

Males with LQT3 are at increased risk regardless of the degree of QT interval prolongation. LQT1 has a better prognosis than other subtypes. Episodes of torsades de pointes and T-wave alternans on Holter monitoring also confer a higher risk.

β-Blockers are highly effective in LQT1 but are less protective in LQT2 and LQT3. Selective high left stellate ganglionectomy (cervical sympathectomy) has been employed successfully in cases with recurrent events despite β-blockers. Permanent pacing at rates of 70 to 80/min, in combination with β-blockers, may also be effective in reducing symptoms but defibrillator implantation is necessary for resistant cases, and is commonly used as first-line therapy if episodes of torsades de pointes have resulted in cardiac arrest or in those thought to be at high risk of sudden death.

Short-QT syndrome

This is a recently described entity with autosomal dominant inheritance characterized by a gain of function mutation in the outward

Table 4.2.13 Congenital long-QT syndromes

Subtype	Chromosome	Gene	Protein	Ion current affected	Frequency
LQT1	11	KCNQ1	KvLQT1	$\downarrow I_{Ks}$	c.50%
LQT2	7	KCNH2	HERG	$\downarrow I_{Kr}$	30–40%
LQT3	3	SCN5A	Nav 1.5	$\uparrow I_{Na}$	5–10%
LQT4	4	ANKB	Ankyrin-B	$\downarrow$ Multiple	Rare
LQT5	21	KCNE1	minK	$\downarrow I_{Ks}$	Rare
LQT6	21	KCNE2	MiRP1	$\downarrow I_{Kr}$	Rare
LQT7	17	KCNJ2	Kir2.1	$\downarrow I_{K1}$	Rare
LQT8	12	CACNA1C	Cav1.2	$\uparrow I_{CaL}$	Rare
LQT9	3	CAV3	Caveolin 3	$\uparrow I_{Na}$	Rare
LQT10	11	SCN4B	Sodium channel β4	$\uparrow I_{Na}$	Rare
LQT11	7	AKAP9	Yotiao	$\downarrow I_{Ks}$	Rare
LQT12	20	SNTA1	Syntrophin α1	$\uparrow I_{Na}$	Rare
LQT13	11	KCNJ5	Kir3.4	$\downarrow I_{Kr}$	Rare

Table 4.2.14 Schwartz score for the diagnosis of long-QT syndrome

	Clinic features		Points
	ECG findings[a]		
A	QTc[b]	≥480 ms	3
		460–479 ms	2
		450–459 ms (male)	1
B	QTc[b] 4th minute of recovery from exercise stress test ≥480 ms		1
C	Torsade de pointes[c]		2
D	T-wave alternans		1
E	Notched T-wave in three leads		1
F	Low heart rate for age[d]		0.5
	Clinical history		
A	Syncope[c]	With stress	2
		Without stress	1
B	Congenital deafness		0.5
	Family history		
A	Family members with definite LQTS[e]		1
B	Unexplained sudden cardiac death <age 30 among immediate family members[e]		0.5
	Score		
	≤1 point: low probability of LQTS		
	1.5–3 points: intermediate probability of LQTS		
	≥3.5 points: high probability of LQTS		

[a] In the absence of medications or disorders known to affect these ECG features.

[b] QTc calculated using Bazett's formula where QTc = QT/√RR.

[c] Mutually exclusive.

[d] Resting heart rate below the 2nd percentile for age.

[e] The same family member cannot be counted in A and B.

Source: Schwartz PJ et al. (1993). Diagnostic criteria for the long-QT syndrome—an update. *Circulation*, **88**, 782–4.

potassium currents (I_{Kr} and I_{Ks}). It produces a markedly shortened QTc, often less than 280 ms, and predisposes to atrial and ventricular fibrillation.

Brugada syndrome

The Brugada syndrome is an autosomal dominant condition which has a risk of sudden cardiac death associated with characteristic ECG abnormalities and a structurally normal heart. There is an unusual pattern of coved ST-segment elevation of at least 2 mm in two of the right precordial leads (Fig. 4.2.43). Mutations of genes encoding the voltage-gated sodium channel (*SCN5A*), causing partial inactivation, have been identified in about 20% of patients. Patients with a history of syncope and spontaneous ECG features should be considered for defibrillator therapy.

Catecholaminergic polymorphic ventricular tachycardia (CPVT)

This is a rare arrhythmia characterized by polymorphic or bidirectional ventricular tachycardia occurring in situations of strenuous exercise, psychological stress, or emotion, often presenting in childhood. It is associated with mutations of genes involved in controlling intracellular calcium handling. Mutations of the cardiac ryanodine receptor have autosomal dominant transmission, whereas mutations of the gene encoding for calsequestrin have autosomal recessive transmission. The resting ECG has no diagnostic features and the heart is structurally normal. β-Blockers may prevent syncope but an ICD may be indicated for recurrent symptoms or high risk of cardiac arrest.

Heart muscle diseases

Hypertrophic cardiomyopathy

Hypertrophic cardiomyopathy has a prevalence of 0.2% in the population, and is associated with a wide range of mutations encoding structural or regulatory proteins of the cardiac myofibrillar apparatus. The mode of inheritance is autosomal dominant in 70%

of cases, with variable penetrance. Although symptoms are often related to impaired haemodynamics, LV hypertrophy and myofibre disarray increase the risk of re-entrant arrhythmias and sudden death. Patients with sustained ventricular tachycardia or fibrillation should be considered for defibrillator therapy. Risk assessment should be performed in all patients with hypertrophic cardiomyopathy. Unexplained syncope, nonsustained ventricular tachycardia, ventricular septal thickness greater than 30 mm, a family history of sudden cardiac death, and a hypotensive response to exercise are all associated with increased risk. An ICD may be considered if one or more high-risk features are present. See Chapter 7.2 for further discussion.

Arrhythmogenic right ventricular cardiomyopathy

Arrhythmogenic right ventricular cardiomyopathy (dysplasia) is an autosomal dominant condition associated with replacement of the right ventricular free wall with fat and fibrous tissue. These patients may have no symptoms or signs of cardiac disease, but typical ECG changes (epsilon wave in V1, or T-wave inversion in the right precordial leads) are associated with variable degrees of dilatation of the right ventricle demonstrable by echocardiography or MRI. This creates a substrate for heart failure or arrhythmia (ventricular tachycardia and fibrillation) and many patients will ultimately require defibrillator therapy.

Dilated cardiomyopathy

This is often used as an umbrella term for cardiomyopathy of nonischaemic aetiology. In some cases, there is an inheritable cause which predisposes to arrhythmia, such as the Lamin A/C, SCN5A, or Titin mutations.

Genetic testing

A strong clinical index of suspicion may warrant targeted genetic testing for certain conditions (e.g. LQTS, CPVT). In many inherited cardiac conditions, genetic testing may be indicated for family

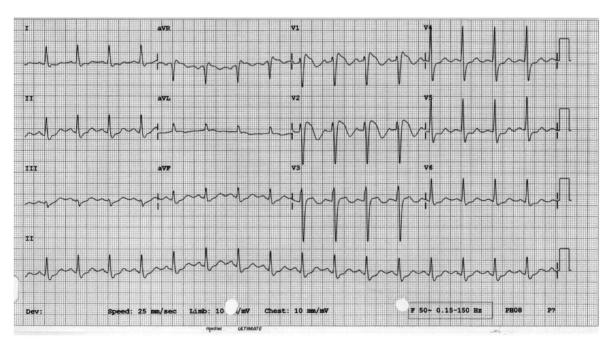

Fig. 4.2.43 Brugada ECG.

members and appropriate relatives once the causative mutation has been diagnosed in the index case.

Further reading

Diagnosis and treatment

Echt DS, *et al.* (1991). Mortality and morbidity in patients receiving encainide, flecainide, or placebo. *N Engl J Med*, **324**, 781–8.

Eckardt L, *et al.* (2006). Approach to wide complex tachycardias in patients without structural heart disease. *Heart*, **92**, 704–11.

Fitzpatrick AP, *et al.* (1994). New algorithm for the localization of accessory atrioventricular connections using a baseline electrocardiogram. *J Am Coll Cardiol*, **23**, 107–16.

Hall MC, Todd DM (2006). Modern management of arrhythmias. *Postgrad Med J*, **82**, 117–25.

Morady F. (1999). Radio-frequency ablation as treatment for cardiac arrhythmia. *N Engl J Med*, **340**, 534–44.

Roden DM. (2000). Antiarrhythmic drugs: from mechanisms to clinical practice. *Heart*, **84**, 339–46.

Bradycardia

Brignole M, *et al.* (2013). ESC guidelines on cardiac pacing and cardiac resynchronization therapy. *Eur Heart J*, **34**, 2281–329.

Fitzpatrick A, Sutton R. (1992). A guide to temporary pacing. *BMJ*, **304**, 365–9.

Gammage MD. (2000). Temporary cardiac pacing. *Heart*, **83**, 715–20.

Healey JS, *et al.* (2006). Cardiovascular outcomes with atrial-based pacing compared with ventricular pacing: meta-analysis of randomized trials, using individual patient data. *Circulation*, **114**, 11–17.

Morley-Davies A, Cobbe SM (1997). Cardiac pacing. *Lancet*, **349**, 41–6.

Atrial arrhythmias

Apostolakis S, *et al.* (2013). Factors affecting quality of anticoagulation control among patients with atrial fibrillation on warfarin: the SAMe-TT2R2 score. *Chest*, **144**, 1555–63.

Banerjee A, *et al.* (2012). Net clinical benefit of new oral anticoagulants (dabigatran, rivaroxaban, and apixaban) versus no treatment in a 'real world' atrial fibrillation population: a modelling analysis based on a nationwide cohort study. *Thromb Haemost*, **107**, 584–9.

Calkins H, *et al.* (2012). HRS/EHRA/ECAS Expert Consensus Statement on Catheter and Surgical Ablation of Atrial Fibrillation: Recommendations for patient selection, procedural techniques, patient management and follow-up, definitions, endpoints, and research trial design. *Europace*, **14**, 528–606.

Camm AJ, *et al.* (2010). Guidelines for the management of atrial fibrillation. Europace, **31**, 2369–2429.

Camm AJ, *et al.* ESC Committee for Practice Guidelines (CPG) (2012). 2012 focused update of the ESC Guidelines for the management of atrial fibrillation: an update of the 2010 ESC Guidelines for the management of atrial fibrillation. *Eur Heart J*, **33**, 2719–47.

Clarkesmith DE, *et al.* (2013). Educational intervention improves anticoagulation control in atrial fibrillation patients: the TREAT randomised trial. *PLoS One*, **8**, e74037.

Cowan C, *et al.* (2013). The use of anticoagulants in the management of atrial fibrillation among general practices in England. *Heart*, **99**, 1166–72.

Haïssaguerre M, *et al.* (1998). Spontaneous initiation of atrial fibrillation by ectopic beats originating in the pulmonary veins. *N Engl J Med*, **339**, 659–66.

Healey JS, *et al.* (2012). Subclinical atrial fibrillation and the risk of stroke. *N Engl J Med*, **366**, 120–9.

Heidbuchel H, *et al.* (2015). Updated European Heart Rhythm Association Practical Guide on the use of non-vitamin K antagonist anticoagulants in patients with non-valvular atrial fibrillation. *Europace*, **17**(10):1467–507. doi: 10.1093/europace/euv309.

Kakkar AK, *et al.* GARFIELD Registry Investigators (2013). Risk profiles and antithrombotic treatment of patients newly diagnosed with atrial fibrillation at risk of stroke: perspectives from the international, observational, prospective GARFIELD registry. *PLoS One*, **8**, e63479.

Lip GYH, Lane DA (2015). Stroke prevention in atrial fibrillation: a systematic review. *JAMA*, **313**(19):1950–62. doi: 10.1001/jama.2015.4369. Review. Erratum in: *JAMA*. 2015 Aug.

Lip GYH, *et al.* (2012). Atrial fibrillation. *Lancet*, **379**, 648–61.

Mant J, *et al.* BAFTA investigators; Midland Research Practices Network (MidReC) (2007). Warfarin versus aspirin for stroke prevention in an elderly community population with atrial fibrillation (the Birmingham Atrial Fibrillation Treatment of the Aged Study, BAFTA): a randomised controlled trial. *Lancet*, **370**, 493–503.

National Clinical Guideline Centre (2014). *Atrial fibrillation: The management of atrial fibrillation*. National Institute for Health and Care Excellence. Draft for consultation.

Olesen JB, *et al.* (2012). The value of the CHA2DS2-VASc score for refining stroke risk stratification in patients with atrial fibrillation with a CHADS2 score 0-1: A nationwide cohort study. *Thromb Haemost*, **107**, 1172–9.

Pisters R, *et al.* (2010). A novel user-friendly score (HAS-BLED) to assess 1-year risk of major bleeding in patients with atrial fibrillation: the Euro Heart Survey. *Chest*, **138**, 1093–100.

Steger C, *et al.* (2004). Stroke patients with atrial fibrillation have a worse prognosis than patients without: data from the Austrian Stroke registry. *Eur Heart J*, 25, 1734–40.

Wijffels MCEF, *et al.* (1995). Atrial fibrillation begets atrial fibrillation: a study in awake chronically instrumented goats. *Circulation*, **92**, 1954–68.

Wolf PA, *et al.* (1991). Atrial fibrillation as an independent risk factor for stroke: the Framingham Study. *Stroke*, **22**, 983–8.

Wyse DG, *et al.* (2002). A comparison of rate control and rhythm control in patients with atrial fibrillation. *N Engl J Med*, **347**, 1825–33.

Supraventricular tachycardias

Blomstrom-Lundquist C, *et al.* (2003). ACC/AHA/ESC guidelines for the management of patients with supraventricular arrhythmias—executive summary: a report of the American College of Cardiology/American Heart Association Task Force on Practice Guidelines and the European Society of Cardiology Committee for Practice Guidelines. *Circulation*, **108**, 1871–909.

Calkins H. (2001). Radiofrequency catheter ablation of supraventricular arrhythmias. *Heart*, **85**, 594–600. [Review of the role of catheter ablation in the management of patients with supraventricular tachycardia.]

Ventricular arrhythmias

Bardy GH, *et al.* (2005). Amiodarone or an implantable cardioverter-defibrillator for congestive heart failure. *N Engl J Med*, **352**, 225–37.

Connolly SJ, *et al.* (2000). Meta-analysis of the implantable cardioverter defibrillator secondary prevention trials. AVID, CASH and CIDS studies. Antiarrhythmics vs Implantable Defibrillator study. Cardiac Arrest Study Hamburg. Canadian Implantable Defibrillator Study. *Eur Heart J*, **21**, 2071–8.

Gupta A, *et al.* (2007). Current concepts in the mechanisms and management of drug-induced QT prolongation and torsade de pointes. *Am Heart J*, **153**, 891–9.

Moss AJ, *et al.* (2002). Prophylactic implantation of a defibrillator in patients with myocardial infarction and reduced ejection fraction. *N Engl J Med*, **346**, 877–83.

Schwartz PJ, *et al.* (1993). Diagnostic criteria for the long QT syndrome—an update. *Circulation*, **88**, 782–4.

Stevenson WG, *et al.* (1998). Radiofrequency catheter ablation of ventricular tachycardia after myocardial infarction. *Circulation*, **98**, 308–14.

Zipes DP, *et al.* (2006). ACC/AHA/ESC 2006 Guidelines for Management of Patients With Ventricular Arrhythmias and the Prevention of Sudden Cardiac Death: a report of the American College of Cardiology/American Heart Association Task Force and the European Society of Cardiology Committee for Practice Guidelines. *Circulation*, **114**, e385–484.

Genetic syndromes

Ackerman MJ, *et al.* (2011). HRS/EHRA expert consensus statement on the state of genetic testing for the channelopathies and cardiomyopathies. *Heart Rhythm*, **8**, 1308–39.

Brugada J, *et al.* (1998). Right bundle branch block and ST-segment elevation in leads V1 through V3: a marker for sudden death in patients without demonstrable structural heart disease. *Circulation*, **97**, 457–60.

Garratt C, *et al.* (2010). Heart Rhythm UK position statement on clinical indications for implantable cardioverter defibrillators in adult patients with familial sudden cardiac death syndromes. *Europace*, **12**, 1156–75.

Kies P, *et al.* (2006). Arrhythmogenic right ventricular dysplasia/cardiomyopathy: screening, diagnosis, and treatment. *Heart Rhythm*, **3**, 225–34.

Maron BJ, *et al.* (2003). American College of Cardiology/European Society of Cardiology clinical expert consensus document on hypertrophic cardiomyopathy. A report of the American College of Cardiology Foundation Task Force on Clinical Expert Consensus Documents and the European Society of Cardiology Committee for Practice Guidelines. *J Am Coll Cardiol*, **42**, 1687–713.

Roden D (2008). Long QT syndrome. *N Engl J Med*, **358**, 169–76.

Shah M, *et al.* (2005). Molecular basis of arrhythmias. *Circulation*, **112**, 2517–29.

Wilde AA, Bezzina CR (2003). Genetics of cardiac arrhythmias. *Heart*, **91**, 1352–8.

Wilde AA, *et al.* (2002). Proposed diagnostic criteria for the Brugada syndrome: consensus report. *Circulation*, **106**, 2514–19.

Cardiac failure

CHAPTER 5.1

Epidemiology and general pathophysiological classification of heart failure

Theresa A. McDonagh and Kaushik Guha

Essentials

Definition and classification

Heart failure is a clinical syndrome caused by cardiac dysfunction, most commonly left ventricular systolic dysfunction (LVSD). Patients with heart failure symptoms or signs and normal or near normal LV function are often classified as having heart failure with preserved ejection fraction (HF-PEF), but there is no clear and generally accepted definition of this condition.

Epidemiology

Estimates of incidence and prevalence are heavily influenced by definition. An echocardiographic study of a random sample of the general population aged 25–74 years in Glasgow (Scotland) estimated a prevalence of heart failure of 1.5%, with a further 1.4% having asymptomatic LVSD. Prevalence rises significantly with age, with a median age of first presentation in the mid seventies. Longitudinal data suggests that the incidence of heart failure has remained fairly stable over the last few decades, but prevalence is increasing as more people survive cardiovascular disease earlier in life.

Aetiology

Determining the aetiology of heart failure in epidemiological studies is difficult: the commonest cause in the developed world is coronary artery disease, followed by hypertension, which predominates in those with a diagnosis of HF-PEF.

Prognosis and morbidity

Data from the United States of America and the United Kingdom show the death rates of those admitted to hospital with a diagnosis of heart failure have a mortality of over 30% at one year. The outcome has improved in recent years, perhaps linked to the increased usage of angiotensin inhibitors and β-blockers. Heart failure accounts for around 5% of all adult general medical admissions, and in developed countries the condition consumes 1 to 2% of health care budgets.

Introduction

Over the last 30 years we have gone from famine to feast for heart failure epidemiological data. The first seminal publication on the natural history of heart failure was from the Framingham Heart Study in 1971, showing a prevalence of heart failure of 0.8% in those aged between 50 and 59 rising to 9.1% in those over 80 years with incidence rates of 0.2% at age 54 and 0.4% at age 85 (Fig. 5.1.1). This was followed by a large European study, 'The Men Born in 1913', which gave similar figures of a prevalence of 2.1% at age 50 and 13% at age 67 and incidence rates of 0.15% and 1% respectively at ages 50 and 67. These landmark studies relied on a clinical diagnosis of heart failure, based on symptoms, signs, and scoring systems to identify cases. More modern epidemiological studies have used definitions of heart failure which include objective measures of cardiac function in their definition, in keeping with the ever-changing definitions of heart failure as we have developed more insight into its pathophysiology and treatment. Initially studies focused on systolic

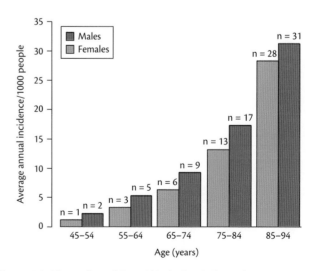

Fig. 5.1.1 Incidence of heart failure within the Framingham cohort.
The natural history of congestive heart failure: the Framingham study. *N Engl J Med*; 1971;**285**;26;1441–6. McKee PA, Castelli WP, McNamara PM & Kannel WB.

dysfunction as they reported at much the same time as the heart failure treatment trials which also enrolled patients with systolic heart failure. More recently attention has turned to describing the epidemiology of heart failure with preserved systolic function. This chapter outlines the contemporary epidemiology of heart failure by describing its prevalence, incidence, aetiology, mortality, and trends.

Current pathophysiological description of heart failure

Most clinical practice guidelines produced by the major international cardiology and heart failure societies have very similar definitions of heart failure. All agree that it is not a diagnosis, per se, but a clinical syndrome: a constellation of symptoms and signs that are ultimately due to cardiac dysfunction. That cardiac dysfunction can be epicardial, myocardial, or endocardial in origin. Most commonly heart failure is attributable to myocardial dysfunction. Of particular importance, due to its main causes being coronary artery disease and hypertension, is the occurrence of left ventricular systolic dysfunction (LVSD). This has added significance, as the main heart failure treatment trials which sealed the place of the neurohormonal antagonists in the therapeutics of heart failure were conducted in those with left ventricular ejection fractions (LVEF) which were less than 40%. Many epidemiology studies therefore focused on characterizing the incidence and prevalence of LVSD, using varying cut points of the normally distributed variable, LVEF, ranging from less than 30% to 50%. This difference in the cut points chosen affects the incidence and prevalence rates which are quoted (see Tables 5.1.1 and 5.1.2). Often studies have classified those with heart failure symptoms and signs with a normal or only mildly reduced left ventricular function to have heart failure with preserved ejection fraction (HF-PEF). In the absence of

Table 5.1.1 Prevalence of symptomatic and asymptomatic LVSD in populations with a calculated prevalence of manifest heart failure where applicable

Authors	Name of Study	Number of patients (no of cases of heart failure)	Location	Age Range	Percentage Symptomatic Left Ventricular Systolic Dysfunction (LVSD)	Percentage Asymptomatic Left Ventricular Systolic Dysfunction (ASLVD)	Prevalence of heart failure < 65 yrs of age	Prevalence of heart failure >65 yrs of age
Parameshwar J et al, 1992	Prevalence of heart failure in 3 GP practices	30,204 (117)	North-West London, UK	5–99	28% had echoes		0.6 per 1000	27.7 per 1000
Murphy NF et al, 2004	National survey of heart failure	307,741 (2186)	Scotland, UK	0–>85	—		7.1 per 1000 (though not <65)	>85–90.1 per 1000
Rutten FH et al, 2003	A questionnaire based survey of heart failure	(202)	Utrecht, Netherlands	40–95	53 % had echoes 97% -LVSD			
McDonagh TA et al, 1997	MONICA	1640 (43)	North Glasgow, UK	25–74	2.9% LVSD	1.4% ALVSD	15 per 1000	
Davies M et al, 2001	ECHOES	3960 (72)	West Midlands, UK		1.8% LVSD 3.5% Preserved EF	0.9% ALVSD	31 per 1000 (>45 yrs of age)	
Kupari M et al, 1997	Helsinki Ageing Study	501 (41)	Helsinki, Finland	75–86	4.1 % HEFPEF 3.9 % LVSD	9% ASLVD		(75–86) – 82 per 1000
Mosterd A et al, 1999	Rotterdam Heart Study	2267 (88)	Rotterdam, Netherlands	55–94	3.7% LSVD	1.4% ASLVD	Men 7 per 1000 (55–64) Women 6 per 1000 (55-64)	Men 37 per 1000 (65–74) 144 per 1000 (75–84) 59 per 1000 (85–94) Women 16 per 1000 (65–74) 121 per 1000 (75–84) 140 per 1000 (85-94)
Morgan S et al, 1999	Poole Heart Study	817 (61)	Poole, Dorset, UK	70–84	7.5 % LVSD	3.9 % ASLVD		

Table 5.1.2 Studies demonstrating incident rates of heart failure within different populations

Study	Name of study	Number of patients	Location	Age range	Mean/Median age of diagnosis	Incidence of heart failure < 65 yrs of age	Incidence of heart failure >65 yrs of age
McKee PA et al, 1971	Framingham		Framingham, US	45–94		2 per 1000 (45–54 years)	40 per 1000 (85–94 years)
Erikkson H et al, 1989	The men born in 1913	973	Gothenburg, Sweden	67			10 per 1000
Cowie MR et al, 1999	Hillingdon Heart Study	151,000	Hillingdon, North West London, UK	29–95	76 years	0.02 per 1000 (25–34 years) 0.2 per 1000 (35–44 years) 0.2 per 1000 (45–54 years) 1.2 per 1000 (55–64 years)	3 per 1000 (65–74 years) 7.4 per 1000 (75–84 years) 11.6 per 1000 (85–94 years)
Murphy NF et al, 2004	GP database, Continuous morbidity recording scheme	307,741 (2186 cases)	Scotland, UK	45–85	—	1.3 per 1000 (45–64 years)	6.1 per 1000 (65–74) 16 per 1000 (75–84 years)
De Giuli F et al, 2005	GP Research Database	696,884 (6478 cases)	United Kingdom	45–101	77 years	3.4 per 1000 (55–64 years)	25.5 per 1000 (75–84 years)
Kalogeropoulos A et al, 2009	ABC Study	2934 (258)	Pittsburgh, & Memphis, Tennesee US	70–79	73.6 years		13.6 per 1000
Bibbins-Domingo K et al	CARDIA Study	5115 (27)	Birmingham, Alabama, Chicago, Illinois, Minneapolis, Oakland, California, US	18–30	39.1 years	African American Male (Cumulative Incidence) -0.9% African American Female (Cumulative Incidence) -1.1% Caucasian Male (Cumulative Incidence)- 0% Cacuasain Female (Cumulative Incidence) −0.08%	—-

any convincingly positive drugs trials for this end of the spectrum of heart failure, no unifying definition of HF-PEF has emerged and been applied to community-based studies. The latest definitions of HF-PEF, in addition to symptoms and or signs of heart failure and a relatively preserved ejection fraction, also require evidence of structural heart disease (usually left ventricular hypertrophy, increased left atrial size/volume and Doppler or tissue Doppler evidence of diastolic dysfunction). Rigorous population-based studies with these more modern definitions have yet to appear.

Prevalence studies

Community-based studies

Many studies have been conducted in primary care or across geographical healthcare communities. One of the first was in northwest London where 30 204 case records were reviewed, yielding a crude prevalence of 3.8/100 cases in the general population with a marked rise from those under 65 to those above 65 years of age, where the rate rose from 0.6 per 1000 to 28.0 per 1000.

More recent data is available from the Scottish Continuous Morbidity scheme, which covers 57 general practices in Scotland and uses GP Read codes for heart failure in 307 741 patients. This results in a calculated prevalence of heart failure within the general population in Scotland of 7.1 per 1000, increasing to 90.1 per 1000 in the population above 85 years old. The population identified in the primary care setting were more elderly and had more comorbidities than in population-based studies or clinical trial populations. These findings have been corroborated in a European study based in Utrecht, Netherlands where patients with heart failure who were under the supervision of a cardiologist were more likely to be male, in their sixties, and have an ischaemic aetiology. When considering such data it should be remembered that the signs and symptoms of heart failure are neither sensitive nor specific. Studies evaluating referrals from primary care, when compared to expert cardiology assessment, have revealed only approximately 30% of patients actually have heart failure.

Population-based studies using echocardiography

Systolic dysfunction

The North Glasgow MONICA study was the first to report on the prevalence of left ventricular dysfunction (LVD) in a random sample of the general population of 2000 men and women aged 25–74 years. In this cohort 2.9% had significant systolic dysfunction, and of these just over half had symptoms of breathlessness or were taking a loop diuretic. The estimated prevalence of heart failure in this population was therefore 1.5% with 1.4% having the important precursor of heart failure, asymptomatic systolic dysfunction (ASLVD). The prevalence rose with age and was higher in men than in women (Fig. 5.1.2).

Many studies have reported since both in Europe and in the United States of America. Data from these cohorts is fairly consistent for the general population. Prevalence rates for LVSD were 1.8–3.5% in the ECHOES study from the English Midlands, with 50% of the left ventricular dysfunction being asymptomatic, and in the US Olmsted county study 2.2% had heart failure validated using the Framingham criteria and of these 56% had systolic dysfunction.

When we look at population-based studies which have included much older subjects the prevalence rates increase markedly. In the Helsinki Ageing Study of 501 subjects aged 75–86 years, clinical heart failure was found to be 8.2% overall, 2.3% had systolic dysfunction, and 9% had ASLVD. In the Rotterdam Study of 2267 men and women aged 55–95, 3.7% had fractional shortening of 25% or less (5.5% men and 2.2% women) and 2.2% had asymptomatic left ventricular dysfunction (Fig. 5.1.3). Similar findings were reported in a UK study of 817 subjects aged 70–84 years from Poole (southern England) which demonstrated that 7.5% had LVSD (12.2% of men and 2.9% of women) and 52% were undiagnosed.

Heart failure with preserved systolic function

Many of the population-based studies them have also by default or design been able to comment on the prevalence of HF-PEF. Hogg *et al.* reviewed the epidemiological data for HF-PEF and found that the prevalence ranged from 1.5% to 4.8% depending on the study. There was a definite increase in the proportion of heart failure due to this in cohorts which studied more elderly subjects. In the ECHOES study of the general population, 1.1% had definite heart failure and a LVEF greater than 50%, whereas in the Helsinki Ageing Study, 72% of all the heart failure identified occurred with a normal LVEF. In the United States of America, the Rochester Epidemiology Project in a random sample of 2042 subjects over 45 years of age reported similar findings with 44% of subjects having heart failure with a LVEF greater than 50%.

Even higher prevalence rates have been found in a recent large cross-sectional study from Portugal: 16.1% in the population above

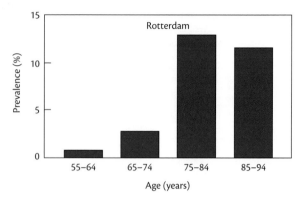

Fig. 5.1.3 Prevalence of left ventricular systolic dysfunction within the Rotterdam Study.
Mosterd A, Hoes AW, de Brunye MC, Deckers JW, Linker DT, Hofman A, Grobbee DE. Prevalence of heart failure and left ventricular dysfunction in the general population; the Rotterdam study. *Eur Heart J*;1999;**20**;6;447–455.

80 years old had heart failure. The prevalence was split roughly equally between preserved and reduced ejection fraction. These studies all confirm one thing, that heart failure is common and increases exponentially with age (Fig. 5.1.3). It is unsurprising, therefore, that heart failure affects 15 million Europeans and more than 5 million Americans.

Incidence

Contemporary studies of incidence are far fewer than those for prevalence. In the west London district of Hillingdon all incident cases of heart failure were identified via either a specialist referral clinic or emergency hospital admission (Fig. 5.1.4). The population served was 151 000, and 220 new cases were identified. Participants had a full clinical assessment, standard investigations including a chest radiograph, electrocardiogram, and echocardiography; 99% of the study population had an echocardiogram. The gold standard diagnosis was made by a panel of three cardiologists. The incidence rose from 0.02/1000 per year in the 25–34 age group to 11.6/1000 in those aged over 85. Most had LVSD. This study confirmed that heart failure is predominantly a disease of the elderly with a median age of first presentation of 76 years.

Incidence data for the United States of America are also reported from the Cardiovascular Health Study, showing a rate of 19.3/1000 person-years in 5.5 years of follow-up. In the United Kingdom data are also available for incidence from general practice from the General Practice Research Database (GPRD): 696 884 potential patients aged above 45 years old were identified. The records were interrogated and categorized on the basis of clinical data and medication prescription patterns. Using this approach, 6478 patients had definite heart failure, 14 050 possible heart failure and 6076 were treated with diuretics but a non-heart-failure diagnosis was assigned. The overall incidence of definite heart failure was 9.3/1000 per year but when possible heart failure was included the figure increased to 20.2/1000 per year. The mean age of the definite heart failure population was 77 years.

More recently data from the Scottish Continuous Morbidity Recording (CMR) data set showed an overall incidence of 2/1000 population per year; it was 25/1000 per year in men over the age of 85 years.

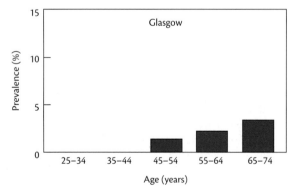

Fig. 5.1.2 Prevalence of left ventricular systolic dysfunction in the North Glasgow MONICA cohort.
Reprinted from *The Lancet*, **350**, McDonagh TA, Morrison CE, Lawrence A, Ford I, Tunstall-Pedoe H, McMurray JJ, Dargie HJ. Symptomatic and Asymptomatic left ventricular systolic dysfunction in an urban population. *Lancet*; 829–833; 1997, with permission from Elsevier.

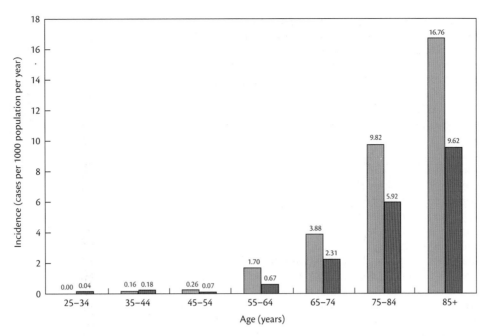

Fig. 5.1.4 Incidence of heart failure by sex and age group in Hillingdon Heart Failure Study.
Cowie MR, Wood DA, Coats AJC, Thompson SG, Poole-Wilson PA, Suresh V & Sutton GC. *Eur Heart J*;1999;**20**;421–428.

Trends in incidence and prevalence

Data from the Framingham Heart Study have not shown any increase in incidence since the 1970s, dispelling the theory that we are experiencing an epidemic of heart failure. Similarly, data from Medicare records show a slight reduction in incidence from 57.5/1000 to 48.4/1000 person-years in the 80–84 year age group in the period 1994–2003. However, despite the slight reduction in incidence, the prevalence rate rose markedly from 90/1000 to 120/1000. These trends will continue with the changing demography of most Western populations, with more elderly people and a greater number of survivors from cardiovascular disease earlier in life.

Aetiology

Determining the exact aetiology of patients with heart failure in epidemiological studies is difficult. The commonest cause within the Western world currently is coronary artery disease. This represents a change in aetiology over time. When the Framingham study first reported, the main factor was hypertension. Over time in this study the influence of coronary heart disease has increased by 40% in men and 20% in women.

In the North Glasgow MONICA study over 95% of patients with symptomatic LVSD had some evidence of prior ischaemic heart disease (IHD), although hypertension was also prevalent in this group, occurring in 68%. Other data from prevalence studies show similar results. In the ECHOES study, 53% of those with systolic dysfunction had evidence of IHD and 42% had hypertension, and in the Helsinki Ageing Study it was 54% for hypertension and for IHD. In the United States of America data from the Cardiovascular Health Study confirm similar results, with the population attributable risk for heart failure for coronary heart disease being 13.1% and for hypertension 12.8%. Both are clearly important aetiological factors.

In the original Hillingdon study of incident heart failure, 41% of the heart failure cohort was due to coronary artery disease and a much smaller number, 6%, had hypertension. A subsequent study carried out in Bromley (south London) looked into putative ischaemic aetiologies in more depth. All incident cases of heart failure were identified and referred to a specialist dedicated clinic or identified by tracking the patient during their hospitalization. Using the diagnostic criteria, 332 patients had been identified and 99 of the 136 cases under 75 years of age also underwent coronary angiography. An ischaemic aetiology was eventually attributed to 52% of the 136 cases.

Hypertension as a cause of heart failure still seems to predominate in those HF-PEF patients where ischaemic heart disease seems less prominent. These patients tend to be older and there is a higher proportion of women than men. Both diseases are still common: a recent study by Zile showed a prevalence rate of 82% for hypertension and 45% for coronary heart disease in patients with HF-PEF.

Comorbidities

Heart failure is predominantly a disease of elderly people and is therefore associated with multiple comorbidities, which include renal impairment, anaemia, diabetes mellitus, obstructive sleep apnoea, and chronic obstructive pulmonary disease. These all have an adverse impact on survival when associated with heart failure.

Anaemia was present in 51% of patients with heart failure in the Rochester Epidemiology Project. Severely impaired renal function was present in 10%. These rates are increased in patients presenting with acute heart failure syndromes: renal dysfunction occurred in 20% of those admitted with decompensated heart failure in the Euroheart Failure Survey II.

Prognosis

The 32-year follow-up of the Framingham study highlighted the substantial mortality rate of heart failure: 62% for men and 42% for women at 5 years of follow-up from incident diagnosis. However, data from the Framingham study have shown consistent improvements in survival over time for both men and women. In Europe, the mortality of incident heart failure also seems to be falling. In the initial Hillingdon study, 25% of patients were dead at 6 months, but in the more recent cohort of this study from 2004–5 this figure had dropped to 14%. This was independent of confounding variables and linked to the increased usage of angiotensin inhibitors and β-blockers.

Although mortality is higher in studies of incident heart failure, it is also poor in prevalent cases (Fig. 5.1.5). In the ECHOES study, the 5-year survival rate was 53% for those with heart failure due to systolic function. Survival for those with HF-PEF was a little better, at 62%. This is in contrast to the Mayo Clinic data which showed that survival in the community with heart failure was similar for those with systolic and nonsystolic heart failure. However, more recently the Mayo Clinic group reported on 4596 patients of whom 47% had preserved left ventricular function between 1987 and 2001. The survival rate was slightly better within the population with preserved systolic function. However, rates of mortality declined in the population with systolic dysfunction over the study period, whereas patients with normal ventricular function had no change in mortality rates throughout the study period.

The mortality rates for left ventricular dysfunction in the population are also high—21% dead at 4 years in the North Glasgow MONICA cohort—with no significant difference between those with symptoms of heart failure and those with ALVD. This underscores the need for early detection and treatment of this precursor phase of heart failure.

Data from hospitalized patients in Scotland also show a trend to towards improved survival (Fig. 5.1.6). Between 1986 and 2003 median survival after a first admission to hospital with heart failure

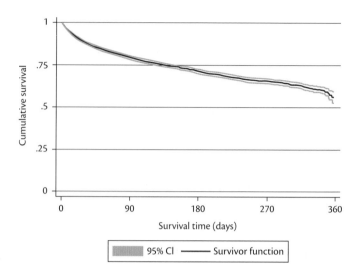

Fig. 5.1.5 Overall annual mortality from the Echocardiographic Heart of England Screening Study (ECHOES).

Hobbs FD, Roalfe AK, Davis RC, Davies MK et al. Prognosis of all-cause heart failure and borderline left ventricular systolic dysfunction: 5 year mortality follow-up of the Echocardiographic Heart of England Screening Study (ECHOES). *Eur Heart J*;2007;**28**;9;1128–1134.

improved in men from 1.3 to 2.3 years and in women from 1.3 to 1.8 years. Overall survival remains poor, with 50% of men dead at 2.3 years and 50% of women dead at 1.7 years after a first admission for heart failure.

This poorer survival between those with acute heart failure syndromes requiring admission, compared to population-based surveys of prevalence, is now well described. Data from large European and US registries show consistent findings. In the Euro

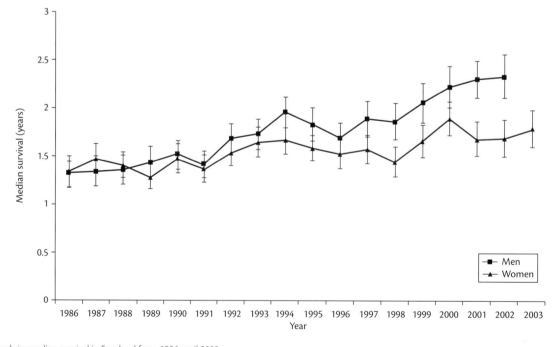

Fig. 5.1.6 Trends in median survival in Scotland from 1986 until 2003.

Jhund PS, McIntyre K, Simpson CR, Lewsey JD, Stewart S, Redpath A, Chalmers JT, Capewell S, McMurray JJV. Long term trends in first hospitalization for heart failure and subsequent survival between 1986 and 2003: A study of 5.1 million people. *Circulation*;2009;**119**;515–523.

Heart Failure II survey, in-hospital mortality was 6.6%. This varied with presentation but was nearly 40% in those presenting with cardiogenic shock. In-hospital mortality in the United States of America is better, running at 4% in the OPTIMISE heart failure registry.

However, the picture is probably bleaker when we look to data sources that try to capture consecutive admissions to hospital with heart failure. One of the world's largest single-country audits of acute hospital admissions has been running in the United Kingdom since 2008. Inpatient case fatality rates for those admitted to hospital with a primary diagnosis of heart failure are high; they were 11.1% in 2011/12 and fell slightly to 9.8% in 2012/13. Worryingly, US and UK data show concordant death rates of those admitted to hospital with heart failure of over 30% at 1 year.

Morbidity and hospitalizations

Part of the enormous morbidity incurred by heart failure patients relates to frequent hospitalizations. In advanced heart failure, patients who have been hospitalized experience rehospitalization rates at 6 months of 36–45%. In the 1990s studies in the Netherlands, Scotland, the United States of America, and Sweden documented increasing trends of admissions relating to heart failure. The rise in hospital admissions was accompanied with increasing expenditure. In Scotland, 0.2% of the population were hospitalized per annum and heart-failure-related admissions accounted for more than 5% of all adult general medical admissions. Some evidence has now emerged that heart failure admissions may have peaked in certain European countries during the mid-1990s. Data from Scotland on 116 556 patients identified from hospital discharge records during the period 1986–2003 showed that rates of admission rose and peaked in the mid-1990s and subsequently fell by 2003 (Fig. 5.1.6) This is also the case in the Netherlands (Fig. 5.1.7).

The most recent American data, however, initially seems to contradict this finding. Using the period between 1979 and 2004, heart failure admissions were recorded using the National Hospital Discharge Survey. The rate of admission tripled from 1 274 000 in 1979 to 3 860 000 in 2004. However, lengths of stay and mortality have reduced in the United States of America according to data from the ADHERE registry.

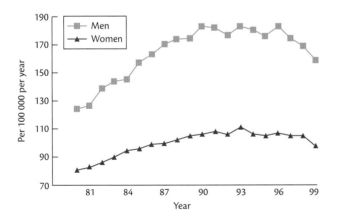

Fig. 5.1.7 Heart failure hospitalization rate in the Netherlands from 1980 to 1999. Reproduced from *Heart*, Mosterd A & Hoes AW. 2007;**93**;9;1137–1146 with permission from BMG Publishing Group.

Health economics

The high prevalence and frequent and recurrent hospitalizations place a large economic burden on healthcare budgets. In the United States of America, total expenditure on heart failure in 2007 was more than $33 billion (£21 billion, €24 billion). The statistics are mirrored in European settings. Within the United Kingdom heart failure consumes 1–2% of the National Health Service budget, which is approximately £1.2 billion (€1.3 billion, $1.8 million). It is the leading cause of hospitalization within the elderly population in the United Kingdom. Approximately 60% of the total expenditure on heart failure in the United Kingdom is spent on hospital admissions. Figures are similar in continental Europe, with heart failure consuming approximately 1% of healthcare budgets. The length of stay also contributes to the expense, with median stay in Europe of 9 days. These estimates of cost are likely to be underestimates as true costs should include all primary care consultations, secondary care referrals, diagnostics, prescribing habits, further therapies including devices and care networks, and surgical intervention including transplantation.

Conclusions

Despite the advances which have been made in its treatment over the course of the last 20 years, which have seen mortality rates for those in clinical trials of heart failure therapies fall to less than 10% per annum, epidemiological studies still indicate that heart failure remains a common, lethal, disabling, and expensive condition. This is hardly surprising as most of the reduction in mortality is due to advances in treatment for a subset of heart failure patients, those with chronic heart failure due to LVSD. We still have much to do. The increasing prevalence of heart failure, and the lack of advances to date for patients presenting acutely to hospital or those with HF-PEF, mean that heart failure still remains a 'malignant' condition.

Further reading

Cleland JG, *et al.* on behalf of the National Heart Failure Audit Team for England and Wales (2011). The national heart failure audit for England and Wales 2008–2009. *Heart*, **97**, 876–86.

Cowie MR, Wood DA, Coats AJC, *et al.* (1999). Incidence and aetiology of heart failure: a population-based study. *Eur Heart J*, **20**, 421–8.

Davies M, Hobbs F, Davis R, *et al.* (2001). Prevalence of left-ventricular systolic dysfunction and heart failure in the Echocardiographic Heart of England Screening study: a population based study. *Lancet*, **358**, 439–44.

Fonarow GC, Heywood JT, Heidenreich PA, *et al.* (2007). Temporal trends in clinical characteristics, treatments, and outcomes for heart failure hospitalizations in 2002–2004: findings from the ADHERE registry. *Am Heart J*, **153**, 1021–8.

Gottdiener JS, Arnold AM, Aurigemma GP, *et al.* (2000). Predictors of congestive heart failure in the elderly: the Cardiovascular Health Study. *J Am Coll Cardiol*, **35**, 1628–37.

Ho KKL, Anderson KM, Kannel WB, Grossman W, Levy D. (1993). Survival after the onset of congestive heart failure in Framingham Study subjects. *Circulation*, **88**, 107–15.

Hogg K, Swedberg K, McMurray J. (2004). Heart failure with preserved left ventricular systolic function: epidemiology, clinical characteristics and prognosis. *J Am Coll Cardiol*, 43, 317–27.

McDonagh TA, Morrison CE, Lawrence A, *et al.* (1997). Symptomatic and asymptomatic left ventricular systolic dysfunction in an urban population. *Lancet*, **350**, 829–33.

McDonagh TA, Cunningham AD, Morrison CE, *et al.* (2001). Left ventricular dysfunction, natriuretic peptides, and mortality in an urban population. *Heart*, **86**, 21–6.

McKee PA, Castelli WP, McNamara PM, Kannel WB (1971). The natural history of congestive heart failure: the Framingham study. *N Engl J Med*, **285**, 1441–6.

McMurray JJ, Adamopoulos S, *et al.* (2012). ESC guidelines for the diagnosis and treatment of acute and chronic heart failure 2012: The Task Force for the Diagnosis and Treatment of Acute and Chronic Heart Failure 2012 of the European Society of Cardiology. Developed in collaboration with the Heart Failure Association (HFA) of the ESC. *Eur J Heart Fail*, **14**, 803–69.

Mehta PA, Dubrey SW, McIntyre HF, *et al.* (2009). Improving survival in the 6 months after diagnosis of heart failure in the past decade: population based data from the UK. *Heart*, **95**, 1851–6.

Nieminen MS, Brutsaert D, Dickstein K, *et al.* (2006). EuroHeart Failure Survey II (EHFS II): a survey on hospitalized acute heart failure patients: description of population. *Eur Heart J*, **27**, 2725–36.

Senni M, Tribouilloy CM, Rodeheffer RJ, et al. (1998). Congestive heart failure in the community: a study of all incident cases in Olmsted County, Minnesota, in 1991. *Circulation*, **98**, 2282–9.

The National Heart Failure Audit 2011/12 and 12/13. www.ucl.ac.uk/nicor

CHAPTER 5.2

Acute cardiac failure: definitions, investigation, and management

Andrew L. Clark and John G. F. Cleland

Essentials

Presentation

Presentations of acute heart failure fall into three overlapping categories: (1) acute breathlessness and pulmonary oedema, (2) chronic fluid retention and peripheral oedema (anasarca), and (3) cardiogenic shock.

Examination features include tachycardia, hypotension, a raised venous pressure, basal crackles, and peripheral oedema. Auscultation may reveal a third heart sound or features of precipitating valvular heart disease. Initial management focuses on confirming the diagnosis and identification of the immediate precipitant (e.g. arrhythmias, myocardial infarction, decompensating valvular heart disease).

Investigations

Initial investigations include a 12-lead electrocardiogram (ECG), chest radiograph, full blood count, biochemical screen, troponin and thyroid function. Natriuretic peptides (NP) are useful in confirming the diagnosis where clinical features are present and a normal NP is helpful in excluding the diagnosis. All patients should undergo echocardiographic assessment early in the course of a hospital admission to assess left ventricular function and to look for underlying valvular heart disease.

Management

In patients with acute pulmonary oedema investigation and management should proceed simultaneously. Intravenous loop diuretics and nitrates are commonly used therapies and may be combined with ventilatory support with oxygen and continuous positive airways ventilation. Mechanical support may be appropriate as a bridge to definitive therapy in potentially reversible causes. Inotropes are often used but without convincing evidence that they improve outcome.

In patients with features are of peripheral oedema and low cardiac output, fluid retention (usually >5 litres) is the predominant feature. Management is principally with bed rest, loop diuretics (usually by intravenous infusion), and, where appropriate, aldosterone antagonists. Thiazide diuretics can be added in resistant cases. Prophylactic low molecular weight heparin should be prescribed. Careful monitoring of fluid balance with daily weights and daily electrolytes is essential. Angiotensin converting enzyme (ACE) inhibitors and

subsequently β-blockade can be introduced once a satisfactory diuresis has been achieved.

Management of cardiogenic shock is usually determined by the cause. Fluid status should be assessed and an adequate left ventricular filling pressure ensured by the administration of intravenous fluids where required (particularly in the case of right ventricular infarction). Revascularization is the mainstay of therapy in acute myocardial infarction. Circulatory support with intra-aortic balloon counter-pulsation (IABP), inotropic agents, ventricular assist devices (VADs), and extracorporeal membrane oxygenation should be considered for reversible causes (e.g. ventricular septal rupture, papillary muscle rupture, acute myocarditis and postpartum cardiomyopathy).

Prognosis

Hospital admission with acute heart failure caries a poor prognosis with an average in-hospital mortality of 10–15% rising to up to 60% at 30 days in cases of cardiogenic shock.

Definitions

Although the term 'acute heart failure' often conjures up an image of a patient with acute pulmonary oedema, *in extremis*, struggling to breathe and producing pink, frothy sputum, such a dramatic presentation is not common. Admissions to hospital for heart failure, on the other hand, are extremely common, and most patients admitted are not breathless at rest, only becoming breathless on mild exertion. It is better to think of acute heart failure as being a worsening of symptoms and/or signs leading the patient, carer, or primary care physician to seek urgent expert advice—leading, in turn, to an urgent admission to hospital for investigation and/or treatment. Many patients will be able to walk, albeit slowly, from their wheelchair to their hospital bed.

Patients admitted with heart failure usually have a problem with oedema: that is, fluid in the wrong place. The old-fashioned term 'anasarca' describes a state of severe generalized oedema. It is helpful to think of patients as being on a spectrum between pulmonary oedema at one end, in which the fluid is predominantly in the lung, and anasarca on the other, in which patients have an absolute excess of fluid, usually manifesting as peripheral oedema. This notion is similar to the classification system used for patients with chronic airways disease and

Table 5.2.1 The spectrum of acute heart failure ranges from patients with acute pulmonary oedema, perhaps 15% of patients presenting to hospital with acute pulmonary oedema, to those with fluid retention. Differences between the two groups are highlighted

	Pulmonary oedema	Anasarca
Syndrome	Puffers	Bloaters
Acute precipitant	Yes	Usually no
Oedema	In lungs	Predominantly peripheral
Absolute fluid excess	No	Yes
Time course	Minutes to hours	Days to weeks

emphysema: patients with pulmonary oedema can be termed 'puffers', and those with anasarca as 'bloaters' or having dropsy (Table 5.2.1).

Patients with pulmonary oedema usually present with a short history of deterioration. There is often an obvious acute precipitating factor such as acute coronary syndrome or atrial fibrillation, particularly with a rapid ventricular response. They often have hypertension and a high peripheral vascular resistance. The patient has had no time to retain a substantial excess of body fluid. In contrast, patients with dropsy ('bloaters') usually have a history of deterioration over a period of weeks and no acute precipitating factors (although the development of atrial fibrillation with a slow ventricular response, anaemia, and chronic kidney disease (CKD) could be considered chronic precipitants). They have a low blood pressure and have had time to retain many litres (sometimes ≥20 litres) of excess fluid. The distinction is important in interpreting the results of clinical trials: an agent that is designed to improve acute breathlessness, but given to someone who is already comfortable at rest (perhaps rendered so by standard background therapy) is likely to appear ineffective, even if it is highly effective in the appropriate patient at the appropriate time.

There is little evidence from randomized controlled trials in acute heart failure syndromes to guide management. The European Society of Cardiology (ESC) produced guidelines in 2012 which are helpful; but it is noteworthy that the only treatment to receive a class I, level A recommendation was the use of prophylaxis against thromboembolism. Much of what follows in terms of management advice thus reflects the balance of expert opinion rather than definitive recommendations.

The lack of evidence reflects a constellation of difficulties. The reasons for hospital admission may be misunderstood and patients often present at inconvenient hours of the night when it is least likely they will encounter people with the time or inclination to do research (funding nocturnal research can be expensive). Protocol procedures often cause delays which allow standard therapies to be effective before a new intervention can be started. Indeed, the effectiveness of oxygen, nitrovasodilators, and diuretics for the short-term management of symptoms suggests that the needs for managing acute pulmonary oedema are largely satisfied.

The big problems for 'acute' heart failure really appear 2–3 days after admission when it is clear that diuretics alone have not solved the immediate problem. For most patients, the problem then is peripheral oedema and exertional breathlessness rather than breathlessness at rest. In the longer term, the big problems are recurrent exacerbations and death. Thankfully, the vast majority of patients who survive to discharge attain a reasonable quality of life in the intervening period.

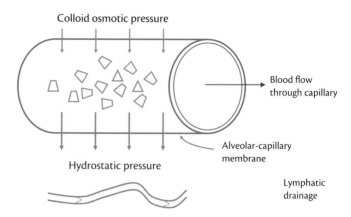

Fig. 5.2.1 The forces acting on fluid in a pulmonary capillary.

Cardiogenic pulmonary oedema
Pathophysiology

In patients with pulmonary oedema, fluid from the lung capillaries collects in the extravascular spaces of the lung. The Starling equation describes the forces acting on fluid in the pulmonary capillaries (Fig. 5.2.1). Hydrostatic pressure tends to force fluid out of the capillaries while the colloid osmotic pressure (largely provided by proteins) tends to maintain the fluid within the capillary. The balance between the forces varies between arteriole and venule: however, there is net filtration along the length of the capillary. Some resistance to fluid movement is provided by the alveolar–capillary membrane and any fluid entering the interstitium is removed by the lymphatics.

Problems with any of these components can lead to (or worsen) pulmonary oedema. Pulmonary lymphatic flow may increase substantially in heart failure, reducing the risk of pulmonary oedema. However, the lymphatics drain into the venous circulation and so a rise in venous pressure may inhibit lymphatic clearance. Lymphatic occlusion, as occurs in lymphangitis carcinomatosa, and disruption to the alveolar capillary membrane, as happens in adult respiratory distress syndrome, can cause pulmonary oedema. Hypoalbuminaemia causes peripheral oedema and reduces the hydrostatic pressure at which pulmonary oedema occurs.

In the normal circulation, the Frank–Starling relation describes the relation between the load on the left ventricle at the end of diastole, usually expressed as the end-diastolic pressure, and the work subsequently performed by the ventricle during systole. The end-diastolic pressure is the same as the left atrial and hence pulmonary venous pressure. In patients with heart failure, the curve relating the two is shifted to the right: for any given cardiac output, the filling pressure required is greater in the failing ventricle (see Fig. 5.2.2). An acutely failing ventricle needs a higher and higher filling pressure to maintain cardiac output. The rising end-diastolic pressure is reflected in a rise in left atrial, pulmonary venous, and pulmonary capillary pressure, resulting in faster rates of fluid filtration. Ultimately, fluid is filtered faster than the rate at which the lymphatics can remove it, and pulmonary oedema results.

This sequence cannot be quite the full explanation: a rise in pressure (including left ventricular filling pressure) can only arise from an input of energy. In acute pulmonary oedema, the energy for the rise in left ventricular pressure can only come from the right heart. When the left ventricle fails, there is a fall in left ventricular stroke

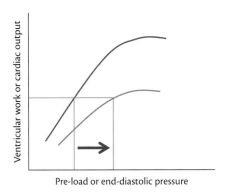

Fig. 5.2.2 The Frank-Starling relation. As pre-load increases, so does cardiac output. In the failing ventricle, the relation is shifted to the right so that to deliver any given cardiac output, the ventricle requires a higher filling pressure.

volume and consequent mismatch between left and right ventricular stroke volumes. The higher right ventricular stroke volume causes the increase in left ventricular filling pressure and restoration of cardiac output, but an inevitable consequence is some accumulation of fluid in the pulmonary circulation. The greater the fall in stroke volume of the left in relation to the right ventricle, the higher the left ventricular filling pressure will be and the greater the pulmonary fluid volume.

Note that the total amount of fluid in the body does not increase and the effect is brought about by fluid moving to the 'wrong' body compartment. The fluid extravasation into the alveoli results in a reduction in blood volume during acute pulmonary oedema, which then increases back to normal levels during successful treatment.

The fluid accumulation in the lungs starts with peribronchial swelling/oedema, followed by distension of the alveolar walls; only then does fluid enter the alveoli, initially at the alveolar angles, and eventually flooding the alveoli. The accumulation starts at the lung bases as the hydrostatic pressure is greatest here.

Clinical presentation

Acute pulmonary oedema is a dramatic medical emergency. The typical patient presents with very severe shortness of breath that has developed abruptly over minutes or hours. He or she has to sit upright (and might indeed die if forced to lie flat) and may be unable to speak or gasp only a few words. Patients are usually very frightened and often certain that they are dying. Coughing may be prominent and will often produce blood-tinged oedema fluid. There may be some clues in the history as to the precipitant of pulmonary oedema.

Sympathetic nervous system activation usually results in a tachycardia and a rise in blood pressure; the skin is white, cold, and clammy. The patient usually exhibits central cyanosis. Heart sounds may be inaudible but a gallop rhythm is common. The lung fields are usually filled with crackles and sometimes wheezes (so-called 'cardiac asthma').

Given how sick the patient with pulmonary oedema is, the initial investigations and management have to be carried out at speed. The ESC guidelines for the management of heart failure emphasize the need to investigate and treat simultaneously (Fig. 5.2.3). There are three strands: making the diagnosis, identifying the immediate precipitant, and initiating treatment. Identifying precipitating factors is particularly important as it will influence subsequent management (see Table 5.2.2).

Initial investigation

A 12-lead electrocardiogram (ECG) will often show grossly abnormal QRS complexes, including evidence of acute myocardial infarction, or abnormal heart rhythm, including atrial fibrillation with a rapid ventricular response and ventricular tachycardia (see Fig. 5.2.4).

A chest radiograph gives vital information. At early stages in the development of pulmonary oedema, the patient may have septal (or Kerley B) lines (Fig. 5.2.5), fluid in the lung fissures, and pleural effusions. There is peribronchial cuffing and upper lobe blood diversion. As oedema worsens, confluent shadows spreading out from the hila develop (Fig. 5.2.6).

Near-patient testing for cardiac markers is becoming more widely available. Natriuretic peptide (NP) measurement can be helpful in making the diagnosis where there is clinical uncertainty: a patient with a normal NP level is extremely unlikely to have heart failure. A raised troponin suggests that there might be an acute coronary syndrome (ACS) in progress, but troponin is commonly raised in acute heart failure even in the absence of ACS.

A full blood count, biochemical screen, and thyroid function are important investigations. Anaemia is common, often due to iron deficiency but exacerbated by plasma volume expansion. Glucose is very commonly raised due to the high sympathetic drive, and does not necessarily mean that diabetes is present. Other appropriate investigations may include CT pulmonary angiography and a septic screen.

Echocardiographic assessment early in the course of admission is very useful in confirming the cause of presentation and guiding subsequent therapy.

Management

Patients with acute pulmonary oedema should be managed in a high-dependency unit. Whether this should be cardiac care or a unit where intubation and ventilation is available will depend upon the degree of respiratory distress.

Ventilatory support

The lowest dose of oxygen needed to restore normal oxygenation should be used. Care should be taken in patients with chronic airways disease who are at risk of developing CO_2 retention (which may be exacerbated by the use of opiates). In a patient who is tiring or whose gas exchange is worsening despite treatment, positive pressure ventilation provides immediate relief. Noninvasive ventilation should be tried first: there is good evidence that both continuous positive airway pressure ventilation and bilevel positive airway pressure ventilation are safe.

Medical treatment

Opiates are commonly prescribed to relieve the distress of acute pulmonary oedema. However, there is no evidence that they are safe, and some data to suggest that their use is associated with adverse outcomes. They should be used cautiously, if at all.

Diuretics are almost universally used in patients with acute pulmonary oedema, although trials to prove efficacy are lacking. As patients are usually not fluid overloaded, diuretics may not be the most logical therapy, although by reducing circulating volume, they do reduce filling pressure and relieve oedema. There is a firmly held view that furosemide is a vasodilator, but its haemodynamic effects coincide with the onset of diuresis.

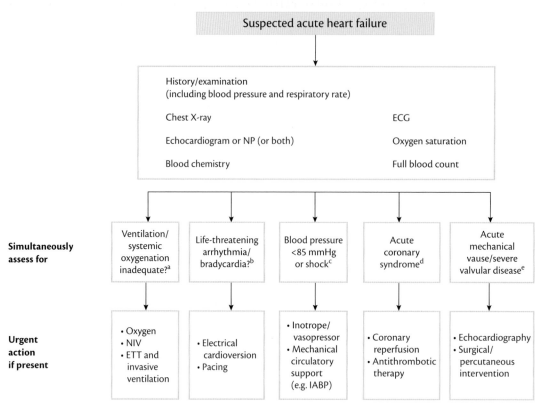

Suspected acute heart failure

History/examination
(including blood pressure and respiratory rate)

Chest X-ray   ECG

Echocardiogram or NP (or both)   Oxygen saturation

Blood chemistry   Full blood count

Simultaneously assess for

| Ventilation/ systemic oxygenation inadequate?[a] | Life-threatening arrhythmia/ bradycardia?[b] | Blood pressure <85 mmHg or shock[c] | Acute coronary syndrome[d] | Acute mechanical vause/severe valvular disease[e] |

Urgent action if present

| • Oxygen • NIV • ETT and invasive ventilation | • Electrical cardioversion • Pacing | • Inotrope/ vasopressor • Mechanical circulatory support (e.g. IABP) | • Coronary reperfusion • Antithrombotic therapy | • Echocardiography • Surgical/ percutaneous intervention |

ECG = electrocardiogram; ETT = endotracheal tube; IABP = intra-aortic balloon pump; NIV = non-invasive ventilation; NP = natriuretic peptide.
[a]For example, respiratory distress, confusion SpO$_2$ <90%, or PaO$_2$ < 60 mmHg (8.0 kPa).
[b]For example, ventricular tachycardia, third-degree atrioventricular block.
[c]Reduced peripheral and vital orgen perfusion—patients often have cold skin and urine output ≤15 ml/h and/or disturbance of consciousness.
[d]Percutaneous coronary revascularization (or thrombolysis) indicated if ST-segment elevation or new left bundle branch block.
[e]Vasodilators should be used with great caution, and surgery should be considered for certain acute mechanical complications (e.g. inter-ventricular septal rupture, mitral value papillary muscle rupture).

Fig. 5.2.3 The treatment algorithm recommended by the European Society of Cardiology. Note that investigations and active management have to be undertaken simultaneously.

Table 5.2.2 Common precipitants of acute pulmonary oedema, helpful investigations, and possible immediate treatment options. ECG is electrocardiogram; CXR is chest X ray; (N)STEMI is (non) ST elevation myocardial infarction

Precipitant	Examples	Investigation	Immediate management
Acute ischaemia	STEMI NSTEMI	ECG, troponin[#]	Immediate cardiology review
Arrhythmia	Atrial fibrillation Ventricular tachycardia	ECG	DC cardioversion
Mechanical disaster	Rupture of: Inter-ventricular septum Mitral papillary muscle Sinus of Valsalva	Echocardiogram	Cardiac surgery
Hypertensive crisis	Renal artery stenosis Salt load	*During recovery*	Vasodilators
Intercurrent illness	Pneumonia Urinary infection Sepsis	CXR, septic screen	As appropriate
Pulmonary embolus		CT pulmonary angiogram	Thrombolysis, anticoagulation
Environment	Lack of compliance with medication/diet High salt intake	History	Education

[#] often elevated in acute or chronic heart failure in the absence of any other evidence of ACS. An elevated troponin in patients with heart failure is a bad prognostic sign.

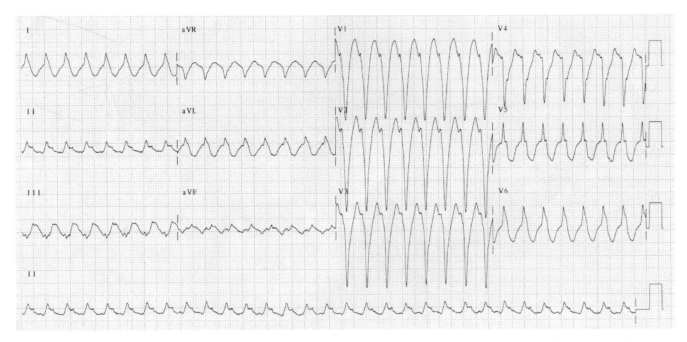

Fig. 5.2.4 A 12 lead electrocardiogram from a 76 year old man presenting with acute pulmonary oedema. His ventricular tachycardia had been precipitated by an acute coronary syndrome.

Nitrovasodilators are a more logical approach to the treatment of pulmonary oedema. They reduce both preload and afterload as well as helping to relieve any myocardial ischaemia. Small studies suggest that nitrates may be more helpful than diuretics, but the evidence is not definitive. Clinical surveys suggest that they are only used in a minority of patients.

Other vasodilators have been tried. Nesiritide, human recombinant B-type natriuretic peptide, was shown to have no overall effect on outcome in a large trial, and no patient subset obtained a striking benefit. Serelaxin, human recombinant relaxin (a vasoactive peptide produced in pregnancy) may improve symptoms and markers of cardiovascular function in the days following admission and might improve long-term outcome after acute administration. Further trials of this promising therapy are awaited.

Inotropic support is often used, particularly as a 'last ditch' attempt to help very sick patients, more in despair than hope. What evidence exists from randomized trials suggests that all positive inotropic drugs working through adrenergic pathways are associated with an adverse outcome. Investigational approaches include cardiac myosin activators and inhibitors of sarcoplasmic calcium re-uptake.

Mechanical support

In selected patients, there may be a role for intra-aortic balloon pumping to buy time, particularly when there is a potentially

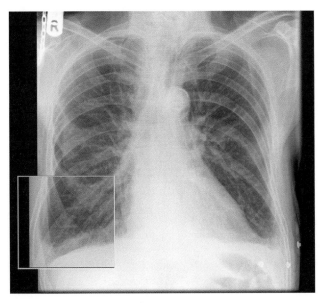

Fig. 5.2.5 A plain postero-anterior chest X ray in a breathless patient showing Kerley B lines – multiple short horizontal lines visible towards the lung peripheries. There are also small pleural effusions.

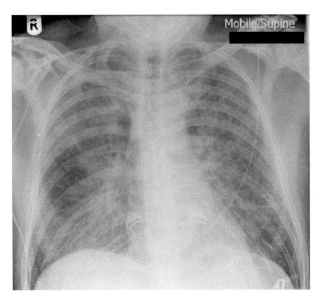

Fig. 5.2.6 More severe pulmonary oedema on supine antero-posterior film showing confluent shadowing spreading out from the hila. Note the relatively small heart shadow suggesting that this is an acute event in a previously normal heart.

reversible cause for the pulmonary oedema. Similarly, a left ventricular assist device and extracorporeal membrane oxygenators may have a role when there is a potential either for recovery or for heart transplantation.

Clinical course and recovery

The recovery from pulmonary oedema is in part an active process in which cells take up fluid and return it to the capillary or lymphatic circulation. Novel agents designed to enhance this process are being developed.

The clinical course of acute pulmonary oedema is usually very brisk: the patient usually recovers rapidly after treatment, or deteriorates rapidly and dies. Overall, in-hospital mortality is around 15% but strongly age-related; it is less than 10% in those aged less than 65 years and much higher in those aged more than 85 years. However, these figures do not include those dying before reaching hospital.

Cardiogenic anasarca

Pathophysiology

At the other end of the scale from pulmonary oedema are patients with fluid retention. Two processes result in oedema: the retention of sodium and water, and the transfer of fluid into the tissues. To take the second first: fluid collects in the tissues as a consequence of a rise in intravascular hydrostatic pressure or fall in osmotic pressure. As with the lungs, there is continuous filtration of fluid from the capillaries to the tissues: if extravasation exceeds lymphatic drainage, oedema develops. The effect of gravity means that the hydrostatic pressure is highest in the feet, so ankle swelling is usually the first sign of fluid retention. In a patients confined to bed, though, the fluid will collect around the sacrum.

The reasons why the body retains water are less certain. Sodium and water are retained by the kidneys, presumably in response to decreased renal perfusion or deviation from the kidney's set-point for renal perfusion pressure (i.e. the blood pressure the kidney 'wants'). The consequence is renin production by the juxtaglomerular apparatus leading to conversion of angiotensinogen to angiotensin I and ultimately to aldosterone production, which in turn causes salt and water retention by the kidney. In addition, antidiuretic hormone (ADH, or arginine vasopressin) is released in increased quantities, stimulating fluid retention and, importantly, thirst, and thus greater fluid intake. However, antagonists of each of these systems, even when used in combination, do not seem sufficient to prevent salt and water retention and do not obviate the need for diuretics, although they might reduce the dose required.

The stimulus leading to neuroendocrine activation is not clear. A common assumption is that it is a fall in blood pressure due to the failing heart. The body responds in the same way as it would to any other cause of a fall in blood pressure, such as dehydration or haemorrhage, with avid salt and water retention to maintain blood pressure. Although some patients have a normal or high blood pressure compared to healthy people, this blood pressure may be below their individual set-point. If the set-point could be changed, then perhaps salt and water retention would not occur.

Clinical presentation

The typical picture is of a patient with gradual weight gain, often in the context of previous coronary disease, hypertension, atrial fibrillation, and CKD. Around 5 litres of fluid (weighing 5 kg) are needed before oedema first appears. As the process is often very gradual, patients will often present only once they have retained many litres of fluid and have pitting oedema affecting the abdominal wall, and sometimes even the thoracic wall. Pleural and pericardial effusions and ascites are common in this situation. In some patients, the oedema causes obvious ballooning of the ankles. However, in many patients the oedema does not grossly distort the shape of the leg, and oedema of the trunk may develop and go unobserved by the patient or a careless doctor. Symptoms such as 'I can't get my shoes on' or 'I have had to loosen my belt' or 'I have increased a waist size' in a patient with increasing breathlessness should alert the clinician to the possibility of oedema.

The oedema is usually very obvious on examination. Cardiogenic oedema is pitting. The highest level of pitting oedema should be sought. The jugular venous pressure will be raised: however, when it is very high, the top of the column of the blood may not be visible in the neck, even with the patient sitting upright.

There is usually a tachycardia and often hypotension. The apex beat is displaced and dyskinetic and there is almost always a third sound or gallop rhythm. Mitral regurgitation is very common. There are commonly signs of ascites and pleural effusions, with basal crackles in some patients who have pulmonary congestion.

Differential diagnosis

It is important to consider the differential diagnosis of peripheral oedema (Table 5.2.3). Once a firm diagnosis of cardiogenic oedema is made, the next step is to consider the possible causes of the 'right heart' failure. Although the commonest cause is left heart failure, other cardiac conditions, particularly constrictive pericarditis, can result in severe fluid overload and be difficult to diagnose (see Table 5.2.4). Pulmonary hypertension leading to right ventricular dysfunction appears increasingly common in frail elderly patients with right heart failure, many of whom also have lung and left heart disease.

Initial investigations

Patients presenting with anasarca should be investigated as patients presenting with chronic heart failure (see Chapter 5.3) with the aim of making the diagnosis, unmasking any treatable cause, and identifying any associated comorbidities.

Table 5.2.3 Differential diagnosis of peripheral oedema. Note that anasarca is easily overlooked without careful examination

Oedema fluid	Cardiogenic
	hypoalbuminaemia
Fluid overload	Pregnancy
Lymphatic obstruction	Idiopathic
Medicines	Dihydropyridines/glitazones
Venous insufficiency	Varicose veins
	Previous DVT
Chronic stasis	
Fat	(Obesity)

Table 5.2.4 Differential diagnosis of cardiogenic peripheral oedema

Possible cause	Examples
Raised left atrial pressure (left heart failure)	Impaired left ventricular ◆ Contraction • Ischaemic heart disease (IHD) • Dilated cardiomyopathy ◆ Relaxation • Left ventricular hypertrophy (hypertension) • Hypertrophic cardiomyopathy • Amyloid Mitral valve disease
Raised right atrial pressure (right heart failure)	Chronic left atrial hypertension Pumonary hypertension IHD Tricuspid valve disease (often tricuspid regurgitation due to dilated right ventricle) Right ventricular cardiomyopathy
Congenital heart disease	Left-to-right shunts Right ventricle in systemic position
Pulmonary hypertension	Chronic left atrial hypertension Lung disease (cor pulmonale) Thromboembolic disease
Pericardial disease	Constrictive pericarditis

- Common ECG abnormalities include previous myocardial infarction, left bundle branch block, atrial fibrillation.

- A chest radiograph will show a large heart shadow and evidence of pulmonary venous congestion. It may also exclude other causes of breathlessness.

- Urinary dipsticks will help pick up infection and gross proteinuria.

- Anaemia is common in anasarca due to heart failure. Patients may benefit from an iron infusion should they have iron deficiency.

- Renal dysfunction and electrolyte abnormalities are common in patients with heart failure and major determinants of outcome. Regular testing during treatment (see below) is vital.

- NP levels are usually grossly raised.

- An echocardiogram is essential (see Fig. 5.2.7). The key elements to look at are:
  - Left atrial size—mitral valve disease or chronic elevation in left ventricular filling pressure will cause left atrial dilatation. It is probably the best guide to the chronic health of the left heart but may not be enlarged with severe acute-onset disease.
  - Left ventricular size and contractility—the left ventricle is commonly dilated with reduced systolic function but sometimes small, hypertrophied, and 'stiff'. Regional wall motion abnormalities suggest a possible underlying diagnosis of ischaemic heart disease.
  - Valve disease

- More sophisticated investigation may reveal pulmonary hypertension, right ventriclar disease, and dilated vena cava. Ultrasound can also be used to identify 'lung comets' indicating pulmonary congestion.

Management

The problem is one of an absolute excess of fluid, and initial management is directed at fluid removal. General care is important: the patient should be managed with bed rest with prophylactic low molecular weight heparin used to reduce the (high) risk of venous thrombosis. The only way to monitor progress accurately is with strict fluid balance monitoring and daily weights. The urea and electrolytes should be measured at least daily, and the patient should be reviewed daily by an experienced member of the team.

Oedema is due to retention of water, not salt: in 1 litre of oedema fluid, there are 991 g of water and 9 g of salt. There is no good evidence that sodium restriction is useful, although restricting a very high intake may be useful in the occasional patient. Salt restriction may lead to hyponatraemia. Aquaresis may be greater (and hyponatraemia less likely) when moderate salt intake is allowed. Fluid intake is often restricted to around 1.5 litres per day, but the evidence for this is weak. The aim should be to try and induce a net diuresis of around 2 litres per day.

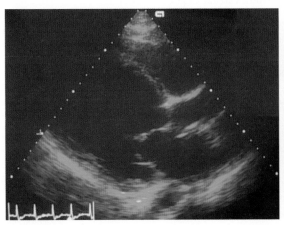
Diastole: mitral valve open

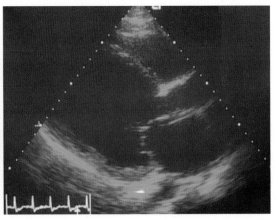
Systole: mitral valve shut

Fig. 5.2.7 Echocardiogram of a patient presenting with anasarca. Long axis parasternal view. The left ventricular internal diameter is approximately 8 centimetres, and there is little difference between systolic and diastolic frames.

Diuretic management is key. Diuretics work by preventing the reabsorption of some of the filtered sodium from the tubular lumen.

• Loop diuretics block the sodium–potassium–chloride co-transporter in the thick ascending loop of Henle. As they reach their site of action from the lumen of the nephron, they only work if there is at least some glomerular function. Once their effects are over, the kidney goes into overdrive to restore the lost salt and water.

• Thiazide diuretics work at the distal convoluted tubule. They induce a small but persistent diuresis; over a 24-hour period loop and thiazide diuretics may have the same natriuretic effect.

• Mineralocorticoid antagonists block the effects of aldosterone at the sodium–potassium exchanger in the distal convoluted tubule, resulting in potassium retention.

A typical approach is to use intravenous loop diuretic. Oral absorption is very erratic in patients with cardiogenic oedema because of bowel oedema. An infusion of 10 mg per hour of furosemide is often used. Data from small studies suggests that an infusion causes a greater natriuresis than repeated boluses to the same dose, but the biggest study of infusion versus bolus dosing showed no difference between the two strategies.

Particularly after chronic loop diuretic usage, the cells of the distal convoluted tubule hypertrophy and increase their capacity to reabsorb sodium. The addition of a thiazide will block the distal convoluted tubule (so-called 'progressive nephron blockade') which may lead to a profound diuresis. Metolazone is often used for this purpose although there is no convincing evidence that it is more potent than other thiazides. Combination therapy can be very helpful, but patients having the two diuretics must be monitored very closely.

Potentially nephrotoxic drugs, such as nonsteroidal anti-inflammatory drugs (including aspirin) should be stopped. It is not certain whether pre-existing β-blocker (or ACE inhibitor) therapy should be stopped: the evidence available suggests that those patients whose pre-existing therapy is not stopped are less likely to be discharged without these life-saving treatments.

Towards the end of intravenous therapy, ACE inhibitors and β-blockers should be started simultaneously at low doses. If not already being used, a mineralocorticoid (aldosterone) receptor antagonist (MRA) should also be started (see Fig. 5.2.8). The dose of ACE inhibitor should be titrated rapidly to target with careful monitoring of blood pressure and renal function. β-Blockers are titrated more slowly and often only after discharge.

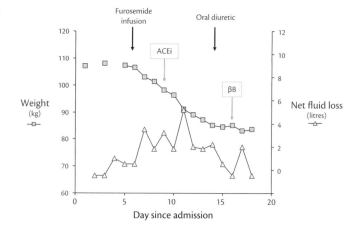

Fig. 5.2.8 Time course of diuresis for a patient presenting with approximately 25 litres of anasarca. Note the brisk response once the furosemide infusion was started, and the timing of introduction of long-term medication. ACEi is angiotensin converting enzyme inhibitor and βB is beta adrenoceptor antagonist.

Intravenous diuretic therapy should be continued until the oedema has resolved unless an oral diuretic regimen is clearly having the desired results. It is not uncommon for renal function to improve following diuresis and diuretic therapy should not be withheld or reduced in patients with impaired renal function at the time of presentation where there is clear evidence of fluid overload. For some patients, however, complete resolution of oedema cannot be achieved due to worsening renal impairment and a balance has to be struck between some peripheral oedema and a raised creatinine. Ideally, a patient finishing intravenous therapy will be monitored for 48 h to make sure that the fluid does not re-accumulate immediately.

Some patients may fail to respond adequately to intravenous diuretics. It is important to reconsider the diagnosis: Has constrictive pericarditis been missed? Is there some correctable cause of renal dysfunction, such as renal artery stenosis?

Other therapeutic options include the use of digoxin, which has a diuretic effect, although the evidence base for its use in acute heart failure is poor. Positive inotropic drugs, particularly in hypotensive patients, are sometimes used. There is no evidence to support the practice, and no evidence that 'renal dose dopamine' has anything to offer. Serelaxin might be useful in this setting but appropriate studies are lacking.

Ultrafiltration can be used to remove fluid rapidly from patients with anasarca (see Table 5.2.5). Veno-venous filtration is possible

Table 5.2.5 Diuretics commonly used in the management of anasarca. DCT is distal, and PCT, proximal, convoluted tubule. MRA is mineralocorticoid antagonist

Class	Example	Route	Site of action	Comments	
Loop	Furosemide Bumetanide	Intravenously	Na$^+$/K$^+$/Cl$^-$ co-transporter in thick ascending loop of Henle	High ceiling; short duration of action	Shorter half life than thiazides
Thiazide	Bendroflumethiazide	By mouth	DCT	Low ceiling; longer period of action	Combined with loop may cause profound diuresis
"Thiazide-like"	Metolazone	By mouth	DCT (and PCT)		Combined with loop may cause profound diuresis
MRA	Spironolactone Eplerenone	By mouth	DCT – aldosterone antagonists		Essential component of long term management

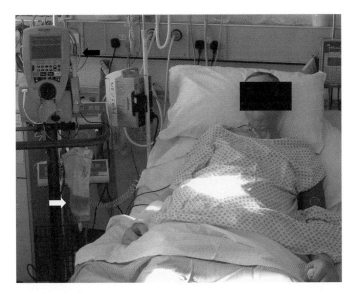

Fig. 5.2.9 A patient receiving ultrafiltration. There is a two-lumen right internal jugular venous line from which blood is continuously removed, pumped through a filter (black arrow) and then returned to the body. Filtrate is seen collecting in the bag (white arrow).

in a cardiac care unit setting with small devices. There is conflicting evidence as to its value: in one study, its use was associated with a reduction in the need for subsequent emergency care, but in patients with worsening renal function, a second study suggested that ultrafiltration was associated with worse renal outcomes. Although its role in routine practice is still uncertain, there is no doubt that as much as 5 litres can safely be removed from a patient in 24 h, and it is useful in selected patients who are unresponsive to combined diuretic therapy or when diuresis is limited by renal dysfunction (Fig. 5.2.9).

Cardiogenic shock

Shock occurs when there is tissue hypoperfusion despite adequate ventricular filling. There is no blood pressure level that can be used to define shock, with the consequence that the incidence and prognosis quoted varies from study to study.

Pathophysiology

Cardiogenic shock most commonly arises from an acute myocardial insult which results in sufficient reduction in cardiac output that the perfusion to vital organs is insufficient to maintain organ function. By far the commonest cause is acute myocardial infarction, although patients with acute presentation of cardiomyopathy, including peripartum cardiomyopathy, may develop shock.

The result is massive sympathetic nervous system activation as the body tries to restore blood pressure. The consequent increase in afterload cannot be met by the failing left ventricle. Reduced coronary artery perfusion results in worsening myocardial function, perpetuating the problem.

Clinical presentation

The patient is hypotensive, usually tachycardic, pale, and sweaty. Reduced cerebral perfusion results in confusion and agitation, and the patient becomes oliguric or anuric. Except for those patients with predominant right ventricular infarction, some degree of pulmonary oedema is invariably present.

Differential diagnosis and investigations

Making the correct diagnosis is fundamental: investigations should be directed at finding any reversible cause for the patient's state.

Making certain that the left ventricle is adequately filled is essential to make the diagnosis of shock: if the left ventricle is underfilled, then fluid replacement should result in rapid resolution of symptoms. If there is doubt, then fluid challenges with rapid infusion of 100–200 ml fluid can be helpful. In some cases, pulmonary artery catheterization is used to determine the pulmonary capillary wedge pressure and hence confirm adequate filling. There is no evidence that using the catheter to guide further management is helpful.

An ECG with right-sided leads will help make the diagnosis of a predominantly right-sided myocardial infarct. An echocardiogram to confirm the extent of left and right ventricular damage and to exclude a mechanical problem (free wall rupture, papillary muscle rupture, ventricular septal rupture) is a vital early investigation.

Bladder catheterization will confirm that the patient is genuinely oliguric rather than confused due to retention of urine. Sepsis should be excluded.

Management

Dealing with any treatable cause of shock is the most important step. Revascularization in patients presenting with acute myocardial infarction may relieve shock, although if shock develops following or despite a successful procedure, the outlook is particularly poor.

Patients with mechanical problems tend to have smaller and more localized infarctions than those without: although it is very high risk, early surgery may be life-saving. For those patients with right ventricular infarction as the cause, fluid loading may improve the patient's condition, but at a cost of high central venous pressure.

Trying to sustain the circulation in patients with no readily reversible cause is rarely successful.

- Positive inotropic drugs, such as catecholamines and phosphodiesterase inhibitors, may improve cardiac output and blood pressure: however, their use has not been shown to improve prognosis. Indeed, dobutamine in randomized trials is associated with a worse outcome.

- Intra-aortic balloon counter-pulsation (IABP) can improve the situation, at least temporarily. Trial evidence suggests that the IABP does not improve prognosis in patients with cardiogenic shock due to acute infarction, but it can certainly help patients with acute mechanical causes such as septal rupture and mitral regurgitation. In some patients with potentially reversible causes, such as peripartum cardiomyopathy, IABP has been used successfully to sustain the circulation for many weeks.

- Advanced therapies with ventricular assist devices (VADs), extracorporeal membrane oxygenation (ECMO) and even heart transplantation have been successful in selected patients. VADs and ECMO are only available in the United Kingdom in transplant centres, but there is a move to make them more widely available as a temporizing measure before patients are transferred to the centres.

The prognosis of cardiogenic shock is bleak. Unless there is a readily correctable cause, the mortality rate approaches 60% at 30 days. Once treatable causes of shock have been excluded, conservative management and an easy death may be preferred rather than transfer to the intensive care unit for valiant, desperate, protracted, but ultimately futile, intervention.

Further reading

Chen HH, Anstrom KJ, Givertz MM, *et al.* for the NHLBI Heart Failure Clinical Research Network (2013). Low-dose dopamine or low-dose nesiritide in acute heart failure with renal dysfunction: the ROSE acute heart failure randomized trial. *JAMA*, **310**, 2533–43.

Clark AL, Cleland JG (2013). Causes and treatment of oedema in patients with heart failure. *Nat Rev Cardiol*, **10**, 156–70.

Costanzo MR, Guglin ME, Saltzberg MT, *et al.* UNLOAD Trial Investigators (2007). Ultrafiltration versus intravenous diuretics for patients hospitalized for acute decompensated heart failure. *J Am Coll Cardiol*, **49**, 675–83.

Gray A, Goodacre S, Newby DE, *et al.* 3CPO Trialists (2008). Noninvasive ventilation in acute cardiogenic pulmonary edema. *N Engl J Med*, **359**, 142–51.

Harris P (1983). Evolution and the cardiac patient. *Cardiovasc Res*, **17**, 313–319, 373–378, 437–345

MacIver DH, Dayer MJ, Harrison AJ (2013). A general theory of acute and chronic heart failure. *Int J Cardiol*, **165**, 25–34.

McMurray JJ, Adamopoulos S, Anker SD, *et al.* ESC Committee for Practice Guidelines (2012). ESC Guidelines for the diagnosis and treatment of acute and chronic heart failure 2012: The Task Force for the Diagnosis and Treatment of Acute and Chronic Heart Failure 2012 of the European Society of Cardiology. Developed in collaboration with the Heart Failure Association (HFA) of the ESC. *Eur Heart J*, **33**, 1787–847.

Teerlink JR, Cotter G, Davison BA, *et al.* RELAXin in Acute Heart Failure (RELAX-AHF) Investigators (2013). Serelaxin, recombinant human relaxin-2, for treatment of acute heart failure (RELAX-AHF): a randomised, placebo-controlled trial. *Lancet*, **381**, 29–39.

Tharmaratnam D, Nolan J, Jain A (2013). Management of cardiogenic shock complicating acute coronary syndromes. *Heart*, **99**, 1614–23.

Thiele H, Zeymer U, Neumann FJ, *et al.* IABP-SHOCK II Trial Investigators (2012). Intraaortic balloon support for myocardial infarction with cardiogenic shock. *N Engl J Med*, **367**, 1287–96.

CHAPTER 5.3

Chronic heart failure: definitions, investigation, and management

John G. F. Cleland and Andrew L. Clark

Essentials

Heart failure is a common clinical syndrome, often presenting with breathlessness, fatigue and peripheral oedema. It is predominantly a disease of older people. The prevalence is increasing, exceeding 2% of the adult population in developed countries.

Pathophysiology

The pathophysiology of heart failure is complex. A common feature is salt and water retention, possibly triggered by a relative fall in renal perfusion pressure. Common aetiologies include ischaemic heart disease, hypertension, and valvular heart disease.

Investigation

The early diagnosis of heart failure relies on a low threshold of suspicion and screening of people at risk before the onset of obvious symptoms or signs. In patients with suspected heart failure, routine investigation with electrocardiography and blood tests for urea and electrolytes, haemoglobin and BNP/NT-proBNP are recommended. Low plasma concentrations of BNP/NT-proBNP exclude most forms of heart failure. Intermediate or high concentrations should prompt referral for echocardiography to identify possible causes of heart failure and the left ventricular ejection fraction (LVEF). Patients can be classified as reduced (<40%) LVEF (HFrEF), normal (>50%) LVEF (HFnEF), or borderline (40–50%) LVEF (HFbEF). Currently HFbEF and HFnEF are managed similarly by current guidelines.

Treatment

Treatable causes for heart failure (e.g. valvular disease, tachyarrhythmias, thyrotoxicosis, anaemia or hypertension) should be identified and corrected. Patients with heart failure will generally benefit from lifestyle advice (diet, exercise, vaccination). Pharmacological therapy is given to improve symptoms and prognosis. Diuretic therapy is the mainstay for control of congestion and symptoms; it may be life-saving for patients with acute heart failure but its effect on long-term prognosis is unknown. For patients with HFrEF, either angiotensin converting enzyme (ACE) inhibitors, angiotensin receptor blockers, or, more recently, angiotensin receptor neprilysin inhibitors, combined with β-blockers and mineralocorticoid receptor antagonists (triple therapy) provide both symptomatic and prognostic benefit. Ivabridine may be added for those in sinus rhythm where the heart rate remains above 70 bpm. Whether digoxin still has a role in contemporary management is uncertain.

Cardiac resynchronization therapy is appropriate for symptomatic patients with HFrEF if they are in sinus rhythm and have a broad QRS (>140 ms). Implantable defibrillators provide additional prognostic benefit in selected patients with an ejection fraction below 35%. For patients with HFnEF, treatments directed at comorbid conditions (e.g. hypertension, atrial fibrillation) and congestion (e.g. diuretics and mineralocorticoid receptor antagonists) are appropriate but there is no robust evidence that any treatment can improve prognosis. Heart transplantation or assist devices may be options for highly selected patients with endstage heart failure; many others may benefit from palliative care services. Effective management of chronic heart failure requires a coordinated multidisciplinary team, including heart failure nurse specialists, primary care physicians, and cardiologists.

Prognosis

New treatments have improved the prognosis of heart failure substantially over the past two decades. The annual mortality is now probably less than 5% for patients with HFrEF receiving good contemporary care whose symptoms are stable and controlled. For patients with recurrent or recalcitrant congestion requiring admission to hospital, the prognosis is much worse. In-patient mortality is about 5% for those aged less than 75 years but threefold higher for older patients; mortality in the year after discharge ranges from 20% to 40% depending on age.

Introduction

Heart failure is the most common malignant disease in the United Kingdom. Heart failure, in its various manifestations, now causes or complicates twice as many hospital admissions (about half a million deaths and discharges each year in the United Kingdom) as do all cancers or acute coronary syndromes combined. This is likely to be a gross underestimate of total activity as the diagnosis of heart failure is often missed or ignored during admission. In the community, heart failure syndromes are almost as common as diabetes mellitus and far more deadly. Considering the enormous size of the problem, the effort expended in identifying and managing heart failure is pitiful; the current mainstay for the management of most patients is neglect.

For some cardiac phenotypes (e.g. left ventricular systolic function), treatment is often highly effective and may even be curative. However, diagnostic awareness is low and care, when given, is often fragmented and disorganized. Only a lucky minority receive the benefits of a high standard of care from someone with appropriate expertise.

The reasons for the current clinical neglect of heart failure are not entirely clear but may reflect the lack of a robust definition, the difficulty and uncertainties of its clinical diagnosis, the relative complexity of its treatment, all combined with ageism and fatalism, on the part of both the clinician and patient. Ultimately, heart failure may just be too large a problem for health services to have the energy and will to tackle.

Definition

No consensus has been reached on a simple, practical universal definition of heart failure. Indeed, it may be better to consider the diagnosis of heart failure across a spectrum of certainty based on clinical acumen supported by blood tests (particularly natriuretic peptides) and cardiac imaging.

Until now, most experts and guidelines have required that the patient should have symptoms before a diagnostic label of heart failure is applied. Of course, a sedentary lifestyle and liberal use of diuretics may mask symptoms. Simply asking the patient to take a walk will often reveal how poor the patient's effort tolerance is, and stopping diuretics, if you dare, will often lead to the diagnosis becoming obvious.

Other specialities use biochemical definitions to define organ failure (kidney, pancreas, liver). Central to the concept of heart failure is congestion, indicating that the heart is unable to sustain a normal filling (atrial) pressure for the required cardiac output. Cardiac output is usually fairly normal at rest until the late stages of heart failure. How then should congestion be measured? Natriuretic peptides, hormones that are secreted by the stressed heart and designed to counter sodium retention, provide a simple objective method of detecting congestion, even before it becomes clinically overt (Fig. 5.3.1). Thus, heart failure could be considered

cardiac dysfunction leading to an increase in natriuretic peptides. Natriuretic peptides are now an essential tool for the early detection and confirmation of a diagnosis of heart failure in a modern health service.

Broadening the definition of heart failure has many consequences, the most obvious being a great increase in the number of patients. About 3% of the adult population is taking loop diuretics for no obvious reason other than symptoms or signs suggestive of heart failure. Currently, most cases of heart failure are diagnosed during a hospital admission, suggesting that the diagnosis is usually missed until the problem is bad enough to provoke severe symptoms. The onset of symptomatic heart failure may well be precipitated by an acute event but usually on a background of chronic cardiac dysfunction. Earlier diagnosis will increase identification in the community before the onset of severe symptoms and at a time when therapy might be more effective.

Clinical physiology

Heart failure can be considered as a sequence of unfortunate events (Fig. 5.3.2), starting with cardiac (usually left ventricular) dysfunction leading to haemodynamic changes that are often initially subtle, including a rise in atrial pressures and a fall in blood pressure below the set-point for renal sodium retention. This triggers activation of neuroendocrine systems such as the renin–angiotensin–aldosterone and sympathetic nervous system in an attempt to restore blood pressure by vasoconstriction and blood volume expansion. This has long-term deleterious effects on the heart. Fortunately, there is also activation of counter-regulatory mechanisms, most notably the natriuretic peptides, which attempt to prevent sodium retention and delay the onset of symptomatic congestion. Eventually, counter-regulatory systems are overwhelmed and clinical evidence of congestion appears, manifest either as breathlessness (loosely related to left atrial pressure) or peripheral oedema (loosely related to right atrial pressure). The treatment of heart failure revolves around preventing or reversing congestion and avoiding sudden death due either to arrhythmias or vascular events.

Cardiac (imaging) phenotypes

Cardiac phenotype is strongly linked to the aetiology of cardiac dysfunction and is a key determinant of management. For some cardiac phenotypes there is little evidence that treatment alters outcome. Few patients have a single pure phenotype; most patients manifest several phenotypes but usually one is dominant (Table 5.3.1).

When heart failure is associated with a reduced left ventricular ejection fraction (LVEF) this is often termed HFrEF or left ventricular systolic dysfunction (LVSD). Patients with heart failure and a normal or preserved LVEF are termed HFnEF, HFpEF. Left ventricular diastolic dysfunction (LVDD) is a subset of HFnEF as it is possible to have HFnEF without LVDD (e.g. patients with isolated right ventricular dysfunction).

Various authorities suggest different LVEF thresholds for defining HFnEF, with the cutoff ranging from less than 40% to over 50%. Since echocardiographers usually refer to a LVEF of under 50% as LVSD the terminology is confusing and some believe that patients with an LVEF of 40 to 50% should be considered a separate group HFbEF (heart failure with a borderline LVEF), which

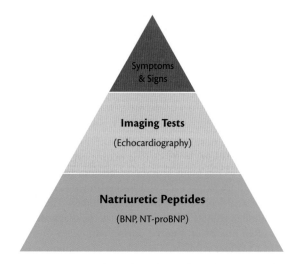

Fig. 5.3.1 Natriuretic peptides are the earliest and most sensitive sign of congestion but do not distinguish between cardiac and renal causes. Cardiac imaging is less sensitive and accurate (i.e. abnormal cardiac function may not cause congestion) for detecting congestion but, along with tests for heart rhythm and renal function, it helps to determine the cause of congestion. Symptoms and signs are late manifestations of congestion and usually only first detected when they have deteriorated sufficiently to precipitate a hospital admission.

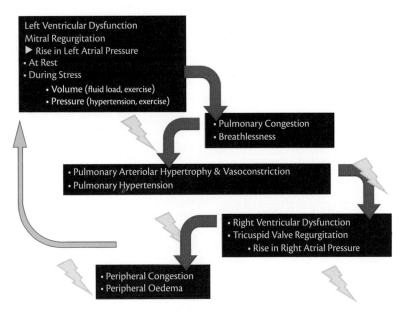

Fig. 5.3.2 Development and progression of heart failure. Lightning bolts signify the risk of sudden (arrhythmic) death.

seems a helpful concept. LVEF measured by conventional echocardiography is only accurate to within about 10%, although more advanced imaging techniques, such as cardiac MRI (CMRI), may have greater precision.

Each of the phenotypes is heterogeneous, particularly HFnEF (Fig. 5.3.3). HFrEF is the predominant cardiac phenotype in men and patients aged <75 years and is often due to ischaemic heart disease. HFnEF is the predominant phenotype in older women and is often due to hypertension. In patients with HFrEF, it is important to consider to what extent contractile dysfunction is due to dysfunction of viable myocardium, which may be reversible, or to consolidated scar that is likely to be irreversible using existing technology. The relative contribution of extra-cellular matrix and fibrosis and impaired cardiac myocyte relaxation to HFnEF is uncertain; the therapeutic target at the myocardial level is unclear. Heart failure due to valve disease may occur at any age but degenerative valve disease is an increasingly common cause in older people.

Table 5.3.1 Common cardiac phenotypes in heart failure

	HFrEF	HFbEF	HFpEF / HFnEF
LVEF	<40%	40-50%	>50%
Ischaemic Heart Disease	XXX	XX	X
Hypertension	X	XX	XXX
Atrial Fibrillation	XX	XX	XXX
Dilated Cardiomyopathy	XXX	?	NA
Aortic Stenosis	X	XX	XXX
Mitral Regurgitation	XX	XX	XX

Number of crosses reflects strength of association (although not necessarily proportion affected or prevalence).

HFrEF = heart failure with a reduced left ventricular ejection fraction.

HFbEF = heart failure with a reduced left ventricular ejection fraction.

HFpEF / HFnEF = heart failure with a preserved or normal left ventricular ejection fraction.

Risk factors and aetiology

The most important risk factor for heart failure is age. It is likely that everyone will develop heart failure if they live long enough. Biological rather than chronological age may account for the link between physical frailty and the risk of developing heart failure. Currently, one in five people is expected to develop heart failure before they die. This may be a gross underestimate given the diagnostic gap outlined above.

The most important medical risk factors for developing heart failure are hypertension and ischaemic heart disease and their combination may confer more than additive risk (Table 5.3.1). Both may go undetected and untreated for years; the onset of symptoms of heart failure may be the first time the patient seeks help. There is a wealth of evidence that hypertension, even when detected, is often poorly managed. Alarmingly, studies suggest that most myocardial infarctions, perhaps especially among older people, do not provoke symptoms sufficient for the person to seek immediate medical assistance. Good treatment of hypertension and other risk factors for coronary artery disease will undoubtedly delay the onset of disease. Poor lifestyle and inferior medical care probably account for the association between social deprivation and the onset of heart failure at an earlier age.

Among patients aged under 50 years, cardiomyopathies and congenital heart disease account for a large proportion of heart failure. In patients aged over 50 years, ischaemic heart disease is the dominant cause of HFrEF and hypertension the dominant cause of HFnEF. There are many rarer causes of heart failure (Table 5.3.2) but as a group these affect a substantial number of patients.

Diagnosis

Most heart failure is first diagnosed at a late stage in the disease subsequent to a hospital admission. Until screening the population at risk with natriuretic peptides becomes routine, this is unlikely to change.

Table 5.3.2 Some rarer causes of heart failure

Causes	Comments	Phenotype & Specific Therapy
Amyloidosis	Due to plasma cell expansion / myeloma (AL), transthyretin (ATTR) gene mutation or chronic infection/inflammation (AA). TTR mutations may cause 10% of HFpEF in older people.	Increased LV wall thickness, HFbEF or HFpEF. Often atrio-ventricular conduction delay. Poor prognosis for AL . Most patient die within a year of diagnosis. ATTR better prognosis. Specific therapies in discovery (eg:- tafamidis).
Haemochromatosis	High serum ferritin and transferrin saturation. Often diabetic. Affects ~0.05% of Northern Europeans	HFrEF or HFbEF. Often a restrictive picture. Treat with phlebotomy and iron chelation therapy. Early detection important
Haemosiderosis	Usually associated with multiple blood transfusions due to haemolytic or aplastic anaemia	
Carcinoid Syndrome	Caused by hepatic or more rarely pulmonary metastasis of serotonin secreting tumours	Tricuspid regurgitation and pulmonary stenosis leading to low output and peripheral congestion.
Sarcoid Heart Disease	Often associated with pulmonary disease.	HFrEF or HFpEF. Arrhythmias and conduction defects common.
Tachy-cardiomyopathy	Ventricular rate usually persistently >150bpm. Usually supra-ventricular but rarely ventricular tachycardia. Lower rates suggest that tachycardia is a consequence of heart failure.	Dilated cardiomyopathy. Resolves usually within a few weeks when arrhythmia is corrected.
Thyrotoxicosis	May be iodine / amiodarone induced. Weight loss, tachycardia and other features of thyroid hormone excess	High output
Phaeo-chromocytoma	Due to catecholamine secreting tumours – usually adrenal	HFrEF. Care with the use of adrenergic antagonists. Requires surgical correction
Genetic DCM	More than a dozen genetic mutations, notably of the titin gene.	HFrEF
Lamin A/C gene mutation	Rare	HFbEF. Atrio-ventricular conduction defects, ventricular arrhythmias and sudden death
Muscular Dystrophy	Duchenne, Becker and Myotonic Dystrophy	HFrEF often with conduction defects
Hypertrophic Cardiomyopathy	May be genetic or sporadic	HFpEF or HFbEF
Left Ventricular Non-Compaction	May be familial.	HFrEF or HFbEF
Endomyocardial Fibrosis	Usually a tropical disease possibly due to parasitic disease. Consider if eosinophilia	HFpEF or HFbEF. Restrictive defect.
Iatrogenic	Cancer chemotherapy, radiation, calcium channel blockers, hypoglycaemic therapies	Anthracycline and radiation induced damage may be irreversible. Maybe HFrEF or HFpEF
Nutritional Deficiency	Thiamine, iron, selenium	Rare unless severe deficiency
Peripartum Cardiomyopathy	Usually in last trimester or within a few weeks of delivery	May only be recognized when severe. Usually recovers if patient survives. May recur with further pregnancy.
Myocarditis	May be viral, including HIV, or due to borrelia (Lyme disease) or trypanosomiasis (Chaga's Disease). Giant cell myocarditis has a particularly poor prognosis.	HFrEF. HIV – often pulmonary hypertension. Chaga's disease – arrhythmias Borrelia – consider doxycycline Giant Cell – steroids? / immunosuppression?

There are six diagnostic steps:

Step 1: Case ascertainment

The first and most important step is suspecting that something might be wrong. The patient may complain of breathlessness, but this is a late manifestation of disease in a sedentary population. By the time orthopnoea, paroxysmal nocturnal dyspnoea, or breathlessness on mild exertion has developed, the disease is far advanced. Walking with the patient at a brisk pace may well provoke symptoms but does not lend itself to the organization of conventional clinics in primary or secondary care. Ankle oedema due to rising systemic venous pressure is also a late manifestation of disease and also carries low specificity. Symptoms and signs may be abolished by diuretic therapy but concerns exist that such treatment may accelerate the progression of disease by activating deleterious neuroendocrine system. Earlier detection of heart failure

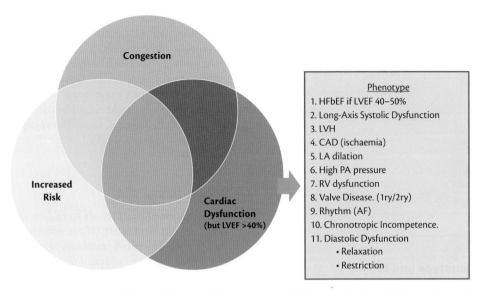

Fig. 5.3.3 Heterogeneity of heart failure with normal left ventricular ejection fraction. Conceptually, the diagnosis of heart failure requires evidence of congestion: for example, elevated natriuretic peptides, evidence of a cardiac abnormality, and (retrospectively) an increased risk of cardiovascular events.

requires a provocative test of cardiac reserve (e.g. a corridor walking test) or identification of activated compensatory mechanisms (e.g. natriuretic peptides) in patients deemed at risk of heart failure by virtue of age or medical risk factors. Any patient prescribed a loop diuretic should be presumed to have heart failure until proven otherwise.

Step 2: Proving that cardiac dysfunction and heart failure are present

Once heart failure is suspected, objective evidence of cardiac dysfunction is required. Breathlessness and ankle swelling are not specific to heart failure. Signs of heart failure, such as jugular venous distension, are relatively specific but insensitive, often difficult to elicit and are not easily recorded in a way that convinces colleagues who are uncertain of your skills. Chest radiography is no longer regarded as essential. A normal chest radiograph is not uncommon in patients with heart failure and radiographic cardiomegaly is frequently a spurious finding. The electrocardiogram (ECG) is almost universally abnormal in heart failure and if genuinely normal places the diagnosis in doubt.

Until recently, echocardiography was considered the practical gold-standard measure for cardiac dysfunction and focused almost exclusively on identifying valve disease and HFrEF. However, there is growing awareness of the limitations of echocardiography, especially when not interpreted by experts. Reproducibility of LVEF is poor and measurements of diastolic function are complex and often contradictory. Probably the best echocardiographic guide to cardiac dysfunction, at least when chronic, is atrial volumes.

Natriuretic peptides provide a simple alternative approach to diagnosis and are more closely associated with atrial volumes than many other measures of cardiac dysfunction. They are not only more sensitive than cardiac imaging but a better guide to the patient's prognosis. Natriuretic peptides are also more specific than imaging when the question is 'Does this patient have serious disease requiring further investigation?' rather than 'Does this patient have cardiac dysfunction?' A normal plasma concentration of a

natriuretic peptide in the absence of a diuretic effectively excludes heart failure with one uncommon exception; constrictive pericarditis. Gross obesity is associated with somewhat lower plasma concentrations of natriuretic peptides and diuretics may reduce them as they improve congestion. The N-terminal fragment of pro brain natriuretic peptide (NT-proBNP) is stable for days in blood samples and therefore can be measured easily and inexpensively in primary or secondary care. Interpretation of results requires additional information. Atrial fibrillation and renal dysfunction are other common reasons for an increase in plasma natriuretic peptides concentrations. Clinical acumen supported by a measurement of natriuretic peptide is usually sufficient to make or refute a diagnosis of heart failure (see Fig. 5.3.3).

Step 3: Differential diagnosis

If a patient has symptoms, merely excluding or diagnosing heart failure is not enough. Alternative causes of symptoms should be sought. The common differential diagnoses for breathlessness are lung disease, obesity, and being unfit, all of which may coexist with heart failure. Determining how much each is contributing to symptoms will help guide use of diuretics; dehydrating patients with lung disease is unlikely to make them better and may make them worse. Spirometry may help identify lung disease but low values may reflect general frailty and poor technique rather than lung disease. Natriuretic peptides can help; a slim patient who is very breathless but only has moderately elevated NT-proBNP is likely to have lung disease as the dominant pathology. Cardiopulmonary exercise testing aids differential diagnosis but requires special equipment and expertise. In particular, a diagnosis of HFnEF made on the isolated echocardiographic finding of diastolic dysfunction should always be made with caution and only following exclusion of alternative pathology. Echocardiographic evidence of mild diastolic dysfunction is very common in elderly people and heart failure can be readily over-diagnosed. Conditions that in isolation or in combination that may masquerade as 'diastolic heart failure' are listed in Table 5.3.3.

Table 5.3.3 Conditions masquerading as diastolic heart failure

COPD/Cor pulmonale (without RV dysfunction)
Obesity-hypoventilation syndrome
Obstructive sleep apnoea
Severe renal disease
Anaemia
Thyrotoxicosis
Nephrotic syndrome
Silent myocardial ischaemia
Venous insufficiency
Lymphatic obstruction

Step 4: Cardiac phenotype and cause(s) of cardiac dysfunction

Clinical acumen combined with natriuretic peptides may be enough to make a diagnosis of heart failure but is a poor guide to cardiac phenotype. The workhorse of cardiac phenotyping is the echocardiogram. The echocardiogram provides an approximate guide to LVEF and therefore differentiates HFrEF from HFnEF, identifies abnormal heart valves, and quantifies atrial volumes. Of the many parameters of diastolic function increased left atrial size is probably the simplest and most reliable and is an important prognostic indicator regardless of baseline left ventricular function. For patients with HFrEF, the amount of myocardial scar is an important determinant of the response to treatment and is best assessed by CMRI. However, many heart failure services have little access to this investigation. Radionuclear imaging is an alternative.

A diagnosis of coronary disease can usually be made based on the clinical history or, failing that, by CMRI, stress echo, or radionuclear imaging. In the absence of symptomatic angina there is no evidence that revascularization improves outcome in patients with chronic heart failure. The presence or absence of coronary disease should have little influence on the choice of pharmacological or device treatment; there is no evidence that antiplatelet agents are safe or effective in this setting. Angiography should therefore be reserved for patients with limiting angina despite pharmacological therapy and in those presenting with heart failure in the context of an acute coronary syndrome. CT angiography can be used if it is felt necessary to exclude left main-stem or other proximal coronary artery disease. There is little information to be gained from heart catheterization that cannot be obtained more pleasantly, safely and at lower cost by noninvasive methods that may also supply information that the angiogram cannot.

Step 5: Comorbidity—what other problems might exacerbate or complicate heart failure?

Patients rarely only have heart failure. Identifying important cardiovascular and noncardiovascular comorbidity provides additional therapeutic targets (Table 5.3.4).

Step 6: Diagnostic tests required to achieve therapeutic aims

The therapeutic goals should first be defined. If it is palliative care, then only treatments designed to control symptoms are appropriate

(this may include diuretics, ACE inhibitors, mineralocorticoid antagonists (MRA), cardiac resynchronization therapy, and possibly digoxin and intravenous iron). If the goal is to improve prognosis through 'disease-modifying' interventions then β-blockers, ivabradine, and implantable cardiac defibrillators should be added to the list. Preventing patients with atrial fibrillation from developing the misery of a stroke might be considered appropriate regardless of other therapeutic aims. The small amount of information (ten items) routinely required to use these agents safely and effectively is shown in Table 5.3.5.

Prognosis

The prognosis of heart failure should be separated into four broad categories: incident heart failure (which is associated with a 30% mortality at 6 months), mortality during readmission for worsening heart failure (which is about 10–15%), mortality in the 6 months after discharge from a readmission (which is 15–25%), and annual mortality of chronic stable patients (which may now be <5% per annum). Age is an important determinant of mortality (Figure 5.3.4).

Readmission rates are also high; most patients will be admitted at least once in a 3 year period and following a readmission, 15 to 25% will have a further readmission within 30 days without expert support. Age is not such a good predictor of readmission, perhaps because older people have a higher mortality and because death prevents readmission.

Diagnostic assessment also provides important prognostic information. A pragmatic prognostic scoring system for chronic heart failure exist (<http://www.heartfailurerisk.org/>) that may be improved by adding some simple pieces of information, such as whether the patient has had a recent exacerbation of symptoms, the dose of diuretic, and plasma concentration of NT-proBNP. Knowing prognosis can help with management both in terms of advice to the patient and choice of therapy.

Treatment

Modern management of patients with heart failure requires the coordinated input of a multidisciplinary team of dedicated cardiologists, specialist heart failure and rehabilitation nurses, primary care physicians, and palliative care specialists. The key to the successful management of these patients is prompt identification in the community and following admission to hospital, and access to follow-up and management by a specialist team.

Lifestyle

Patients with heart failure should be advised to lead a healthy lifestyle, avoiding smoking and excessive alcohol consumption, eating a balanced diet, and taking regular exercise (<http://www.heartfailurematters.org/en_GB>). There is little evidence that such advice makes a difference to prognosis, but it probably improves well-being. Attention to psychological health is important. Keeping socially active, taking holidays (with adequate health insurance; <http://www.bhf.org.uk/heart-health/living-with-a-heart-condition/living-with-heart-failure.aspx>) and investing in hobbies and recreations are more important than pharmacological treatments for anxiety and depression that are, however, mostly safe. There is no evidence that complementary medicine can alter

Table 5.3.4 Common problems (comorbidities) complicating the diagnosis and management of heart failure

Problem	Comment
Obesity (and lack of fitness)	Alternative cause for breathlessness creating diagnostic uncertainty and problems with judging diuretic dose. Diuresis will not help breathlessness due to obesity. Obesity is consistently associated with a better prognosis in a broad spectrum of patients with cardiovascular disease, including heart failure
Cachexia	Ominous sign in heart failure. Exclude cancerous malignant disease. If patient is a candidate for transplant or mechanical assist, consider urgent referral.
COPD	Alternative cause for breathlessness creating diagnostic uncertainty and problems with judging diuretic dose. Diuresis will not help breathlessness due to COPD. Patients with heart failure and COPD have a worse prognosis
Atrial Fibrillation	AF may cause heart failure and vice versa. Optimal ventricular rate control may be about 80bpm at rest. Need for anti-coagulation.
Ischaemic Heart Disease	Common cause of a reduced LVEF. Little evidence that revascularisation improves prognosis. Coronary angiography only indicated if patient has angina. Ongoing research into revascularisation of viable myocardium but randomised controlled trials neutral so far.
Hypertension	A sign that the left ventricle still has some reserve. Most treatments for heart failure reduce blood pressure. So hypertension is a good sign!
Hypotension	Often limits amount of pharmacological treatment. Bad prognostic sign. Cardiac resynchronisation will increase systolic blood pressure in appropriately selected patients.
Anaemia	Often associated with iron deficiency although not always corrected by oral or even intravenous iron. Some anaemia is dilutional (plasma volume expansion) and some caused by renal dysfunction and deficient erythropoiesis. Folate and B12 are rarely important causes of anaemia in heart failure.
Diabetes Mellitus	Indicates a worse prognosis, possibly because of associated renal problems. Treatment for diabetes may make heart failure worse. Optimal HbA1c in patients with heart failure being treated for diabetes may be around 7.5% (lower if 'pre-diabetic').
Chronic Kidney Disease	Often due to pre-existing renal damage and exacerbated by hypotension and low renal blood flow. Often limits the doses of medication that can be given. Renal function is a powerful prognostic marker (more powerful than LVEF)
Stroke	Related mainly to pre-existing hypertension, atherosclerosis and atrial fibrillation.
Dementia	Age often brings deterioration in cognitive as well as cardiac function. Dementia reduces ability for self-care and adherence to advice and medication. Worsening heart failure may impair cognitive function
Aortic Stenosis	Common in older people. Diuretics may reduce congestion and symptoms but other medication may be of little help and may cause hypotension. Consider aortic valve surgery or transcutaneous procedure.
Mitral Regurgitation	Common in all forms of heart failure. May improve with treatments that reduce ventricular volume, especially cardiac resynchronization. Patient selection for surgery often difficult. Transcutaneous repair may be considered.

the course of heart failure but, provided the patient is not tempted to stop conventional therapy, it may provide them with a psychological support. Patients should know what medication to take and have a system to ensure it is done.

Excessive dietary salt and fluid consumption should be avoided but there is scant evidence that severe restriction of dietary salt is helpful and it might do harm. Fluid restriction (to <1.5 litres/day) may be required in patients with advanced, diuretic-resistant heart failure. The ideal body mass index for a patient with heart failure is probably about 30 kg/m². Dieting to lose weight might improve symptoms but there is no evidence that it will improve prognosis and it may be harmful. Patients with severe heart failure may develop cachexia (in the context of heart failure, this may mean achieving a normal body mass index) that may be partly due to reduced calorie intake. Trying to improve appetite seems reasonable although of uncertain prognostic value and may not reverse weight loss. There is no evidence that supplementing the diet with vitamins or trace elements helps.

Patients with heart failure are at increased risk of dying from influenza and pneumococcal pneumonia and should receive these vaccinations although there is no specific evidence that they alter outcome in patients with heart failure.

It is important to be sensitive to the patient's view of their illness. Many patients will not want to discuss how they are likely to die, others will. Developing counselling skills that allow patients to raise issues such as death and identifying when a patient has run out of therapeutic options and requires palliative care is an important part of a heart failure service.

It is also important to address the worries and concerns of carers and the patient's social network as this may help them to support the patient with issues such as adherence to medicine, keeping appointments or doing monitoring tests.

Treatment of HFrEF

The change in prognosis exerted by pharmacological and device therapy for patients with HFrEF (Table 5.3.5) is among the most remarkable success stories for any malignant disease in the last quarter century (see Fig. 5.3.4).

Loop and thiazide diuretics

Diuretics are the most effective method of dealing with congestion, regardless of cardiac cause. They are also the most abused and least evaluated class of medication for heart failure. They are generally given at a fixed daily dose but many patients can do without their

Table 5.3.5 Indications for therapy and information required for choosing and monitoring key treatments in heart failure

	HISTORY	EXAMINATION		ELECTROCARDIOGRAM			BLOOD TESTS			ECHOCARDIOGRAM (evidence base for use)	
	SOB (NYHA CLASS)	BP	OEDEMA	HR	AF	QRS	K	GFR	BNP	HFrEF	HFpEF (>40%)
Loop Diuretics	II - IV	X	X				X	X		Symptomatic	Symptomatic
ACE/ARB	II - IV	X					X	X		Symptomatic/Prognostic	Symptomatic
ARNI	II - IV	X					X	X	X	Symptomatic/Prognostic	?
β - Blocker	II - IV	X		X	X					Prognostic	?
MRA	II - IV	X					X	X		Symptomatic/Prognostic (<35%)	?
Ivabridine	II - IV			X	X					Symptomatic/Prognostic (<35%)	?
Digoxin	III-IV	X		X	X		X	X		Symptomatic	?
Hydralazine/ Nitrates	III - IV	X								Symptomatic/Prognostic	?
ICD	I - III					>120 msec				Prognostic (<35%)	?
CRT	II - IV			X	X	>120 msec/ LBBB				Symptomatic/Prognostic (35%)	

ARNI – angiotensin receptor nepilysin inhibitor; MRA – mineralocorticoid receptor antagonist; ICD – implantable cardiodefibrillator; CRT – cardiac resynchronisation therapy; X indicates where information is required to guide treatment.

diuretics for several days at a time and others for much longer. Some advocate adjusting the diuretic dose to maintain an ideal weight; this suits some patients. Diuretic-free days may allow the patient greater freedom of activity. Reliable daily weight monitoring with accurate scales, potentially as part of a telemonitoring programme, may facilitate this strategy.

In most countries, diuretics acting on the loop of Henle, which produce a powerful diuresis lasting a few hours, are preferred. Once the diuresis is over, avid renal salt and water retention occur. In some countries, thiazide diuretics acting on the distal convoluted tubule are preferred first-line agents. They produce a less powerful but much longer natriuresis. This may result in similar 24 h sodium excretion to loop diuretics, but some patients will complain of an increase in nocturia and the rate of hyperkalaemia and hyponatraemia may be higher. Thiazides are said to be ineffective when renal function is substantially impaired. In patients with hypertension, thiazide diuretics have repeatedly been shown to reduce myocardial infarction, stroke, heart failure, and death. Similar evidence for loop diuretics is lacking.

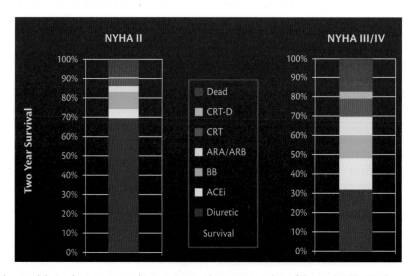

Fig. 5.3.4 Cumulative effect of drugs and device therapy on mortality in patients with symptomatic heart failure and LVEF <40% between the ages of 50 and 70 years (baseline mortality represented by that on diuretic therapy only).

Typically, a patient will be initiated on 40 mg of furosemide or 1 mg of bumetanide per day. The patient should be warned that the first few doses are likely to provoke a marked diuresis but that this will subside as pathophysiological signals for salt and water retention intensify (the 'braking' effect). Diuretics may provoke urinary retention in patients with prostatic disease. Serum electrolytes and renal function should be monitored. If serum potassium drops below 4.0 mmol/litre then a potassium-sparing diuretic should be given; usually an MRA.

Patients with severe congestion may be treated with high doses of loop diuretics or with a combination of loop and thiazide diuretics. It is unclear which is the better strategy. An MRA may be added to either combination to prevent hypokalaemia and further enhance natriuresis.

Angiotensin converting enzyme inhibitors, angiotensin receptor blockers, and renin inhibitors

ACE inhibitors are one of the cornerstones of contemporary therapy for HFrEF. The onset of heart failure provokes the production of renin and, in turn, angiotensin II which stimulates AT1 receptors that cause vasoconstriction, secretion of aldosterone, and sodium retention. Activation of the renin–angiotensin–aldosterone system (RAAS) is subtle until diuretics are given. ACE inhibitors block the production of angiotensin II. The ACE is also responsible for the breakdown of bradykinin, which may be responsible for side effects such as cough (much more common in women) and angioneurotic oedema. Persistent cough should be investigated radiologically to identify any underlying pulmonary pathology. Bradykinin also stimulates the production of prostacyclin, which may be an important part of the mode of action of ACE inhibitors. Aspirin blocks the production of prostacyclin and may detract from benefit.

ACE inhibitors improve symptoms and exercise capacity, have favourable effect on ventricular remodelling (disease progression), reduce the risks of atrial fibrillation and hospitalization for heart failure, and delay death by reducing the rate of both sudden death and death from progressive heart failure. In addition to idiosyncratic side effects such as cough and angioneurotic oedema, they will usually reduce blood pressure and increase serum potassium and creatinine, each of which may be dose limiting. In patients with renal artery stenosis, the rise in serum creatinine may be marked.

ACE inhibitors are contraindicated in pregnancy or during breastfeeding and in patients with a history of angioneurotic oedema. They should be used with caution in patients with a low blood pressure, high serum potassium, or marked renal dysfunction.

ACE inhibitors should be started at a low dose, typically enalapril 2.5 mg bd or ramipril 1.25 mg bd. If the patient has well-maintained blood pressure and renal function and frequent monitoring is possible (e.g. in hospital), then doses may be doubled every 48 h up to a target of 10–20 mg bd for enalapril or 5 mg bd for ramipril. Patients who do not achieve guideline target doses quickly may never achieve them unless the continuity of care is excellent. For more fragile patients, titration of ACE inhibitors at 2 week intervals with a blood test at each step is recommended. Dose-ranging studies of ACE inhibitors failed to show a striking advantage to higher doses, although patients at the milder end of the spectrum may benefit more from higher doses, perhaps because they can tolerate them. Asymptomatic low blood pressure should not deter attaining guideline target doses, but excessive increases in potassium and creatinine require dose reduction or may occasionally prevent use of ACE inhibitors. See section on blood pressure in 'Practical aspects of monitoring and management' for further details.

ARBs inhibit the binding of angiotensin II to the AT1 receptor. The AT2 receptor is not blocked and there is some evidence that this may be beneficial. Bradykinin degradation is not blocked and therefore ARBs do not cause cough or angioneurotic oedema. Overall, ARBs appear to have similar benefits to ACE inhibitors but the evidence is somewhat less convincing and so they are a second choice (e.g. for patients who have troublesome cough with an ACE inhibitor). It is possible that ARBs are only effective when used in high doses. There may be some benefit to adding an ARB on top of an ACE inhibitor, but ACE inhibitors combined with MRAs are now preferred; triple therapy with ACE inhibitor, MRA, and ARB should be avoided.

The results of a large trial of a renin inhibitor used as an alternative or in addition to an ACE inhibitor should report in 2015 but currently there is no role for these agents in heart failure.

Angiotensin receptor–neprilysin inhibitors (ARNI)

LCZ696 (valsartan/sacubitril) is the first of a new class of drug which is a hybrid of an ARB (valsartan) and a neutral endopeptidase or neprilysin inhibitor, an enzyme responsible for inhibiting the degradation of both natriuretic peptides and bradykinin. At the time of writing, a clinical trial comparing LCZ with enalapril in more than 8000 patients has just been stopped due to substantial benefit on morbidity and mortality (about double that of an ACE inhibitor alone). Potentially, this will lead to a revolution in care, sweeping aside both ACE inhibitors and ARBs for patients with HFrEF and increased plasma concentrations of natriuretic peptides (e.g. NT-proBNP >600 ng/litre), although it may not be available for prescription until 2016. Cost-effectiveness may be the key factor driving uptake. A large trial in HFpEF is now under way.

Mineralocorticoid receptor antagonists

Addition of an MRA to either an ACE inhibitor or an ARB has become another cornerstone of the contemporary management of HFrEF. Although ACE inhibitors and ARBs reduce the secretion of aldosterone, suppression is incomplete. MRAs block the effects of aldosterone much more effectively. MRAs improve symptoms and reduce hospitalizations and death due to worsening heart failure, reduce the incidence of atrial fibrillation presumably by treating congestion, and reduce the risk of sudden death, possibly by preventing hypokalaemia. All the benefits of MRAs may be explained by their ability to reduce urinary potassium and increase urinary sodium excretion and the associated fall in blood pressure. However, some believe that MRAs may also reduce myocardial fibrosis but there is little evidence that MRAs improve underlying myocardial function or remodelling. Spironolactone stimulates oestrogen receptors that may cause gynaecomastia and testicular atrophy that become clinically problematic in about 10% of men. Eplerenone is more selective and does not cause these problems.

MRAs should not be given to patients with a serum potassium greater than 4.9 mmol/litre and should be used with caution in patients with substantial renal dysfunction or low blood pressure, and in frail elderly patients.

Spironolactone and eplerenone should generally be started at 25 mg/day. Lower initial doses may be appropriate in older patients with impaired renal function (e.g. 25 mg on Monday, Wednesday, Friday—daily doses are unnecessary and splitting tablets can be problematic). The dose should be adjusted according to the effects on serum potassium, renal function, and blood pressure. The ideal serum potassium is around 4.5 mmol/litre. Doses of MRA should be increased to get serum potassium to this target but reduced if potassium rises above 4.9 mmol/litre. Titration at 2 week intervals is generally appropriate unless the serum potassium is below 3.5 mmol/litre, in which case more urgent action is required.

β-Blockers

Addition of a β-blocker to ACE inhibitor or ARB and an MRA (triple therapy) is the third cornerstone of the contemporary management of HFrEF. Typically, an ACE inhibitor and β-blocker will be started in low doses at the same time. The dose of ACE inhibitor will be increased every day, week, or fortnight but the β-blocker more slowly at 2 to 4 week intervals. MRAs are then added sooner if potassium is low or congestion is severe or if not, later, once titration of the ACE inhibitor and β-blocker are complete.

The sympathetic nervous system is activated in heart failure leading to increases in heart rate, cardiac myocyte dysfunction, and weight loss (cachexia). Blockade of adrenergic receptors reduces heart rate and reverses cardiac myocyte dysfunction, often leading to a remarkable recovery in myocardial function (although not scar) and may retard, prevent, or reverse the development of cardiac cachexia. These effects lead to a reduction in mortality from worsening heart failure. Adrenergic receptor blockade also reduces the risk of supraventricular and ventricular arrhythmias, coronary events, and sudden death. How much of the benefit of β-blockers is mediated by reduction in heart rate or by other mechanisms is unclear. Recent analyses suggest that β-blockers may not be effective in patients with HFrEF and atrial fibrillation (see section on heart rate in 'Practical aspects of monitoring and management').

β-Blockers are contraindicated in patients with bradycardia, impaired atrioventricular conduction (unless the patient has a pacemaker), asthma (although not in most patients with chronic lung disease, who have little reversibility with sympathomimetic bronchodilators), and in patients with severe uncontrolled congestion. Initiation of a β-blocker may cause some initial worsening of congestion and symptoms. Overcautious clinicians are probably a major reason for patient side effects and intolerance.

Many β-blockers are available but only four have been shown to be effective for HFrEF. Three are selective for the β_1-receptor— bisoprolol, metoprolol succinate (not available in the UK) and nebivolol. There is one nonselective agent, carvedilol. There is some evidence that carvedilol may be superior and it is the best studied in trials.

β-blockers should be started at a low dose (e.g. carvedilol 3.125 mg bd or bisoprolol 1.25 mg once daily) and titrated upwards at 2 to 4 week intervals to target doses (carvedilol 25–50 mg bd or bisoprolol 10 mg/day). In sinus rhythm the optimal resting heart rate appears to be 50–60 bpm, and doses should be adjusted to try to achieve this target. Achieving optimal heart rate appears more important than the dose of β-blocker. Low doses of β-blocker may confer most of their benefits but may be insufficient to optimize heart rate. In atrial fibrillation, a ventricular rate of 75–85 bpm is associated with the best prognosis. If a β-blocker is used in atrial fibrillation then aggressive titration should be avoided. Fatigue and hypotension, or perhaps prescribing inertia on the part of doctors, prevents many patients from achieving target doses.

Ivabradine

Ivabradine slows the rate of discharge of the sinus node and, so far, has been shown to have very few other effects. It slows heart rate only when the patient is in sinus rhythm. In patients with HFrEF and a resting sinus rate in excess of 70 bpm, ivabradine improves cardiac function and symptoms and reduces hospitalization and death from worsening heart failure. It does not reduce arrhythmias or prevent sudden death.

Ivabradine is indicated only when β-blocker have failed to reduce sinus rate below 70 bpm. Many patients are perceived to be intolerant of doses of β-blockers required to control heart rate but this can often be overcome by extra care and persuasion. Most patients with chronic lung disease tolerate β-blockers. Unlike β-blockers, ivabradine does not reduce blood pressure and has little or no effect on atrioventricular conduction. Younger patients with dilated cardiomyopathy may obtain larger benefits from ivabradine. Ivabradine is effective in patients who are unable to tolerate β-blockers. However, patients should be strongly encouraged to take at least a low dose of β-blocker in addition. The channels that ivabradine acts on are also present in the retina. Distortion of colour vision, especially while driving at night, may occur but usually settles in a few weeks. Ivabradine is conventionally started at 5 mg bd and adjusted down to 2.5 mg bd or up to 7.5 mg bd to attain a resting heart rate of 50–60 bpm.

Alternative vasodilators

There is no certain place for other vasodilator agents in patients with heart failure. Although venous and arteriolar vasodilatation may have beneficial haemodynamic effects there is little evidence that this improves symptoms or outcome. Vasodilatation may provoke further renal sodium retention and merely shunt blood through tissues, thereby reducing the useful work of the heart. For instance, there is evidence that both sildenafil and endothelin antagonists may increase pulmonary shunting in patients with heart failure, leading to a fall in arterial oxygen saturation. Similar shunting of blood may occur through peripheral tissues.

Neither nitrates nor hydralazine used alone has been shown to improve symptoms or outcome in patients with heart failure. However, when used in combination there is some evidence of benefit similar to that of ACE inhibitors but potentially with less adverse effects on renal function. Some doctors use this combination as an alternative to ACE inhibitors in patients with severe renal dysfunction (for instance eGFR <20 ml/min). Few patients in trials or clinical practice were able to tolerate the high doses intended.

A study in patients of African-American origin suggested an improvement in morbidity and mortality when added to contemporary medical therapy including ACE inhibitors, β-blockers, and MRA. This study has not been repeated in other racial groups.

Vasodilator calcium antagonists have also failed to improve outcome and other agents of this class, such as diltiazem and verapamil, have an adverse effect on outcome.

Inotropic agents

There is no firm place for any inotropic agent in patients with chronic heart failure. Whether digoxin has a role in the contemporary management of heart failure is uncertain since the trials of digoxin demonstrating modest benefit were conducted before the widespread introduction of β-blockers and MRA. These agents might have rendered digoxin obsolete but also might have made it safer and more effective. Digoxin has vagomimetic effects, slowing sinus rate and prolonging atrioventricular conduction and therefore ventricular rate in patients with sinus rhythm or atrial fibrillation. It is also a diuretic. It does not drop and may increase blood pressure. For digoxin-naive patients with severe heart failure, an initial loading dose that does not need to be adjusted for renal dysfunction is appropriate. Maintenance doses should be adjusted according to renal function, erring on the side of caution in older people. The contemporary fashion is to use lower maintenance doses of digoxin, typically 125 micrograms/day for a standard-sized, middle-aged patient with good renal function and 62.5 micrograms/day for older, frailer patients. Monitoring of serum digoxin is rarely necessary. Prevention of hypokalaemia that increases the risk of digoxin-induced arrhythmia is important.

Antiarrhythmic agents

Amiodarone and dronedarone should only be given after expert advice and should be discontinued unless there is a clear need. In patients with moderate or severe heart failure and HFrEF addition of these agents to contemporary therapy increases mortality. They have a limited role in maintaining sinus rhythm in atrial fibrillation and for the symptomatic treatment of ventricular tachycardia. Side effects such as pulmonary fibrosis or hepatitis are rare provided the maintenance dose of amiodarone is 200 mg/day or less. Photosensitivity and hypothyroidism are problems with long-term treatment. In iodine deficiency, initiation of amiodarone may cause a thyrotoxic storm. Other antiarrhythmic agents should generally be avoided in heart failure as they have adverse effects on cardiac function and prognosis.

Lipid-modifying therapies

There is no established role for lipid-modifying therapies in patients with heart failure. Two large trials of rosuvastatin failed to show a reduction in mortality, although some reduction in hospitalizations was observed. Considering all of the evidence, it is likely that patients with less severe cardiac dysfunction (e.g. NT-proBNP <1000 ng/litre) do benefit from statins but that patients with more advanced disease do not. Some argue that treatment should be rationalized and statins withdrawn. Others argue that there is no evidence of harm and some evidence for a reduction in morbidity and that they should be continued. Informed patients may wish to express an opinion. Both neutral trials used rosuvastatin. There might be differences in effect among agents. One large trial suggested a small reduction in mortality with the addition of omega-3 fatty acids to contemporary heart failure therapy. This awaits confirmation.

Anticoagulants and antiplatelet agents

Patients with heart failure and paroxysmal or persistent atrial fibrillation should be anticoagulated. Warfarin has been the mainstay for many decades but newer agents that do not require therapeutic monitoring may be less likely to cause intracranial bleeding. Antiplatelet therapies are not effective in reducing emboli and markedly increase the risk of bleeding when used concomitantly with anticoagulants. They should usually be withdrawn when anticoagulants are introduced unless the patient has had a recent cardiac procedure.

There is no evidence that anticoagulant or antiplatelet agents, including aspirin, improve outcome in patients with heart failure in sinus rhythm whether or not the patient has coronary artery disease. There are theoretical concerns about the safety of aspirin in patients with heart failure but no robust evidence to refute or support its use. Aspirin might be partly responsible for the epidemic of iron deficiency anaemia now observed in heart failure.

Medicines to avoid

Some medicines should be avoided because evidence of benefit is lacking. Aspirin, statins, and omega-3 fatty acids might fall into this category. Other agents are harmful. For patients with HFrEF, rate-limiting calcium channel blockers increase morbidity and mortality. Oral hypoglycaemic agents may cause fluid retention, probably by increasing renal insulin sensitivity, or exacerbate heart failure in other ways. Metformin is relatively contraindicated in renal dysfunction in heart failure because of an increased risk of lactic acidosis, although this is rare. Non-steroidal anti-inflammatory drugs, including aspirin, may cause worsening renal function and hyperkalaemia. Paracetamol and opioids are the preferred analgesics. Many cancer chemotherapies are associated with cardiac toxicity. Amiodarone and dronedarone should be avoided unless there is a clear indication.

Other medicines in development

The failing heart has a shortened ejection time. Omecamtiv mecarbil is a cardiac myosin activator that prolongs the duration of systole and therefore increase stroke volume and efficiency. Large clinical trials are just getting under way.

The effects of adding to background therapy (usually including aspirin) a low dose of rivaroxaban, a factor Xa antagonist, on vascular events and mortality in patients with heart failure is being studied.

Soluble guanylate cyclase inhibitors and stimulators, novel MRAs, vaptans, nitroxyl donors, ryanodine channel stabilizers, agents acting on the mitochondrial respiratory chain, and superabsorbent polymers are among a substantial array of compounds under investigation.

Gene therapy and stem cells

The potential to improve cardiac myocyte function by transfecting cells with the SERCA2a (to improve calcium uptake of the sarcoplasmic reticulum) or ribonucleotide reductase (to increase synthesis of dATP) genes is being explored. Administering a variety of stem cells has met with little success so far. Small molecules that activate the patient's own stem cells are another avenue of research.

Devices used to treat HFrEF

Implantable cardioverter–defibrillators

Most patients with mild to moderate heart failure will die suddenly rather than progress to terminal disease. Sudden death is often due to a ventricular arrhythmia, either spontaneous or provoked by myocardial ischaemia or infarction. Implantable cardioverter–defibrillators (ICDs) deliver pacing and shock therapy to terminate ventricular arrhythmias. They reduce the rate of sudden death by about 70% but, as might be expected, patients then often die for other reasons. Overall ICDs exert a 1 to 2% absolute annual reduction in all-cause mortality. A patient has to avoid dying of other things for quite a long time before benefiting substantially from an ICD! ICDs do not improve and may impair symptoms and quality of life. The risk of inappropriate shocks has declined dramatically after much longer device-diagnostic delays were introduced prior to delivering ICD therapy. Forcing ICDs to hesitate before they intervene has revealed that most ventricular tachycardia self-terminates. The ideal candidate for an ICD has mild heart failure, a low ejection fraction and a QRS duration exceeding 120 ms, which is rather similar to the criteria for implanting a cardiac resynchronization therapy (CRT) device. Indeed, it is possible that patients who are not candidates for CRT have little to gain from an ICD. Implanting a CRT device rather than an ICD in an appropriate patient may increase the benefit of the ICD component of therapy, although CRT alone can reduce sudden death. In summary, there is no statistical doubt that ICDs reduce sudden death and all-cause mortality but there are grave doubts about their cost-effectiveness in the absence of a concomitantly implanted CRT.

Cardiac resynchronization therapy

CRT in appropriately selected patients improves ventricular function, reduces mitral regurgitation, raises blood pressure, improves symptoms and quality of life, reduces recurrent hospitalization for heart failure, and increases longevity substantially by reducing the rate of both sudden death and endstage heart failure. Adding an ICD function to a CRT device may prevent some sudden deaths and provide modest incremental benefit to CRT alone. Current evidence suggests that patients with HFrEF (up to an LVEF of 40%) in sinus rhythm with a QRS duration of more than 140 ms, who have been stabilized on optimal medical therapy, are likely to benefit from CRT regardless of the severity in symptoms. Patients with a QRS duration between 130 and 140 ms may get some benefit, but patients with a QRS duration of less than 130 ms may be harmed by CRT. Patients with ischaemic heart disease have less improvement in cardiac function than patients with dilated cardiomyopathy but similar prognostic benefit. It is not clear whether QRS morphology is important, although left bundle branch block is associated with longer QRS duration which is, in turn, associated with a better response to CRT. Whether patients with atrial fibrillation (AF) benefit from CRT is controversial, although some advocate CRT with atrioventricular node ablation. Many uncertainties exist about the optimal programming of devices. Expert advice should be sought for patients who have had a disappointing response to CRT.

Comorbidity and its impact on drug therapy

Valve disease

Valve repair or replacement should be considered for all patients with heart failure and substantial mitral or aortic valve disease. Pharmacological treatment, other than for the treatment of congestion, will make little difference to symptoms, disease progression, or prognosis in the presence of substantial aortic or mitral stenosis. Patients with aortic stenosis should be considered for aortic valve surgery or trans-arterial aortic valve implantation (TAVI). Mitral regurgitation is often functional due to left ventricular dysfunction. Although severe mitral regurgitation due to structural disease may benefit from surgical repair, the results of surgery for functional mitral regurgitation are less certain. Transcutaneous procedures to reduce mitral regurgitation have met with some success. On the other hand, surgical correction of tricuspid regurgitation is of dubious benefit and carries substantial risk. Pulmonary valve disease is not common. Diuretics may relieve the symptoms of congestion in patients with aortic or mitral regurgitation for long periods, allowing the disease to progress beyond the optimal timing of surgery.

Renal dysfunction

Renal dysfunction is a bad prognostic sign in heart failure and yet many agents that improve prognosis cause a decline in glomerular filtration rate. Clearly, at some point there will be a trade-off between the benefits of therapy and their adverse effect on renal function. Precisely where that point lies is unknown. Patients with renal dysfunction are prone to developing hyperkalaemia.

Renal dysfunction often precedes the development of heart failure and reflects the damage that hypertension has done to both heart and kidney. Many patients will have renal artery atheroma. Low arterial and high venous pressures conspire to produce a low net renal perfusion pressure, which is a major determinant of renal function.

The introduction of an ACE or angiotensin II often causes a rise in serum creatinine, and an increase of up to 50% may be acceptable provided renal function subsequently stabilizes. A rise in creatinine may occur also on starting the MRA spironolactone, reflecting in part inhibition of active secretion of creatinine by the renal tubules rather than a decline in GFR.

Many medicines are excreted by the kidney and therefore lower doses are required to obtain plasma concentrations similar to those in people with normal renal function.

Improving the net renal perfusion pressure, avoiding NSAIDs (including aspirin), stopping non-ACE/ARB antihypertensive agents, and if this fails allowing efferent renal arteriolar tone to increase by reducing or stopping ACE inhibitors or ARBs are the best hope of improving renal function. Methods of increasing blood pressure are discussed later in the chapter. Diuretics and nitrates can reduce both arterial and venous pressure and their effects on renal function are rather unpredictable but usually adverse unless venous pressure is high and falls substantially with treatment. In practice, if congestion is not severe, reducing the dose of diuretic should be the first response to declining renal function. Only if this fails or is inappropriate should the dose of ACE inhibitor/ARB be reduced or stopped.

Ultrafiltration or renal dialysis can be used to lower serum creatinine and potassium but neither intervention prolongs survival, although they bridge a patient to a definitive procedure (e.g. mechanical circulatory support). Temporary extracorporeal mechanical circulatory support can also improve renal function when this is due to severe heart failure and may be used as a bridge to a more permanent solution.

Respiratory disease

Patients who have a definite diagnosis of asthma should avoid β-blockers; ivabradine may be similarly effective to β-blockers for patients in sinus rhythm. Most patients with chronic obstructive pulmonary disease tolerate and benefit from β-blockers. Monitoring of airways obstruction by spirometry may be appropriate when in doubt. This may also provide an opportunity to withdraw un-needed bronchodilator therapy. Patients with pulmonary fibrosis may have persistent fine crepitations at the lung bases that may be confused with pulmonary oedema leading to overaggressive diuretic therapy.

Sleep-disordered breathing

Patients with heart failure are prone to both obstructive and central sleep apnoea and many will have both. The severity of sleep-disordered breathing may vary according to the severity of congestion or the reduction in cardiac output, sleeping posture, or the effects of alcohol or hypnotic or anxiolytic agents. Simple ambulatory equipment is available for diagnosis. Arterial oxygen desaturation is probably the key manifestation of important disease but arrhythmias induced by airways obstruction may also be important. Studies of continuous positive airways pressure ventilation were disappointing, possibly because high intrathoracic pressures can reduce cardiac output and increase right-sided congestion. Studies using adaptive servoventilation, which is less likely to cause such problems, are nearing completion.

Angina and myocardial ischaemia

There is no evidence that revascularization reduces morbidity or mortality in patients with heart failure and coronary artery disease. Pharmacological treatment of angina is appropriate in the first instance. This may include β-blockers, ivabradine, and short- and longer acting nitrates. Ranolazine may also be used although the evidence base is limited. Vasodilator calcium antagonists should be used cautiously and avoided if blood pressure is low. For patients with persistent, limiting angina, coronary angiography and revascularization should be considered. There is anecdotal evidence that revascularization of silent myocardial ischaemia or viable but dysfunctional myocardium may have striking benefits of cardiac dysfunction and symptoms of heart failure, but two randomized trials have failed to show that this strategy is generally superior to pharmacological therapy. There is no imperative, based on current evidence, to investigate for ischaemia or to do a coronary angiogram that may set in train a series of events that the patient and clinician may regret.

Atrial fibrillation

About 50% of patients with AF also have heart failure and at least 25% of patients with heart failure have AF. Patients with AF and heart failure should be anticoagulated (see 'Anticoagulants and antiplatelet agents', earlier).

Clinical trials show no benefit from β-blockers in patients with AF and HFrEF, perhaps due to excessive reduction in ventricular rate. The optimal resting ventricular rate (measured at clinic rather than by ambulatory monitoring) in AF may be 75–85 bpm. Digoxin can improve ventricular rate control but is rarely required. Its vagomimetic properties provide better resting and nocturnal ventricular rate control, while β-blockers reduce the rise in ventricular rate during exercise.

There is little evidence to support pulmonary vein ablation to restore sinus rhythm in chronic heart failure. Nor is there good evidence that CRT is effective when AF is present. These patients cannot benefit from atrioventricular (AV) resynchronization. Patients who require a pacemaker or a defibrillator should be considered for AV node ablation and biventricular pacing, although the evidence for this strategy is not robust. CRT should be considered an intervention of last resort in the setting of AF.

Anaemia

Anaemia in heart failure is often due to iron deficiency. Ferritin is often normal in the presence of iron deficiency because it is also a marker of inflammation, increasingly recognized as part of the heart failure syndrome. Measurement of serum iron alone or with transferrin saturation is a better test. A transferrin saturation in excess of 35% excludes iron deficiency.

The reasons for iron deficiency are unclear and may be related to reduced absorption (less gastric acidity due to proton pump inhibitors or increased hepatic secretion of hepcidin) or increased gastrointestinal losses (perhaps exacerbated by aspirin). It is unclear whether oral supplements correct iron deficiency. New intravenous iron preparations are safe and easy to administer and appear to improve symptoms. Large outcome studies are under way.

Anaemia is rarely due to folate or B_{12} deficiency. Many patients have impaired renal function and are either deficient in or resistant to erythropoietin or have plasma volume expansion leading to 'dilutional' anaemia. Administration of darbepoeitin increases haemoglobin and exerts a modest improvement in quality of life but does not reduce morbidity or mortality. Whether darbepoeitin would work better if administered with iron is unknown.

Gout

Gout is common in patients receiving diuretics for heart failure. Acute attacks of gout should be treated with colchicine. NSAIDs should be avoided if at all possible. High-dose paracetamol or even opiates are preferred analgesics. Steroids may be used to treat an acute attack. Once the acute attack has settled, allopurinol may be used to reduce the formation of uric acid and the risk of recurrent attacks. However, allopurinol may initially increase the risk of gout attacks. Prophylactic colchicine may reduce this risk. NSAIDs should be avoided.

Endstage heart failure

For patients with severe intractable heart failure, palliative care, mechanical circulatory support with left ventricular assists devices or heart transplantation should be considered. Early referral of patients potentially appropriate for such therapy to an expert centre is warranted. Usually, these patients will be aged less than 70 years with no other serious, irreversible disease. Always consider the following:

- Review pharmacological and device therapy; ensure optimal treatment and withdraw what is unnecessary or harmful
- Check for anaemia and iron deficiency
- Consider adding digoxin (a rapid loading dose may be appropriate)
- Opiates might improve breathlessness.

Exacerbation of chronic heart failure

Heart failure is often portrayed as an inexorably progressive condition with a poor prognosis. This is no longer true for many patients receiving modern treatment. Stabilization for a decade or more, remission and, for a lucky few, medical cure is now well documented. However, many patients do deteriorate, even if well managed. The reasons are diverse and often remediable.

Sudden acute deterioration in a previously stable patient may be due to infection, myocardial ischaemia or infarction, arrhythmias (especially AF), or, more rarely, catastrophic failure of a heart valve. Failure to comply with advice on diet or to take prescribed medicines, anaemia, renal dysfunction or poorly controlled hypertension are more often subacute and should be detected long before the patient reaches an acute crisis.

Treatment of heart failure with a normal ejection fraction (HFnEF)

No treatment has been conclusively shown to alter the natural history of HFnEF. However, diuretics relieve congestion and congestion can kill. Indeed, treatments directed predominantly at congestion, such as ACE inhibitors and MRA, may produce similar benefits in patients with HFnEF and HFrEF, provided the patient with HFnEF has evidence of congestion (i.e. a raised plasma concentration of natriuretic peptides). The same may not be true of β-blockers: reduction in heart rate will increase the duration of diastole that may be advantageous when the problem is impaired cardiac myocyte relaxation, but deleterious when the problem is myocardial fibrosis and restriction. There is some evidence that digoxin reduces the risk of hospitalization for heart failure. There is little evidence for the safety or efficacy of calcium channel blockers. Hypertension and anaemia are common in this population and therapeutic targets. The effects of LCZ696, soluble guanylate cyclase inhibitors, and inter-atrial septal shunt devices and many other interventions are currently being explored in this population.

Practical aspects of monitoring and management

Regular monitoring of symptoms, weight, and vital signs is essential to good management especially in sicker, unstable patients. Patient should be encouraged to do this for themselves, potentially assisted by a home telemonitoring system linked to expert clinical surveillance and advice and supported by family and informal carers. Serum electrolytes and renal function should be measured at least every 6 months and much more frequently in patients with advanced or unstable disease. QRS duration and haemoglobin should be measured on at least an annual basis. There is little evidence to support routine serial echocardiography. There is some evidence to support serial monitoring of natriuretic peptides to identify patients who are in need of more intensive therapy.

Symptoms

The clinical trials on which guidelines are based focus on morbidity and mortality, but symptoms are usually the reason why the patient seeks medical help. Fortunately, treatment can usually control symptoms for most patients for most of the time. Patients with severe endstage symptoms represent less than 5% of patients with heart failure at any time; most of these patients either improve or die within a few weeks.

Heart rate

A reduction in parasympathetic and increase in sympathetic tone are responsible for the increase in heart rate in heart failure. β-blockers and digoxin will reduce ventricular rate regardless of heart rhythm; ivabradine only if the patient is in sinus rhythm. For patients with HFrEF, the target range for resting heart rate in sinus rhythm is 50–60 bpm but for AF it is 75–85 bpm.

Blood pressure

High blood pressure is an important risk factor for developing heart failure, especially HFnEF. Low blood pressure is a bad prognostic sign, perhaps because it reflects more severe impairment in the pumping action of the heart (cardiac power output). Many medicines that reduce morbidity and mortality also lower blood pressure. Identifying the appropriate blood pressure for the individual patient, and achieving it, is a key aspect of managing heart failure.

For most patients, treatment of heart failure will reduce systolic blood pressure below 140 mmHg. Treatment of hypertension may cause the features of heart failure to disappear and may account for much of the confusion and uncertainty surrounding HFnEF as a clinical entity. A patient may be admitted in florid heart failure with a systolic blood pressure greater than 200 mmHg, but after treatment, usually with diuretics and ACE inhibitors, there may be little residual evidence for heart failure even when diuretics are withdrawn.

A low blood pressure that is not causing problems should not deter the patient or clinician from titrating medication to guideline-indicated doses. Patients often tolerate a systolic blood pressure of 80 mmHg or less but presumably a point must be reached where the benefits of treatment are outweighed by the reduction in blood pressure. Low blood pressure may cause postural hypotension and reduce renal perfusion and glomerular filtration. When low blood pressure is a problem then treatments for heart failure that increase blood pressure may be added or treatments that reduce blood pressure reduced in dose or withdrawn. If the patient's symptoms and signs of heart failure are well controlled, the preferred action is to reduce the dose of diuretic. If symptoms and signs are not well controlled then digoxin or CRT, if the patient is indicated, will increase systolic blood pressure. If the above are inappropriate or fail, then reducing the dose of disease-modifying therapies should be considered, with the potential benefits and risks explained to the patient. If the patient is oedematous, then the dose of β-blocker should be reduced allowing heart rate to rise to *c.*80 bpm if in AF or, if in sinus rhythm, using ivabradine to keep resting heart rate at 50–60 bpm. If serum creatinine is in excess of 200 µmol/litre then the dose of ACE inhibitor should be reduced. If serum potassium is in excess of 5 mmol/litre then the dose of MRA should be reduced. If appropriate, referral for assessment for mechanical circulatory support or heart transplantation may be considered.

Blood tests

Patients with heart failure receiving diuretics should have a blood test at intervals not exceeding 6 months.

Serum potassium

Many laboratories have an excessively wide 'normal' range for serum potassium. For patients with HFrEF, mortality climbs steeply when potassium drops below 4.0 mmol/litre or rises above 4.9 mmol/litre. Aiming for a serum potassium of about 4.5 mmol/litre, usually by manipulating the dose of MRA, appears ideal. Potassium supplements are rarely necessary and should be used only short term. Patients with HFnEF may benefit similarly from this strategy.

Renal function

Serum urea and creatinine are stronger markers of prognosis than measures of cardiac dysfunction such as LVEF. As noted above, most treatments that improve the prognosis of heart failure cause a decline in renal function. Advice on manipulation of therapy to optimize renal function is provided in the section on blood pressure.

Haemoglobin

Anaemia, often due to iron deficiency, is common in patients with heart failure and indicates a poor prognosis. Treatment may improve symptoms and perhaps prognosis. Haemoglobin should be measured at least annually.

Table 5.3.6 Example care plan context: recovering in hospital from episode of worsening heart failure

Mandatory information (Unchanging)		Discharge	Target
◆ Date of Birth:- 07/01/1943	Carvedilol	3.125 mg bd	25 mg bd
◆ Sex; Women	Enalapril	2.5 mg bd	5 mg bd
◆ Height: 160cm	Spironolactone	25 mg/d	25 mg/d
	Bumetanide	1 mg/d	1 mg/d
Mandatory information (Most recent with date)	Aspirin	75 mg/d	stop
◆ Aetiology:- Ischaemic Heart Disease	Clopidogrel	—	75 mg/d
◆ Most Recent MI: Yes: Anterior 09/11/2005	Metformin	500 mg bd	500 mg bd
◆ Co-morbidity: Type 2 Diabetes, Arthritis	Lansoprazole	30 mg/d	stop
◆ LVEF: 32% (HFrEF)	Ferrous sulfate	200 mg tid	re-assess
◆ Mitral regurgitation: moderate			Exercise for 10 min x 3/wk
◆ Other important valve disease: no			

	Now	Target
Symptoms (NYHA Class)	Recent IV	I/II
Resting heart rate (bpm)	73	55–65
Systolic BP (mmHg)	114	110–130
Weight (Kg)	68.7	67.0–69.0
Potassium (mmol/L)	4.5	4.0–4.9
Creatinine (µmol/L)	134	<150

Mandatory information (Most recent with date) continued:
- ◆ Heart rhythm: sinus
- ◆ PR interval: 210 msec
- ◆ QRS duration: 110 msec
- ◆ Device: None
- ◆ FEV1: 2.1 (83% of predicted)
- ◆ FEV1/FVC: 75%
- ◆ Haemoglobin: 10.8 g/dL
- ◆ Haematinic screen: to be done
- ◆ HbA1c: 7.4%
- ◆ Sodium: 138 mmol/L
- ◆ Potassium: 4.0 mmol/L
- ◆ Urea: 11.5 mmol/L
- ◆ Creatinine: 137 umol/L
- ◆ Albumin: 44 g/dL
- ◆ NT-proBNP: 3,742 ng/L

Instructions

- ◆ Double carvedilol every 2 wks until target achieved
  - Delay titration if heart rate <65 bpm or systolic BP <110 mmHg
  - Down titrate if heart rate <55 bpm
- ◆ Add ivabradine 5mg bd if heart rate remains >70 bpm despite achieving carvedilol target
- ◆ Double enalapril in one week to achieve target
  - Reduce dose if systolic BP <90 mmHg
  - Check renal function and electrolytes in 10 days. Reduce dose if serum creatinine >180 µmol/L (~30% increase). Re-check in 10 days if >150 µmol/L (~10% increase)
  - If serum potassium >5.5 mmol/L stop spironolactone and re-check potassium in 10 days. Re-initiate at half-dose if potassium <5 mmol/L
- ◆ Stop ferrous sulfate in 3 months and re-check haemoglobin and iron status.
- ◆ Advise on diet and exercise
- ◆ Increase bumetanide in one month if
  - Systolic BP not at target and the patient is not at dry weight
  - Remains symptomatic and the patient is not at dry weight
  - Reverse this decision if patient does not like the change
- ◆ Further cardiology review in six weeks

The electrocardiogram

Most patients with HFrEF will have a QRS duration greater than 100 ms and each year a proportion of these will develop a QRS duration greater than 140 ms, indicating the need for CRT. Treatment with β-blockers will often mask the onset of AF, requiring anticoagulation and a change in strategy of heart rate control. Patients should generally have an annual ECG.

Organization of care

Good management requires great organization to ensure that appropriate treatment is delivered safely and effectively in order to

* gain and maintain clinical stabilization

* recognize when patients are deteriorating and do something about it before they reach a crisis

* identify patients who need more specialized services.

This is greatly facilitated by the use of electronic health records (EHRs), especially if they are enhanced by decision support systems. EHRs and home telemonitoring have a synergistic role in improving health care. Increasingly, patients, their carers, and their social network are becoming involved with long-term care and any good organization will use them as part of the care team. Delivering good care requires a care plan that is shared with the patient and all the services that support them. These should provide enough information about the patient to deliver the treatments and doses specified in the care plan safely and effectively.

Further reading

Kotecha D, *et al.* on behalf of the Beta-Blockers in Heart Failure Collaborative Group (2014). Efficacy of β blockers in patients with heart failure plus atrial fibrillation: an individual-patient data meta-analysis. *Lancet*, **384**(9961), 2235–43.

McMurray JJ, *et al.* ESC Committee for Practice Guidelines (2012). ESC guidelines for the diagnosis and treatment of acute and chronic heart failure 2012: The Task Force for the Diagnosis and Treatment of Acute and Chronic Heart Failure 2012 of the European Society of Cardiology. Developed in collaboration with the Heart Failure Association (HFA) of the ESC. *Eur J Heart Fail*, **14**, 803–69. Erratum in: *Eur J Heart Fail*, 2013, **15**, 361–2.

McMurray JJ, *et al.* the PARADIGM-HF Investigators and Committees (2014). Angiotensin-neprilysin inhibition versus enalapril in heart failure. *N Engl J Med*, **371**, 993–1004.

CHAPTER 5.4

Cardiorenal syndrome

Darren Green and Philip A. Kalra

Essentials

Concurrent renal and cardiovascular disease is common. Renal disease is a potent cardiovascular risk factor and consequently cardiovascular disease is the most important cause of mortality in patients with end-stage renal disease. This increased risk is mediated by vascular disease (coronary calcification, endothelial dysfunction, dyslipidaemia, etc.), left ventricular hypertrophy, risk of arrhythmias and left ventricular systolic and diastolic dysfunction. These interactions are further complicated by the presence of anaemia in advanced renal disease.

The coexistence of renal disease and heart failure presents a major therapeutic challenge and requires careful attention to fluid status and renal function. Diuretic resistance is common and the important prognostic benefit of angiotensin converting enzyme (ACE) inhibition in this high-risk group is often neglected. Cardiovascular drugs, in particular antiarrhythmic agents such as digoxin, sotalol, and flecainide, should be used with caution in patients with renal disease. Patients with severe cardiac and renal disease require a multidisciplinary approach to their management.

What is the cardiorenal syndrome?

The term 'cardiorenal syndrome' was first introduced to describe the frequent finding of worsening renal function in response to acute decompensation of heart failure or the up-titration of nephrotoxic agents used in its treatment.

This definition of cardiorenal syndrome is criticized for focusing only on a small subgroup of patients in whom specific diseases of the heart and kidney lead to concurrent morbidity in the other organ. Indeed, the majority of patients who have evidence of adverse cardiorenal interaction will not fall into this category, and likewise acute kidney injury (AKI) will not be a precipitant to major cardiac morbidity in most patients with this condition.

Further attempts to classify different interactions of renal failure and heart disease into subtypes of cardiorenal syndrome have yielded the Acute Dialysis Quality Initiative classification system found in Table 5.4.1. It acknowledges the wider spectrum of cardiac disease that may be precipitated by renal impairment, such as sudden cardiac death (SCD) and the impact of heart failure on chronic kidney disease (CKD) as well as AKI. However, its use in clinical practice is very limited as it provides no mechanistic, therapeutic, or prognostic guidance, and does not accommodate the complex interactions of acute and chronic illness when coexisting. For this reason, both clinical and experimental terms and definitions relating to cardiorenal syndrome are likely to change as understanding of this medical field evolves.

In this chapter, rather than simply outlining the purported different types of cardiorenal syndrome (1–5) that have been repeatedly described elsewhere, we instead concentrate on the important structural abnormalities and pathophysiological interactions which result from the interplay of diseased kidneys, heart, or both.

Epidemiology of concurrent cardiac and renal disease

Difficulties in classifying CRS arise from the broad disease categories implicated and their overlapping interactions. Cardiovascular

Table. 5.4.1 Acute Dialysis Quality Initiative classification of cardiorenal syndrome

Type	Onset	Precipitant		Secondary effect		Examples
1	Acute	CARDIAC	Acute cardiac dysfunction	RENAL	AKI	Cardiogenic shock causing rapid rise in serum creatinine, decompensated heart failure leading to AKI
2	Chronic		Chronic cardiac dysfunction		CKD	Chronic heart failure leading to long-term decline in eGFR
3	Acute	RENAL	Acute kidney injury	CARDIAC	Acute cardiac event	Acute glomerulonephritis with oliguria leading to pulmonary oedema, AKI causing hyperkalaemia leading to arrhythmia
4	Chronic		CKD		Cardiac remodelling	Renal artery stenosis and CKD leading to LVH, CKD associated vascular calcification with chronic ischaemia
5	Secondary	OTHER	Systemic condition	BOTH	Cardiac and renal dysfunction	Diabetes mellitus, hypertension, SLE

AKI, acute kidney injury; CKD, chronic kidney disease; LVH, left ventricular hypertrophy; SLE, systemic lupus erythematosus.

Table. 5.4.2 Comparison of event rates for sudden cardiac death (SCD) in the general population and high-risk clinical groups including patients with heart failure and receiving dialysis

SCD events (per 1000 patient years)	
General population <85 years	1–2
General population >85 years	40
Post-myocardial infarction	40
Heart failure, ejection fraction <35%	90–200
Pre-dialysis CKD	7
CKD on dialysis	70–120

CKD, chronic kidney disease.

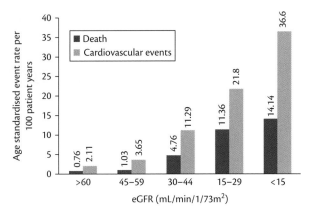

Fig. 5.4.1 The increasing cardiovascular burden of declining renal function. Adapted from Go et al. *Circulation*. 2006;113:2713–2723.

mortality is disproportionate in CKD compared to the general population. Annual mortality for dialysis patients is 15% in Europe and 19% in North America, and 46% of these deaths are due to cardiovascular disease. The most common cause of death in dialysis patients is SCD, likely due to arrhythmia. The event rate far exceeds that of the general population (70–120 versus 1–2 events per 1000 patient years, see Table 5.4.2), and accounts for a greater proportion of all deaths (26% vs 11%).

The period of highest mortality is actually the first 6 months after initiation of chronic haemodialysis therapy. Left ventricular hypertrophy (LVH) is present in 74% of new haemodialysis patients, and reduced ejection fraction is present in 36%. That these abnormalities are already present at the initiation of dialysis indicates that the high cardiovascular risk to which these patients are exposed is a function of progression of cardiac disease during pre-dialysis CKD as well as an effect of dialysis itself.

The increased risk of cardiovascular events and death persists after renal transplant, albeit at a reduced event rate. New-onset coronary artery disease after transplant occurs at approximately 10 events per 1000 patient years, and cardiovascular death accounts for more than 50% of all post-transplant mortality. This risk is greatest in diabetic transplant recipients, who have a threefold greater risk of cardiovascular disease than their non-diabetic counterparts. Indeed, in the latter group, post-transplant infection and malignancy cause more deaths than cardiovascular disease.

Renal disorders are also common in patients presenting with cardiac disease. Only 17% of patients seen in heart failure clinics will have normal renal function, and up to 55% will have CKD stage 3 to 5 (for CKD stages see Table 5.4.3) and mortality risk increases

Table 5.4.3 The stages of chronic kidney disease

Stage	eGFR (ml/min/1.73m²)
1	>90[a]
2	60–89
3a	45–60
3b	30–44
4	15–29
5	<15

Suffix T = transplant ; suffix D = dialysis.

[a] Evidence of damage without change in function, e.g. proteinuria.

as renal function worsens (Fig. 5.4.1). Similarly, AKI occurs in 27 to 45% of hospitalizations for decompensated heat failure depending on definition. Inpatient mortality, critical care admission, and total length of stay are all independently associated with AKI in this population. Although definitions of AKI have differed between studies this is a consistent finding, even after a fall in serum creatinine of just 9 µmol/litre. In one study of 1007 nonelective hospital heart failure admissions the relative risks of adverse outcomes if AKI supervened compared to normal renal function were 7.5 for death, 2.1 for major complication, and 3.2 for length of stay greater than 10 days (here, AKI was defined as an increase in serum creatinine >26.5 µmol/litre).

The predictive power of AKI to recognize adverse outcome in decompensated heart failure has a high degree of specificity (>80%) but is poorly sensitive (<70%). In fact, AKI is as predictive of adverse outcome in acute heart failure as left ventricular ejection fraction and blood pressure. AKI is also most common in heart failure patients with pre-existing CKD. A summary of factors predisposing to AKI after decompensation of heart failure is found in Box 5.4.1.

Haemodynamic effects of cardiorenal interaction in disease

Systemic blood pressure is dependent on the actions of both the heart and kidneys, which regulate body fluid volumes by changes in vascular tone, diuresis, and natriuresis. Dysregulation of one may lead to dysfunction of the other. For example, a fall in blood pressure associated with heart failure will activate the renin–angiotensin–aldosterone (RAAS) pathway to retain salt and water, and increase vascular tone via sympathetic pathways. Subsequent volume expansion will help maintain renal perfusion but may paradoxically lead to further decompensation of heart failure. Activation of the RAAS system will also have other deleterious actions such as increasing oxidative stress, inflammation, and tissue fibrosis.

Reduced cardiac output may also in turn lead to reduced cardiac filling and increased central venous pressures. Should such pressures increase in the renal vasculature, glomerular filtration may become compromised by a reduction in the pressure difference between afferent and efferent vessels. This will lead to CKD or AKI. This vicious cycle of worsening chronic cardiorenal deterioration is summarized in Fig. 5.4.2.

Box 5.4.1 Risk factors for acute kidney injury in hospital admissions for heart failure

- ◆ Laboratory parameters
  - Underlying CKD
  - Anaemia
  - Hyponatraemia
  - Echocardiographic parameters
  - Diastolic dysfunction
  - Pulmonary hypertension
  - Atrioventricular valvular incompetence
- ◆ Haemodynamic factors
  - Hypotension on admission
  - Underlying hypertension
- ◆ Comorbidities
  - Older age
  - Diabetes
  - Previous acute heart failure admissions
  - Previous AKI or dialysis
  - Nephrotoxic polypharmacy

Other factors implicated in cardiorenal syndrome are the relationship between nitric oxide and reactive oxygen species, both of which affect haemodynamic regulation and endothelial function, and both of which are under partial control by the heart and kidneys. The relative importance of each factor is unknown and is likely to be different in different cardiorenal syndrome settings. This complexity of pathways leading to cardiorenal syndrome means that the search for biomarkers of cardiorenal syndrome risk or a common signalling pathway, such as interleukin-6, has thus far not been fruitful.

Nephrotoxicity and other adverse drug effects

The problem of mechanism is further confounded by the effect of external factors, most notably prescribed medication. Perhaps most obviously, AKI may be caused directly by contrast agents used in coronary angiography. This risk can be quantified based on weighted scoring of risk factors for contrast nephropathy, as shown in a cohort study of 8357 patients (Table 5.4.4). This is a useful tool in clinical decision-making and for the process of obtaining informed consent.

The use of RAAS blockade, particularly angiotensin converting enzyme (ACE) inhibitors, is associated with improved survival in heart failure. ACE inhibitors are also known to affect glomerular filtration and may lead to AKI during decompensated heart failure with resultant uncertainty as to how best manage these drugs during the episode. However, the extent to which ACE inhibitors are implicated in AKI may be overstated. In the Studies of Left Ventricular Dysfunction (SOLVD) trial, 16% of patients treated with enalapril (mean daily dose 16.6 mg) developed a rise in serum creatinine in excess of 44 µmol/litre. However, the figure for the placebo arm was 12%. Also, such studies do not usually report improvements in GFR but it is estimated that 10% may have comparable improvements in renal function due to improved cardiac output. Furthermore, as demonstrated in Fig. 5.4.2, RAAS overactivation may lead to acute

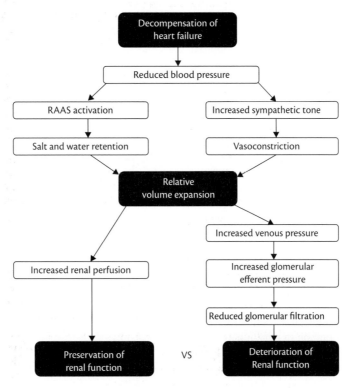

Fig. 5.4.2 The competing haemodynamic response to heart failure in causing and preventing deterioration in renal function.

Table 5.4.4 Risk prediction for nephropathy after intravenous contrast for coronary angiography

Factor		Component score
NHYA III/IV HF		5
Hypotension <80 mmHg/invasive support		5
Diabetes mellitus		3
Age >75 years		4
Anaemia (haematocrit <39%[M], <36% [F])		3
IV contrast (per 100 ml contrast used)		1
eGFR (ml/min/1.73m^2)	40–60	2
	20–40	4
	<20	6

Combined score	Risk (%)	
	Nephropathy	**Dialysis**
0–5	8	0.04
6–10	14	0.12
11–16	26	1.09
17+	57	12.6

Reprinted from the *Journal of the American College of Cardiology*, Vol 44, Issue 7, Mehran *et al.*, A simple risk score for prediction of contrast-induced nephropathy after percutaneous coronary intervention: development and initial validation. 1393–1399. Copyright (2004) with permission from Elsevier.

worsening of both cardiac and renal function and so cessation of ACE inhibitors is of possible detriment in such cases.

Fear of deteriorating renal function is often a reason for under-prescribing ACE inhibitors for cardioprotection in CKD patients. However, ACE inhibition is protective against renal deterioration even in CKD stage 4 and deterioration in the presence of renovascular disease is much less common than anticipated at approximately 11%. A rise in creatinine with the introduction of ACE inhibitors in patients with heart failure of up to 50% above baseline or to a creatinine of 200 µmol/litre is accepted in some guidelines provided renal function subsequently stabilizes.

Long-term monitoring of renal function in patients with CKD on ACE inhibitors is vital, as is adequate counselling about the risk of AKI and the importance of seeking medical advice in the event of a dehydrating illness such as diarrhoea. There are now reports of medico-legal disputes involving such cases, akin to those relating to anticoagulation and chemotherapeutic agents.

There is also a reluctance to prescribe high-dose loop diuretics in patients with renal disease. This is based on a fear of renal toxicity and prerenal failure due to intravascular volume depletion. It is frequently not appreciated that in fluid-overloaded patients with heart failure the adverse effects on renal function due to an elevated right atrial pressure and renal congestion are greater than the impact of reduced cardiac output. Inducing a significant diuresis with high-dose diuretics in this situation may result in a significant improvement rather than deterioration in renal function. Key to the assessment of the likely impact of diuretic therapy on renal function in these patients is a careful assessment of the intravascular volume status of the patient.

Determining the most appropriate action in respect of these drugs is poorly evidence based, but the key message is that monitoring of renal function is vital in both chronic and acute care of cardiac disease, and although suspension of ACE inhibitors during acute illness is often the safest action, their timely reintroduction is also necessary.

As noted above, the most common cause of mortality in CKD is SCD, and a number of drugs commonly prescribed in nephrology clinics have the potential to exacerbate arrhythmia. The three most common pathways for this are (1) electrolyte disturbances, (2) drugs affecting repolarization manifesting as QT prolongation, or (3) altered metabolism of antiarrhythmic drugs leading to toxicity. Table 5.4.5 summarizes familiar drugs implicated in each of these scenarios.

Antiarrhythmic therapy is further complicated in dialysis patients, as many of these drugs are not removed from the body by dialysis. Those that would normally be excreted via the kidneys can therefore accumulate in such patients, and the timing of dosing of short-acting drugs may need to accommodate the timing of haemodialysis sessions. Managing antiarrhythmic drugs may require the input of a specialist renal pharmacist. Certain drugs, such as sotalol, ought to be avoided completely in dialysis patients where possible. Sotalol may predispose to QT$_c$ prolongation and torsades de pointes in toxic doses. It is over 90% absorbed after oral intake, undergoes almost no hepatic first-pass metabolism, and is excreted via the kidneys.

Table 5.4.5 Prescribed medication that may exacerbate cardiorenal disease via arrhythmia

Cardioprotective drugs that cause hyperkalaemia	
Renin–angiontensin blockade	Causes hypoaldosteronism and reduced eGFR
Digoxin	Impairs renal excretion and prevents cellular uptake
β-Blockade	Supresses cellular uptake of potassium mediated by β$_2$ receptors
Unfractionated heparin	Hypoaldosteronism
Low molecular weight heparin	Mechanism not certain
Drugs that cause QTc prolongation	**Indication for use**
Calcineurin inhibitors	Transplant immunosuppression
Midodrine	Refractory hypotension
Quinolones	Antibiotics
Macrolides	Antibiotic
Benzodiazepines	Anxiolytic
SSRIs	Antidepressant
Potentially arrhythmogenic drugs requiring dose adjustment in dialysis	
Flecanide	Use 50% normal dose
Sotalol	Avoid in CKD5D, use at 25% normal dose in eGFR <15 ml/min
Digoxin	Start at 62.5 micrograms daily

Diuretic resistance in chronic renal disease

The use of thiazide diuretics in patients with cardiovascular disease is usually limited to hypertension in the elderly and patients with heart failure. Thiazides are effective in inducing a natriuresis in patients with a GFR less than 30 ml/min. Patients with a GFR below this level will usually require loop diuretics to achieve a satisfactory diuresis. Loop diuretics are progressively less effective at lower GFR and proportionately higher doses given in a once-daily regimen are required to induce a diuresis. Activation of the RAAS in conjunction with distal tubular cell hypertrophy induces diuretic resistance. A combination of thiazide diuretic and loop diuretic may be helpful in overcoming diuretic resistance in these patients. Diuretic resistance is particularly prominent in diabetic proteinuric renal disease where protein binding of loop diuretics within the renal tubules reduces bioavailability.

Arrhythmia in chronic kidney disease

SCD is the most common cause of death in dialysis patients. Although this is presumed to be predominantly due to ventricular tachyarrhythmia as for SCD in the general population, there is emerging evidence that bradycardia and asystole are implicated more often than is the case in nonrenal patients. Medications commonly prescribed in CKD that may predispose to arrhythmia are listed in Table 5.4.5. There is also a high prevalence of ECG conduction abnormalities that may indicate risk. In one cross-sectional analysis of 323 prevalent dialysis patients, 34% had QRS duration in excess of 100 ms, 19% first-degree heart block, and 10% atrial fibrillation or flutter. Other studies have shown high rates of QT_c prolongation and increased QT dispersion as well as loss of heart rate variability in CKD populations. Such abnormalities are associated with worse outcome. The best ECG predictor of mortality appears to be left bundle branch block, with an increased hazard ratio for death of 4.6 compared to normal QRS morphology. Equally, the impact of supraventricular arrhythmia on mortality cannot be overstated. The absence of sinus rhythm on ECG is associated with an 89% increased risk of death in diabetic dialysis patients, and atrial fibrillation is associated with an 80% 5 year mortality in dialysis patients. Importantly, current evidence suggests that anticoagulation with warfarin leads to worse outcome for dialysis patients with atrial fibrillation, albeit that this evidence comes from observational studies and not randomized trials. The increased risk is thought to result from increased bleeding and vascular calcification.

The substrates for arrhythmia in CKD are manifold and Fig. 5.4.3 summarizes these. Myocardial ischaemia is likely to play a role via coronary atheroma, medial calcification, and poor coronary perfusion due to diastolic dysfunction and pathological LVH with fibrosis and capillary rarefaction. The process of haemodialysis also induces arrhythmia but it is not clear whether this is directly due to dialysis-induced myocardial ischaemia, autonomic effects, or the rapid electrolyte and fluid shifts that occur during dialysis. The role of LVH is likely to be an important one as endomyocardial biopsies from dialysis patients demonstrate abnormal remodelling with interstitial fibrosis and myocyte hypertrophy. These changes affect conduction through the myocardium and potentially will lead to arrhythmia.

Vascular calcification

Although 40% of dialysis patients have coronary artery disease, lipid-lowering drugs are less efficacious in this setting than in the wider population. One reason is that arterial disease in CKD is not typically due to atheroma: 50% of CKD patients have significant diffuse medial arterial calcification at the initiation of chronic dialysis. There is a fivefold increase in calcification of the coronary arteries in dialysis patients compared to non-CKD patients with coronary atheroma where calcification tends to be focal and found in the intimal layer.

Calcification in CKD is associated with hyperphosphataemia, hypercalcaemia, and hyperparathyroidism, all of which can stimulate calcification of vascular smooth muscle cells and matrix. CKD also leads to a reduction in endogenous inhibitors of calcification, such as fetuin A. Vascular calcification and renal bone abnormalities are together termed 'chronic kidney disease–mineral bone disorder' (CKD-MBD), acknowledging the wide spectrum of associated disease.

Aortic stiffness, a surrogate of calcification, can be measured noninvasively with pulse wave velocity (PWV). An increase in PWV is associated with LVH and increased left ventricular myocardial infarction (and with reduced coronary filling), all of which may eventually predispose to heart failure. Indeed, increased PWV

Autonomic imbalance
Sympathetic overactivity

LVH
Fibrosis
Reduced systolic function
Reduced capillary density
Aberrant conduction

Concurrent diabetes
Hypoglycaemia
Reduced ischaemia tolerance
CAD
Myocardial fibrosis.

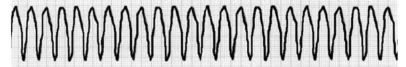

CKD-MBD
LVH via FGF-23
Increased vascular stiffness
Coronary artery calcification

Dialysis
Myocardial ischaemia
Rapid electrolyte shifts
Rapid fluid shift

Reduced eGFR
Chronic inflammation
Interstitial fibrosis
Oxidative stress
Pericarditis/myocarditis
Hyperkalaemia

Fig. 5.4.3 Potential triggers to sudden cardiac death in chronic kidney disease.

Table 5.4.6 Suggested indicators for referral to renal services for cardiology patients with chronic kidney disease, and investigations to request on referral

Problem	Diagnosis	Investigations
Diuretic resistant peripheral or pulmonary oedema/recurrent acute decompensation of heart failure	Renal artery stenosis; consider peritoneal dialysis for heart failure therapy	Renal tract ultrasound
Unexplained anaemia	Renal anaemia	Rule out gastrointestinal bleeding, ferritin, Fe/TIBC/B-vitamins, PTH, CRP,
Electrolyte or acid–base disturbance	Tubular or pararenal disease, renal adverse drug effects	Serum bicarbonate, chloride, calcium, magnesium, urine salts
Hyperphosphataemia (particularly with valvular annular calcification on echocardiography or radiographic evidence of aortic/arterial calcification)	CKD-MBD	Serum phosphate, calcium, PTH, food diary
Protenienuria or haematuria	Nephropathy/glomerulonephritis not cause by vascular disease	Urine microscopy, urine culture, urine PCR, renal tract ultrasound, electrophoresis, ESR, HIV, HCV, autoantibody screen if haematuria (ANA, ANCA, GBM, C3, C4)
Progressive decline in eGFR	Drug effect, renal artery stenosis/occlusion, progressive CKD, approaching dialysis, ? palliation	Send full medication list/dose changes and historical eGFR with referral

ANA, antinuclear antibody; ANCA, antineutrophil cytoplasmic antibody; C3, C4, complement components; CKD, chronic kidney disease; CKD-MBD, chronic kidney disease–mineral bone disorder; CRP, C-reactive protein; ESR, erythrocyte sedimentation rate; GBM, glomerular basement membrane; HCV, hepatitis C virus; PCR, polymerase chain reaction; PTH, parathyroid hormone; TIBC, total iron binding capacity.

has been shown to be more important than hypertension in the development of LVH in CKD.

Left ventricular hypertrophy

The mechanism of LVH development in CKD is likely to be multifactorial but evidence is emerging that the association of vascular stiffness with LVH may be concurrent pathological manifestations of CKD-MBD as well as demonstrating a cause and effect response to increased afterload. Fibroblast growth factor 23 (FGF-23) is produced by osteocytes as renal function declines. Its role in this setting is to induce phosphaturia and to inhibit hydroxylation of vitamin D to its active form. Elevated FGF-23 levels are independently associated with LVH in CKD, intracardiac administration of FGF-23 leads to LVH in wild type mice, and *in vitro* administration of FGF-23 to isolated rat myocytes results in pathological hypertrophy.

LVH may yet become a therapeutic target in CKD given its high prevalence and implications for worse outcome. The relative risk of cardiac death in dialysis patients with LVH is 2.7 compared to those without. Above a mean arterial pressure of 106 mmHg, small increases in blood pressure are associated with significant increases in the rate of *de novo* heart failure in CKD. On a more optimistic note, tight control of blood pressure is associated with regression of LVH, slowing progression of CKD may slow progression of LVH, and tight control of CKD-MBD is also likely to positively impact on pathological cardiac remodelling.

Multidisciplinary approach to renal disease in cardiac patients

The high prevalence of coexistent cardiac and renal disease, and the high risk of major morbidity this combination brings, will often necessitate referral to nephrology services outside the usual guidelines. A list of potential circumstances triggering referral is listed in Table 5.4.6. Importantly, such referrals provide access to a multidisciplinary team beyond renal physicians, such as anaemia services, specialist psychologists, dietetic services, pharmacists, palliative care teams, and dialysis-planning specialist nurses, each of whom can provide care which may improve the quality of life and prognosis for patients. Indeed, being aware of and monitoring for the possibility of these problems in the likes of heart failure clinics may lead to earlier diagnosis and intervention for significant renal disease in many cases.

Summary

The interaction between heart and kidneys in acute and chronic disease leads to poorer survival and greater hospitalization for patients. The pathophysiology of the cardiorenal illness differs according to clinical scenario and between cases, from CKD-induced arrhythmia to decompensated heart failure causing dialysis-dependent AKI. The management of each scenario is further complicated by potential nephrotoxicity and altered renal drug clearance. This means that a general guideline for care in cardiorenal syndrome is not applicable, and patients must be assessed on a case-by-case basis.

Further reading

Bongartz LG, *et al.* (2005). The severe cardiorenal syndrome: 'Guyton revisited'. *Eur Heart J*, **26**(1), 11–17.
Braam B, *et al.* (2014). Cardiorenal syndrome—current understanding and future perspectives. *Nat Rev Nephrol*, **10**(1), 48–55.
Faul C, *et al.* (2011). FGF 23 induces left ventricular hypertrophy. *J Clin Invest*, **121**(11), 4393–4408.
Green D, Kalra PA (2012). The heart in atherosclerotic renovascular disease. *Front Biosci*, **4**, 856–864.

Green D, *et al.* (2011). Sudden cardiac death in hemodialysis patients: an in-depth review. *Am J Kidney Dis*, **57**(6), 921–929.

McCullough PA, *et al.* (2013). A DQI consensus on AKI biomarkers and cardiorenal syndromes. *Contrib Nephrol*, **182**, 82–98.

Mehran R, *et al.* (2004). A simple risk score for prediction of contrast-induced nephropathy after percutaneous coronary intervention. *J Am Coll Cardiol*, **44**(7), 1393–1399.

Roberts PR, Green D (2011). Arrhythmias in chronic kidney disease. *Heart*, **97**(9), 766–73.

Ronco C, *et al.* (2008). Cardiorenal syndrome. *J Am Coll Cardiol*, **52**(19), 1527–1539.

CHAPTER 5.5

Cardiac transplantation and mechanical circulatory support

Jayan Parameshwar and Steven Tsui

Essentials

Cardiac transplantation

Cardiac transplantation is the treatment of choice for selected patients with advanced heart failure: median survival exceeds 10 years and recipients enjoy an excellent quality of life, but availability is severely limited by shortage of donor organs. The need for lifelong immunosuppression is associated with side effects, including an increased incidence of malignancy. Newer immunosuppressive agents offer promise in reducing nephrotoxicity of conventional regimens and in delaying the onset of (currently inevitable) cardiac allograft vasculopathy.

Mechanical circulatory support

Ventricular assist devices (VADs) are mechanical blood pumps that work in parallel or series with the native ventricles. First-generation volume-displacement pulsatile VADs have largely been superseded by rotary blood pumps that generate continuous flow. Significant complications include bleeding, thromboembolism, and infection.

Temporary support—several devices are available for use in patients who require support for days to weeks in the intensive care unit: these are invaluable in postcardiotomy cardiogenic shock and in patients who present *in extremis* with uncertain viability.

Chronic support—implantation of a durable VAD in patients with chronic heart failure can either be as a bridge to heart transplantation or as permanent support, sometimes referred to as destination therapy (DT). The REMATCH study (Randomized Evaluation of Mechanical Assistance for the Treatment of Congestive Heart Failure) randomized patients with endstage heart failure to best medical therapy or the implantation of the first-generation HeartMate I VAD: survival was improved in the device group (52% vs 25% at 1 year; 23% vs 8% at 2 years). A subsequent study randomizing similar heart failure patients between a newer continuous-flow left ventricular assist device (LVAD) (the HeartMate II) and the pulsatile HeartMate XVE showed that survival with continuous-flow VAD was even better (58% vs 24% at 2 years).

Heart transplantation

In 1964 James Hardy transplanted a chimpanzee heart into a 68-year-old man with ischaemic heart failure, but the patient did not survive surgery. The first human-to-human heart transplant was performed in Cape Town on 3 December 1967 by Christiaan Barnard; the patient died 18 days afterwards of infective complications. By the end of 1968, 102 patients had received heart transplants in 50 hospitals in 17 countries: mean survival was only 29 days and there was widespread disenchantment with the procedure. Only a few institutions continued clinical cardiac transplantation during the 1970s, the team at Stanford University under the leadership of Norman Shumway being pre-eminent among them. By the late 1970s 1-year survival at Stanford had increased to 65%, establishing the place of heart transplantation. The introduction of new immunosuppressive drugs in the 1980s led to further improvement in outcome and an explosion of activity around the world. During the 1990s there was a decline in the number of heart transplants performed owing to a shortage of donor organs.

Before transplantation

Recipient selection

Heart transplantation is the treatment of choice for selected patients with endstage heart failure. However, the limited number of available donor hearts restricts this treatment to a small fraction of potential recipients. Careful selection of patients is therefore crucial to make best use of this scarce resource. Patients with New York Heart Association (NYHA) class IIIB and class IV heart failure are best discussed with the local heart failure/transplant centre to optimize medical management and to consider high-risk non-transplant cardiac surgery where appropriate (see Chapter 13.6). Patients with chronic heart failure should be referred before they develop significant end-organ dysfunction (renal and hepatic) or irreversible secondary pulmonary hypertension. Box 5.5.1 summarizes criteria used to select patients for transplantation. The use of cardiopulmonary exercise testing to objectively quantify functional capacity and to estimate prognosis is an important part of the assessment process. Box 5.5.2 outlines the important contraindications.

Matching of donor and recipient

Donor and recipient blood groups need to be compatible. Appropriate size matching is also generally thought to be necessary to minimize the risk of donor organ failure. HLA matching is not routinely carried out, but there is some evidence that HLA-DR matching results in fewer episodes of acute rejection. The presence of pre-formed antibodies to HLA antigens is an important consideration; selection of an appropriate donor includes ruling out those with the relevant HLA antigens. The waiting time for heart transplantation in sensitized patients can be much longer.

Box 5.5.1 Indications for heart transplantation

- Persistent symptoms of heart failure at rest or minimal exertion despite optimal medical therapy. Functional capacity measured by peak oxygen uptake on exercise $<14\,ml\,kg^{-1}\,min^{-1}$ (or 50% predicted). For patients receiving β-blockers a value of $<12\,ml\,kg^{-1}\,min^{-1}$ has been recommended

- History of recurrent hospital admissions for worsening heart failure

- Recurrent symptomatic ventricular arrhythmia associated with severe impairment of ventricular function

- Refractory ischaemia not amenable to revascularization associated with severe impairment of left ventricular function

---

After transplantation

Most patients spend 2 to 3 weeks in hospital after a heart transplant and are fit to return to work after 4 to 6 months. In the first year they need to return to the transplant centre at set intervals to monitor immunosuppression, and to have surveillance endomyocardial biopsies to screen for acute rejection, although recent studies suggest that—at least for low-risk patients—a noninvasive monitoring strategy involving gene-expression profiling of peripheral blood mononuclear cells may be a safe alternative to endomyocardial biopsy.

Immunosuppression

Immunosuppression is commenced at surgery and continued for life. The intensity of immunosuppression is greatest early post-transplant, with a staged reduction in the dosage of drugs over the first year. Box 5.5.3 lists the agents commonly used for maintenance immunosuppression: some units routinely deploy induction therapy with an antibody for the first few days after the transplant. At

---

Box 5.5.2 Relative contraindications to heart transplantation

- Active infection including chronic viral infections, e.g. HIV, hepatitis B. (Patients with undetectable viral titres and no organ damage other than the heart may be considered.)

- Symptomatic cerebral or peripheral or vascular disease

- Diabetes mellitus with end-organ damage, e.g. nephropathy, neuropathy, proliferative retinopathy

- Coexistent or recent neoplasm

- Severe lung disease—FEV_1 and FVC <50% predicted and evidence of parenchymal lung disease

- Renal dysfunction with creatinine clearance less than $40\,ml\,min^{-1}$

- Recent pulmonary thromboembolism

- Pulmonary hypertension - pulmonary artery systolic pressure >60 mmHg, transpulmonary gradient ≥15 mmHg and/or pulmonary vascular resistance >5 Wood units

- Psychosocial factors including history of noncompliance with medication, inadequate support, drug or alcohol abuse

- Obesity (body mass index >35 or weight >140% of ideal body weight

---

Box 5.5.3 Immunosuppressive agents

- Calcineurin inhibitor: ciclosporin or tacrolimus

- Antimetabolites: mycophenolate mofetil or azathioprine

- Corticosteroid: usually prednisolone

- Target of rapamycin (TOR) inhibitor: sirolimus or everolimus

- Antibody therapy: anti-thymocyte globulin (ATG), basiliximab, alemtuzumab

---

least 50% of patients can be safely weaned off prednisolone in the first 2 years after heart transplant. Episodes of acute rejection (usually confirmed by endomyocardial biopsy) are treated with intravenous methylprednisolone and are almost always reversible. The importance of antibody-mediated rejection has been increasingly recognized in recent years; while there is a growing consensus on the diagnosis of this entity, there is little evidence for the efficacy of the various treatments that have been tried. When antibody-mediated rejection is associated with ventricular dysfunction, medium-term prognosis is compromised.

Outcome

Figure 5.5.1 shows the survival of patients after heart transplantation. Median survival now exceeds 10 years in most large centres. Annual mortality after the first year is approximately 3.5% per year. Most patients enjoy an excellent quality of life after a heart transplant, with minimal or no functional limitation. Successful pregnancy is possible after heart transplantation: management requires close collaboration between transplant and obstetric teams. Maternal morbidity is higher than in the general population and there is a higher incidence of small-for-date babies. Teratogenicity does not seem to be a significant problem with the immunosuppressive regimens used in the 1980s and most of the 1990s (steroids, azathioprine, calcineurin inhibitors), but the same cannot be said of many of the newer agents.

Complications

General complications related to immunosuppression include an increase in opportunistic infection and malignancy, in particular squamous cell carcinoma of the skin and non-Hodgkin's B-cell lymphoma (which affects 2 to 4% of heart transplant recipients). Calcineurin inhibitors can cause headaches, tremor, hypertension, nephropathy, and peripheral neuropathy, and exacerbate myalgia/myositis associated with statin use. Corticosteroids are associated with osteoporosis and diabetes. Ciclosporin can cause hirsutism and gum hypertrophy. Issues particular to cardiac transplantation are described below.

Hyperlipidaemia

Abnormalities in lipid levels have been reported in up to 80% of patients on standard immunosuppressive drug regimes. Pre-transplant abnormalities are common in patients transplanted for ischaemic cardiomyopathy. Use of statins early post-transplant has been shown to delay the onset of cardiac allograft vasculopathy thus increasing late survival, and is now standard practice in most units.

Renal dysfunction

The most serious side effect of calcineurin inhibitors (CNI) is renal toxicity. Data from the International Society for Heart and

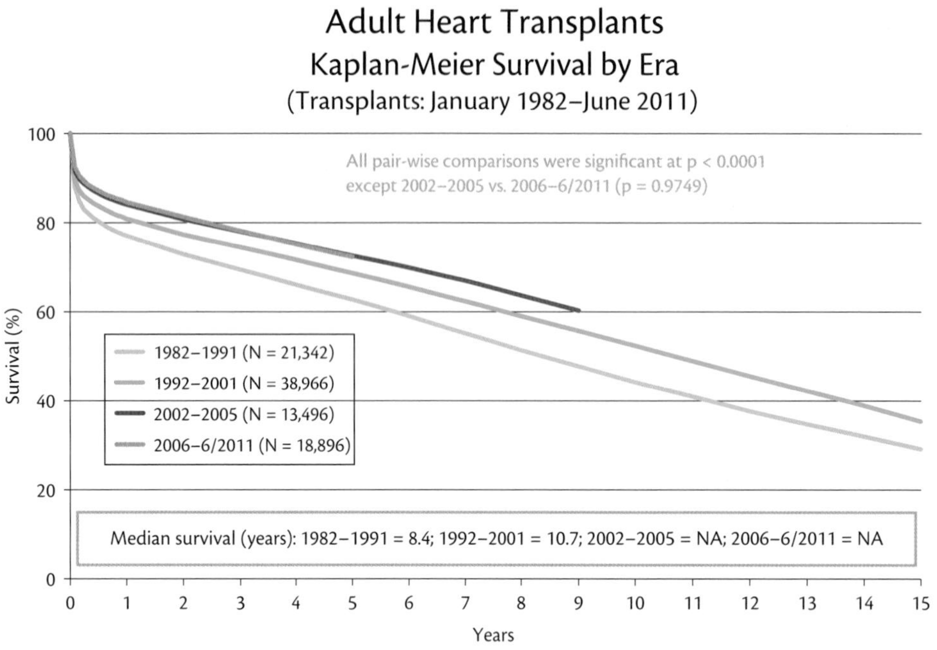

Adult Heart Transplants
Kaplan-Meier Survival by Era
(Transplants: January 1982–June 2011)

All pair-wise comparisons were significant at p < 0.0001
except 2002–2005 vs. 2006–6/2011 (p = 0.9749)

1982–1991 (N = 21,342)
1992–2001 (N = 38,966)
2002–2005 (N = 13,496)
2006–6/2011 (N = 18,896)

Median survival (years): 1982–1991 = 8.4; 1992–2001 = 10.7; 2002–2005 = NA; 2006–6/2011 = NA

Survival (%)

Years

Fig. 5.5.1 Survival was calculated using the Kaplan–Meier method, which incorporates information from all transplants for whom any follow-up has been provided. Since many patients are still alive and some patients have been lost to follow-up, the survival rates are estimates rather than exact rates because the time of death is not known for all patients. The median survival is the estimated time point at which 50% of all of the recipients have died. Survival rates were compared using the log-rank test statistic. Adjustments for multiple comparisons were done using Scheffe's method.

Lung Transplantation indicate that about 20% of patients have some degree of renal dysfunction at 1 year after transplantation. Afferent renal arterial vasoconstriction is believed to be the cause of early renal dysfunction and is reversible. Late renal dysfunction is related to tubular damage and tends to be progressive, even when the offending drug is discontinued. At least 5 to 6% of heart transplant recipients progress to require renal replacement therapy in the first 10 years post-transplant, and their prognosis on dialysis is poor. Judicious use of CNI-free regimes slows the progression to endstage renal disease and, if introduced early, renal function may improve significantly. Selected heart recipients who have developed renal failure but maintained good cardiac allograft function can be considered for renal transplantation.

Cardiac allograft vasculopathy

This term is used to describe concentric narrowing of the coronary arteries (and sometimes veins) of the transplanted heart. It is believed to be an immune-mediated disease and is also referred to as 'chronic rejection', although nonimmune mechanisms probably contribute to pathogenesis. It is the commonest cause of late death after heart transplantation but occasionally presents as a fulminant process that causes death within the first year. Conventional risk factors like smoking and hyperlipidaemia are associated with earlier disease, but cardiac allograft vasculopathy occurs in children and in the absence of other risk factors.

The basic pathological lesion is a diffuse and progressive thickening of the intima that occurs in epicardial and intramyocardial arteries (Fig. 5.5.2). The disease tends to affect the arterial tree diffusely, although there is heterogeneous involvement of different parts of the arteries. The degree of intimal thickening that occurs in the first year (measured by intravascular ultrasonography) is a predictor of the development of angiographic disease and death or

retransplantation for cardiac allograft vasculopathy, risk factors for which are shown in Box 5.5.4.

Most patients with cardiac allograft vasculopathy present with signs and symptoms of heart failure, although angina can be experienced despite denervation. The disease is commonly first seen during surveillance coronary angiography. Revascularization is rarely feasible because the disease is diffuse, but occasionally patients have focal proximal lesions that are amenable to angioplasty.

Intravascular ultrasonography (IVUS) is the most sensitive technique for diagnosis of early disease and most clinical trials of new immunosuppressive drugs include IVUS-derived parameters as an endpoint. The only definitive treatment for cardiac allograft

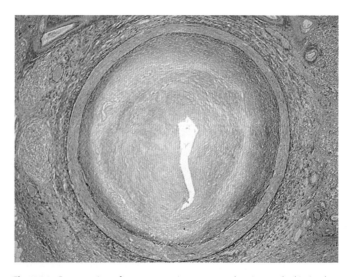

Fig. 5.5.2 Cross-section of coronary artery at autopsy showing marked intimal hyperplasia and obliteration of the lumen.

Box 5.5.4 Risk factors for cardiac allograft vasculopathy

Immunological

◆ Number of episodes of acute rejection

◆ HLA-DR mismatch between donor and recipient

◆ Anti-HLA antibodies in the recipient (associated with the deposition of antibody and complement in the vasculature of the allograft)

Nonimmunological

◆ Donor age

◆ Recipient age and gender

◆ Coronary artery disease as the cause for transplantation in the recipient

◆ Cytomegalovirus infection

◆ Smoking

◆ Obesity

◆ Hyperlipidaemia

Box 5.5.5 Guidelines for the use of LVAD as a bridge to transplantation

Inclusion criteria

◆ The patient is a candidate for transplantation, or is likely to become a candidate after a period of mechanical circulatory support (bridge to candidacy)

◆ Haemodynamics (usually on IV inotropic therapy; cardiac index <2.0 litres min^{-1} m^{-2}; systolic blood pressure <80 mmHg; pulmonary capillary wedge pressure >20 mmHg)

◆ Progressive end-organ dysfunction (renal or hepatic) due to reduced perfusion

◆ >2 heart failure hospitalizations in previous 12 months without an obvious precipitating cause

Exclusion criteria

◆ Active endocarditis

◆ Multiorgan failure

◆ *Life-limiting comorbidities:* Systemic disease that limits 1-year survival, e.g. advanced or irreversible pulmonary disease, advanced hepatic disease (cirrhosis and portal hypertension), severe peripheral vascular disease, metastatic cancer, and irreversible neurological or neuromuscular disorders

◆ Severe right ventricular failure (would need BIVAD)

Factors increasing the risk of perioperative complications

◆ Age

◆ Prolonged prothrombin time or raised INR

◆ Hypoalbuminaemia

◆ Era of implantation (lower mortality for implants after May 2007)

◆ Centre experience (>15 implants associated with decreased mortality).

---

vasculopathy is retransplantation, which—given the shortage of donor organs—is an option for only a few patients. Target of rapamycin (TOR) inhibitors may delay the onset and slow the progression of cardiac allograft vasculopathy.

Mechanical circulatory support (MCS)

The concept of arterial counterpulsation to unload the heart in systole was introduced in the early 1960s. This led to the development of the intra-aortic balloon pump, which was first applied clinically by Kantrowitz in 1967. In 1966 DeBakey reported the first successful clinical application of a true ventricular assist device (VAD) in a 37-year old woman who could not be weaned from cardiopulmonary bypass following aortic and mitral valve replacement. In 1969 Cooley supported a patient with a total artificial heart for 64 h until a donor heart was available. In 1984 Stanford University reported the first successful heart transplant following bridging with a left ventricular assist device (LVAD).

VADs are mechanical blood pumps that work in parallel or series with the native ventricle. An LVAD draws oxygenated blood from the left atrium or ventricle and returns it to the aorta; a right ventricular assist device (RVAD) draws venous blood from the right atrium or ventricle and returns it to the pulmonary artery.

Contexts for using mechanical circulatory support

Bridge to transplantation

Successful cardiac transplantation provided the stimulus for the development of devices that could be used to support patients until a suitable donor organ became available. The availability of donor hearts is unpredictable, hence the patient with acute haemodynamic deterioration requires other means of circulatory support when intravenous inotropic therapy cannot maintain adequate perfusion to vital organs. Renal and hepatic function improve on mechanical support, pulmonary vascular resistance falls, nutritional status and muscle strength recover. This buys time for the patient until a suitable donor heart is identified and reduces the risk

of subsequent transplantation. Box 5.5.5 outlines guidance for use of a LVAD as a bridge to transplantation and factors affecting risk of perioperative complications.

Permanent support

Depending on definition, the prevalence of severe heart failure between the ages of 65 and 75 years is 0.5 to 1.2%. Most of these patients will not be candidates for heart transplantation by virtue of age and comorbidity. VADs were originally developed as a long-term treatment for heart failure and patients who are not transplant candidates can be considered for this form of therapy.

The REMATCH study (Randomized Evaluation of Mechanical Assistance for the Treatment of Congestive Heart Failure) randomized patients with endstage heart failure to best medical therapy or the implantation of the pulsatile HeartMate assist device. Survival at 1 year was 52% in the device group and 25% in the medical group; at 2 years it was 23% and 8% respectively. Quality of life was significantly improved at 1 year in the device group, but with a higher frequency of serious adverse events. In the more recently completed HeartMate II study, patients with endstage heart failure were randomized to undergo implantation of the pulsatile HeartMate XVE or a continuous-flow LVAD (HeartMate II). The quality of life and functional capacity improved significantly in both groups. Patients implanted with the continuous-flow LVAD had superior actuarial survival rates at 2 years (58% vs 24%, p = 0.008) and significantly lower adverse event rates. This provides compelling evidence that LVAD therapy can increase life expectancy and quality of life in selected patients with advanced heart failure.

Bridge to recovery

Patients dying from fulminant myocarditis can be supported with mechanical circulatory support and it is not uncommon to see recovery of myocardial function to the point where the device can be removed. Recovery has also been reported in patients with idiopathic dilated cardiomyopathy. LVADs unload the ventricle to a degree that cannot be achieved by drug therapy, and there is a considerable body of evidence to show that the myocardium recovers at the cellular and molecular level with mechanical circulatory support. Structural improvement detectable by echocardiography occurs much less frequently, and clinical recovery to the point where the device can be removed safely is rarer still (<10% of patients in most series, although there are intriguing reports of higher rates of clinical recovery from a few centres). Studies are ongoing, but at present implantation of a device in patients with chronic heart failure should be viewed as a bridge to heart transplantation or as permanent support.

Short-term support

Several devices are available for use in patients who need support for days or weeks. These are invaluable in post-cardiotomy cardiogenic shock and in patients who present *in extremis* with multiorgan failure. In the latter group a short-term device may be a bridge to a longer-term device or to heart transplantation, but occasionally patients may improve to the point where the device can be removed and they can be stabilized on medical therapy. This is sometimes

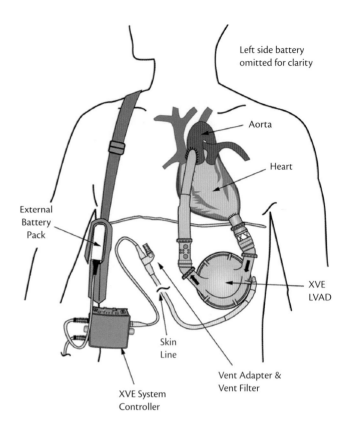

Fig. 5.5.3 Stylized picture of a patient with a HeartMate XVE LVAD. Courtesy of Thoratec.

described as 'bridge to decision'. To support patients for periods of a few weeks to several months, the CentriMag device has been widely used with reasonable success. Veno-arterial extracorporeal membrane oxygenation (ECMO) can be introduced at the bedside in critically ill patients to maintain systemic circulation and to afford the opportunity to assess the appropriateness of further therapy. It may also be used to stabilize patients for transport to an advanced heart failure centre for ongoing support. Patients with any of these devices are confined to critical care or a high-dependency area and cannot be discharged from hospital.

Types of ventricular assist devices

There are many devices available for clinical use. Box 5.5.6 shows a classification of devices and examples of each type: a brief description of selected devices in each category follows.

Pulsatile devices

The first generation of VADs were pulsatile devices, also referred to as volume-displacement VADs. An inflow cannula carries blood from the apex of the left ventricle to the device, while the outflow graft is anastomosed to the ascending aorta. The Thoratec HeartMate I (Fig. 5.5.3), which was used in the REMATCH trial, was by far the most successful first-generation LVAD with over 5000 implants worldwide before it was superseded by continuous-flow devices.

Rotary ventricular assist devices

Rotary devices deploy an impeller spinning at high speed to generate blood flow. They are smaller, have a limited blood contact surface,

---

Box 5.5.6 Classification of devices for MCS

Temporary devices

- Thoratec CentriMag
- Impella 2.5; 4.0; 5.0
- TandemHeart
- Venoarterial Extra Corporeal Membrane Oxygenatinon (VA-ECMO)

Long-term devices

Pulsatile (volume displacement)

- BerlinHeart Excor
- Abiomed BVS 5000

Continuous flow

- Jarvik 2000
- Berlin Incor
- HeartMate II and HeartMate III
- HeartWare HVAD and HeartWare MVAD

(a)

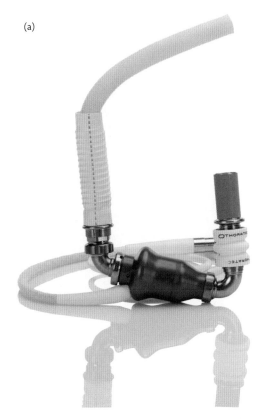

Fig. 5.5.4a HeartMate II.

Courtesy of Thoratec.

(b)

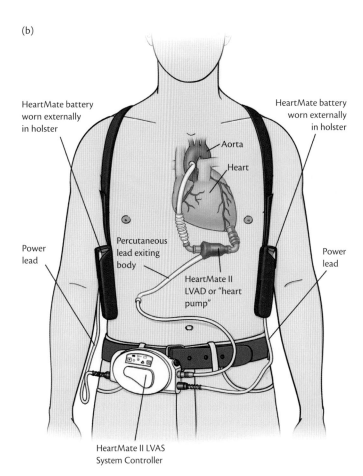

Fig. 5.5.4b Stylized picture of a patient with a HeartMate II LVAD.
Courtesy of Thoratec.

with a single moving part, and are silent in operation. Newer pump designs have eliminated mechanical bearings altogether with the hope that these will be even more durable. Implantation is generally easier and infections are less common because of the less invasive surgery and thinner drive line.

They provide continuous flow and are therefore not 'physiological'; patients usually do not have a palpable pulse, and blood pressure measurement with a sphygmomanometer requires a Doppler probe to detect blood flow. Rotary pumps are preload dependent and afterload sensitive. Adequate left ventricular filling is required to ensure sufficient preload and avoid ventricular 'suckdown'. The absence of valves makes them simpler to operate. However, in the event of pump stoppage, free regurgitation from the ascending aorta back into the left ventricle may occur. Depending on native left ventricular function, some pulsatility may be seen as more blood is delivered to the VAD during ventricular systole. The impeller spinning at speed results in high sheer stress to blood components which can cleave the von Willebrand factor, resulting in an acquired von Willebrand disease. Pump thrombosis is another potential complication of continuous-flow devices and all rotary pumps currently require anticoagulation with warfarin and antiplatelet agents.

The Thoratec Heartmate II (Fig. 5.5.4) is a second-generation device which consists of an axial-flow blood pump with a percutaneous lead that connects the pump to an external computer controller and power source. The blood pump is a 12 mm diameter straight tube made of titanium alloy containing an internal rotor

with helical blades that curve around a central shaft. When the rotor spins on its axis, blood is drawn from the left ventricular apex through the pump and into the ascending aorta. The pump requires a pump pocket in the anterior abdominal wall, has an implant volume of 63 ml and weighs 350 g. It operates at approximately 8000 to 10 000 rpm and can generate up to 10 litres of flow per minute. The controller and two batteries are wearable, providing 4 to 6 h of power. The HeartMate II is approved for clinical use in Europe and the United States of America for bridging to transplant as well as for destination therapy. It has been implanted in over 20 000 patients worldwide, representing the benchmark against which other continuous-flow devices are being compared.

The HeartWare HVAD (Fig. 5.5.5) is a third-generation centrifugal blood pump which contains a wide-bladed impeller with a hydrodynamic suspension. This pump weighs only 160 g, has an implant volume of 70 ml, and does not require an abdominal pump pocket, allowing intrapericardial placement. It operates at 2400 to 3800 rpm and can generate flows of up to 10 litres/min. The HeartWare HVAD is approved for clinical use in Europe and for bridging to transplant in the United States of America. The HeartWare HVAD has been implanted in nearly 10 000 patients worldwide and has produced very favourable clinical outcomes.

Outcome of ventricular assist device treatment

Clinical outcomes of patients treated with implantable VADs have improved significantly over the last decade. This is a result

(a)

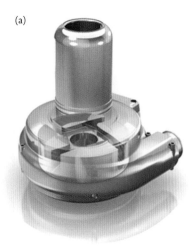

Fig. 5.5.5a The HeartWare HVAD.

(b)

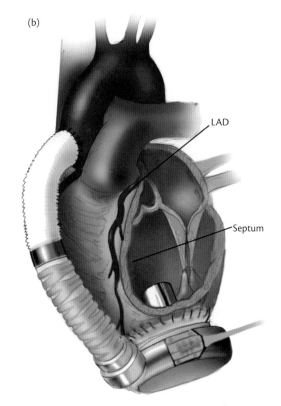

LAD

Septum

of better understanding of patient selection criteria, the development of clinical strategies to minimize perioperative complications, and improvements in device technology. Algorithms have been developed to risk stratify patients preoperatively, allowing targeted medical optimization of high-risk patients before VAD implantation. The introduction of the INTERMACS registry in the United States of America created a template for rigorous data monitoring and audit. Actuarial survival following implantation of continuous-flow LVADs is 80% at 1 year and 70% at 2 years

Fig. 5.5.5b Stylized picture of a HeartWare HVAD showing inflow drainage from left ventricular apex and outflow graft anastomosed to ascending aorta. Courtesy of HeartWare Inc.

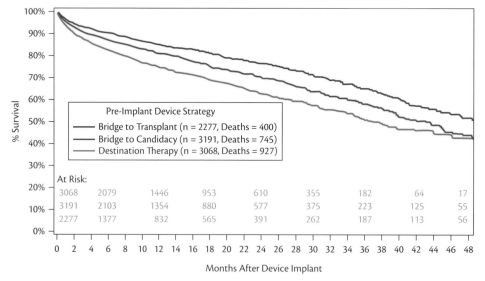

INTERMACS-Kaplan-Meier Survival for Continuous Flow LVADs (with or without RVAD implant at time of LVAD operation) by Pre-Implant Device Strategy Primary Prospective Implants: June 23, 2006 to September 30, 2013

Shaded areas indicate 70% confidence limits
p (log-rank) = <.0001
Event: Death (censored at transplant or recovery)

Fig. 5.5.6 Kaplan–Meier survival for continuous-flow LVADs (with or without RVAD implant at time of LVAD operation) by pre-implant device strategy. Primary prospective implants: 23 June 2006 to 30 September 2013.
From INTERMACS Registry.

across all indications (Fig. 5.5.6). The commonest causes of 30-day mortality are right ventricular failure, multiorgan failure, and neurological events. In the longer term, device-related infection emerges as the most important cause of death. Multivariate analysis identified older age, greater severity of right ventricular failure, cardiogenic shock at implant, and the use of a pulsatile VAD as risk factors for death.

Complications of ventricular assist devices

With long-term requirement for anticoagulation therapy and the need for a percutaneous driveline, bleeding and infection remain the most common adverse events following LVAD implant. Other common complications include arrhythmias, respiratory failure, renal dysfunction, and right heart failure. Patients receiving continuous-flow devices appear to experience significantly reduced incidences of device malfunction, infection, hepatic dysfunction, and neurological events. However, there appears to be a significantly increased risk of gastrointestinal bleeding with the use of rotary devices, which may be associated with an acquired form of von Willebrand's disease and reduced pulsatility of the systemic circulation.

Further reading

Barnard CN (1967). A human cardiac transplant: an interim report of a successful procedure performed at Groote Schuur Hospital, Cape Town. *S Afr Med J*, 41, 1271–4.

Berry GJ, *et al.* (2013). The 2013 International Society for Heart and Lung Transplantation Working Formulation for the standardization of nomenclature in the pathologic diagnosis of antibody-mediated rejection in heart transplantation. *J Heart Lung Transplant*, 32, 1147–62.

Billingham ME (1992). Histopathology of graft coronary disease. *J Heart Lung Transplant*, 11, S38–44.

Birks EJ, *et al.* (2006). Left ventricular assist device and drug therapy for the reversal of heart failure. *N Engl J Med*, 355, 1873–84.

Cowger J, *et al.* (2013). Predicting survival in patients receiving continuous flow left ventricular assist devices: the HeartMate II risk score. *J Am Coll Cardiol*, **61**, 313–21.

Hill DJ, *et al.* (2006). Positive displacement ventricular assist devices. In Frazier OH, Kirklin JK (eds) *Mechanical circulatory support*, pp. 537–6. Elsevier, Philadelphia.

Kapadia SR, *et al.* (1998). Development of transplantation vasculopathy and progression of donor-transmitted atherosclerosis. *Circulation*, 98, 267–78.

Kirklin J, *et al.* (2013). Fifth INTERMACS annual report: Risk factor analysis from more than 6,000 mechanical circulatory support patients. *J Heart Lung Transplant*, 32, 141–56.

Leitz K, *et al.* (2007). Outcomes of left ventricular assist device implantation as destination therapy in the post-REMATCH era: implications for patient selection. *Circulation*, 116, 497–505.

Lund LH, *et al.* (2013). The Registry of the International Society for Heart and Lung Transplantation: Thirtieth Official Adult Heart Transplant Report-2013. *J Heart Lung Transplant*, **32**, 951–64.

Mancini DM, *et al.* (1991). Value of peak oxygen consumption for optimal timing of cardiac transplantation in ambulatory patients with heart failure. *Circulation*, 83, 778–86.

Mehra MR, *et al.* (2006). Listing criteria for heart transplantation: International Society for Heart and Lung Transplantation Guidelines for the Care of Cardiac Transplant Candidates—2006. *J Heart Lung Transplant*, 25, 1024–42.

Pham MX, *et al.* (2010). Gene-expression profiling for rejection surveillance after cardiac transplantation. *N Engl J Med*, 362, 1890–900.

Rose EA, *et al.* (2001). Long-term use of a left ventricular assist device for end-stage heart failure. *N Engl J Med*, 345, 1435–43.

Slaughter M, *et al.* (2009). Advanced heart failure treated with continuous-flow left ventricular assist device. *N Engl J Med*, 361, 1–11.

Stevenson LW, *et al.* (2009). INTERMACS profiles of advanced heart failure: the current picture. *J Heart Lung Transplant*, 28, 535–41.

Heart valve disease

CHAPTER 6.1

Valvular heart disease

Michael Henein

Essentials

Rheumatic valve disease remains prevalent in developing countries, but over the last 50 years there has been a decline in the incidence of rheumatic valve disease and an increase in the prevalence of degenerative valve pathology in northern Europe and North America. In all forms of valve disease, the most appropriate initial diagnostic investigation is almost always the echocardiogram.

Mitral stenosis

The most common cause is rheumatic valve disease. Other causes include mitral annular calcification, congenital mitral stenosis, infective endocarditis (very rarely), and systemic lupus erythematosus (SLE) (Liebman–Sachs endocarditis).

The important consequences of mitral stenosis are its effect on left atrial pressure, size, and the pulmonary vasculature; it commonly causes atrial fibrillation. Presenting symptoms are typically exertional fatigue and breathlessness; systemic embolism can occur. Characteristic physical signs are irregular pulse, tapping apex beat, loud first heart sound, opening snap, and an apical low-pitched rumbling mid-diastolic murmur.

Management—the only medical treatments in mitral stenosis are (1) prophylactic measures against rheumatic fever and endocarditis; (2) anticoagulation to prevent systemic thrombo-embolism; and (3) diuretics for raised left atrial pressure. Patients who are symptomatic need intervention by either surgical valvotomy or catheter–balloon valvuloplasty, whether or not they have pulmonary hypertension. Early intervention—before the development of atrial fibrillation and an enlarged left atrium—is recommended, provided a conservative operation is possible. Mitral valve replacement is reserved for cases where the mitral valve cannot be repaired.

Mitral regurgitation

The most common causes are ischaemic myocardial dysfunction, mitral valve prolapse, and dilated cardiomyopathy. Other causes include congenital valve disease, infective endocarditis, endomyocardial fibrosis, and connective tissue diseases (including Marfan's syndrome).

Mitral regurgitation is an isolated volume overload on the left ventricle, providing the physiological equivalent of afterload reduction so that a normal forward cardiac output is maintained by the combination of increased ejection fraction and higher preload. Patients with mild regurgitation may not have any symptoms: those with severe regurgitation are likely to present with dyspnoea. Characteristic physical signs are an apex beat that may be prominent and displaced, an apical pansystolic murmur, and a third heart sound (in severe cases). The loudness of the murmur generally correlates with severity of regurgitation. The cardinal signs of mitral prolapse are a mid-systolic click followed by a murmur.

Endocarditis prophylaxis may be recommended to high-risk patients with regurgitation. Patients in atrial fibrillation should be given anticoagulants. The development of symptoms suggests the need for surgical correction to avoid development of irreversible left ventricular dysfunction. Assessment during routine follow-up should identify those likely to need surgical intervention even in the absence of symptoms, with an effective regurgitant orifice of over 40 mm^2 being one proposed indication. It is generally considered that a left ventricular end-systolic dimension more than 50 mm indicates a poor prognosis and that surgical intervention is unlikely to be of benefit. If technically possible, mitral valve repair results in a much better clinical outcome than does valve replacement, but mitral replacement by a mechanical valve or bioprosthesis is the only option for irreparable valves.

Aortic stenosis

Aortic stenosis may be at subvalvar, valvar, or supravalvar level, the commonest being valvar stenosis. Age-related degenerative calcific disease is the commonest cause in western Europe and the United States of America. Other causes include congenital bicuspid aortic valve and rheumatic disease (always associated with aortic regurgitation, 'mixed aortic valve disease', and usually with rheumatic mitral disease).

With the increase in outflow tract resistance in aortic stenosis, left ventricular wall stress increases and hypertrophy develops, preserving overall ventricular systolic function, but potentially at the expense of subendocardial ischaemia. Patients with mild disease may be asymptomatic, and even severe stenosis may be silent, but breathlessness, angina, and syncope are typical. Characteristic physical signs are a slowly rising, low-amplitude pulse, a narrow pulse pressure, a sustained apex beat, and a long and harsh ejection systolic murmur that is loudest at the base (second right intercostal space, also known as the aortic area) of the heart, and in most cases radiates to the carotids (where a thrill may be palpable).

Management—patients with moderate or severe disease should be advised to avoid strenuous exercise. Prophylaxis against endocarditis may be recommended to high-risk patients. Asymptomatic patients with mild or moderate aortic stenosis require follow-up; those with severe disease (pressure gradient >70 mmHg) need aortic valve replacement.

Aortic regurgitation

Aortic regurgitation is caused by leaflet disease or aortic root dilatation, the commonest causes being isolated medionecrosis, rheumatic disease, infective endocarditis, and Marfan's syndrome.

The left ventricular stroke volume is significantly increased, which is accommodated by an increase in left ventricular cavity size. As disease progresses, end-systolic volume increases out of proportion to stroke volume, and eventually these changes lead to irreversible damage. The onset of symptoms, particularly breathlessness, coincides with the onset of left ventricular disease. Characteristic physical signs of chronic severe aortic regurgitation are a large amplitude 'collapsing' pulse (which when severe can induce pulsations in many parts of the body), a low diastolic blood pressure (<50 mmHg) and/or a high pulse pressure (>80 mmHg), an apex beat that is sustained and/or displaced, and an early diastolic, decrescendo murmur, loudest at the left sternal border. Acute aortic regurgitation causes the patient to be cold and shut down, with tachycardia, hypotension, and a short early diastolic murmur that is easily missed.

Management—medical treatment of chronic aortic regurgitation includes angiotensin converting enzyme (ACE) inhibitors and/or calcium channel blockers to reduce afterload. Patients with a dilated aortic root should be given β-blockade with ACE inhibition/angiotensin receptor blockers. Prophylaxis against endocarditis may be recommended to high-risk patients. Although patients with severe chronic aortic regurgitation may remain asymptomatic, valve replacement should be offered when there is progressive increase in left ventricular end-systolic dimension, which should not be allowed to reach more than 40 mm.

Right heart valve disease

Many of the conditions that cause right-sided valve diseases are congenital, and are excluded from further discussion here (see Chapter 12).

Tricuspid stenosis—this is rare, but most often caused by rheumatic disease that almost invariably simultaneously affects the mitral valve. Symptoms include fatigue, dyspnoea, and fluid retention. On auscultation at the left or right sternal edge, a mid-diastolic murmur is heard and a tricuspid opening snap may be present. Diuretics can help to minimize fluid retention. Severe tricuspid stenosis needs surgical repair, or replacement if additional regurgitation is present.

Tricuspid regurgitation—significant disease is most commonly secondary to pulmonary hypertension and/or right heart dilatation; the commonest noncongenital primary cause is infective endocarditis. Symptoms include fluid retention and hepatic congestion. A raised venous pressure with prominent V-wave is expected. Other signs include a pansystolic murmur at the left or right sternal edge (in one-third of cases), expansile pulsation of the liver (in most), and peripheral oedema/ascites. Diuretics and ACE inhibitors may reduce systemic venous pressure and right ventricular size, even restoring valve competence in some cases. Valve repair or replacement may be advised in some cases.

Pulmonary stenosis—a rare condition usually caused by rheumatic disease or carcinoid syndrome. Fatigue and dyspnoea are the main symptoms. Characteristic physical signs are a prominent venous 'a' wave in the neck and an ejection systolic murmur loudest at the upper left sternal edge. Balloon valvuloplasty is the procedure of choice if intervention is warranted.

Pulmonary regurgitation—significant disease is rare, but usually caused by rheumatic disease, carcinoid, and endocarditis. The characteristic physical sign is a soft early diastolic murmur in the left upper parasternal region. Arrhythmia or progressive right ventricular dilatation are indications for surgery, using homograft or conduit and valve.

Introduction

Over the last 50 years there has been a significant shift in the causes of heart valve disease in northern Europe and North America, with a decline in the incidence of rheumatic valve disease and an increase in the prevalence of degenerative valve pathology. Rheumatic valve disease remains prevalent in the developing countries, particularly in areas with limited clinical services. The commonest valve involved with rheumatic pathology is the mitral valve, but the aortic and tricuspid valves can also be involved. The apparent increase in the diagnosis of valve disease could be due either to ageing of the population or to the extensive use of echocardiography in cardiology clinics. Age affects the valves, making leaflets thicker with fibrous strands and adipose tissue deposition at the closure lines of the leaflets. Isolated myxomatous changes may also occur in the valve fibrosa. In patients with a suspected diagnosis of endocarditis these changes can add to diagnostic difficulty since they may look like small vegetations, and they also need to be distinguished from papillary muscle fibroelastoma.

Medical treatment of valve disease is limited, focusing mostly on prophylaxis against endocarditis and ventricular dysfunction as well as optimizing haemodynamics. Although surgical repair is the main conventional treatment of severe valve disease, the need for this is 5 to 10 times less than that for coronary artery disease.

Valve-related mortality is more common in aortic valve disease than mitral valve disease, largely due to the frequent development of left ventricular dysfunction that causes congestive heart failure. Other causes of death in valve disease are additional pathologies such as coronary artery disease, endocarditis, or arrhythmia.

The mitral valve

Normal mitral valve anatomy and function

Optimum function of the mitral valve depends on the intact function of all its components—leaflets, chordae, annulus, and papillary muscles, in addition to the left atrium and the left ventricle. A normal mitral valve does not close passively. In addition to the pressure difference between the ventricle and atrium in systole, the annular contraction and papillary muscle contraction play an important role in the competence of the mitral valve. The anterior mitral valve leaflet represents a continuation of the posterior aortic root wall. The annular fibrous ring is located mainly posteriorly; it is usually D-shaped but there is significant variability in different individuals. The normal diameter of the mitral annulus is around 3 cm with a circumference of 8 to 9 cm: it is not a passive structure, so in addition to its normal movement towards the apex in systole, the contraction of the posterior myocardial muscle shortens its diameter by 25%, with such movement being a very important component in the mechanism of mitral valve competence.

Change in the size and shape of the left atrial cavity is a cause for incompetence of the mitral valve by enlarging the annular diameter. Loss of atrial mechanical function may contribute significantly to the development of mitral regurgitation in patients with atrial fibrillation. Likewise, atrial fibrillation itself has been shown to contribute to the enlargement of the left atrium and consequently the development of mitral regurgitation.

The two leaflets of the mitral valve meet at the medial and lateral commissures. The area of the U-shaped anterior leaflet is larger than that of the posterior leaflet, which is wider and shorter than the anterior leaflet. The posterior leaflet is made up of a number of scallops, commonly three. The two leaflets coapt at the zone of apposition, leaving an overlapping segment 5 mm long.

The chordal anatomy of the mitral valve is complicated, with around 12 primary chordae rising from each papillary muscle. These divide into secondaries and numerous tertiary branches that attach themselves to the margins of the two leaflets. In addition, a number of basal chordae also attach themselves to the ventricular surface of the leaflets and to the commissures. The location of the chordae follows that of the papillary muscles anterolaterally and posteromedially. Any rupture or redundancy of the chordae or extra tissue in the leaflets results in mitral regurgitation.

Mitral stenosis

Causes

The most common cause of mitral stenosis, which affects women more than men (2:1), is rheumatic valve disease. The rheumatic process involves not only the leaflets but may also affect the chordae and the annulus, causing fibrosis and superimposed calcification. The rheumatic leaflets become thickened and fibrosed, and the commissures fuse. The end result of this pathology is a reduction in mitral valve area, the rigid movement of the leaflets and the commissural fusion together contributing to the limited flow across the mitral valve orifice and hence stenosis. It is not uncommon for the fibrotic process to involve the subvalvar region in an aggressive way, thus causing flow to be limited at the level of the subvalvar apparatus. In such cases the chordae become short and the inflow tract of the left ventricle becomes tunnel-like.

Mitral annular calcification is another cause of raised filling velocities: this is seen in older people with the calcification limited to the annulus and the proximal segments of the leaflets, but the leaflets themselves are normal. A very uncommon cause of mitral stenosis is congenital mitral stenosis, which may be associated with other cardiac abnormalities. Infective endocarditis with bulky vegetations may rarely cause restriction of mitral flow, and patients with systemic lupus erythematosus (SLE) can develop fibrosis of the mitral cusps with commissural fusion following Liebman–Sachs endocarditis.

Pathophysiology and complications

The important consequence of mitral stenosis is its effect on left atrial pressure and size and on the pulmonary vasculature. As the valve area falls progressively, left atrial pressure rises, its size increases, and the pulmonary venous pressure also increases. In most patients with rheumatic mitral valve disease the left ventricle is normal in size and systolic function unless the valve stenosis is severe and making the ventricle under filled.

With a mild degree of mitral stenosis, reduced orifice area is compensated by increased flow during atrial systole. As the valve stenosis becomes more severe, the left atrial pressure increases, the pressure difference between the atrium and the ventricle increases, and the filling occurs throughout diastole. In severe mitral stenosis the pressure difference may be as high as 25 to 30 mmHg. Long-standing disease may result in irreversible pulmonary

hypertension secondary to the raised left atrial pressure. Atrial fibrillation also develops, with loss of mechanical atrial function.

The area of a normal mitral valve area is of the order of 5 cm^2, compared to less than 1 cm^2 in a patient with severe mitral stenosis. Effective mitral valve area changes very little with increase in heart rate compared to aortic valve area (which increases), the reason probably being the smaller number of commissures that assist opening of the mitral valve compared to the aortic valve. During exercise, particularly in atrial fibrillation, diastolic time falls and the fixed valve area causes raised left atrial pressure and pulmonary venous pressure.

Left atrial dilatation

Progressive reduction in mitral valve orifice area causes progressive increase in left atrial pressure and size and pulmonary venous pressure. Left atrial dilatation is associated with reduction in its mechanical function that slows down intra-atrial blood circulation (swirling). With progressive disease and development of atrial fibrillation, the circulation in the atrium becomes very sluggish and echocardiography may demonstrate spontaneous echo-contrast, particularly on transoesophageal images. Such patients are given anticoagulants in order to avoid clot formation and hence the risk of transient ischaemic attacks (TIA) or strokes. Almost one-fifth of the patients undergoing surgery for mitral stenosis have left atrial thrombus, and in one-third of them the thrombus is restricted to the atrial appendage.

Atrial fibrillation

This is the most common complication of mitral stenosis and its prevalence increases with age; it is found in 70% of patients in their thirties and in 80% of those in their fifties. The presence of pulmonary hypertension raises the prevalence of atrial fibrillation. The Framingham study estimated a 20-fold increase in risk of stroke in patients with atrial fibrillation and mitral stenosis compared to only 5-fold increase in those without mitral valve disease. Left atrial thrombus may also form in patients with a dilated left atrium with spontaneous echo-contrast who are in sinus rhythm. The loss of left atrial appendage mechanical function has been proposed as a possible mechanism behind blood stagnation and thrombus formation.

Left ventricular dysfunction

Although in most cases of mitral stenosis the left ventricle is normal in size and systolic function, in some patients diastolic function may be impaired and end-diastolic pressure raised. This could be related to additional pathology (e.g. systemic hypertension and diabetes). The left ventricle is dilated only in the presence of additional coronary artery disease. Primary rheumatic myocardial disease was proposed years ago, but no convincing evidence has ever come to light.

Pulmonary hypertension

With the increase in left atrial pressure, the pulmonary venous pressure increases and hence pulmonary arterial pressure also rises. Although pulmonary artery pressure corresponds to the degree of increase in left atrial pressure, a discrepancy between the two may reflect a raised pulmonary vascular resistance. A normal pressure drop across the pulmonary bed is of the order of 10–15 mmHg. The pulmonary hypertension is not always reversible after valve surgery. For any degree of mitral stenosis patients can display a wide range of pulmonary pressures, but it is very rare for secondary pulmonary hypertension to develop with left atrial pressure less than 20 mmHg in the setting of isolated mitral stenosis.

Right heart disease

With the development of pulmonary hypertension the right ventricle becomes hypertrophied and its cavity dilates. This is also reflected in right atrial size. Patients with rheumatic mitral valve disease may have additional tricuspid valve involvement in particular, the annulus dilating and causing significant tricuspid regurgitation. Patients with severe tricuspid regurgitation may complain of fluid retention that needs careful management in order to maintain the left-sided cardiac output and obtain tissue perfusion. Long-standing significant tricuspid regurgitation and raised right atrial pressure may cause further deterioration of right ventricular function and congestive heart failure. By that stage the damage is usually irreversible despite any successful mitral valve surgery.

Clinical presentation

Symptoms

Patients may remain asymptomatic with mild mitral stenosis. As the disease progresses, early symptoms are exertional fatigue and breathlessness. With severe mitral stenosis shortness of breath is accompanied by orthopnoea and paroxysmal nocturnal dyspnoea. With the development of pulmonary hypertension, right ventricular dysfunction, and tricuspid regurgitation, patients may present with fluid retention as well as recurrent chest infection. Atrial fibrillation may be an early symptom in patients with mitral stenosis, particularly palpitations on exercise. Major systemic embolus can also be a presenting symptom, and the condition may be detected for the first time during pregnancy as patients complain of disproportionate dyspnoea.

Physical examination

Long-standing mitral stenosis characteristically causes weight loss and a malar flush. The pulse character is normal, but pulse volume may be reduced and atrial fibrillation is likely. The jugular venous pressure is usually normal unless there is tricuspid regurgitation and/or pulmonary hypertension. The apex is not displaced, but the first heart sound is sometimes palpable ('tapping apex'), and less frequently the opening snap is also.

The characteristic auscultatory features of rheumatic mitral stenosis are an opening snap in early diastole, a mid-diastolic murmur, and a loud first heart sound. The opening snap is caused by the abrupt tension that develops in the fibrosed leaflets at the termination of the opening movement. It is best heard at the lower left sternal edge or apex, becoming closer to the second heart sound as left atrial pressure rises, and it is absent with leaflet calcification. The diastolic murmur is low pitched and maximal at the apex. It is caused by increased blood flow velocity between the left atrium and left ventricle and is accentuated in late diastole by atrial contraction in patients in sinus rhythm. The loud first heart sound is associated with fibrosis of the anterior leaflet and is lost with leaflet calcification. Many patients with mitral stenosis have some degree of mitral regurgitation, which is not significant in the presence of severe stenosis.

In the presence of pulmonary hypertension the jugular venous pressure is raised, there may be a palpable right ventricular heave, and the second heart sound is usually loud. In patients with significant tricuspid regurgitation, whether secondary to pulmonary hypertension or due to rheumatic tricuspid valve, there is a clear V-wave and deep Y descent in the jugular venous pulse, and expansile pulsation of the liver. The murmur of tricuspid regurgitation is not usually prominent.

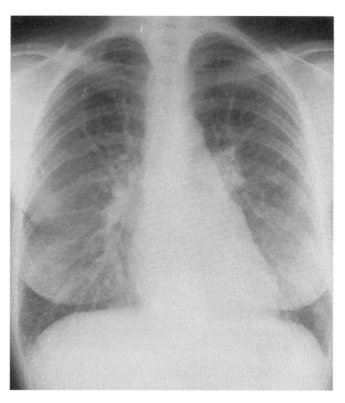

Fig. 6.1.1 Chest radiograph from a patient with pure mitral stenosis. The heart size is normal, but the left atrial appendage is enlarged. The upper lobe vessels are dilated and there are Kerley lines at both bases.

Investigations

Chest radiograph and electrocardiogram

Early in the disease a chest radiograph may show a completely normal cardiac silhouette. Later, as the disease progresses, left atrial enlargement appears and a prominent left atrial appendage contour becomes very evident (Fig. 6.1.1). Left atrial double-density and elevation of left main bronchus may also be evident. In patients with raised left atrial pressure, pulmonary vascular redistribution manifest as 'dilated upper lobe veins' and interstitial pulmonary oedema ('Kerley B lines') may be seen. The central pulmonary arteries become prominent as pulmonary hypertension develops, and upper lobe deviation is also seen. Finally, right-sided dilatation may also be seen as tricuspid regurgitation develops.

The electrocardiogram can show a broad and notched P-wave due to left atrial hypertrophy and enlargement ('P mitrale') as a classical finding in mitral stenosis, and its progressive broadening predicts the occurrence of atrial fibrillation, which is common in mitral stenosis.

Echocardiography

Echocardiography is the investigation of choice in mitral valve disease. A typical picture of rheumatic valve disease is a short, fibrosed, and stiff posterior leaflet; a fibrosed anterior leaflet that bows down towards the ventricle in diastole; and narrow valve area (Fig. 6.1.2). Short-axis images clearly demonstrate the fused commissures and two-dimensional images show the extent of chordal fibrosis. Planimetry of the mitral valve area in diastole gives an estimate of the degree of stenosis. Continuous-wave Doppler assesses the blood flow velocity across the valve. In mild stenosis, transmitral Doppler demonstrates a peak velocity in late diastole compared to in early

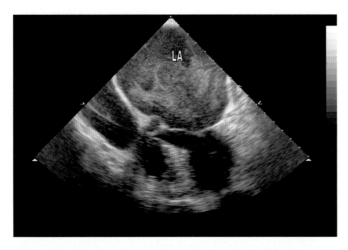

Fig. 6.1.2 Transoesophageal echocardiogram from a patient with severe rheumatic mitral stenosis showing a dilated left atrium (LA) with spontaneous echo-contrast.

diastole in severe stenosis. With atrial fibrillation there is a single early diastolic filling component to the left ventricle. A transmitral mean pressure gradient of more than 4 mmHg suggests a moderate degree of stenosis (Fig. 6.1.3), and a mean pressure gradient of more than 8 mmHg suggests severe stenosis. Colour-flow Doppler can provide a quantitative approach for assessing mitral stenosis severity using the proximal isovelocity surface area (PISA) method or the vena contracta method (the vena contracta being the narrowest region of the stenotic jet, just downstream of the valve orifice and reflecting the size of that orifice). Although the latter is easy to use it has its limitations since it varies more with deformation of the mitral orifice area and shape. Colour-flow Doppler will also show any mitral regurgitation jet and give some indication of its severity.

Echocardiography also assesses any involvement of the aortic valve or the tricuspid valve by the same or other pathologies.

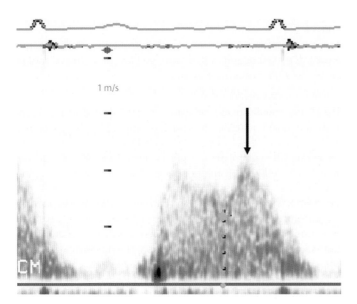

Fig. 6.1.3 Continuous-wave Doppler of left ventricular filling from a patient with mitral stenosis, showing raised velocities (>2 m/s, arrowed) across the mitral valve as the ventricle fills in diastole. A mean velocity of more than 1.3 m/s at the mitral valve leaflet tips is abnormal.

It is now common practice that most patients with mitral valve disease are studied by transoesophageal echo because this provides more detailed assessment of the mitral valve, the subvalvar apparatus, and the presence of left atrial spontaneous contrast and appendage clots.

Cardiac catheterization

Echocardiography has replaced cardiac catheterization in making the diagnosis of mitral stenosis. Catheterization may provide additional information on pulmonary vascular resistance and coronary artery disease before surgery.

Differential diagnosis

The diagnosis of mitral stenosis is usually straightforward on the basis of clinical findings supported by echocardiography, which should distinguish the presence of an Austin–Flint murmur caused by aortic regurgitation and the rare conditions of left atrial myxoma (see Chapter 10) and cor triatriatum (see Chapter 12).

Management

There is a significant time lag between the acute event of rheumatic fever and the presentation of mitral stenosis with mild symptoms, which could be up to 15 years. Patients may need another 10 years to develop signs and symptoms of severe stenosis. The likely reason behind this delay is the time needed for rheumatic leaflet fibrosis and calcification to develop and cause raised left atrial pressure. This time lag between acute rheumatic fever and clinical presentation varies significantly between developed and developing countries. In Europe and North America patients need valve surgery for mitral stenosis in their fifties, whereas those in developing countries need it in their thirties. The clinical outcome of patients with unoperated rheumatic mitral stenosis has changed significantly over time, with 20-year follow-up mortality dropping from historically 85% to recently 44% in those who refuse surgery.

Medical

The only medical treatments in mitral stenosis are the prophylactic measures against rheumatic fever (penicillin prophylaxis, see Chapter 9.1) and endocarditis (considered for high-risk cases, see Chapter 9.2), anticoagulation to prevent systemic embolism, and diuretics for raised left atrial pressure. There is no medication that has a direct effect on slowing disease progress.

Patients with mitral stenosis should be followed up clinically using noninvasive investigations, particularly Doppler echocardiography. The frequency of follow-up should be tailored according to individual patient's clinical condition and the severity of disease: this could be every 2 years in a patient with mild stenosis and regurgitation, but closer attention is required for the patient with severe stenosis and evidence of pulmonary hypertension. Particularly close follow-up is advised for pregnant women who have mitral stenosis.

In patients who develop atrial fibrillation, attempts to restore sinus rhythm are usually unsuccessful unless associated with surgery. To maintain sinus rhythm the organic mitral lesion should be dealt with either interventionally or surgically. In addition to heart rate control, digoxin may keep a patient with a modestly dilated left atrium in sinus rhythm. However, once atrial fibrillation is established, attention should be diverted to rate control with digoxin, β-blockers, or calcium channel blockers. With persistent atrial fibrillation anticoagulation is essential and INR level should be monitored and maintained at 2.5 to 3.5. Patients recommended for percutaneous mitral valvuloplasty should receive stable anticoagulation therapy for at least 3 months before the procedure and transoesophageal echo should exclude left atrial clot. Those who need surgical intervention may receive a maze procedure as a means for restoring the sinus rhythm, which involves surgically creating a single electrical pathway from the sinus node to the atrioventricular node, while isolating the abnormal electrical activity of the left and right atrial tissue. Recently, electrophysiological mapping with isolation of pulmonary veins has offered an alternative procedure. The success of the maze procedure varies considerably, ranging between 25% and 80% even after an initially successful procedure. See Chapter 4 for further discussion.

Patients who are symptomatic need intervention by either surgical valvotomy or catheter balloon valvuloplasty, whether or not they have pulmonary hypertension. Early intervention is highly recommended before the development of atrial fibrillation and an enlarged left atrium, provided a conservative operation is possible. The percutaneous mitral valvuloplasty procedure involves inserting an Inoue balloon into the mitral valve orifice and inflating it until an increase in mitral valve area is achieved (Fig. 6.1.4). Contraindications to this procedure are left atrial appendage thrombus, calcified subvalvar apparatus, and/or mitral regurgitation. Early results of this technique are satisfactory, particularly if patients are well selected, e.g. those with relatively mobile, noncalcified leaflets that are not greatly thickened, and without subvalvular thickening. Mitral stenosis may recur following this procedure after the healing period of the split of the fused commissures.

Surgical

Closed mitral valvotomy has been replaced by percutaneous mitral valvuloplasty, but its results are not optimal in low-workload centres in developed countries. There is thus still room for surgical repair of the mitral valve. This is better suited to patients with minimal calcification and those with short chordae. The technique offers the advantage of avoiding replacement of the mitral valve, which has effects on left ventricular function. However, in a patient with an irreparable mitral valve the only remaining option is mitral valve replacement.

Closed mitral commissurotomy

This historic procedure aimed at opening the mitral valve by applying a dilator through the ventricular apex, with the surgeon using a finger to feel the valve leaflets and orifice to judge when the desired valve area was achieved. The first successful operations were carried out in 1948. It has been intensively used in the United Kingdom and other countries, with an average mortality of 3 to 4%.

Open mitral valvotomy

This operation requires the use of an extracorporeal circulation and aims at direct visualization of the mitral valve through a medial sternotomy, with careful dissection of the fused commissures under direct vision. In contrast to the closed operation, the surgeon is able to deal with the subvalvar apparatus and the fused chordae, and correct chordal shortening if required. The left atrial appendage can also be visualized, and if there is thrombus present it can be removed. With appropriate patient selection and preoperative evaluation open commissurotomy is feasible in most patients, with an operative mortality of approximately 1%; however, most cases not suitable for balloon valvotomy require mitral valve replacement.

Mitral valve replacement

Mitral valve replacement involves either a mechanical or a tissue valve substitute. Surgical mortality varies according to other comorbidities: it is of the order of 3% in patients with isolated mitral valve stenosis but can be as high as 12% in patients with additional pulmonary hypertension. The life of biological mitral valve substitutes, particularly porcine xenografts, is limited to less than 10 years in most adults, hence their use tends to be restricted to very elderly patients. Cryopreserved mitral homografts have been proposed recently as a better option, as has the use of a pulmonary autograft in a Dacron tube, but experience is limited.

Mitral regurgitation

Causes

The most common causes of mitral regurgitation are ischaemic myocardial dysfunction, mitral valve prolapse, and dilated cardiomyopathy. Other causes are given in Table 6.1.1.

Ischaemic mitral regurgitation

The posteromedial papillary muscle is predisposed to ischaemic dysfunction and infarction because it is supplied by a single branch of the posterior descending artery and tends to have only a few collaterals. The anterolateral papillary muscle receives blood from branches of both the left anterior descending artery and the circumflex artery, so it is less susceptible to ischaemia. Ischaemic disturbances of left ventricular function contribute to the development of mitral regurgitation through a number of mechanisms: (1) regional wall motion abnormalities with adverse ventricular remodelling and systolic tenting of the valve leaflets, (2) left ventricular dilatation and shape change that alters normal alignment of the papillary muscles and results in leaflet tethering and inadequate closure, and (3) annular dilatation leading to inadequate annular contraction. These mechanisms may contribute to further enlargement of the left ventricle and deterioration of its function, which itself would add to the severity of mitral regurgitation. Four clinical presentations are seen in ischaemic mitral regurgitation: acute myocardial infarction,

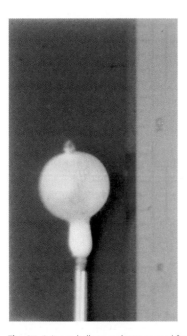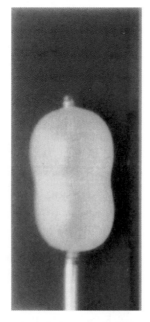

Fig. 6.1.4 Inoue balloon catheter, as used for mitral valvuloplasty, partially (left) and completely (right) inflated.

Table 6.1.1 Common causes of mitral regurgitation

Structure primarily affected	Anatomical defect	Cause
Valve cusps	Congenital cleft	Primary atrial septal defect
		Isolated
	Redundant cusp	Mitral valve prolapse
		Marfan's syndrome
	Perforation	Infective endocarditis
	Scarring	Rheumatic fever
		Ergot-derived dopamine receptor agonists
Chordae	Redundant	Mitral valve prolapse
		Marfan's syndrome
		Other connective tissue disease
	Rupture	Acute myocardial infarction
		Mitral valve prolapse
		Marfan's syndrome
		Other connective tissue disease
		Infective endocarditis
		Rheumatic fever
	Shortening	Rheumatic fever
		Endomyocardial fibrosis
Papillary muscle	Dysfunction	Ischaemia
Valve annulus	Dilatation	Severe left ventricular disease of any cause—'dilated cardiomyopathy'

papillary muscle rupture, reversible ischaemic myocardial dysfunction in the presence of preserved left ventricular systolic function, and endstage ischaemic cardiomyopathy with reduced function.

Acute myocardial infarction

Significant mitral regurgitation complicates 3 to 16% of acute myocardial infarctions. Most present within the obvious context of acute myocardial infarction, but some with pulmonary oedema from the acute development of mitral regurgitation. Most patients presenting with myocardial infarction complicated by mitral regurgitation have right and circumflex coronary artery disease that causes inferior wall dysfunction. Mitral regurgitation does not therefore seem to be related to infarct size, but to the extent of ischaemic dysfunction and involvement of the posteromedial papillary muscle. The resulting poor support to the posterior leaflet, referred to as tethering, causes lack of leaflet coaptation and valve incompetence. When severe mitral regurgitation develops it carries a poor prognosis, with mortality rising to 25% at 30 days and over 50% at 1 year. The effect of reperfusion on mitral regurgitation remains controversial.

Papillary muscle rupture

Complete papillary muscle rupture causes severe mitral regurgitation and cardiogenic shock that is usually fatal (70% within 24 h without emergency surgery). Surgical repair of the papillary muscle is not feasible in most cases because tissues are necrotic: valve replacement is necessary, with risk influenced by other factors including the severe left ventricular disease that is usually present.

Ischaemic mitral regurgitation in a normal left ventricle

Patients with long-standing ischaemic myocardial dysfunction usually have exertional reversible ischaemia. If this affects the posterior wall of the left ventricle it leads to further deterioration of posterior wall function and consequently the posterior leaflet function with the development of mitral regurgitation. Exertional breathlessness in these patients does not always have to be due to raised end-diastolic pressure and may be caused by a sudden increase in left atrial pressure through the development of mitral regurgitation with exercise, particularly in those with a dilated left atrium. Stress echocardiography is ideal for demonstrating the stress-induced ischaemic ventricular dysfunction and the development of mitral regurgitation and raised left atrial pressure, when antianginal therapy and afterload reduction may be beneficial. Patients who develop significant mitral regurgitation with stress and who are accepted for coronary artery bypass surgery should receive mitral valve repair and a ring insertion at the time of surgical revascularization.

Ischaemic mitral regurgitation in ventricular dysfunction

Mitral regurgitation is very common in patients with long-standing ischaemic left ventricular dysfunction and/or endstage ventricular disease. Since the valve leaflets appear morphologically normal, the mitral regurgitation is described as 'functional'. However, three-dimensional echocardiographic assessment of the mitral valve proves that it is not entirely normal, with long-standing progressive changes in the interleaflet relations and subvalvar apparatus. Reducing ventricular pressures may improve left ventricular geometry, and lowering blood pressure may reduce mitral regurgitation severity.

Mitral valve prolapse

Mitral valve prolapse is a genetic connective tissue disorder that affects the mitral leaflets, chordae, and annulus, with an autosomal dominant pattern of inheritance and variable penetrance. Histologically the leaflets show thickening of the spongiosa and disruption of the fibrosa with fragmentation. Collagen is also abnormal with high rate of synthesis, deficiency in type III collagen, and splitting of collagen with fibre disarray. The cause has not yet been identified: defects in a collagen gene or in a gene encoding a component of microfibrils, similar to that involved in Marfan's syndrome, have obviously been considered. The condition is common: 1.5 to 6% of adults have mitral prolapse, depending on definition, and screening of first-degree family members demonstrates prolapse in approximately 30% of cases.

Mitral prolapse can be classified into two types: a benign condition seen in young people, commonly women, that does not always progress; and the 'myxomatous mitral valve disease' seen in older people, often causing significant mitral regurgitation that needs surgical repair. Overall survival in patients with mitral prolapse is 97% at 6 years and 88% at 8 years, but those with myxomatous mitral valve disease and a flail leaflet have a 10-year survival much less. With posterior leaflet myxomatous prolapse, progressive chronic mitral regurgitation is associated with progressive dilatation of the left atrium and left ventricle.

The commonest site for posterior mitral prolapse is the middle scallop (P_2). Significant mitral regurgitation occurs in less than 10% of patients with posterior prolapse compared to 25% of those with anterior leaflet prolapse. In contrast, the incidence of atrial fibrillation and heart failure is significantly higher in posterior leaflet prolapse than in anterior leaflet prolapse. In general severe mitral regurgitation is associated with redundant leaflets, a longer posterior leaflet, and a larger annulus. Chordal distribution may also be abnormal, and there may be a relative scarcity of chordae to the central scallop of the posterior leaflet, increased chordal division or a higher incidence of chordal rupture.

There is a clear relationship between mitral valve prolapse, arrhythmia, and sudden death. The annual rate of sudden death in mitral prolapse is approximately 2%, which significantly falls after surgical repair. The risk of endocarditis is estimated at three to eight times that of the general population, the substrate being that leaflet prolapse causes significant turbulence of the blood flow across the valve orifice, disrupting platelet and fibrin deposition on the valve surface and subsequently resulting in vulnerability to infection. There is controversy regarding the relationship between mitral prolapse and embolic events.

Dilated cardiomyopathy

Mitral regurgitation is common in dilated nonischaemic cardiomyopathy. Dilatation of the left ventricle disturbs the normal closure of the mitral valve, the leaflets fail to coapt, and hence mitral regurgitation occurs.

Pathophysiology and complications
Regurgitant orifice and jet

The regurgitant volume of mitral regurgitation is calculated as the regurgitant flow over the regurgitant area. The flow velocity through the orifice is related to the ventricular–atrial systolic pressure difference. A high left ventricular systolic pressure, e.g. systemic hypertension, increases mitral regurgitation volume, and low left ventricular pressure reduces it. Left atrial pressure in acute mitral regurgitation is raised, with a V-wave in late systole due to the increased volume and the velocity of blood entering it (although the absence of such a wave on the left atrial or pulmonary wedge pressure trace does not exclude the diagnosis of severe mitral regurgitation).

Mitral regurgitation is often a dynamic lesion, with the size of the regurgitant orifice and regurgitant volume varying with the pressure gradient across the valve and with changes in left ventricular volume and geometry. The use of medical therapy to reduce left ventricular volume and improve its systolic function may therefore assist in reducing the severity of mitral regurgitation.

Left atrium

Left atrial volume increases in patients with mitral regurgitation in response to the increase in its pressure, to the transmission of the mitral regurgitation kinetic energy to the left atrial wall, and also to the development (in some cases) of atrial fibrillation. These effects balance those of the mitral regurgitation jet on left atrial pressure, which is normal in compensated patients. In contrast to mitral stenosis, the fast regurgitant jet in the left atrium reduces the risk of thrombus formation.

Afterload

Mitral regurgitation is an isolated volume overload on the left ventricle, providing the physiological equivalent of afterload reduction so that a normal forward cardiac output is maintained by the combination of increased ejection fraction and higher preload. Therefore, unlike the situation with pressure overload, the coronary blood flow is normal and the increase in myocardial oxygen consumption in mitral regurgitation is only mild. Left ventricular dysfunction, manifest by increased end-systolic diameter, is one of the most important determinants of outcome.

Right heart

The risk of right heart disease and dysfunction in mitral regurgitation is very similar to that in mitral stenosis. The raised left atrial pressure and pulmonary venous pressure are directly reflected on right ventricular systolic pressure. Right ventricular dysfunction as a complication of pulmonary hypertension is an important determinant of outcome.

Clinical presentation
Symptoms

Patients with mild mitral regurgitation may not have any symptoms: those with severe regurgitation are likely to present with dyspnoea. It is sometimes reported that mitral valve prolapse may be associated with nonspecific symptoms such as chest pain and fatigue, but this is debatable.

Physical examination

The patient with nonrheumatic mitral regurgitation is usually in sinus rhythm, but with severe mitral regurgitation of any cause patients may present in atrial fibrillation. The pulse is likely to be of normal character, but is sometimes reported as 'jerky', meaning of normal amplitude but rapid upstroke. The venous pressure is normal unless there is significant pulmonary hypertension or associated tricuspid disease.

The apex beat may be prominent and displaced, it may be double due to a palpable third heart sound, and there may be a palpable systolic thrill in severe cases. A palpable left parasternal heave may be due to systolic expansion of the left atrium and/or right ventricular hypertrophy.

The first heart sound is normal or soft, the most prominent findings on auscultation being an apical pansystolic murmur and a third heart sound. The loudness of the murmur generally correlates with severity of regurgitation, a murmur of less than grade 2/6 (meaning that it can be heard only with special effort) indicating mild disease, with the notable exception that no murmur may be audible with acute mitral regurgitation (when the mitral valve may effectively be absent). The cardinal signs of mitral prolapse are the mid-systolic click, due to the backward movement of the mitral leaflet into the left atrium, and the late systolic mitral regurgitation that occurs after the click. The murmur extends throughout systole as mitral regurgitation becomes severe.

The radiation of a mitral regurgitant murmur depends on the direction of the regurgitant jet. A posterolateral jet—seen in ischaemic mitral regurgitation, anterior leaflet disease and dilated cardiomyopathy—radiates from the apex to the axilla, and even to the back. An anterosuperior jet due to posterior leaflet prolapse is heard better at the lower left sternal edge or cardiac base (second right intercostal space, also known as the aortic area), and even on the carotids.

Other physical signs depend on the severity of mitral regurgitation and possible complications, e.g. pulmonary hypertension.

Investigations
Chest radiography and electrocardiogram

The chest radiograph reflects the haemodynamic disturbance (Fig. 6.1.5). The overall heart size is often normal or only moderately enlarged, with selective enlargement of the left atrium, although not to the same extent as with mitral stenosis (see Fig. 6.1.1). However, considerable cardiac enlargement develops due to secondary left ventricular disease if mitral regurgitation is severe and long-standing.

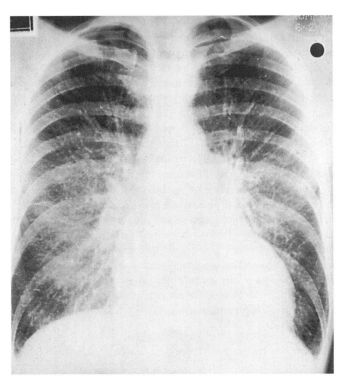

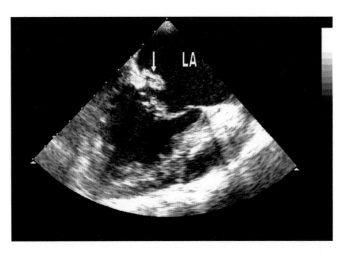

Fig. 6.1.6 Transoesophageal echocardiogram from a patient with posterior mitral leaflet prolapse (arrow). LA, left atrium.

Fig. 6.1.5 Chest radiograph showing acute pulmonary oedema due to acute mitral regurgitation resulting from ruptured chordae tendinae.

The electrocardiograph (ECG) usually shows sinus rhythm. There may also be evidence of left atrial hypertrophy, left ventricular hypertrophy, and frequent ventricular ectopic beats.

Echocardiography

Two-dimensional echocardiography provides a thorough assessment of the anatomy and function of the mitral valve apparatus, including the leaflets and annular diameter, as well as left ventricular size and function, left atrial size, and pulmonary artery pressure. The echocardiographic criterion for mitral prolapse is the presence

of at least 2 mm of late systolic posterior displacement of the leaflets across the mitral annular plane (Fig. 6.1.6). Severe myxomatous degeneration is associated with thickening of the leaflets and the appearance of extensive folding or redundancy of the leaflets in diastole, chordal elongation, and systolic anterior motion of the leaflets. Secondary mitral prolapse can easily be distinguished from primary prolapse in patients such as those with Marfan's syndrome, where the leaflets (particularly the anterior) are thin and long, and also in hypertrophic cardiomyopathy, with long leaflets and anterior motion of the mitral valve. Transthoracic echocardiography is perfectly adequate, but transoesophageal echocardiography is recommended if images are limited in quality.

Because it is noninvasive, echocardiography is an ideal tool for the follow-up of patients to allow early identification of worsening of regurgitation or deterioration in ventricular function. Many echocardiographic methods for determining the severity of regurgitation have been described (Fig. 6.1.7), three-dimensional reconstruction of the mitral regurgitation jet being a very promising

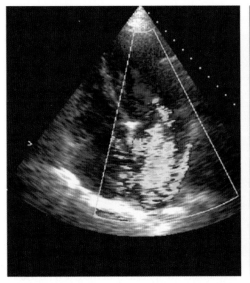

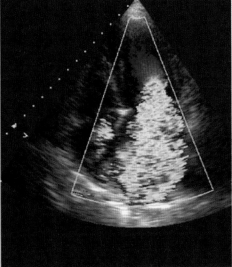

Fig. 6.1.7 Apical four-chamber views from a patient with coronary artery disease and ischaemic mitral regurgitation at rest (left) and stress (right). Note the significant increase in mitral regurgitation severity with stress as the ventricle became ischaemic.

tool for obtaining accurate regurgitant volume assessment since it avoids the conventional cross-sectional limitations. The extent of left ventricular cavity activity directly reflects the severity of volume overload, thus limiting the accuracy of using ejection fraction as a measure of ventricular function in such patients, hence changes in left ventricular end-systolic volume or dimensions should be taken as a marker of ventricular dysfunction. Patients recommended for surgical repair need detailed transthoracic and transoesophageal echocardiographic assessment of the anatomy of the valve and sub-valvular apparatus to assist surgeons in planning.

Findings that support pulmonary hypertension, in particular enlargement of the right side of the heart and increase in the retrograde pressure drop across the tricuspid valve, are easily obtained from a conventional Doppler echocardiographic study. Tricuspid leaflet prolapse is seen in 20% of patients with mitral valve prolapse, but aortic involvement is much less frequent.

Cardiac catheterization

This is not indicated for diagnostic purposes but may be required for preoperative assessment of the coronary arteries.

Differential diagnosis

Mitral regurgitation needs to be distinguished from ventricular septal defect (VSD), aortic valve disease, and tricuspid regurgitation.

Congenital VSDs are discussed in Chapter 12, but the commonest scenario in adult practice where distinction between mitral regurgitation and VSD needs to be made is the patient who deteriorates shortly after a myocardial infarction and is found to have a pansystolic murmur. It is impossible to distinguish reliably between the two by physical examination, although if the murmur is heard over the back VSD is most likely. Echocardiography and/or right heart catheterization with measurement of oxygen tension in the various cardiac chambers are required (see Chapter 13.5).

The systolic murmur of aortic valve disease can radiate to the apex, and sometimes be louder there than at the base (aortic area). The latter can lead to misdiagnosis of mitral valve disease, and the former can lead to confusion as to whether both aortic and mitral valves are diseased. Aside from looking for other evidence of aortic valve disease, the key thing is to establish the precise timing of the murmur. Mitral valve disease should only be diagnosed if the murmur is pansystolic, extending right up to and even obliterating the second heart sound (or right up to the onset of the early diastolic murmur of aortic regurgitation).

The murmur of tricuspid regurgitation is typically loudest at the lower left sternal border, is loudest during inspiration, and is associated with elevation of the venous pressure with systolic waves.

Management

Patients with chronic mitral regurgitation may survive for a long time with no limiting symptoms. Once symptoms develop they suggest the need for surgical correction of valve regurgitation to avoid development of irreversible left ventricular dysfunction. Assessment during routine follow-up identifies those likely to need surgical intervention even in the absence of symptoms, with an effective regurgitant orifice of over 40 mm^2 being the cut-off recommended value. Although patients with acute regurgitation secondary to papillary muscle rupture need emergency surgery, this does not necessarily apply to those with ruptured chordae or chronic ischaemic regurgitation. Such patients need to be stabilized and other risk factors and comorbidities identified and optimally managed.

Medical

There is no medical therapy that cures mitral regurgitation or mitral valve prolapse. Endocarditis prophylaxis is recommended for high-risk patients with regurgitation, although isolated mitral prolapse in the absence of regurgitation might not be counted as a definite indication. Symptomatic supraventricular arrhythmia needs optimum therapy, usually with β-blockers, and patients with ventricular tachycardia and syncope should be evaluated for implantable defibrillator (see Chapter 4). Those in atrial fibrillation should be given anticoagulants and INR adjusted at 2.5 to 3.5.

Appropriate pacing for dilated cardiomyopathy has been reported as reducing the severity of mitral regurgitation. Vasodilators improve prognosis and also reduce preload and the venous return, which improves leaflet coaption and reduces mitral regurgitation. Their effect on the afterload improves the forward flow and also reduces the retrograde flow across the mitral valve. Carvedilol has been shown to reduce long-axis length over diameter ratio ('cardiac index') and reduce mitral regurgitation severity. Similar findings have been documented in patients receiving ACE inhibitors or angiotensin receptor antagonists.

Surgical

A number of factors predict surgical outcome after correction of mitral regurgitation. As might be expected, the more complex the surgical procedure the higher the surgical risk. Age-related operative mortality is of the order of 12% in patients over 75 years of age and 1% in younger patients. Symptoms related to mitral regurgitation are important predictors: patients in New York Heart Association (NYHA) classes I and II carry a mortality of 0.5%, but for those in classes III and IV it is 10% or more. The aetiology of mitral regurgitation is another determinant, with 1 to 3% mortality in rheumatic mitral valve disease, compared to 9% in ischaemic mitral regurgitation.

Ventricular dysfunction adds to the surgical risk, in particular having an end-systolic dimension greater than 45 to 50 mm. However, recent data suggest that even significant left ventricular dysfunction should not be used as an exclusion criterion for correction of mitral regurgitation, although the general belief remains that a systolic dimension of more than 50 mm indicates a poor prognosis and that surgical intervention is unlikely to be of benefit. Pulmonary hypertension is another important predictor of outcome that carries a poor prognosis: correction of mitral regurgitation does not always guarantee normalization of pulmonary artery pressure, particularly if long-standing, which indicates that surgical intervention should be considered before development of this complication.

Mitral valve prolapse accounts for approximately 25% of mitral valve surgical procedures. The benefit of surgical intervention and ring insertion into patients with dilated cardiomyopathy remains controversial.

Mitral valve repair

The intention of mitral valve repair is to preserve the integrity of the valve, which—if successful—results in a much better clinical outcome for patients with mitral regurgitation than does valve replacement. Preservation of the chordal attachment is crucial, keeping the continuity between the mitral leaflets and the papillary muscles which control the long-axis function of the left ventricle. This itself also affects the sphericity of the left ventricle and hence overall performance of the cavity.

Mitral valve repair avoids the use of anticoagulants that are needed for life in patients with mechanical prostheses, and even those who develop atrial fibrillation from mitral valve repair might not need the higher dose of anticoagulants necessary for those who receive a mechanical valve. The risk of endocarditis is much lower from mitral valve repair compared to replacement.

As for any operation, patient selection for mitral valve repair is important. Although historical results of mitral valve repair for rheumatic regurgitation showed a success rate of 50%, better results have been reported recently, with a reoperation in approximately 20% of patients at 10 years. Surgical repair for rheumatic mitral valve disease is also affected by rheumatic aortic and tricuspid valve disease.

The most common procedure is the quadrilateral resection of the posterior leaflet, removing excess valve tissue, reapproximating the scallops, and reducing the annulus, with or without mitral annuloplasty. The success rate of this technique is of the order of 90%. Although historically anterior leaflet repair was not so easy as that of the posterior leaflet, recent advances have made it as successful. An alternative approach (not widely accepted in the surgical community) is the Alfieri repair, which involves suturing the posterior and anterior leaflets together in the central section and creating a double-orifice mitral valve.

Nonsurgical mitral-clip insertion has emerged as a replacement for repair procedures where the surgical risk is high. This procedure involves transcatheter implantation of a clip that hooks the tips of the anterior and posterior leaflets, thus creating a double-orifice mitral valve and reducing the extent of regurgitation. Early post-procedure results are satisfactory, but patients may continue to complain of breathlessness secondary to left ventricular stiffness rather than mitral regurgitation.

It is now routine practice to use intraoperative transoesophageal echocardiography to provide detailed assessment and detect signs of valve dysfunction immediately on completion of surgery on the valve: residual regurgitation can be dealt with before closure of the chest.

In addition to mitral repair, patients with atrial fibrillation may be considered for arrhythmia ablation—surgically or by radiofrequency—to restore sinus rhythm. Results of the combined procedure have been satisfactory, even with chronic atrial fibrillation before surgery.

Mitral valve replacement

Mitral valve replacement has a higher operative mortality than aortic valve replacement for aortic stenosis or regurgitation, or conservative operation for mitral stenosis. Although survival from mitral valve replacement surgery has improved significantly over the years, probably because of the better selection, improved myocardial preservation, and surgical techniques, it remains of concern, particularly in patients with ischaemic mitral regurgitation, where 5-year survival is 75%.

The ideal valve would be a homograft in the mitral position, but this can only be achieved by use of a composite including the mitral valve and related structures and placing it attached to the annulus, which avoids cutting the papillary muscle heads and the chordae and preserves the continuity between the mitral valve apparatus and the left ventricle. However, such attempts have proved uniformly unsuccessful. Pulmonary autograft has been used in the mitral position with satisfactory results, but in only a small group of patients in one or two centres.

Mitral replacement by a mechanical valve or bioprosthesis is the only option for irreparable valves. It has a very satisfactory success rate, particularly when papillary muscles and chordae are preserved. Bileaflet or tilting disc are currently the most commonly used mechanical valves.

Mixed mitral valve disease

Mixed mitral disease is nearly always due to rheumatic valve disease. In general, it occurs in older patients than pure mitral stenosis, and the valve is more likely to be calcified with limited cusp mobility and scarred subvalve apparatus. The mitral regurgitation is not usually severe, but the increased stroke volume increases the diastolic pressure drop across the valve.

Symptoms are the same as for mitral stenosis or regurgitation. On examination the first heart sound is not palpable or loud, the pansystolic murmur is usually loudest towards the axilla, and there is a mid-diastolic murmur.

The chest radiograph (Fig. 6.1.8) may show more advanced changes than in pure mitral stenosis (see Fig. 6.1.1): the left atrium can be extremely large. Echocardiography is likely to show thickened cusps with reduced motion in addition to mitral regurgitation. When symptoms merit, valve replacement is usually required.

Aortic valve disease

Aortic stenosis

Causes

Aortic stenosis is caused by congenital, rheumatic, or senile disease. It may be at subvalvar, valvar, or supravalvar level, the commonest being valvar stenosis.

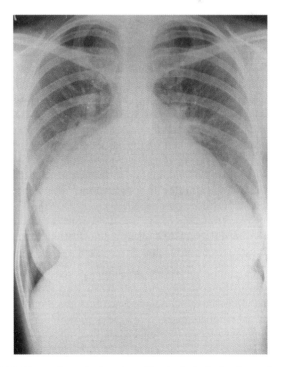

Fig. 6.1.8 Chest radiograph of a patient with mixed mitral valve disease, showing gross cardiac enlargement, mainly due to dilatation of the left atrium.

Age-related degenerative calcific disease is now the commonest cause of aortic stenosis in western Europe and the United States of America. The commonest congenital valvar aortic disease is the bicuspid aortic valve, which may remain completely silent for years, but as age advances the leaflets become thickened and calcified resulting in significant reduction in valve area, raised transvalvar velocities, and pressure drop (gradient) across the valve. Rheumatic aortic stenosis is nearly always associated with aortic regurgitation ('mixed aortic valve disease') and with rheumatic mitral disease. Symptomatic valvar aortic stenosis is more prevalent in men.

Subvalvar aortic stenosis is caused by a membrane (shelf) or a hypertrophied upper septal segment bulging into the outflow tract. Subaortic membrane is a congenital anomaly that commonly progresses with age. Hypertrophy of the upper septum is an acquired syndrome that affects older people, particularly those with long-standing hypertension. Supravalvar aortic stenosis is rare: when found it is commonly part of Williams' syndrome (OMIM 194050; 'elfin' facies with low nasal bridge, unusual behaviours and mental retardation, transient hypercalcaemia; supravalvar aortic stenosis).

Pathophysiology and complications

In addition to the anatomical narrowing of the aortic valve, left ventricular function plays an important role in determining the transvalvar velocities. Patients with severe aortic stenosis and poor left ventricular function may have underestimated velocities and pressure drop. By contrast, those with mild valve narrowing but a hyperactive ventricle (e.g. hyperdynamic circulation) may present with overestimated velocities across the valve; in particular, significant aortic regurgitation can lead to overestimation of the degree of valve stenosis because of increased stroke volume. Despite various attempts to determine the most sensitive marker of aortic stenosis, valve gradient (pressure drop) remains the most appropriate measure in clinical practice.

Left ventricular response

With the increase in outflow tract resistance in aortic stenosis, left ventricular wall stress increases and hypertrophy develops. This compensatory mechanism preserves overall ventricular systolic function. Most patients develop concentric left ventricular hypertrophy and increased mass, which regresses after removal of the stenosis. Patients with untreated aortic stenosis may present very late with left ventricular cavity dilatation, reduced ejection fraction, and dyssynchrony. Left ventricular subendocardial ischaemia may result from long-standing ventricular hypertrophy and outflow tract obstruction, and diastolic left ventricular function also become impaired, resulting in increased end-diastolic pressure and left atrial pressure. Most patients with aortic stenosis who are allowed to reach this degree of ventricular dysfunction complain of progressive breathlessness and finally pulmonary oedema.

Coronary circulation

Even in the absence of significant coronary artery disease (atherosclerosis), the coronary circulation plays an important role in the pathophysiology and clinical presentation of aortic stenosis. Proximal coronary artery size is often increased, probably as a compensatory mechanism for the increased myocardial oxygen demand because of left ventricular hypertrophy, but coronary flow reserve remains suboptimal. This limited coronary flow reserve is manifested in the subendocardium, which may become irreversibly damaged, and the more severe the aortic stenosis, the greater the impairment of subendocardial function. Furthermore, left ventricular relaxation is usually prolonged in left ventricular hypertrophy, which further reduces coronary flow. The combination of hypertrophy-related altered coronary flow and increased myocardial work probably contributes to the angina-like symptoms, even in the absence of epicardial coronary disease. Regression of left ventricular hypertrophy after aortic valve replacement improves coronary flow reserve.

Clinical presentation

Symptoms

Mild aortic stenosis does not give any symptoms, and even severe stenosis may be silent. Breathlessness or exercise intolerance is the most common symptom. Progressive deterioration of left ventricular function and increased end-diastolic pressure leads to acute pulmonary oedema and florid heart failure. Angina is the second most frequent symptom, but less common than breathlessness. When it happens it represents a significant mismatch between myocardial oxygen supply and demand, and it may be exercise limiting even in the absence of epicardial coronary artery disease. The third symptom is syncope, which in some patients is clearly related to exertion. This can be caused by reduced cardiac output due to outflow tract obstruction, or by arrhythmia (transient atrioventricular block, ventricular arrhythmia, and carotid sinus hypersensitivity have all been described), with exercise-induced peripheral vasodilatation in the face of a fixed cardiac output the likely explanation for those who collapse when exercising.

Physical examination

The physical signs of significant aortic stenosis are very characteristic. Proper examination of the character of the pulse is crucial: a slowly rising, low-amplitude carotid (or brachial) pulse has high specificity for diagnosing severe aortic stenosis, and there may be a carotid thrill. Arterial pulse pressure is narrow.

The venous pressure is usually normal until late in the disease, but a small 'a' wave is often present. This is known as a Bernheim 'a' wave and appears to be related in some poorly understood way to the presence of left ventricular hypertrophy and atrial crosstalk: it should not be taken in isolation as evidence of pulmonary hypertension.

The apex beat is often sustained and may be double, due to an additional left atrial impulse. On palpation of the precordium there may be a systolic thrill over the aortic area in severe cases.

On auscultation the first heart sound is normal or soft, and may be preceded by a fourth heart sound. The characteristic long and harsh ejection systolic murmur is loudest at the base (second right intercostal space, also known as the aortic area) of the heart, and in most cases it radiates to the carotids. The murmur is often heard at the lower left sternal border, and in a minority the ejection systolic murmur may also be referred to the apex. A systolic ejection click may be heard, typically in patients with an uncalcified bicuspid valve. The second heart sound in aortic stenosis is typically single because of the limited cusp movement in a heavily calcified valve, but in young patients with severe aortic stenosis and mobile leaflets the splitting of the second sound is reversed. A normal split second heart sound is a reliable sign for mild aortic stenosis. A third heart sound may be heard when left ventricular cavity dilatation and raised left atrial pressure have developed. A soft early diastolic murmur is often present, which does not necessarily imply haemodynamically significant aortic regurgitation.

It is important to note these physical signs are modified as ventricular disease progresses and stroke volume falls. Pulse volume drops and the pulse loses its slow rising quality, the systolic murmur becomes shorter and softer and may even disappear, and a functional mitral regurgitant murmur can appear along with a third heart sound. Such 'silent' but critical aortic stenosis cannot be diagnosed reliably on the basis of physical signs: a high index of suspicion and a good-quality echocardiogram are required to prevent misdiagnosis of 'congestive cardiomyopathy, cause unknown'.

Investigations

Chest radiograph and electrocardiogram

The chest radiograph may be completely normal in patients with uncomplicated aortic stenosis. Poststenotic dilatation of the ascending aorta may be seen. Associated left ventricular disease leads to pulmonary venous congestion.

In most patients the ECG shows evidence of left ventricular hypertrophy based on voltage criteria, but in some cases it can be completely normal. Advanced hypertrophy may be associated with nonspecific T-wave changes. With progressive left ventricular dysfunction QRS duration broadens and left bundle branch block may develop. Inverted U wave may be seen in patients with severe left ventricular disease.

Echocardiography

Echocardiography is the investigation of choice for patients with aortic stenosis, providing comprehensive information on valve anatomy and function and left ventricular size and function, as well as other associated cardiac abnormalities that may contribute to patient's symptoms, e.g. mitral valve regurgitation. Transthoracic echocardiography is mandatory in all patients with suspected aortic stenosis. Transoesophageal echocardiography may assist in examining the aortic root and the proximal ascending aorta.

The most clinically valuable measure of severity of aortic stenosis is transvalvular velocity using continuous-wave Doppler. The blood flow sounds under two-dimensional echocardiographic guidance assist in deciding on the optimum positioning of the probe for velocity recordings, with the beam as parallel as possible to the jet direction. Peak velocities across the aortic valve are converted into a pressure drop (pressure gradient) using the modified Bernoulli equation, $P = 4V2$.

Timing of peak velocity across the valve is a good indicator of the degree of aortic stenosis: in mild stenosis velocities peak in early systole, but in severe stenosis velocities peak in mid-systole, in parallel with the rise in aortic pressure.

Aortic stenosis can be quantified as valve area, which can be calculated from Doppler velocity data using the continuity equation based on the fact that the flow rate across the stenotic valve and the normal subvalvar area are equal. Valve area is therefore calculated from the relative increase in blood velocity across the aortic valve with respect to the subvalvar region, in conjunction with an estimate of the subvalvar cross-sectional area. Thus, an increase in peak velocity across the aortic valve by five times that of subvalvar velocity, with a pressure gradient of at least 35 mmHg, is consistent with a fivefold drop in aortic valve area and suggests severe aortic stenosis (Fig. 6.1.9).

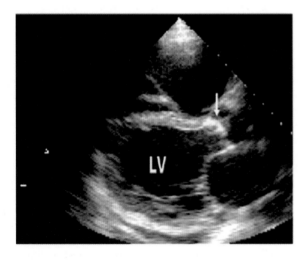

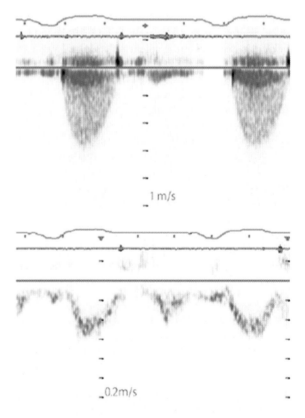

1 m/s

0.2m/s

Fig. 6.1.9 Parasternal long-axis views from a patient with severe calcific aortic stenosis (arrow) and poor left ventricular function showing a dilated cavity with increased end-systolic dimension (LV). Transvalvar peak velocity of 3.0 m/s (upper right panel) and subvalvar velocity of 0.6 m/s (lower right panel).

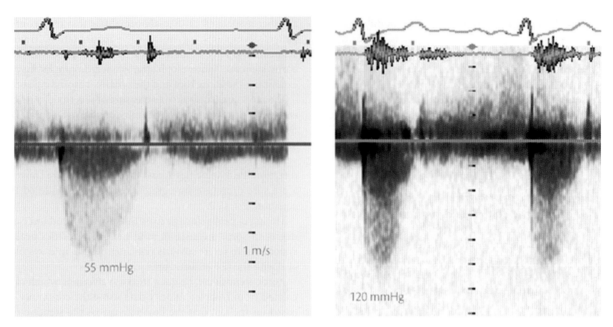

Fig. 6.1.10 Continuous-wave Doppler of transaortic valve velocities at rest (left panel) and peak stress (right panel) showing significant increase in velocities and consequently gradient from 55 to 120 mmHg.

An important application of this principle is seen in patients who have a moderate aortic pressure drop and in whom it is not clear whether this is simply because stenosis is not severe, or because stroke volume is low due to impaired left ventricular function. Stress echocardiography is a useful investigation in these circumstances (Fig. 6.1.10). With increase in heart rate the increased blood flow across the valve differentiates between severe valve narrowing and severe left ventricular disease. A significant increase in transvalvular velocities and pressure gradient reflects fixed valve area and hence the diagnosis of severe aortic stenosis. By contrast, failure of aortic velocities to increase significantly with stress suggests impaired left ventricular function as the cause of the low cardiac output and symptoms rather than aortic stenosis.

Colour-flow Doppler will reveal the presence of mild aortic regurgitation in most patients with aortic stenosis, and in those with impaired left ventricular function and raised end-diastolic pressure Doppler recordings of aortic regurgitation should be assessed carefully to avoid overestimating the degree of regurgitation because of raised left ventricular end-diastolic pressure.

Echocardiography can also provide accurate measurements of left ventricular dimensions and systolic function, as well as left ventricular hypertrophy and mass, from which mass index can be calculated. Left ventricular filling pattern guides the assessment of left atrial pressure. Most patients with aortic stenosis and left ventricular hypertrophy have a small early diastolic filling component and a dominant late-diastolic one. With progressive left ventricular disease and increase in end-diastolic pressure, the left atrial pressure increases and ventricular filling becomes of the restrictive pattern, with a dominant early diastolic filling component with short deceleration time and a very small late-diastolic filling component with flow reversal in the pulmonary veins. Most patients presenting with this pattern of physiology have a dilated left atrium and some may even present with atrial arrhythmia. The extent of the commonly found mitral regurgitation can also be assessed, and other parameters enable estimation of the presence and degree of pulmonary hypertension. Mitral annular calcification is a very common finding in patients with severe aortic stenosis but rarely contributes to any increase in atrial pressure or results in mitral stenosis.

Cardiac catheterization

High-standard echocardiographic estimation of the severity of aortic stenosis is clinically very reliable and does not need to be reconfirmed by catheterization. The traditionally measured aortic pressure gradient during cardiac catheterization, using a pull-back technique to record the difference between peak left ventricular and aortic pressure, is a less satisfactory measure than that possible echocardiographically because the two peaks do not occur simultaneously. A further problem with estimation of aortic gradient by cardiac catheterization occurs because left ventricular pressure may not be uniform, hence the measured pressure difference depends on the location of catheter tip in the ventricle, particularly in the presence of significant hypertrophy as in most cases of aortic stenosis. The difficulty increases since aortic pressure also depends on its distance from the valve leaflets and the aortic wall, as well as the pressure recovery process in the aortic root. Such estimates should thus be regarded as semiquantitative.

Cardiac catheterization is needed only to assess possible coronary artery disease, which frequently accompanies aortic stenosis. CT coronary angiography can now provide similar information.

Differential diagnosis

The commonest differential diagnosis that needs to be considered is aortic sclerosis, when examination of an elderly patient reveals an ejection systolic murmur at the cardiac base or left sternal edge. Other features of aortic stenosis—slow rising pulse, narrow pulse pressure, radiation of the murmur to the carotids, presence of a thrill—are not present.

Most often in a younger patient the possibility of hypertrophic cardiomyopathy needs to be considered, but here the carotid pulse is normal or jerky rather than slow rising (see Chapter 7.2). Fixed subaortic stenosis also needs to be considered in children and young adults (see Chapter 12).

All of these differential diagnoses can be distinguished from aortic stenosis by echocardiography.

Management

Progression of aortic stenosis is generally slow. Symptoms are variable but overall reflect left ventricular disease. Patients with a congenital bicuspid aortic valve tend to develop symptoms at an average age of 50 years, whereas those with senile valve disease do so at the age of 70 to 80 years. Patients with significant congenital aortic valve stenosis may develop symptoms earlier in life. Some 50% of patients with severe aortic stenosis die suddenly.

Raised aortic velocities and gradient, and the rate of increase in velocities over time, are the most accurate predictors of outcome, the rate of deterioration being faster in senile disease than rheumatic aortic stenosis. Once symptoms develop the outcome is poor without surgical intervention, with 5-year survival less than 50%. Autopsy series showed that the average time from symptom development to death is 2 years in patients with exertional syncope, 3 years in those with dyspnoea, and 5 years in those with angina. It should be highlighted that prognosis is much better in patients with a high valve gradient rather than those with low gradient due to severe left ventricular disease. Recent data suggests that patients presenting with an ejection fraction below 20% fail to thrive even after successful aortic valve replacement surgery.

Approximately 50% of adults with aortic stenosis who need surgery have additional coronary artery disease. Patients with angina-like symptoms who have only mild aortic stenosis are likely to have significant epicardial coronary disease, but a new onset of angina in patients with severe aortic stenosis may reflect a further deterioration of the degree of aortic stenosis and subendocardial ischaemia. A particularly difficult group of patients to manage is those with moderate aortic stenosis and angina-like symptoms.

Medical

There is no medical treatment for aortic stenosis that will stop disease progression. Asymptomatic patients with mild or moderate aortic stenosis require follow-up; those with severe aortic stenosis need aortic valve replacement. It is prudent to advise those with moderate or severe disease to avoid strenuous exercise. A pressure gradient of more than 70 mmHg across the aortic valve is a good indication for surgery, particularly in those who are symptomatic. Patients with severe aortic stenosis and left ventricular disease who present with heart failure should be stabilized before referral for surgery: diuretics are important, as well as β-blockers for controlling the heart rate; vasodilators, including ACE inhibitors, are contraindicated. Once a patient develops raised left atrial pressure and pulmonary hypertension the outcome is less than satisfactory, even with surgery.

Instructions on endocarditis prophylaxis and the use of antibiotics before dental and surgical procedures should be given to high-risk patients. Patients with other comorbidities and risks, in particular hyperlipidaemia, should have these addressed. The effect of statins on the rate of progression of aortic stenosis seems to be negligible.

Surgical

Recent advances in aortic valve surgery—earlier intervention, changes in the procedures used, improved methods of myocardial preservation—have resulted in a significant fall in surgical mortality, to 2.7 to 8.3% in adults under 70 years of age. Concurrent coronary artery disease, ventricular dysfunction, and pulmonary hypertension are important surgical risks. Older patients with aortic stenosis, particularly those over the age of 80 years, tend to have a higher mortality, but age is not a contraindication to surgery. Surgical intervention in octogenarians has been shown to provide improvement in quality of life, with a 5-year postoperative survival compared to only 1 year for the unoperated.

Aortic valve repair. In young people aortic valvotomy is an acceptable procedure, but the option of valve repair in adults remains uncertain. It may provide a medium-term solution for a clinical problem, but further surgical intervention will definitely be required in the long term.

Tissue valves. Tissue valves do not need anticoagulants in the absence of atrial fibrillation. Although their durability is significantly lower than that of mechanical valves, indications for their use are clear: older people, young pregnant women, and patients with limited access to anticoagulant therapy. Over the years the durability of tissue valves has significantly improved: for patients over the age of 60, modern, third-generation, glutaraldehyde-preserved valves provide 90% survival at 15 years. Stentless tissue valves have better durability and are associated with faster recovery of ventricular function, but they are more difficult to implant.

The best option to replace a native valve is a human valve (homograft), but availability is limited. An aortic valve homograft replacement is particularly indicated in patients with endocarditis that involves the aortic root and is associated with abscess formation, because a mechanical valve replacement in this scenario compromises eradication of the infection. Aortic homograft implantation techniques have evolved from a two-layer subcoronary implantation to conduit implantation, which involves replacing the valve and sinus of Valsalva by a full root and valve. This still is considered more challenging than mechanical or tissue valve implantation. Under the age of 30 years aortic homografts tend to fail within 10 years: in older patients the mean survival of the valve is 15 to 18 years.

An alternative procedure is the pulmonary autograft or 'Ross procedure'. This goes back to 1967 when Donald Ross transferred a patient's own living pulmonary valve to the aortic position and inserted a homograft in the pulmonary position. In children these autograft valves, unlike any other valve substitute, are capable of growth. A pulmonary homograft is placed in the right ventricular outflow tract, where because of the lower pressures on the right side of the circulation the mean survival of the valve is 20 years. More recently, percutaneous replacement of the aortic valve (transcutaneous aortic valve implantation procedure, TAVI; see 'Transcutaneous aortic valve implantation and' Chapter 13.6) has become an alternative for patients at high surgical risk, with satisfactory results worldwide.

Mechanical valves. Over the years technical improvement in valve design has been remarkable, providing larger orifice area and greater resistance to thrombosis. In the long term the commonest problem, affecting less than 5% of patients with mechanical prostheses, is paravalvular dehiscence. While this may not always be haemodynamically significant, it may be responsible for haemolytic anaemia due to shear stress on red blood cells, and it is a focus for infective endocarditis. Valve dysfunction due to subvalvar tissue ingrowth that influences valve opening and closure remains a problem.

Transcutaneous aortic valve implantation. A transcatheter stent-mounted bioprosthesis has recently been developed as an alternative to surgical aortic valve replacement in patients with impaired left ventricular function, prior coronary artery bypass surgery, or other comorbidities (e.g. renal impairment or chronic obstructive pulmonary disease). The procedure has proved a great success in patients with heavily calcified aortic root and valve. Long-term clinical results of the TAVI procedure are similar to those of surgical aortic valve replacement, despite a slightly higher prevalence of stroke.

Aortic regurgitation

Causes

Aortic regurgitation is caused by either leaflet disease or aortic root dilatation (Table 6.1.2), the commonest causes being isolated medionecrosis, rheumatic disease, infective endocarditis, and Marfan's syndrome.

Pathophysiology and complications

The left ventricular stroke volume, which equals the forward stroke volume plus the regurgitant volume, is significantly increased in aortic regurgitation. This is accommodated by an increase in left ventricular cavity size, a process that is progressive in a similar fashion to mitral regurgitation, although the degree of ventricular dilatation is greater. Another difference between the two conditions is the peripheral vascular resistance, which is significantly raised only in patients with aortic regurgitation. This combination of volume overload and raised peripheral resistance results in a progressive increase in left ventricular wall thickness and mass. In uncomplicated aortic regurgitation, the left ventricular ejection fraction is maintained, but as the disease progresses end-systolic volume increases out of proportion to stroke volume, and eventually these

Table 6.1.2 Causes of aortic regurgitation

Structure primarily affected	Anatomical defect	Cause
Cusp	Distortion	Rheumatic
		Rheumatoid
		Ergot-derived dopamine receptor agonists—pergolide, cabergoline (treatments for Parkinson's disease)
		Fenfluramine, phentermine (appetite suppressants)
	Perforation	Infective endocarditis
Root disease	Dilatation	Isolated medionecrosis
		Marfan's syndrome
		Syphilis
		Ankylosing spondylitis or other connective tissue disease
Loss of support		Dissecting aneurysm of aortic root
		Subaortic ventricular septal defect

changes lead to irreversible damage which persists even after surgical correction of the aortic regurgitation.

Whether or not aortic regurgitation is accompanied by some degree of aortic stenosis due to intrinsic valve leaflet disease, the increase in stroke volume causes high systolic velocities across the aortic valve. Pressure relations between the aorta and the left ventricle in diastole are of great importance, in particular the end-diastolic pressure difference that depends not only on aortic but also on left ventricular end-diastolic pressure: the higher the left ventricular end-diastolic pressure the lower the pressure difference across the valve.

In mild aortic regurgitation the pressure drop between the aorta and the left ventricle is maintained throughout diastole. By contrast, with acute aortic regurgitation the pressure difference between the aorta and the left ventricle falls to 15 mmHg or even less before end of diastole, either because of the very low resistance at the valve level or because the left ventricle is stiff, hence a relatively small regurgitant volume causes a disproportionate left ventricular diastolic pressure rise. This disturbed physiology has major implications because the aortic–left ventricular diastolic pressure gradient is the pressure head supporting the coronary flow. Coronary autoregulation stops at a perfusion pressure difference between the aorta and the left ventricle of 40 mmHg, and with acute aortic regurgitation—or even severe chronic aortic regurgitation—the gradient is less than this, resulting in significant myocardial ischaemia and progressive ventricular dysfunction. This disturbed physiology may be tolerated in chronic severe aortic regurgitation, but in acute severe aortic regurgitation it may contribute to rapid clinical deterioration.

The limitation of coronary flow by a raised ventricular end-diastolic pressure is further exacerbated by the increased oxygen demand of the myocardium as a result of the hyperdynamic ventricular state, as well as (in chronic regurgitation) the hypertrophy resulting from the volume overload. This causes subendocardial ischaemia, particularly with stress.

Clinical presentation
Symptoms

Patients with aortic regurgitation may remain asymptomatic for a long time. The onset of symptoms, particularly breathlessness, coincides with the onset of left ventricular disease, a significant rise in end-diastolic pressure, and development of pulmonary venous hypertension. Angina is an uncommon symptom in chronic aortic regurgitation, but when it occurs it should suggest significant subendocardial ischaemia as a result of the mismatch between the coronary artery flow and myocardial mass. It is more common in those with acute aortic regurgitation. Any sudden worsening of symptoms may reflect acute deterioration of the degree of aortic regurgitation or impairment of left ventricular function.

Physical examination

The physical signs of significant chronic aortic regurgitation are characteristic. The pulse has large amplitude and is 'collapsing' in nature ('water hammer', Corrigan's pulse) due to the increased stroke volume and rapid fall-off in aortic pressure during diastole. When severe, this can induce pulsations in many parts of the body, generating many eponyms that describe what is effectively a single physical finding. Amongst the better known of these are Quincke's capillary pulsations (best demonstrated by blanching a portion of a fingernail by applying gentle pressure and observing the pulsating border between the white and the red segments), de Musset's sign (bobbing of the head in time with the arterial pulse, named after the French poet who had the condition), and pulsations of various organs or their parts (uvula—Muller's sign, retinal arteries—Becker's sign).

The same pathophysiology underlies two peripheral arterial signs. Pistol shot sounds are short, loud sounds that can be heard over large peripheral arteries if the stethoscope is lightly applied: they occur because of sudden expansion and tensing of the walls during systole. Duroziez's sign is a double to-and-fro (systolic and diastolic) murmur heard over the brachial or femoral artery if the stethoscope is firmly applied: the diastolic component results from reversal of flow in the artery during diastole.

A diastolic blood pressure of less than 50 mmHg and/or a pulse pressure of 80 mmHg or more suggest moderate or severe regurgitation in patients who have a characteristic murmur (but are of no significance with regard to the aortic valve if no murmur is present). The venous pressure is normal until late in the course of disease, although a dominant Bernheim 'a' wave may be seen. The apex beat is sustained and/or displaced because of the left ventricular hypertrophy and/or dilatation.

On auscultation the classical murmur of aortic regurgitation is diastolic, starting immediately after the second heart sound, decrescendo in nature, and loudest at the left sternal border. It may be short, or extend throughout diastole. It may radiate to the right sternal border if it is caused by aortic root dilatation, and rarely it is loudest at the apex or even in the left axilla. The louder the murmur, the more severe is the regurgitation. The heart sounds may not demonstrate any specific change in aortic regurgitation, or—as with aortic stenosis—the aortic component of the second heart sound may be absent. An ejection systolic murmur due to increased stroke volume is nearly always present. At the apex a low-pitched mid-diastolic murmur (Austin–Flint murmur) mimicking that of mitral stenosis may be heard: it is usually assumed that this is due to the aortic regurgitant jet striking the anterior leaflet of the mitral valve, but other hypotheses have been advanced.

In acute aortic regurgitation—usually caused by infective endocarditis, thoracic aortic dissection, or disintegration of a tissue valve replacement—the physical signs are quite different, based on the fact that the stroke volume in acute regurgitation does not increase by the same magnitude as in chronic regurgitation. The patient is cold and shut down due to a low cardiac output, with tachycardia, a low systolic blood pressure and low pulse pressure, and a short early diastolic murmur that is easily missed. The apex is not displaced and peripheral signs are absent. There may be a loud third heart sound.

Investigations

Chest radiograph and electrocardiogram

The chest radiograph may show increased cardiothoracic ratio and dilatation of the aortic root (Fig. 6.1.11). In isolation these appearances cannot be taken as diagnostic, but they are very useful for follow-up of a known case.

The 12-lead ECG may demonstrate increased voltage and a 'strain' pattern that correlates with increase in left ventricular cavity dimensions, hypertrophy, and wall stress. The voltage pattern may fall significantly after correction of the aortic regurgitation and regression of left ventricular mass. Nonspecific T-wave changes may occur with exercise, reflecting either the development of subendocardial ischaemia or increase in systolic left ventricular

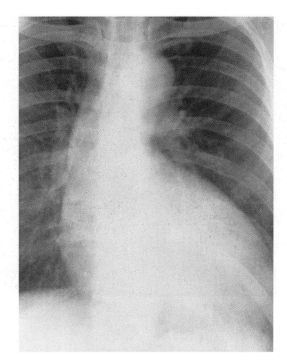

Fig. 6.1.11 Chest radiograph of a patient with chronic aortic regurgitation showing cardiac enlargement and dilatation of the ascending aorta.

volume. Increased QRS duration is a marker of left ventricular disease. A long PR interval may indicate aortic root abscess, particularly in those with other clinical suspicion of endocarditis.

Echocardiography

Doppler echocardiography is an invaluable investigation in the assessment of patients with aortic regurgitation (Fig. 6.1.12). Two-dimensional images can identify the exact cause of regurgitation, revealing the valve anatomy, leaflet number, calcification, or evidence of infection. The diameter of the aortic root and proximal ascending aorta can also be measured. Transoesophageal examination is always recommended if this is not achievable on transthoracic images, particularly in patients with Marfan's syndrome or those presenting with suspected dissection. Left ventricular size, dimensions, wall thickness, and ejection fraction can easily be measured, and muscle mass calculated using simple formulae. Colour Doppler detects the presence of aortic regurgitation and gives some idea of its severity: the finding of large vena contracta, a large regurgitant orifice area, and jet diameter more than 50% of the aortic root diameter are all consistent with significant regurgitation. Continuous-wave Doppler is ideal for assessing regurgitation severity as well as pressure differences between the aorta and the left ventricle (Fig. 6.1.13): in general, the faster the pressure decline on the aortic regurgitation trace, the more severe is the regurgitation likely to be, although this does not apply in patients with raised end-diastolic pressure. Doppler can also confirm severity of aortic regurgitation by demonstrating flow reversal in the descending aorta or femoral arteries. In patients with symptoms disproportionate to the degree of aortic regurgitation, a diagnosis of left ventricular disease should be considered, e.g. hypertension or coronary heart disease.

In acute aortic regurgitation echocardiography demonstrates clearly the cause of the disease; endocarditis with its complications or disintegrating homograft or bioprosthesis. M-mode

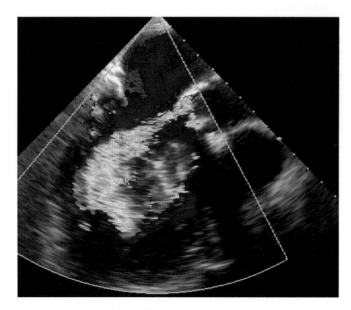

Fig. 6.1.12 Transoesophageal echocardiogram from a patient with aortic regurgitation on colour-flow Doppler.

echocardiography shows premature mitral valve closure which, together with the left ventricular activity, support the diagnosis of acute aortic regurgitation.

Cardiac catheterization

Cardiac catheterization is not needed to assess the severity of aortic regurgitation: it is only needed to confirm the presence of additional coronary artery disease, particularly before surgical intervention.

Differential diagnosis

It can sometimes be difficult to distinguish the early diastolic murmur of aortic regurgitation from that caused by pulmonary regurgitation (Graham–Steell murmur). In this circumstance no other features of aortic regurgitation are expected, and pulmonary regurgitation is usually associated with other signs indicating the presence of significant pulmonary hypertension (including a large pulmonary artery on the chest radiograph).

Other causes of aortic run-off, including persistent ductus arteriosus, ruptured sinus of Valsalva aneurysm, and coronary arterio-venous fistula, can also produce auscultatory findings that can be confused with aortic incompetence. However, they all cause a continuous murmur, rather than one confined to diastole.

Management

It is uncommon for mild aortic regurgitation to progress rapidly to severe regurgitation, hence the importance of Doppler echocardiography in the follow-up of patients. Identification of the cause of aortic regurgitation helps in determining how often patients should be reviewed: those with mild aortic regurgitation due to aortic root or ascending aorta disease should be followed up more closely than those with stable valve disease. Patients with moderate or severe aortic regurgitation may have no symptoms for years. As symptoms always reflect ventricular dysfunction, a progressive increase in end-systolic dimension/volume should be taken as an indication for serious consideration of surgery, even in the absence of symptoms. Ejection fraction cannot be taken as a marker of ventricular function in aortic regurgitation because of the volume overload and overestimation of the ejection performance: an end-systolic dimension up to 40 mm carries a good prognosis, whereas a dimension more than 50 mm is associated with 20% possibility of developing

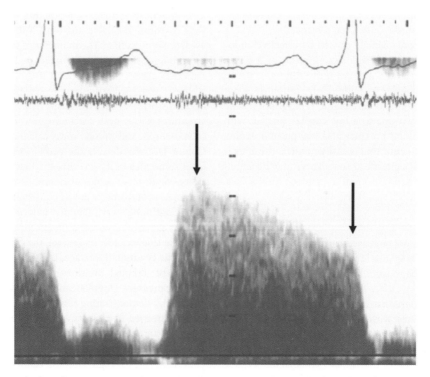

Fig. 6.1.13 Continuous-wave Doppler from the same patient as shown in Fig. 6.1.12, showing significant regurgitation based on the rate of transvalvar pressure decline in diastole (between the arrows)

ventricular dysfunction, symptoms, or even death over a course of 5 years.

In the same way that patients with aortic regurgitation secondary to aortic valve disease are managed, those with aortic regurgitation associated with or causing aortic root dilatation should be followed up to assess the aortic root dimensions, with the aim of preventing progressive dilatation and the potential risk thereof. Some patients with a bicuspid aortic valve develop progressive dilatation of the aortic root and ascending aorta because of the eccentric jet, as well as the accompanying aortopathy. Another group of patients who need regular follow-up and careful aortic root assessment are those with Marfan's syndrome, in whom aortic root aneurysmal dilatation and dissection are the major causes of morbidity and mortality. In addition to using conventional Doppler echocardiography, CT scanning and MRI can play a useful role in the follow-up of patients with aortic root or ascending aorta disease, and three-dimensional echocardiography for assessment of left ventricular size and function (see Chapters 3.2 and 3.3 for further discussion).

Medical

Medical management in aortic regurgitation aims at slowing down its progression, supporting the left ventricle, and determining the optimal time of surgical intervention. The increased afterload in patients with aortic regurgitation should be managed medically to reduce the wall stress and the diastolic driving pressure across the valve. Doing so decreases the pressure and the volume overload on the left ventricle and prevents progressive left ventricular dilatation and systolic dysfunction, and can delay the need for surgery. This effect has been demonstrated using ACE inhibitors and calcium channel blockers, the choice of the pharmacological agent for left ventricular afterload reduction depending on the other comorbidities, e.g. coronary artery disease, as well as patient tolerance.

Patients with aortic root dilatation should not be treated with vasodilators alone. In this instance β-blockers are recommended because they decrease aortic wall stress, blood pressure, and the rate of pressure increase in systole. Although patients with Marfan's may remain completely asymptomatic, the rate of aortic root dilatation is the most important risk factor. It may be that the combination of β-blockade with ACE inhibition/angiotensin receptor blockers (possibly acting through inhibition of TGF-β signalling) may prove effective in retarding or even preventing dilatation. However, when dilatation does occur, previous guidelines have suggested that aortic root dimension larger than 55 mm is a good indication for surgical intervention, although recent recommendations have advocated an earlier surgical approach, particularly in the presence of family history of dissection. See Chapter 11 for further discussion.

As is the case with all valve disease, oral hygiene should be encouraged in patients with aortic regurgitation and prophylactic antibiotics prescribed to cover dental, proctological, urological, and gynaecological surgeries for patients at risk.

Surgical

Although patients with severe chronic aortic regurgitation may remain asymptomatic, surgical intervention should be offered when there is progressive increase in systolic dimension. A left ventricular end-systolic dimension of 40 mm is a cut-off value for preserved left ventricular systolic function, particularly for an active ventricle. Predictors of outcome after valve surgery are severe aortic regurgitation, age, severe symptoms, exercise intolerance, and evidence for left ventricular hypertrophy on echocardiography. Raised left ventricular end-diastolic pressure and the ratio of wall thickness to chamber dimension have also been identified as potential predictors of outcome. An additional risk is the presence of coronary artery disease. These patients should be carefully evaluated by preoperative cardiac catheterization and receive myocardial revascularization surgery and coronary grafting at the same setting with aortic valve replacement surgery. There is evidence to suggest that patients with aortic regurgitation and ventricular dysfunction develop faster reverse remodelling and fall of left ventricular mass index following successful valve replacement if they receive a stentless rather than a stented valve. Details of surgical procedures for aortic regurgitation are as described in the preceding section on aortic stenosis.

Acute aortic regurgitation, irrespective of its aetiology, should be managed as an emergency with surgical intervention. While diagnostic evaluation is in progress the patient should be treated with afterload reduction. Aortic balloon counter pulsation is contraindicated because it increases afterload. Cases caused by infective endocarditis should receive optimal antibiotic therapy following blood culture and emergency valve replacement, which could be life-saving.

Mixed aortic disease

Mild to moderate aortic regurgitation often accompanies aortic stenosis but does little to alter the overall clinical picture. The combination can result from a bicuspid aortic valve or chronic rheumatic heart disease, or be the result of endocarditis or conservative surgery on a stenosed valve. The main haemodynamic disturbance is increased resistance to ejection, but the superimposition of even a moderately increased stroke volume due to regurgitation on the small, stiff left ventricle of pure aortic stenosis can lead to high filling pressures, left atrial enlargement, and even pulmonary hypertension. Breathlessness and chest pain are the most prominent symptoms. The arterial pulse is bisferiens, and typical ejection systolic and early diastolic murmurs are expected. Patients with symptoms are likely to require valve replacement.

Right heart valve disease

Many of the conditions that affect right-sided valves are congenital: these are discussed in detail in Chapter 12. Particular pulmonary and tricuspid valve diseases that develop later in life are discussed here, after general discussion of effects of abnormal right-sided haemodynamics on right heart function and diagnostic techniques.

Pathophysiology and complications

Right ventricular response to valve disease

The right ventricle responds to chronic pressure overload, e.g. caused by pulmonary stenosis or pulmonary hypertension, by hypertrophy and early dilatation. With increased afterload and right ventricular dilatation the ventricle adapts by making the intraventricular septum function as part of the right heart. This can be identified by studying septal movement during various phases of the cardiac cycle using M-mode echocardiography, revealing that it becomes reversed in systole and in diastole. Right ventricle dilatation includes the tricuspid annulus and results in tricuspid regurgitation. Eventually right ventricular systolic function deteriorates, and this may become irreversible even after correcting the volume or pressure overload. With right ventricular volume overload the ventricle is very active, readily apparent on recording its free-wall movement at the level of the tricuspid ring. However, assessing right ventricular ejection fraction and overall systolic function is difficult because of its complex anatomy, being made up of an inlet portion and an outlet portion that are at a significant angle to each other, and a trabecular portion at the apex.

Assessment of right ventricular size and function

A three-dimensional approach to the assessment of right ventricular systolic function is the ideal method, but other cross-sectional echocardiographic and MRI techniques have developed over the years and proved sensitive in assessing right ventricular ejection fraction. Right ventricular inlet diameter can be used as a marker of cavity dilatation. Free-wall long-axis movement studied by M-mode and tissue Doppler imaging from the lateral angle of the tricuspid annulus is an easy measure of systolic function and correlates closely with right ventricular ejection fraction. Likewise, right ventricular outflow tract diameter has been shown a sensitive measure of systolic function. In patients with reversed septal movement it is crucial to exclude any shunt as a cause for volume overload in the right ventricle.

Estimation of pulmonary artery pressure is an essential component in the evaluation of patients with right-sided valve disease. The retrograde flow velocity across the tricuspid valve gives an indication of systolic right ventricular pressure by use of the simplified Bernoulli equation. In all patients systolic pulmonary artery pressure equals the retrograde peak pressure drop across the tricuspid valve added to the estimated right atrial pressure, according to the collapsibility of the inferior vena cava. These measurements are clinically useful in patients without pulmonary stenosis.

Investigation of valve stenosis and regurgitation

The methods used in clinical practice for investigating possible tricuspid and pulmonary valve stenosis and regurgitation are the same as those used in assessment of conditions affecting the left side of the heart. Colour Doppler detects the level at which there are increased velocities as a sign of valve narrowing, which can be confirmed by continuous-wave Doppler. In patients with valve regurgitation colour Doppler assesses the jet diameter, direction, and area which, with respect to the right atrial area in cases of tricuspid regurgitation, gives some indication of the severity of tricuspid regurgitation. Transoesophageal echo images, particularly in tricuspid valve disease, provide detailed assessment of valve pathology.

Transthoracic images of the pulmonary valve can be somewhat limited technically, but in most cases Doppler studies can exclude significant valve disease based on forward and backward velocities and pressure drop. Transoesophageal echo provides a clearer image of the pulmonary valve and so is best suited for determining the level of valve stenosis. The degree of pulmonary stenosis and regurgitation severity is assessed by continuous-wave Doppler, with timing of reversal of regurgitant pulmonary flow being another confirmation of its severity. Mild pulmonary regurgitation occupies the whole of diastole, while in severe regurgitation there is early pressure equalization between the two chambers. A jet diameter of 7 mm or more also supports the diagnosis of severe pulmonary regurgitation.

MRI is another good noninvasive technique for assessment of right-sided chamber size and valve function, in particular the pulmonary valve. The level of narrowing can easily be determined, the degree of stenosis by velocity mapping, and severity of regurgitation by estimating the regurgitant volume.

Tricuspid stenosis

Tricuspid stenosis is a rare condition, most often caused by rheumatic disease, which almost invariably simultaneously affects the mitral valve. Other (even rarer) causes are carcinoid disease, infective endocarditis, and Whipple's disease. A right atrial myxoma or extension of hypernephroma into the inferior vena cava and right atrium can in very rare instances present with signs and symptoms of right ventricular inflow tract obstruction, similar to tricuspid stenosis.

Symptoms include fatigue, dyspnoea, and fluid retention. In patients with chronic rheumatic heart disease the problem is to recognize that the tricuspid valve has been affected in addition to the mitral valve (and perhaps the aortic valve as well). If the patient is in sinus rhythm there may be an 'a' wave in the venous pulse, which would be unusual in the presence of pulmonary hypertension and mitral stenosis alone (when the patient is very likely to be in atrial fibrillation). On auscultation at the left or right sternal edge a mid-diastolic murmur (usually higher in pitch than the murmur of mitral stenosis) is heard, and a tricuspid opening snap may be present (later in the cardiac cycle than a mitral opening snap, and varying in timing in relation to P2 with respiration), although it is not possible to differentiate this reliably from the mitral opening snap that is likely to coexist.

The chest radiograph shows a large right atrium with normal pulmonary artery size and clear lung fields. Echocardiography shows a dilated right atrium and demonstrates clearly the valve anatomy and function, as well as other intracardiac pathologies. The echocardiographic signs of rheumatic tricuspid disease are similar to those of the mitral valve, including commissural fusion, fibrosed leaflets that dome in diastole, short and fibrosed chordae, and raised transtricuspid forward flow velocities.

Tricuspid valve disease progresses very slowly and needs careful follow-up. Medical treatments are not satisfactory: diuretics can help to minimize fluid retention, but at the expense of reduced cardiac output if pushed too hard. Mild and moderate tricuspid stenosis is generally tolerated; severe tricuspid stenosis needs surgical repair, or replacement if additional regurgitation is present.

Tricuspid regurgitation

Mild tricuspid regurgitation is found in 50% of normal individuals. Causes of significant tricuspid regurgitation are shown in Table 6.1.3, the commonest being secondary to either pulmonary hypertension or right heart dilatation.

Endocarditis is commonly caused by intravenous access, either in those who abuse drugs intravenously, or in patients who required prolonged right heart catheters for medical therapy. Endomyocardial fibrosis, which is prevalent in tropical Africa, causes fibrosis of the papillary muscle tips and thickening and shortening of tricuspid valve leaflets and chordae. Permanent pacemaker wires across the tricuspid valve may rarely cause leaflet adhesions and dysfunction. Blunt trauma to the chest may be complicated by tricuspid regurgitation through the papillary muscle or chordal lacerations. Metastatic carcinoid tricuspid valve disease is rare, but echocardiographic findings of carcinoid involvement of the tricuspid valve are very characteristic, showing short, fibrosed, and thickened leaflets resulting in larger areas of

Table 6.1.3 Causes of tricuspid regurgitation

Cause	Type of condition	Disease
Primary	Congenital	Ebstein's anomaly
		Atrioventricular defect
		Prolapsing cusp
	Acquired	Rheumatic fever
		Infective endocarditis
		Permanent pacemaker wires
		Endomyocardial fibrosis
		Blunt trauma to the chest
		Carcinoid syndrome
		Ergot-derived dopamine receptor agonists
		Following radiotherapy to the chest
Secondary	'Functional'	Pulmonary hypertension or right heart dilatation
		Ischaemic right ventricular disease

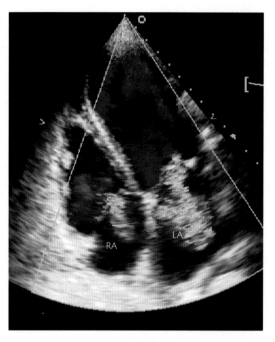

Fig. 6.1.14 Apical four-chamber view from a patient with tricuspid regurgitation secondary to left-sided dilated cardiomyopathy and mitral regurgitation: regurgitation into both left atrium (LA) and right atrium (RA) can be seen.

incomplete coaption and severe tricuspid regurgitation. Tricuspid valve prolapse is occasionally seen in patients with mitral valve prolapse.

The symptoms of tricuspid regurgitation are usually nonspecific. When it develops in a patient with mitral stenosis it is often associated with increased fatigue rather than breathlessness. Some patients will present with increasing peripheral oedema, and hepatic congestion may cause nausea or upper abdominal pain exacerbated by exercise. Diarrhoea caused by a protein-losing enteropathy (thought to be secondary to venous congestion of the gut) has been reported.

The main physical sign is a raised venous pressure with prominent V-wave, without which the diagnosis of significant tricuspid regurgitation is very difficult to sustain. In about one-third of cases a pansystolic tricuspid regurgitation murmur can be heard at the left or right sternal edge: this tends to increase in intensity with inspiration as the venous return increases, and it can radiate into the epigastrium. Expansile pulsation of the liver is present in most cases, but hepatic fibrosis (and jaundice) can occur if regurgitation is long-standing and this physical sign then disappears. Most patients with severe regurgitation have peripheral oedema, ascites, or both.

The findings on a chest radiograph depend mainly on whether or not the patient has any other cardiac disease, but there may be enlargement of the heart shadow towards the right. The ECG may show right atrial hypertrophy. Echocardiography is the best way to make the diagnosis (Fig. 6.1.14). Cardiac catheterization is not required for assessment of tricuspid regurgitation but may be indicated for diagnosis or assessment of other concurrent heart disease.

Many patients tolerate tricuspid regurgitation for a long time, but some present with symptoms that significantly limit their exercise capacity and lifestyle. Medical treatment with diuretics and ACE inhibitors may reduce systemic venous pressure and right ventricular size, even restoring competence to the tricuspid valve in some cases. Attempts should be made to treat pulmonary hypertension if this is the primary cause of right ventricular dilatation and tricuspid regurgitation. If fluid retention is severe and

refractory to medical treatment, careful consideration should be given to surgical correction of tricuspid regurgitation before the patient develops irreversible right ventricular damage. Repair and replacement of the tricuspid valve are problematic operations, with the former sometimes failing to prevent regurgitation and the latter leading to a significant diastolic pressure drop between the right atrium and ventricle, creating a problem of iatrogenic tricuspid stenosis, but in specialist centres the current approach is less conservative than it used to be.

Tricuspid valvuloplasty is often performed at the time of mitral valve surgery for rheumatic disease. Annuloplasty involves a full ring, incomplete ring, or suture plication of the annulus. A semicircular ring has the advantage of maintaining annular flexibility and avoiding conduction disturbances, but residual tricuspid regurgitation occurs less often with a circular angioplasty ring than with a semicircular one. Tricuspid valve replacement by a mechanical prosthesis has a potential risk for endocarditis, particularly in drug abusers. Bioprostheses have a much lower thrombogenicity and resistance to flow in the tricuspid position and are therefore the preferred choice.

The surgical mortality of tricuspid valve surgery depends particularly on the degree of preoperative hepatic congestion. Survival following tricuspid valve replacement is not purely related to the surgical procedure itself or to valve function, but is significantly affected by right ventricular dysfunction that is almost always masked by the volume overload before surgery.

Pulmonary stenosis

Pulmonary stenosis is congenital in 95% of cases (see Chapter 12): rarely it is caused by rheumatic valve disease or carcinoid syndrome. Patients can tolerate moderate pulmonary stenosis (gradient <50 mmHg) for years, fatigue and dyspnoea due to reduced cardiac output being the main symptoms in those with severe disease. Physical examination reveals a prominent venous 'a' wave in the neck and an ejection systolic murmur at the upper left sternal edge that radiates to the suprasternal notch and left side of the neck. With severe pulmonary stenosis the pulmonary component of the second sound may be delayed, but it is often inaudible. An ejection click may be heard at the upper left sternal edge. Echocardiography and MRI show the level of stenosis. Doming leaflets are consistent with congenital valve disease. MRI imaging is particularly good for demonstrating supravalvar stenosis. Event-free survival is related to the pressure gradient across the pulmonary valve.

Balloon valvuloplasty is the procedure of choice for children and adults with significant pulmonary stenosis. On average transpulmonary gradient drops by two-thirds of the baseline value without development of significant pulmonary regurgitation. Additional subvalvar stenosis may underestimate the success of the procedure. Surgical valvotomy may be considered if balloon valvuloplasty fails, and valve replacement may be needed for those with iatrogenic significant pulmonary regurgitation, especially after repair of tetralogy of Fallot. Homograft replacements might be advantageous to avoid anticoagulation and thrombogenicity.

Pulmonary regurgitation

A small amount of pulmonary regurgitation is common. Significant pulmonary regurgitation is very rare and most commonly preceded by intervention to the pulmonary valve during childhood. Although the outcome of repair of tetralogy of Fallot is excellent in most cases, many of its complications are related to pulmonary regurgitation. Rare causes of pulmonary regurgitation are rheumatic disease, carcinoid, and endocarditis. Many patients with pulmonary hypertension and dilatation of the right ventricular outflow tract will demonstrate some degree of pulmonary regurgitation.

The typical murmur of pulmonary regurgitation is a soft early diastolic murmur that is best heard in the left upper parasternal region. It begins after the pulmonary component of the second sound and may be accompanied by an ejection systolic murmur caused by increased stroke volume. Most patients have enlarged neck veins and other evidence of pulmonary hypertension.

Most patients with mild pulmonary regurgitation remain completely asymptomatic for years. Although those with severe regurgitation may remain asymptomatic, correction of valve incompetence may save them irreversible damage of the right ventricle. Arrhythmia or progressive right ventricular dilatation are indications for surgery, using homograft or conduit and valve. Normalization of right ventricular size and function following pulmonary homograft insertion occurs in some but not all patients, probably depending on preoperative ventricular dysfunction that could be masked by volume overload.

Further reading

Henein MY, *et al.* (2004). *Clinical echocardiography.* Springer.

Henein MY (2009). *Valvular heart disease in clinical practice.* Springer.

Mitral valve diseaseAlpert JS (1999). Mitral stenosis. In: Alpert JS, Dalen JE, Rahimtoola SH (eds) *Valvular heart disease.* Lippincott Williams & Wilkins, Philadelphia.

Bonow RO, *et al.* (2006). ACC/AHA 2006 guidelines for the management of patients with valvular heart disease: a report of the American College of Cardiology/American Heart Association Task Force on Practice Guidelines (writing committee to revise the 1998 guidelines for the management of patients with valvular heart disease) developed in collaboration with the Society of Cardiovascular Anesthesiologists endorsed by the Society for Cardiovascular Angiography and Interventions and the Society of Thoracic Surgeons. *J Am Coll Cardiol,* **48**, e1–148.

Bonow RO, *et al.* (2008). American College of Cardiology/American Heart Association Task Force on Practice Guidelines. *J Am Coll Cardiol,* **52**, e1–142. [2008 focused update incorporated into the ACC/AHA 2006 guidelines for the management of patients with valvular heart disease: a report of the American College of Cardiology/American Heart Association Task Force on Practice Guidelines (Writing Committee to revise the 1998 guidelines for the management of patients with valvular heart disease). Endorsed by the Society of Cardiovascular Anesthesiologists, Society for Cardiovascular Angiography and Interventions, and Society of Thoracic Surgeons.]

Breithardt OA, *et al.* (2003). Acute effects of cardiac resynchronization therapy on functional mitral regurgitation in advanced systolic heart failure. *J Am Coll Cardiol,* **41**, 765–70.

Devereux RB (1995). Recent developments in the diagnosis and management of mitral valve prolapse. *Curr Opin Cardiol,* **10**, 107–16.

Devereux RB, Kramer-Fox R, Kligfield P (1989). Mitral valve prolapse: causes, clinical manifestations, and management. *Ann Intern Med,* **111**, 305–17.

Duren DR, Becker AE, Dunning AJ (1988). Long-term follow-up of idiopathic mitral valve prolapse in 300 patients: a prospective study. *J Am Coll Cardiol,* **11**, 42–7.

Enriquez-Sarano M, *et al.* (2005). Quantitative determinants of outcome in asymptomatic mitral regurgitation. *N Engl J Med,* **352**, 875–83.

Horstkotte D, Niehues R, Strauer BE (1991). Pathomorphological aspects, aetiology and natural history of acquired mitral valve stenosis. *Eur Heart J,* **12** Suppl, 60.

Rothlisberger C, *et al.* (1993). Results of percutaneous balloon mitral valvotomy in young adults. *Am J Cardiol,* **72**, 73–7.

Sharma SK, *et al.* (1992). Clinical, angiographic and anatomic findings in acute severe ischemic mitral regurgitation. *Am J Cardiol,* **70**, 77–280.

Waller BF (1988). Etiology of mitral stenosis and pure mitral regurgitation. In: Waller BF (ed.) *Pathology of the heart and great vessels,* pp. 101–48. Churchill Livingstone, New York.

Wan B, *et al.* (2013). A meta-analysis of MitraClip system versus surgery for treatment of severe mitral regurgitation. *Ann Cardiothorac Surg,* **2**, 683–92.

Aortic valve diseaseBorer JS, *et al.* (1998). Prediction of indications for valve replacement among asymptomatic or minimally symptomatic patients with chronic aortic regurgitation and normal left ventricular performance. *Circulation,* **97**, 525–34.

Cohn LH, Narayanasamy N (2007). Aortic valve replacement in elderly patients: what are the limits?. *Curr Opin Cardiol,* **22**, 92–5.

Enriquez-Sarano M, Tajik AJ (2004). Clinical practice. Aortic regurgitation. *N Engl J Med,* **351**, 1539–46.

Frank S, Johnson A, Ross J, Jr. (1973). Natural history of valvular aortic stenosis. *Br Heart J,* **35**, 41–6.

Généreux P, *et al.* (2012). Vascular complications after transcatheter aortic valve replacement: Insights from the partner (placement of aortic transcatheter valve) trial. *J Am Coll Cardiol,* **60**, 1043–52.

Kodali SK, *et al.* (2012). Two-year outcomes after transcatheter or surgical aortic-valve replacement. *N Engl J Med,* **366**,1686–95.

Kvidal P, *et al.* (2000). Observed and relative survival after aortic valve replacement. *J Am Coll Cardiol,* **35**, 747–56.

Leon MB, Smith CR, Mack M, *et al.* PARTNER Trial Investigators (2010). Transcatheter aortic-valve implantation for aortic stenosis in patients who cannot undergo surgery. *N Engl J Med,* **363**, 1667–8.

Lombard JT, Selzer A (1987). Valvular aortic stenosis. A clinical and hemodynamic profile of patients. *Ann Intern Med,* **106**, 292–8.

Malouf JF, *et al.* (2002). Severe pulmonary hypertension in patients with severe aortic valve stenosis: clinical profile and prognostic implications. *J Am Coll Cardiol,* **40**, 789–95.

Marsalese DL, *et al.* (1989). Marfan's syndrome: natural history and long-term follow-up of cardiovascular involvement. *J Am Coll Cardiol*, **14**, 422–8.

O'Brien MF, *et al.* (2001). The homograft aortic valve: a 29-year, 99.3% follow up of 1,022 valve replacements. *J Heart Valve Dis*, **10**, 334–44.

Otto CM, *et al.* (1997). Prospective study of asymptomatic valvular aortic stenosis. Clinical, echocardiographic, and exercise predictors of outcome. *Circulation*, **95**, 2262–70.

Pohle K, *et al.* (2001). Progression of aortic valve calcification: association with coronary atherosclerosis and cardiovascular risk factors. *Circulation*, **104**, 1927–32.

Richards AM, *et al.* (1984). Syncope in aortic valvular stenosis. *Lancet*, **ii**, 1113–16.

Rosenhek R, *et al.* (2000). Predictors of outcome in severe, asymptomatic aortic stenosis. *N Engl J Med*, **343**, 611–17.

Ross DN (1967). Replacement of aortic and mitral valves with a pulmonary autograft. *Lancet*, **ii**, 956–958.

Smith CR, *et al.* (2011). Transcatheter versus surgical aortic-valve replacement in high-risk patients. *N Engl J Med*, **364**, 2187–98

Vahanian A, *et al.* (2008). Transcatheter valve implantation for patients with aortic stenosis: a position statement from the European Association of Cardio-Thoracic Surgery (EACTS) and the European Society of Cardiology (ESC), in collaboration with the European Association of Percutaneous Cardiovascular Interventions (EAPCI). *Eur J Cardiothorac Surg*, **34**, 1–8.

Tricuspid and pulmonary valve diseaseHansing CE, Rowe GG (1972). Tricuspid insufficiency. A study of hemodynamics and pathogenesis. *Circulation*, **45**, 793–799.

Lindqvist P, Calcutteea A, Henein M.(2008). Echocardiography in the assessment of right heart function. *Eur J Echocardiogr*, **9**, 225–34.

Pellikka PA, *et al.* (1993). Carcinoid heart disease. Clinical and echocardiographic spectrum in 74 patients. *Circulation*, **87**, 1188–96.

Weinreich DJ, *et al.* (1985). Isolated prolapse of the tricuspid valve. *J Am Coll Cardiol*, **6**, 475–81.

EndocarditisHabib G, Hoen B, Tornos P, *et al.* ESC Committee for Practice Guidelines (2009). Guidelines on the prevention, diagnosis, and treatment of infective endocarditis (new version 2009): the Task Force on the Prevention, Diagnosis, and Treatment of Infective Endocarditis of the European Society of Cardiology (ESC). Endorsed by the European Society of Clinical Microbiology and Infectious Diseases (ESCMID) and the International Society of Chemotherapy (ISC) for Infection and Cancer. *Eur Heart J*, **6**, 475–81.

SECTION 7

Diseases of heart muscle

CHAPTER 7.1

Myocarditis

Jay W. Mason

Essentials

Myocarditis has many infectious and noninfectious aetiologies; in most regions, viral infections are the main cause, with notable exceptions such as Chagas myocarditis in South America. The condition often results in congestive heart failure and is a common cause of chronic dilated cardiomyopathy, and it can also present with chest pain and/or ventricular arrythmias.

Patients with lymphocytic myocarditis are usually young (average age in the forties) and often report an antecedent viral illness. The disease can be diagnosed specifically by demonstration of lymphocyte infiltration and adjacent myocyte damage on endomyocardial biopsy. Detection of viral genomic material and tissue markers of immune activation in biopsy specimens, MRI and other imaging techniques, and presence of circulating biomarkers are also helpful in establishing the diagnosis. Adverse immune activation is the primary cause of myocardial damage in most cases.

Appropriately timed immunosuppressive therapy, most commonly with a steroid (prednisolone), may improve outcome in some cases, but efficacy is limited to special cases. Other immunomodulatory therapies and antiviral therapies have also been used, usually in patients who are deteriorating, but without proof of benefit. Specific forms of myocarditis include peripartum myocarditis, Lyme carditis, cardiac sarcoidosis, giant cell myocarditis, and Chagas carditis, each of which requires specific diagnostic and therapeutic measures.

Introduction

Myocarditis has captured the interest of clinicians and scientists because of its varied aetiology, its diagnostic and therapeutic challenges, and the possibility that myocarditis may be the primary cause of dilated cardiomyopathy. Scientific study of myocarditis is facilitated by the availability of numerous easily manipulated animal models of the disease and by new molecular probes.

Clinical features

Myocarditis affects young people: the average age of patients in the United States Myocarditis Treatment Trial was 42 years. There was a slight male predominance (62%) in that trial, but other series have not demonstrated a sex predilection. The true incidence of myocarditis is unknown: autopsy studies have reported figures of up to 3%, but varying histological criteria were used, and myocarditis may occur as an incidental complication of other fatal illnesses. About 10% of patients with influenzal infections have electrocardiographic abnormalities, but it is not known if these are the result of myocarditis. The incidence of fatal myocarditis was estimated in a retrospective review of United States Air Force recruits undergoing boot camp training: there were 8 such deaths over 1 606 167 person days, which yields an estimate of 4/100 000 per year in people aged 17 to 28 years. This incidence is probably greater than would be expected in the general population in the United States of America, who would not be exposed to similar levels of intense exercise or high probability of transmission of viral illnesses.

In Europe and North America most cases of myocarditis present with congestive heart failure of unknown cause. In many cases there is a history of recent upper respiratory tract infection or of a 'flu-like' illness. This is followed by symptoms of cardiac decompensation, usually fatigue, breathlessness, and cough. Chest pain occurs in a substantial minority of patients, and, when combined with regional ST-segment shifts on the electrocardiogram (ECG), can mimic acute myocardial infarction. A few patients present with ventricular tachyarrhythmias and minimal or no cardiac dilatation. Typically, the duration of symptoms due to infection is brief, less than 1 month in approximately 50% of patients and nearly always less than 1 year. Myocarditis should always be suspected when a patient presents with unexplained congestive heart failure with a rapid onset, especially if there is a viral prodrome. In adults under the age of 40, the combination of typical chest pain and a significant rise in troponin I is more likely due to myocarditis than to myocardial infarction, and fever or a viral prodrome are usually reported by those with myocarditis.

Clinical examination typically reveals signs of cardiac failure. The ECG may show conduction abnormalities, ST/T-wave changes (including persistent ST-segment elevation that does not proceed to Q-wave development), or arrhythmias (atrial or ventricular). The chest radiograph shows cardiomegaly and pulmonary oedema. The echocardiogram reveals four-chamber dilatation and reduced contractility, and is notable for the fact that valvular disease is absent or minimal. Cardiac scintigraphy with indium-111 antimyosin antibodies and single photon emission computed tomography (SPECT) have been used to detect myocarditis. Cardiac MRI is the most reliable noninvasive method for diagnosis, and can be used to distinguish acute myocardial infarction, acute myocarditis, and healed myocarditis. Contrast-enhanced MRI allows assessment of the regional extent of myocardial involvement. Detection of a pericardial effusion on the MRI increases the probability of a diagnosis of myocarditis, and injection of fluorine-19, which is taken up by inflammatory cells, is a promising method for MRI detection of localized inflammation due to myocarditis. Should coronary angiography be performed, the vessels are normal or show only minor abnormalities. The role of myocardial biopsy is discussed later; see

Fig. 7.1.2 and related text). Elevation of serum cardiac biomarkers (e.g. troponin, creatine phosphokinase) is common.

Although viruses are thought to be the most common cause of myocarditis, viral titres are rarely useful in diagnosis and treatment. Although the cardiotrophic enteroviruses, including echoviruses and coxsackieviruses, are the predominant aetiological agents, dozens of viruses have been implicated and many more undoubtedly cause myocarditis in humans. Thus, it is impractical to exclude them all. Some patients may present in the acute phase of the viral illness, as has recently been described in patients with influenza A (H1N1), but they usually present a substantial length of time after the viral infection has cleared, making it difficult or impossible to document an acute rise in titre. Knowledge of a specific virus, or any virus, as the cause in a given case of myocarditis has little, if any, therapeutic relevance, excepting for patients with acute presentation with influenza A. Even if viricidal therapy (which is not yet a proven treatment; see 'Treatment of postviral and nonspecific lymphocytic myocarditis') is being considered, negative titres for the common viral agents do not exclude a viral aetiology.

A small number of patients, perhaps about 10%, present with a secondary form of myocarditis: these special presentations are discussed below.

Aetiology and pathogenesis

The most common form of myocarditis in Europe and North America is known as lymphocytic myocarditis or nonspecific lymphocytic myocarditis. Other frequently applied terms are viral or postviral myocarditis, because an antecedent viral infection is common (Table 7.1.1). Indeed, some experts believe that nearly all lymphocytic myocarditides are the result of viral infections, presumed to be subclinical in those patients with no awareness of a viral prodrome.

In animal models enteroviruses, such as coxsackie B3, can cause two phases of myocarditis. The first is the result of direct injury of myocytes by replicating virus and the resulting acute immune response. A delayed immune response brings about the second phase, and it is this that is thought to be the more common cause of overt congestive heart failure. The underlying mechanisms are complex and incompletely understood, but most hypotheses suggest that autoimmune phenomena play a major role. In some instances molecular mimicry may be involved, in which the similarity of a viral antigen to a myocardial protein triggers an autoimmune reaction. In others an autoimmune response to cellular proteins released during the viral replication phase may occur, and myosin has been implicated in this regard. Cytokines arising from immune activation and cellular necrosis probably play a role in some cases, bringing about further cellular damage, such as through activation of matrix metalloproteinases. Viral persistence appears to induce a chronic adverse immune response and, as a result, to correlate with a poor prognosis. Although all of these mechanisms have been well delineated in murine models, they have not been proven to cause myocarditis in humans, nor has their delineation generated proven therapies.

Myocarditis may result from a hypersensitivity reaction to a drug or other agent (see Table 7.1.1). In these cases eosinophils accompany the inflammatory lymphocytic infiltrate. A number of other specific causes of myocarditis, each with differing pathogeneses and presentations, are discussed below.

Table 7.1.1 Aetiologies of myocarditis

Infection	
Viruses	
	Adenovirus
	Arbovirus
	Arenavirus
	Coronavirus
	Coxsackievirus (A, B)
	Cytomegalovirus
	Echovirus
	Encephalomyocarditis
	Epstein–Barr
	Hepatitis B
	Hepatitis C
	Herpes simplex
	Human immunodeficiency
	Influenza (A, B)
	Junin
	Parvovirus (B19)
	Mumps
	Polio
	Rabies
	Respiratory syncytial virus
	Rubella (German measles)
	Rubeola (measles)
	Vaccinia
	Varicella-zoster virus
	Variola
Bacteria, spirochaetes, and bacteria-like organisms	
	β-Haemolytic streptococci
	Borrelia burgdorferi (Lyme disease)
	Brucella spp.
	Campylobacter jejuni
	Chlamydia psittaci (psittacosis)
	Chlamydia trachomatis (trachoma)
	Clostridia spp.
	Corynebacterium diphtheriae
	Francisella tularensis (tularaemia)
	Gonococcus
	Haemophilus influenzae
	Legionella pneumophila
	Leptospira spp.

(continued)

Table 7.1.1 Continued

Infection		
	Listeria monocytogenes	
	Mycobacterium spp.	
	Mycoplasma pneumoniae	
	Neisseria meningitidis	
	Salmonella typhi	
	Streptococcus pneumoniae	
	Staphylococcus spp.	
	Treponema pallidum (syphilis)	
	Tropheryma whippleii	
Rickettsia		
	Coxiella burnetii (Q fever)	
	Orientia tsutsugamushi (scrub typhus)	
	Rickettsia rickettsii (Rocky Mountain spotted fever)	
	Rickettsia prowazekii (typhus)	
Protozoa		
	Entamoeba histolytica	
	Leishmania spp.	
	Toxoplasma gondii	
	Trypanosoma cruzi (Chagas disease)	
Helminths		
	Cysticerus	
	Echinococcus spp.	
	Schistosoma spp.	
	Toxocara spp.	
	Trichinella spp.	
Fungi		
	Actinomyces spp.	
	Aspergillus spp.	
	Blastomyces dermatitides	
	Candida spp.	
	Coccidioides immitis	
	Cryptococcus neoformans	
	Fusarium	
	Oxysporum	
	Histoplasma capsulatum	
	Mucor	
	Nocardia spp.	
	Sporothrix schenckii	
Drugs and chemicals		
Toxicity		
	2-Interferon	
	Amphetamines	

Table 7.1.1 Continued

Infection		
	Animal and insect toxins	
	Anthracyclines	
	Arsenic	
	Catecholamines	
	Cocaine	
	5-Fluorouracil	
	Interleukin 2	
	Lithium	
	Paracetamol	
Hypersensitivity		
	Aminophylline	
	Ampicillin	
	Azithromycin	
	Benzodiazepines	
	Digoxin	
	Ephedrine	
	Furosemide	
	Hydrochlorthiazide	
	Methyldopa	
	Penicillin	
	Phenytoin	
	Tetracycline	
	Tricyclic antidepressants	
Autoimmunity		
	Antigenic mimicry	
	Autoimmune disease associated	
	Cardiac myosin	
	Cytokines	
	Dressler's syndrome	
	Post-cardiotomy syndrome	
	Post-infection	
	Post-radiation	

Relationship to idiopathic dilated cardiomyopathy

Classic lymphocytic myocarditis usually resolves, with resultant improvement in cardiac function over weeks or months. In the United States Myocarditis Treatment Trial, the mean left ventricular ejection fraction improved during the year after initial presentation by more than 10 ejection fraction units (from 24% to 36%; normal >55%). However, residual cardiac dilatation and dysfunction were common, and mortality was high, reaching 55% at 5 years. In those patients who do not recover fully, the ensuing clinical picture cannot be distinguished from that of idiopathic dilated cardiomyopathy. The possibility that myocarditis may occur without an obvious viral prodrome therefore raises the interesting possibility that viral myocarditis may be a common covert cause of idiopathic dilated cardiomyopathy. In the United States trial, only 10% of patients with suspected myocarditis had positive biopsies. Hence, the fact that endomyocardial biopsy does not reveal myocarditis in patients with idiopathic dilated cardiomyopathy may be the result of timing of the biopsy after resolution of the lymphocytic infiltrate, sampling error, or absence of a lymphocytic response in some patients. The presence of viral genomic material in some of these negative biopsies lends support to the viral aetiology hypothesis. Absence of viral genome in the rest of them does not eliminate postviral autoimmune processes, proceeding despite complete viral clearing, as a possible aetiology. The fact that immunomodulatory therapy may improve cardiac function in patients with dilated cardiomyopathy but without lymphocytic myocardial infiltrates adds indirect evidence that idiopathic dilated cardiomyopathy has an inflammatory origin in some cases.

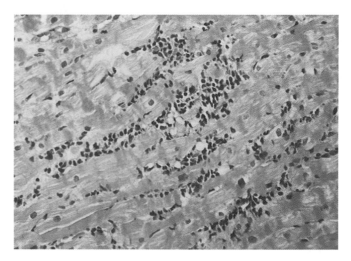

Fig. 7.1.1 An example of acute myocarditis, with lymphocytic infiltration adjacent to frayed myocytes.

Treatment of postviral and nonspecific lymphocytic myocarditis

As stated above, nonspecific lymphocytic myocarditis is believed by most to have a viral aetiology, even in the absence of a clinically apparent viral prodrome. In the acute phase of viral myocarditis, the direct cytolytic effect of viral myocyte infection may lead to congestive heart failure, although this is uncommon. In this early phase, the immune response is likely, on balance, to be beneficial. Thus, antiviral therapy might be expected to be helpful, but on theoretical grounds immunosuppressive therapy would not. However, though antiviral therapies have shown promise, none have been adequately tested in humans with acute myocarditis, although it is routine practice to administer neuraminidase inhibitors such as oseltamivir to those with influenza A.

In the second stage of myocarditis, thought to result from an adverse immune response to previous infection, immunosuppressive therapy has appeared to be beneficial in uncontrolled trials. However, no benefit was demonstrated in the United States Myocarditis Treatment Trial, the only prospective randomized trial performed in patients with myocarditis defined histologically. In that trial the 'Dallas' criteria defined myocarditis histologically as a lymphocytic infiltrate with associated myocyte necrosis (Fig. 7.1.1). Treatment with prednisone combined with either ciclosporin or with azathioprine did not improve outcome, as defined by change in left ventricular ejection fraction. However, it is appropriate to consider other diagnostic criteria, such as presence of viral genomic material and human leucocyte antigen (HLA) up-regulation on biopsy, circulating antiheart antibodies, and imaging in the diagnosis and treatment of myocarditis. RNA microarray analysis on biopsy specimens has been found to be highly sensitive and specific in differentiation of myocarditis from idiopathic dilated cardiomyopathy, myocardial infarction, and other myocardial disorders associated with inflammation.

An algorithm for the diagnosis and treatment of suspected myocarditis is shown in Fig. 7.1.2. This algorithm differs somewhat from recently published recommendations of the European Society of Cardiology (ESC), primarily in the use of endomyocardial biopsy, which is more liberally applied in the ESC consensus statement. Spontaneous improvement in left ventricular function can be anticipated in many patients. In most cases it is reasonable to use standard therapy for congestive heart failure, without performing a biopsy or administering steroids, and to observe the patient, using echocardiography to monitor left ventricular function. However, in patients who deteriorate, or who present in cardiogenic shock, an endomyocardial biopsy should be performed. Many experts would also base a diagnosis of myocarditis on proven imaging techniques, such as contrast-enhanced MRI, in combination with a circulating biomarker such as cardiac-specific antibodies. If myocarditis is present, immunosuppressive therapy should be administered, typically beginning with prednisone at 1.25 mg/kg per day, tapering to 0.15 mg/kg per day over 1 month. It must be admitted, however, that the efficacy of such treatment has not been proved. If the patient worsens despite this therapy, antiviral or immunomodulatory therapy can be offered in an investigative setting. Direct antiviral treatments that have been tested or proposed include aciclovir, ganciclovir, foscarnet, and amantadine. Immunomodulatory treatments include immunoadsorptive apheresis, interferons, immune globulins, pentoxifylline, and cytokines such as interleukin-6.

Management of ventricular tachyarrhythmias in patients with myocarditis

Lymphocytic myocarditis, with or without a viral prodrome, may present with ventricular tachyarrhythmias and little or no cardiac dilatation and dysfunction. An endomyocardial biopsy should be considered in all cases of ventricular tachycardia of recent onset if no aetiology is apparent, because the presence of myocarditis can substantially change treatment strategy. Since myocarditis is often a self-limited disorder, the patient's risk of recurrent ventricular tachyarrhythmias may resolve, and it may be unnecessary to subject the patient to electrophysiological study and/or cardioverter–defibrillator implantation. If arrhythmia does not improve spontaneously, a trial of immunosuppressive therapy should be considered. In such cases it is difficult to know how long to continue with antiarrhythmic drugs. The risks of ventricular arrhythmia should not be underestimated, but nor should those of long-term treatment with agents such as amiodarone. If 24-h ECG monitoring at 6 months shows no sinister abnormalities, then many would withdraw antiarrhythmic treatment at that point, but others

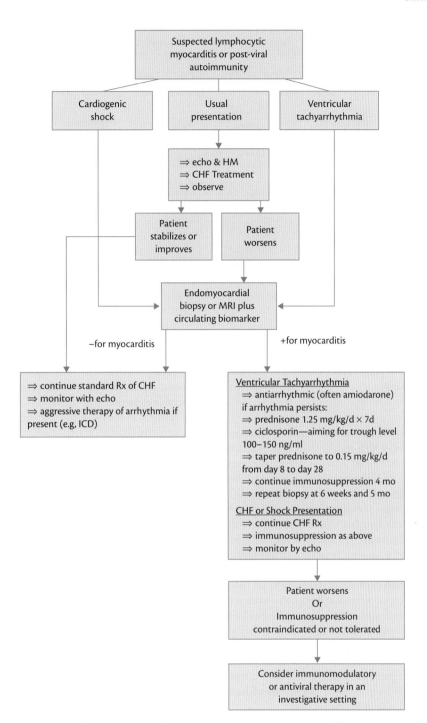

Fig. 7.1.2 Algorithm for diagnosis and treatment of suspected myocarditis. ACE, angiotensin converting enzyme; CHF, congestive heart failure; echo, echocardiogram; HM, Holter monitor; ICD, implantable cardioverter–defibrillator.

advocate repeat endomyocardial biopsy to document complete resolution of myocarditis before taking this step.

Specific forms of myocarditis

Specific forms of myocarditis are shown in Fig. 7.1.3.

Peripartum myocarditis

Dilated cardiomyopathy developing during the last trimester of pregnancy or within 6 months of delivery is known as peripartum or postpartum cardiomyopathy. In some series the dominant cause is myocarditis. When heart failure develops rapidly in the first few weeks after delivery, myocarditis is more likely to be found on endomyocardial biopsy than when the onset is insidious and delayed, and patients with early, rapid onset are more likely to recover quickly and completely. While steroid therapy has been used and is recommended by some, its efficacy has not been proved, and spontaneous resolution of peripartum cardiomyopathy is well documented. The usual prohibition against future pregnancy has been debated; it is very clear that some women risk recurrent heart

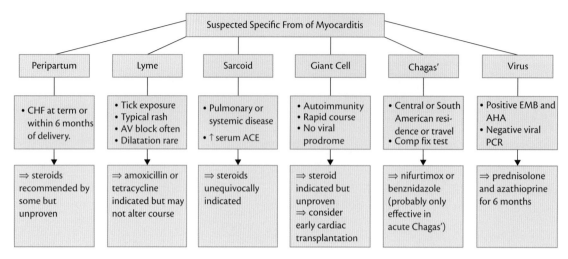

Fig. 7.1.3 Suspected specific forms of myocarditis.
ACE, angiotensin converting enzyme; CHF, congestive heart failure; Comp fix, complement fixation; EMB, endomyocardial biopsy; AHA, antiheart antibody; PCR, polymerase chain reaction.

failure, while others do not. In those women in whom severe heart failure persists, cardiac transplantation is an appropriate therapy. After transplantation, successful pregnancies have occurred without recurrence of cardiomyopathy.

Lyme carditis

Borrelia burgdorferi, a spirochaete, infects humans following **Ixodes** tick bites. Lyme disease, which results from this infection, has been reported in 48 of the 50 United States as well as in Europe and Asia (see Chapter 7.6.32). It is characterized by an erythema migrans rash and flu-like symptoms, followed by arthritis, carditis, and neurological disorders in some patients. Carditis is detected in approximately 8% of cases. Both lymphocytic infiltration and the bacterium itself can be demonstrated by endomyocardial biopsy. The usual cardiac manifestation is varying degrees of atrioventricular block. Infrequently, cardiac dilatation occurs. Atrioventricular block is usually transient, though permanent complete heart block has been reported. The site of block appears to be the atrioventricular node in most cases, but block within the His bundle has been documented by electrophysiological study, and the common occurrence of intraventricular conduction delays suggests that bundle branch block may also occur. Temporary pacing is usually sufficient, though recovery of antegrade conduction may take a week or longer. Lyme carditis should be considered in any case of heart block of unknown cause, especially in young people.

Antibiotic therapy is recommended in Lyme carditis, but it is not known if this alters the course of carditis and atrioventricular block.

Cardiac sarcoidosis

Less than 10% of patients with pulmonary or systemic sarcoidosis have clinically manifest cardiac involvement, ranging from conduction disturbances and arrhythmias to cardiac dilatation. Endomyocardial biopsy reveals typical sarcoid granulomas. The most serious complications of cardiac sarcoidosis are complete heart block, ventricular tachyarrhythmias, and dilated cardiomyopathy. Cardiac sarcoidosis accounts for as much as 19% of all cases of unexplained atrioventricular block requiring pacemaker implantation in adults under 55 years of age. The relatively high incidence of sudden death in patients with sarcoidosis is thought

to result from sudden complete heart block or ventricular fibrillation. Patients with sarcoidosis who develop significant conduction disease, arrhythmias, or congestive heart failure should receive steroids. Occasionally, cardiac involvement will occur without detectable systemic manifestations of sarcoidosis. Thus, cardiac sarcoidosis is in the differential diagnosis of any undiagnosed ventricular arrhythmia, dilated cardiomyopathy, or atrioventricular block. See Chapter 7.3 for further discussion.

Giant cell myocarditis

Early recognition of this rapidly progressive form of myocarditis is required, as it has a prognosis considerably worse than that of nonspecific lymphocytic myocarditis. The endomyocardial biopsy is distinguished by the presence of multinucleated giant cells and scattered lymphocytic infiltrates with eosinophils. The aetiology of giant cell myocarditis is unknown, but thought to be autoimmune, given its association with myasthenia gravis, thymoma, Crohn's disease, and other immune disorders. It should be suspected in patients—particularly those with a history of an autoimmune condition—who present with disease which progresses unusually rapidly, without viral prodrome, and who do not respond to standard therapy of congestive heart failure. Endomyocardial biopsy should be performed if giant cell myocarditis is suspected, because immunosuppressive therapy appears to be helpful, though not yet proved. Patients with giant cell myocarditis should be considered for early cardiac transplantation if they do not respond to therapy. Giant cell infiltration can be isolated to the atria, producing atrial enlargement and arrhythmias; this form of the disease is more benign.

Chagas disease

Chagas disease, caused by *Trypanosoma cruzi*, is the leading cause of myocarditis and dilated cardiomyopathy in some Central and South American countries, but uncommon in the United States of America (see Chapter 7.8.11). Overt acute myocarditis with congestive heart failure, arrhythmias, and conduction disease may develop, but cardiac involvement in early Chagas disease is usually subclinical. Years later, chronic Chagas disease may develop and may involve the heart. In the chronic phase, right bundle branch block and biventricular failure are present, and right heart failure predominates. Myocarditis occurs in both the acute and chronic phases, when immune mediation of myocyte injury is well documented. Antiprotozoal treatment with nifurtimox or benznidazole is beneficial in the acute phase. These agents are also indicated in the chronic phase, but—while they do reduce or eliminate serological immune markers of disease—it is not known if they improve outcome.

Virus-negative myocarditis

An entity known as virus-negative myocarditis is defined as chronic systolic heart failure with histological and immunochemical evidence of lymphocytic inflammation, but without evidence of a viral aetiology, as determined by negative comprehensive polymerase chain reaction detection of RNA or DNA of known cardiotropic viruses on endomyocardial biopsy tissue. Frustaci and colleagues showed recently in a randomized trial that immunosuppression with prednisolone and azathioprine improved left ventricular size and performance in virus-negative myocarditis. This result supports the hypothesis that inefficacy of immunosuppression in previous studies resulted from exacerbation of disease in the subset of patients with ongoing viral infection, and it provides a rationale for rigorously excluding the presence of inflammation in patients with chronic heart failure.

Likely future developments

The use of endomyocardial histology for diagnosis of myocarditis will be replaced gradually by other methods, including molecular assessments of biopsy tissue and noninvasive methods. In addition to diagnosis, new techniques will identify more accurately subsets of patients likely to respond to specific therapies. Relevance of animal models to clinical forms of myocarditis will be improved by a fuller analysis and understanding of the disorder in humans. The most important advances will lead to prevention of the causative infections through vaccination and other prophylactic measures. These developments could profoundly reduce the incidence of dilated cardiomyopathy throughout the world.

Further reading

Aretz HT, *et al.* (1987). Myocarditis. A histopathologic definition and classification. *Cardiovasc Pathol*, **1**, 3–14.

Baughman KL (2006). Diagnosis of myocarditis: death of Dallas criteria. *Circulation*, **113**, 593–5.

Blauwet LA, Cooper LT (2010). Myocarditis. *Prog Cardiovasc Dis*, **52**, 274–88.

Caforio, ALP, *et al.* (2013). Current state of knowledge on aetiology, diagnosis, management, and therapy of myocarditis: a position statement of the European Society of Cardiology Working Group on Myocardial and Pericardial Diseases. *Euro Heart J*, **34**, 2636–48.

Cooper LT (2009). Myocarditis. *N Engl J Med*, **360**, 1526–38.

Cooper LT, Berry GJ, Shabetai R (1997). Idiopathic giant-cell myocarditis—natural history and treatment. *N Engl J Med*, **336**, 1860–6.

Felker GM, *et al.* (2000). Myocarditis and long-term survival in peripartum cardiomyopathy. *Am Heart J*, **140**, 785–91.

Frustaci A, *et al.* (2003). Immunosuppressive therapy for active lymphocytic myocarditis: virological and immunologic profile of responders versus nonresponders. *Circulation*, **107**, 857–63.

Frustaci A, et al. (2009). Randomized study on the efficacy of immunosuppressive therapy in patients with virus-negative inflammatory cardiomyopathy: The TIMIC study. *Eur Heart J*, **30**, 1995–2002.

Gauntt CJ, *et al.* (1995). Molecular mimicry, antcoxsackievirus B3 neutralizing monoclonal antibodies, and myocarditis. *J Immunol*, **154**, 2983–95.

Lurtz P, *et al.* (2012). Diagnostic performance of CMR imaging compared with EMB in patients with suspected myocarditis. *JACC Cardiovasc Imaging*, **5**, 513–24.

Mason JW (2013). Basic research on myocarditis: superb but unrequited. *J Am Coll Cardiol*, **62**, 1746–7.

Mason JW, *et al.* (1995). A clinical trial of immunosuppressive therapy for myocarditis. *N Engl J Med*, **333**, 269–75.

Matsumori A, Sasayama S (2001). The role of inflammatory mediators in the failing heart: immunomodulation of cytokines in experimental models of heart failure. *Heart Fail Rev*, **6**, 129–36.

McManus BM, *et al.* (1993). Direct myocardial injury by enterovirus: a central role in the evolution of murine myocarditis. *Clin Immunol Immunopathol*, **68**, 159–69.

McNamara DM, *et al.* (2001). A controlled trial of intravenous immune globulin in recent-onset dilated cardiomyopathy. *Circulation*, **103**, 2254–9.

Muller JG, *et al.* (2000). Immunoglobulin adsorption in patients with idiopathic dilated cardiomyopathy. *Circulation*, **101**, 385–91.

Rose NR, Hill SL (1996). The pathogenesis of postinfectious myocarditis. *Clin Immun Immunopath*, **80**, S92–S99.

Skouri HN, *et al.* (2006). Noninvasive imaging in myocarditis. *J Am Coll Cardiol*, **48**, 2085–93.

Wojinicz R, *et al.* (2001). Randomized, placebo-controlled study for immunosuppressive treatment of inflammatory dilated cardiomyopathy: two-year follow-up results. *Circulation*, **104**, 39–45.

Yajima T, Knowlton KU (2009). Viral myocarditis from the perspective of the virus. *Circulation*, **119**, 2615–24.

CHAPTER 7.2

The cardiomyopathies: hypertrophic, dilated, restrictive, and right ventricular

William J. McKenna, Perry Elliott, and Oliver Guttmann

Essentials

The term cardiomyopathy is used to describe heart muscle disease unexplained by abnormal loading conditions (hypertension, valve disease, etc.), congenital cardiac abnormalities, and ischaemic heart disease. The current classification is based on the predominant phenotype, i.e. hypertrophic, dilated, arrhythmogenic right ventricular, restrictive, and unclassifiable (including left ventricular noncompaction), and—where possible—incorporating inheritance and genotype. Cardiomyopathies associated with systemic diseases are described in Chapter 7.3.

Hypertrophic cardiomyopathy

The diagnosis of hypertrophic cardiomyopathy is based on the demonstration of unexplained myocardial hypertrophy, defined as a wall thickness measurement exceeding two standard deviations above normal for gender and age. In practice, in an adult of normal size, the presence of a left ventricular myocardial segment of 1.5 cm or greater in thickness is diagnostic. Less stringent criteria should be applied to first-degree relatives of an unequivocally affected individual. Ninety per cent of patients have familial disease, usually with autosomal dominant inheritance. Mutations in genes encoding proteins of the cardiac sarcomere are most common (60% of cases).

Symptomatic presentation may be at any age, with breathlessness on exertion, chest pain, palpitation, syncope, or sudden death. In children and adolescents, the diagnosis is most often made during screening of siblings and offspring of affected family members. In most patients the physical examination is unremarkable, but characteristic features include a rapid upstroke arterial pulse, a forceful left ventricular cardiac impulse with palpable atrial beat, an ejection systolic murmur, and a fourth heart sound.

Investigation and diagnosis—the 12-lead ECG is the most sensitive diagnostic test, with ST-segment depression and T-wave changes being the most common abnormalities, usually associated with voltage changes of left ventricular hypertrophy and/or deep S waves in the anterior chest leads V1 to V3. Echocardiography reveals left ventricular hypertrophy that may be symmetric or asymmetric and localized to the septum or the free wall, but most commonly to both the septum and free wall with relative sparing of the posterior wall.

Management—β-adrenoceptor blockers and calcium antagonists (verapamil, diltiazem) are the mainstay of symptomatic pharmacological therapy. Surgery is considered for patients with left ventricular outflow-tract obstruction (typically, resting left ventricular outflow-tract gradient >50 mmHg) and/or mitral valve abnormalities, the commonest operation being removal of a segment of the upper anterior septum (myectomy) via a transaortic approach. Injection of alcohol into the septal artery that supplies the septal muscle is an alternative percutaneous technique that can be used in patients with suitable cardiac and coronary anatomy.

Prognosis—overall annual cardiovascular mortality is 1 to 2%/year, with sudden cardiac death (c.1%), heart failure (c.0.5%), and thromboembolism (c.0.1%) the main causes. The risk of death and other disease-related complications varies between individuals. Prevention of sudden death relies on risk factor stratification to identify high-risk individuals and targeted therapy with implantable cardioverter–defibrillators (ICD).

Dilated cardiomyopathy

Dilated cardiomyopathy is defined by dilatation and impaired systolic function of the left or both ventricles not attributable to coronary artery disease, valvular abnormalities, or pericardial disease. Up to 50% of cases are familial, with a large number of disease-causing gene mutations described.

Initial presentation is usually with symptoms of cardiac failure, but other presentations include arrhythmia, systemic thromboembolism, or the incidental finding of an electrocardiographic or radiographic abnormality. Physical examination may reveal cardiac enlargement and signs of congestive heart failure.

Investigation and diagnosis—on echocardiography, the presence of ventricular end-diastolic dimensions greater than two standard deviations above the mean and fractional shortening less than 25% is generally sufficient to make the diagnosis.

Management—symptomatic therapy involves the treatment of heart failure with diuretics, angiotensin converting enzyme (ACE) inhibitors, and β-blockers. Anticoagulation with warfarin is advised in patients in whom an intracardiac thrombus is identified echocardiographically, or those with a history of thromboembolism. ICDs are warranted if sustained or symptomatic ventricular arrhythmias are documented and for primary prophylaxis in selected high-risk patients. Cardiac resynchronization therapy (CRT) can improve symptoms and prognosis in selected patients with broad QRS duration, and cardiac transplantation may be appropriate for those with progressive deterioration.

Restrictive cardiomyopathy

Restrictive cardiomyopathies are defined by restrictive ventricular physiology in the presence of normal or reduced diastolic volumes of one or both ventricles, normal or reduced systolic volumes, and normal ventricular wall thickness. In developed countries amyloidosis is the commonest cause; in the tropics it is endomyocardial fibrosis. Familial restrictive cardiomyopathy is usually caused by sarcomere protein gene mutations, with the full spectrum of restrictive cardiomyopathy and hypertrophic cardiomyopathy sometimes seen within individual families.

Presentation is usually insidious. Left-sided disease may present with symptoms of pulmonary congestion and/or mitral regurgitation; right-sided disease presents with raised jugular venous pressure, hepatomegaly, ascites, and tricuspid regurgitation. Atrial fibrillation is common. Echocardiography confirms the diagnosis, typically showing that ventricular dimensions and wall thickness are normal, but the atria are grossly enlarged.

Congestive symptoms from raised right atrial pressure can be improved with diuretics, though too great a reduction in ventricular filling pressure will lead to a reduction in cardiac output. Prognosis of advanced disease is poor.

Arrhythmogenic right ventricular cardiomyopathy

Arrhythmogenic right ventricular cardiomyopathy is a heart muscle disease characterized by progressive fibro-fatty replacement of right ventricular myocardium, associated with ventricular arrhythmia, heart failure, and sudden cardiac death. It is inherited and caused by mutations in desmosomal genes in at least 50% of cases.

Symptomatic presentation is usually with palpitation and/or syncope from sustained ventricular arrhythmia, but the first presentation of the disease may be with sudden cardiac death. There is no single diagnostic test, and the diagnosis is based on the presence of criteria encompassing structural, histological, electrocardiographic, arrhythmic, and genetic parameters. The most common electrocardiographic abnormality is T-wave inversion in leads V1 to V3 in the absence of right bundle branch block. Typical echocardiographic findings include right ventricular dilatation, regional hypokinesia or dyskinesia, and aneurysms.

Management—patients with symptomatic, non-life-threatening ventricular arrhythmias are treated empirically with β-blockers, amiodarone, or sotalol. Those with a history of sustained, haemodynamically compromising ventricular arrhythmia should be offered an ICD.

Introduction

Cardiomyopathies are defined as heart muscle disorders unexplained by abnormal loading conditions (hypertension, valve disease, etc.), congenital cardiac abnormalities, and ischaemic heart disease. The current classification is based on the predominant phenotype and, when feasible, assessment of the familial and genetic basis. Heart muscle disease associated with systemic or extracardiac diseases are described in more detail in Chapter 7.3.

Hypertrophic cardiomyopathy

Definition

Hypertrophic cardiomyopathy (HCM) is defined clinically by the presence of increased myocardial thickness in the absence of loading conditions (hypertension, valve disease, etc.) sufficient to cause the observed degree of hypertrophy. Historically, ventricular thickening caused by systemic diseases such as amyloidosis and glycogen storage disease has been excluded from the definition in order to separate conditions in which there is myocyte hypertrophy from those in which left ventricular mass and wall thickness are increased by interstitial infiltration or intracellular accumulation of metabolic substrates. In everyday clinical practice, however, it is frequently impossible to differentiate these two entities using noninvasive imaging, and hence metabolic and infiltrative disease should be considered in the differential diagnosis of hypertrophic cardiomyopathy.

Causes

Pedigree analysis reveals familial disease in 40 to 50% of patients, but when cardiovascular evaluation of first-degree relatives using electrocardiography (ECG) and echocardiography is performed, up to 90% of patients are found to have familial disease. In most cases, the inheritance is autosomal dominant.

Approximately 60% of patients with familial hypertrophic cardiomyopathy have mutations in genes encoding proteins of the cardiac sarcomere: specifically cardiac β-myosin heavy chain, cardiac myosin-binding protein C, essential and regulatory myosin light chain, α-tropomyosin, cardiac troponin T and I, cardiac actin, titin, and α-myosin. Most mutations involve a single base-pair change in exons encoding highly conserved regions that result in amino acid substitutions. *De novo* mutations occur, but appear to account for less than 10% of cases. Some 5–10% of patients carry multiple sarcomeric mutations, with compound heterozygotes presenting with more severe disease at an earlier age. Several genes related to the sarcomere Z-disc and calcium handling have been associated with hypertrophic cardiomyopathy, but are relatively uncommon.

Variable clinical expression and incomplete penetrance is common, even within families bearing the same gene defect, but some phenotypes do seem to associate with particular mutations. β-Myosin heavy chain mutations that are fully penetrant are associated with worse prognosis (such as Arg403Glu or Arg453Cys), while disease complications are uncommon in patients with mutations that cause mild or no clinical expression (such as Leu908Val). This contrasts with troponin T disease, which although associated with mild hypertrophy and few symptoms can still cause premature sudden death. Mutations in myosin-binding protein C cause 20 to 30% of disease; most are major deletions rather than single base-pair changes. Disease expression can occur later in life, sometimes associated with mild hypertension. Once disease expression occurs (abnormal ECG and/or echocardiogram), patients are at the same risk from symptoms and disease-related complications as patients with disease onset in early life. The expression of disease in patients with troponin I mutations is variable and mutations in this gene may also cause restrictive cardiomyopathy.

Table 7.2.1 Nonsarcomeric causes of left ventricular hypertrophy at age 3 years or less

Metabolic	Pompe's disease (GSD II)
	Forbes' disease (GSD III)
	Total lipodystrophy
	Hurler's syndrome
	Infant of a diabetic mother
Hypertrophic cardiomyopathy with associated syndromes	Noonan's syndrome
	LEOPARD syndrome
	Friedreich's ataxia
	Beckwith–Wiedemann syndrome
	Mitochondrial myopathy
	MELAS
	MERFF
	NADH–coenzyme Q reductase deficiency
	Cytochrome *b* deficiency
Miscellaneous causes	Hypertension
	In utero ritodrine HCl exposure
	Swyer's syndrome (46, XY pure gonadal dysgenesis)

GSD, glycogen storage disorder; MELAS, myopathy, encephalopathy, lactic acidosis, stroke-like episodes; MERFF, myoclonic epilepsy and ragged red fibres.

Many inborn errors of metabolism and congenital syndromes are associated with HCM. Most are inherited as autosomal recessive traits, but a few are X-linked. The most common metabolic disorders in adults with HCM are Anderson–Fabry disease (0.5–1% of patients older than 35–40 years), and disease caused by mutations in the gene encoding the γ_2 subunit of the adenosine monophosphate-activated protein kinase *(PRKAG2)* (1%). LAMP-2 mutations that cause Danon disease occur in 0.7% to 2.7%. Although still rare, metabolic disorders account for a greater proportion of disease in children and adolescents (Table 7.2.1).

Pathology

Hypertrophic cardiomyopathy may involve the left or both ventricles (Fig. 7.2.1). Hypertrophy in the left ventricle is usually asymmetric, involving the anterior and posterior septum and the free wall to a greater extent than the posterior wall. Right ventricular hypertrophy is seen in up to 30% of patients but isolated right ventricular hypertrophy (in the absence of pulmonary hypertension or right ventricular outflow obstruction) rarely if ever occurs. Many patients have structural abnormalities of the mitral valve, including increased leaflet area and length, and malposition or anomalous insertion of the papillary muscles. A common macroscopic finding is a patch of endocardial thickening just below the aortic valve, which results from contact of the septum with the anterior mitral leaflet in patients with dynamic left ventricular outflow-tract obstruction.

The histological findings in hypertrophic cardiomyopathy are distinctive and provide the basis for the pathological diagnosis. Affected myocardium shows interstitial fibrosis with gross disorganization of the muscle bundles resulting in a characteristic whorled pattern. The cell-to-cell orientation of muscle cells is lost (disarray) and there is disorganization of the myofibrillar architecture within cells. Myocardial cells are broad, short, and often bizarre in shape. Foci of disorganized cells are often interspersed among areas of hypertrophied muscle cells that are otherwise normal in appearance. Such changes are not completely specific: small amounts of myofibre disarray may be seen in congenitally abnormal hearts and in secondary left ventricular hypertrophy; disarray is also present at the junction of the septum with the anterior and posterior walls of the left ventricle in normal subjects. However, the extent of myocyte disarray in normal subjects rarely exceeds 5%, while in hypertrophic cardiomyopathy up to 40% of the myocardium may be involved. As well as contributing to diastolic and systolic dysfunction, the disorganized myocardial architecture provides a substrate for electrical instability.

Pathophysiology

Diastolic dysfunction

Diastolic abnormalities caused by myocardial hypertrophy, myocardial ischaemia, myocyte disarray, and fibrosis are common but variable in severity. Typically, left ventricular end-diastolic pressure and atrial pressures are elevated as a consequence of abnormal left ventricular diastolic filling and reduced compliance. The isovolumic relaxation time is prolonged, left ventricular filling is slow, and the proportion of filling volume that results from atrial systolic contraction (while still preserved) may be increased. Occasionally, there is rapid early filling with restrictive physiology similar to that seen in constrictive pericarditis or endocardial fibrosis (see Chapter 8).

Systolic function and dynamic outflow-tract obstruction

Most patients with hypertrophic cardiomyopathy have rapid and near-complete ventricular emptying resulting in a high ejection fraction but the stroke volume, particularly during exercise is frequently reduced. 'Endstage' hypertrophic cardiomyopathy—characterized by severe impairment of contractile performance, restrictive left ventricular physiology, and heart-failure symptoms—is uncommon (>5%), but can develop at any age including childhood and adolescence. In most, the time from onset of symptoms to diagnosis of severe systolic impairment is long (a mean of 14 years).

Approximately 30% of patients have a gradient between the body and outflow tract of the left ventricle at rest; an additional 20 to 25% develop such a gradient following manoeuvres that increase myocardial contractility or that reduce ventricular afterload or venous return. The presence and magnitude of a gradient is determined by the size and geometry of the left ventricular outflow tract, which are in turn a function of the severity of septal hypertrophy, mitral leaflet morphology, and papillary muscle size and position. The conventionally accepted mechanism of the gradient is that Venturi forces from increased ejection velocity in the narrowed outflow tract draw the anterior and/or posterior mitral leaflets towards the septum. More recent data suggest that the abnormally positioned mitral valve leaflets are 'driven' rather than sucked into the septum.

Myocardial ischaemia

Patients with hypertrophic cardiomyopathy have reduced coronary flow reserve and evidence for myocardial ischaemia during rapid atrial pacing and pharmacological stress. Myocardial ischaemia is almost certainly a major cause of exertional symptoms and

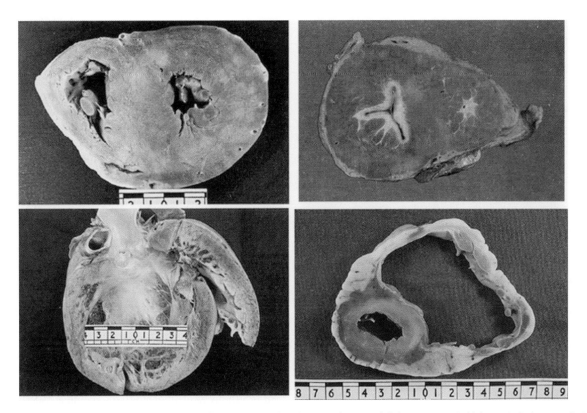

Fig. 7.2.1 Transverse short-axis section through the ventricles from patients with cardiomyopathy. Upper left shows symmetrical left ventricular hypertrophy in hypertrophic cardiomyopathy. Upper right shows dense white fibrous tissue obliterating the apex of both ventricles in endomyocardial fibrosis. Lower left shows a globular, dilated left ventricle in a child with dilated cardiomyopathy. Lower right shows a grossly dilated right ventricle with adipose infiltration of the right ventricular free wall in arrhythmogenic right ventricular dysplasia.
Davies MJ, 1986, *Colour atlas of cardiovascular pathology*, Oxford University Press.

may be a trigger for ventricular arrhythmia. However, detection of ischaemia in everyday clinical practice is challenging because conventional markers of ischaemia such as ST-segment change and reversible perfusion abnormalities on single photon emission computed tomography (SPECT) imaging correlate poorly with objective biochemical markers of ischaemia.

Diagnosis

Left ventricular hypertrophy in the absence of moderate to severe hypertension and valve disease occurs in about 1 in 500 adults. The prevalence of HCM in children is unknown, but population-based studies report an annual incidence of 0.3 to 0.5 per 100 000 (range 0.005–0.07%). The diagnosis of HCM is based on the demonstration of unexplained myocardial hypertrophy, defined as a wall thickness measurement exceeding two standard deviations for gender and age. In practice, in an adult of normal size the presence of a left ventricular myocardial segment of 1.5 cm or greater in thickness is diagnostic. Less stringent criteria should be applied to first-degree relatives of an unequivocally affected individual, where the probability of carrying the disease gene is 1 in 2 (Table 7.2.2).

Problems in diagnosis may arise in patients with moderate to severe hypertension. The determinants of the hypertrophic response in a patient with hypertension are unknown, but are partly influenced by racial origin, with a greater increase in left ventricular mass in African-Caribbean individuals. In general, however, hypertrophic cardiomyopathy should be suspected in any individual with

hypertension and a wall thickness in excess of 1.5 cm, particularly if the ECG shows widespread repolarization abnormalities or there is evidence of good blood pressure control.

The physiological changes of athletic training can rarely mimic hypertrophic cardiomyopathy. Athletes who participate in events that combine both isometric and isotonic activities (e.g. rowing and cycling) have the greatest increases in left ventricular wall thickness. Pure strength training is associated with an increase in left ventricular mass and wall thickness relative to the left ventricular cavity size, but is rarely associated with an increase in absolute wall thickness (unless the athlete also uses anabolic steroids). A diagnosis of hypertrophic cardiomyopathy in an elite athlete is likely when left ventricular wall thickness exceeds 1.6 cm in males and 1.4 cm in females and when they are symptomatic or have a family history of HCM. In athletes, the ECG frequently displays voltage criteria for left ventricular hypertrophy, sinus bradycardia, and sinus arrhythmia. Abnormal Q waves or marked repolarization abnormalities are rare in elite athletes and should raise suspicion of myocardial disease. Echocardiographic features favouring hypertrophic cardiomyopathy include small left ventricular cavity dimensions, left atrial enlargement, left ventricular outflow gradients, and diastolic impairment.

Clinical features

History

Symptomatic presentation may be at any age with breathlessness on exertion, chest pain, palpitation, syncope, or sudden cardiac

Table 7.2.2 Major and minor criteria for the diagnosis of hypertrophic cardiomyopathy in adult members of affected families. Criteria are fulfilled if (1) one major echocardiographic, or (2) two minor echocardiographic, or (3) one minor echocardiographic plus two minor electrocardiographic abnormalities are seen

Major criteria	Minor criteria
Echocardiography	
Left ventricular wall thickness ≥13 mm in the anterior septum or posterior wall or ≥15 mm in the posterior septum or free wall	Left ventricular wall thickness of 12 mm in the anterior septum or posterior wall or of 14 mm in the posterior septum or free wall
Severe SAM (septal–leaflet contact)	Moderate SAM (no septal–leaflet contact)
	Redundant mitral valve leaflets
Electrocardiography	
Left ventricular hypertrophy + repolarization changes (Romhilt and Estes)	Complete bundle branch block or (minor) interventricular conduction defect (in LV leads)
T-wave inversion in leads I and aVL (≥3 mm) (with QRS–T-wave axis difference ≥30°), V3–V6 (≥3 mm) or II and III and aVF (≥5 mm)	Minor repolarization changes in LV leads
Abnormal Q (>40 ms or >25% R wave) in at least two leads from II, III, aVF (in absence of left anterior hemiblock), V1–V4; or I, aVL, V5–V6	Deep S in V2 (>25 mm)
Clinical	
There are no clinical major criteria	Unexplained chest pain, dyspnoea, or syncope

LV, left ventricular; SAM, systolic anterior motion of the mitral valve.

Reproduced from *Heart*, McKenna WJ *et al*, 77, 130–2. Copyright 1997 with permission from the BMJ Publishing Group.

death. HCM is occasionally found at autopsy in a stillborn baby or presents during infancy with cardiac failure, which is usually fatal. In children and adolescents, the diagnosis is most often made during screening of siblings and offspring of affected family members. Paroxysmal symptoms or mild impairment of exercise tolerance are often present, but in the absence of a murmur may not prompt cardiac evaluation.

About 50% of adults present with symptoms; in the remainder the diagnosis is made during family screening or following the detection of an unsuspected abnormality on physical, electrocardiographic, or echocardiographic examination. Dyspnoea is common (>50%) as a consequence of elevated left atrial and pulmonary capillary wedge pressures resulting from impaired left ventricular relaxation and filling, and about 50% complain of chest pain, which is exertional, atypical, or both in similar proportions of patients. Atypical pain may have no obvious precipitant; more commonly it follows exercise- or anxiety-related tachycardia, when it persists for up to several hours after the stress has been removed without enzymatic evidence of myocardial damage. Syncopal episodes occur in 15 to 25%, but in only a few are there findings suggestive of an arrhythmia or evidence of overt conduction disease: in most patients, the

mechanism cannot be determined. Patients rarely present with paroxysmal nocturnal dyspnoea, ascites, or peripheral oedema.

Physical examination

In most patients with hypertrophic cardiomyopathy the physical examination is unremarkable. There may be a rapid upstroke arterial pulse reflecting dynamic left ventricular emptying. In about one-third, the jugular venous pulse may demonstrate a prominent 'a' wave, reflecting diminished right ventricular compliance secondary to right ventricular hypertrophy. Many patients have a forceful left ventricular cardiac impulse, best appreciated on full-held expiration in the left lateral position, when there may be a palpable atrial beat reflecting forceful atrial systolic contraction that may or may not be associated with significant forward flow of blood.

The first and second heart sounds are usually normal, and—unless the patient is in atrial fibrillation—there is likely to be a loud fourth heart sound, reflecting increased atrial systolic flow into a noncompliant ventricle. However, in those patients (20–30%) who have a resting left ventricular outflow-tract gradient, the most obvious physical sign is an ejection systolic murmur. This murmur starts well after the first heart sound and ends well before the second. It is best heard at the left sternal border, radiating towards the aortic and mitral areas, but not into the neck or the axilla. The intensity varies with changes in ventricular volume; it can be increased by physiological and pharmacological manoeuvres that decrease afterload or venous return (amyl nitrate, standing, Valsalva, etc.), and decreased by manoeuvres that increase afterload and venous return (squatting, phenylephrine, etc.). Occasionally there is an ejection sound at the onset of the systolic murmur.

Most patients with a left ventricular outflow-tract gradient also have mitral regurgitation. Doppler examination reveals that mitral regurgitation usually begins just before (30–40 ms) the onset of the gradient and continues for the duration of systole. Radiation of the systolic murmur to the axilla is often the best auscultatory clue to the presence of coexistent mitral regurgitation, which may be moderate to severe, either alone or in association with a left ventricular outflow-tract gradient. A mid-diastolic rumble may sometimes result from increased transmitral flow in patients with severe mitral regurgitation.

Early diastolic murmurs of aortic incompetence may develop following surgical myectomy or infective endocarditis involving the aortic valve. Although such murmurs are rare in the absence of such complications, they appear to occur more commonly than would be expected by chance and may reflect traction on the noncoronary cusp of the aortic valve by the septum. An ejection systolic murmur in the pulmonary area, reflecting right ventricular outflow-tract obstruction, is also rare; when present, it is usually associated with severe biventricular hypertrophy in the young or in those with coexistent Noonan's syndrome and a dysplastic pulmonary valve (see Chapter 12.1).

Prognosis

Patients with hypertrophic cardiomyopathy experience slow progression of symptoms and gradual deterioration of left ventricular function, and are at risk of sudden cardiac death throughout life. Annual mortality rates are in the range of 1 to 2%, but the risk of death and other disease-related complications varies between individuals and within individuals during the course of the disease.

Severe heart failure symptoms may develop in association with progressive myocardial wall thinning caused by myocardial fibrosis and severe reduction in left ventricular systolic performance and/or diastolic filling. The development of systolic failure is associated with a poor prognosis, with rapid progression from onset to death or transplantation, and an overall mortality rate of up to 11% per year.

Atrial dilatation and the development of atrial fibrillation/flutter are important features in the clinical course, leading to a risk of acute deterioration and thromboembolic stroke. Onset of atrial fibrillation is part of the evolution of patients with diastolic dysfunction, and with appropriate management need not represent a major cause of morbidity or mortality. A few patients who experience such deterioration present with a clinical picture resembling restrictive cardiomyopathy, with grossly enlarged atria, signs of right heart failure, and relative preservation of left ventricular systolic performance.

Left ventricular hypertrophy develops during childhood and adolescence, but is not progressive in adults. The trigger and other determinants of disease expression in late-onset disease are uncertain.

Investigations

Cardiological evaluation of patients with hypertrophic cardiomyopathy is performed to confirm the diagnosis, to guide symptomatic therapy, and to assess the risk of complications, particularly that of sudden death.

Electrocardiography

The 12-lead ECG is the most sensitive diagnostic test, although occasionally normal (c.5%), particularly in the young. At the time of diagnosis 5 to 10% of patients are in atrial fibrillation. Many have an intraventricular conduction delay and 20% have left-axis deviation, but complete right bundle or left bundle branch block is uncommon (c.5%). The latter may develop following surgery and is occasionally seen in elderly patients. ST-segment depression and T-wave changes are the most common abnormalities and are usually associated with voltage changes of left ventricular hypertrophy and/or deep S waves in the anterior chest leads V1 to V3. Isolated repolarization changes or giant negative T waves are occasionally seen. Voltage criteria for left ventricular hypertrophy are rare in the absence of repolarization changes. About 20% of patients have abnormal Q waves, either inferiorly (II, III, and aVF), or less commonly in leads V1 to V3. P-wave abnormalities of left and/or right atrial overload are common. The distribution of the PR interval is similar to that in the normal population, but occasionally a short PR interval may be associated with a slurred upstroke to the QRS complex, similar to that seen in the Wolff–Parkinson–White syndrome. At electrophysiological study, such changes are not usually associated with evidence of pre-excitation, although patients with hypertrophic cardiomyopathy and accessory pathways have been described. Despite the many electrocardiographic abnormalities, there is no ECG that is typical of HCM; a useful rule is to consider the diagnosis whenever the ECG is bizarre, particularly in younger patients.

The incidence of arrhythmias during 48-h ambulatory electrocardiographic monitoring increases with age. Nonsustained ventricular tachycardia is detected in 20 to 25% of adults and, although usually asymptomatic, is associated with an increased risk of sudden cardiac death. Supraventricular arrhythmias are also common in adults and can be poorly tolerated if sustained (>30 s) unless the ventricular response is controlled and carry an increased risk of thromboembolism. By contrast, most children and adolescents are

in sinus rhythm, and arrhythmias during ambulatory electrocardiographic monitoring are uncommon. The increased incidence of supraventricular arrhythmias with age is related to increased left atrial dimensions and increased left ventricular diastolic pressure. The aetiology of ventricular arrhythmias is not known, but may relate to myocyte loss and myocardial fibrosis. Documented sustained ventricular tachycardia is uncommon, but is a recognized complication in patients with an apical aneurysms, which may develop as a consequence of midventricular obstruction.

Chest radiography

The chest radiograph may be normal or show evidence of left and/or right atrial or left ventricular enlargement; if left atrial pressure has been chronically elevated, there may be evidence of redistribution of blood flow to upper lung zones. Mitral valve annular calcification is seen, particularly in elderly patients.

Echocardiography

Left ventricular hypertrophy may be symmetric or asymmetric and localized to the septum or the free wall, but most commonly to both the septum and free wall with relative sparing of the posterior wall (Fig. 7.2.2). Isolated apical hypertrophic cardiomyopathy occurs in about 10% of patients and may be more common in Japan. Approximately one-third of patients also have hypertrophy of the right ventricular free wall, the presence and severity of which is strongly related to the severity of left ventricular hypertrophy. Typically, left ventricular end-systolic and end-diastolic dimensions are reduced, and the left atrial dimension is increased. Indices of systolic function such as ejection fraction may be increased, but systolic function is often impaired, which may be best appreciated by measurement of long-axis rather than short-axis function.

Colour Doppler provides a sensitive method of detecting left ventricular outflow-tract turbulence (Fig. 7.2.3), and when combined with continuous-wave Doppler the peak velocity (V_{max}) of left ventricular blood flow can be measured and left ventricular outflow-tract gradients calculated. Doppler gradients (pressure gradient (mmHg) = $4 V_{max}^2$) are seen in 20 to 30% of patients and

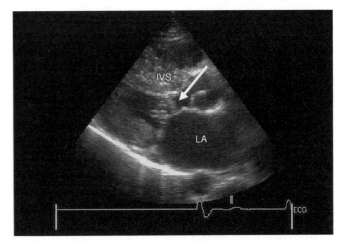

Fig. 7.2.2 An echocardiogram (parasternal long-axis view) of a patient with hypertrophic obstructive cardiomyopathy demonstrating hypertrophy of the interventricular septum (IVS), enlargement of the left atrium (LA), and systolic anterior motion of the mitral valve, bringing it into contact with the septum (arrow).

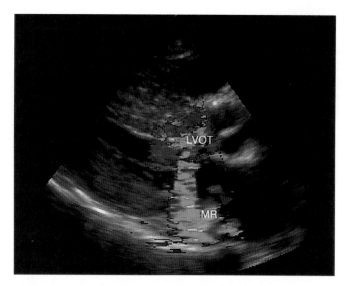

Fig. 7.2.3 Colour-flow Doppler image (parasternal long-axis view) of the same patient as shown in Fig. 7.2.2, demonstrating left ventricular outflow tract (LVOT) turbulence and mitral regurgitation (MR) with a posteriorly directed jet.

correlate well with those measured invasively. Systolic anterior motion of the mitral valve is usually present when the calculated outflow-tract gradient is more than 30 mmHg, and early closure or fluttering of the aortic valve leaflets is often seen in association with such motion. A posteriorly directed mitral regurgitant jet is seen in association with and related to the magnitude of the outflow-tract gradient (Fig. 7.2.3). An anterior regurgitant jet or mitral regurgitation in the absence of obstruction suggests the coexistence of structural mitral valve abnormalities.

Other imaging techniques

Good-quality echocardiography suffices for diagnostic and therapeutic purposes in most patients with hypertrophic cardiomyopathy, but cardiac MRI is useful in selected cases to assess right ventricular, apical, and lateral left ventricular involvement. Gadolinium-enhanced cardiac MRI permits detection of myocardial fibrosis, the extent of which may predict evolution to the burnt-out phase.

Cardiac catheterization

Two-dimensional echo/Doppler evaluation has replaced invasive haemodynamic measurements and angiography as the method of assessing left ventricular structure and function in hypertrophic cardiomyopathy. Cardiac catheterization is not necessary for diagnosis and is rarely indicated unless symptoms are refractory and direct measurement of cardiac pressures is potentially informative, particularly in assessing the severity of mitral regurgitation. Coronary arteriography may be necessary to exclude coexistent coronary artery disease in older patients who have significant angina or ST-segment changes during exercise. The left coronary arteries are usually large in calibre. The left anterior descending and septal perforator arteries may demonstrate narrowing during systole in the absence of fixed obstructive lesions, but such changes do not appear to relate to symptoms. Left ventricular angiography is rarely indicated, but recognition of the abnormally shaped ventricle, which typically ejects at least 75% of its contents in association with mild mitral regurgitation, may provide a valuable diagnostic

clue when hypertrophic cardiomyopathy was not suspected before catheterization.

Exercise testing

Maximal exercise testing in association with respiratory gas analysis provides useful functional and prognostic information, which can be monitored serially. Oxygen consumption at peak exercise (peak Vo_2) is usually moderately reduced, even in patients who do not complain of exertional symptoms. Continuous measurement of the blood pressure during upright treadmill or bicycle exercise reveals that about one-third of younger patients (<40 years) have an abnormal blood pressure response, with either a drop of more than 10 mmHg from peak recordings or a failure to rise by 20 mmHg or more despite an appropriate increase in cardiac output. Such changes are usually asymptomatic but are associated with an increased risk of sudden death. The mechanism of the hypotensive response during exercise in hypertrophic cardiomyopathy varies, but may relate to myocardial mechanoreceptor activation and altered baroreflex control causing inappropriate drops in systemic vasculature resistance, to a poor cardiac output response, or to exercise-induced left ventricular outflow-tract obstruction. ST-segment depression of up to 2 mm from baseline is documented in 25% of patients, but appears not to be of prognostic significance.

Electrophysiological studies

Electrophysiological studies may occasionally be necessary in patients with sustained, rapid palpitation to identify associated accessory pathways or aid management of sustained monomorphic ventricular tachycardia. Conventional, programmed ventricular stimulation does not aid the identification of high-risk patients (see 'Risk stratification').

Tests for specific causes of hypertrophic cardiomyopathy

A number of clinical features that suggest particular causes of hypertrophic cardiomyopathy are listed in Table 7.2.3; the presence of such clues should trigger appropriate biochemical and genetic testing.

Management

Pharmacological

The goal of therapy is to improve symptoms and prevent complications, in particular sudden death. β-Adrenoreceptor blockers and calcium antagonists, especially verapamil, are the mainstay of symptomatic pharmacological therapy. Both drugs have several potentially beneficial actions, including a decrease in myocardial oxygen consumption and blunting of the heart rate response during exercise, thereby increasing time for filling. Both agents exert a negative inotropic effect, thereby reducing hyperdynamic systolic function and left ventricular gradients, and they may improve diastolic function, verapamil by improving relaxation and β-blockers by increasing compliance. The side effects of propranolol are rarely serious, but the suppressant effect of verapamil on atrioventricular nodal conduction may cause problems in patients with unsuspected pre-existing conduction disease, and its vasodilatory and negative inotropic effects can result in acute pulmonary oedema and death in symptomatic patients with severe obstruction and pulmonary hypertension.

Endocarditis is a rare complication of hypertrophic cardiomyopathy, occurring predominantly in patients with left ventricular outflow tract turbulence and/or mitral regurgitation. Current

Table 7.2.3 Clinical features suggesting the aetiology of hypertrophic cardiomyopathy

Clinical feature	Examples
Symptoms	Acroparaesthesiae, tinnitus, deafness (Anderson–Fabry disease)
	Skeletal muscle weakness (desminopathy, mitochondrial cytopathy, etc.)
Physical examination	Retinitis pigmentosa (mitochondrial, Danon disease, etc.)
	Postural hypotension (amyloid)
	Angiokeratoma (Anderson–Fabry disease)
	Lentigines (LEOPARD syndrome)
	Facial morphology (Noonan, Anderson–Fabry disease, etc.)
Electrocardiogram	Pre-excitation/premature conduction disease (AMP kinase)
	Low-voltage/infarct pattern (amyloid)
Echocardiography	Concentric/biventricular hypertrophy (infiltrative, metabolic disease, etc.)
	Valve thickening (Anderson–Fabry disease, amyloid, etc.)
Family history	X-linked inheritance (Anderson–Fabry disease, Danon, etc.)
	Diabetes, epilepsy, and deafness (mitochondrial)
Biochemistry	Creatine kinase (glycogen storage disease, mitochondrial, etc.)
	Lactate (mitochondrial)
	Renal dysfunction (Anderson–Fabry disease, mitochondrial, etc.)
	Paraproteinaemia (amyloid)
Exercise testing	Severe premature acidosis (mitochondrial)

guidelines no longer support the previous recommendation of antibiotic prophylaxis in patients with outflow-tract obstruction or intrinsic valve disease.

Surgical

Surgery is a therapeutic option in patients with obstruction and/or mitral valve abnormalities. The conventional indication for surgery is a resting left ventricular outflow-tract gradient of more than 50 mmHg in patients refractory to medical therapy, and the commonest operation is the removal of a segment of the upper anterior septum (myectomy) via a transaortic approach. Transventricular approaches have been used, but these are associated with a higher incidence of late complications, particularly of cardiac failure. Mitral valve repair and papillary muscle remodelling may be required, and mitral valve replacement has also been advocated; excellent results have been achieved, particularly in elderly patients with severe mitral regurgitation. Specialist hypertrophic cardiomyopathy centres report perioperative mortality of 1% or less, with 90% success in abolishing gradients and improving symptoms.

Alcohol septal ablation

Injection of alcohol into the septal artery that supplies the septal muscle has been developed as a percutaneous, nonpharmacological approach to gradient reduction. Most experienced centres have reported symptomatic improvement in 70% of patients. As for surgery and dual-chamber (DDD) pacing (see below), patient selection—in particular, regarding the mechanism of the gradient—and technical considerations are important determinants of outcome. The major complication has been the need for a pacemaker in up to 20%, and concerns remain about long-term left ventricular function and arrhythmia risk. At present, alcohol septal ablation offers a therapeutic option in older patients with suitable anatomy who are refractory to drugs.

Pacing

Alteration of the ventricular activation sequence by pacing the right ventricular apex may result in reduction of gradients and filling pressures and improved symptoms in selected patients. The role of atrioventricular synchronous pacing (DDD pacing) in symptomatic management of obstruction has been evaluated in two randomized multicentre trials, demonstrating symptomatic improvement and gradient reduction (50%), but no change in exercise capacity. However, the placebo effect of the procedure was considerable. Nevertheless, pacing offers a therapeutic option in patients with obstruction that is refractory to drug treatment, and in whom surgery is either not acceptable or inappropriate. It appears that elderly patients with localized septal hypertrophy and without significant free wall involvement or mitral regurgitation may be the most likely to respond.

Clinical approach to individual symptoms

Dyspnoea

Dyspnoea most often occurs in patients who also experience chest pain or discomfort. Treatment depends on the predominant mechanism. In patients with dyspnoea who have slow filling that continues throughout diastole, β-blockers and verapamil are appropriate. Conversely, those with rapid, early filling may benefit from a relative tachycardia and do better without negative chronotropic agents. When dyspnoea is associated with significant obstruction, β-blockers, disopyramide, and (failing these) myectomy or the other nonpharmacological options may be beneficial. Disopyramide should be used in the maximum tolerated dose (anticholinergic side effects may limit higher doses) in conjunction with a conventional β-blocker. Occasionally, dyspnoea is associated with severe mitral regurgitation and responds well to mitral valve repair or replacement.

Chest pain

Exertional chest pain usually responds to therapy with propranolol or verapamil, and when refractory can respond to very high doses of these agents (propranolol at 480 mg daily, verapamil at 720 mg daily). Short-acting nitrates, diuretics, and high-dose verapamil may be useful in selected patients, perhaps by reducing filling pressures and improving coronary flow to subendocardial layers. Atypical chest pain may persist long after the initial stimulus has been removed.

Arrhythmia

Arrhythmias are a common complication of hypertrophic cardiomyopathy. The overall prevalence and annual incidence of atrial fibrillation are around 23% and 3%, respectively in a recent systematic review. Treatment with anticoagulants and verapamil or β-blockers is appropriate once atrial fibrillation is established, the aims being to control the ventricular response and prevent emboli. Most patients who develop atrial fibrillation during electrocardiographic monitoring are unaware of changes from sinus rhythm to atrial fibrillation as long as the ventricular response is well controlled. However, in a few cases the loss of atrial systolic contribution to filling volume is important, when electrical cardioversion can be facilitated by prior therapy (4–6 weeks) with amiodarone (300 mg daily) if pharmacological cardioversion does not occur first.

Sustained (>30 s) episodes of paroxysmal atrial fibrillation or supraventricular tachycardia can cause haemodynamic collapse and systemic emboli. Low-dose amiodarone (1000–1400 mg weekly) is effective in suppressing such episodes and also provides control of the ventricular response should breakthrough occur. The threshold for anticoagulation should be low as embolic complications are common, even when atrial dimensions are only moderately increased.

Nonsustained episodes of supraventricular arrhythmia are common, and although often asymptomatic, they are a marker (albeit of low positive predictive accuracy) for the subsequent development of established atrial fibrillation. The threshold to introduce amiodarone, with or without anticoagulation, should be low if they occur in the presence of atrial enlargement. Episodes of nonsustained ventricular tachycardia are common but are rarely symptomatic: therapy is warranted only if it can be shown to improve prognosis.

Prevention of sudden cardiac death

Sudden cardiac death is a consequence of multiple interacting mechanisms. The histological abnormalities—particularly myocyte disarray, small-vessel disease, and replacement scarring—contribute to the underlying substrate. Events may be triggered by haemodynamic alterations, myocardial ischaemia, and arrhythmias, including ventricular tachycardia, atrial fibrillation, atrioventricular block, and rapid conduction of a supraventricular arrhythmia via an accessory pathway. Intense physical exertion may also contribute to the above triggers. The interaction of triggers and substrate may be modified by inappropriate peripheral vascular responses and the development of myocardial ischaemia.

Risk stratification

Prevention of sudden death relies on risk factor stratification to identify a high-risk cohort who will benefit from an implantable cardioverter–defibrillator (ICD). Several adverse features that can be elicited from the clinical history and noninvasive evaluation have been identified (Box 7.2.1). Their relative importance varies with age; for example, the finding of nonsustained ventricular tachycardia on 24-h electrocardiographic monitoring in children and adolescents is uncommon (<5%), but is associated with an eightfold increased risk of sudden death, whereas in adults this arrhythmia is common (20–25%), but in isolation confers only a twofold increased risk.

In young people (<25 years) the finding of nonsustained ventricular tachycardia, severe and extensive left ventricular hypertrophy, unexplained syncope (particularly if recurrent or exertional), or a family history where a high proportion of affected individuals experienced premature (<40 years) sudden death warrants prophylactic treatment. Such patients usually also exhibit abnormal blood pressure responses to exercise; indeed, the finding of a normal exercise blood pressure response appears to identify the low-risk

---

> **Box 7.2.1** Risk factors for sudden death
>
> - Family history of sudden death (≥1 premature (<40 years) sudden death)
> - Unexplained syncope within previous year
> - Abnormal exercise blood pressure
> - Nonsustained ventricular tachycardia (≥3 beats at ≥120 beats/min)
> - Severe left ventricular hypertrophy (>3 cm)
> - Severe left ventricular outflow-tract obstruction (>90 mmHg)
> - Cardiac arrest (or sustained ventricular tachycardia)

---

younger (<40 years) patient (negative predictive accuracy 97%), allowing appropriate reassurance that is also clinically important. In adults aged 25 to 60 years, the positive predictive accuracy for each of the risk factors is much lower (15–20%): prophylactic treatment is advised for those with two or more risk factors who will have a predicted risk of sudden death of at least 3% per year. Those with a single risk factor have an annual sudden death risk of 1%, but the confidence limits range from 0.2 to 2%, indicating that some but not all single risk factor patients may benefit from an ICD.

Recently, a large multicentre longitudinal cohort study of 3675 patients (HCM-RISK SCD) developed and validated a statistical sudden cardiac death risk prediction model, which provides individualized risk estimates. This model uses left atrial diameter, peak left ventricular outflow-tract gradient, and patient age, together with the same major risk factors recommended in previous guidelines (with the exception of abnormal blood pressure response) to estimate the risk of sudden cardiac death at 5 years. It is important to consider risk in all patients, even those who are asymptomatic or who have mild echocardiographic features of hypertrophic cardiomyopathy. Although children and adolescents with severe congestive symptoms may be at greater risk, the data reveals that the severity of chest pain, dyspnoea, and exercise limitation are not reliable predictors of the risk of sudden death in adults. In addition, it is recognized that most patients who die suddenly have mild (1.5–2.0 cm) or moderate (2.0–2.5 cm) left ventricular hypertrophy, while some genetic defects (e.g. cardiac troponin T) may cause sudden death in the absence of symptoms or hypertrophy.

The presence of a left ventricular outflow-tract gradient is also associated with sudden death. The management of symptomatic patients should be focused on gradient reduction; in asymptomatic patients, severe left ventricular outflow-tract obstruction should be considered in the overall risk profile of the patient. Diastolic impairment with abnormal Doppler filling patterns and atrial enlargement is associated with symptomatic limitation and poor prognosis, but not with premature sudden death.

Some investigators have suggested that the induction of sustained ventricular arrhythmias during programmed electrophysiological stimulation is associated with a higher risk of sudden death. However, the predictive accuracy is low, and as most high-risk patients can be identified using noninvasive clinical markers, the inherent risks and inconvenience associated with programmed stimulation dictate that it should not be used routinely to assess risk in hypertrophic cardiomyopathy.

Dilated cardiomyopathy

Definition

Dilated cardiomyopathy is a heart muscle disorder defined by dilatation and impaired systolic function of the left ventricle or both ventricles in the absence of coronary artery disease, valvular abnormalities, or pericardial disease. A number of different cardiac and systemic diseases are associated with left ventricular dilatation and impaired contractility (see Chapter 7.3). When no identifiable cause is found, the condition is referred to as idiopathic dilated cardiomyopathy.

Dilated cardiomyopathy has been described in Western, African, and Asian populations, affecting both genders and all ages. In North America and Europe, symptomatic dilated cardiomyopathy has an incidence and prevalence of 20 and 38 per 100 000, respectively, and is the commonest indication for cardiac transplantation.

Causes

Pedigree analysis reveals familial disease in at least 25% of cases; a further 20 to 30% of relatives have mild abnormalities of left ventricular performance that evolve into dilated cardiomyopathy in about one-third. Inheritance is usually autosomal dominant with incomplete penetrance, with a smaller number of families having X-linked transmission. Penetrance is age dependent and has been estimated to be 10% in those aged less than 20 years, 34% in young adults aged 20 to 30 years, 60% in adults aged 30 to 40 years, and 90% in those over 40 years. Guidelines for the diagnosis of familial disease based on the identification of major and minor criteria are shown in Box 7.2.2. The diagnosis of familial dilated cardiomyopathy is fulfilled in a first-degree relative of a proband in the presence of one major criterion, or left ventricular dilatation plus one minor criterion, or three minor criteria.

> **Box 7.2.2** Major and minor criteria for the diagnosis of familial dilated cardiomyopathy in adult members of affected families (see text for details)
>
> **Major criteria**
>
> - A reduced ejection fraction of the left ventricle (<45%) and/or fractional shortening (<25%) as assessed by echocardiography, radionuclide scanning, or angiography
> - An increased left ventricular end-diastolic diameter corresponding to >117% of the predicted value corrected for age and body surface area
>
> **Minor criteria**
>
> - Unexplained supraventricular or ventricular arrhythmia
> - Ventricular dilatation (>112% of the predicted value)
> - An intermediate impairment of left ventricular dysfunction
> - Conduction defects
> - Segmental wall motion abnormalities in the absence of intraventricular conduction defect or ischaemic heart disease
> - Unexplained sudden death of a first-degree relative or stroke before 50 years of age

Disease-causing mutations are reported in numerous genes, most of which are important in maintaining myocyte cytoskeletal integrity, including dystrophin, metavinculin, cardiac actin (autosomal dominant), lamin A/C (associated with premature conduction disease and sudden death), desmin, myosin-binding protein C, troponin T and C, β-myosin heavy chain, and Z-line associated protein (ZASP). Lamin A/C mutations also cause Emery–Dreifuss and limb-girdle muscular dystrophy and familial partial lipodystrophy; desmin may cause conduction disease with restrictive cardiomyopathy; dystrophin mutations cause childhood (Duchenne) and adult (Becker) forms of muscular dystrophy. A further gene mutation implicated in the development of dilated cardiomyopathy (DCM) is titin (*TTN*), which is a connectin linking the Z-line to the M-line in the sarcomere. The frequency of *TTN* mutations is higher in subjects with dilated cardiomyopathy (27%) than in HCM (1%), but they are also found in some normal individuals.

Different patterns of disease expression are recognized. Disease progression appears to be slow (over decades) in most cases, and conduction disturbance is a late complication related to disease severity. However, in some families (<10%), particularly those with mutations in the lamin A/C gene, the early stages are characterized by progressive conduction disease, and left ventricular dilatation and impairment are later manifestations, in the 4th to 6th decade. Sudden death in the absence of severe left ventricular impairment is seen in disease caused by mutations in lamin A/C or desmosomal genes.

Pathology and pathophysiology

Macroscopic examination of hearts with dilated cardiomyopathy reveals dilated cardiac chambers (see Fig. 7.2.1), mural thrombi, and platelet aggregates with normal extra- and intramural coronary arteries. Myocardial mass is increased, but ventricular wall thickness is normal or reduced. Histology is nonspecific with patchy perimyocyte and interstitial fibrosis, various stages of myocyte death, as well as myocyte hypertrophy and often extensive myofibrillary loss, resulting in a vacuolated appearance of the myocytes. An interstitial T-lymphocyte infiltrate and focal accumulations of macrophages associated with individual myocyte death are common.

The identification of disease-causing mutations in genes encoding various components of the cardiac myocyte cystoskeletal and sarcomeric contractile apparatus shows that the pathogenesis of dilated cardiomyopathy is heterogeneous. Two models have been proposed to explain ventricular remodelling in dilated cardiomyopathy. In the 'final common pathway' hypothesis, dilated cardiomyopathy reflects a nonspecific degenerative state, which may result from a variety of stimuli, including genetic mutations, viral infections, toxins, and volume overload. The alternative hypothesis suggests that a number of distinct, independent, pathways can remodel the heart and cause dilated cardiomyopathy—in other words, the different causes of dilated cardiomyopathy share a common histopathology, but their molecular biology is distinct. The final common pathways resulting in dilated cardiomyopathy include altered myocyte energetics and calcium handling.

Clinical features

History

Initial presentation is usually with symptoms of cardiac failure (fatigue, breathlessness, decreased exercise tolerance, etc.), but arrhythmia (atrial fibrillation, ventricular tachycardia, atrioventricular block), systemic embolism, or the incidental finding of an ECG or radiographic abnormality during routine screening may prompt earlier diagnosis.

Physical examination

Physical examination may be entirely normal or may reveal evidence of myocardial dysfunction with cardiac enlargement and signs of congestive heart failure. Systolic blood pressure is often low, with a narrow pulse pressure and a low-volume arterial pulse. Pulsus alternans may be present in patients with severe left ventricular failure, and the jugular veins may be distended, with a prominent V wave reflecting tricuspid regurgitation. In such patients, the liver may be engorged and pulsatile, and there is usually peripheral oedema and ascites. The precordium often reveals a diffuse and dyskinetic left (and occasionally right) ventricular impulse. The apex is usually displaced laterally, reflecting ventricular dilatation. The second heart sound is usually normally split, but paradoxical splitting may be present when there is left bundle branch block, which occurs is about 15% of patients. With severe disease and the development of pulmonary hypertension, the pulmonary component of the second heart sound may be accentuated. Characteristically, a presystolic gallop or fourth heart sound is present before the development of overt cardiac failure. However, once cardiac decompensation has occurred, ventricular gallop or third heart sound is often present. When there is significant ventricular dilatation, systolic murmurs are common, reflecting mitral and (less commonly) tricuspid regurgitation.

The development of unexplained cardiac failure in the last month of pregnancy or 5 months postpartum is termed peripartum cardiomyopathy. There is usually uncertainty whether the cardiac failure is acute or chronic and exacerbated by the haemodynamic stress of pregnancy and labour. When the heart failure is acute and there is persistence of left ventricular chamber dilatation or impaired systolic performance, the diagnosis of peripartum cardiomyopathy can legitimately be made. An abnormally cleaved prolactin producing a raised 16 kDa prolactin level (normal prolactin is 23 kDa) has been identified in some patients with peripartum cardiomyopathy and, in a pilot study, treatment with the prolactin inhibitor bromocriptine improved left ventricular function and outcome. The diagnostic utility of urinary 16 kDa prolactin, its potential genetic basis, and the spectrum of therapeutic utility of bromocriptine remain to be determined. For further discussion of cardiac disease in pregnancy, see Chapter 18.

Prognosis

The natural history of dilated cardiomyopathy is uncertain because the diagnosis is usually not made until clinical features, which are late manifestations of the disease, become obvious. Follow-up of asymptomatic first-degree relatives suggests that disease progression is insidious over decades. An upper respiratory tract infection or a salt or fluid load can precipitate clinical presentation. Symptoms develop when filling pressures rise or when stroke volume diminishes sufficiently to cause salt and water retention and oedema. Once clinical symptoms and signs of impaired ventricular performance are apparent, prognosis is related to the degree of left ventricular dilatation and impaired contractile performance but. survival has been substantially improved by early recognition of mild disease, and by modern management with angiotensin converting enzyme (ACE) inhibitors, β-blockade, mineralocorticoid antagonists, aggressive treatment of arrhythmias, and cardiac transplantation.

Arrhythmia

Atrial arrhythmias, particularly atrial fibrillation, are common and associated with the severity of symptoms, left ventricular dysfunction, and poor prognosis, but atrial fibrillation is not an independent predictor of disease progression or sudden death. Occasionally, however, persistent atrial tachycardia or atrial fibrillation may cause gradual deterioration in left ventricular function, resembling dilated cardiomyopathy ('tachycardiomyopathy'): systolic function usually returns to normal with control of the arrhythmia.

Ventricular arrhythmias are common and like supraventricular arrhythmias are markers of disease severity. Nonsustained ventricular tachycardia during ECG monitoring is seen in about 20% of asymptomatic or mildly symptomatic patients and in up to 70% of those who are severely symptomatic. The prognostic significance of this arrhythmia is controversial: its presence early in the course of disease, when left ventricular function is relatively preserved, is probably an independent marker of sudden death risk, whereas in general markers of haemodynamic severity (such as ejection fraction, left ventricular end-diastolic dimension, or filling pressures) are more predictive of disease-related mortality and sudden death. Risk of sudden death in patients with severe disease (New York Heart Association, NYHA class III or IV) increases approximately threefold when syncope is present.

Investigation

Electrocardiography

The electrocardiographic features of dilated cardiomyopathy are nonspecific and highly variable. Sinus tachycardia is common (particularly in children and infants); nonspecific ST-segment and T-wave changes may be seen, most commonly in the inferior and lateral leads; and pathological Q waves may be present in the septal leads in patients with extensive left ventricular fibrosis. Atrial enlargement is common, and in advanced disease may be associated with bundle branch block. All degrees of atrioventricular block may also be seen and should raise the possibility of mutations in the lamin A/C gene if associated with relatively mild impairment of left ventricular function, or when present in a young patient.

Chest radiography

The chest radiograph is usually abnormal in patients with dilated cardiomyopathy, except in a rare subset of patients with acute viral myocarditis associated with left ventricular systolic impairment and preserved cavity dimensions. An increased cardiothoracic ratio (>0.5) is typically seen, reflecting left ventricular and left atrial dilatation. Increased pulmonary vascular markings and pleural effusions may be present in patients with elevated left ventricular filling pressures.

Echocardiography

Echocardiography is used to identify the presence of left ventricular cavity dilatation and systolic impairment, which are the typical features of the condition. In general, the presence of ventricular end-diastolic dimensions more than two standard deviations above body surface area-corrected mean values and fractional shortening less than 25% are sufficient to make the diagnosis (Fig. 7.2.4). Two-dimensional echocardiography is also used to determine whether intracavitary thrombus is present in the ventricles.

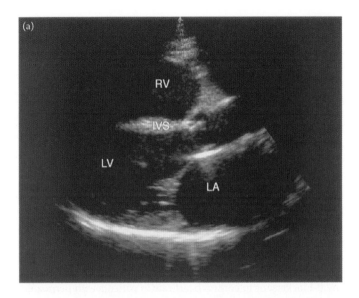

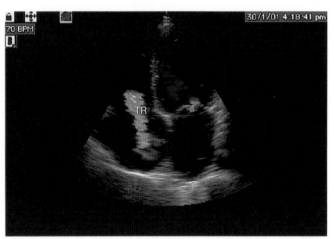

Fig. 7.2.5 Colour-flow Doppler image of the same patient as shown in Fig. 7.2.4a demonstrating a regurgitant tricuspid jet (TR).

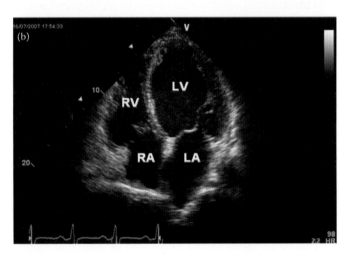

Fig. 7.2.4 Echocardiographic appearances of two patients with familial dilated cardiomyopathy. (a) Parasternal long-axis view showing significant left atrial (LA) and biventricular dilatation with a thin intraventricular septum (IVS). (b) Apical four-chamber view demonstrating a globular dilated left ventricle. LA, left atrium; LV, left ventricle; RA, right atrium; RV, right ventricle.

Colour-flow Doppler may be used to determine the presence and quantify the severity of functional mitral (and/or tricuspid) regurgitation (Fig. 7.2.5). Pulsed-wave and-continuous-wave Doppler can be used to estimate pulmonary artery pressures. Patients with dilated cardiomyopathy usually have abnormalities of diastolic left ventricular function in addition to systolic impairment: these can be assessed using mitral inflow, pulmonary vein, and tissue Doppler parameters.

Cardiac biomarkers

Serum creatine kinase should be measured in all patients with dilated cardiomyopathy because this simple test may provide an important clue to the aetiology of the condition (e.g. muscular dystrophy, lamin A/C defect, etc.). Other cardiac biomarkers, e.g. troponin I and troponin T, may also be elevated in dilated cardiomyopathy, particularly in association with an inflammatory cause. Plasma natriuretic peptide levels are elevated in chronic heart failure and predict mortality.

Many of the systemic diseases that are associated with heart muscle disorders have typical clinical, immunological, and biochemical features (see Chapter 7.3), and in the absence of clinical clues to suggest a systemic disease an exhaustive 'routine screen' is probably not cost-effective. There are, however, several potential reversible secondary causes of heart muscle disorder that may simulate dilated cardiomyopathy, and basic screening tests should include serum phosphorus (hypophosphataemia), serum calcium (hypocalcaemia), serum creatinine and urea (uraemia), thyroid function tests (hypothyroidism), and serum iron/ferritin (haemochromatosis).

Exercise testing

Symptom-limited exercise testing (treadmill or bicycle) combined with respiratory gas analysis is a useful technique to assess functional limitation in patients with dilated cardiomyopathy and provides a means of objectively evaluating disease progression. The detection of respiratory markers of severe lacticacidaemia during metabolic exercise testing may suggest a mitochondrial or other metabolic cause for dilated cardiomyopathy. Assessment of exercise capacity is essential in the assessment of patients prior to cardiac transplantation.

Cardiac catheterization

Cardiac catheterization is performed to exclude coronary artery disease as a cause of impaired systolic function. Haemodynamic assessment of left ventricular end-diastolic and pulmonary artery pressures is performed as part of cardiac transplant work-up. Endomyocardial biopsy may be diagnostic for myocarditis and may be considered when the presentation suggests myocarditis, i.e. acute chest pain in the absence of coronary artery disease, new-onset (days up to 3 months) or worsening of dyspnoea at rest or exercise, with or without left and/or right heart-failure signs, unexplained arrhythmia and/or aborted sudden cardiac death or unexplained cardiogenic shock, in the presence of biochemical markers of cardiac damage or compatible cardiac imaging features.

Cardiac MRI

Cardiac MRI may be a useful alternative imaging technique in patients with poor echocardiographic windows. In addition, the detection of fibrosis with gadolinium contrast enhancement may provide additional prognostic and diagnostic information.

A nontransmural, patchy or epi/mid-myocardial distribution of late gadolinium may help exclude myocardial infarction as the cause of left ventricular dysfunction. Cardiac MRI is also helpful in suspected myocarditis.

Electrophysiological testing

Programmed electrical stimulation is of limited clinical value in the identification of high-risk patients. Polymorphic ventricular tachycardia is inducible in up to 30% of cases, but this is a nonspecific finding. Approximately 10% of patients have inducible sustained monomorphic ventricular tachycardia; about one-third of these die suddenly, but most (75%) who die in this way do not have inducible ventricular tachycardia during programmed stimulation. In some patients (as many as 40% in one series), ventricular tachycardia arises as the consequence of bundle branch re-entry. This tachycardia is typically rapid (mean cycle length 280 ms) and uses a macro re-entrant circuit that involves the His–Purkinje system, usually with right bundle branch anterograde conduction and left bundle branch retrograde conduction. Differentiation from myocardial ventricular tachycardia is confirmed by the presence of a His or right bundle branch potential preceding each QRS: diagnosis is important since catheter ablation of either the left or right bundle branch is usually curative.

Management

Management in dilated cardiomyopathy aims to improve symptoms, to attenuate disease progression, and prevent arrhythmia, stroke, and sudden death.

Pharmacological treatment

Symptomatic therapy is the treatment of heart failure with reliance on diuretics, ACE inhibitors, and β-blockers (see Chapter 5.1).

Diuretics

Loop and/or thiazide diuretics should be used in all patients with fluid retention to achieve a euvolaemic state, but they should never be used as monotherapy as they exacerbate neurohormonal activation, thereby worsening disease progression. The aldosterone antagonist, spironolactone, reduces the overall risk of death by 30% in adults with severe heart failure (NYHA class IV and ejection fraction <35%): side effects include hyperkalaemia (infrequent in the presence of normal renal function) and painful gynaecomastia.

ACE inhibitors and angiotensin receptor blockers

Activation of the renin–angiotensin–aldosterone system is central to the pathophysiology of heart failure, regardless of the underlying aetiology, and ACE inhibitors should be considered in all patients with dilated cardiomyopathy. Many clinical trials have shown that ACE inhibitors improve symptoms, reduce hospitalizations, and reduce cardiovascular mortality in adults with symptomatic heart failure, and reduce the rate of disease progression in asymptomatic patients. ACE inhibitors are usually well tolerated, the most common side effects being cough and symptomatic hypotension.

The angiotensin receptor blockers (ARBs) have similar haemodynamic effects to ACE inhibitors. Clinical trials in adults with heart failure have shown similar haemodynamic effects, efficacy, and safety to ACE inhibitors, such that ARBs are currently recommended in adults who are intolerant of ACE inhibitors. Combination treatment with ACE inhibitors and ARBs may be more beneficial at preventing ventricular remodelling than either drug alone, but with little additional benefit on overall survival.

β-Blockers

Excess sympathetic activity contributes to heart failure and numerous multicentre placebo-controlled trials—using carvedilol, metoprolol, and bisoprolol—have shown substantial reductions in mortality (both sudden death and death from progressive heart failure) in adults with NYHA class II and III heart-failure symptoms. β-Blockers are usually well tolerated, but side effects include bradycardia, hypotension, and fluid retention, and they are generally contraindicated in asthma. β-Blockers should be started at low doses and slowly up-titrated; they should not be started in patients with decompensated heart failure.

Digoxin

Digoxin improves symptoms in patients with heart failure, but no survival benefit has been demonstrated in large study cohorts. High serum digoxin levels may be associated with increased mortality in some patients. Digoxin should be used only in patients who remain symptomatic in spite of treatment with diuretics, ACE inhibitors, and β-blockers, or to control heart rate in patients with permanent atrial fibrillation.

Anticoagulation

The prevalence of intramural thrombi and systemic thromboembolism ranges between 3% and 50%, with an incidence between 1.5% and 3.5% per year. Anticoagulation with warfarin is, therefore, advised in patients in whom an intracardiac thrombus is identified echocardiographically, or those with a history of thromboembolism. There are no trial data to guide prophylactic anticoagulation in dilated cardiomyopathy, but patients with severe ventricular dilatation and moderate to severe systolic impairment may also benefit from warfarin therapy.

Treatment of arrhythmia in dilated cardiomyopathy

If sustained or symptomatic arrhythmias are documented during 24-h ECG monitoring or exercise testing, conventional treatment is warranted (see Chapter 4.1). Many commonly prescribed antiarrhythmic agents should be avoided or used with caution because of their negative inotropic and proarrhythmic effects. Data on amiodarone are contradictory, but the Sudden Cardiac Death in Heart Failure Trial (SCD-HeFT) showed that amiodarone had no beneficial effect on survival when compared with implantable cardioverter–defibrillators. It can, however, be used safely to prevent or treat atrial arrhythmias.

Nonpharmacological treatment

Permanent pacing can correct two important intracardiac conduction abnormalities. First, a small subset of patients who have marked PR interval prolongation (>220 ms), usually secondary to atrioventricular nodal disease, experience deleterious effects on left ventricular haemodynamics with reduction in diastolic ventricular filling time and the development of end-diastolic tricuspid and mitral regurgitation. Correction of PR interval prolongation with short atrioventricular delay dual-chamber pacing may increase stroke volume and blood pressure, thus decreasing mitral regurgitation with dramatic clinical improvement. Second, patients with marked intraventricular conduction delay (left bundle branch block >150 ms) have dyssynchronous contraction of the left ventricular free wall and interventricular septum (which may decrease ejection fraction) and late activation of the anterolateral papillary muscle (which may increase functional mitral regurgitation). Biventricular or left ventricular pacing with specialized leads via the coronary sinus can correct both problems and has been shown to improve symptoms and prognosis in randomized trials. In addition, the resultant increase in blood pressure and pacemaker maintenance of the desired minimum heart rate permits use of higher doses of β-blockade and ACE inhibition with potential secondary benefit. Cardiac transplantation may be appropriate in patients with progressive deterioration. In addition, improvements in left ventricular assist devices and artificial heart technology provide alternatives that are now reasonably seen as viable future treatment options. These issues are discussed in Chapter 5.2.

Restrictive cardiomyopathy

Definition

Restrictive left ventricular physiology is characterized by a pattern of ventricular filling in which increased stiffness of the myocardium causes ventricular pressure to rise precipitously with only small increases in volume. The definition of restrictive cardiomyopathy has been confusing because this pattern can occur with a wide range of different pathologies. For the purposes of this chapter, restrictive cardiomyopathies are defined by restrictive ventricular physiology in the presence of normal or reduced diastolic volumes of one or both ventricles, normal or reduced systolic volumes, and normal ventricular wall thickness. Historically, systolic function was said to be preserved in restrictive cardiomyopathy, but it is rare for contractility to be truly normal.

Causes

Though restrictive physiology is often seen in hypertrophic cardiomyopathy and dilated cardiomyopathy, restrictive cardiomyopathy, as defined above, is uncommon. There are many causes including infiltrative and storage disorders, and endomyocardial disease including Loffler's endocarditis with hypereosinophilia. In the Western world amyloidosis is the commonest cause in adults, with some familial cases caused by mutations in the transthyretin gene. In the tropics, endomyocardial fibrosis is the commonest cause in adults, and probably also in children.

Rare reports of familial restrictive cardiomyopathy associated with autosomal dominant skeletal myopathy, autosomal recessive musculoskeletal abnormalities, and Noonan's syndrome have been described in children. Mutations in the gene encoding desmin (an intermediate filament protein) cause restrictive cardiomyopathy associated with skeletal myopathy and, in some cases, abnormalities of the cardiac conduction system. Familial restrictive cardiomyopathy is increasingly recognized as a specific phenotype within the spectrum of hypertrophic cardiomyopathy caused by sarcomere mutations, particularly troponin I and β-myosin heavy chain. Families are described in which restrictive cardiomyopathy and asymmetric hypertrophy are seen alone and in combination in carriers of affected genes.

Pathology

Restrictive cardiomyopathy is best regarded as a heterogeneous group of conditions with different aetiologies rather than a single disease entity. Macroscopically, restrictive cardiomyopathy is characterized by marked biatrial dilatation in the presence of normal heart weight, a small ventricular cavity, and no left ventricular hypertrophy. The histological features of idiopathic restrictive cardiomyopathy are usually nonspecific, with patchy interstitial fibrosis that may range in extent from very mild to severe. There may also be fibrosis of the sinoatrial and atrioventricular nodes. Myocyte disarray is not uncommon in patients with pure restrictive cardiomyopathy, even in the absence of macroscopic ventricular hypertrophy, consistent with restrictive cardiomyopathy being a clinically unrecognized manifestation of hypertrophic cardiomyopathy caused by sarcomere protein gene mutations.

When restrictive cardiomyopathy is caused by endomyocardial fibrosis the cardiac pathology is distinctive, with endocardial fibrosis and overlying thrombosis involving the inflow tracts and the apices, but sparing the outflow tracts of one or both ventricles. Necrotic, thrombotic, and fibrotic stages have been defined in patients with endomyocardial fibrosis and hypereosinophilia. In the necrotic stage, there is an acute inflammatory reaction characterized by eosinophilic abscesses in the myocardium, with associated necrosis and arteritis. The endocardium is often thickened and mural thrombi may develop. The thrombotic stage is characterized by endocardial thrombus formation that may be severe, with massive intracavitary thrombosis causing restriction to ventricular filling and a low-output state with high filling pressures. There is a risk of systemic emboli. During the necrotic and thrombotic stages the disease may mimic a hyperacute rheumatic carditis (see Chapter 9.1). If the patient survives, healing by fibrosis with hyaline fibrous tissue occurs. There is no further evidence of inflammation and the impact of the disease is caused by the effect of the dense fibrous tissue on ventricular filling volume and atrioventricular valve function.

Clinical features and investigation

Disease onset is usually insidious. Left-sided disease may present with symptoms of pulmonary congestion and/or mitral regurgitation; right-sided disease with raised jugular venous pressure, hepatomegaly, ascites, and tricuspid regurgitation. Radiographic and electrocardiographic appearances are nonspecific, showing evidence of raised left and/or right atrial pressure and cardiomegaly with left ventricular hypertrophy. Pulmonary infiltrates, nonspecific repolarization changes, and fascicular blocks may be seen.

Two-dimensional echocardiography confirms the diagnosis, allowing visualization of the structural abnormalities involving the endocardium and atrioventricular valves as well as demonstration of the abnormal physiology with restriction to filling (Fig. 7.2.6). There may be intracavitary thrombus with apical cavity obliteration, or bright echoes from the endocardium of the right or left ventricle with tethering of the chordae and reduced excursion of the posterior mitral valve leaflet. Typically, ventricular dimensions and wall thickness are normal, whereas the atria are grossly enlarged. Left ventricular filling terminates early and is followed by a plateau phase coincident with the third heart sound.

Diagnosis and management

Idiopathic restrictive cardiomyopathy

Demonstration of diagnostic features requires detailed imaging and may involve haemodynamic measurements at cardiac catheterization. Endomyocardial biopsy may be required to exclude storage and infiltrative diseases. It is particularly important to differentiate idiopathic restrictive cardiomyopathy from constrictive pericarditis, where surgical therapy may be curative (see Chapter 8.1). The clinical course of idiopathic restrictive cardiomyopathy is

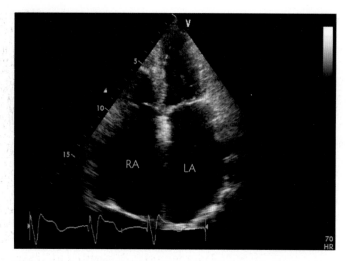

Fig. 7.2.6 Two-dimensional echocardiogram (apical four-chamber view) showing normal-sized ventricles with massive dilatation of left (LA) and right (RA) atria.

protracted (one to two decades), but once congestive symptoms develop, time to transplant or death is typically less than 5 years.

Endomyocardial fibrosis

The principal haemodynamic consequence of endomyocardial scarring is a restriction to normal filling. Early diastolic pressures are normal, but there is a rapid mid-diastolic rise (square root sign), which plateaus and is not associated with impairment of systolic performance. A similar functional haemodynamic abnormality is seen in pericardial constriction (see Chapter 8.1), but in the latter condition end-diastolic pressures are usually similar within the two ventricles, whereas in endomyocardial fibrosis there is usually inequality of the end-diastolic pressures. Mitral and tricuspid regurgitation may be severe and both ventricles appear abnormal in shape on angiography due to obliteration of the apices. This may be particularly marked in the right ventricle in which the infundibulum is hypertrophied and hypocontractile. In addition, the fibrotic process results in smoothing of the internal architecture of the ventricle with loss of the normal trabeculae. The presence of intracavitary thrombi in the left ventricle may give rise to the erroneous diagnosis of a cardiac tumour.

The structural and physiological abnormalities that can be demonstrated with two-dimensional echocardiography or during cardiac catheterization result from the thrombotic and fibrotic stages of the disease. Diagnosis may be difficult during the early acute phase, when the appearances of the left and right ventricle are far less abnormal, and may require confirmation by endomyocardial biopsy. In later stages, however, the diagnosis should be readily apparent and the risk of biopsy is excessive.

There is no good medical treatment for advanced disease and the prognosis is poor, with 35 to 50% 2-year mortality. Congestive symptoms from raised right atrial pressure can be improved with diuretics, though too great a reduction in ventricular filling pressure will lead to a reduction in cardiac output. Arrhythmias are common, but their prognostic significance is uncertain and they should not be treated unless they are sustained or associated with symptoms. Antiarrhythmic drugs that significantly slow the heart rate may be deleterious because of the small stroke volume. Digoxin may be helpful to control the ventricular response in atrial

fibrillation, but cannot be expected to improve congestive symptoms as systolic function is usually well preserved. Anticoagulants may help to prevent venous thrombosis and systemic emboli; both warfarin and antiplatelet drugs are advised.

Surgery with either mitral and/or tricuspid valve replacement, with or without decortication of the endocardium, has been carried out in some patients with endomyocardial fibrosis. Good long-term results have been obtained, but there is significant perioperative mortality (15–20%).

Arrhythmogenic right ventricular cardiomyopathy

Definition

Arrhythmogenic right ventricular cardiomyopathy (which replaces the older term 'arrhythmogenic right ventricular dysplasia') is a heart muscle disease characterized by progressive fibro-fatty replacement of right ventricular myocardium, initially with regional and later with global right and left ventricular involvement, associated with ventricular arrhythmia, heart failure, and sudden cardiac death, with as many as 20% of such deaths in young individuals and athletes attributable to the condition. Arrhythmogenic right ventricular cardiomyopathy occurs worldwide in all ethnic groups. The prevalence is unknown, but is conservatively estimated to be between 1 in 1000 and 1 in 5000.

Causes

Systematic family studies have shown that arrhythmogenic right ventricular cardiomyopathy is inherited in at least 50% of cases. The mode of transmission is usually autosomal dominant with variable penetrance, but rare autosomal recessive forms have provided the first insights into the genetic basis of the condition. Two autosomal recessive syndromes characterized by arrhythmogenic right ventricular cardiomyopathy, woolly hair, and palmoplantar keratoderma (Naxos disease, OMIM 601214; Carvajal–Huerta syndrome, OMIM 605676) are caused by mutations in the genes encoding plakoglobin and desmoplakin, respectively. These proteins are important components of the desmosome, with key roles in cell-to-cell adhesion and transduction of mechanical stress. Analysis of these and similar proteins in families with the more common autosomal dominant form of disease have revealed mutations in desmoplakin, plakophilin, desmoglein, and desmocollin. There are isolated reports of nondesmosomal gene mutations in arrhythmogenic right ventricular cardiomyopathy involving the ryanodine-2 receptor (more typically associated with catecholaminergic polymorphic ventricular tachycardia) transforming growth factor β, and lamin AC.

Pathology and pathophysiology

Segmental disease is usual in arrhythmogenic right ventricular cardiomyopathy, with involvement of the diaphragmatic, apical, and infundibular regions of the right ventricular free wall (the 'triangle of dysplasia'). Evolution to more diffuse right ventricular involvement and left ventricular abnormalities with heart failure are more common than the earlier literature suggested. Macroscopic examination of the heart may show diffuse thinning of the right ventricular wall, with aneurysms present in up to 50% of cases. The fibro-fatty replacement of the myocardium may be focal or widespread, usually involves the subepicardial layer of the right ventricular free wall and, when severe, may appear transmural. Isolated and predominantly left ventricular disease caused by desmosomal mutations is not uncommon. Histologically, arrhythmogenic right ventricular cardiomyopathy is characterized by replacement myocardial fibrosis with thinning and discrete bulges of the ventricular apices and of the right ventricular free wall, often in association with lymphocytic infiltrates surrounding degenerating or necrotic myocytes. Animal and *in vitro* studies support the hypothesis that mutations in plakoglobin or analogous genes involved in cell adhesion may cause myocytes under mechanical stress to detach and die, with subsequent fibro-fatty replacement.

Suggested arrhythmic mechanisms include re-entry circuits arising from fibro-fatty myocardial replacement and heterogeneous conduction resulting from destabilization of cell-adhesion complexes and gap junctions.

Clinical features

Symptomatic presentation is usually with palpitation and/or syncope from sustained ventricular arrhythmia, but the first presentation of the disease—especially in young people—may be with sudden cardiac death in an individual who was previously asymptomatic. Occasionally, the victim will have experienced syncope in the months preceding their death (particularly during exercise). Other symptoms are presyncope and chest pain. Features of right and later biventricular failure may be present, including dyspnoea on exertion, as the disease progresses. 'Hot phases' are recognized, during which previously stable patients may suffer repeated episodes of ventricular arrhythmia and be prone to sudden death.

Investigation

There is no single diagnostic test for arrhythmogenic right ventricular cardiomyopathy, and the diagnosis is based on the presence of major and minor criteria encompassing structural, histological, electrocardiographic, arrhythmic, and genetic factors (Table 7.2.4). The diagnosis of arrhythmogenic right ventricular cardiomyopathy is fulfilled in the presence of two major criteria, or one major plus two minor criteria, or four minor criteria from different categories. The recently revised criteria reflect family studies which (1) show that at least 30% of patients have left ventricular involvement in the form of regional or global left ventricular dysfunction, and many have subclinical left ventricular fibrosis (evident on magnetic resonance) affecting particularly the posterolateral segments, and (2) show that first-degree relatives of affected individuals may have minor cardiac abnormalities, which—although not fulfilling the above diagnostic criteria—are likely to represent disease expression in the context of an autosomal dominant disease.

Electrocardiography

The most common electrocardiographic abnormality is T-wave inversion in leads V1 to V3 in the absence of right bundle branch block (but note that this is a normal finding in children and therefore cannot be used as a diagnostic criterion) (Fig. 7.2.7). Other electrocardiographic features include QRS dispersion (localized prolongation of the QRS complex in the right ventricular leads, with a difference in QRS duration of at least 40 ms between right and left precordial leads), right intraventricular conduction delay (progressing to right bundle branch block in some patients) and the presence of an epsilon wave (a terminal notch in the QRS complex), typically seen in lead V1. Ventricular tachycardia is of left bundle branch block morphology suggesting a right ventricular origin. The signal-averaged ECG is used to detect late potentials which predict susceptibility to ventricular arrhythmia and disease progression.

Exercise testing

The role of exercise testing in arrhythmogenic right ventricular cardiomyopathy is primarily to detect ventricular arrhythmias induced by physical activity. Ventricular ectopy and nonsustained ventricular tachycardia of right ventricular origin have been described in young patients. Cardiopulmonary exercise testing may be useful as an objective measure of functional capacity in patients with advanced disease.

Echocardiography

Echocardiography is used to confirm the diagnosis and to exclude congenital heart disease, which may present as a differential diagnosis for arrhythmogenic right ventricular cardiomyopathy. Typical echocardiographic findings include right ventricular dilatation, regional hypokinesia or dyskinesia, free wall aneurysms, increased echogenicity of the moderator band, and right ventricular apical hypertrabeculation. Left ventricular involvement with posterior wall hypokinesia or ventricular dilatation may be seen in up to 30% of cases. In patients in whom the right ventricle is difficult to visualize adequately using standard two-dimensional echocardiography, injection of echocardiographic contrast may provide improved definition of the right ventricular endocardial border.

Cardiac MRI

Assessment of the right ventricle using echocardiography is challenging, even in experienced hands. Cardiovascular MRI has the advantage that it is a three-dimensional technique with no limitations imposed by acoustic windows (Fig. 7.2.8). When performed with a dedicated protocol by experienced operators, in both children and adults, the technique has a high sensitivity for detecting right ventricular abnormalities in individuals who fulfil conventional diagnostic criteria. Assessment of right ventricular fat, gadolinium late enhancement, and wall thinning on MRI are not considered to be adequately robust measures for inclusion in the revised diagnostic criteria. Left ventricular late enhancement, which often involves the epi- and mid-myocardial segments of the posterolateral wall, may provide the earliest nonelectrical manifestation of desmosomal disease and be observed with otherwise normal left ventricular structure and function.

Endomyocardial biopsy

Although a histological diagnosis of arrhythmogenic right ventricular cardiomyopathy may be definitive, the sensitivity of endomyocardial biopsies is low because (1) the disease is segmental in nature, (2) the amount of tissue usually obtained is insufficient to differentiate fibro-fatty replacement from islands of adipose tissue that are not infrequently seen between myocytes in the right ventricle of normal subjects, and (3) samples are usually taken from the septum, a region that is less frequently involved. The complication rate—which includes cardiac perforation and tamponade because of thinning of the right ventricular wall—is also relatively high, hence endomyocardial biopsies are no longer considered part of the routine diagnostic work-up for the condition.

Table 7.2.4 Revised Task Force criteria

I. Global or regional dysfunction and structural alterations[a]

Major	By 2D echo:
	Regional RV akinesia, dyskinesia, or aneurysm
	and 1 of the following (end diastole):
	◆ PLAX RVOT ≥32 mm (corrected for body size [PLAX/BSA] ≥19 mm/m^2)
	◆ PSAX RVOT ≥36 mm (corrected for body size [PSAX/BSA] ≥21 mm/m^2)
	◆ *or* fractional area change ≤33%
	By MRI:
	Regional RV akinesia or dyskinesia or dyssynchronous RV contraction
	and 1 of the following:
	◆ Ratio of RV end-diastolic volume to BSA ≥110 mL/m^2 (male) or ≥100 mL/m^2 (female)
	◆ *or* RV ejection fraction ≤40%
	By RV angiography:
	◆ Regional RV akinesia, dyskinesia, or aneurysm
Minor	By 2D echo:
	Regional RV akinesia or dyskinesia
	and 1 of the following (end diastole):
	◆ PLAX RVOT ≥29 to <32 mm (corrected for body size [PLAX/BSA] ≥16 to <19 mm/m^2)
	◆ PSAX RVOT ≥32 to <36 mm (corrected for body size [PSAX/BSA] 18 to <21 mm/m^2)
	◆ *or* fractional area change >33% to ≤40%
	By MRI:
	Regional RV akinesia or dyskinesia or dyssynchronous RV contraction
	and 1 of the following:
	◆ Ratio of RV end-diastolic volume to BSA ≥100 to <110 mL/m^2 (male) or ≥90 to <100 mL/m^2 (female)
	◆ *or* RV ejection fraction >40% to ≤45%

II. Tissue characterization of wall

Major	Residual myocytes<60% by morphometric analysis (or <50% if estimated), with fibrous replacement of the RV free wall myocardium in ≥1 sample, with or without fatty replacement of tissue on endomyocardial biopsy
Minor	Residual myocytes 60% to 75% by morphometric analysis (or 50% to 65% if estimated), with fibrous replacement of the RV free wall myocardium in ≥1 sample, with or without fatty replacement of tissue on endomyocardial biopsy

III. Repolarization abnormalities

Major	Inverted T waves in right precordial leads (V1, V2, and V3) or beyond in individuals >14 years of age (in the absence of complete RBBB QRS ≥120 ms)
Minor	Inverted T waves in leads V1 and V2 in individuals >14 years of age (in the absence of complete RBBB) or in V4, V5, or V6
	Inverted T waves in leads V1, V2, V3, and V4 in individuals >14 years of age in the presence of complete RBBB

IV. Depolarization/conduction abnormalities

Major	Epsilon wave (reproducible low-amplitude signals between end of QRS complex to onset of the T-wave) in the right precordial leads (V1–V3)
Minor	Late potentials by SAECG in ≥1 of 3 parameters in the absence of a QRS duration of ≥110 ms on the standard ECG
	Filtered QRS duration (fQRS) ≥114 ms
	Duration of terminal QRS <40 μV (low-amplitude signal duration) ≥38 ms
	Root-mean-square voltage of terminal 40 ms ≤20 μV
	Terminal activation duration of QRS ≥55 ms measured from the nadir of the S wave to the end of the QRS, including R′, in V1, V2, or V3, in the absence of complete RBBB

V. Arrhythmias

Major	Nonsustained or sustained ventricular tachycardia of left bundle branch morphology with superior axis (negative or indeterminate QRS in leads II, III, and aVF and positive in lead aVL)
Minor	Nonsustained or sustained ventricular tachycardia of RV outflow configuration, LBBB morphology with inferior axis (positive QRS in leads II, III, and aVF and negative in lead aVL) or of unknown axis
	>500 ventricular extrasystoles per 24 h (Holter)

(continued)

Table 7.2.4 Continued

VI. Family history	
Major	ARVC/D confirmed in a 1st-degree relative who meets current Task Force criteria
	ARVC/D confirmed pathologically at autopsy or surgery in a 1st-degree relative
	Identification of a pathogenic mutation[b] categorized as associated or probably associated with ARVC/D in the patient under evaluation
Minor	History of ARVC/D in a first-degree relative in whom it is not possible or practical to determine whether the family member meets current Task Force criteria
	Premature sudden death (<35 years of age) due to suspected ARVC/D in a 1st-degree relative
	ARVC/D confirmed pathologically or by current Task Force criteria in 2nd-degree relative

[a]VF, augmented voltage unipolar left foot lead; aVL, augmented voltage unipolar left arm lead; BSA, body surface area; LBBB, left bundle branch block; PLAX, parasternal long-axis view; PSAX, parasternal short-axis view; RBBB, right bundlee branch block; RVOT, RV outflow tract.

Diagnostic terminology for revised criteria: definite diagnosis: 2 major or 1 major and 2 minor criteria or 4 minor from different categories; borderline: 1 major and 1 minor or 3 minor criteria from different categories; possible: 1 major or 2 minor criteria from different categories.

[b] A pathogenic mutation is a DNA alteration associated with ARVC/D that alters or is expected to alter the encoded protein, is unobserved or rare in a large non-ARVC/D control population, and either alters or is predicted to alter the structure or function of the protein or has demonstrated linkage to the disease phenotype in a conclusive pedigree.

From Marcus FI, McKenna WJ, Sherrill D, et al. (2010). Diagnosis of arrhythmogenic right ventricular cardiomyopathy/dysplasia: proposed modification of the Task Force Criteria. *Eur Heart J*, **31**, 806–14.

Management

Treatment in arrhythmogenic right ventricular cardiomyopathy is individualized according to the presence of symptoms, arrhythmia, and perceived risk of sudden death. Patients with symptomatic, non-life-threatening ventricular arrhythmias are treated empirically with β-adrenoreceptor blockers, amiodarone, or sotalol. β-Blockers are particularly veffective at treating symptoms related to exercise-induced arrhythmia, and sotalol suppresses ventricular arrhythmia in most patients. Those with a history of sustained, haemodynamically compromising ventricular arrhythmia should be offered an implantable cardioverter–defibrillator (ICD). Studies in such patients have shown a high rate of appropriate device discharges, ranging from

15% to 22% per year. More problematic is the prevention of sudden death in patients without such a history. A number of markers of increased risk have been proposed, including unexplained syncope, symptomatic ventricular tachycardia, family history of sudden death, young age, left ventricular involvement, and diffuse right ventricular dilatation. However, population-based survival studies are needed to evaluate the significance of these and other factors (such as asymptomatic nonsustained ventricular tachycardia).

Patients with severe right ventricular or biventricular involvement should be treated according to current heart-failure treatment guidelines, including the use of diuretics, ACE inhibitors, and anticoagulation. Patients with advanced disease are candidates for cardiac transplantation (see Chapters 5.1 and 5.2).

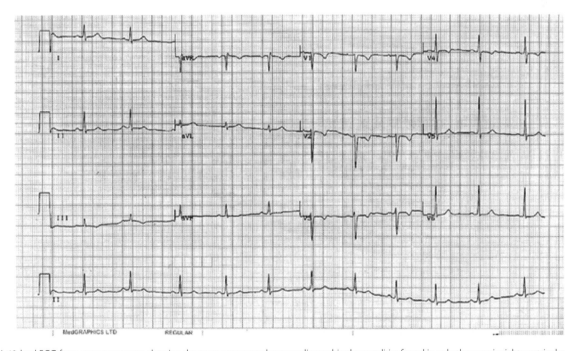

Fig. 7.2.7 A 12-lead ECG from a young woman showing the most common electrocardiographic abnormalities found in arrhythmogenic right ventricular cardiomyopathy with low voltage and T-wave inversion in the precordial leads V1–V4.

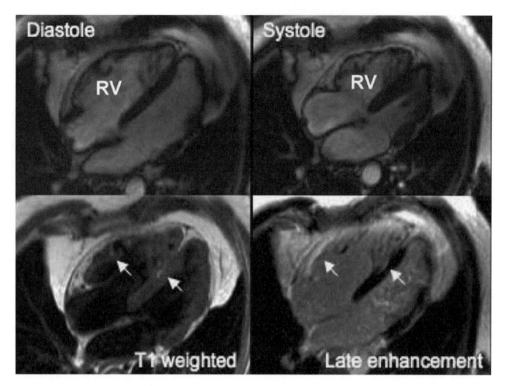

Fig. 7.2.8 Arrhythmogenic right ventricular cardiomyopathy. On the cine images (top) the right ventricle (RV) is globally dilated with multiple RV wall motion abnormalities. There are two areas of LV involvement with wall thinning (free wall, apex). On T1-weighted imaging, fat can be seen in the septum and RV trabeculae (arrows). After contrast, late enhancement representing fibrosis is also seen (arrows).

Evaluation, genetic testing, and follow-up of asymptomatic patients

It is now possible to offer genetic testing to individuals with unequivocal cardiomyopathy, particularly with highly penetrant disease in large families and in families affected by a sudden cardiac death. If a disease-causing mutation is identified, relatives can be offered predictive genetic testing, but this should only be done after appropriate genetic counselling and informed consent obtained by a trained health care professional working within a multidisciplinary team. This is to ensure understanding of the psychological, social, professional, ethical, and legal implications of a genetic disease.

In children and adolescents with a sarcomeric protein gene mutation, ECG and echocardiographic manifestations of myocardial hypertrophy often develop during growth. For this reason, young people should be assessed annually during adolescence. The earliest clinical manifestations of hypertrophic cardiomyopathy are electrocardiographic, while diastolic dysfunction and altered biomarkers of collagen synthesis may precede the development of left ventricular hypertrophy and also provide early markers of disease. In adults, *de novo* development of unexplained left ventricular hypertrophy is uncommon, but it does occur, particularly in patients with myosin-binding protein C gene mutations. In dilated cardiomyopathy follow-up of asymptomatic first-degree relatives suggests that disease progression is slow (over decades). The same applies to arrhythmogenic right ventricular cardiomyopathy.

Asymptomatic normal adults with a family history of cardiomyopathy but no identifiable mutation should be offered rescreening every 5 years, or sooner should they develop symptoms. This includes a clinical evaluation with ECG and echocardiography. Rescreening should be guided by the age of onset and severity of cardiomyopathy within the family. Individuals with nondiagnostic clinical features that could represent early disease should be seen more frequently.

Athletes, sports, and cardiomyopathy

Differentiation between pathological changes of HCM and physiological hypertrophy in athletes is required by many governing bodies prior to participation in competitive exercise. Careful assessment is needed and often a detraining period of 3 months is recommended. Presence of a family history of HCM or sudden cardiac death, symptoms (palpitations, syncope), and ECG changes such as Q waves, ST depression, deep T-wave inversions in inferolateral leads, all favour a diagnosis of HCM rather than athlete's heart. Other important clues to a diagnosis of HCM include low aerobic capacity, a maximal wall thickness of more than 13 mm, and diastolic dysfunction (Box 7.2.3).

The upper limits of left ventricular wall thickness used to discriminate physiological left ventricular hypertrophy from HCM are established in white athletes. Left ventricular hypertrophy with a wall thickness of more than 15 mm can be physiological in black athletes. The most extreme increase in left ventricular wall thickness have been observed in isotonic or endurance exercise such as rowing, cycling, or swimming. Female athletes have smaller left ventricular diastolic cavity dimension and smaller wall thickness than males.

International guidelines advise against competitive exercise in HCM in view of a potential increased risk of sudden cardiac death.

Box 7.2.3 Features favouring a diagnosis of pathological versus physiological hypertrophy in athletes with mild left ventricular hypertrophy (≥12 mm)

- Family history of HCM or sudden cardiac death in first-degree relative(s) ≤40 years

- Female gender

- Palpitations, syncope

- ECG: Abnormal Q waves in at least two leads, ST depression, deep T-wave inversion in inferolateral leads

- Peak Vo_2 <100% of predicted

- MWT ≥14 mm

- Small left ventricle cavity size (left ventricular end-diastolic diameter <45 mm)

- Diastolic dysfunction

- Reduced longitudinal left ventricular function

- No response to detraining for 3 months

- Left atrial enlargement >50 mm

- Myocardial fibrosis on cardiac MRI

Adapted from Elliott PM, Lambiase PD, Kumar D (2011). *Inherited cardiac disease*. Oxford University Press, Oxford.

Some evidence implicates physical exercise in increased disease progression and risk of sudden death in arrhythmogenic right ventricular cardiomyopathy. Data on exercise in dilated cardiomyopathy is very limited and controversial.

Further reading

Hypertrophic cardiomyopathy

Davies MJ, McKenna WJ (1995). Hypertrophic cardiomyopathy: pathology and pathogenesis. *Histopathology*, **26**, 493–500.

Elliott P, McKenna WJ (2004). Hypertrophic cardiomyopathy. *Lancet*, **363**, 1881–91.

Elliott P, et al. (2008). Classification of the cardiomyopathies: a position statement from the European Society of Cardiology Working Group on Myocardial and Pericardial Diseases. *Eur Heart J*, **29**, 270–6.

Jacoby D, McKenna WJ (2012). Genetics of cardiomyopathy. *Eur Heart J*, **33**, 296–304.

Maron BJ (2002). Hypertrophic cardiomyopathy. A systematic review. *JAMA*, **287**, 1308–20.

Maron BJ, et al. (2003). American College of Cardiology Foundation Task Force on Clinical Expert Consensus Documents; European Society of Cardiology Committee for Practice Guidelines. American College of Cardiology/European Society of Cardiology Clinical Expert Consensus Document on Hypertrophic Cardiomyopathy. A report of the American College of Cardiology Foundation Task Force on Clinical Expert Consensus Documents and the European Society of Cardiology Committee for Practice Guidelines. *Eur Heart J*, **24**, 1965–91.

O'Mahony C, et al. (2014). A novel clinical risk prediction model for sudden cardiac death in hypertrophic cardiomyopathy (HCM Risk-SCD). *Eur Heart J*, **35, 2010–20.**

Richard P, et al. (2003). Hypertrophic cardiomyopathy: distribution of disease genes, spectrum of mutations, and implications for a molecular diagnosis strategy. *Circulation*, **107**, 2227–32.

Wang L, Seidman JG, Seidman CE (2010). Narrative review: harnessing molecular genetics for the diagnosis and management of hypertrophic cardiomyopathy. *Ann Intern Med*, **152**, 513–20, W181.

Dilated cardiomyopathy

Caforio AL, et al. (2007). Prospective familial assessment in dilated cardiomyopathy: cardiac autoantibodies predict disease development in asymptomatic relatives. *Circulation*, **115**, 76–83.

Herman DS, et al. (2012). Truncations of titin causing dilated cardiomyopathy. *N Engl J Med*, **366**, 619–28.

Hershberger RE, Morales A, Siegfried JD (2010). Clinical and genetic issues in dilated cardiomyopathy: A review for genetics professionals. *Genet Med*, **12**, 655–71.

Jefferies JL, Towbin JA (2010). Dilated cardiomyopathy. *Lancet*, 375, 752–62.

Sliwa K, et al. (2010). Evaluation of bromocriptine in the treatment of acute severe peripartum cardiomyopathy: a proof-of-concept pilot study. *Circulation*, **121**, 1465–73.

Restrictive cardiomyopathy

See Chapter 7.2.

Arrhythmogenic right ventricular dysplasia

Corrado D, Basso C, Thiene G (2009). Arrhythmogenic right ventricular cardiomyopathy: an update. *Heart*, **9**, 766–73.

Delmar M, McKenna WJ (2010). The cardiac desmosome and arrhythmogenic cardiomyopathies: from gene to disease. *Circ Res*, **107**, 700–14.

Marcus FI, et al. (2010). Diagnosis of arrhythmogenic right ventricular cardiomyopathy/dysplasia: proposed modification of the Task Force Criteria. *Eur Heart J*, **31**, 806–14.

Quarta G, et al. (2011). Familial evaluation in arrhythmogenic right ventricular cardiomyopathy: impact of genetics and revised Task Force Criteria. *Circulation*, **123**, 2701–9.

CHAPTER 7.3

Specific heart muscle disorders

William J. McKenna, Perry Elliott, and Oliver Guttmann

Essentials

Autoimmune rheumatic disorders and the vasculitides

Cardiovascular involvement is very common, but may be occult and often goes undetected. Any anatomical structure in the heart can be involved, hence patients may present with pericarditis, myocarditis, endocarditis, or coronary vasculitis. There is usually no correlation between the extent of systemic disease and cardiac involvement.

Systemic lupus erythematosus (SLE)—more than 50% have cardiovascular involvement at some time; 30% have clinical pericarditis; myocarditis can occasionally present with heart failure or arrhythmias; marantic endocarditis can be identified in at least 30% at autopsy, but is rarely clinically significant; neonates born to mothers with SLE who have anti-Ro/anti-La antibodies frequently develop complete heart block; atherosclerosis is the leading cause of late death in SLE.

Systemic sclerosis—symptomatic cardiac involvement is uncommon (10%), but is frequently detected at autopsy (60%), when the most common features are chronic pericarditis and myocardial fibrosis; pulmonary hypertension is common, usually secondary to lung involvement, and has a very poor prognosis.

Rheumatoid arthritis—10 to 15% have clinical cardiac involvement, 60% on echocardiography: pericarditis is most frequent, with up to 40% having an effusion on echocardiography; myocarditis is frequent at autopsy but rarely causes symptoms; vasculitis affecting epicardial arteries, nonspecific valvitis, and conduction disturbances are reported.

Seronegative arthropathies—associated with pancarditis, proximal aortitis, aortic incompetence, and varying degrees of conduction abnormalities.

Takayasu's arteritis—proximal coronary arteries are involved in 15 to 20%; dilatation of the aortic root may cause aortic regurgitation; pulmonary artery aneurysms and stenoses are common; involvement of the renal arteries can cause malignant hypertension; aortic, coronary, pulmonary, and bronchial arterial fistulae are reported.

Kawasaki disease—myocarditis is frequent (35%) in the acute stage, often in association with a pericardial effusion; coronary artery involvement occurs in 20%, resulting in aneurysm formation and thrombotic occlusion, such that—in the longer term—patients can present with myocardial ischaemia.

Other conditions

Amyloid—in systemic AL (primary) amyloidosis up to 50% have cardiac involvement; systemic AA (secondary) amyloidosis is almost never associated with clinical cardiac amyloidosis; the heart is frequently involved in familial amyloid polyneuropathy caused by mutations in the transthyretin gene. The clinical picture most frequently mimics hypertrophic cardiomyopathy with restrictive physiology. The ECG may show diminished voltages, loss of R waves in precordial leads, and Q waves in the inferior leads. Echocardiography may show a characteristic 'sparkling' appearance to the myocardium, thickening of the heart valves and the interatrial septum, and pericardial effusions. Symptomatic heart disease typically occurs late in the course of amyloidosis and is an ominous feature.

Sarcoidosis—cardiac involvement is clinically apparent in less than 10% of cases, but sudden (presumed arrhythmic) death is not infrequent amongst these.

Endocrine disorders—diabetes is associated with an increased risk of developing heart failure; hyperthyroidism can cause a high-output state with symptoms of heart failure and echocardiographic demonstration of dilated cardiomyopathy and systolic dysfunction; hypothyroidism frequently causes pericardial effusion, but heart failure generally represents exacerbation of pre-existing cardiac disease by thyroid deficiency.

Neuromuscular disorders—myocardial dysfunction is common in the muscular dystrophies. In Duchenne and Becker muscular dystrophy (dystrophin gene mutations) the commonest abnormality is dilated cardiomyopathy; in laminopathies (lamin AC gene mutations) atrial arrhythmia, heart block, dilated cardiomyopathy and sudden cardiac death are frequent.

Inherited metabolic disorders—hereditary haemochromatosis causes thickening of the ventricular walls, dilatation of the ventricular chambers, and heart failure; cardiac disease is particularly important in lysosomal and glycogen storage diseases, including hypertrophic and dilated cardiomyopathy, arrhythmia, and valvular disease.

Cardiac disease in autoimmune rheumatic disorders

The autoimmune rheumatic disorders (connective tissue diseases) are a heterogeneous group of conditions with multisystem involvement. Cardiovascular involvement is very common, although it may be occult and often goes undetected. As any anatomical structure in the heart may be involved, patients may present with one or more features consistent with pericarditis, myocarditis, endocarditis, and vasculitis. There is usually no correlation between the

Table 7.3.1 Cardiac manifestations of autoimmune rheumatic diseases and the vasculitides

Disease	Cardiac manifestation
Systemic lupus erythematosus	Accelerated atherosclerosis
	Noninfective endocarditis (Libman–Sacks)
	Myocarditis
	Pericarditis
Rheumatoid arthritis	Coronary arteritis
	Aortic and mitral regurgitation
Seronegative arthropathies—ankylosing spondylitis, Reiter's syndrome, psoriatic arthritis, ulcerative colitis, Crohn's disease	Pancarditis
	Proximal aortitis
	Conduction disease
Systemic sclerosis	Myocarditis
	Pericarditis
	Arrhythmias
Wegener's granulomatosis	Constrictive pericarditis
	Atrioventricular block
Churg–Strauss syndrome	Congestive cardiac failure
	Pericarditis
	Coronary arteritis/myocardial infarction
	Arrhythmias
Polyarteritis nodosa	Hypertension
	Congestive heart failure
	Partial or complete coronary artery occlusion
	Pericarditis
	Arrhythmias
Takayasu's syndrome	Pericarditis
	Aortic arch vasculitis
	Heart failure

extent of systemic disease and cardiac involvement. For details of the cardiac manifestations of autoimmune rheumatic diseases and the vasculitides, see Tables 7.3.1 and 7.3.2.

Systemic lupus erythematosus

Systemic lupus erythematosus (SLE) is a multisystem immune disorder characterized by the formation of autoantibodies to various cell antigens. The prevalence of cardiovascular involvement at some time in the illness is more than 50%. The pericardium is most commonly affected, with as many as 30% of patients having clinical pericarditis at some stage, and up to 80% affected at autopsy. Progression to constrictive pericarditis or tamponade is extremely rare.

Clinically evident myocardial involvement occurs less frequently, but is reported in 40 to 50% of patients at autopsy: signs and symptoms are uncommon, but patients may occasionally present with heart failure or arrhythmias. Other factors that may contribute to

ventricular dysfunction in SLE include atherosclerosis, hypertension, and drugs (e.g. chloroquine).

As many as one-third of patients with SLE have systolic murmurs, which are usually caused by hyperdynamic flow. The classic verrucous vegetations adherent to the endocardium described by Libman and Sacks in 1924 (marantic endocarditis) can be identified in 30% or more at autopsy. These lesions most commonly affect the mitral valve but are rarely clinically significant.

Neonates born to mothers with SLE who have anti-Ro/anti-La antibodies frequently develop complete heart block (see Chapter 14.14). Various degrees of heart block and bundle branch block can be seen in adults, but complete heart block is rare. Arrhythmias such as atrial fibrillation and flutter may also occur, particularly in association with pericarditis.

Myocardial infarction is very uncommon in patients with SLE, but accelerated or premature atherosclerosis is the leading cause of late death in SLE. Its cause is unknown, but suggested contributory factors include chronic inflammation, immune complex deposition, antiphospholipid antibodies, hypertension, dyslipidaemia, and hyperglycaemia (caused by chronic steroid administration).

Death from the cardiac complications of lupus is rare. Mild pericardial disease may respond to nonsteroidal anti-inflammatory drugs, heart failure is treated conventionally, and conduction defects may require pacing. Coronary vasculitis and/or lupus myocarditis are usually treated with steroids and other immunosuppressants, but there are no trials to guide therapeutic decision-making in these rare conditions.

Antiphospholipid syndrome

The antiphospholipid syndrome is recognized both in patients without SLE (primary) and with SLE. It is a thrombophilic disorder characterized by arterial and venous occlusions, recurrent fetal loss, thrombocytopenia, and increased maternal complications of pregnancy, and is associated with persistently raised titres of anticardiolipin antibodies. Anticoagulation is indicated in patients with thrombotic symptoms and prevents miscarriage in pregnant women. In refractory cases plasmapheresis can be used (see Chapter 15.14 for further information).

Systemic sclerosis

Systemic sclerosis is characterized by abnormal collagen deposition in various organ systems. Symptomatic cardiac involvement is uncommon (10%), but is frequently detected at autopsy (60%), when the most common features are chronic pericarditis (70%) and myocardial fibrosis (37%). Clinically these cause heart failure, ventricular arrhythmia, and conduction disease. Rare cases of tamponade are reported. Valve involvement is less common, except for tricuspid regurgitation, which occurs in 40% of patients and is usually associated with pulmonary hypertension. Pulmonary hypertension is present in 47% of patients, usually secondary to lung involvement, and is associated with a 1-year survival of only 50%. Involvement of the large epicardial blood vessels is not a feature of systemic sclerosis, but microvascular dysfunction is common and may contribute to myocardial ischaemia and patchy myocardial fibrosis. In the limited form of systemic sclerosis (formerly known as CREST syndrome) the overall prognosis is more favourable: pulmonary hypertension without severe lung disease occurs in 10 to 15%, and subclinical left ventricular dysfunction is reported.

Table 7.3.2 Cardiac involvement in the more common autoimmune rheumatic disorders

	Pericardial involvement	Myocardial involvement	Valvular involvement	Coronary/arteritis	Conduction system involvement
Rheumatoid arthritis	16–40% at autopsy 10–15% clinical pericarditis	4–20% at autopsy Symptomatic in <5%	>50% valvulitis at autopsy Symptoms rare	11–20% involvement of coronary vessels at autopsy Vasculitis affecting the aorta rare	Any part of conduction system involved Varying degrees of heart block in 0.1%
SLE	45–66% at autopsy 20–30% clinical pericarditis	30% at autopsy Symptomatic in <10%	Libman–Sacks lesions in 30% at autopsy	Coronary vessels involved in <10% Vasculitis affecting the aorta rare	Any part of conduction system involved Varying degrees of heart block in <1%
Systemic sclerosis and variants	70% at autopsy 7–15% clinical pericarditis	Up to 60% at autopsy Symptoms rare	Rare, AR and MVP described Symptoms in <10%	Reversible perfusion defects in up to 40% Vasculitis demonstrated rarely	Any part of conduction system involved; Abnormal ECG in 50%
Polymyositis/ dermatomyositis	Clinical involvement rare (usually in children with dermatomyositis)	Up to 25% at autopsy Symptoms in 13–26%	MVP common Other lesions rare		Any part of conduction system involved Symptoms extremely rare
Seronegative spondyloarthro pathies	<1% incidence of pericarditis in AS and Reiter's	Myocardial involvement/ dysfunction common on echo in AS Symptoms rare	Aortic incompetence most common: 1–10% in AS, 1–15% in Reiter's MR very rare	Aortitis: 1–10% in AS, 1–15% in Reiter's	Heart block: 8% in AS, 8% in Reiter's, rare in other forms of spondyloarthropathy

AR, aortic regurgitation; AS, ankylosing spondylitis; MR, mitral regurgitation; MVP, mitral valve prolapse; SLE, systemic lupus erythematosus.

Rheumatoid arthritis

Cardiac involvement is found in up to 60% of patients on echocardiography, but in only 10 to 15% clinically. The presence of cardiac disease correlates with the severity of joint disease and the presence of rheumatoid nodules, male gender, age, high titres of rheumatoid factor, and other systemic markers of disease activity. Histological changes consist of a nonspecific inflammatory infiltrate, myocyte necrosis, and fibrosis affecting any part of the heart. Rheumatoid nodules may accompany this, and the heart may be affected rarely 5% by secondary amyloidosis. Myocarditis is reported in up to 40% at autopsy, but symptoms are uncommon. Pericarditis occurs more frequently, and up to 40% of patients have an effusion on echocardiography, but progression to constrictive pericarditis or tamponade is rare. Acute vasculitis involving the larger epicardial arteries has been reported but is uncommon. Nonspecific valvitis may affect the mitral and particularly the aortic valve: this may eventually lead to scarred, hyalinized, and even incompetent valves. Rheumatoid nodules may occasionally deform the mitral valve and lead to valvular incompetence. Conduction disturbances may be secondary to infiltration by rheumatoid nodules: the commonest ECG abnormality is first-degree heart block, but left bundle branch block and complete heart block are also described. Although pericarditis is usually responsive to steroids, it is unclear whether steroids or disease-modifying drugs alter the other cardiac manifestations.

Seronegative arthropathies

This group of disorders is characterized by the absence of rheumatoid factor and includes ankylosing spondylitis, Reiter's syndrome, and psoriatic and gastrointestinal arthropathies. These may all be associated with cardiac involvement, in particular pancarditis, proximal aortitis, aortic incompetence, and varying degrees of conduction abnormalities. They may also result in amyloid deposition. On occasion cardiac disease may present before joint disease. Treatment is empirical and based on symptomatology.

Polymyositis and dermatomyositis

Cardiac symptoms in polymyositis or dermatomyositis are rare, but post-mortem and clinical studies suggest that left ventricular diastolic dysfunction and conduction disturbances are present in 40 to 50% of cases. When cardiac symptoms are present they are associated with a poor prognosis. Rare cases of cardiac tamponade are reported. Interstitial lung disease, found in 5 to 30% of cases, may lead to right heart failure. Treatment is symptomatic.

Cardiac disease in the vasculitides

Takayasu's arteritis

Takayasu's arteritis is a rare inflammatory arteritis that predominantly affects the thoracic aorta and the proximal portions of its major branches, the pulmonary arteries and the coronary vessels. Asians are affected more than other ethnic groups, with a 10:1 female to male ratio. The disease typically evolves from an early inflammatory stage to a fibrotic obliterative phase with arterial aneurysms, stenoses, and occlusions. The proximal coronary arteries are involved in 15 to 20% of cases. Dilatation of the aortic root may cause aortic regurgitation. Pulmonary artery aneurysms and stenoses are common and can cause pulmonary hypertension, right heart failure, and pulmonary haemorrhage. Involvement of the renal arteries can cause malignant hypertension. Aortic, coronary, pulmonary and bronchial arterial fistulae are reported. Subclinical myocardial involvement, in the absence of coronary lesions, is reported in up to 50% of patients. Pericarditis is rare.

Polyarteritis nodosa

Classic polyarteritis nodosa (PAN) is a rare, nongranulomatous, necrotizing arteritis of small and medium-sized vessels without microscopic angiitis or glomerulonephritis. The most typical cardiovascular complication is malignant hypertension caused by renal artery vasculitis. Coronary vasculitis causing aneurysms, myocardial infarction, and cardiomyopathy are reported, but they are probably rare. Pericarditis and clinically important conduction system involvement is uncommon. Valve disease appears not to be a feature.

Giant cell (temporal) arteritis

Giant cell arteritis is a granulomatous arteritis of the aorta and its major branches, in particular the carotid artery. It usually affects people older than 50 years of age. Five to ten per cent of patients have cardiac involvement, the most common lesions being thoracic aortic aneurysms and aortic regurgitation. Coronary involvement is rare.

Kawasaki's disease

Kawasaki's disease (or mucocutaenous lymph node syndrome) is an acute vasculitis of small and medium-sized vessels that typically presents in children aged less than 5 years, with a peak at 1 year and a small male predominance (1.5:1). In the acute stage, myocarditis is frequent (35%), often in association with pericardial effusions, treatment being with aspirin and high-dose gammaglobulin. Coronary artery involvement occurs in 20%, resulting in aneurysm formation and thrombotic occlusion, such that in the longer term patients can present with acute coronary syndromes and myocardial ischaemia, which are managed conventionally. See Chapter 19.11.8 for further discussion.

Microscopic polyangiitis

Microscopic polyangiitis is a disorder of capillaries, venules, and arterioles with occasional involvement of medium-sized vessels. In one series, 50% of patients had cardiac involvement in the form of pericarditis, heart failure, and myocardial infarction.

Wegener's granulomatosis

Wegener's granulomatosis is a necrotizing vasculitis of medium and small vessels associated with granulomatous lesions in the upper and lower respiratory tract. Pericarditis and valvulitis are the most frequently reported abnormalities, but their frequency varies substantially between series. Coronary arteritis is relatively common at post-mortem, but rarely causes myocardial infarction. Myocarditis and complete heart block are rare (2%).

Behçet's disease

Behçet's disease is a relapsing inflammatory disorder characterized by oral and genital ulceration, uveitis, and arterial and venous thrombosis. The disease is common in the eastern Mediterranean and eastern Asia. Cardiac disease, including myocarditis, atrioventricular block, pericarditis, and valve disease, is present in less than 5% of patients. Coronary artery disease is very rare (<1%) but poses

challenges for revascularization because of tissue fragility and pseudoaneurysm formation. Aneurysms may also be seen in the pulmonary (Hugues–Stovin syndrome), coronary, and other arteries.

Amyloidosis

Amyloidosis describes a group of diverse diseases (see Chapter 12.12.3) that is characterized by extracellular insoluble fibrils derived from the aggregation of various misfolded proteins.

AL amyloidosis is the most commonly diagnosed form of systemic amyloidosis and occurs equally between the genders. As many as 50% of patients have cardiac involvement, which will manifest clinically in up to one-half of these. Multiorgan involvement causing neuropathy and nephropathy is typical. Some 'benign' gammopathies are implicated in the pathogenesis, but any B-cell dyscrasia can be the cause.

Systemic AA (secondary) amyloidosis, a complication of chronic inflammatory conditions, is almost never associated with clinical cardiac amyloidosis.

The heart is frequently involved in familial amyloid polyneuropathy. This is the most common type of hereditary amyloidosis and is caused by one of more than 70 mutations in the transthyretin (*TTR*) gene. Senile amyloidosis caused by deposition of wild-type *TTR* is extremely common; indeed, almost all individuals over the age of 80 years will have scattered deposits of amyloid, particularly affecting the aorta: clinical involvement is variable, depending on the extent of deposition. In patients with severe cardiac involvement, there is a large male predominance, and the condition is almost exclusive to individuals older than 65 years of age. The disease is slowly progressive with a median survival of about 75 months.

The extracellular deposition of amyloid results in a firm, thickened, noncompliant myocardium. Deposition occurs throughout the atrial and ventricular muscle and in the specialized conduction tissue: fibrosis of these structures may occur. Valvular function is rarely affected, although thickening of cardiac valves is common. Intramural coronary arteries and veins frequently contain deposits, which can occasionally compromise the lumina of these vessels.

Amyloid heart disease most frequently mimics hypertrophic cardiomyopathy with restrictive physiology. The reduced compliance of the myocardium produces the characteristic diastolic dip and plateau (square root sign) in the ventricular pressure waveform. An impaired rate of early diastolic filling is characteristic and systolic dysfunction may also occur, leading to congestive heart failure.

Arrhythmias are common, in particular ventricular premature beats and atrial fibrillation. Complex ventricular arrhythmias may be harbingers of sudden death. Progressive atrioventricular conduction delay is common and infiltration of the autonomic nervous system results in orthostatic hypotension in 10% of cases.

The chest radiograph may show cardiomegaly in patients with systolic dysfunction but is often normal in those with restrictive cardiomyopathy, although pulmonary congestion may be prominent. Electrocardiography (CG) shows diminished voltages in about 50% of patients, and loss of R waves in precordial leads; the presence of Q waves in the inferior leads may simulate myocardial infarction. Echocardiography reveals an increased thickness of the ventricular walls with small ventricular chambers, dilated atria, intra-atrial septal thickening, left ventricular dysfunction, and a characteristic 'sparkling' appearance to the myocardium.

The pattern of hypertrophy is usually concentric but may be asymmetrical septal. In hereditary transthyretin-related amyloidosis ^{99m}Tc-3,3-diphosphono-1,2-propanodicarboxylic acid (DPD) scintigraphy can identify myocardial infiltration. Serum amyloid protein (SAP) scintigraphy is useful to assess extracardiac but not cardiac involvement in AL amyloidosis. Cardiac MRI with gadolinium contrast agents has a characteristic pattern of late enhancement once there is left ventricular hypertrophy and/or systolic impairment. In AL cardiac amyloidosis, troponin T and B-natriuretic peptide (BNP) plasma concentrations are usually elevated and relate to prognosis.

Diagnosis can be confirmed histologically from rectal, salivary gland, subcutaneous fat, or (if necessary) cardiac biopsy; all forms of amyloid show an amorphous proteinaceous substance that demonstrates apple green birefringence under polarized light when stained with Congo Red. Genetic testing can be used to confirm hereditary TTR amyloidosis.

Symptomatic heart disease typically presents late in the course of amyloidosis and the presence of clinical signs is an ominous feature, with mortality approaching 100% at 2 years for AL amyloidosis. Treatment is supportive in combination with measures to suppress the underlying amyloidogenic condition. Chemotherapy or peripheral autologous stem cell therapy may be appropriate in some cases of AL amyloidosis. Orthotopic liver transplantation or combined heart and liver transplantation have shown promising results, particularly in selected cases of TTR-related familial amyloidosis. Anticoagulation is important in patients with atrial arrhythmia due to the high incidence of thromboembolism. Digoxin and calcium channel antagonists should be avoided as they selectively bind to amyloid fibrils, enhancing their effect. Patients with symptomatic conduction system disease require a pacemaker. Diuretics and vasodilators should be used cautiously as they may aggravate hypotension. Cardiac transplantation is feasible in selected cases, but is a palliative procedure without treatment of the underlying process

Sarcoid

Sarcoid is a multisysytem granulomatous disorder of unknown aetiology. The overall prevalence is about 20 per 100 000 population. Myocardial involvement is seen in 20 to 30% of patients at autopsy, but is clinically apparent in less than 10% of cases. Primary cardiac involvement is extremely rare.

Noncaseating granulomas may involve any region of the heart, although the left ventricular free wall and interventricular septum are the most commonly affected sites. The granulomas can be localized or widespread, and healing may result in the formation of scars. The ventricular muscle eventually becomes increasingly noncompliant, leading to defects in contractile function as well as wall motion. Replacement of large portions of the ventricle by sarcoid tissue may lead to aneurysm formation. Granulomas and fibrosis may also extend to involve nodal or conducting tissue. Isolated pericardial involvement is rare, although pericardial effusions are commonly seen on echo. Valvular dysfunction occurs in less than 5% of patients and may be the result of infiltration of papillary muscles or direct valvular involvement, which is less common.

Clinical manifestations of myocardial sarcoidosis are shown in Table 7.3.3. Chest pain has been described in up to 28% of patients, and since about one-half of these will have abnormal thallium

Table 7.3.3 Clinical manifestations in myocardial sarcoidosis

Abnormality	Reported percentage of patients affected
Atrioventricular block	41–52
Ventricular ectopics	31–47
Congestive heart failure	12–19
Sudden death	21–38
Bundle branch block	26–34
Supraventricular tachycardia	11–25
Ventricular tachycardia	12–23
Simulating myocardial infarction on ECG	14–18
Pericarditis/pulmonary embolism	4–8

perfusion scans despite arteriographically normal coronary arteries, this is thought to be secondary to microvascular dysfunction.

Sudden death secondary to ventricular tachycardia and fibrillation occurs in some cases. The presence of a ventricular aneurysm may be associated with resistant ventricular arrhythmias and necessitate its resection. Conduction disturbances such as complete heart block are a frequent occurrence, particularly in the acute phase of the disease. The electrocardiogram is frequently abnormal, with T wave abnormalities and varying degrees of intraventricular or atrioventricular block. Pathological Q waves may simulate myocardial infarction when myocardial involvement becomes extensive. Echocardiography shows features which may mimic dilated, restrictive or arrhythmogenic cardiomyopathy with systolic and/or diastolic dysfunction, regional wall motion abnormalities and aneurysms. Gallium or fluorodeoxyglucose (FDG) positron emission tomography (PET), single photon emission computed tomography (SPECT), and MRI with gadolinium late enhancement have all been used to detect affected areas of myocardium. Endomyocardial biopsy can be diagnostic, but may be negative due to the patchy nature of the disease.

Steroids can improve symptoms as well as electrocardiographic and echocardiographic features and myocardial perfusion defects, but there is a lack of randomized trial data. Steroid-sparing agents such as methotrexate and azathioprine may be used in relapsing or refractory disease. Amiodarone may be of benefit in resistant arrhythmia, and the insertion of an implantable defibrillator (ICD) may protect against sudden death in susceptible patients. Transplantation may improve prognosis and quality of life in patients who remain symptomatic despite these measures, although recurrence in the graft has been documented.

Cardiac disease in endocrine disorders
Diabetes

A man with diabetes has a relative risk of developing heart failure that is 2.4 times higher than that of a man without diabetes, and the equivalent relative risk for a woman is 5:1. The risk has been shown to be independent of age, systolic blood pressure, serum cholesterol, and weight. People with diabetes have elevated end-diastolic pressures, reduced ejection fractions, left ventricular dilatation, and hypertrophy, even in the absence of coronary artery disease. Diastolic dysfunction as well as a diffuse hypokinesis of the myocardium has also been demonstrated. Implicated mechanisms include small-vessel disease and autonomic neuropathy.

The most prominent histopathological finding is myocardial fibrosis. Occasionally a picture resembling restrictive heart disease is seen, with a small left ventricular chamber and reduced compliance of the left ventricle.

The treatment of heart failure is the same as in patients without diabetes, although β-blockers with intrinsic sympathomimetic activity are preferred. Preload and afterload reducing agents should be used cautiously because of autonomic dysfunction. It is unclear whether tight glucose control affects the progression of diabetic cardiomyopathy, but it is clearly prudent for other reasons to optimize control as well as to reduce obesity and control hypertension.

Hyperthyroidism

In general, excess thyroid hormone results in a high-output state with tachycardia, increased cardiac contractility, and peripheral vasodilatation. In the long term this can result in ventricular hypertrophy and an increase in ejection fraction. However, some patients may develop a low-output state with symptoms of heart failure and echocardiographic demonstration of dilated cardiomyopathy and systolic dysfunction. These changes may be a result of long-standing tachycardia and increased cardiac work, but thyroxine (T_4) itself may directly alter the expression of cardiac proteins involved in cardiac function, and there is also some evidence that direct autoimmune myocardial damage may occur in Graves' disease.

Typical cardiac symptoms of hyperthyroidism include angina-like chest pain, fatigue, palpitations, and exertional dyspnoea. Cardiac findings include sinus tachycardia and atrial flutter or fibrillation in 17 to 20%. These may be complicated by thromboembolism in up to 40%; also by congestive heart failure. Mitral valve prolapse has been reported in patients with Graves' disease.

Control of the ventricular rate in atrial fibrillation should be achieved with digoxin, β-blockers, or calcium channel antagonists. The increased metabolic clearance of digoxin may necessitate a higher maintenance dose. Attempts at cardioversion should generally be deferred until the patient is euthyroid, at which time they may have spontaneously reverted to sinus rhythm. The presence of an already dilated vascular bed means that diuretics should be used with caution and vasodilators are generally contraindicated.

Hypothyroidism

Patients suffering from hypothyroidism, whether in its mild form or myxoedema, present a wide variety of symptoms. Complaints of fatigue, lethargy, mental slowness, and cold intolerance usually dominate. Less frequently, symptoms suggestive of cardiac dysfunction such as dyspnoea on exertion, syncope, or angina-like chest pain may be prominent. The most common cardiac abnormality is pericardial effusion, which is usually asymptomatic but reported in at least 30% of untreated patients. Heart failure generally represents exacerbation of pre-existing cardiac disease by the superimposed haemodynamic consequences of thyroid deficiency—bradycardia, diminished myocardial contractility, and increased peripheral vascular resistance. Rarely, hypothyroidism alone can closely resemble cardiomyopathy and be severe enough to cause heart failure. Echocardiographic evidence of asymmetric thickening of the interventricular septum as well as reduced dimensions of the left ventricular outflow tract has been reported. The characteristic ECG

findings are sinus bradycardia, prolongation of the QT interval, and a reduction in voltages if there is an associated pericardial effusion.

The management of heart failure involves the identification of any coexisting cardiac disease and thyroid hormone replacement. Levothyroxine significantly enhances myocardial performance within 1 week but in patients with known or suspected coronary artery disease it should be initiated at a lower dose than usual, typically 25 micrograms/day, and increased slowly at 4- to 6-week intervals until the thyroid-stimulating hormone is within the normal range. Tri-iodothyronine (T_3) may be preferable in severe cases as clinical improvement occurs sooner. β-Blockade can be used prophylactically or added if treatment with thyroxine exacerbates ischaemic heart disease.

Cardiac disease in neuromuscular disorders

Myocardial dysfunction is particularly common in the muscular dystrophies, a group of disorders characterized by progressive skeletal and cardiac muscle involvement (Table 7.3.4). Dystrophic effects on skeletal muscle result in fibre necrosis, followed by fibrosis and fatty replacement. These structural and functional changes, which occur in the ventricles, can lead to the development of cardiomyopathy, in particular dilated cardiomyopathy and heart failure. The effect on the specialized conducting tissue may lead to bradyarrhythmias, conduction defects, malignant arrhythmias, and sudden death.

Duchenne and Becker muscular dystrophy are progressive disorders arising from abnormalities (deletion, duplication, or point mutation) in the genes coding for the extrasarcomeric cytoskeletal protein dystrophin. In addition to defects in dystrophin, other defects that cause muscular dystrophy and dilated cardiomyopathy include those affecting the genes for the intracellular proteins emerin (a transmembrane protein that is embedded in the inner nuclear cell membrane) and lamin A/C (filament-like proteins that form a proteinaceous mesh underlying and attached to the inner nuclear membrane). Mutations in desmin, a type III intermediate filament protein, cause dilated cardiomyopathy, restrictive cardiomyopathy, and progressive distal myopathy.

By the age of 13 years more than 50% of boys with Duchenne muscular dystrophy (OMIM 310220) have an abnormal echocardiogram (hypertrophic or dilated cardiomyopathy). ECG abnormalities (poor R wave amplitude, axis deviation, and Q waves) are found in more than 90% from an early age. There is some evidence that angiotensin converting enzyme (ACE) inhibitors delay progression of dilated cardiomyopathies in Duchenne muscular dystrophy.

Cardiac death occurs in up to 50% of patients with Becker muscular dystrophy (OMIM 300376). ECG and echocardiography are abnormal in most patients, and it is noteworthy that the severity of cardiomyopathy is not related to the degree of skeletal muscle involvement.

Autosomal dominant Emery–Dreifuss muscular dystrophy (OMIM 181350) and limb girdle muscular dystrophy type 1B (OMIM 159001) are caused by mutation in lamin A/C. Heart block is common and patients require pacing at a mean age of 32 years. About 35% of patients will have early-onset dilated cardiomyopathy (age 19–55 years). ICD implantation is often indicated as pacemakers do not prevent sudden cardiac death.

Myotonic dystrophy type I (OMIM 160900) is an autosomal dominant disease caused by expanding CTG repeats in the *DMPK*

Table 7.3.4 Cardiovascular abnormalities in neuromuscular disorders

Condition	Inheritance	Cardiac disease	Noncardiac manifestations	Genetic defects
Duchenne	X-linked 1:3500 male births HCM and DCM reported Symptoms uncommon	Begins in first decade, 62% have ECG changes by age 10 years: short PQ, prolonged QT, tall R in V1 Conduction system anomalies/dependency by age 12 Death in adolescence	Severe muscle weakness, proximal-girdle distribution at 2–5 years in males Calf pseudohypertrophy, mild cognitive impairment, high CPK Wheelchair	Xp21; dystrophin gene mutations
Becker	X-linked 1:15 000 male births	High incidence of clinical cardiac involvement, heart failure is the most common cause of death DCM seen ECG usually abnormal: reduced R wave or prominent Q in 1, AVL and V6 Arrhythmias and heart block in <10%	Mild to moderate muscle weakness, proximal-girdle distribution from childhood, and ambulation preserved at least until late teens Calf pseudohypertrophy, high CPK Lifespan usually dependent on severity of cardiac involvement	Xp21; dystrophin gene mutations
X-linked dilated cardiomyopathy	X-linked (rare)	2nd or 3rd decade onset of CM and heart failure, rapid cardiac progression Milder variants possible Heart block not reported, arrhythmias in <10%	No muscular weakness. Muscle cramps, myalgias CPK usually elevated	Xp21; altered or selective loss of cardiac dystrophin
Limb girdle	AD	Variable degrees of AV block, AF, with high degree block, bradycardia, palpitations, and syncope	Mild to moderate muscle weakness, proximal limb girdle distribution. CPK elevated	Lamin A/C gene, 1q11–21
1B	AD	DCM in 35% 19–55 yrs, 90% conduction anomalies by 30 yrs, SCD in 50% (despite pacing)	Childhood onset of contractures, mild muscle weakness in humeroperoneal distribution Lower extremities affected first CPK elevated moderately May be little evidence of skeletal myopathy	Allelic to AD-EDMD and isolated cardiomyopathy with conduction system disease mapped to 1q
2A	AR	Cardiac involvement rare	Muscle weakness, proximal-girdle distribution CPK elevated	15q15 Calpain-3 (calcium activated neutral protease)
with sarcoglycan deficiency	AR	DCM reported Arrhythmias uncommon	Proximal-girdle distribution of muscle weakness Calf pseudohypertrophy. CPK elevated Severity varies from Duchenne to Becker-like	α-Sarcoglycan, 17q12 β-Sarcoglycan, 4q12 γ-Sarcoglycan, 13q12 δ-Sarcoglycan, 5q3
Myotonic (1:8000)	AD	Conduction defects and arrhythmias common yet most remain asymptomatic ECG changes in 23–80%: prolonged PR and QRS intervals Left and right bundle branch block, AF, a flutter and bradycardias MVP common DCM and HCM detected rarely	Muscle weakness, may be associated with frontal balding, cataracts, hypogonadism, and myotonia	19q13.3 Myotonin-protein kinase gene mutations (unstable CTG trinucleotide repeats)
Emery–Dreifuss	X-linked	AV block is the most common feature, high incidence of sudden death (pacemaker advised) Sinus node disease as well as tachyarrhythmias are common DCM is rare	Childhood onset of contractures, mild muscle weakness in humeroperoneal distribution Lower extremities affected first CPK elevated moderately No calf pseudohypertrophy	Xq28 defect of nuclear transmembane protein emerin

Table 7.3.4 Continued

Condition	Inheritance	Cardiac disease	Noncardiac manifestations	Genetic defects
Desminopathies	AD (actually more common than X-linked) AD, AR	DCM associated with conduction system disease commonly seen Ventricular fibrillation reported despite pacing Restrictive cardiomyopathy Cardiac conduction blocks Arrhythmias Echo/MRI changes of DCM	Same as X-linked form May be little evidence of skeletal myopathy Progressive distal myopathy CPK elevated	1.q11–21 Lamin A/C mutation (allelic to LGMD1B) DES 2q35

AD, autosomal dominant; AR, autosomal recessive; AF, atrial fibrillation; AV, atrioventricular; CM, cardiomyopathy; CPK, creatinine phosphokinase; DCM, dilated cardiomyopathy; EDMD, Emery–Dreifuss muscular dystrophy; HCM, hypertrophic cardiomyopathy; MVP, mitral valve prolapse.

Table adapted from Cox et al. (1997). Dystrophies and heart disease. *Current Opinion in Cardiology*, **12**, 329–42.

gene. Cardiomyopathy is rare, but cardiac involvement in the form of distal atrioventricular conduction disturbance is very common (90%). Bradycardia, PR interval prolongation, atrioventricular block, bundle branch block, and atrial arrhythmias are described. Sudden cardiac death occurs in 10 to 33% of patients. An electrophysiology study should be considered in patients with first-degree atrioventricular block or with evidence of arrhythmia and syncope/near syncope. Implantation of a permanent pacemaker is indicated if the HV interval is greater than 70 ms. Therapy with ICD can be considered in patients with symptomatic ventricular arrhythmia. Myotonic dystrophy type II (OMIM 602668) is similar to type I, but less severe, with cardiac involvement in about 20% of patients.

Cardiac disease in inherited metabolic disorders

Haemochromatosis

Hereditary haemochromatosis (OMIM 235200) is the most common single-gene disorder in people of northern European origin, where approximately 3 to 5 persons per 1000 are homozygous for the condition. It results in excessive and inappropriate mucosal absorption of iron, which is then deposited predominantly in the heart, liver, gonads, and pancreas. Clinical involvement of the heart is uncommon, but thickening of the ventricular walls together with dilatation of the ventricular chambers and heart failure is described. Histopathologically, myocardial degeneration and fibrosis occur over time and may extend to involve the conducting system of the heart.

The ECG most commonly reveals changes in ST and T waves. Supraventricular arrhythmias are characteristic, with atrioventricular conduction defects and ventricular arrhythmias being less common. Echocardiography typically shows a mixed dilated and restrictive cardiomyopathy with thickened ventricular walls, ventricular chamber enlargement, systolic and/or diastolic dysfunction. Endomyocardial biopsy may be useful to confirm the diagnosis. Treatment involves repeated phlebotomy and/or iron chelators.

Lysosomal diseases

Cardiac disease is particularly important in lysosomal storage disorders. They are categorized into mucopolysaccharidoses, mucolipidoses, glycoproteinoses, and glycosphingolipidoses (Anderson–Fabry disease, OMIM 301500). The prevalence of lysosomal storage disorders is about 1 in 7000. With the exception of Anderson–Fabry, Danon's (OMIM 300257), and Hunter's syndrome (OMIM 309900), which are X-linked, all are autosomal recessively inherited. Cardiac involvement is characterized by substrate accumulation within the myocardium and heart valves. This results in structural abnormalities and arrhythmias. Management requires a multidisciplinary approach in view of the chronic and progressive nature of these diseases. Treatment options (depending on the particular disorder) include substrate inhibition therapy, surgical intervention, bone marrow transplantation to replace enzyme deficiencies, and enzyme replacement therapy (available at very considerable cost for mucopolysaccharidoses I, II, and VI, Pompe's (OMIM 232300), Gaucher's (OMIM 230800), and Anderson–Fabry disease).

Mucopolysaccharidoses

Mucopolysaccharidosis type I (Hurler's syndrome, OMIM 607014; Hurler–Scheie syndrome, OMIM 607015, and Scheie's syndrome, OMIM 607016) is a progressive childhood disorder with skeletal and cardiopulmonary involvement. Cardiac involvement consists of systolic and diastolic dysfunction and progressive aortic and mitral valve disease. Mucopolysaccharidosis type II (Hunter's syndrome, OMIM 309900) is characterized by later onset, similar cardiomyopathy and valvular involvement as in mucopolysaccharidosis type I. Sudden cardiac death due to atrioventricular block has been described.

Anderson–Fabry disease (angiokeratoma corporis diffusum universale)

Anderson–Fabry disease is an X-linked condition with a population prevalence of 1 in 40 000 to 117 000 live births. It is caused by mutations in the gene encoding the lysosomal enzyme α-galactosidase A, which leads to intralysosomal accumulation of neutral glycosphingolipids, mainly globotriaosylceramide (Gb_3), in various organ systems. The disease is characterized by progressive clinical manifestations and premature death from renal disease, stroke, and cardiac disease. The ECG often shows left ventricular hypertrophy, a short PR interval, conduction defects, and arrhythmias. Echocardiography usually demonstrates increased thickness of the left ventricle, which may simulate hypertrophic cardiomyopathy. Differentiation from other hypertrophic or restrictive processes may require MRI or endomyocardial biopsy. A low leucocyte α-galactosidase activity is diagnostic in males.

Gaucher's disease

Gaucher's disease is the most common sphingolipidosis, caused by a deficiency in β-glucocerebrosidase that leads to lysosomal accumulation of glucocerebroside within macrophages. Lipid-laden macrophages (Gaucher cells) accumulate within the reticuloendothelial system resulting in hepatosplenomegaly, bone marrow replacement, anaemia, and thrombocytopenia. Valvular and aortic calcification, heart failure, and pericarditis are reported, but the heart is not involved in most patients. Pulmonary hypertension occurs in up to 30% of untreated patients, with enzyme replacement treatment reducing the prevalence to 7.4%.

Glycogen storage diseases

Glycogen storage diseases affect the storage, synthesis and breakdown of glycogen. Glycogen storage disease types II (Pompe's disease), IIb (Danon's disease), III, IV and VI, IX, and 0 affect the heart, causing left ventricular hypertrophy, restrictive cardiomyopathy, dilated cardiomyopathy and conduction disease.

Pompe's disease presents in neonates and infants with short PR interval, QT dispersion, and extreme left ventricular hypertrophy on ECG. On echocardiography severe concentric biventricular hypertrophy, small left ventricular cavity, left ventricular outflow tract obstruction, and diastolic dysfunction are evident. The adult-onset form presents with few cardiac features. Conduction abnormalities are common.

Danon's disease presents in boys with hypertrophic cardiomyopathy, conduction disease and skeletal muscle weakness; female carriers present later in adulthood with dilated cardiomyopathy.

Disease caused by mutations in the *PRKAG2* (AMP kinase) gene (OMIM 602743) is characterized by biventricular hypertrophy, impaired systolic function, high-grade atrioventricular conduction system disease, and ventricular pre-excitation.

Mitochondrial diseases

Defects affecting mitochondrial DNA are maternally inherited. Prevalence studies suggest that mitochondrial DNA defects affect 9.2 in 100 000 adults aged less than 65 years. Neurological sequelae usually present before cardiac manifestations. Conduction defects (Kearns–Sayre syndrome, OMIM 530000), left ventricular hypertrophy, and dilated cardiomyopathy are presenting features. Ocular myopathy with large mitochondrial DNA deletions (OMIM 258450) can be associated with ECG abnormalities.

Arrhythmias, in particular ventricular tachycardia, may occur in about 10% of patients. Second- or third-degree atrioventircular block necessitates cardiac pacing, and sudden death can occur. The serum creatine kinase may be mildly elevated and the blood lactate high. Management consists of supportive care and surveillance in addition to genetic counselling and pharmacological therapies for mitochondrial disease.

Takotsubo cardiomyopathy

Transient left ventricular apical ballooning syndrome, takotsubo cardiomyopathy, is a cardiac syndrome characterized by transient left ventricular dysfunction. It is associated with ECG changes that can mimic acute myocardial infarction. The left ventricular angiogram usually reveals a hyperkinetic base and a hypokinetic apex, mimicking the shape of a round-bottomed, narrow-necked pot used to catch octopus in Japan (tako-tsubo).

Coronary spasm, microvascular dysfunction, or cardiotoxicity due to catecholamines have been postulated as causes. Most cases (up to 88%) occur in postmenopausal women (mean age 58–77 years).

The onset of symptoms is frequently preceded by physical or emotional stress. The most common presentation is with chest pain and dyspnoea, but cardiogenic shock and ventricular arrhythmias are reported in 4.2% and 1.5% of patients respectively. Between 21% and 49% of patients will have ST-segment elevation at the time of presentation, typically in the precordial leads. Reciprocal inferior ST depression is less likely when compared to patients with anterior ST elevation myocardial infarction. Most patients recover fully and the left ventricular impairment usually improves swiftly in a period of days to weeks. The prognosis is generally very good, with a recurrence in few patients (3–5%) and a mortality of about 1%.

There are no randomized controlled studies on therapy of takotsubo cardiomyopathy. Empirical supportive treatment is advised with use of diuretics and vasodilators. In view of the potential role of catecholamines and sympathetic activation, β-blockers have been recommended as well. Patients with haemodynamic instability may require mechanical support.

Hypereosinophilia and the heart

Hypereosinophilic syndromes are defined by a persistent blood eosinophilia ($>1.5 \times 10^9$/L) lasting for more than 6 consecutive months, associated with evidence of eosinophil-induced organ damage in the absence of other causes of hypereosinophilia, such as allergy, parasitic infection, or malignancy. Hypereosinophilia is a feature of some vasculitides, in particular Churg–Strauss syndrome. Some cases of hypereosinophilia (OMIM 607685) are caused by stem cell mutations that lead to expression of fusion genes (mainly *FIP1L1-PDGFRA*) with constitutive tyrosine kinase activity that cause overproduction of interleukin-5 by activated T-cell subsets.

Clinically, hypereosinophilia syndromes can be classified into chronic eosinophilic leukemia, lymphocytic hypereosinophilic syndrome, myeloproliferative hypereosinophilic syndrome, and idiopathic hypereosinophilic syndrome. The term organ-restricted eosinophilic disease is used when disease is confined to a specific organ or tissue. Löeffler's fibroplastic endocarditis with eosinophilia refers to cardiac disease caused by direct toxicity of circulating eosinophils.

Hypereosinophilic heart disease is characterized by endocardial thickening and apical obliteration caused by large mural thrombi. A restrictive left ventricular filling pattern is typical. Gadolinium delayed-enhanced cardiac MRI identifies regions of myocardial fibrosis and thrombosis. Diffuse myocardial involvement may lead to heart failure, ventricular remodelling and dilated cardiomyopathy. Involvement of the atrioventriclar valves can lead to severe mitral and tricuspid regurgitation. General therapy includes anticoagulation and heart failure therapy. Patients with the *FIP1L1-PDGFRA* fusion gene chromosomal rearrangement are treated with the tyrosine kinase inhibitor imatinib, often following pretreatment with corticosteroids. For patients without the *FIP1L1-PDGFRA* fusion gene, corticosteroids are the usual first-line therapy; steroid-sparing and second-line drugs include hydroxycarbamide, interferon alfa, and imatinib. The prognosis is generally poor even if the hypereosinophilia is resolved, due to high mortality from heart failure, sudden death. or thromboembolism, depending on the underlying cause and end-organ damage.

Further reading

Bargout R (2004). Sarcoid heart disease: clinical course and treatment. *Int J Cardiol*, **97**, 173–82.

Benson MD (1997). Aging, amyloid, cardiomyopathy. *N Engl J Med*, **336**, 502–4.

Braunwald E (ed.) (1998). *Heart disease: a textbook of cardiovascular medicine*, 5th edition, pp. 1427–35. WB Saunders, Philadelphia.

Cox GF, Kunkel LM (1997). Dystrophies and heart disease. *Curr Opin Cardiol*, **12**, 329–42.

Dubrey SW, Comenzo RL (2012). Amyloid diseases of the heart: current and future therapies *Q J Med*, **105**, 617–31.

Gianni M (2006). Apical ballooning syndrome or takotsubo cardiomyopathy: a systematic review. *Eur Heart J*, **27**, 1523–9.

Gotlib J (2014). World Health Organization-defined eosinophilic disorders: 2014 update on diagnosis, risk stratification, and management. *Am J Hematol*, **89**, 325–37.

Guertl B, Noehammer C, Hoefler G (2000). Metabolic cardiomyopathies. *Int J Exp Pathol*, **81**, 349–72.

Landerson PW (1990). Recognition and management of cardiovascular disease related to thyroid dysfunction. *Am J Med*, **88**, 638–41.

Lofiego C (2005). Ventricular remodeling in Loeffler endocarditis: implications for therapeutic decision making. *Eur J Heart Fail*, 7, 1023–6.

Shabina H, Isenberg DA (1999). Autoimmune rheumatic diseases and the heart. *Hospl Med*, **60**, 95–9.

Shammas RL (1993). Sarcoidosis of the heart. *Clin Cardiol*, **16**, 462–72.

Wicks E, Elliott P (2012). Genetics and metabolic cardiomyopathies. *Herz*, **37**, 598–610.

SECTION 8

Pericardial disease

CHAPTER 8.1

Pericardial disease

Michael Henein

Essentials

The most common clinical presentations of pericardial disease are pericarditis, effusion, tamponade, and constriction.

Acute pericarditis

The most common proven causes are viral infection or as a complication of myocardial infarction, but a wide range of other conditions including autoimmune rheumatic disorders and tuberculosis need to be considered. No firm cause is established in many cases, which are regarded as 'idiopathic' (presumed viral).

The main clinical features are chest pain, the presence of a pericardial rub, and widespread ST segment elevation on the ECG. Idiopathic disease is self-limiting: treatment is with analgesics and/ or nonsteroidal anti-inflammatory agents and colchicine.

Pericardial effusion

Acute rapid collection is usually caused by traumatic injury, iatrogenic ventricular puncture, or aortic dissection. Presentation is with pericardial tamponade.

Chronic fluid accumulation is most commonly caused by viral infection, uraemia, autoimmune rheumatic disease, myocardial infarction, myxoedema, or malignancy. Patients may remain asymptomatic despite the presence of a large volume of fluid in the pericardium due to corresponding increase in the capacity of the pericardial cavity. Examination may reveal distant heart sounds and increase in the area of cardiac dullness to percussion. The chest radiograph typically shows a large globular heart and clear lung fields. Echocardiography is the investigation of choice for confirming the presence of effusion and for assessing its volume.

Pericardial tamponade

Pericardial tamponade is a condition of haemodynamic instability caused by chamber compression because increased intrapericardial pressure is greater than the filling pressure of the right and left ventricles.

Presentation is typically with shortness of breath or circulatory collapse. The key physical findings are tachycardia, pulsus paradoxus (an exaggeration of the normal fall in systolic blood pressure on inspiration) of greater than 10 mmHg, and elevation of the venous pressure. Echocardiography is the most important investigation, providing clear evidence of fluid collection around the heart and presence of diastolic right ventricular or right atrial collapse. Immediate management is by pericardial aspiration.

Pericardial constriction

A stiff pericardium loses its stretching ability to accommodate normal changes in intracardiac pressures. Most patients present with leg or abdominal swelling and dyspnoea. The key physical findings are elevated venous pressure (with a characteristic 'M' or 'W' waveform), a pericardial knock, hepatomegaly, ascites, and oedema.

Investigation and diagnosis—Doppler echocardiography is the best noninvasive investigation. Cardiac catheterization demonstrates a difference of less than 5 mmHg between end-diastolic pressures in the two ventricles, persisting with respiration and fluid loading; a peak right ventricular pressure of less than 50 mmHg; and a ratio of end-diastolic to peak right ventricular pressure of more than 0.33.

Management—fluid retention in early pericardial constriction can be managed by diuretics, with pericardiectomy recommended for patients who are resistant.

Anatomy and physiology

The pericardium consists of two layers, a visceral layer lined by mesothelial cells and a parietal or fibrous layer also lined by mesothelial cells, but with attached fat and fibrous tissue. The mesothelial layer secretes about 50 ml of clear pericardial fluid that allows both surfaces to slide together during the cardiac cycle. The innermost layer of the visceral pericardium is adherent to the outer myocardial layer, the epicardium. The fibrous layer is usually 1 mm in thickness, and the visceral layer is a transparent membrane on the surface of the heart. The fibrous pericardium attaches the heart to the diaphragm below and the great vessels above.

Intrapericardial pressure normally ranges between −2 and +2 mmHg, thus it is less than that of the right heart. It falls with the intrapleural pressure during inspiration, resulting in a fall in right-sided cardiac pressures. This causes a modest increase in right heart filling velocities with inspiration. These effects are often exaggerated in patients with clinically significant pericardial disease.

The most common clinical presentations of pericardial disease are pericarditis, effusion, tamponade, and constriction.

Pericarditis

Causes

Infection

The most common causes of acute viral pericarditis are coxsackie B, flu, mumps, hepatitis B, rubella, echovirus 8, and HIV. The typical presentation is with 'flu-like' upper respiratory tract infection along with chest pain that is related to breathing. Sending blood tests for viral titres is not usually conclusive in routine clinical practice. The condition is usually self-limiting.

Bacterial infection (other than tuberculous) is a very rare cause of pericarditis, usually caused by staphylococci, pneumococci, or streptococci spreading directly from the lungs or pleura, particularly in patients with impaired immunity.

Tuberculous infection is an important cause of bacterial pericardial disease, particularly in developing countries. It may take the form of acute pericarditis, pericardial effusion, or constriction. The primary response is an acute pericarditis due to allergic reaction. Chronic pericardial effusion and constriction both reflect granulomatous disease complicated by fibrosis and calcification. Both parietal and visceral layers of the pericardium may be involved, including the epicardial layer of the myocardium. In sub-Saharan Africa most patients (>80%) with tuberculous pericarditis will be HIV positive. This needs to be established before treatment: antituberculous chemotherapy is the first line of management for all, but if there is pericardial effusion or constriction steroids are used for the first few weeks to limit the development of adhesions and hence the need for pericardiectomy in those who are HIV-negative.

Actinomycosis, coccidioidomycosis, histoplasmosis, and hydatid disease can rarely cause pericarditis in endemic areas.

Myocardial infarction

This may be complicated by acute pericarditis in 15% of cases, particularly in patients with transmural infarction, when electrocardiography (ECG) demonstrates ST and T-wave changes that are more generalized than the segmental distribution of the infarct. A friction rub may be heard and a small effusion may be seen on transthoracic echocardiographic examination. A delayed response 3 to 4 weeks after an acute infarct may present as Dressler's syndrome, with fever and pericardial rub. Although this condition is self-limiting it may respond to nonsteroidal anti-inflammatory medications (NSAIDs) and (if needed) steroids.

Autoimmune diseases

Pericardial involvement can be a serious manifestation of rheumatoid disease, systemic lupus erythematosus, systemic sclerosis, and Churg–Strauss syndrome. Presentation can be with pericardial pain, effusion, or even constriction. A small pericardial effusion is seen in most cases of rheumatic fever, but this hardly ever develops into a significant problem. If adhesions develop they may later mature in the form of constriction, a pathology which can be confirmed at the time of valve surgery.

Other medical conditions

Inadequately treated chronic renal failure may be complicated by pericarditis and pericardial effusion. Pericardial tamponade may develop if the effusion remains untreated. Hypothyroidism may be complicated by pericarditis, usually accompanied by a small fluid collection that is unlikely to require drainage.

Irradiation

Irradiation can cause pericarditis soon after treatment, with typical ECG presentation, fluid collection or even constriction. Late presentation can be seen years after irradiation, when the pericardium is thickened and fibrosed.

Clinical features and management

There are three main features of the clinical syndrome of acute pericarditis—chest pain, pericardial rub, and ECG changes.

The chest pain occurs at rest and varies with posture and respiration. It is typically sudden in onset (although often preceded by the nonspecific symptoms of a viral illness), retrosternal, continuous, sharp or 'raw' in character, worse on inspiration, radiating to the trapezius ridge, and relieved by sitting up. It needs to be distinguished from ischaemic cardiac pain (particularly in the context of recent myocardial infarction), oesophageal pain, and musculoskeletal pain.

On examination the main feature is the presence of a pericardial rub. This scratching or creaking sound, variably described as being like 'walking on fresh snow' or the 'creaking of new leather', is usually loudest at the left sternal border, but may be heard anywhere in the chest. It often changes with posture, may be louder with inspiration, and can be fleeting, recurring in hours. In isolated pericarditis, other elements of the cardiovascular examination are usually normal unless pericarditis is associated with the presence of significant pericardial fluid to cause tamponade, or with pericardial constriction.

The typical ECG change is generalized ST elevation, usually concave upwards, by 1 mm or more. The extent of ST change (unlike that of myocardial infarction) does not usually conform to a single coronary artery territory. Similar ECG features may be seen in individuals with early repolarization and in cases without a typical presentation it is important to repeat the ECG in the convalescent phase to ensure that the changes are not fixed to avoid over diagnosis of the condition. Depression of the PR segment is a subtle but characteristic feature. Nonspecific T-wave changes may follow after the acute episode has resolved. ST changes usually resolve, but T-wave changes may persist for years afterwards in some cases. A minor troponin rise reflecting myocardial involvement is not uncommon. Inflammatory markers—C-reactive protein (CRP) and erythrocyte sedimentation rate (ESR)—are also commonly raised.

The chest radiograph is not usually helpful in diagnosis: it may show cardiac enlargement, but may be completely normal. Echocardiography is the best technique to show any fluid collection around the heart and to assess its physiological significance. Similar findings can be shown by cardiac MRI, if available.

Although the underlying cause of pericarditis should always be sought, the final diagnosis is often 'idiopathic' or 'presumed viral'. Idiopathic pericarditis is self-limiting and needs only analgesics. Small effusions due to other causes rarely need drainage, but with symptoms the patient may benefit from NSAIDs. Colchicine is traditionally used as second line therapy in patients with recurrent or persistent pericarditis. However recent evidence suggests that the use of colchicine as a first line agent (at a dose of 0.5 mg twice daily for 3 months for patients weighing >70 kg or 0.5 mg once daily for patients weighing ≤70 kg) may also reduce the rate of symptom persistence and recurrence.

Pericardial effusion

The diagnosis of pericardial effusion is only made when the volume of the fluid in the pericardial space is more than the physiological amount of 50 ml. Two-dimensional echocardiography can detect 100 ml fluid in the pericardial space.

Pericardial effusion can be secondary to cardiac or non-cardiac causes. Acute rapid collection is usually caused by traumatic injury, iatrogenic ventricular puncture, or aortic dissection. The common

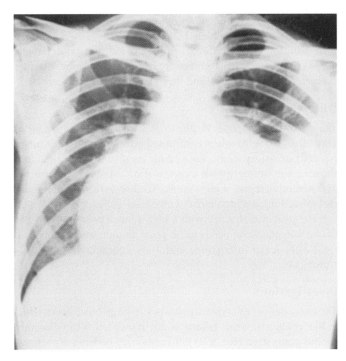

Fig. 8.1.1 Posteroanterior chest radiograph of a patient with a large pericardial effusion. The heart shadow is greatly enlarged and globular in shape. Those parts of the lung fields that can be seen are normal.

causes of chronic fluid accumulation are viral infection, uraemia, autoimmune rheumatic disease, myocardial infarction, myxoedema, and malignancy. Conditions associated with generalized salt and water retention such as congestive cardiac failure, renal failure, and hepatic cirrhosis may also be complicated by pericardial effusion.

A small, rapidly accumulated effusion may result in raised pericardial pressure and development of symptoms (see 'Pericardial tamponade'), whereas with a slowly accumulating effusion patients may remain asymptomatic despite the presence of a large volume of fluid because of the corresponding increase in the capacity of the pericardial cavity. Symptoms in uncomplicated pericardial effusion are nonspecific—reduced exercise tolerance or dull aching chest pain—but patients may develop symptoms of mediastinal syndrome: cough caused by bronchial compression, dyspnoea due to lung compression, or hoarseness of voice caused by recurrent laryngeal nerve compression.

On examination distant heart sounds and increase in the area of cardiac dullness to percussion may be the only physical signs until tamponade develops.

The chest radiograph does not always confirm the presence of pericardial effusion if it is less than 250 ml, but when the effusion is large there is an increased cardiothoracic ratio and the cardiac shadow is globally enlarged (Fig. 8.1.1). The ECG may show low-voltage QRS complexes, and electrical alternans may be present if

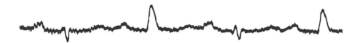

Fig. 8.1.2 ECG from a patient with a massive malignant pericardial effusion. All QRS complexes are sinus beats with a constant PR interval, but the QRS axis alternates, hence the term 'electrical alternans'.

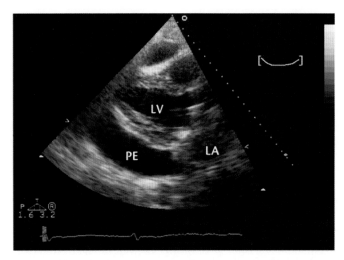

Fig. 8.1.3 Parasternal long axis echocardiographic view from a patient with a large pericardial effusion (Pe), located mostly posteriorly to the left ventricle (LV). LA, left atrium.

the effusion is large, with the heart swinging to and fro within it (Fig. 8.1.2).

Echocardiography is the investigation of choice for confirming the presence of pericardial effusion and for assessing its volume (Fig. 8.1.3). An echo-free space in the pericardium, on both M-mode and two-dimensional images, should be distinguished from anterior pericardial fat pad. Quantitation of pericardial effusion is quite reliable from two-dimensional echocardiographic images: a 1-cm global collection around the heart suggests an approximate amount of 200 ml. With localized effusion, a comparative assessment of the effusion size with that of the left ventricle gives a rough estimation of the collection volume. The haemodynamic effects of pericardial effusion depend on the pressure–volume relation of the pericardium, the speed of fluid collection and the volume of the effusion. Changes in ventricular compliance may also influence the haemodynamic effects of pericardial effusion in patients with ventricular disease.

Pericardial tamponade

Pericardial tamponade is a condition of haemodynamic instability caused by chamber compression because increased intrapericardial pressure is greater than the filling pressure of the right and left ventricles.

Pathophysiology

Provided the pericardium can stretch slowly, more than 2000 ml of fluid can be accumulated without a significant increase in pressure, but rapid accumulation of as little as 200 ml increases pericardial pressure. Inability of the pericardium to distend acutely causes its pressure to rise above right atrial pressure, followed by right ventricular pressure, and eventually results in right ventricular collapse. Intrapericardial and intrapleural pressures normally fall equally during inspiration, but with tamponade intrapericardial pressure does not fall as much, resulting in a reduced pressure gradient between intrathoracic pressure/pulmonary veins and left atrium/left ventricle. This results in reduced left-sided filling velocities during inspiration and hence stroke volume. On the right side of the heart the normal increase in right ventricular dimensions during inspiration enhances right-sided filling and ejection. Progressive increase in pericardial pressure and right ventricular pressure may affect the left heart further, adding to the compromise of its filling during inspiration and exacerbating reduction in stroke volume. The combined effect of these two mechanisms eventually compromises cardiac output.

Pericardial pressure greater than 10 mmHg results in right ventricular collapse and raised diastolic pressures of both ventricles as well as increased capillary wedge pressure. This leads to inspiratory fall of aortic pressure and hence hypotension with pulsus paradoxus (see 'Clinical features'). Left ventricular and left atrial collapse are much less commonly seen with tamponade.

Causes

The most common cause of tamponade is malignant effusion or acute fluid collection after cardiac surgery. Intrapericardial clot formation after cardiac surgery or as a complication of an interventional procedure, e.g. trans-septal puncture, may result in signs of tamponade due to the rapid increase in intrapericardial pressure, even in the absence of a significantly large fluid volume. Left ventricular invagination caused by localized collection around the free wall has been reported after open heart surgery. Significant localized posterior effusion is usually caused by anterior adhesions between the right ventricle, the right atrium, and pericardium.

Clinical features

Patients with cardiac tamponade present with shortness of breath or circulatory collapse. The key physical findings to make the diagnosis are tachycardia, pulsus paradoxus of more than 10 mmHg, and elevation of the venous pressure.

Tachycardia (>100 beat/min) is almost invariable, but clearly not specific for tamponade. Pulsus paradoxus describes an exaggeration of the normal fall in systolic blood pressure (up to 10–12 mmHg) on inspiration. With the patient breathing normally, the best way to detect this sign is to stop deflation of the blood pressure cuff as soon as the first Karotkoff sound is heard, in which case in the presence of pulsus paradoxus the sound will disappear on every inhalation and reappear on every exhalation. After noting the systolic pressure reading, the cuff is then gradually deflated until the Karotkoff sound is heard throughout the respiratory cycle, at which point the pressure is again noted—the difference between the two readings is the measurement of the amount of paradox. A pulsus paradoxus greater than 10 mmHg is found in 98% of patients with tamponade, greater than 20 mmHg in 78%, greater than 30 mmHg in 49%, greater than 40 mmHg in 38%, and total (pulse not palpable on inspiration) in 23%. The most common reason for pulsus paradoxus to be absent in tamponade is compromised stroke volume. However, although pulsus paradoxus is a sensitive sign of tamponade, it must be noted that it is not specific: it can be seen not infrequently in severe asthma, also (uncommonly) in constrictive pericarditis, right ventricular infarction, and pulmonary embolism.

The venous pressure is always high in cardiac tamponade: if it is not, then the diagnosis is wrong. Usually it is very high, which can make it difficult to see the top. The venous pressure normally falls on inspiration because right heart pressures drop as intrathoracic pressure decreases. Kussmaul's sign is an increase in venous pressure during inspiration, which can be observed (infrequently if at all in most series) in tamponade because of the inability of the right atrium and ventricle to accommodate greater influx of blood.

Abnormalities of the venous wave form are not helpful in making the diagnosis of tamponade.

In addition to tachycardia, pulsus paradoxus, and elevated venous pressure, patients with tamponade will usually have tachypnoea and cool peripheries, and they may have a pericardial rub.

Differential diagnosis

The main requirement is for the doctor to consider the diagnosis, even if only briefly, when confronted with any patient in unexplained circulatory shock. Tamponade must be distinguished from the common causes of such a presentation, namely hypovolaemia, overwhelming sepsis, severe ventricular disease (e.g. acute myocardial infarction), and pulmonary embolism.

If the patient is shocked with a high venous pressure, then particular consideration needs to be given to pulmonary embolism, right ventricular infarction, and (less commonly) pericardial constriction.

Investigations

The chest radiograph typically shows a large globular heart, which unlike congestive heart failure, is not associated with pulmonary venous congestion (Fig. 8.1.1): if pulmonary oedema is present it suggests additional myocardial disease. The ECG shows tachycardia, often with low-voltage QRS complexes, and may reveal electrical alternans (Fig. 8.1.2).

Echocardiography is the most important investigation. It provides clear evidence for fluid collection around the heart, which is usually large with tamponade (Fig. 8.1.3), and is likely to show evidence for diastolic right ventricular or right atrial collapse. Right ventricular collapse is a sensitive (92%) and highly specific (100%) diagnostic sign for tamponade, reflecting transient negative transmural early diastolic pressure as pericardial pressure exceeds right ventricular pressure. Right atrial collapse is less sensitive (82%) but equally specific (100%). In the absence of a haemodynamically significant pericardial effusion, right ventricular diastolic collapse

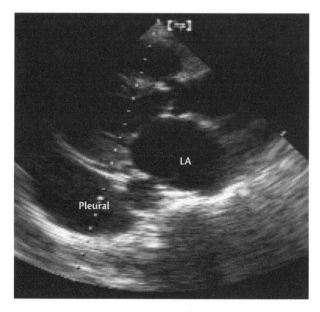

Fig. 8.1.4 Parasternal long axis view showing pleural effusion posterior to the left ventricle.

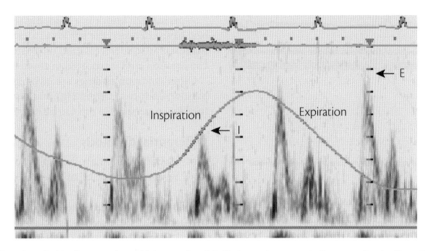

Fig. 8.1.5 Transmitral pulsed Doppler velocities from a patient with large pericardial effusion and tamponade demonstrating significant fall in left ventricular filling velocities with inspiration (arrow, I) compared to expiration (arrow, E).

may be caused by bilateral large pleural effusions (Fig. 8.1.4). Right ventricular collapse may be delayed by myocardial hypertrophy, pulmonary hypertension, or free wall adhesions, commonly associated with malignant effusions. Swinging of the heart inside the pericardial fluid may be seen. Doppler recordings of right and left cardiac filling and ejection show inspiratory dominance in the right with reciprocal changes in the left (Fig. 8.1.5). Finally, echocardiography can exclude the presence of large pleural effusion as a potential cause of the clinical and physiological disturbances: it is essential for the echocardiographer to identify the high-intensity echo of the fibrous pericardium posterior to the left ventricle on the left parasternal image—a pericardial effusion is inside this layer and a pleural effusion outside it.

Management

Pericardial tamponade is a medical emergency, particularly when there is clear evidence for arterial paradox, or if the effusion is collecting rapidly. Pericardial aspiration should be performed in an area where resuscitation facilities are available. Echocardiography is used to determine where to insert the needle and to estimate the depth and direction of advancement. The subcostal route is the most popular because it avoids possible injury to the coronary artery (left anterior descending). After administration of a local anaesthetic a larger needle or polythene cannula is introduced into the effusion, followed by a pigtail catheter inserted over a guide wire. An injection of agitated saline through the drain can help to confirm that it is in the pericardial space. A maximum of 500 ml of fluid is removed initially to relieve haemodynamic instability: rapid withdrawal of a larger volume can provoke cardiovascular collapse. Continuous drainage is then commenced and the rest of the effusion drained over the next few hours.

Many pericardial effusions are heavily bloodstained, particularly those that are malignant. The aspirated fluid can be distinguished from blood (usually to the great relief of the doctor performing the procedure) by its colour (dark because very desaturated) and failure to clot (because defibrinated). Fluid should be sent for culture and cytological analysis. Biochemical analysis (glucose and protein) can sometimes be useful but is diagnostically less reliable than for pleural effusions.

Surgical creation of a pericardial window (usually with video-assisted thoracoscopy) is recommended for recurrent or rapidly accumulating effusions and permits therapeutic pressure relief, fluid drainage, and pericardial biopsy (for culture and histological examination).

Constrictive pericarditis

Pericardial constriction is a pathological condition characterized by pericardial thickening and fibrosis that results in adhesion of its two layers. Chronic constrictive pericarditis frequently proves to be 'idiopathic'; a (presumed) viral aetiology is frequently invoked when no other cause is found. Tuberculosis is currently an uncommon cause, particularly in developed countries. Other causes include radiation, autoimmune rheumatic disease, chronic renal failure, neoplastic disease, and previous cardiac surgery.

Pathophysiology

The stiff pericardium loses its stretching ability to accommodate normal changes in intracardiac pressures. This is demonstrated by equalization of a raised end-diastolic pressures in the right and left ventricles, with the dip–plateau pattern a cardinal sign for diagnosing pericardial constriction (see Fig. 3.4.1).

Pericardial constriction also leads to characteristic abnormalities in the venous pressure waveform, with prominent 'x' and 'y' descents. The 'x' descent, which occurs after atrial contraction ('a' wave), is caused by two processes: (1) right atrial relaxation (followed by a positive 'c' wave that is not visible on inspection) and (2) the atrioventricular tricuspid valve ring moving downwards during systole, increasing the volume of the right atrium. A fibrosed and unstretchable pericardium, being adherent to the epicardial layer of the myocardium, can limit its normal movement during the cardiac cycle along the ventricular transverse axis, particularly in systole. It cannot, however, affect shortening and lengthening of the longitudinal myocardial fibres that are located in the subendocardium, hence the downward displacement of the tricuspid ring and valve in systole is preserved, allowing a column of blood to enter the atrium rapidly, thereby producing a characteristic exaggerated 'x' descent (Fig. 8.1.6). Following the 'x' descent the 'v' wave represents right atrial filling, with the 'y' descent beginning the moment

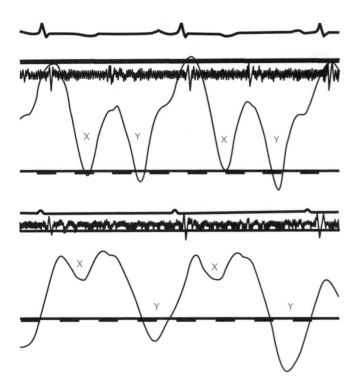

Fig. 8.1.6 Systemic venous pulse from a patient with constrictive pericarditis before (top) and after (bottom) pericardiectomy. Note the 'M' or 'W' pattern, with deep 'x' descent that disappears after pericardiectomy.

that the tricuspid valve opens at the beginning of diastole and allows blood to enter the ventricle. In pericardial constriction the 'y' descent is prominent because, from a high venous pressure, diastolic filling is not impaired at the beginning of diastole, only when the relaxing ventricle meets the rigid pericardium. Similar features can be seen in the left heart physiology.

It should be noted that simply the presence of a thickened pericardium on imaging techniques (echo or MRI) is not a sufficient diagnostic criterion for constrictive physiology. Furthermore, in rare cases of rapidly increasing ventricular volumes, as in dilated cardiomyopathy, the pericardium may be completely normal and yet demonstrate an external constricting effect, thus adding to the deterioration of the clinical condition.

Clinical features

Most patients with constrictive pericarditis present with leg or abdominal swelling and dyspnoea. Rarely the patient can present with jaundice, or with features of nephrotic syndrome or protein-losing enteropathy. The key physical findings are elevated venous pressure, a pericardial 'knock', hepatomegaly, ascites, and oedema.

As with pericardial tamponade, the venous pressure is always high; if it is not, then the diagnosis is almost certainly wrong. However, unlike with pericardial tamponade, the form of the venous waveform is characteristic, with exaggerated 'x' followed by 'y' descent (for reasons explained above) that create two conspicuous dips per cardiac cycle, making the waveform appear to follow an 'M' or 'W' pattern with each arterial pulse (Fig. 8.1.6). Kussmaul's sign (an increase in venous pressure during inspiration) is seen in 50% of cases. Sometimes the changes in venous pressure are transmitted to the liver, which then pulses twice with each cardiac cycle.

A pericardial knock is a loud, high-frequency sound, typically best heard between the left lower sternal border and the apex. It is caused by sudden cessation of ventricular filling as it meets the constriction, and is reported in about 50% of cases in most series.

Other common findings are atrial fibrillation, a mild degree of pulsus paradoxus (≤20 mmHg), and systolic retraction of the apical impulse. A pericardial rub can be heard in some cases.

Differential diagnosis

The main differential diagnosis of constrictive pericarditis is restrictive myocardial disease (see Chapters 7.2 and 7.3). Distinction between these can be difficult. In restriction, ventricular filling becomes limited to early diastole, with high acceleration and deceleration frequently associated with right-sided third heart sound. Respiratory variation of ventricular filling and ejection velocities may be present in constriction but is absent in restrictive right ventricular disease. Imaging can help to determine if the main abnormality is likely to be pericardial or myocardial.

Pericardial constriction also needs to be distinguished from other causes of raised venous pressure, including obstruction of the superior vena cava, tricuspid stenosis, or tricuspid regurgitation.

Investigations

The chest radiograph is usually normal but may show pericardial calcification, either as multiple plaques or as a rim covering the diaphragmatic and anterior surfaces of the heart. The ECG is not diagnostic, but can show low-voltage QRS complexes and nonspecific T-wave changes. On CT or MRI the pericardium may appear thickened, but this is an insensitive marker for constriction.

Doppler echocardiography is the best noninvasive investigation to demonstrate the systolic descent in the jugular venous pressure and systolic filling of the right atrium from the superior and inferior vena cavae during ventricular systole. Ventricular filling is nonspecific, depending on additional myocardial disease. In constrictive pericarditis there is less intracardiac than extracardiac respiratory variation, particularly on the right side, when compared to that seen with pericardial tamponade. A raised right atrial pressure during inspiration (Kussmaul's sign) and dilated inferior vena cava are nonspecific signs of constriction. Spontaneous contrast in the inferior vena cava, resulting from the limited venous return, may also be an additional finding in favour of constrictive pericarditis.

Cardiac catheterization demonstrates the following diagnostic features for constriction:

- a difference of less than 5 mmHg between end-diastolic pressures in the two ventricles, persisting with respiration and fluid loading

- a peak right ventricular pressure of less than 50 mmHg

- a ratio of end-diastolic to peak right ventricular pressure of more than 0.33.

Management

Fluid retention in early pericardial constriction can be managed by diuretics, with pericardiectomy recommended for patients who are resistant. After surgical removal of the pericardium, which is often very difficult, the venous pressure drops and the 'x' descent disappears from the jugular venous pressure (Fig. 8.1.6). This is not always instantaneous and may take up to few days or even weeks to settle.

Pericardial complications after open heart surgery

Apart from the commonly seen pericardial collection, other significant complications may occur that have a major impact on clinical management.

Pericardial clot

A collection of clot in the pericardial space, with or without pericardial effusion, is often associated with delayed postoperative clinical recovery. It may have an important physiological effect on overall cardiac function, irrespective of the amount present. The clinical presentation is typically with cooling of the peripheries, hypotension, and fall in urine output over minutes to hours, and the condition should be suspected particularly in any patient who has bled rather heavily at operation, especially if the blood flow from the chest drains suddenly falls. There are no specific abnormalities on the chest radiograph or ECG; transthoracic echocardiography rarely gives good images immediately postoperatively; transoesophageal echocardiography may show clot alongside the heart. Reopening the chest to remove the clot surgically is the best management, with early detection and removal securing complete recovery.

'Tight' pericardium

In the absence of postoperative pericardial effusion, intrapericardial pressure may be raised to the extent that it affects right-sided physiology so that superior vena caval flow occurs only during inspiration. This condition mimics left ventricular disease and may lead to inappropriate administration of inotropic agents. The jugular venous pressure is raised and right-sided filling and ejection is predominantly inspiratory. On two-dimensional echocardiographic images there is no evidence for right atrial or ventricular collapse. Although these signs usually resolve with time, delayed sternal closure has proved beneficial when the clinical manifestations are severe. The condition tends to settle within days or weeks after surgery, with complete normalization of venous pressure.

Restrictive pericarditis

This is a rare clinical presentation that has been documented after open heart surgery, presenting with resistant fluid retention and raised venous pressure. Two-dimensional echocardiographic images may not show any specific abnormality, although MRI may demonstrate a thickened pericardium. The underlying pathology seems to be chronic combined pericardial and epicardial inflammation that results in massive fibrosis and adhesions between the two layers, with myocardial involvement. Patients with this condition are usually resistant to medical therapy, demonstrating signs of restrictive physiology on both sides of the heart with a dominant early diastolic filling component and short deceleration time. Cases resistant to medical therapy may respond to surgical decortication of the pericardium.

Pericardial tumours

The commonest tumours of the pericardium are secondaries from elsewhere, most frequently carcinoma of the breast and lung, malignant melanoma, lymphoma, and leukaemia. They invade the pericardium either directly, or via lymphatics, or by haematogenous dissemination. Primary tumours are rare but include malignant mesothelioma and sarcomas. Whereas carcinomas metastasize in the pericardium in the form of localized masses, lymphomas and leukaemia present in the form of uniform pericardial infiltration and thickening, which may cause tumour incarceration of the heart and hence the clinical syndrome of 'constrictive physiology'. A mild degree of pericardial thickening can easily be missed on echocardiography, but the pattern of ventricular wall motion is characteristic. MRI or CT may be better at showing pericardial thickening.

Recurrent pericardial effusion of unknown aetiology should always suggest malignancy until otherwise proved, as should pericardial effusion in the presence of an intracardiac mass.

Congenital pericardial disease

Congenital anomalies of the pericardium are rare. Pleuropericardial defect, either complete or partial (80% of cases), is the most common form. The left side is most commonly involved in the partial form, allowing the left atrial appendage or part of the left ventricle (if the defect is large) to herniate through the defects. The chest radiograph is characteristic, demonstrating a shift of the heart to the left and prominent main pulmonary artery. Defects in the diaphragmatic portion of the pericardium are extremely rare. In most instances pericardial defects are asymptomatic, but about one-third of cases are associated with congenital abnormalities of the heart and lungs.

Pericardial cysts are very rare, difficult to diagnose, and if present do not cause any clinical problem. Their presence can only be confirmed when found surgically and removed.

Pericardial constriction due to fibrosis of unknown cause may contribute to the clinical picture of Mulibrey (muscle, liver, brain, eye) nanism (OMIM 253250), which is an autosomal recessive condition characterized by growth failure, a triangular face (often with a hydrocephalus), hypotonia, a peculiar voice, large liver, and yellowish dots and pigment dispersion in the optic fundi.

Further reading

Bertog SC, et al. (2004). Constrictive pericarditis: etiology and cause-specific survival after pericardiectomy. *J Am Coll Cardiol*, **43**, 1445–52.

Callahan JA, et al. (1985). Two-dimensional echocardiographically guided pericardiocentesis: experience in 117 consecutive patients. *Am J Cardiol*, **55**, 476–479.

Cameron J, et al. (1987). The etiologic spectrum of constrictive pericarditis. *Am Heart J*, **113**, 354–360.

Clare GC, Troughton RW (2007). Management of constrictive pericarditis in the 21st century. *Curr Treat Options Cardiovasc Med*, **9**, 436–42.

Guberman BA, et al. (1981). Cardiac tamponade in medical patients. *Circulation*, **64**, 633–40.

Hatle LK, Appleton CP, Popp RL (1989). Differentiation of constrictive pericarditis and restrictive cardiomyopathy by Doppler echocardiography. *Circulation*, **79**, 357–70.

Henein MY, et al. (1999). Restrictive pericarditis. *Heart*, **82**, 389–92.

Henein MY, et al. (2012). *Clinical echocardiography*, 2nd edition. Springer, London.

Imazio M, et al. (2013). A randomized trial of colchicine for acute pericarditis. *N Engl J Med*, **369**, 1522–8.

Kochar GS, Jacobs LE, Kotler MN (1990). Right atrial compression in postoperative cardiac patients: detection by transesophageal echocardiography. *J Am Coll Cardiol*, **16**, 511–16.

McGee SR (2001). *Evidence-based physical diagnosis*. W B Saunders, Philadelphia.

Price S, *et al.* (2004). Tamponade following cardiac surgery: terminology and echocardiography may both mislead. *Eur J Cardiothorac Surg*, **26**, 1156–60.

Reddy PS, *et al.* (1978). Cardiac tamponade: hemodynamic observations in man. *Circulation*, **58**, 265–272.

Sagrista-Sauleda J, *et al.* (2004). Effusive-constrictive pericarditis. *N Engl J Med*, **350**, 469–75.

Shabetai R, *et al.* (1965). Pulsus paradoxus. *J Clin Invest*, **44**, 1882–98.

Shabetai R, Fowler NO, Guntheroth WG (1970). The hemodynamics of cardiac tamponade and constrictive pericarditis. *Am J Cardiol*, **26**, 480–9.

Singh S, *et al.* (1984). Right ventricular and right atrial collapse in patients with cardiac tamponade—a combined echocardiographic and hemodynamic study. *Circulation*, **70**, 966–71.

Troughton RW, Asher CR, Klein AL (2004). Pericarditis. *Lancet*, **363**, 717–27.

Cardiac involvement in infectious disease

CHAPTER 9.1

Acute rheumatic fever

Jonathan R. Carapetis

Essentials

Acute rheumatic fever is an immunologically mediated multisystem disease induced by recent infection with group A streptococcus. About 5% of people have the potential to develop acute rheumatic fever after infection by a strain of streptococcus with propensity to cause the condition. Most cases (97%) occur in low-income and some middle-income countries, with indigenous populations in some affluent countries also affected. Children aged 5 to 15 years are most commonly affected, and rheumatic heart disease remains the most common acquired heart disease of childhood in the world.

Presentation—after a latent period (1–5 weeks in most cases, but up to 6 months for presentation with chorea) the disease presents with one or more of the following major criteria: (1) carditis—most typically manifest as an apical pansystolic murmur of mitral regurgitation, but subclinical disease (evident only on echocardiogram) is also now recognized; (2) polyarthritis—severe, large-joint, and migratory; (3) chorea; (4) subcutaneous nodules; (5) erythema marginatum. Other minor criteria that can support the diagnosis include fever, polyarthralgia or monoarthritis, elevated C-reactive protein (CRP) or erythrocyte sedimentation rate (ESR), prolongation of the PR interval on the ECG.

Diagnosis—in addition to the criteria described above, evidence of preceding group A streptococcal infection is required: (1) positive throat culture, or (2) elevated or rising anti-streptolysin O or other streptococcal antibody, or (3) rapid antigen test for group A streptococcus. The most recent revision of the Jones criteria for diagnosis of acute rheumatic fever allows subclinical carditis as a major manifestation and more sensitive criteria in populations at moderate or high risk of disease, with monoarthritis and polyarthralgia acceptable as major manifestations and lower grade fever (≥38 °C compared to ≥38.5 °C) and less-elevated ESR (≥30 mm/h compared to ≥60 mm/h) as minor manifestations in those groups.

Prognosis and management—untreated acute rheumatic fever lasts for about 3 months. All patients with acute disease should be given penicillin to eradicate the group A streptococcus that precipitated the attack. Children with arthritis or severe arthralgia should be treated with nonsteroidal anti-inflammatory medication (usually salicylates). For severe carditis, many clinicians use oral prednisone or prednisolone at a dose of 40 to 60 mg/day (1–2 mg/kg per day in children), tapering after 2 or 3 weeks, but benefit is not proven. Important prognostic factors are the severity of the acute carditis and the number of recurrences: 30 to 50% of patients with a first episode of acute rheumatic fever will develop chronic rheumatic heart disease, but more than 70% of those with severe carditis at the first episode, or with recurrent episodes. Recent evidence suggests a benefit of corticosteroids for severe or refractory chorea.

Secondary prophylaxis—every patient with acute rheumatic fever should immediately commence intramuscular benzathine benzyl-penicillin every 3 or 4 weeks (preferable), or twice daily oral phenoxymethylpenicillin. In patients without carditis, this should continue for 5 years or until age 21, whichever comes later (although some organizations recommend a minimum of 10 years from last episode); with mild or healed carditis, for 10 years or until age 21, whichever is longer; those with more severe valvular disease or after valve surgery should have secondary prophylaxis until age 40 or sometimes for life.

Primary prophylaxis—a full course of penicillin treatment commencing within 9 days of the onset of symptomatic group A streptococcal pharyngitis will prevent the subsequent development of acute rheumatic fever in most cases and should be advocated.

Introduction

Acute rheumatic fever is an immunologically mediated multisystem disease induced by recent infection with group A streptococcus. Most medical practitioners in industrialized countries will rarely, if ever, see a case. However, the dramatic decline in incidence of acute rheumatic fever in industrialized countries during the second half of the 20th century was not replicated in many developing countries, or among some indigenous and other populations living in poverty in industrialized countries. Acute rheumatic fever continues largely unabated in many low-income countries, and rheumatic heart disease remains the most common acquired heart disease of childhood in the world.

Epidemiology

It is estimated that 33 million people are affected by rheumatic heart disease, with more than 9 million Disability Adjusted Life Years lost and 275 000 deaths occurring each year as a result. Ninety-seven per cent of acute rheumatic fever cases and deaths occur in developing countries. Although acute rheumatic fever and rheumatic heart disease are relatively common in all developing countries, they occur at particularly high rates in sub-Saharan Africa, Pacific nations, Australasia, and the Indian subcontinent. There have been dramatic declines in incidence in recent decades in many Latin American and Asian countries with improving economic and living conditions.

In most populations with high incidence, the predisposing conditions are those that promote endemicity and high levels of transmission of group A streptococci: these include overcrowded housing, poor personal and community hygiene, poor access to medical services, and, in some circumstances, widespread skin infection and scabies infestation.

Outbreaks of acute rheumatic fever occurred in middle-class areas of the United States during the 1980s and 1990s. These outbreaks arose because of the emergence of virulent strains of group A streptococci, particularly belonging to M serotypes 1, 3, and 18. By contrast, outbreaks of acute rheumatic fever have rarely, if ever, been described from developing countries; most cases appear to arise from the ongoing circulation of pathogenic group A streptococcal strains in the population.

Recurrent episodes are almost as common as primary episodes in many populations with high incidence rates of acute rheumatic fever. These may lead to accumulated cardiac valvular damage and are therefore responsible for many cases of rheumatic heart disease, yet they are almost entirely preventable using secondary prophylaxis.

In many developing countries, females are affected more than males, although this gender association is stronger for rheumatic heart disease (especially mitral stenosis) than for acute rheumatic fever; this may reflect a greater tendency to recurrences among females. Any female preponderance may relate to inherited characteristics, to greater exposure to group A streptococci because of the increased involvement of girls and young women in child-rearing in most cultures, or to reduced access by females to primary and secondary prophylaxis.

The maximum incidence of acute rheumatic fever is between the ages of 5 and 15 years in all populations. Approximately 5% of cases occur in children younger than 5 years, but very rarely are children younger than 3 years affected. This age distribution parallels that of group A streptococcal pharyngitis, and supports the hypothesis that all cases of acute rheumatic fever follow this condition. However, it may be that cases do not occur in infants or very young children because of the need for maturity of the immune system (particularly of cellular immunity), or sensitization of the immune response by prior streptococcal infections. New cases occur occasionally up to age 30, but rarely beyond. Hypotheses to explain the reduced incidence in adulthood include development of non-type-specific immunity to primary group A streptococcal infections, further maturation of immune responses, or reduced sensitization by recurrent streptococcal infections.

Pathogenesis

Despite a century of research, the pathogenesis of acute rheumatic fever remains incompletely understood. The presumed pathogenetic pathway is summarized in Fig. 9.1.1, which suggests that the initial damage may be T-cell mediated, although others postulate antibody-mediated damage as the initial event.

Host factors

Epidemiological evidence suggests that less than 5 to 6% of people have the potential to develop acute rheumatic fever after relevant streptococcal exposure, and that this proportion does not vary substantially between populations. Attack rates of acute rheumatic fever after untreated group A streptococcal pharyngitis vary from less than 1% to 3%. Genetic susceptibility to acute rheumatic fever is suggested by a 44% concordance in monozygotic twins compared to 12% in dizygotic twins, and heritability more recently estimated at 60%.

The basis for genetic susceptibility is not known. Susceptibility has been associated with human leukocyte antigen (HLA) class II alleles, particularly HLA-DR7 and DR4, polymorphisms at the tumour necrosis factor-α locus (TNF-α-308 and TNF-α-238), high levels of circulating mannose binding lectin, and Toll-like receptors. However, it is not yet clear whether or how these associated markers are involved in the pathogenesis of acute rheumatic fever.

Organism factors

The observation that outbreaks of pharyngitis due to certain serotypes of group A streptococcus resulted in high attack rates of acute rheumatic fever, whereas no cases occurred after infection with other serotypes, led to the concept of 'rheumatogenicity'—that only some strains of group A streptococcus have the potential to cause acute rheumatic fever. M serotypes 1, 3, 5, 6, 14, 18, 19, 24, 27, and 29 were most frequently implicated in studies predominantly from the United States of America. However, recent studies from regions with high endemicity of group A streptococcal infections have not found consistent M serotype, or *emm* genotype, associations with acute rheumatic fever. There may be substantial genetic diversity among strains belonging to a particular *emm* type, and not all strains of 'rheumatogenic serotypes' appear to cause acute rheumatic fever. Therefore, rheumatogenicity may be strain specific rather than serotype specific; i.e. any group A streptococcus may acquire the potential to cause acute rheumatic fever.

The pathogenic factor(s) are not known. Parts of the organism have immunological cross-reactivity with human tissue; there is close homology between regions of the M protein and human myosin, tropomyosin, keratin, actin, laminin, vimentin, and N-acetylglucosamine. Other components of group A streptococci, including the hyaluronic acid capsule, the cell-wall associated group-specific carbohydrate, and the cell membrane, cross-react with a variety of human tissues damaged in acute rheumatic fever, including components of heart muscle and valves, joints, and brain. Acute rheumatic fever-associated strains of group A streptococcus also tend to be heavily encapsulated with hyaluronic acid, and not to express opacity factor. Group A streptococci possess components which act as superantigens, selectively stimulating subsets of T cells without the need for antigen presentation. Their role in acute rheumatic fever pathogenesis is not yet clear.

Site of infection

Although it is widely accepted that acute rheumatic fever may result from group A streptococcal infection of the upper respiratory tract, but not of the skin, there is some evidence that this may not always be the case. Upper respiratory tract infection certainly accounts for most, if not all, episodes of acute rheumatic fever in countries with a temperate climate. However, in tropical countries where streptococcal impetigo is highly endemic but group A streptococcal pharyngitis less common, it may be that skin infection accounts for many cases of acute rheumatic fever, either *de novo* or after subsequent throat infection. Determining whether group A streptococcal skin infection may have a role in pathogenesis of acute rheumatic fever would have enormous public health implications, as it may redirect present approaches to primary prevention.

The immune response

Molecular mimicry between group A streptococcal epitopes and human tissue is thought to be the basis for the autoimmune response

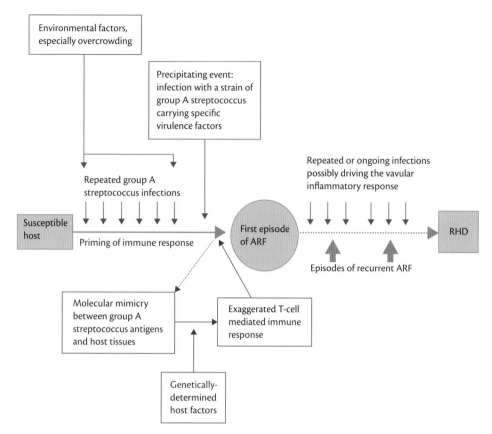

Fig. 9.1.1 Pathogenetic pathway for acute rheumatic fever and rheumatic heart disease. Simplified approach to understanding the pathogenesis of acute rheumatic fever. ARF, acute rheumatic fever; RHD, rheumatic heart disease.

Reprinted from *The Lancet*, Vol. 366, Carapetis JR, McDonald M, Wilson NJ, Acute rheumatic fever, pp. 155–68. Copyright (2005), with permission from Elsevier.

that leads to rheumatic fever. Some models suggest that binding of cross-reactive antibodies to heart valve endothelium leads to activation of the adhesion molecule VCAM-1 and subsequent recruitment of inflammatory cells. The ensuing tissue damage results in the release of peptides such as laminin, keratin, and tropomyosin, which lead to further damage from activation of cross-reactive T cells. Recently, an alternative hypothesis has been suggested proposing that streptococcal invasion of epithelial surfaces leads to binding of streptococcal M protein to type IV collagen through a mechanism not involving molecular mimicry. Overall, it is not entirely clear if the initial damage in rheumatic fever is primarily due to cellular or humoral immunity, but it does appear that ongoing damage is mainly due to T-cell and macrophage infiltration.

Clinical manifestations

There is always a latent period between group A streptococcal infection and the development of acute rheumatic fever. This varies from 1 to 5 weeks in most cases (usually *c.*3 weeks), but may be shorter in recurrences. Chorea may occur up to 6 months after the precipitating streptococcal infection. The preceding infection is asymptomatic in about two-thirds of cases.

The tissues most commonly affected are the heart, joints, and brain. Although the symptoms due to each can be disabling in the short term, only cardiac damage may be permanent and progressive. Therefore, the focus in controlling or treating acute rheumatic fever is always to prevent the development of rheumatic heart disease.

The frequency with which the various clinical manifestations have occurred in recent descriptions of acute rheumatic fever is listed in Table 9.1.1.

Carditis

Although inflammation in acute rheumatic fever may affect the pericardium (causing pericardial rubs and occasionally pleuritic chest pain) or the myocardium (sometimes causing cardiac failure, and evident on biopsy with pathognomonic Aschoff bodies), endocardial inflammation is the most important cause of cardiac damage. If either acute cardiac failure or chronic cardiac disease occurs, it is almost always due to damage to the cardiac valves.

A murmur is the most common evidence of acute valvular disease, usually the apical pansystolic murmur of mitral regurgitation, with or without a low-pitched mid-diastolic (Carey–Coombs) murmur. Occasionally an aortic regurgitant murmur may be heard, mainly in older adolescents or young adults. Murmurs of tricuspid or pulmonary regurgitation are rare and are usually secondary to increased pulmonary venous pressures resulting from mitral regurgitation or stenosis. Sinus tachycardia or gallop rhythms may also be present in acute carditis.

Valves affected by rheumatic carditis may have a characteristic appearance or pattern of regurgitation on Doppler echocardiography (when interpreted by experienced technicians), which may be found even in the absence of a cardiac murmur (subclinical disease). Recent efforts to standardize the echocardiographic diagnosis of rheumatic heart disease have led to publication of an evidence-based guideline

Table 9.1.1 Frequency of clinical manifestations in acute rheumatic fever

Manifestation	Proportion of patients with manifestation (%)	
	Chorea[a] absent	Chorea[a] present
Carditis	40–60	20–30
Polyarthritis	50–75	<10
Erythema marginatum	1–10	0–1
Subcutaneous nodules	1–10	0–1
Fever >37.5 °C	>90	10–25
Arthralgia	<10–20	<5
Elevated acute-phase reactants	>90	10–25
Prolonged PR interval	30–50	5–10

[a] Chorea is present in <10% to >30% of patients with acute rheumatic fever, depending on the population.

by the World Heart Federation, which focuses on features of mitral and aortic regurgitation and valvular morphology that can be considered pathological, and combines these features into criteria for 'definite' and 'borderline' rheumatic heart disease. Although these criteria were devised for rheumatic heart disease rather than acute rheumatic fever, there is accumulating evidence that many similar features are useful in diagnosing acute rheumatic carditis on echocardiography. The recent revision of the Jones criteria identifies the features of regurgitant jets and valvular morphology that can be used to make a diagnosis of acute rheumatic carditis, even in the absence of a significant cardiac murmur (Table 9.1.2)

Mitral or aortic stenosis may develop as later complications of severe and/or recurrent acute carditis due to scarring and contraction following the acute inflammatory process. Rarely, mitral stenosis may occur in young children with acute rheumatic fever—so-called 'juvenile mitral stenosis'—the reasons for the development of this condition are not clear.

Damage to the electrical conduction pathways may result in prolongation of the PR interval on electrocardiography (ECG). Although a subset of healthy people may have this finding, the presence of a prolonged PR interval that resolves over the ensuing few days to weeks may be a useful diagnostic feature in cases where the clinical manifestations are not clear. Occasionally, in the acute phase, second- or third-degree heart block or a nodal rhythm may be present (Fig. 9.1.2).

Arthritis

The characteristic joint manifestation of acute rheumatic fever is severe, large-joint, migratory polyarthritis. The knees, ankles, wrists, and elbows are most commonly involved; only rarely, and usually only when the patient is untreated for several days, are the hips or small joints of the hands or feet inflamed. One joint characteristically becomes exquisitely painful and inflamed as another is waning. Most patients have only one or two joints affected at any one time, and each joint may be involved for just a few hours or up to 1 or 2 days. The arthritis is so responsive to nonsteroidal anti-inflammatory medication (NSAIDs) that its persistence more than 1 or 2 days after commencing high-dose aspirin should lead one to consider alternative diagnoses.

Table 9.1.2 Findings on echocardiography in rheumatic valvulitis

Valve	Doppler findings	Morphological findings
Mitral valve		
	Pathological mitral regurgitation (all 4 met)	**Acute mitral valve changes**
	Seen in at least 2 views	Annular dilation
	Jet length ≥2 cm in at least one view	Chordal elongation
	Peak velocity >3 m/s	Chordal rupture resulting in flail leaflet with severe mitral regurgitation
	Pansystolic jet in at least one envelope	Anterior (or less commonly posterior) leaflet tip prolapse
		Beading/nodularity of leaflet tips
		Chronic mitral valve changes: not seen in acute carditis
		Leaflet thickening
		Chordal thickening and fusion
		Restricted leaflet motion
		Calcification
Aortic valve		
	Pathological aortic regurgitation (all 4 met)	**Aortic valve changes in either acute or chronic carditis**
	Seen in at least 2 views	Irregular or focal leaflet thickening
	Jet length ≥1 cm in at least one view	Coaptation defect
	Peak velocity >3 m/s	Restricted leaflet motion
	Pandiastolic jet in at least one envelope	Leaflet prolapse

Adapted with permission from Gewitz MH, et al. Revision of the Jones criteria for the diagnosis of acute rheumatic fever in the era of Doppler echocardiography: a scientific statement from the American Heart Association Committee on Rheumatic Fever, Endocarditis, and Kawasaki Disease of the Council of Cardiovascular Disease in the Young Endorsed by the World Heart Federation. *Circulation*, **131**, 1806–18.

Arthritis of a single large joint, and polyarthralgia in the absence of clear arthritis, are increasingly described in acute rheumatic fever from regions with high rates of disease. This is sometimes, but not always, due to early administration of anti-inflammatory medication, before the typical migratory pattern has emerged. Other causes of monoarthritis, including septic arthritis, should first be excluded before a diagnosis of acute rheumatic fever is entertained. Arthralgia (joint pain without objective evidence of inflammation) is usually migratory and affects large joints, and like the arthritis of acute rheumatic fever is very responsive to NSAIDs.

Sydenham's chorea

In 1686 the English physician Thomas Sydenham described rheumatic chorea, initially naming it 'St Vitus' dance'. It is the most intriguing manifestation of acute rheumatic fever, particularly as it commonly occurs in the absence of other manifestations, usually

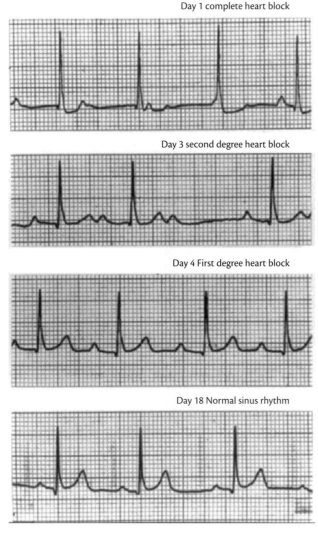

Day 1 complete heart block

Day 3 second degree heart block

Day 4 First degree heart block

Day 18 Normal sinus rhythm

Fig. 9.1.2 ECG changes in a young adult with acute rheumatic fever, showing evolution over 18 days from complete heart block, to second-degree (Wenckebach) block, to first-degree block, and then to normal sinus rhythm.
From: A subtle presentation of acute rheumatic fever in remote Northern Australia, Bishop W et al. *Australian and New Zealand Journal of Medicine*, Vol 26, Issue 2, © 1996 John Wiley & Sons Inc.

follows a prolonged latent period (up to 6 months) after the precipitating group A streptococcal infection, and occurs most commonly in females (and almost never in postpubertal males). The rapid, jerky, involuntary movements affect predominantly the upper limbs and face, may be asymmetrical, and may be sufficiently severe to render the patient unable to eat, drink, walk, or perform other activities of daily living. Mild chorea can sometimes be detected by having the patient join palms above the head to reveal occasional twitches of the arms or the head. Typical signs include the 'milkmaid's grip' (rhythmic squeezing when the patient grasps the examiner's fingers), spooning of extended hands (caused by flexion of the wrists and extension of the fingers), darting of the protruded tongue, and the 'pronator sign' (the arms and palms turn outwards when held above the head). As with other forms of chorea, the disorder usually becomes more evident with anxiety or purposeful movements (such as drinking or writing). Movements may appear semi-purposeful, and symptoms subside during sleep. Sydenham's chorea is often associated with excessive emotional lability or personality changes, which may precede the abnormal movements.

Most patients can be reassured that Sydenham's chorea will resolve completely and leave no long-lasting effects, usually within 6 weeks and almost always within 6 months, but rarely lasting up to 3 years.

Subcutaneous nodules and erythema marginatum

Both of these manifestations are found in less than 2% of patients with acute rheumatic fever, although they were described in up to 10 to 20% of patients in earlier studies from the United States of America and the United Kingdom. Subcutaneous nodules are firm, painless lumps, usually between 0.5 and 2 cm in diameter, commonly found in crops of three or more, and usually appear 2 to 3 weeks after the onset of acute rheumatic fever. They occur mainly over extensor surfaces or bony protuberances, particularly the hands, feet, occiput, and back. The nodules are similar to those found in rheumatoid arthritis, though often smaller, and are most likely to be associated with severe carditis. Nodules usually last from a few days to 2 or 3 weeks.

The characteristic rash, erythema marginatum, appears as a light pink macule that spreads outwards with a serpiginous, well-demarcated edge, while the central portion clears. It appears, disappears, or moves before the observer's eyes. Multiple areas are often involved, usually over the trunk, occasionally over the proximal portions of the limbs, but rarely, if ever, the face. It usually appears together with the other initial symptoms of acute rheumatic fever, but may recur intermittently for weeks or even months. This does not indicate ongoing rheumatic inflammation, and patients can be reassured that the rash will eventually disappear without complications.

Fever

With the exception of those with pure chorea, 90% of patients will have a temperature at presentation higher than 37.5 °C. Although it has been reported that the temperature usually exceeds 39 °C, others have found only 25% of confirmed cases with fever to that level. The recent revision of the Jones criteria specifies that a temperature of 38.5 °C or more is sufficient to be a minor manifestation in low-risk populations while a temperature of 38.0 °C or more is sufficient in moderate- to high-risk populations. As with arthritis, fever is very sensitive to NSAIDs, usually resolving completely within 1 or 2 days of commencing high-dose salicylates.

Elevated acute-phase reactants

Almost all patients, except those with pure chorea, have a dramatically elevated erythrocyte sedimentation rate (ESR) or serum C-reactive protein (CRP). There appears little difference between these measurements in their diagnostic usefulness. The CRP may return to normal more rapidly than the ESR when rheumatic activity subsides. Mild to moderate peripheral leucocytosis is common, although this is a less sensitive marker of rheumatic inflammation and has therefore been removed as a minor manifestation from the most recent revision of the Jones criteria.

Other features

Severe central abdominal pain is found at presentation in a small proportion of patients. It may be associated with other features of acute rheumatic fever; if not, these features usually appear within 1 or 2 days. The pain responds quickly to NSAIDs. Epistaxis was reported frequently in historical accounts of acute rheumatic fever, but does not feature prominently in recent descriptions. Pulmonary infiltrates may be found in patients with acute carditis; this has been labelled 'rheumatic pneumonia' although it is not clear whether the infiltrates represent rheumatic inflammation or another process. There may be microscopic haematuria, pyuria, or proteinuria; also mild elevations of liver transaminases: these are nonspecific and not usually severe.

Associated poststreptococcal syndromes

Poststreptococcal reactive arthritis has been differentiated from rheumatic fever by some authors because it has a shorter incubation period after streptococcal infection, sometimes follows non-group-A β-haemolytic streptococcal infection, may have a different pattern of arthritis (including small joint involvement), and is less responsive to NSAIDs. Because of the lack of cardiac involvement, these patients are said not to require secondary prophylaxis. However, descriptions of patients who have subsequently developed carditis have led other authors to question the distinction between poststreptococcal reactive arthritis and rheumatic fever. If poststreptococcal reactive arthritis is diagnosed, secondary prophylaxis should be prescribed for at least 1 year and discontinued if there is no evidence of carditis. In populations with high incidence rates of acute rheumatic fever, it may be prudent to treat all cases of possible poststreptococcal reactive arthritis as acute rheumatic fever.

The frequent finding of emotional lability, motor hyperactivity, and occasional obsessive–compulsive symptoms in patients with Sydenham's chorea led to the observation that group A streptococcal infections may precipitate or exacerbate other disorders of the basal ganglia. These include tic disorders, Tourette's syndrome, and obsessive–compulsive disorder, and the term PANDAS (paediatric autoimmune neuropsychiatric disorders associated with streptococcal infections) has been coined. A recent follow-up study that failed to find any exacerbations of symptoms associated with streptococcal infections in PANDAS patients has raised questions about the existence of PANDAS as a distinct disease entity.

Diagnosis

Because of the diversity of symptoms and signs, and the nonspecific nature of most of them, in 1944 Dr T Duckett Jones developed a set of criteria to aid in the diagnosis of acute rheumatic fever. The Jones criteria have subsequently been revised and updated a number of times to improve their specificity in an era of declining acute rheumatic fever incidence in high-income countries. Because the Jones criteria were perceived to be overly specific for populations with high incidence of disease, other bodies have recently published their own diagnostic criteria, including the World Health Organization (WHO) and expert groups in Australia and New Zealand. The American Heart Association has responded to these concerns in its latest revision of the Jones criteria, presenting more sensitive criteria for populations at moderate or high risk of acute rheumatic fever (Table 9.1.3).

The manifestations are divided into major, those which are most predictive of acute rheumatic fever, and minor, those which are commonly found in acute rheumatic fever but are less specific. The

Table 9.1.3 Revised Jones criteria (2015 revision)

A. For all patient populations with evidence of preceding group A streptococcal infection:	
Diagnosis—initial ARF	2 major manifestations or 1 major plus 2 minor manifestations
Diagnosis—recurrent ARF	2 major or 1 major and 2 minor or 3 minor

B. Major criteria	
Low-risk populations[a]	Moderate/high-risk populations

Carditis[b]
   Clinical and/or subclinical
	Carditis
	   Clinical and/or subclinical

Arthritis
   Polyarthritis only
	Arthritis
	   Monoarthritis or polyarthritis
	   Polyarthralgia

Chorea	Chorea
Erythema marginatum	Erythema marginatum
Subcutaneous nodules	Subcutaneous nodules

C. Minor criteria	
Low-risk populations[a]	Moderate/high-risk populations
Polyarthralgia	Monoarthralgia
Fever (≥38.5 °C)	Fever (≥38 °C)
ESR ≥60mm/in the first hour and/or CRP ≥3.0 mg/dl[c]	ESR ≥ 30 mm/Hr and/or CRP ≥3.0 mg/dl[c]
Prolonged PR interval (unless carditis is a major criterion)	Prolonged PR interval (unless carditis is a major criterion)

ARF, acute rheumatic fever; CRP, C-reactive protein; ESR, erythrocyte sedimentation rate; RHD, rheumatic heart disease.

[a] Low-risk populations = ARF incidence ≤2 per 100 000 school-aged children or all age RHD prevalence of ≤1 per 1000 population per year.

[b] Subclinical carditis = echocardiographic valvulitis as defined in Table 9.1.2. Erythema marginatum and subcutaneous nodules are rarely 'standalone' major criteria. Additionally, joint manifestations can only be considered in either the major or minor categories but not both in the same patient.

[c] CRP value must be greater than upper limit of normal for laboratory.

Reprinted with permission from Gewitz MH, et al. Revision of the Jones criteria for the diagnosis of acute rheumatic fever in the era of Doppler echocardiography: a scientific statement from the American Heart Association Committee on Rheumatic Fever, Endocarditis, and Kawasaki Disease of the Council of Cardiovascular Disease in the Young Endorsed by the World Heart Federation. *Circulation*, **131**, 1806–18.

diagnosis of an initial episode requires the presence of either two major, or one major and two minor criteria, plus the demonstration of a current or recent group A streptococcal infection. Evidence of group A streptococcal infection is not required for chorea, where the onset may be delayed up to 6 months after streptococcal infection, and late-onset carditis, when low-grade inflammation may persist for prolonged periods after the precipitating infection. Recurrences can be diagnosed with less stringent criteria.

Proof of a recent group A streptococcal infection can include demonstrating the organism in the upper respiratory tract, either by culture or rapid antigen techniques. However, most children with acute rheumatic fever no longer have a group A streptococcus detectable by these methods, and up to 15 to 25% of normal children in temperate climate countries may carry the organism in their throat. Serological techniques are therefore most commonly used, particularly the antistreptolysin O, anti-DNase B, or antihyaluronidase titres. One of any two of these tests will be positive in well over 90% of recent streptococcal infections. Their usefulness is increased by performing more than one serological test, or by demonstrating rising titres in paired sera. Serology is of limited value in regions with high prevalence rates of streptococcal impetigo, where children may have positive antistreptococcal titres most of the time. There is therefore a need for a better diagnostic test of recent streptococcal infection, or an objective diagnostic test for acute rheumatic fever itself.

The most common clinical presentation, that of a child with fever and polyarthritis, raises multiple differential diagnoses that will vary by region. Table 9.1.4 lists some alternative diagnostic possibilities for the three most common major manifestations.

Table 9.1.4 Differential diagnoses of common major presentations of acute rheumatic fever

	Presentation		
	Polyarthritis and fever	Carditis	Chorea
Differential diagnoses	Septic arthritis (including gonococcal)	Innocent murmur	SLE
	Connective tissue and other autoimmune disease[a]	Mitral valve prolapse	Drug intoxication
	Viral arthropathy[b]	Congenital heart disease	Wilson's disease
	Reactive arthropathy[b]	Infective endocarditis	Tic disorder[c]
	Lyme disease	Hypertrophic cardiomyopathy	Choreoathetoid cerebral palsy
	Sickle cell anaemia	Myocarditis—viral or idiopathic	Encephalitis
	Infective endocarditis	Pericarditis—viral or idiopathic	Familial chorea (including Huntington's)
	Leukaemia or lymphoma		Intracranial tumour
	Gout and pseudogout		Lyme disease
			Hormonal[d]

SLE, systemic lupus erythematosus.

[a] Includes rheumatoid arthritis, juvenile chronic arthritis, inflammatory bowel disease, systemic lupus erythematosus, systemic vasculitis, sarcoidosis, among others.

[b] Mycoplasma, cytomegalovirus, Epstein–Barr virus, parvovirus, hepatitis, rubella vaccination, and yersinia and other gastrointestinal pathogens.

[c] Possibly including PANDAS.

[d] Includes oral contraceptives, pregnancy (chorea gravidarum), hyperthyroidism, hypoparathyroidism.

Reprinted from *The Lancet*, Vol. 366, Carapetis JR, McDonald M, Wilson NJ, Acute rheumatic fever, pp. 155–68. Copyright (2005), with permission from Elsevier.

Treatment

If untreated, acute rheumatic fever lasts on average for 3 months. Except in the case of life-threatening acute carditis, there is no evidence that presently available treatments alter the outcome. Most treatments are designed to provide symptomatic relief or are based on theoretical (but unproven) approaches to attenuating the long-term damage.

If practical, all patients with acute rheumatic fever should be admitted to hospital to confirm the diagnosis, perform baseline investigations to ascertain the status of the heart, provide adequate treatment for the acute phase, commence secondary prophylaxis, allow communication of details to personnel responsible for long-term follow-up of the patient, and begin education of the patient and family. The mainstays of treatment are bed rest, penicillin, and salicylates.

Bed rest

Previous recommendations that children with acute rheumatic fever be rested in bed until all signs of active inflammation abated were probably more extreme than is necessary. Once symptoms of arthritis have subsided and any cardiac failure is controlled, the child may begin gentle mobilization, which may be increased as tolerated. There is no evidence that bed rest beyond the period where mobilization leads to exacerbation of pain or cardiac failure has any long-term benefit.

Penicillin

All patients with acute rheumatic fever should be given penicillin to eradicate the group A streptococcus that precipitated the attack. This is based on an early finding that, in some cases, prolonged group A streptococcal infection led to more severe acute rheumatic fever. Although in most cases the precipitating organism cannot be cultured, a treatment course of penicillin is prudent in case the strain remains present in low numbers, and to prevent its transmission to other contacts. As the aim is eradication of group A streptococcal infection, penicillin may be administered either as a single intramuscular injection of benzathine benzylpenicillin at a dose of 1.2 million units (600 000 U for patients <27 kg) into the gluteal or quadriceps muscles, or as a 10-day course of oral phenoxymethyl penicillin (V) at a dose of 500 mg (adolescents and adults) or 250 mg (children) given two times daily or amoxicillin 50 mg/kg (max 1 g) daily. In the case of penicillin allergy, the present recommendation is to use oral erythromycin at 20 to 40 mg/kg per day given two to four times daily for 10 days, although in some regions levels of erythromycin resistance among group A streptococci are increasing.

Salicylates

Children with arthritis or severe arthralgia should be treated with NSAIDs; salicylates have been most widely used. Aspirin at a dose of 50 to 60 mg/kg per day up to a maximum of 80 to 100 mg/kg per day (4–8 g/day in adults), given in 4 to 5 divided doses, usually results in defervescence and resolution of arthritis and arthralgia within 1 to 2 days. Sometimes higher doses lead to nausea or vomiting, which can be minimized by increasing from lower starting doses. After a few days or up to 2 weeks, when the initial symptoms are abating, patients on higher doses can have the dose reduced to 50 to 60 mg/kg per day for the remaining 2 to 4 weeks. Arthritis or arthralgia may return up to 2 to 3 weeks after discontinuation of therapy; this is usually a brief and mild recrudescence, often associated with increased ESR or CRP, and can be managed either with rest and reassurance or a short course of lower-dose NSAIDs.

When the diagnosis is uncertain, salicylates should be withheld for a day or two to look for the development of characteristic migratory polyarthritis. In such cases, paracetamol or codeine can be used to control pain until the diagnosis is confirmed. There is no evidence that salicylates reduce the severity of acute carditis or the risk of chronic cardiac valve damage.

Corticosteroids

For many years, corticosteroids have been used in acute rheumatic fever, particularly for patients with severe carditis. Two meta-analyses have found no evidence that they reduce the risk of long-term valve damage. However, the studies included in these meta-analyses were all conducted more than 40 years ago and used corticosteroid medications not in common usage today. Many clinicians continue to use oral prednisone or prednisolone at a dose of 40 to 60 mg/day (1–2 mg/kg per day in children), tapering after 2 or 3 weeks, in the belief that this might reduce the severity of acute carditis. The role of corticosteroids in chorea is discussed below.

Treatment of cardiac failure

There is no doubting the need to treat cardiac failure. Diuretics, angiotensin converting enzyme (ACE) inhibitors (especially in aortic regurgitation), and fluid restriction are most commonly employed. Digoxin is usually restricted to cases where atrial fibrillation coexists with cardiac failure, often found in older patients with established mitral stenosis.

If medical therapy fails, cardiac surgery should be considered, even during the acute phase. In populations where fulminant acute carditis is relatively common (e.g. South Africa), mitral valve repair or replacement can be life-saving and surgeons have developed techniques for undertaking these procedures despite friable, acutely inflamed valvular and perivalvular tissues. In recent years, there has been a greater tendency to undertake valve repair rather than replacement, or to use homografts or xenografts rather than mechanical prostheses. This is to avoid high rates of thromboembolic complications associated with mechanical prostheses, particularly in populations where compliance with anticoagulation chemotherapy is suboptimal and there are difficulties in monitoring coagulation indices.

Treatment of chorea

Sydenham's chorea always resolves, and in most cases there is no need for medical treatment. However, medications may reduce abnormal movements in moderate or severe chorea. Carbamazepine or sodium valproate are recommended as first line treatment, haloperidol less commonly because of its side-effect profile. Other medications sometimes employed include pimozide, chlorpromazine, or benzodiazepines. All of these medications should be used sparingly and only for limited periods, and the tendency to try multiple medications should be avoided.

Recent evidence suggests that corticosteroids lead to more rapid symptom reduction in chorea, so oral prednisone or prednisolone may be considered for severe or refractory cases (0.5 mg/kg daily, weaning as early as possible, preferably after 1 week if symptoms reduce). Psychotherapeutic interventions have little role in the short to medium term, and may increase the stigma of this self-limited organic disease. However, behavioural therapy should be considered if longer-term behavioural abnormalities persist (e.g. emotional lability, obsessive–compulsive traits).

Newer therapies

Because of the autoimmune nature of acute rheumatic fever, immunomodulatory therapies have been tried. Intravenous immune globulin (IVIG) has been given in some small trials. One study showed no apparent benefit on rate of improvement of clinical, laboratory, or echocardiographic parameters of acute carditis, but another suggested that it may accelerate recovery from chorea. Other therapies have yet to be formally assessed.

Prognosis and follow-up

The most important prognostic factors are the severity of the acute carditis and the number of recurrences. Overall, approximately 30 to 50% of patients with a first episode of acute rheumatic fever will develop chronic rheumatic heart disease. This increases to more than 70% in patients with severe carditis at the first episode, or in those who have had at least one recurrence.

Any patient with acute rheumatic fever requires long-term follow-up. Follow-up assessments should focus on cardiac status, adherence to secondary prophylaxis, early treatment of group A streptococcal pharyngitis, and prevention of streptococcal pyoderma (including hygiene and treatment or prevention of scabies infestation). Patients with evidence of cardiac valve damage should be assessed regularly by specialist physicians and considered for cardiac surgery before substantial left ventricular dysfunction occurs. Vasoactive drugs, particularly ACE inhibitors, may delay the need for operation in asymptomatic patients with chronic aortic regurgitation. Regular echocardiography may be useful to follow the progress of rheumatic heart disease, especially in populations where follow-up may be irregular or in whom communication or cultural differences make clinical assessment difficult.

Recurrences

About 75% of all recurrences occur within 2 years of an episode of acute rheumatic fever. The reasons for this are not known, but are thought to relate to a time-dependent sensitization of the immune response. The clinical features of recurrences tend to mimic those present at the initial episode, particularly in the case of chorea. However, this rule is not absolute, and the risk of developing other manifestations, particularly carditis, increases with each recurrence. The practical implication of this is that the absence of carditis at the first episode does not help to identify patients who may not need secondary prophylaxis.

Prevention of acute rheumatic fever
Secondary prophylaxis

Every patient with acute rheumatic fever should immediately commence secondary prophylaxis: long-term, regular antibiotics to prevent primary group A streptococcal infections. This strategy is proven to reduce the incidence of recurrences and the risk of developing chronic rheumatic heart disease.

The optimal regimen is 1.2 million units of intramuscular benzathine benzylpenicillin every 3 or 4 weeks, and this is commonly given in populations with high incidences of acute rheumatic fever and programmes in place to support the regimen. An alternative strategy is to use oral phenoxymethylpenicillin at a dose of 250 mg twice daily; this is less effective than benzathine benzylpenicillin, and adherence is usually less reliable.

For patients proven to be allergic to penicillin, the present recommendation is to use oral erythromycin at a dose of 250 mg twice daily. Recent trials have shown newer oral cephalosporins to be effective at eliminating upper respiratory tract carriage of group A streptococci. However, none of these antibiotics has been evaluated for the ability to prevent acute rheumatic fever.

The duration of secondary prophylaxis is dictated by the reducing risk of recurrence with increasing age, with time since the last episode, and the possible consequences of recurrences. In patients without carditis, secondary prophylaxis should continue for 5 years following the most recent episode or until age 21 years, whichever comes later. In patients with mild or healed carditis, prophylaxis should be continued for 10 years following the most recent episode or until age 21 years, whichever is longer. Patients with more severe valvular disease or those who have undergone valve surgery should have secondary prophylaxis until age 40 or sometimes for life.

Primary prophylaxis

A full course of penicillin treatment commencing within 9 days of the onset of symptomatic group A streptococcal pharyngitis will prevent the subsequent development of acute rheumatic fever in most cases. After the diagnosis has been confirmed by a throat culture or rapid antigen diagnostic test, the treatment of choice is penicillin, administered either as a single intramuscular injection of benzathine benzylpenicillin (600 000 U for children who weigh <27 kg, or 1.2 million U for larger children and adults) or as a full 10 days of oral phenoxymethylpenicillin (250 mg for children or 500 mg for adults given two times daily) or amoxicillin (50 mg/kg to a maximum of 1 g as a daily dose). The importance completing the 10-day course, even if symptoms abate quickly, should be stressed to patients and parents. Shorter courses of oral penicillin treatment are associated with higher risks of acute rheumatic fever. There has never been a clinical isolate of group A streptococcus that is resistant to penicillin; therefore, the use of other antibiotics for primary prophylaxis should be restricted to patients who are allergic to penicillin.

In the case of penicillin allergy, a 10-day course of erthythromycin or clarithromycin is recommended. First-generation oral cephalosporins may also be considered, as may a 5-day course of azithromycin. However, these agents have not been evaluated in populations with high incidences of acute rheumatic fever.

It is not possible to predict which episodes of group A streptococcal pharyngitis will precipitate acute rheumatic fever, so this treatment must be offered in all cases to be effective. Unlike prevention of recurrent episodes, which is virtually complete using secondary prophylaxis, penicillin treatment of streptococcal pharyngitis will at best prevent only the one-third or so of cases of acute rheumatic fever that follow a sore throat. However, this important intervention may also arrest the spread of pathogenic group A streptococci in the community. Penicillin treatment of group A streptococcal pharyngitis should begin as early as possible in patients with a history of acute rheumatic fever, should they not be taking secondary prophylaxis, but even then may not prevent a recurrence, hence the need for secondary prophylaxis.

In recent years the use of primary prophylaxis has been questioned in some industrialized countries where acute rheumatic fever is now rare. It is argued that the strategy prevents few cases of acute rheumatic fever but contributes to overuse of antibiotics. Similar arguments were raised in the United States of America during the 1970s, but faded somewhat with the resurgence of acute rheumatic fever in that country during the 1980s. Any country considering abandoning primary prophylaxis should first have in place effective surveillance to detect changes in the epidemiology of primary group A streptococcal infections and the appearance of cases of acute rheumatic fever.

Primary prophylaxis is unsuccessful in most developing countries. It requires trained health workers, microbiology laboratories, transportation and communication infrastructure, the availability of penicillin, and a population likely to seek and adhere to treatment for sore throats. Approaches based on diagnosis using clinical algorithms, or an approach of treating all sore throats with intramuscular benzathine benzylpenicillin without further attempts at diagnosis, are being increasingly recommended in resource-poor settings. If primary prophylaxis were to be instituted effectively in developing countries, there would be a substantial impact on acute rheumatic fever incidence, but it would not disappear because most cases do not follow a sore throat.

Other methods of primary prevention are clearly needed in developing countries. Improved living standards, particularly less-crowded housing, and access to primary health care, are priorities. Although streptococcal skin infections may be linked to acute rheumatic fever pathogenesis, there are no trials of impetigo control programmes to prevent acute rheumatic fever. There is a current focus on attempts to develop a group A streptococcal vaccine. Clinical trials of prospective vaccines have begun, but the process will take many years, and recent experience suggests that new vaccines are often beyond the financial reach of most developing countries. For the foreseeable future at least, acute rheumatic fever prevention in many developing countries will depend on improving adherence to secondary prophylaxis and developing new strategies for primary prevention.

Further reading

Anonymous (1995). Strategy for controlling rheumatic fever/rheumatic heart disease, with emphasis on primary prevention: memorandum from a joint WHO/ISFC meeting. *Bull World Health Org*, **73**, 583–7.

Bach JF, *et al.* (1996). 10-year educational programme aimed at rheumatic fever in two French Caribbean islands. *Lancet*, **347**, 644–8.

Bisno AL (1991). Group A streptococcal infections and acute rheumatic fever. *N Engl J Med*, **325**, 783–93.

Bryant P, *et al.* (2014). Susceptibility to acute rheumatic fever based on differential expression of genes involved in cytotoxicity, chemotaxis, and apoptosis. *Infect Immun*, **82**, 753–61.

Carapetis JR, *et al.* (2005). The global burden of group A streptococcal diseases. *Lancet Infect Dis*, **5**, 685–94.

Carapetis JR, McDonald M, Wilson NJ (2005). Acute rheumatic fever. *Lancet*, **366**, 155–68.

Cilliers AM (2006). Rheumatic fever and its management. *BMJ*, **333**, 1153–6.

Cilliers AM, Manyemba J, Saloojee H (2003). Anti-inflammatory treatment for carditis in acute rheumatic fever. *Cochrane Database Syst Rev*, CD003176.

Cunningham MW (2000). Pathogenesis of group A streptococcal infections. *Clin Microbiol Rev*, **13**, 470–511.

Cunningham MW (2004). T cell mimicry in inflammatory heart disease. *Mol Immunol*, **40**, 1121–7.

Dale JB, *et al.* (2013). Group A streptococcal vaccines: paving a path for accelerated development. Vaccine 18, **31 Suppl 2**, B216–22.

Gewitz MH, *et al.* (2015). Revision of the Jones criteria for the diagnosis of acute rheumatic fever in the era of Doppler echocardiography: a scientific statement from the American Heart Association Committee on Rheumatic Fever, Endocarditis, and Kawasaki Disease of the Council of Cardiovascular Disease in the Young Endorsed by the World Heart Federation. *Circulation* , **131**, 1806–18.

Hu MC, *et al.* (2002). Immunogenicity of a 26-valent group A streptococcal vaccine. *Infect Immun*, **70**, 2171–7.

Irlam J, *et al.*, (2013). Primary prevention of acute rheumatic fever and rheumatic heart disease with penicillin in South African children with pharyngitis: a cost-effectiveness analysis. *Circ Cardiovasc Qual Outcomes*, **6**, 343–51.

Kaplan EL (1993). T. Duckett Jones Memorial Lecture. Global assessment of rheumatic fever and rheumatic heart disease at the close of the century. Influences and dynamics of populations and pathogens: a failure to realize prevention? *Circulation*, **88**, 1964–72.

Karthikeyan G, Mayosi BM. (2009). Is primary prevention of rheumatic fever the missing link in the control of rheumatic heart disease in Africa? *Circulation*, **120**, 709–13.

McDonald M, Currie BJ, Carapetis JR (2004). Acute rheumatic fever: a chink in the chain that links the heart to the throat? *Lancet Infect Dis*, **4**, 240–5.

McDonald M, *et al.* (2005). Preventing recurrent rheumatic fever: the role of register-based programs. *Heart*, **91**, 1131–3.

National Heart Foundation of Australia (RF/RHD guideline development working group) and the Cardiac Society of Australia and New Zealand (2006). *Diagnosis and management of acute rheumatic fever and rheumatic heart disease in Australia—an evidence-based review*. National Heart Foundation of Australia, Melbourne.

Quinn RW (1989). Comprehensive review of morbidity and mortality trends for rheumatic fever, streptococcal disease, and scarlet fever: the decline of rheumatic fever. *Rev Infect Dis*, **11**, 928–53.

Remenyi B, *et al.* (2012). World Heart Federation criteria for echocardiographic diagnosis of rheumatic heart disease-an evidence-based guideline. *Nat Rev Cardiol*, **9**, 297–309.

RHDAustralia (ARF/RHD writing group), National Heart Foundation of Australia, and the Cardiac Society of Australia and New Zealand, (2012). *Australian guideline for prevention, diagnosis and management of acute rheumatic fever and rheumatic heart disease*, 2nd edition. Menzies School of Health Research, Darwin. 2012.

Roberts K, *et al.* (2014). Echocardiographic screening for rheumatic heart disease in high and low risk Australian children. *Circulation*, **129**, 1953–61.

Robertson KA, Volmink JA, Mayosi BM (2005). Antibiotics for the primary prevention of rheumatic fever: a meta-analysis. *BMC Cardiovasc Disord*, **5**, 11.

Seckeler MD, Hoke TR (2011) The worldwide epidemiology of acute rheumatic fever and rheumatic heart disease. *Clin Epidemiol*, **3**, 67–84.

Shulman ST, *et al.* (2012). Clinical practice guideline for the diagnosis and management of group A streptococcal pharyngitis: 2012 update by the Infectious Diseases Society of America. *Clin Infect Dis*, **55**, 1279–82.

Steer AC, *et al.* (2002). Systematic review of rheumatic heart disease prevalence in children in developing countries: the role of environmental factors. *J Paediatr Child Health*, **38**, 229–34.

Stollerman GH (2001). Rheumatic fever in the 21st century. *Clin Infect Dis*, **33**, 806–14.

Tubridy-Clark M, Carapetis JR (2007). Subclinical carditis in rheumatic fever: a systematic review. *Int J Cardiol*, **119**, 54–8.

Veasy LG, Tani LY, Hill HR (1994). Persistence of acute rheumatic fever in the intermountain area of the United States. *J Pediatr*, **124**, 9–16.

Wannamaker LW (1973). The chain that links the heart to the throat. *Circulation*, **48**, 9–18.

WHO Expert Consultation on Rheumatic Fever and Rheumatic Heart Disease (2004). *Rheumatic fever and rheumatic heart disease: report of a WHO Expert Consultation, Geneva, 29 October–1 November 2001*. WHO Technical Report Series 923, World Health Organization, Geneva.

CHAPTER 9.2

Endocarditis

James L. Harrison, Bernard D. Prendergast, and William A. Littler

Essentials

Endocarditis predominantly affects the aortic and mitral valves; involvement of the tricuspid valve occurs in approximately one-fifth of cases and pulmonary valve involvement is rare. In the developing world rheumatic heart disease is the most common predisposing factor. In developed countries endocarditis is more common in older people with native valve disease and in patients with prosthetic valves and intracardiac devices (pacemakers and defibrillators). In these countries up to 50% of cases have no predisposing cardiac lesion and more cases are related to intravenous drug abuse and nosocomial infection related to invasive procedures. Mortality remains high (30%) despite advances in antimicrobial therapy and surgery, and at least 50% of cases require valve surgery. Early diagnosis, specialist management, and timely intervention are key to successful outcome.

Clinical features

Presenting symptoms and signs include those of a bacteraemic illness, tissue destruction (heart valve(s) and adjacent structures); phenomena thought to be related to circulating immune complexes, e.g. splinter and conjunctival haemorrhages, Osler's nodes, Janeway lesions, vasculitic rash, Roth spots, and nephritis; and systemic and septic pulmonary emboli in left- and right-sided lesions respectively.

Blood culture is the most important laboratory investigation, with prolonged incubation requested in circumstances where endocarditis is strongly suspected. Serological tests can aid in the identification of organisms that are difficult to isolate. Echocardiography should be performed as soon as possible when endocarditis is suspected: its principal role is to detect vegetations, but it is not sufficiently sensitive to allow the clinician to exclude the diagnosis confidently on the basis of a negative result. Diagnosis is based on pathological criteria (demonstration of microorganisms by culture or histological examination, or histological evidence of active endocarditis) or—more usually—a combination of major and minor clinical criteria, with the major clinical criteria relating to (1) positive blood cultures of 'typical' or 'consistent' organisms, and (2) evidence of endocardial involvement detected on physical examination (new murmur) or with echocardiography.

Causes and management

Worldwide the principal causes of endocarditis are viridans streptococci (up to 58%) and *Staphylococcus aureus* (30% of community-acquired and 46% of hospital-acquired disease) with *Streptococcus*

bovis, enterococcus species, fungi, coagulase-negative staphylococci, and the HACEK group of organisms making up the remainder. However, in developed countries the epidemiological profile has changed in recent decades: rheumatic heart disease is now rare, and with more cases related to prosthetic valves (20% of all cases) device therapy and nosocomial infection, *Staph. aureus* has overtaken oral streptococci as the most common pathogen.

Best management is provided by a multidisciplinary team involving cardiologists, microbiologists, infectious disease specialists, and cardiac surgeons. Bactericidal antibiotics are the mainstay of treatment. Recommended empirical therapy for the patient with suspected native valve endocarditis is amoxicillin or ampicillin (12 g/day IV in four divided doses) plus gentamicin (1mg/kg body weight IV 8-hourly, modified according to renal function), substituting vancomycin for amoxicillin/ampicillin in patients with penicillin allergy. This should be modified to a definitive antibiotic treatment regimen when the pathogen is known. Surgery is required in about 50% of cases, with the main indications being haemodynamic instability, persistent infection, annular or aortic abscesses, and significant residual valve regurgitation once antibiotic therapy is complete.

Prevention

Until recently, antibiotic prophylaxis in at-risk patients—meaning any with a wide variety of cardiac lesions undergoing a wide variety of dental, medical, and surgical procedures—was accepted as reasonable, but there is no good evidence to support this practice. Recommendations from relevant United Kingdom, European, and American professional bodies are now much more restrictive. National Institute for Health and Clinical Excellence (United Kingdom) guidelines state that antibiotic prophylaxis should only be given to high-risk patients (including those with prosthetic cardiac valves or other prosthetic material within their hearts, previous endocarditis, and some forms of congenital heart disease) if they are undergoing a gastrointestinal or genitourinary procedure at a site where there is suspected infection. Most cardiologists feel that this is too restrictive and prefer European and American guidelines that recommend prophylaxis before dental and nondental procedures for patients at high risk.

When prophylaxis is recommended for dental and other procedures, regimens typically include amoxicillin (or clindamycin if penicillin-allergic), with the addition of gentamicin if risks are thought to be high, and substitution of vancomycin (or teicoplanin) for amoxicillin if the patient is penicillin-allergic (or has taken more than a single dose of penicillin in the previous month).

Historical background

Lazerous Riverius recorded the first case of what is now known as endocarditis in 1723. He described a French magistrate with an irregular pulse, oedema, and congestion, who at autopsy had fleshy masses 'the size of hazelnuts' obstructing the aortic ostia. Some 50 years later, Morgani (1769) made the link between infection (fulminating gonorrhoea) and 'whitish polypus concretions on the upper part of the aortic valve near its borders'.

The clinical picture of endocarditis was first described by Jean Baptiste Bouillard, in 1835: 'fever, an irregular pulse, cardiomegaly (by percussion) and a bellows murmur in the heart'. He gave the disease the name 'endocarditis', or an inflammation of the inner membrane of the heart and fibrous tissues of the valve, and was the first to use the term 'vegetations' for the valvular lesions.

Winge used the term 'mycoses endocardi' for the groups of microorganisms that he saw when he examined vegetations under the microscope in 1870. In 1886, Wyssecokowitch cultured *Staphylococcus aureus* from an endocardial vegetation. Lenthartz, in 1901, was the first to use blood cultures in the diagnosis of endocarditis. 'Infective endocarditis' was the term used by Thomas Horder, in 1901, to describe the syndrome consisting of (1) the presence of valvular disease, (2) the occurrence of systemic embolism, and (3) the discovery of microorganisms in the bloodstream.

Epidemiology

Endocarditis was universally fatal before the advent of antibiotic therapy. Despite significant advances in diagnosis and treatment, it remains a dangerous disease, particularly for people at risk (prosthetic valves, congenital heart disease, previous endocarditis), in whom morbidity and mortality approach 50%. About 200 deaths are recorded each year in the United Kingdom, but this is almost certainly an underestimate. A recent review of papers published between 1993 and 2003 found the mean age of patients varied between 36 and 69 years, the median incidence being 3.6 per 100,000 population per year (range 0.3–22.4), increasing from 5 or less per 100,000 population per year in individuals aged younger than 50 years to 15 or more per 100,000 population per year in those older than 65 years. The median in-hospital mortality rate was 16% (range 11–26%). The incidence is greater in men, in those over 65 years of age, and in those with prosthetic heart valves. In intravenous drug users, the incidence of endocarditis is estimated as 150 to 200 per 100,000 person years.

Pathogenesis

Normal vascular endothelium is resistant to microbial infection and very few patients potentially at risk actually develop endocarditis. Bacteraemia may occur spontaneously during chewing, tooth brushing, and other normal activities. Since low-grade bacteraemia occurs frequently in everyone, a defence mechanism must exist that can eradicate microbes adherent to fibrin-platelet aggregates at the site of injured endothelium. Platelets play a pivotal role in the antimicrobial host-defence mechanism and human platelets have been found to contain at least 10 different bactericidal proteins or 'thrombocidins'.

Damage to the endothelial surface of the heart or blood vessels induces platelet and fibrin deposition producing a sterile thrombotic vegetation; endocarditis is initiated by the binding of microbes, discharged into the general circulation from a peripheral site, to these vegetations. These microbes become rapidly encased in further depositions of platelets and fibrin, and multiply.

The pathogenesis of endocarditis involves complex interactions between microbes and the host-defence mechanisms, both circulating and at the site of endothelial damage. An essential step is the activation of the clotting system and the formation of a fibrin clot on the endothelial surface. Experimental evidence suggests that the main pathogens in endocarditis (streptococci and staphylococci) can bind to endothelial cells and induce functional changes within these cells causing monocyte adhesion. The endothelial cells respond to local inflammation by expressing $\beta 1$-integrins which promote the adhesion of pathogens that carry fibronectin-binding proteins on their surface. The combination of damaged endothelial cells, bacteria, and endothelial bound monocytes results in the induction of tissue-factor-dependent procoagulant activity which initiates clot formation. Polymorphonuclear leucocytes which are recruited to the infected endothelial site may be subsequently involved in the disease progression, with the contents of lysosomes released by the activated leucocytes probably causing softening and separation of valve tissue, leading to its destruction.

In endocarditis, the vegetations are found predominately on the left side of the heart (85%). In a large autopsy series of more than 1000 cases reported over 50 years ago, the mitral valve was involved in 86%, the aortic in 55%, the tricuspid in 20%, and the pulmonary valve in only 1%. The predominance of left-sided lesions has led to the belief that the higher pressures and velocities encountered in the left side of the heart and the proximal aorta must impose a greater mechanical stress on the valves and endocardium, which in turn leads to local damage.

Endocarditis is classically associated with 'jet lesions', where blood flowing from a high-pressure area through an orifice to an area of lower pressure produces a high-velocity jet. Vegetations are usually found in the lower-pressure area, e.g. on the atrial surface of the mitral valve in mitral regurgitation, or the ventricular surface of the aortic valve in aortic regurgitation. This particular deposition of vegetations has been explained on the basis of the Venturi effect.

Once a vegetation is established, it determines the subsequent clinical picture by four basic processes: bacteraemia, local tissue destruction, embolization, and the formation of circulating immune complexes.

Clinical features

Early reports of endocarditis described a low-grade, febrile illness caused by viridans streptococci from the mouth in a patient with chronic rheumatic heart disease. Night sweats, anorexia, and weight loss were followed by the development of splinter haemorrhages and Osler nodes, finger clubbing, and splenomegaly. The infection progressed relentlessly with increasing cachexia, and the patient died from cardiac failure or a major embolic episode. The term 'subacute bacterial endocarditis' was used to describe this illness. 'Acute or malignant endocarditis' described an aggressive form of the disease, usually caused by *Staph. aureus* or other virulent bacteria.

During the past 50 years, there has been a striking change in the pattern of endocarditis. The proportion of patients in developed countries with endocarditis who have no known pre-existing cardiac lesion has risen to almost 50%. This change is related both to the decline in rheumatic heart disease and to the increase in extracardiac predisposing factors, including intravenous drug abuse, haemodialysis, and the use of intravascular devices. Prosthetic heart valves are an important predisposing factor and cardiac surgery for complex congenital lesions has increased the lifespan of patients who would previously have died prematurely. Antibiotic-resistant organisms have emerged. The longevity of the populations of developed countries has resulted in an increasing age of patients with endocarditis, with mean age rising from under 40 years before 1940, to 60–70 years today.

For the general physician the diagnosis of endocarditis is dependent upon a high index of suspicion. In the elderly population with a high incidence of degenerative valvular disease an early presentation of endocarditis may often be misdiagnosed and treated as a urinary or upper respiratory tract infection with an incidental finding of a heart murmur. Routine investigation with blood cultures of all patients with a history of valvular heart disease presenting with fever, sepsis, or malaise is therefore recommended.

Features of a bacteraemic illness

Discharge of the infecting agent into the circulation produces constant bacteraemia which may present as pyrexia, rigors, malaise, anorexia, headache, confusion, arthralgia, and anaemia. Some cases of endocarditis, particularly in older people, may present without fever.

Features of tissue destruction

Endocarditis initially affects valve cusps, leaflets, or chordae tendineae. Tissue destruction results in valvular incompetence, cusp perforation, or rupture of the chordae, producing an appropriate cardiac murmur that may change in character during the course of the illness: 80% of patients present with a murmur, and 15–20% develop one during their hospital stay. Large vegetations rarely obstruct a native valve, but mechanical obstruction of prosthetic valves is more common and clinically more difficult to detect.

As the infective process progresses, it may extend beyond the valve into the paravalvular structures. Aortic root abscess is a serious complication: extension through the aortic wall into other tissues or cavities can create a fistula or pseudoaneurysm. Particular problems can include the development of a sinus of Valsalva aneurysm and involvement of the coronary ostia. Septal abscesses can lead to progressive conduction defects evidenced by prolongation of the PR interval on the electrocardiogram (ECG) and, eventually, complete heart block.

Paravalvular abscess is more common in native aortic valve endocarditis than in mitral valve infection. Infection of a mechanical valve involves the sewing ring and may lead to valve dehiscence. In the case of a mechanical aortic valve, where infection is often localized to the junction between the sewing ring and the aortic annulus, a large false aneurysm may develop in this area. Free-wall myocardial abscesses may rupture and cause sudden death.

Features of systemic or pulmonary emboli

Fragments of an infected vegetation may be dislodged into the systemic or pulmonary circulation, producing emboli in 20–40% of cases (up to 50% reported in autopsy series). These may lodge in any part of the circulation and present as a cerebrovascular accident, limb arterial occlusion, myocardial infarction, sudden unilateral blindness, or infarction of the spleen or a kidney. Septic embolism from the left side of the heart may result in the formation of a cerebral abscess. In right heart endocarditis, recurrent septic pulmonary emboli may be misinterpreted as 'pneumonia'.

Mycotic aneurysms arise from embolism of the vasa vasorum that weakens the arterial wall: these have been reported in almost 3% of clinical cases but are found in up to 15% at autopsy. In the cerebral circulation, such aneurysms may produce subarachnoid haemorrhage or intracerebral haemorrhage. The popliteal artery is also a common site for mycotic aneurysms.

Emboli are characteristic of *Staph. aureus* infections and large emboli are a feature in HACEK and fungal endocarditis. They usually occur before or within the first few days after starting antimicrobial therapy. Anterior mitral valve-leaflet vegetations are more likely to embolize than aortic valve vegetations, especially if they are highly mobile. Vegetation size does not predict systemic embolism, but large vegetations (>10 mm) are associated with poor overall outcome.

After an embolic complication, recurrent episodes are likely to follow, especially if vegetations persist on echocardiography. In more than 50% of cases, such recurrence occurs within 30 days of the first episode. The risk of embolism falls rapidly after the initiation of antibiotic therapy but is not reduced by treatment with anticoagulants or antiplatelet therapy: both may increase the risk of bleeding and should be avoided unless they are essential.

Features of circulating immune complexes

The infected vegetation acts as an antigen that triggers an immune response. Chronic antigenaemia stimulates generalized hypergammagloblinaemia such that after several weeks of infection a variety of autoantibodies can be detected. Immune complex deposition probably causes many of the extracardiac manifestations of endocarditis, but these classical signs are relatively uncommon and frequently absent in acute presentations.

- Splinter haemorrhages (5–15% of cases)—found in the nail bed of the fingers and, less commonly, the toes (Fig. 9.2.1).
- Conjunctival haemorrhages.
- Osler's nodes (5–10% of cases)—transient painful erythematous nodules that are found at the ends of fingers and toes and the thenar and hypothenar eminences which may be due to minute infected emboli rather than immune complex deposition (Fig. 9.2.2).
- Janeway lesions—irregular painless erythematous macules found in roughly the same distribution as Osler's nodes (Fig. 9.2.3); they tend to blanch with pressure.
- Vasculitic rash— due to immunoglobulin and complement deposits in the walls of skin capillaries (Fig. 9.2.4).
- Roth spots (5% of cases)—boat-shaped haemorrhages in the retina are often called Roth spots, but true Roth spots are white retinal exudates that may be surrounded by haemorrhage that consist of perivascular lymphocyte collections.

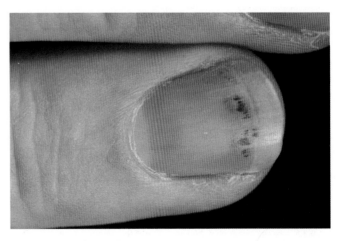

Fig. 9.2.1 Splinter haemorrhages.

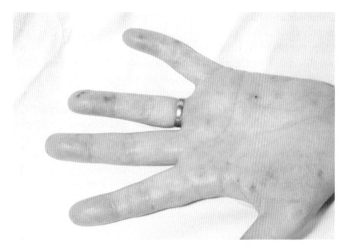

Fig. 9.2.2 Osler's nodes involving the fingers and the thenar and hypothenar eminences.

- Splenomegaly—clinical splenomegaly is less common than was reported in earlier literature (20% of cases); however, abdominal CT scanning demonstrates splenomegaly in at least 50% of cases, often with associated splenic infarcts (Fig. 9.2.5). Splenic abscesses may occur and splenic rupture can be fatal.

- Nephritis (10–15% of cases)—immune complexes can cause glomerulonephritis, manifest as proteinuria, haematuria, and decline in renal function, with immunoglobulin and complement deposition within glomeruli on renal biopsy. Key investigations are simple dipstick testing of the urine (with microscopy if more than 1+ positive for blood and/or protein) and measurement of serum creatinine.

- Arthralgia—joint manifestations may result from immune complex deposition in the synovial membrane.

Other features

Up to 30% of patients with endocarditis present with neurological symptoms: these are most common in staphylococcal infection, in which one-third present with the clinical features of meningitis. Headaches, confusion, and toxic psychosis can be present as well as encephalomyelitis. It is not certain whether some of these

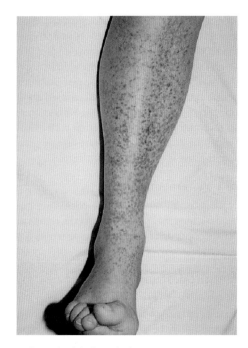

Fig. 9.2.4 Vasculitic rash of the lower limb.

neurological manifestations result from repeated small emboli or from a vasculitic process within the cerebral circulation as a consequence of immune complex deposition. The cerebrospinal fluid can show an increase in white cells, but is usually sterile on culture. Very occasionally it may be positive for staphylococcal infection.

Although immune-mediated glomerulonephritis has been regarded as the typical renal lesion of endocarditis, this assumption was based on small series predating modern treatment regimens. More recent work indicates that the most common histological finding is renal infarction. Circulatory compromise can rarely cause severe renal impairment as a result of renal cortical necrosis.

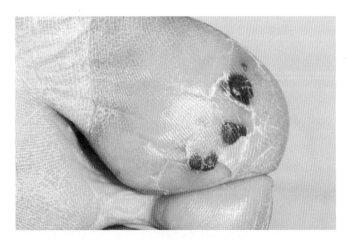

Fig. 9.2.3 Janeway lesions on the under surface of the left big toe.

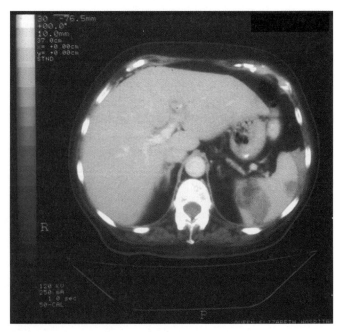

Fig. 9.2.5 CT scan showing multiple splenic infarcts within an enlarged spleen.

Finger clubbing is one of the classical features of endocarditis, usually seen after 1 or 2 months of the illness. It is seldom seen now, but when present is still a useful sign because it rarely occurs in conditions with which endocarditis can be confused.

Specific types or circumstances of endocarditis

Prosthetic valve endocarditis

Patients with prosthetic heart valves have a small, but constant, risk of endocarditis, estimated at 0.2–1.4 events per 100 patient years. The incidence of prosthetic valve endocarditis is about 3% in the first postoperative year, with the highest risk during the first 3 months. Prosthetic valve endocarditis is five times more common in the aortic area than the mitral area and may involve mechanical, xenograft, and homograft valves.

Prosthetic valve endocarditis has been classified as early or late according to its temporal relationship to surgery. Early prosthetic valve endocarditis usually occurs within 60 days of open heart surgery and accounts for 30% of cases. It is caused either by contamination of the prosthetic valve at implantation or by perioperative bacteraemia from intravenous catheters, arterial lines, urethral catheters, or endotracheal tubes. The most common organisms are coagulase-negative staphylococci.

Late prosthetic valve endocarditis accounts for 70% of cases and usually occurs 60 days or more after surgery. The pathogens are those seen in native valve endocarditis, with a preponderance of viridans streptococci and staphylococci, but with a higher incidence of other organisms. Some patients with late prosthetic valve endocarditis will have acquired the infection at the time of surgery, but a bacteraemia is usually the principal cause.

Bacteraemia in a patient with a prosthetic valve must always be taken seriously, but it may not always be the result of endocarditis. The clinical picture of prosthetic valve endocarditis is typically fever, malaise, and weakness, with the more classical signs usually absent. The condition is often insidious and clinically difficult to diagnose. A new murmur may appear, and heart failure and embolic phenomena cause high mortality (20–50%). Infection in a mechanical valve is located in the sewing ring, from which the infection can spread into the host tissues producing annular/myocardial abscesses, paravalvular leak, and prosthetic dehiscence. Infection of a tissue valve usually involves the valve leaflets, resulting in destruction or perforation and valvular incompetence. Vegetations may cause obstruction with all forms of prosthetic valve.

The diagnosis of prosthetic valve endocarditis requires a high index of clinical suspicion, blood cultures, and transoesophageal echocardiography, which is far superior to the transthoracic approach for detecting vegetations and identifying periprosthetic spread of infection. Vegetations are more difficult to identify in patients with mechanical valves than those with bioprostheses.

Right-sided endocarditis

Right-sided endocarditis accounts for only 5% of cases overall, but centres that treat large numbers of intravenous drug users will have a higher incidence. The clinical picture differs significantly from left-sided disease. It is usually associated with intravenous drug addiction or indwelling intravascular devices, including pacemakers, implantable defibrillators, central venous lines of all types, and septal occluder devices. *Staph. aureus* is the most common pathogen and the tricuspid

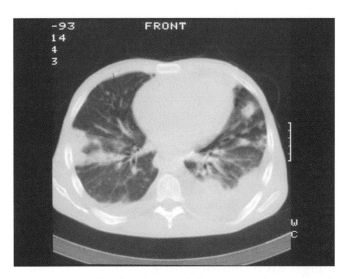

Fig. 9.2.6 CT scan of the chest showing multiple pulmonary infarcts in a case of right-sided endocarditis of the tricuspid valve in an intravenous drug abuser.

valve is more commonly affected (80%) than the pulmonary valve. Fever is almost always present and a cardiac murmur is found in 80% of cases. There may be septic pulmonary emboli (Fig. 9.2.6) and the resultant pulmonary infarcts may cavitate. Symptoms include cough, haemoptysis, and pleuritic chest pain; a chest radiograph shows pulmonary infiltrates, which are often misinterpreted as 'patches of pneumonia'. Renal involvement (most commonly abscess formation or diffuse pyelonephritis) has been described in over one-half of cases. Myocarditis is more common in right-sided involvement than left. Peripheral stigmata, splenomegaly, and central nervous system involvement are rare (no more than 5% of cases). Death is most commonly due to sepsis, rarely to heart failure.

Endocarditis in intravenous drug users

Endocarditis is a serious complication of intravenous drug abuse. The right side of the heart is affected most commonly, but the left may also be involved in a substantial number of patients (37%), and both right and left side in a few (7%). On the left side, mitral and aortic valves are equally infected. A history of previous heart disease is found only in some 25% of cases.

Staph. aureus is responsible for 40% of all cases. Gram-negative bacilli are next most frequent, *Pseudomonas aeruginosa* and *Serratia marcescens* accounting for most of these. Candida can cause endocarditis in intravenous drug users, and polymicrobial endocarditis accounts for 5% of cases.

The skin is the most common site from which pathogens enter the bloodstream via needles. Gram-negative bacilli are rarely recovered from needles or the drug itself, and it has been suggested that these organisms come from tap water, sinks, or lavatory pans.

The clinical picture of endocarditis associated with intravenous drug use depends on which side of the heart is affected. Right-sided disease is described above; left-sided disease behaves like that seen in non-drug cases, with a high incidence of heart failure, arterial embolism, central nervous system involvement, and peripheral stigmata.

The overall mortality depends on when the patient presents: it is high if they present late, reflecting among other things the frequent difficulty in dealing with addicts because of their poor compliance and reluctance to discontinue their drug habit. The principles of management are similar to those in patients who are not drug users. The duration of intravenous antibiotics should be at least 4 weeks, but this is frequently impossible in practice. Furthermore, there are often legitimate concerns regarding the risk of reinfection of a prosthetic valve and surgery requires very careful consideration in this patient group.

Endocarditis in children

Endocarditis does occur in children but is rare, especially in the first decade of life. In the early literature, tetralogy of Fallot was the cardiac problem most commonly associated with endocarditis. Complex cyanotic disease, congenital heart disease corrected with prosthetic material, and small ventricular septal defects now make up the bulk of cases.

Diagnosis of endocarditis

Laboratory methods

Blood culture

This is the most important laboratory investigation in the diagnosis of endocarditis (Table 9.2.1). Isolation of the pathogen enables an effective antibiotic treatment regimen to be devised. Optimal technique is necessary to avoid false-positive cases due to contaminating skin organisms. The recommended regimen for obtaining blood cultures is that three sets of blood cultures should be taken from a separate venepuncture sites over 24h at least 1h apart, with at least 10ml of blood injected into one aerobic and one anaerobic culture bottle. Blood cultures should be taken before antibiotics are given; if they have already been given, cultures should still be done and, if possible, the administration of further antibiotics delayed for a few days. However, previous antibiotics may render the blood sterile for some time, and the chances of recovering the pathogen, particularly when it is a sensitive organism such as viridans streptococcus, are very low. Much mystique has been attached to the number and timing of blood cultures in cases of suspected endocarditis. What is known is that the bacteraemia is usually constant and in most cases all bottles will grow the pathogen whenever the blood is obtained for culture and however many sets are taken. There are, of course, rare exceptions when only a few bottles taken are positive, and this is one reason why it is conventional to take three sets. Another reason for several cultures is to assess the relevance of the common skin contaminants (particularly coagulase-negative staphylococci and corynebacterium) that can cause endocarditis.

In most laboratories, blood culture systems are automated, with continuous monitoring to flag up growth for further investigation. Most cultures become positive within 48h and after this the chances of isolating the pathogen recede (with the exception of fastidious organisms of the HACEK group that may take much longer to recover). In most laboratories, blood cultures are incubated for 5–7 days, but this may not be long enough for the rare fastidious slow grower. The onus is on the clinical microbiologist or clinician to request prolonged incubation for blood cultures from patients in whom endocarditis is strongly suspected, who have not had previous antibiotics, and whose blood cultures are sterile after a week's incubation.

Other routine blood tests

In endocarditis, an elevated erythrocyte sedimentation rate (ESR) and C-reactive protein (CRP) are almost invariable, and these inflammatory markers are used most commonly to monitor the activity of the disease. A normochromic normocytic anaemia is often present and a polymorphonuclear leucocytosis is found in most cases. Hypergammaglobulinaemia and a low serum complement may be present, together with a false-positive rheumatoid factor. Circulating immune complexes may be detected.

Serological tests aid in the identification of organisms that are difficult to isolate, including bartonella, coxiella (Q fever), chlamydia, mycoplasma, legionella, brucella, and fungi. Candida antibodies are of no diagnostic value.

Echocardiography

In suspected cases of endocarditis, transthoracic echocardiography should be performed as soon as possible and interpreted by an experienced cardiologist. Its principal role is to detect vegetations (Fig. 9.2.7), but it is not sufficiently sensitive to allow the clinician to exclude the diagnosis confidently on the basis of a negative result. The sensitivity depends on the size of the vegetations and the time course of the disease: it can resolve vegetations as small as 1–2 mm, but confident identification is more difficult with prosthetic than native valves and more difficult with mechanical than biological prostheses.

Vegetations appear as thick, ragged, non-uniform echoes oscillating on or around a cardiac valve or in the path of a regurgitant jet. They need to be differentiated from other conditions which produce echo-density on cardiac valves, including calcification, myxomatous degeneration, and atrial myxoma. Vegetations do not usually restrict leaflet mobility and exhibit valve-dependent motion. On native valves, vegetations are usually attached to the ventricular side of the aortic valve and the atrial side of the mitral and tricuspid valves (Fig. 9.2.8). Vegetations tend to be larger on the right side and can be demonstrated in 80–100% of cases.

Transoesophageal echocardiography improves the rate of diagnosis of endocarditis over that of transthoracic echocardiography, particularly in the presence of a prosthetic valve. It also makes it easier to recognize many complications of prosthetic valve endocarditis, such as abscesses, fistulae, and paravalvular leak.

Examination of the heart valve and other tissues

Histology

Histology remains the gold standard for explanted valves. When valve replacement is undertaken, valvular tissue (including vegetation) should be examined histologically and cultured for the presence of microorganisms, which may allow postoperative antibiotics to be tailored accordingly. However, the isolation of microorganisms by valvular culture is infrequent: only 15% in one large series, with staphylococci being most common. Fastidious and rare microorganisms have been demonstrated on heart valves by various staining techniques and, more recently using tissue polymerase chain reaction techniques.

Nucleic acid-based techniques

Polymerase chain reaction techniques are now widely used for samples obtained from heart valves, vegetations, and embolic tissue in patients with suspected endocarditis. The intention is to allow identification of the infecting microorganism when blood cultures are negative due to prior antibiotic therapy, or the causative organism is fastidious or cannot be cultured. This is not yet routine practice for the following reasons: (1) bacterial DNA is present within heart

Table 9.2.1 Microbiological diagnosis of endocarditis

Organism	Estimated incidence	Relevant clinical history	Blood cultures	Serology
Staphylococcus aureus	30% of community community-acquired 46% of hospital-acquired	IVDU/IV access devices	Usually positive	Under development (lipid S)
Coagulase-negative staphylococci	5% of native valve endocarditis	Vasectomy/angiography/ haemodialysis/IVDU	Usually positive	In progress
Viridans streptococci	Up to 58%	Dental abscess/poor oral hygiene	Positive, if no previous antibiotics	In progress
Streptococcus bovis	Up to 12%	Gastrointestinal malignancy/ presumed normal heart valves/ older patient population	Positive, if no previous antibiotics	None
HACEK	3%	Dental treatment/URTI/IVDU	Most positive in 6 days with high CO_2 concentrations	None
Fungal	Up to 10%	Prosthetic valves/IVDU/ immunosuppression/long-term IV lines Should be performed if multiple risk factors for fungal endocarditis	Filamentous fungi rarely positive, candida commonly positive	Fungal serology not validated for endocarditis
Enterococcus spp.	Up to 10%	Urinary catheter insertion/ gastrointestinal malignancy	Positive, if no previous antibiotics	In progress
Brucella spp.	1–4%	Endemic area/contaminated milk consumption	Positive in 80%. May need prolonged incubation	Reference assay = tube agglutination
Coxiella burnetii (Q fever)	3–5%	Farming background/exposure to domestic ruminants/raw milk consumption/previous valvulopathy/endemic area	Rarely positive. Tissue cell culture reported as optimal method	Major criteria for modified Duke criteria: Anti-phase 1 IgG >800 and IgA antibody >100 is highly sensitive Reference assay = microimmunofluorescence
Bartonella	Up to 3%	Homelessness/alcoholism/ exposure to cats	Rarely positive	Reference assay = microimmunofluorescence
Legionella	<1%	Usually an outbreak/institution Role unclear for prosthetic valves/pneumonia	Rarely positive IE. Urinary antigen. Bronchial washings/sputum	High antibody levels Reference assay = microimmunofluorescence
Chlamydia	Unknown due to cross-reactivity with bartonella	Pneumonia Significance is controversial	Rarely positive. Needs tissue cell culture	Cross-reaction with *Bartonella* spp. Reference assay = microimmunofluorescence

IV, intravenous; IVDU, intravenous drug use; URTI, upper respiratory tract infection.

Reprinted from *Journal of Infection*, Vol 47, Watkin et al., The microbial diagnosis of infective endocarditis, pp. 1–11. Copyright (2003), with permission from Elsevier.

valves for many months and possibly years following successful treatment; (2) contamination of samples with any bacterial DNA leads to false-positive results; (3) false-negative results can occur due to polymerase chain reaction inhibitory factors present within blood and other bodily fluid.

Criteria for the diagnosis of endocarditis

In 1994, Durack and colleagues introduced criteria for the diagnosis of endocarditis that have been accepted as the 'Duke criteria' and categorize patients into definite, possible, and rejected groups. Although these criteria have been shown to be superior to previous diagnostic tools, they have limitations: in particular, there is a possibility of misclassification when blood cultures remain negative or

echocardiography is inconclusive. Negative blood cultures occur in 5 to 31% of cases of endocarditis, commonly due to prior antibiotic therapy, but also as a result of infection with fastidious and atypical microorganisms. Transthoracic echocardiography visualizes vegetations in only about 50% of cases: transoesophageal echocardiography has a higher sensitivity for detection on both native and prosthetic valves, but will only be diagnostic in 50–94% of cases. These issues mean that the number of patients who may be incorrectly diagnosed as having possible endocarditis, as opposed to definite, could be as high as 24%.

Modification of the Duke criteria to increase their sensitivity has been suggested by several authors (Table 9.2.2). Positive serology for typical microorganisms and the use of polymerase chain reaction

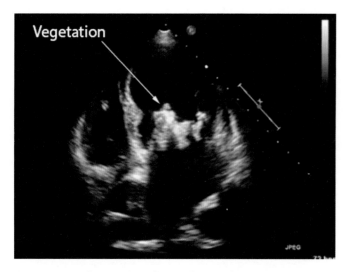

Fig. 9.2.7 A transthoracic echocardiogram showing a large vegetation involving the mitral valve.

techniques have been suggested as major criteria, and the following additional minor criteria have been proposed—newly diagnosed clubbing, splenomegaly, splinter haemorrhages and petechiae, microscopic haematuria, a high ESR or CRP, and the presence of central nonfeeding lines and peripheral lines.

Microbiology

Although almost any microorganism can cause endocarditis, particularly when this involves a prosthetic valve, certain species do so much more commonly than others. The predominant species involved in the infection have not changed significantly in their incidence in the past three decades. Overall, viridans streptococci and staphylococci account for about two-thirds of cases. However, endocarditis cannot be considered as a microbiologically homogeneous entity as the incidence of any specific organism depends (1) on the patient, whether an intravenous drug user or not; (2) on the valve, whether native or prosthetic—and if native, whether previously abnormal or not, and if prosthetic whether mechanical or a bioprosthesis, and whether the infection was acquired early or late; and (3) where (and how) the infection was acquired,

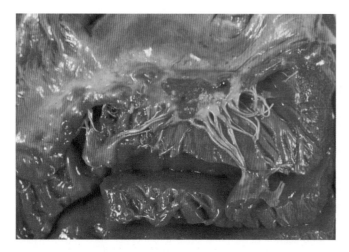

Fig. 9.2.8 Bacterial vegetations on the mitral valve—the patient had died as a result of a large cerebral embolism.

whether in the community or (as increasingly these days) in hospital, usually via an infected intravascular device.

The more common species encountered are considered individually.

Streptococci

The genus *Streptococcus* includes species of differing virulence and pathogenicity as well as differing normal habitat in humans.

Viridans streptococci

For many years, it has been conventional to refer to a group of streptococci that produce greening (α-haemolysis) on blood agar as viridans streptococci; indeed, many still refer (inaccurately) to a microbe 'Streptococcus viridans'. Although most of these streptococci are virtually specific to the normal oropharyngeal flora and are rarely encountered at other sites, some are not found in the oropharynx at all, e.g. *Strep. bovis*, and others are found at many sites including the oropharynx, e.g. the milleri group of streptococci. The most common species of the viridans streptococci specific to the oropharynx are *Strep. sanguis*, *Strep. oralis*, and *Strep. mutans*, but there are others. Dextran formation may be a virulence factor in these streptococci. Contrary to popular belief, they do not require a dental extraction to enter the bloodstream and cause frequent bacteraemias after chewing, tooth brushing, etc. They are organisms of low virulence and thus usually only infect previously abnormal heart valves. Whereas *Strep. oralis* and *Strep. sanguis* are occasionally isolated from blood cultures of patients who do not have endocarditis, the isolation of *Strep. mutans* from the blood is virtually synonymous with endocarditis.

Streptococcus bovis

This streptococcus, which may appear 'viridans' on blood agar, is part of the normal intestinal flora, but may initially be mistaken for an oral streptococcus. In common with the enterococci, it bears the Lancefield group D antigen and thus can also be mistaken for *Enterococcus faecalis*, though it is sensitive to penicillin whereas the latter is resistant. There is a significant association between *Strep. bovis* bacteraemia (and hence endocarditis) and colonic pathology, and any patient with *Strep. bovis* endocarditis thus warrants appropriate investigation. *Strep. bovis* endocarditis is much less common than that caused by oral streptococci.

Pyogenic streptococci

These organisms, often referred to as β-haemolytic streptococci, cause endocarditis less frequently than the viridans streptococci, but are more aggressive microbes and likely to affect (and often rapidly destroy) a previously normal valve. The commonest pyogenic streptococcus to cause endocarditis is the Lancefield group B β-haemolytic streptococcus (GBS), sometimes referred to as *Strep. agalactiae*. This organism is found as normal flora in the genital and gastrointestinal tracts. As with *Staph. aureus*, any patient with community-acquired group B β-haemolytic streptococcus bacteraemia should be assumed to have infection in bone, joint, or on a heart valve until proved otherwise. Groups C and G β-haemolytic streptococci occasionally cause endocarditis, and group A even more rarely. The milleri group of streptococci are best regarded as pyogenic streptococci: they form part of the normal flora of all mucous membranes and occasionally cause endocarditis, though much more often cause abscesses at many different sites. The milleri group consists of three species, *Strep. constellatus*, *Strep. intermedius*, and *Strep. anginosus*.

Table 9.2.2 Duke criteria for the diagnosis of endocarditis and proposed modifications

Duke criteria	Suggested modifications
Pathological criteria	
Microorganisms demonstrated by culture or histological examination	
Active endocarditis demonstrated by histological examination	
Major criteria	
Positive blood cultures	To be added:
Typical microorganisms consistent with endocarditis from two separate blood cultures	Positive serology for *Coxiella burnetii*
Microorganisms consistent with endocarditis from persistently positive blood cultures	Bacteraemia due to *Staph. aureus*
	Positive molecular assay for specific gene targets and universal loci for bacteria and fungi
	Positive serology for *Chlamydia psittaci*
	Positive serology for *Bartonella* spp.
Evidence of endocardial involvement	
Echocardiography—oscillating structures, abscess formation, new partial dehiscence of prosthetic valve	
Clinical—new valvar regurgitation	
Minor criteria	
Predisposing heart disease	To be omitted:
Fever >38 °C	Suspect echocardiography (no major criterion)
Vascular phenomena	To be added:
Immunological phenomena	Elevated CRP, elevated ESR, splenomegaly, haematuria, clubbing, splinter haemorrhages, petechiae, purpura
Microbiological evidence (no major criterion)	Identified IE organism from metastatic lesions
Suspect echocardiography (no major criterion)	
Categories	
Definite:	
Pathological criteria positive	
or 2 major criteria positive	
or 1 major and 2 minor criteria positive	1 major and 1 minor criterion positive
or 5 minor criteria positive	3 minor criteria positive
Possible:	
All cases which cannot be classified as definite or rejected	
Rejected:	
Alternative diagnosis	
Resolution of the infection with antibiotic treatment for <4 days	
No histological evidence	

CRP, C-reactive protein; ESR, erythrocyte sedimentation rate.

Reproduced from *Heart*, Prendergast B. D, Vol 92, pp. 879–885. The changing face of infective endocarditis. Copyright (2006) with permission from BMJ Publishing Group Ltd.

Streptococcus pneumoniae (pneumococcus)

Pneumococcal endocarditis accounted for about 10% of cases of endocarditis in the pre-antibiotic era, but is now rarely seen, although it is sometimes diagnosed at autopsy of patients with fatal pneumococcal infection. The pneumococcus is a virulent pathogen and attacks normal heart valves. Patients with endocarditis generally have pneumonia and sometimes meningitis.

Enterococci

Enterococci form part of the normal gastrointestinal flora. They are more virulent than viridans streptococci and more resistant to antibiotics. The incidence of enterococcal endocarditis is increasing, particularly in older people, but this infection is still much less common than that caused by viridans streptococci. Whilst there are many species of enterococci, those causing endocarditis are usually

E. faecalis and occasionally *E. faecium*. Most cases are community acquired, but the infection can sometimes be acquired in hospital as a result of urological instrumentation. Any patient admitted from the community with *E. faecalis* in the blood should be investigated for endocarditis.

Staphylococci

Staphylococci now account for about one-third of cases of community-acquired endocarditis and are the most common cause of hospital-acquired endocarditis. Most of these staphylococci are *Staph. aureus*, but an increasing proportion are now coagulase-negative staphylococci. All staphylococci are skin organisms and patients become infected from their own skin flora, or in the case of meticillin-resistant *Staph. aureus* (MRSA) from that of others by cross-infection.

Staphylococcus aureus

Staph. aureus is an important and aggressive pathogen in community-acquired native valve endocarditis. Sometimes a trivial skin lesion can be identified as the source of the organism, but there is often no obvious lesion. *Staph. aureus*, and increasingly now MRSA, is the most common cause of hospital-acquired endocarditis. Prosthetic valves can become infected with *Staph. aureus*, both early as result of sternal wound sepsis and late as with native valves. *Staph. aureus* is the commonest pathogen causing endocarditis in intravenous drug users.

Coagulase-negative staphylococci

Although still regarded by many as pathogens of prosthetic rather than native valves, coagulase-negative staphylococci also cause native valve infection. This has become more common, or certainly more commonly recognized, in the last two decades. The infecting species is most often *Staph. epidermidis*, but in many reports the designation '*Staph. epidermidis*' tends to be used for any unspecified coagulase-negative staphylococcus. As in community-acquired *Staph. aureus* endocarditis, there is sometimes a presumptive predisposing skin lesion. Most patients have a pre-existing cardiac abnormality. Many of these staphylococci (particularly *Staph. lugdunensis*) can be as virulent as *Staph. aureus* and share some of the same virulence factors.

Other organisms

A wide variety of organisms account for the few cases of endocarditis that are not caused by streptococci, staphylococci, or enterococci: only a few warrant specific mention.

HACEK group

These are fastidious, slow-growing species that are oropharyngeal commensals and have a predilection for heart valves such that their presence in blood cultures is virtually synonymous with this infection. The group consists of *Haemophilus aphrophilus/paraphrophilus*, *Actinobacillus actinomycetemcomitans*, *Cardiobacterium hominis*, *Eikenella corrodens*, and *Kingella kingae*. *A. actinomycetmecomitans*, in particular, seems more likely to infect prosthetic

Table 9.2.3 Recommendations for empirical therapy of suspected endocarditis

Antimicrobial	Dose/route	Comment
1. NVE—indolent presentation		
Amoxicillin[a] AND (optional)	2 g q4h IV	If patient is stable, ideally await blood cultures
		Better activity against enterococci and many HACEK microorganisms compared with benzylpenicillin
		Use Regimen 2 if genuine penicillin allergy
Gentamicin[a]	1 mg/kg ABW	The role of gentamicin is controversial before culture results are available
2. NVE, severe sepsis (no risk factors for Enterobacteriaceae, *Pseudomonas*)		
Vancomycin[a] AND	Dosed according to local guidelines	In severe sepsis, staphylococci (including) need to be covered
		If allergic to vancomycin, replace with daptomycin 6 mg/kg q24h IV
Gentamicin[a]	1 mg/kg IBW q12h IV	If there are concerns about nephrotoxicity/acute kidney injury, use ciprofloxacin in place of gentamicin[a]
3. NVE, severe sepsis AND risk factors for multiresistant Enterobacteriaceae, *Pseudomonas*		
Vancomycin[a] AND	Dosed according to local guidelines, IV	Will provide cover against staphylococci (including MRSA), streptococci, enterococci, HACEK, Enterobacteriaceae and *P. aeruginosa*
Meropenem[a]	2 g q8h IV	
4. PVE pending blood cultures or with negative blood cultures		
Vancomycin[a] AND	1 g q12h IV	
Gentamicin[a] AND	1 mg/kg q12h IV	
Rifampicin[a]	300–600 mg q12h po/IV	Use lower dose of rifampicin in severe renal impairment

ABW, actual body weight; IBW, ideal body weight; IV, intravenous; MRSA, meticillin-resistant staphylococci; NVE, native valve endocarditis; PVE, prosthetic valve endocarditis; po, orally; q4h, every 4 h; q8h, every 8 h; q12h, every 12 h.

[a] Doses require adjustment according to renal function.

Gould et al. (2012). Guidelines for the antibiotic treatment of endocarditis in adults: report of the Working Party of the British Society for Antimicrobial Chemotherapy. *Antimicrob Chemother*, **67**, 269–89. Reproduced with permission from the British Society for Antimicrobial Chemotherapy.

than native valves. The large vegetations thought to be characteristic of HACEK organisms in native valve infection may be the result of diagnostic delay and prolonged illness rather than any inherent property of the microbes.

Organisms that cannot be cultured by routine techniques

Endocarditis is a rare (and late) sequel of acute *Coxiella burnetii* (Q fever) infection, mostly in middle-aged men with pre-existing valve disease. The reservoir of the organism is usually sheep or cattle, but the source and mode of transmission in many cases is unknown. The diagnosis is usually made serologically, although *C. burnetii* can be recovered from the blood and excised valves by special techniques. The disease is almost certainly underdiagnosed, with some cases labelled culture-negative endocarditis.

Bartonella infection is usually diagnosed by serology, although these bacteria can be recovered from the blood and excised valves by special culture techniques and their presence detected by polymerase chain reaction.

Fungi

Fungal endocarditis is very rare and more likely to occur on prosthetic than native valves, except in intravenous drug users. Most cases are hospital-acquired and associated with infection at intravascular access sites and prior use of broad-spectrum antibiotics. Candida species, usually *Candida albicans*, are the most common fungi, but aspergillus and more exotic genera have also been reported. Blood cultures are only likely to be positive with candida, and often only intermittently; for other fungi, the diagnosis must be made by serology and culture of the fungus from the excised valve or detection on valve histology.

Culture-negative endocarditis

The possibility that an illness is not due to endocarditis should always be entertained when blood cultures are repeatedly negative. However, the blood cultures will be negative in 5 to 31% of definite cases of endocarditis. The most common explanation for this is previous administration of antibiotics. In a few cases the pathogen will be recovered from another site, including the excised valve, excised emboli, or—specifically in right-sided endocarditis—respiratory specimens. Other causes of negative blood cultures are infection with organisms that cannot be grown by conventional blood culture methods, and infections that are diagnosed by serology such as *C. burnetii*, bartonella, and chlamydia.

Table 9.2.4 Summary of treatment options for streptococcal endocarditis

Regimen	Antimicrobial	Dose and route	Duration (weeks)	Comment
Treatment options for streptococci (penicillin MIC ≤0.125 mg/litre)				
1.	Benzylpenicillin[a] monotherapy	1.2g q4h IV	4–6	Preferred narrow-spectrum regimen, particularly for patients at risk of *C. difficile* or high risk of nephrotoxicity
2.	Ceftriaxone monotherapy	2g once a day IV/IM	4–6	Not advised for patients at risk of *C. difficile* infection; suitable for OPAT
3.	Benzylpenicillin[a] AND	1.2g q4h IV	2	Not advised for patients with PVE, extracardiac foci of infection, any indications for surgery, high risk of nephrotoxicity or at risk of *C. difficile*
	Gentamicin	1mg/kg q12h IV	2	
4.	Ceftriaxone AND	2g once a day IV/IM	2	Not advised for patients with PVE, extracardiac foci of infection, any indications for surgery, high risk of nephrotoxicity or at risk of *C. difficile*
	Gentamicin	1mg/kg q12h IV	2	
Treatment of streptococci (penicillin MIC >0.125 to ≤0.5 mg/litre)				
5.	Benzylpenicillin[a] AND	2.4g q4h IV	4–6	Preferred regimen, particularly for patients at risk of *C. difficile*
	Gentamicin	1mg/kg q12h IV	2	
Treatment of *Abiotrophia* and *Granulicatella* spp. (nutritionally variant streptococci)				
6.	Benzylpenicillin[a] AND	2.4g q4h IV	4–6	Preferred regimen, particularly for patients at risk of *C. difficile*
	Gentamicin	1mg/kg q12h IV	4–6	
Treatment of streptococci penicillin MIC >0.5 mg/litre				
Treatment of streptococci in patients with significant penicillin allergy				
7.	Vancomycin AND	1g q12h	4–6	Or dosed according to local guidelines
	Gentamicin	1mg/kg q12h IV	≥2	
8.	Teicoplanin AND		4–6	Preferred option when high risk of nephrotoxicity
	Gentamicin	1mg/kg IV q12h	≥2	

IM, intramuscularly; IV, intravenously; OPAT, outpatient antimicrobial therapy; PVE, prosthetic valve endocarditis; q4h, every 4 h; q12h, every 12 h.

All drug dosages to be adjusted in renal impairment; gentamicin, vancomycin, and teicoplanin levels to be monitored.

[a] Amoxicillin 2g every 4–6h may be used in place of benzylpenicillin 1.2–2.4g every 4h.

From Gould et al. (2012). Guidelines for the antibiotic treatment of endocarditis in adults: report of the Working Party of the British Society for Antimicrobial Chemotherapy. *Antimicrob Chemother*, **67**, 269–289 Reproduced with permission from the British Society for Antimicrobial Chemotherapy.

Treatment

Initial therapy

The treatment of endocarditis should ideally be undertaken by a multidisciplinary team involving cardiologists, microbiologists, infectious disease specialists, and cardiac surgeons. Where possible, patients should be treated in cardiac centres that undertake cardiac surgery. Bactericidal antibiotics are the mainstay of treatment. The choice and duration of treatment depend on the type of microorganism and its susceptibility profile, whether infection involves a native or prosthetic valve, and whether the patient is allergic to any antimicrobials.

In those patients who have been ill for many weeks, antibiotic treatment can be deferred until the blood cultures are positive and the pathogen known. Antibiotic treatment should be started immediately after taking blood cultures in patients who are acutely ill, using a broad-spectrum combination that can be adjusted when the pathogen is known. However, endocarditis is often not suspected initially in many patients who are acutely ill with native valve infection: there may be no obvious signs of this and antibiotics are started for 'septicaemia'. When meticillin-resistant staphylococci (whether *Staph. aureus* or coagulase-negative staphylococci) are likely pathogens, vancomycin or teicoplanin is an essential component of any combination. If empirical therapy is indicated the choice of antimicrobial agent should be dictated by the type of presentation, whether or not there is an intracardiac prosthesis in place, and the likely causative organism as suggested by the clinical picture (Table 9.2.3).

Definitive therapy

There are various international guidelines for the treatment of specific organisms. It is important to realize that these are based on

Table 9.2.5 Recommended regimens for treatment of staphylococcal endocarditis

Agent	Dose/route	Duration (weeks)	Comment
NVE, methicillin-susceptible *Staphylococcus* spp.			
Flucloxacillin	2g every 4–6h IV	4	Use q4h regimen if weight >85 kg
NVE, methicillin-resistant, vancomycin-susceptible (MIC ≤2 mg/litre) rifampicin-susceptible *Staphylococcus* or penicillin allergy			
Vancomycin AND	1g IV q12h	4	Or dose according to local guidelines. Modify dose according to renal function and maintain pre-dose level 15–20 mg/litre
Rifampicin	300–600mg q12h po	4	Use lower dose of rifampicin if creatinine clearance <30 ml/min
NVE, methicillin-resistant, vancomycin-resistant (MIC >2 mg/litre), daptomycin-susceptible (MIC ≤1mg/litre) *Staphylococcus* spp. or patient unable to tolerate vancomycin			
Daptomycin AND	6 mg/kg q24h IV	4	Monitor creatine phosphokinase weekly. Adjust dose according to renal function
Rifampicin OR	300–600 mg q12h po	4	Use lower dose of rifampicin if creatinine clearance <30 ml/min
Gentamicin	1 mg/kg IV, q12h	4	
PVE, methicillin, rifampicin-susceptible *Staphylococcus* spp.			
Flucloxacillin AND	2 g every 4–6h IV	6	Use q4h regimen if weight >85 kg
Rifampicin AND	300–600 mg q12h po	6	Use lower dose of rifampicin if creatinine clearance <30 ml/min
Gentamicin	1 mg/kg IV, q12h	6	
PVE, methicillin-resistant, vancomycin-susceptible (MIC ≤2 mg/litre), *Staphylococcus* spp. or penicillin allergy			
Vancomycin AND	1g IV q12h	6	Or dose according to local guidelines. Modify dose according to renal function and maintain pre-dose level 15–20 mg/litre
Rifampicin AND	300–600 mg q12h po	6	Use lower dose of rifampicin if creatinine clearance <30 ml/min
Gentamicin	1 mg/kg q12h IV	≥2	Continue gentamicin for the full course if there are no signs or symptoms of toxicity
PVE, methicillin-resistant, vancomycin-resistant (MIC >2 mg/litre), daptomycin-susceptible (MIC ≤1 mg/litre) *Staphylococcus* spp. or patient unable to tolerate vancomycin			
Daptomycin AND	6 mg/kg q24h IV	6	Increase daptomycin dosing interval to 48 hourly if creatinine clearance <30 ml/min
Rifampicin AND	300–600 mg q12h po	6	Use lower dose of rifampicin if creatinine clearance <30 ml/min
Gentamicin	1 mg/kg q12h IV	≥2	Continue gentamicin for the full course if there are no signs or symptoms of toxicity

IV, intravenously; NVE, native valve endocarditis; PVE, prosthetic valve endocarditis; po, orally; q12h, every 12 h; q24h, every 24 h.

From Gould et al. (2012). Guidelines for the antibiotic treatment of endocarditis in adults: report of the Working Party of the British Society for Antimicrobial Chemotherapy. *Antimicrob Chemother*, **67**, 269–289 Reproduced with permission from the British Society for Antimicrobial Chemotherapy.

consensus, because there are no randomized controlled trials to show the efficacy of any particular regimen. It is conventional to estimate the minimum inhibitory concentration (MIC) of the antibiotic for the pathogen, but in practice routine disc sensitivity tests are satisfactory in many cases. Although it is widely believed that prosthetic endocarditis requires a longer duration of antibiotic treatment than native valve infection, there are few data to support this.

Recommendations for the treatment of the most common causative organisms are taken from guidelines published by the British Society for Antimicrobial Chemotherapy (Tables 9.2.4, 9.2.5, 9.2.6).

HACEK endocarditis

Treatment should be with a β-lactamase-stable cephalosporin, or with amoxicillin if the organism is sensitive, plus gentamicin 1mg/kg body weight according to renal function (for the first 2 weeks only) and with regular monitoring of drug levels. An alternative agent is ciprofloxacin.

Other uncommon causes of endocarditis

Treatments for uncommon culture-negative causes of endocarditis are shown in Table 9.2.7.

Fungal endocarditis

For candida, micafungin, caspofungin or anidulafungin are first-line therapies. For aspergillus, voriconazole is first-line treatment. Expert advice on dosing should be sought.

Monitoring of treatment

Serum bactericidal titres against the infecting organism are no longer recommended. There was always great variation in the monitoring methods used for these tests and in the interpretation of their results. At best, they could only predict bacteriological not clinical cure, and bacteriological failure is very rare. The most useful laboratory test for monitoring the response to treatment (which is usually obvious clinically) is serial estimation of CRP; this is of greater use than the ESR, which is much slower to fall.

If there is a relapse of endocarditis, this usually occurs within 2 months of cessation of treatment. The relapse rate is lowest for patients with native valve endocarditis caused by penicillin-sensitive viridans streptococci. Relapse rate in prosthetic valve endocarditis is 10 to 15%.

Prevention and prophylaxis

Until recently, antibiotic prophylaxis in at-risk patients, including those with native valve disease undergoing a wide variety of dental, medical, and surgical procedures, was accepted as reasonable. This was largely based on indirect data from *in vitro* studies, experimental animal models, and studies of clinical bacteraemia, but there were many uncertainties about its value, and data confirming its clinical effectiveness were lacking. This lack of evidence has led international bodies to propose more restrictive guidelines in recent years.

The most controversial area for the use of prophylactic antibiotics concerns dental treatment. Innovative French guidelines published in 2002 challenged conventional practice, suggesting prophylaxis only for those with the highest benefit to risk ratio, and emphasizing the importance of oral hygiene. A working party of the British Society of Antimicrobial Chemotherapy recommended in 2006 that the practice of giving antibiotics to all patients with cardiac abnormalities before dental treatment should be stopped, except for those with a history of previous endocarditis, prosthetic heart valves, or surgically constructed conduits. Many other groups vigorously opposed this recommendation, not least because some cases of endocarditis that involve dental procedures have resulted in litigation, and in most of these legal cases, endocarditis was judged to be caused by dental manipulations on the basis of the dental procedure, cardiac pathology, infecting microorganism, and the temporal link between the onset of endocardial infection and the dental manipulation.

In 2007 the American Heart Association (AHA) revised its guidelines limiting the use of antibiotic prophylaxis to the highest-risk patients who were undergoing the highest-risk procedures

Table 9.2.6 Recommended regimens for treatment of enterococcal endocarditis

Regimen	Antimicrobial	Dose and route	Duration (weeks)	Comment
1.	Amoxicillin OR	2 g q4h IV	4–6	For amoxicillin-susceptible (MIC ≤4 mg/litre), penicillin MIC ≤4 mg/litre AND gentamicin-susceptible (MIC ≤128 mg/litre) isolates
	Penicillin AND	2.4 g q4h IV	4–6	Duration 6 weeks for PVE
	Gentamicin[a]	1 mg/kg q12h IV	4–6	
2.	Vancomycin[a] AND	1 g q12h IV or dosed according to local guidelines	4–6	For penicillin-allergic patient or amoxicillin- or penicillin-resistant isolate; ensure vancomycin MIC ≤4 mg/litre
	Gentamicin[a]	1 mg/kg IBW q12h IV	4–6	Duration 6 weeks for PVE
3.	Teicoplanin[a] AND	10 mg/kg q24h IV	4–6	Alternative to Regimen 2, see comments for Regimen 2; ensure teicoplanin MIC ≤2 mg/litre
	Gentamicin[a]	1 mg/kg q12h IV	4–6	
4.	Amoxicillin[a,B]	2 g q4h IV	≥6	For amoxicillin-susceptible (MIC ≤4 mg/litre) AND high-level gentamicin resistant (MIC >128 mg/litre) isolates

IBW, ideal body weight; IV, intravenously; PVE, prosthetic valve endocarditis; q4h, every 4 h; q12h, every 12 h; q24h, every 24 h.

[a] Amend dose according to renal function.

[b] Streptomycin 7.5 mg/kg every 12 h intramuscularly can be added if isolate is susceptible.

From Gould et al. (2012). Guidelines for the antibiotic treatment of endocarditis in adults: report of the Working Party of the British Society for Antimicrobial Chemotherapy. *Antimicrob Chemother*, **67**, 269–289 Reproduced with permission from the British Society for Antimicrobial Chemotherapy.

Table 9.2.7 Management of known causes of culture-negative endocarditis

Pathogen	Proposed treatment
Brucella	Doxycycline plus rifampicin or cotrimoxazole (>3 months treatment)
Coxiella burnetti	Doxycycline plus hydroxychloroquine or doxycycline plus quinolone (>18 months treatment)
Bartonella	β-Lactams or doxycycline plus aminoglycoside (>6 weeks treatment)
Chlamydia	Doxycycline or new fluoroquinolones (long-term treatment, optimum duration unknown)
Mycoplasma	Doxycycline or new fluoroquinolones (>12 weeks treatment)
Legionella	Macrolides plus rifampicin or new fluoroquinolones (>6 months treatment)
Tropheryma whipplei	Co-trimoxazole or β-lactam plus aminoglycoside (long-term treatment; optimum duration unknown)

From *Heart*, Prendergast B. D, 92:879–885. Copyright (2006) with permission from BMJ Publishing Group Ltd.

(Tables 9.2.8 and 9.2.9); in the case of dental treatment these were manipulation of gingival tissue or the periapical region of teeth, or perforation of the oral mucosa. More recently the American College of Cardiology (ACC)/AHA Task Force on Practice Guidelines has downgraded the recommendation for antibiotic prophylaxis for high-risk patients from Class 1 (mandatory) to Class 2 (reasonable practice).

The National Institute for Health and Care Excellence (NICE) developed guidelines in 2008 for adoption by the National Health Service in England, Wales, and Northern Ireland. Based on its findings that (1) there is no consistent association between having an interventional procedure and endocarditis, (2) that the clinical effectiveness of antibiotic prophylaxis is not proven, (3) that the risk of antibiotic-associated adverse effects exceeds the benefits, and (4) that prophylaxis is not cost-effective, NICE concluded that antibiotic prophylaxis should not be given to any at-risk patients undergoing an interventional procedure. NICE made one exception; namely in patients undergoing a gastrointestinal or genitourinary procedure where there is suspected pre-existing infection, who should receive an antibiotic that covers endocarditis causative organisms. NICE have reiterated the same advice in guidelines published in 2015.

In 2009 the European Society of Cardiology also suggested restricting prophylaxis to those with the highest risk of endocarditis undergoing the highest-risk procedures and have reiterated the same advice in guidelines published in 2015. Dental procedures requiring prophylaxis mirror the AHA guidelines.

Not surprisingly these departures from established practice have met with mixed reaction; the dental profession in the United Kingdom has welcomed the NICE proposals, but many British cardiologists and cardiovascular surgeons have opposed them. A sensible approach would appear to be to allow individual doctors to do what they feel is best for their patients and to be encouraged to discuss their reasons for taking a particular stance on antibiotic prophylaxis with them. Patients themselves should be taught the importance of good oral hygiene and to recognize symptoms that might indicate endocarditis and when to seek expert help. Suitable prophylactic antibiotic regimens are described in Table 9.2.9.

Table 9.2.8 Guidelines for antibiotic prophylaxis in endocarditis

	American Heart Association, 2007	National Institute for Health and Clinical Excellence, 2008 and 2015	European Society of Cardiology, 2009 and 2015
High-risk patients	Previous IE	Previous IE	Previous IE
	Prosthetic valve	Prosthetic valve	Prosthetic valve or prosthetic material used for valve repair
	Unrepaired or incompletely repaired cyanotic congenital heart disease	Acquired valvular heart disease with stenosis or regurgitation	Cyanotic congenital heart disease (without surgical repair or with residual defects, palliative shunts, or conduits)
	Congenital heart disease repaired with prosthetic material (for 6 months after the procedure)	Structural congenital heart disease, including surgically corrected or palliated structural conditions; excluding isolated ASD, fully repaired VSD/PDA, endothelialized closure devices	Congenital heart disease repaired with prosthetic material (for 6 months if complete repair, indefinite if residual defect)
	Valve disease in cardiac transplant recipients	Hypertrophic cardiomyopathy	
Procedures requiring prophylaxis	Dental procedures involving manipulation of gingival tissue, the periapical region of teeth, or perforation of the oral mucosa	Gastrointestinal and genitourinary procedures where there is suspected pre-existing infection	Dental procedures requiring manipulation of the gingival or periapical region of the teeth or perforation of the oral mucosa
	Invasive procedures of the respiratory tract needing incision or biopsy of the mucosa		

ASD, atrial septal defect; IE, infective endocarditis; PDA, patent arterial duct; VSD, ventricular septal defect.

Adapted from Harrison JL, Prendergast BD, Habib G (2009). The European Society of Cardiology 2009 guidelines on the prevention, diagnosis, and treatment of infective endocarditis. Key messages for clinical practice. *Pol Arch Med Wewn*, **119**, 773–6.

Table 9.2.9 Prevention of endocarditis in patients with known cardiac risk

Situation	Antibiotic	Adults	Children
		Single dose 30–60 min before procedure	
No allergy to penicillin or ampicillin	Amoxicillin or ampicillin[a]	2 g PO or IV	50 mg/kg PO or IV
Allergy to penicillin or ampicillin	Clindamycin	600 mg PO or IV	20 mg/kg PO or IV

IV, intravenous; PO, by mouth.

Cephalosporins should not be used in patients with anaphylaxis, angio-oedema, or urticaria after intake of penicillin and ampicillin.

[a] Alternatively cephalexin 2 g IV or 50 mg/kg IV for children, cefazolin or ceftriaxone 1 g IV for adults or 50 mg/kg IV for children.

From: 2015 ESC Guidelines for the management of infective endocarditis: The Task Force for the Management of Infective Endocarditis of the European Society of Cardiology (ESC) Endorsed by: European Association for Cardio-Thoracic Surgery (EACTS), the European Association of Nuclear Medicine (EANM). Habib G *et al. Eur Heart J.* 2015 **36**:3075–128.

Surgical treatment of endocarditis

Surgery is required in about 50% of cases. Since surgery may be required at any time during an episode of endocarditis, it is essential to involve a cardiac surgeon in the overall management from the outset, which in practice means transferring the patient to a centre with cardiac surgery whenever possible. Surgery for endocarditis carries a 10 to 25% mortality risk, and up to 10% of patients develop a paravalvular leak requiring a further operation. The main predictive factors for mortality associated with surgery are prosthetic valve endocarditis, infections due to staphylococci or candida, perioperative shock, or late referral.

The timing of surgery is all-important and demands experience and clinical judgement. The main indications are haemodynamic instability, persistent infection, and annular or aortic abscesses. In such cases surgery should never be delayed, even if only hours or days of antibiotic treatment have been given. The primary goals of the surgeon are to remove all infected material and to reconstruct the heart and/or restore valvular function at the lowest operative risk. An understanding of the surgical anatomy of endocarditis is a precondition for surgical success, which means the involvement of an experienced surgical team. Wherever possible, surgeons now strive to preserve the native valve, either by removal of the vegetation(s) or by valve repair. In prosthetic valve endocarditis, removal of all foreign material is mandatory. Actuarial survival figures indicate a 75% survival at 5 years and a 61% survival at 10 years after cardiac surgery for endocarditis.

There are several unresolved issues with regard to the surgical treatment of endocarditis. First, the use of surgery when embolism has already taken place remains controversial. Recurrent emboli, persistent vegetation after a major systemic embolus, and vegetation size (>10 mm) have all been put forward as indications, but there are no controlled trials to support a firm recommendation. Secondly, the optimal timing of surgery in patients who have had a cerebrovascular accident, either as a result of an embolic stroke or from haemorrhage due to a ruptured mycotic aneurysm: as a general rule, delay of at least 4 weeks is suggested if haemorrhage is detected by CT scanning, but surgery can be undertaken within 72 h if no haemorrhage is present. Thirdly, the duration of antibiotic treatment postoperatively: a short postoperative course is appropriate if the excised valve is sterile, whereas continuation for 4 to 6 weeks seems reasonable if the pathogen is isolated from the excised valve.

Further reading

Cohen PS, Maguire JH, Weinstein L (1980). Infective endocarditis caused by gram negative bacteria: a review of the literature 1945–1977. *Prog Cardiovasc Dis*, **22**, 205–41.

Gould FK, *et al.* (2012). Guidelines for the antibiotic treatment of endocarditis in adults: report of the Working Party of the British Society for Antimicrob Chemotherapy, *J Antimicrob Chemother*, **67**, 269–89.

Habib G, *et al.* (2015). ESC Guidelines for the management of infective endocarditis. *Eur Heart J*, **36**, 3075–128.

Hoen B, *et al.* (1995). Infective endocarditis in patients with negative blood cultures: analysis of 88 cases from a one year nationwide survey in France. *Clin Infect Dis*, **20**, 501–6.

Kang DH, *et al.* (2012). Early surgery versus conventional treatment for infective endocarditis. *N Engl J Med*, **366**, 2466–73.

Moreillon P, Que Y-A (2004). Infective endocarditis. *Lancet*, 363, 139–49.

Mylonakis E, Calderwood SB (2001). Infective endocarditis in adults. *N Engl J Med*, **345**, 1318–29.

NICE (2015). *Prophylaxis against infective endocarditis*. Clinical Guideline 64.1. www.nice.org.uk

Prendergast BD (2006). The changing face of endocarditis. *Heart*, **92**, 879–85.

Prendergast BD, Tornos P. (2010). Surgery for infective endocarditis: who and when? *Circulation*, **121**, 1141–52.

Rick A, et al. (2008). ACC/AHA 2008 guideline update on valvular heart disease: focused update on infective endocarditis. *Circulation*, **118**, 887–96.

Task Force on the Prevention, Diagnosis, and Treatment of Infective Endocarditis of the European Society of Cardiology (2009). Guidelines on the prevention, diagnosis, and treatment of infective endocarditis (new version 2009). *Eur Heart J*, **30**, 2369–413.

Watkin R, *et al.* (2003). The microbiological diagnosis of infective endocarditis. *J Infect*, **47**, 1–11.

Wilson W, Taubert KA, Gewitz M, et al. (2007). Prevention of Infective Endocarditis. Guidelines From the American Heart Association. A guideline from the American Heart Association Rheumatic Fever, Endocarditis, and Kawasaki Disease Committee, Council on Cardiovascular Disease in the Young, and the Council on Clinical Cardiology, Council on Cardiovascular Surgery and Anesthesia, and the Quality of Care and Outcomes Research Interdisciplinary Working Group. *Circulation*, **116**, 1736–54.

CHAPTER 9.3

Cardiac disease in HIV infection

Peter F. Currie

Essentials

Symptomatic heart disease can affect up to 10% of HIV-positive patients and cause death in around 2%. Echocardiographic screening is recommended.

In resource-poor countries where access to antiretroviral drugs is limited the typical manifestations are (1) HIV heart muscle disease—this occurs in the late stages of HIV infection, with dilated cardiomyopathy having a dismal prognosis, the median survival after diagnosis being about 100 days; angiotensin converting enzyme (ACE) inhibitors and β-blockers may produce unacceptable side effects; and (2) pericardial effusion—a common finding, but most are symptomless; significant effusions are often due to mycobacterial infection or malignant infiltration, particularly with non-Hodgkin's lymphoma.

In the developed world premature coronary artery disease is more common in patients with HIV than in controls. There is a two- to three-fold increase in the incidence of acute coronary events in HIV patients treated with highly active antiretroviral therapy (HAART), which is thought to be related to HIV lipodystrophy, an ill-defined syndrome that resembles the non-HIV metabolic syndrome and is found in up to 35% of patients after 12 months of protease inhibitor therapy. Isolated pulmonary hypertension is a rare, noninfectious complication of HIV infection and has a grave prognosis (50% survival at 1 year). HAART and specific pulmonary hypertension therapies may be beneficial.

Sudden death due to cardiac rhythm abnormalities is well recognized in HIV infection and may account for 20% of cardiac-related deaths.

Introduction

Cardiovascular manifestations of HIV infection are well recognized and have been reported in up to 40% of autopsies and about 25% of echocardiographic studies performed on patients with AIDS. Although most of these lesions are minor, symptomatic heart disease can affect up to 10% of HIV-positive patients and cause death in around 2%.

Heart muscle disease was previously the dominant cardiac complication of HIV infection in the developed world. However, the development of highly active antiretroviral therapy (HAART) has significantly altered the course of HIV infection and has most likely reduced the incidence of, but not abolished, many forms of heart disease in AIDS. However, HAART-induced dyslipidaemia has become an important factor for the development of premature coronary artery disease, which is becoming increasingly common. Despite significant progress in providing HAART to increasing numbers of patients in the developing world, HIV heart muscle disease, pericardial effusion, and pulmonary hypertension continue to predominate in resource-poor countries where access to antiretroviral drugs is limited. A large-vessel vasculopathy may also be emerging as a specific complication of HIV infection in young African males.

The common cardiovascular manifestations of HIV infection are listed in Table 9.3.1.

HIV/AIDS and the pericardium

Pericardial effusion was found frequently in early autopsy studies, often in association with generalized fluid retention and advanced HIV infection. Small effusions remain common, but most are symptomless. Cardiac tamponade is rare, but the finding of unexplained breathlessness, raised jugular venous pressure, or radiographic cardiomegaly should prompt early echocardiographic assessment (see Chapter 8.1).

In Africa up to 72% of patients with serosanguinous effusions have been found to be HIV positive, and *Mycobacterium tuberculosis* or

Table 9.3.1 Cardiovascular manifestations of HIV/AIDS

Pericardial effusion	Idiopathic
	Infectious (viral, bacterial—especially tuberculous, and fungal)
	Neoplastic (Kaposi's sarcoma and non-Hodgkin's lymphoma)
Heart muscle disease	Myocarditis (idiopathic/lymphocytic, specific infections, toxins)
	Dilated cardiomyopathy
Left ventricular dysfunction	
Isolated right ventricular dysfunction	
Endocarditis	Marantic (nonbacterial thrombotic endocarditis)
	Infective
Pulmonary hypertension	Primary
	Secondary (recurrent bronchopulmonary infections, thromboembolism)
Premature atherosclerosis and coronary artery disease	
Adverse drug effects	Hyperlipidaemia
	Induction of arrhythmia
Vascular disease	Coronary artery disease
Autonomic dysfunction	Sudden death

M. avium-intracellulare pericarditis is common. Appropriate antituberculous and antiviral therapies may be helpful, but it is not clear if corticosteroids are beneficial in this situation and they are generally avoided. Herpes simplex virus, cytomegalovirus, and other unusual organisms may clinically be implicated, but significant pericardial effusions are often due to malignant infiltration, particularly with non-Hodgkin's lymphoma.

Pericardiocentesis and pericardiectomy can be used to treat tamponade in HIV infection, but surgical intervention may not be appropriate in patients with very advanced disease. Clearly, however, culture of pericardial biopsy or fluid from symptomatic effusions may be useful in identifying treatable opportunistic infections or malignancy.

Cardiac tumours in HIV/AIDS

In AIDS patients, Kaposi's sarcoma is a disseminated visceral disease with cardiac involvement in up to 25% of cases. Isolated cardiac Kaposi's sarcoma is rare. The tumour often invades the subpericardial fat around coronary arteries and may infiltrate the pericardium or myocardium. However, despite this, Kaposi's sarcoma is not usually associated with cardiac symptoms and significant effusion is rare. The prevalence of cardiac Kaposi's sarcoma in HIV/AIDS appears to be falling.

Primary cardiac lymphoma is extremely rare in HIV-negative individuals, although disseminated lymphoma may involve the myocardium more frequently. Both patterns of malignant cardiac involvement occur in AIDS patients, and non-Hodgkin's lymphoma in particular, may involve the pericardium or myocardium. In contrast to Kaposi's sarcoma, cardiac lymphoma is commonly associated with tamponade, symptomatic heart failure, and conduction abnormalities. This diagnosis should therefore be considered in AIDS patients with rapidly progressive cardiovascular symptoms, unexpected arrhythmias or heart block.

Endocardial disease in HIV/AIDS

Marantic or nonbacterial thrombotic endocarditis was a frequent finding in early AIDS post-mortem series. Noninfectious systemic thromboembolism was a common sequel and hence the condition is associated with significant morbidity and mortality. It is now rarely described as a complication of AIDS.

Although AIDS patients are susceptible to bacterial infections, infective endocarditis rarely occurs in HIV infection outwith the setting of injection drug use (see Chapter 9.2). Asymptomatic HIV infection *per se* appears to have little effect on the susceptibility to, or the mortality from, the condition, although bacterial endocarditis runs a more fulminant course in the late stages of AIDS. In particular, a CD4 count of less than 200 cells/µl is associated with a poor prognosis in these circumstances. As with infective endocarditis in patients who are HIV negative, in intravenous drug users the tricuspid valve is most commonly involved and *Staphylococcus aureus* or *Streptococcus viridans* are the most frequently isolated organisms. *Aspergillus fumigatus, Pseudallescheria boydii*, and other forms of bacterial and fungal endocarditis occur in endstage AIDS.

Just as for patients without AIDS, adequate bacteriological investigations are required when endocarditis is suspected in HIV-positive individuals, but initial 'best guess' antimicrobial treatment (see Chapter 9.2) may have to be widened, particularly if fungal endocarditis is suspected. Valvular heart surgery has been described in HIV-positive intravenous drug users with endocarditis, but continued drug use often results in a poor prognosis.

Heart muscle disease

HIV heart muscle disease occurs in the late stages of HIV infection and is associated with low CD4 counts. Before HAART, symptomatic congestive cardiac failure was found in around 5% of HIV patients. However, the signs and symptoms of heart failure were frequently mistakenly attributed to anaemia or bronchopulmonary infection. Left ventricular systolic dysfunction—either isolated or in the form of a dilated cardiomyopathy—could be found echocardiographically in 10 to 15% of patients with AIDS previously and currently in up to 3% of patients treated with HAART.

The cause or causes of HIV heart muscle disease remain unknown, but are almost certainly complex. It is likely that an autoimmune lymphocytic myocarditis plays a key pathogenic role, in line with current thinking on the pathogenesis of idiopathic dilated cardiomyopathy in HIV-negative patients. Some form of myocarditis can be found by biopsy or at autopsy in up to 40% of patients with AIDS, and rarely specific organisms may be identified, e.g. *Toxoplasma gondii* or cytomegalovirus, usually in the setting of disseminated infection. Some *in situ* hybridization studies have suggested that HIV-1 may be present in the myocardium of patients with HIV heart muscle disease, although clear evidence for a primary HIV myocarditis is still lacking. It is possible that the myocarditis is secondary to an autoimmune reaction mediated through cytokines or circulating cardiac autoantibodies, but other potential cofactors include specific micronutrient deficiencies (especially selenium) or the cardiotoxic side effects of antiretroviral agents. An acute, lymphocytic myocarditis with intractable ventricular arrythmia, has also recently been described as part of the immune reconstitution inflammatory syndrome (IRIS).

HIV-related dilated cardiomyopathy has a dismal prognosis, with median survival after diagnosis being about 100 days (Fig. 9.3.1). Conventional anti-heart-failure treatment is used, but vasodilating agents such as ACE inhibitors are often poorly tolerated and β-blockers may produce unacceptable side effects. Diuretics, digoxin, and aldosterone antagonists may be more useful. Although successful cardiac transplantation, with or without a left ventricular assist device as a bridging therapy, has been reported in two HIV-positive patients, the latest report relates to the diagnosis of cardiomyopathy in a subject with a normal CD4 count, undetectable viral load, and no history of opportunistic infection. Such treatment may therefore applicable to only a very small minority of HIV patients with heart muscle disease. The incidence of myocarditis, heart muscle disease, and symptomatic heart failure appears to have decreased in the HAART era.

Right ventricular dysfunction and pulmonary hypertension in HIV/AIDS

Right ventricular dysfunction may occur as part of HIV heart muscle disease but can occur in isolation, without pulmonary hypertension, and is of unknown significance (Fig. 9.3.1). Bronchopulmonary infections should be treated aggressively and intravenous drug use, which may result in microvascular emboli, should be discouraged.

Isolated pulmonary hypertension (Fig. 9.3.2) is a rare noninfective complication of HIV infection and has a grave prognosis, with a 50% survival at 1 year. HAART has had no impact on the incidence of this devastating condition, which has little correlation with CD4 counts and may be related to the action of viral proteins

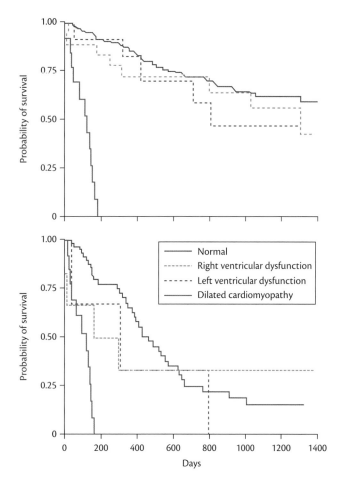

Fig. 9.3.1 Top: Survival curves for 296 patients who were HIV positive with structurally normal hearts or cardiac dysfunction. Bottom: Survival time to death related to AIDS in 81 subjects with CD4 cell count <20 × 10⁶/litre.
Reproduced from *BMJ*, Currie *et al.*, 309:1605–1607. Copyright (1994) with permission from BMJ Publishing Group Ltd.

or cytokines on the endothelial cell. Characteristic pathological lesions including intimal fibrosis and plexiform lesions confirm its similarity to non-HIV primary pulmonary hypertension. Right heart catheterization may be worthwhile to determine if pulmonary hypertension is reversible. Oxygen, calcium channel antagonists, vasodilators, phosphodiesterase V inhibitors, and nitric oxide therapy may be considered, but are unproven therapies in this circumstance and do not necessarily improve prognosis, although HAART itself may prove beneficial in terms of outcome.

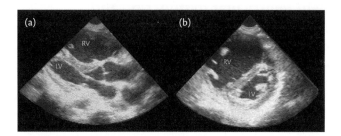

Fig. 9.3.2 (a) Long-axis and (b) short-axis parasternal view of a two-dimensional echocardiogram from an HIV-positive intravenous drug user with idiopathic pulmonary hypertension illustrating dilatation of the right ventricle and flattening of the interventricular septum. LV, left ventricle; RV, right ventricle.

Coronary artery disease in HIV infection

HIV lipodystrophy is an ill-defined syndrome that resembles the non-HIV metabolic syndrome and includes dyslipidaemia and insulin resistance. Although it is dependent on the type and duration of antiretroviral therapy, and can be found in up to 35% of patients after 12 months of protease inhibitor therapy, it has also been suggested that HIV itself is a pro-atherogenic virus with specific effects on cellular cholesterol management.

The significant changes in lipid metabolism noted in the recipients of protease inhibitors have led to fears of an epidemic of premature atherosclerotic disease in this population. The first cases of acute myocardial infarction in treated HIV patients emerged in the late 1990s. Acute myocardial infarction appears to be the commonest presentation of coronary heart disease in HIV populations and it is plausible that—because acute coronary syndromes involve low-volume, lipid-rich plaques—HAART may promote development of vulnerable lesions or influence plaque rupture. Similarly, most HIV patients with coronary symptoms will have been diagnosed with AIDS, which raises the possibility that opportunistic infections may also be involved in this process. A case of coronary arteritis due to HIV has been described, but acute coronary events are not clearly related to HIV replication as one-third of patients have undetectable plasma HIV RNA at the time of symptoms.

Coronary angiography can be carried out safely in patients with HIV and frequently reveals proximal vessel involvement and single vessel disease. Percutaneous coronary intervention is a reasonable therapy, with use of drug-eluting stents advocated by some because of concerns over the possibility of aggressive restenosis. Fibrinolysis and coronary artery bypass have also been used with acceptable survival rates, hence it is reasonable that the clinical situation should determine the use of coronary treatments in the same manner as for the non-HIV population. However, as the non-nucleoside reverse transcriptase inhibitor etravirine inhibits CYP2C19 and can reduce the antiplatelet activity of clopidogrel and ticagrelor, the prescription of these drugs is not recommended. Prasugrel may be a suitable alternative antiplatelet agent for use in these circumstances.

It may be necessary to consider drug treatment for hyperlipidaemia, particularly if antiretroviral treatment cannot be changed or interrupted. Like protease inhibitors, most HMG CoA reductase inhibitors (statins) are metabolized through the cytochrome P450 system. Coprescription of these drugs may therefore result in competitive inhibition, significantly increased plasma statin levels, and increased risk of myopathy and rhabdomyolysis. Pravastatin is metabolized by a different pathway and for this reason it is recommended that hypercholesterolaemia in HIV patients receiving protease inhibitors is initially treated with pravastatin 20 mg daily, with careful monitoring of virological parameters and creatine kinase levels. Rosuvastatin, a more powerful statin, metabolized in a similar manner, may only be used in low dose and with care in some cases. Bile acid sequestrants, although attractive from the point of view of drug interactions, may have adverse effects on serum triglyceride levels or impair absorption of antiretrovirals.

Sudden death and cardiac arrhythmia

Sudden death due to cardiac rhythm abnormalities is well recognized in HIV infection and may account for 20% of cardiac-related deaths in this population. Arrhythmia may be secondary to other cardiac pathology or be a consequence of some forms of treatment,

PATIENT CHARACTERISTICS   CARDIOVASCULAR INVESTIGATIONS

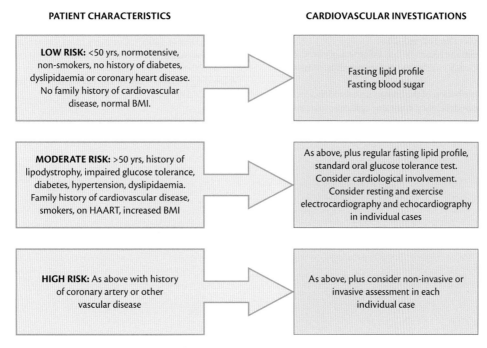

Fig. 9.3.3 An approach to cardiovascular assessment in patients with HIV.

especially in the setting of electrolyte disturbance. Atrial fibrillation is becoming more common as the HIV population is now ageing. It can be found in 2.6% of patients and caution is required as there are important interactions between anticoagulants, anti-arrhythmics, and HAART (see <www.hiv-interaction.org>).

Cardiovascular assessment of the patient with HIV/AIDS

Echocardiography

The usefulness of echocardiographic assessment of patients with HIV has been demonstrated in many studies. It can easily identify many cardiac conditions common in HIV-positive patients that are associated with a poor outcome, including useful information on the appearance of the right ventricle, an indirect assessment of pulmonary pressures, and regional wall motion abnormalities suggestive of coronary artery disease. Any HIV-positive patient at high risk of developing cardiovascular disease, or with any potential clinical manifestation of it, should therefore have an echocardiogram performed, with repeated imaging every 1 to 2 years. It may be justifiable to perform a baseline study at the time of diagnosis of HIV in any patient, with 1- to 2-yearly examination of asymptomatic patients and closer monitoring on discovery of cardiovascular abnormalities or in those with significant viral infection or unexplained pulmonary symptoms.

Assessment of cardiovascular risk

Traditional cardiovascular risk profiling has become more important in the care of HIV-positive patients. The prevalence of heavy cigarette smoking in HIV-infected patients is as high as 40%. Diabetes mellitus requiring treatment is common, and HIV patients appear to be at higher risk of developing hypertension at a younger age than the general population, such that blood pressure screening is recommended. A careful history should also identify a family history of premature vascular disease, recreational drug use, poor diet, and lack of physical exercise. A risk score may be calculated to help guide investigation and treatment (Fig. 9.3.3), but it may also be useful to consider HIV infection and HAART in themselves as specific risk factors for premature atherosclerosis.

Further reading

Calabrese LH, et al. (2003). Successful cardiac transplantation in an HIV-1-infected patient with advanced disease. N Engl J Med, **348**, 2323–8.

Cecchia EJ, et al. (2007). Infective endocarditis in drug addicts: role of HIV infection and the diagnostic accuracy of Duke criteria. J Cardiovasc Med, **8**, 169–75.

Cerrato E, et al. (2013). Cardiac dysfunction in pauci symptomatic human immunodeficiency virus patients: a meta-analysis in the highly active antiretroviral therapy era. Eur Heart J, **34**, 1432–6.

Currie PF, et al. (1994). Heart muscle disease related to HIV infection: prognostic implications. BMJ, **309**, 1605–7.

D'Ascenzo F, et al. (2012). Acute coronary syndromes in human immunodeficiency virus patients: a meta-analysis investigating adverse event rates and the role of antiretroviral therapy. Eur Heart J, **33**, 875–80.

Farrugia PM, et al. (2005). Human immunodeficiency virus and atherosclerosis. Cardiol Rev, **17**, 211–15.

Hsu JC, et al. (2003). Atrial fibrillation and atrial flutter in human immunodeficiency virus—infected persons. J Am Coll Cardiol, **61**, 2288–95.

Hsue PY, Waters DD (2005). What a cardiologist needs to know about patients with human immunodeficiency virus infection. Circulation, **112**, 3947–57.

Huang L, et al. (2006). Intensive care of patients with HIV infection. New Engl J Med, **355**, 173–81.

Janda S, et al. (2010). HIV and pulmonary arterial hypertension: a systematic review. HIV Med, **11**, 620–34.

Knudsen A, et al. (2013). Angiographic features and cardiovascular risk factors in human immunodeficiency virus-infected patients with first-time acute coronary syndrome. Am J Cardiol, **111**, 63–7.

Krishan K, et al. (2012). Successful left ventricular assist device bridge to transplantation in a patient with end-stage heart failure and human immunodeficiency virus. Artif Organs, **36**, 759

Nahass RG, *et al.* (1990). Infective endocarditis in intravenous drug users: a comparison of human immunodeficiency virus type 1–negative and positive patients. *J Infect Dis*, **162**, 967–70.

Rogers JS, *et al.* (2008). Immune reconstitution inflammatory syndrome and human immunodeficiency virus-associated myocarditis. *Mayo Clin Proc*, **83**, 1275–9.

Sliwa K, *et al.* (2012). Contribution of the human immunodeficiency virus/acquired immunodeficiency syndrome epidemic to *de novo* presentations of heart disease in the Heart of Soweto Study Cohort. *Eur Heart J*, **33**, 866–74.

Vittecoq D, *et al.* (2003). Coronary heart disease in HIV-infected patients in the highly active antiretroviral treatment era. *AIDS*, **17 Suppl 1**, S70–6.

Volberding PA, *et al.* (2003). The Pavia consensus statement. *AIDS*, **17 Suppl 1**, S170–9.

CHAPTER 9.4

Cardiovascular syphilis

Krishna Somers

Essentials

Clinicians need to be aware of cardiovascular syphilis in patients at risk of infection, with the time taken from initial infection to clinical manifestation ranging from 10 to 25 years, although this is accelerated in patients with HIV infection. Inadequate or interrupted antibiotic therapy may confound the development of cardiovascular syphilis and make diagnosis difficult.

Presentation may be with (1) asymptomatic aortitis; (2) aortic regurgitation—the commonest manifestation resulting from annular dilatation of the aortic ring and eventually affecting 70% of patients with untreated syphilis; (3) coronary ostial stenosis; (4) aneurysm of the aorta; or (5) a combination of these. Syphilitic aortitis must be included in the differential diagnosis of aortic regurgitation in older people and those with predisposing factors.

Diagnosis—serological testing is the mainstay: latent or inadequately treated syphilis should be suspected with the finding of a positive nonspecific treponemal serological test (e.g. rapid plasma reagin, RPR) and a positive specific treponemal antibody test (e.g. *Treponema pallidum* haemagglutination, TPHA), but negative serology does not absolutely exclude infection with *T. pallidum*, particularly in an immunocompromised host.

Management—parenteral penicillin remains the treatment of choice for cardiovascular syphilis: the World Health Organization and European and United States guidelines recommend benzathine benzylpenicillin 2.4×10^6 units administered once weekly for 3 weeks by the intramuscular route. Modern imaging technology with MRI and three-dimensional CT enables innovative surgical approaches in the repair of syphilitic aortitis.

Introduction

At the beginning of the 20th century cardiovascular syphilis accounted for 5 to 10% of deaths due to cardiovascular disease. The institution of public health measures—early recognition of syphilis and treatment with penicillin since the 1940s—produced a sharp decline in its incidence and hence in the tertiary manifestations and mortality from cardiovascular and neurosyphilis.

The rarity of syphilitic aortitis in recent times has led to publication of a succession of case reports describing challenges in diagnosis and management. With the re-emergence of syphilis in both developed and developing countries, particularly in South East Asia and sub-Saharan Africa, delayed cardiovascular complications of syphilis are likely to be seen with increasing frequency. Syphilis remains a major cause of ascending aortic aneurysm.

An increased rate of infection with the causative organism, *Treponema pallidum*, prevails in sexually promiscuous individuals, intravenous drug abusers, men who have unsafe sex with men, sex workers trafficked from 'east to west', clients of sex workers, and so-called bridging populations, such as men who have both male and female sexual partners. Increase in syphilis infection rates amongst homosexual men is well documented in several cities in the United States of America and also in Europe, Canada, and Australia. As the syphilis epidemic continues to develop it is anticipated that increasing numbers of patients will present with cardiovascular or neurological tertiary syphilis in future decades.

Clinicians need to be aware of cardiovascular syphilis in groups considered to have been at risk of infection. Inadequate or interrupted antibiotic therapy may confound the development of cardiovascular syphilis and make diagnosis difficult.

Pathogenesis and pathology of cardiovascular syphilis

Syphilis is spread through body fluids and is usually acquired by sexual contact with an infected person. Men who have sex with men need to be aware that syphilis can be transmitted through oral sex. In the preantibiotic era, 50 to 75% of partners of persons with primary or secondary syphilis were liable to become infected. Spontaneous healing of the early lesions of primary and secondary syphilis is followed by a long latent period, the time taken from initial infection to clinical manifestation of cardiovascular syphilis, ranging from 10 to 25 years. The 2-year mortality rate after diagnosis of untreated syphilitic aneurysm is about 80%.

T. pallidum has a predilection for small vessels, especially in the aorta and the nervous system. In tertiary syphilis, obliterative endarteritis of the vasa vasorum of the media and the adventitia of the aorta is characterized by the presence of an inflammatory cuff composed of lymphocytes and plasma cells around the affected vessels, causing ischaemic necrosis of collagen and elastic tissue in the aortic media. Syphilis classically involves the proximal ascending aorta, presumably because the vasa vasorum are more plentiful in that region.

The pathological hallmark of syphilitic aortitis is 'tree-barking', a description of longitudinal wrinkling of the aortic intima resulting from contraction of fibrous scars in the aortic media. Fibrosis of the media in the proximal ascending aorta results in dilatation of the aortic root and aneurysm formation, leading to aortic regurgitation, the most common complication of syphilitic aortitis afflicting 20 to 30% of patients. A rarer form of cardiovascular syphilis is 'gummatous' myocarditis, which is usually diagnosed post-mortem.

Clinical presentation

Cardiovascular syphilis may present in one of four forms, but the features may be mixed.

- Asymptomatic aortitis—the most prevalent form, and usually diagnosed at necropsy with the unexpected finding of characteristic 'tree-barking' of the aortic intima.

- Aortic regurgitation—the commonest manifestation of cardiovascular syphilis that results from annular dilatation of the aortic valve ring in syphilitic aortitis affecting the ascending aorta (the valve cusps remain normal); 70 to 80% of patients with untreated syphilis eventually develop aortic regurgitation.

- Coronary ostial stenosis—occurs in up to 30% of cases of cardiovascular syphilis, and frequently coexists with aortic regurgitation as a complication of aortitis affecting the proximal ascending aorta.

- Syphilitic aneurysm of the aorta—the least common manifestation of cardiovascular syphilis, occurring in 10 to 15% of patients with untreated syphilis; usually saccular but may be fusiform, and can occur as solitary aneurysm anywhere along the aorta, with characteristic radiographic appearance of dilatation.

Aortic regurgitation

With typical location of syphilitic disease in the ascending aorta, the murmur of syphilitic aortic regurgitation may be more prominent along the right sternal edge, in contrast to the left side in rheumatic aortic regurgitation. Transthoracic echocardiography will demonstrate that the aortic regurgitation is a result of dilatation of the aortic root (Fig. 9.4.1). Patients with syphilitic aortitis of the ascending aorta die of heart failure resulting from aortic valve regurgitation.

Coronary ostial stenosis

Angina or acute myocardial infarction may be the first presentation of syphilitic heart disease, even in younger patients (Fig. 9.4.2), and may also result from associated coronary atherosclerosis. In the South African literature in the 1980s there were several reports of acute myocardial infarction and death due to syphilitic ostial stenosis (see 'Syphilis and HIV infection' below), hence patients found at coronary angiography to have bilateral coronary ostial stenosis but no distal coronary disease should be screened for syphilis, especially if they have known risk factors.

Syphilitic aneurysm

Nearly one-half of the cases of syphilitic aneurysm occur in the ascending aorta, 30 to 40% in the aortic arch, and the remainder in the descending aorta. Mural thrombus, often with calcification, may obliterate the lumen of an aneurysm. Aneurysm of the aortic arch may compress and erode contiguous structures, such as a bronchus, resulting in pulmonary atelectasis; great veins, with presentation of superior mediastinal obstruction; the left recurrent laryngeal nerve, causing cough and hoarseness; and the vertebral bodies or sternum, causing pain. Aneurysm of the aortic arch may also produce tracheal tug, stridor, and dysphagia. Sternal erosion may be an early manifestation of syphilitic aortitis, as the junction between the ascending aorta and the aortic arch is near to the sternum, and massive aortic aneurysm may present as a pulsatile swelling in the right anterior thoracic cage. Rupture of an aortic aneurysm (70% of cases) into a bronchus—resulting in massive and fatal haemoptysis—or into the pleural space or pericardium may be the first clinical manifestation of syphilitic aneurysm.

Although extremely rare, tertiary syphilis should be considered in the differential diagnosis of thoracic aneurysms, even in the setting of atherosclerotic disease in older subjects. Patients with syphilitic aneurysm of the thoracic aorta, if untreated, have a mean life expectancy of 6 to 9 months from the onset of symptoms.

Aneurysm of the abdominal aorta due to syphilitic aetiology is rare and (if asymptomatic) of unknown prognosis, but it may present with lumbar or abdominal pain and—extremely rarely—as spontaneous aortocaval fistula.

Diagnosis

A high index of suspicion is required to make the diagnosis in a patient found to have aortic regurgitation or aortic aneurysm, but syphilitic disease should be considered, especially if the patient belongs to a group at high risk of syphilitic infection or is elderly with a suggestive background risk factor, such as birth in a country where diagnosis and treatment of syphilis are likely to have been inadequate. With appropriate questioning a history of syphilis and its treatment may be obtained, but patients will often not volunteer such information. The diagnosis of syphilitic aortitis is often overlooked because atherosclerosis has greatly surpassed it as a cause of aortic aneurysm (Fig. 9.4.3).

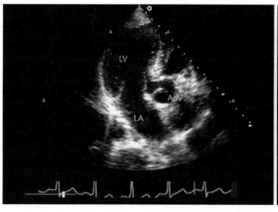
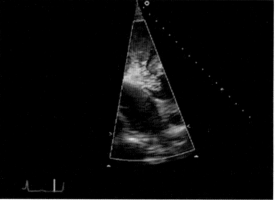

Fig. 9.4.1 Transthoracic echocardiography of a 61-year-old woman with syphilitic aortitis. (a) Apical long-axis view of the left ventricle in mid-diastole. The aortic valve leaflets are closed. The diameter of the ascending aorta is 4.8 cm (normal <3 cm) with the dilatation extending to the arch. AoV, aortic valve; LA, left atrium LV, left ventricle. (b) Apical long-axis colour Doppler study in mid-diastole showing severe aortic regurgitation.

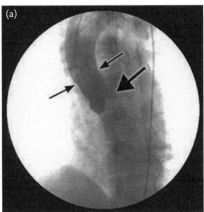
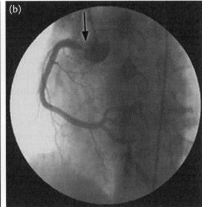

Fig. 9.4.2 Coronary angiogram of a 40-year-old Indonesian man who presented with severe, central chest pain. Note tapering of the aortic root (a, thin arrows), left main coronary artery stump (a, large arrowhead), and 90% ostial lesion of the right coronary artery (b, arrow). Emergency coronary artery grafting was performed. Serology obtained afterwards proved positive for syphilis.
From Tong SYC, *et al.* (2006). *MJA*, **184**, 241–3. © Copyright 2006. The Medical Journal of Australia.

Laboratory investigation

Serological testing is the mainstay of diagnosis. Rapid plasma reagin (RPR) is currently the most widely available nonspecific treponemal test: if positive in high titre, it may indicate latent or inadequately treated disease and be used to gauge response to treatment, but false positives are not uncommon: it is always positive in patients with nonvenereal treponematosis, and it may be negative in cardiovascular syphilis. Specific treponemal antibody tests such as *T pallidum* haemagglutination (TPHA) detect antibodies to *T. pallidum*-specific antigen and are almost always positive in cardiovascular syphilis, indicating prior infection with this organism. However, negative serology does not absolutely exclude infection with *T. pallidum*, particularly in an immunocompromised host. Latent syphilis, defined by the presence of positive serological tests in the absence of clinical evidence of syphilis, may progress to cardiovascular and gummatous manifestations of tertiary syphilis. Even when confirmatory tests are not readily available, treatment should be initiated on suspicion of diagnosis.

The diagnostic gold standard remains direct identification of *T. pallidum* in clinical specimens obtained at surgery. Polymerase chain reaction (PCR) assay can provide definite diagnosis of spirochaetal infection when biopsy material is available. Syphilitic aortitis is often diagnosed on histological examination of the aneurysmal wall in patients who undergo resection of an ascending aortic aneurysm.

Between 10 and 20% of patients with cardiovascular syphilis have coexisting neurosyphilis, hence cerebrospinal fluid examination is recommended.

Recent case-based reports propose the usefulness of ^{18}F-fluorodeoxyglucose positron emission spectroscopy (FDG-PET)/CT for the assessment of extent of disease and response to treatment in syphilitic aortitis.

Syphilis and HIV infection

Syphilis promotes the transmission of HIV infection, and these infections can interact with each other. Cardiovascular syphilis develops more quickly in patients who are HIV seropositive (40 months from the time of primary infection) compared to those who are HIV seronegative (102 months), suggesting that coinfection with HIV hastens progression to late syphilis, perhaps due to immunosuppression. Even though new cases of cardiovascular syphilis remain rare, it has been suggested that the decline of tertiary syphilis in males in the 1990s could be attributed to mortality from AIDS. But at the same time, there has been an increase in the prevalence of infectious syphilis, with many cases undiagnosed.

As a general principle, consideration of one sexually transmissible infection should lead to consideration of another. After appropriate consent, any person with syphilis should be studied for antibodies to HIV and hepatitis B virus, and vice versa, and contacts traced for evidence of infection.

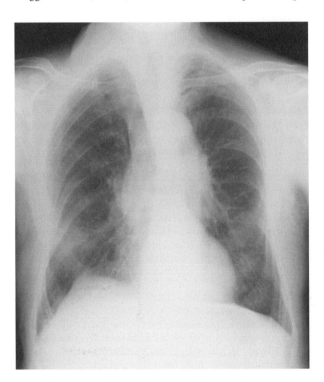

Fig. 9.4.3 Chest radiograph showing aneurysm of the ascending aorta in an elderly man with cardiovascular syphilis. Note the typical linear calcification in the wall of the dilated ascending aorta. Atherosclerotic aneurysm of the ascending aorta in diffuse atherosclerotic disease may present a similar picture, although calcification—when present—is usually limited to the aortic knuckle and descending aorta.

Medical treatment

In spite of discrepancies in dosage regimens, international consensus supports the use of parenteral penicillin as first-line treatment for all stages of syphilitic infection. *T. pallidum* has remained sensitive to penicillin despite more than 60 years of its use in the treatment of syphilis. A standard course cures most patients, although some authorities have recorded serological failure rates as high as 25%.

It is thought that tertiary syphilis requires a longer course of treatment than early syphilis, since the treponemes may be dividing very slowly in the later stage of infection. The World Health Organization and European and United States guidelines recommend treatment of cardiovascular syphilis with benzathine benzylpenicillin 2.4×10^6 units administered once weekly for 3 weeks by the intramuscular route. United Kingdom guidelines propose 750 mg procaine benzyl penicillin once daily for 17 days by the intramuscular route. The Australian recommendation for the treatment of all forms of tertiary syphilis is benzylpenicillin 1.8 g intravenously 4-hourly for 15 days. Doxycycline, 100 mg by mouth twice daily for 28 days, is recommended by the United States Centers for Disease Control in those with penicillin allergy; United Kingdom guidelines suggest that doxycycline 200 mg twice daily for 28 days is preferable.

An unusual feature in the antibiotic treatment of syphilis is the Jarisch–Herxheimer reaction. The mechanism of the reaction, which takes the form of malaise and fever within 24 h of penicillin treatment, is uncertain and may be due to release of endotoxins from the massive death of treponema. In patients with cardiovascular syphilis, the Jarisch–Herxheimer reaction can be avoided by prednisolone 10 to 20 mg three times daily for 3 days, starting 24 h before commencement of penicillin therapy. Established aortic aneurysm and aortic regurgitation cannot be reversed or halted by medical treatment.

All patients with cardiovascular syphilis require clinical and serological follow-up 6 and 12 months after treatment. Syphilis serology is often difficult to interpret after treatment, as post-treatment treponemal tests usually remain positive even after completion of successful treatment. Treatment failure could be indicated by failure of nonspecific treponema antibody titres to decline fourfold within 6 months of treatment. There is a higher rate of syphilis treatment failure in HIV-positive patients.

Surgical treatment

Digital subtraction aortography, MRI, or three-dimensional CT scanning enables visualization of the anatomy of syphilitic aortitis and can inform surgical strategy (Fig. 9.4.4). The aortic valve, if it is involved, may be replaced by a prosthetic valve if there is normal aortic tissue upstream. Alternatively, a Bentall procedure, which involves replacement of the ascending aortic arch, may be the surgical treatment of choice. Coronary ostial lesions have been conventionally treated, with favourable results, using internal mammary grafts or in combination with saphenous vein grafting.

Isolated aortic aneurysm may be treated with endovascular stent-graft repair, especially in patients with comorbidities who may be at high risk for open surgery, provided the lesion is considered anatomically suitable with adequate proximal and distal vessels. Conventional surgery, combined with endovascular repair, may be tried in the patients with syphilitic aortic aneurysm involving the

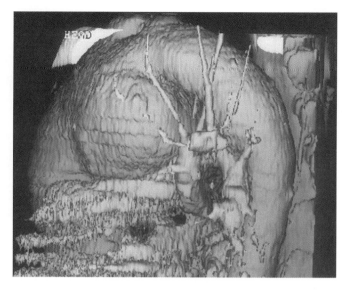

Fig. 9.4.4 Three-dimensional left-profile reconstruction of the thoracic aorta and adjacent structures in a 51-year-old man with the finding, on routine chest radiography, of an aortic aneurysm that proved to be syphilitic.
From de Cannière D, *et al.* (1999). 21st century imaging for a 19th-century disease, *Circulation*, **100**, 884–5.

aortic arch and the descending thoracic aorta, with the 30-day mortality of such intervention ranging from 5 to 10%.

Further reading

Bodhey NK, *et al.* (2003). Early sternal erosion and luetic aneurysms of thoracic aorta. *Eur J Cardiothorac Surg*, **28**, 499–501.

Cheng TO (2001). Syphilitic aortitis is dying but not yet dead. *Catheter Cardiovasc Interv*, **52**, 240–1.

Feier H, *et al.* (2012). Coronary ostial stenosis in a young patient. *Circulation*, **125**, e367–8.

Goh BT (2005). Syphilis in adults. *Sex Transm Infect*, **81**, 448–52.

Golden MR, Marra CM, Holmes KK (2003). Update on syphilis: resurgence of an old problem. *JAMA*, **290**, 1510–14.

Goldstein B, Carroccio A, Ellozy SH (2003). Combined open and endovascular repair of a syphilitic aortic aneurysm. *J Vasc Surg*, **38**, 1422–5.

Jackman JD, Radolf JD (1989). Cardiovascular syphilis. *Am J Med*, **87**, 425–33.

Kennedy JLW, Barnard JJ, Prahlow JA (2006). Syphilitic coronary ostial stenosis resulting in acute myocardial infarction and death. *Cardiology*, **105**, 25–9.

Maharajan M, Sampath Kumaar G (2005). Cardiovascular syphilis in HIV infection: a case-controlled study at the Institute of Sexually Transmitted Diseases, Chennai, India. *Sex Transm Infect*, **81**, 361.

Parkes R, *et al.* (2004). Review of current evidence and comparison of guidelines for effective syphilis treatment in Europe. *Int J STD AIDS*, **15**, 73–88.

Roberts WC, *et al.* (2015). Syphilis as a cause of thoracic aortic aneurysm. *Am J Cardiol*, **116**, 1298–1303.

Tomey MI, Murthy VL, Beckman JA (2011). Giant syphilitic aneurysm: A case report and review of the literature. *Vasc Med*, **16**, 360–4.

Tong SYC, Haqqani H, Street AC (2006). A pox on the heart: five cases of cardiovascular syphilis. *MJA*, **184**, 241–3.

Treglia G, Taralli S, Maggi F, Coli A, Lauriola L, Giordano A (2013). Usefulness of 18F-FDG PET/CT in disease extent and treatment response assessment in a patient with syphilitic aortitis. *Clin Nucl Med*, **38**, e185–7.

Tumours of the heart

CHAPTER 10.1

Tumours of the heart

Thomas A. Traill

Essentials

Cardiac myxoma

Cardiac myxomas are rare benign tumours that grow in the lumen of the atria, usually the left. Most are sporadic, but they can be associated with the Carney complex, where unusual freckling is typically the most obvious clinical clue.

Symptoms and signs most commonly mimic those of mitral stenosis. Systemic emboli occur in about 40% of cases. Constitutional effects predominate in a few patients who present with what seems to be an obscure multisystem disorder. In many patients, specific cardiovascular signs are inconspicuous or absent: an audible 'tumour plop' in early diastole, analogous to a mitral opening snap, is often reported only after the diagnosis is established.

The diagnosis is almost always made by echocardiography. Treatment is by urgent surgical removal. Recurrence is uncommon, provided excision has been complete, except in Carney complex.

Other tumours of the heart

The most common tumour seen in adult patients is the benign papillary fibroelastoma, which should be surgically removed only if it has been discovered in the search for a source of otherwise unexplained embolism.

Primary cardiac sarcomas are found more often in the right heart than in the left. Surgical resection is often attempted for obstructive symptoms, but recurrence and metastasis are common, and long-term outcome is very poor.

Microscopic secondary deposits within the myocardium can often be found in patients who die of metastatic cancer, but these are rarely of clinical importance. Intraluminal spread of cancer to the heart by direct extension up the inferior vena cava is a particular feature of renal cell carcinoma.

Cardiac myxoma

Cardiac myxomas are benign, typically golfball-sized, tumours that grow in the lumen of the atria, usually the left, attached by a stalk to the atrial septum. They are not common, but are important because they can present in a number of ways to general physicians, and because most can straightforwardly and permanently be removed by heart surgery. They are easily demonstrated by conventional transthoracic echocardiography, and it is usually the echocardiographer who makes the diagnosis; seldom has the patient been referred with this possibility in mind. Estimates of the prevalence of such a rare

condition are necessarily approximate and range from 1 to 5 per 10 000 in autopsy series, or 2 per 100 000 in the general population, with a sex ratio of 2:1 in favour of women. As a cause of left atrial obstruction, myxomas are 200 to 400 times less common than mitral stenosis. Most patients are between 30 and 60 years of age, but there are reports of tumours occurring in infants and in older people.

Most myxomas are sporadic, unassociated with other diseases, but there is at least one Mendelian syndrome involving myxoma, best named the Carney complex. This is caused by mutation in the protein kinase A regulatory subunit-1-alpha gene (Carney complex type 1, OMIM 160980) or mutations in other genes and characterized by lentiginosis, multiple myxomas (most of them cardiac), skin fibromas, and various kinds of endocrine overactivity, which has included Cushing's syndrome caused by pigmented adrenocortical hyperplasia, acromegaly, and Sertoli cell tumour. Unlike the usual kind of atrial myxoma, myxomas in Carney's syndrome may arise anywhere in the heart, are commonly multiple, and frequently recur. Inheritance of this rare disease is autosomal dominant, with centrofacial freckling as the most obvious outward marker of the phenotype. This freckling often involves unusual areas, for instance the lips, conjunctiva, and vulva.

Pathology

Cardiac myxomas are benign. Local invasion is unknown and metastatic growth is exceptional, despite the lesions' situation in the bloodstream. They take the form of polypoid masses arising from a stalk, ranging in size from 3 cm to as much as 10 cm or more, with a smooth or lobulated surface and gelatinous consistency. They are frequently covered with more or less adherent thrombus. More than 75% occur within the left atrium, with the base of the pedicle arising from the fossa ovalis or its rim. Occasionally, they arise from the base of the mitral valve leaflets, from the posterior part of the left atrium, or from within the right atrium. Sometimes they grow in both atria, in the form of a dumbbell. Ventricular myxomas are exceptional and seen almost exclusively as part of Carney's syndrome. Left atrial myxomas are not generally as large as those in the right atrium at the time they are first detected. The latter may almost fill the right atrium before they begin to obstruct systemic venous return.

The histology is that of a loosely woven, sparsely cellular, connective tissue tumour with very infrequent mitotic figures. Several cell types are identifiable, including undifferentiated stellate and polygonal cells, as well as smaller numbers of fibroblasts, smooth muscle cells, and endothelial cells. Among these are found macrophages and plasma cells, and rarely other mesodermal tissues, including bone. Cytogenetic studies fit with the general presumption that these indolent masses are indeed neoplastic, but immunohistochemical studies of differentiation markers do not clearly define the cell type of origin. It is suggested that the source is a primitive multipotential mesenchymal cell and that the predilection of these tumours for the atrial septum reflects the abundance of such cells in this region.

Clinical features

Left atrial obstruction

The most common symptoms and signs mimic those of mitral stenosis, with left ventricular inflow obstruction as the chief pathophysiological change. The presenting symptoms are progressive breathlessness, orthopnoea, paroxysmal nocturnal dyspnoea, fluid retention, and atrial arrhythmias. Examination suggests rheumatic heart disease, and before the routine use of ultrasonography a few such patients were referred for mitral valve surgery and the lesion was first diagnosed at operation. Some patients may develop pulmonary hypertension before the diagnosis becomes apparent.

Systemic embolism

Systemic emboli occur in about 40% of patients and are frequently the first manifestation of disease. In contrast to mitral stenosis, such emboli often occur while patients are in sinus rhythm. Emboli may be sizeable, large enough even to occlude the aortic bifurcation, and, besides thrombus, they frequently contain tumour material, hence histological examination may be diagnostic. When systemic emboli are removed from patients, they should always be sent for histological analysis. Typically, patients with systemic embolism are referred for echocardiography, and the diagnosis is then easily made.

Constitutional effects

Constitutional effects of the neoplasm predominate in a few patients who present with what seems to be an obscure multisystem disorder. Symptoms and signs include fever, weight loss (which is more conspicuous than in mitral stenosis and often occurs without severe left atrial obstruction), Raynaud's phenomenon (rare), finger clubbing (rare), a raised erythrocyte sedimentation rate (present in about 60% of patients), and abnormal serum proteins with elevated immunoglobulin levels. These changes are usually attributed to abnormal proteins secreted by the tumour, although the nature of these has not been determined. Other haematological abnormalities include anaemia, which may be due to mechanical haemolysis, polycythaemia, associated particularly with right atrial tumours, leucocytosis, and thrombocytopenia. Such constitutional changes may prompt an initial diagnosis of infective endocarditis in patients who have heart murmurs, or lead to the suspicion of autoimmune rheumatic or vasculitic disease, or of occult cancer.

Physical signs

In many patients, specific cardiovascular signs of myxoma are inconspicuous or absent. In others, they vary from a prominent first heart sound to obvious changes similar to those of mitral valve disease. These include apical systolic murmurs, somewhat more common than diastolic rumbles, and—in some patients—signs of pulmonary hypertension, with accentuated pulmonary closure and tricuspid regurgitation. Some may have an audible 'tumour plop' in early diastole, analogous to a mitral opening snap, but this is often reported only after echocardiographic diagnosis. On combined echocardiographic and phonocardiographic recordings, the plop is seen to coincide with the end of the tumour's downward movement into the ventricle, usually a short time after mitral valve opening. A rare but specific feature of the condition is variation of the auscultatory findings with change in posture; this may be particularly obvious in right atrial tumours.

Investigations

Chest radiography and electrocardiography do not help to distinguish myxoma from mitral valve disease. Left atrial enlargement is common but seldom marked, and signs of pulmonary venous hypertension are infrequent. Calcification within the tumour is rarely demonstrable. Myxomas may be identified as filling defects on CT examinations of the chest .

Echocardiography

While the first account of left atrial myxoma diagnosed during life was not until 1951, it is now exceptional for the diagnosis to be made first at autopsy. This is chiefly attributable to the wide availability of echocardiography, which has proved itself both reliable and specific for recognizing these tumours. It is no accident that the echocardiographic appearance of these lesions was among the first clinical reports by ultrasonographers in 1959. Figure 10.1.1 illustrates a typical two-dimensional echocardiogram from a patient with left atrial myxoma. A video recording would demonstrate the mobility of the mass as it flops to and fro within the atrium, restrained only by its peduncle.

Transoesophageal echocardiography affords the opportunity to examine the tumour and its attachment with great precision; generally this extra clarity is unnecessary, but on occasion the transoesophageal technique is helpful if there is difficulty in differentiating tumour from an atrial thrombus.

The differential diagnosis of left atrial myxoma is seldom difficult. Large masses may occasionally be difficult to distinguish from left atrial ball thrombus—a lesion that is even rarer than myxoma. Smaller left atrial masses may be papillary fibroelastomas or infective vegetations caused by endocarditis. These can usually be distinguished by their clinical context. Masses in the right atrium may also be due to thrombus, sometimes propagated from the inferior vena cava, or occasionally venous extension of abdominal cancers, particularly renal cell cancer. In a few patients, abundant strands

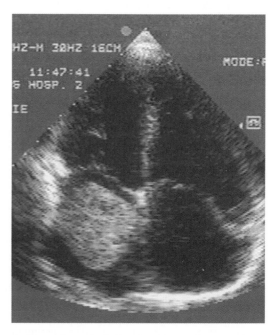

Fig. 10.1.1 Echocardiogram in the four-chamber view showing a myxoma occupying much of the left atrium.

of the Chiari network of right atrial trabeculation may give rise to similar echocardiographic appearances. Myxoma is the only neoplasm of the heart to be found within its lumen: other cardiac neoplasms grow within the walls.

Cardiac catheterization

The echocardiographic appearance is so characteristic that angiography no longer has a role in diagnosis of myxoma, although it may be required as a prelude to surgery in the older patient in whom there is, or might be, coronary artery disease.

Treatment and prognosis

Atrial myxoma is treated by urgent surgical removal. The risk is low, comparable to that of surgery for mitral valve disease. It is important to ensure complete removal of the base by excising a full-thickness button of the atrial septum, the resulting defect being repaired with a small patch.

Functional results of surgery are good. Some patients are left with mitral regurgitation, but this is seldom severe. Recurrence is uncommon, provided excision has been complete, except in Carney's syndrome. In these patients, regular echocardiographic follow-up is required, at intervals of 6 months. The rare occurrence, after excision, of the usual kind of myxoma generally occurs within the first 2 years; thereafter, follow-up can safely be infrequent.

Other tumours of the heart

Although each individually is rare, taken together the other tumours of the heart have an incidence that roughly equals that of myxoma. They include benign lesions, seen especially in children; sarcomas; and secondary involvement by metastasis or direct tumour extension. They are generally first recognized or suspected during echocardiography. MRI, or occasionally echo-directed transvenous biopsy, usually yields the diagnosis.

Benign cardiac tumours

Papillary fibroelastoma

The most common tumour seen in adult patients is the papillary fibroelastoma, a small pedunculated mass that hangs off one of the left-sided valve leaflets, usually the mitral valve. Its echocardiographic appearance is very characteristic. The size of the mass and presence of a peduncle distinguish this small tumour from the usual kind of Lambl's excrescence, but histologically they are identical and, like Lambl's excrescences, papillary fibroelastomas probably arise through organization of fibrinous material that collects at the trailing edges of the valve leaflets. Their importance lies in the fact that they have been labelled as a potential source of systemic embolism, and that some authors have recommended they should be removed as a matter of routine. The evidence to support this view is thin, and the author's recommendation is to remove them only if they have been discovered in the search for a source of otherwise unexplained embolism. If they are an incidental echocardiographic finding, then it is safe to leave them alone; aspirin treatment is recommended.

Fibroma, rhabdomyoma, hamartoma, and haemangioma

These are tumours of childhood, rhabdomyoma being the characteristic cardiac tumour in patients with tuberous sclerosis. In contrast to myxomas and fibroelastomas, they grow within the myocardium, not into the lumen of the heart. Rhabdomyomas are usually asymptomatic, and when they are they should be left alone, since most regress spontaneously. Fibromas and hamartomas are both very rare, presenting with arrhythmias (particularly ventricular hamartomas or Purkinje cell tumours) or with haemodynamic abnormalities caused by their mass effect. They require surgical excision, and when this is feasible the long-term results of treatment are very good. Haemangiomas, also very rare, tend to grow and to develop multiple feeding vessels, so that surgical excision is usually recommended.

Cardiac sarcoma

Primary cardiac sarcomas are found more often in the right heart than in the left, and can have one of several cell types. Haemangiosarcoma is the most common, typically developing in the right atrium. Rhabdomyosarcoma may develop in the ventricular septum or in the right ventricular outflow tract, as may the still rarer osteosarcoma, or tumours that are undifferentiated. Since these tumours often present with mechanical effects, typically obstruction at the atrial or outflow tract level, surgical resection is often attempted. However, recurrence and metastasis are common, and long-term outcome is very poor.

Cardiac involvement by other malignancies

Microscopic secondary deposits within the myocardium can often be found in patients who die of metastatic cancer, but intramyocardial secondaries of a size large enough to be of clinical importance are very rare. By contrast, pericardial involvement by lymphoma, or by cancers of the lung, breast, pancreas, and other tumours is not uncommon, and may sometimes be the first presentation of the tumour (see Chapter 8.1). Treatment is analogous to that of malignant pleural effusions, with drainage, creation of a window, or intrapericardial chemotherapy, depending on the rest of the clinical situation.

Intraluminal spread of cancer, by direct extension up the inferior vena cava, is a particular feature of renal cell carcinoma. Diagnosis by echocardiography is generally obvious, as the tumour has a very characteristic appearance as it waves like seaweed in the right atrium and even dangles through the rest of the right heart. It may prove possible to resect the cava, along with the kidney and the tumour mass, under circulatory arrest.

Further reading

Cardiac myxoma

Casey M, *et al.* (2000). Mutations in the protein kinase A R1alpha regulatory subunit cause familial cardiac myxomas and Carney complex. *J Clin Invest*, **106**, R31–8.

Greenwood WF (1968). Profile of atrial myxoma. *Am J Cardiol*, **21**, 367–75.

Pucci A, Gagliardotto P, Zanini C, *et al.* (2000). Histopathologic and clinical characterization of cardiac myxoma: review of 53 cases from a single institution. *Am Heart J*, **140**, 134–8.

Schaff HV, Mullany CJ (2000). Surgery for cardiac myxomas. *Semin Thorac Cardiovasc Surg*, **12**, 77–88.

Wilkes D, McDermott DA, Basson CT (2005). Clinical phenotypes and molecular genetic mechanisms of Carney complex. *Lancet Oncol*, **6**, 501–8.

Other tumours of the heart

Burke A, Jeudy J Jr, Virmani R (2008). Cardiac tumours: an update. *Heart*, **94**, 117–23.

Cardiac involvement in genetic disease

CHAPTER 11.1

Cardiac involvement in genetic disease

Thomas A. Traill

Essentials

Many clinicians find themselves faced, from time to time, with a patient who has a family history of a known disorder, such as Marfan's syndrome, or who has noncardiac features that suggest a syndrome.

Syndromic congenital heart disease

Down's syndrome—25 to 50% have congenital heart disease, most characteristically atrioventricular canal defect.

Turner's syndrome—causes two principal abnormalities of the aorta: coarctation and congenital abnormalities of the aortic valve (usually bicuspid).

Noonan's syndrome—the most common heritable syndrome that characteristically causes congenital heart disease. Mutations in an intracellular signalling molecule protein tyrosine phosphatase SHP-2 account for 40% of cases. Characteristics include short stature, with a facies that is variously described as elfin or triangular, ocular hypertelorism, ears that are set low and rotated forwards, and webbing of the neck (the most obvious of the features that may lead to confusion with Turner's syndrome). The most typical cardiac lesion is pulmonary stenosis.

Williams' syndrome—caused by macrodeletions of chromosome 7 that include the elastin gene; includes the cardiovascular features of familial supravalvar aortic stenosis along with a characteristic facial appearance, with round, blue eyes, a distinctive stellate pattern of the irises, depression of the nasal bridge, outwards tilting of the nostrils, abnormal dentition, and big lips.

Other conditions—many other genetic syndromes have significant cardiac and vascular manifestations.

Connective tissue disorders

Marfan's syndrome—caused by mutations of the fibrillin-1 gene (*FBN1*); characteristic cardiovascular findings are aneurysmal dilatation of the aorta, and occasionally other large arteries, and floppy mitral valve. Diagnosis is based on the presence of particular major or minor criteria, the major criteria being (1) aortic aneurysm, (2) lens subluxation, (3) characteristic skeletal abnormalities, and (4) dural ectasia. Aortic dissection and rupture are the commonest causes of death in untreated cases. β-Blockers are commonly given to slow the progression to aneurysm, but the benefit is probably modest and recent work suggests that angiotensin-II receptor blockers may be much more effective. Surgical replacement of the

aortic root is generally recommended when the maximum measurement across the aorta reaches 5 cm.
Other conditions—the Ehlers–Danlos syndromes and many other genetic disorders have significant cardiac and vascular manifestations.

Introduction

Picking out a few of the more prominent Mendelian disorders seen by cardiologists may seem a somewhat arbitrary basis for a chapter, especially in an age when we are exploring the molecular genetic basis for so many more of the common heart diseases, but it works in practice. Many clinicians find themselves faced, from time to time, with a patient who has a family history of a known disorder, such as Marfan's syndrome, or who has noncardiac features that suggest a syndrome, perhaps Noonan's. They may wonder how to make the diagnosis, what else to look for, and how to screen family members.

Inherited diseases of the contractile machinery and energy regulation of the heart-muscle cell, which lead to familial hypertrophic and dilated cardiomyopathy, are covered in Chapters 7.2 and 7.3. Ion-channel mutations that underlie long-QT syndromes and other inherited causes of paroxysmal ventricular tachycardia and other arrhythmias are covered in Chapter 4. Heritability of cardiomyopathy and the tendency to arrhythmia is increasingly picked up clinically as awareness of their genetic basis becomes more widespread.

The first part of this chapter deals with developmental syndromes that include congenital cardiac defects, with coverage restricted to a few relatively common disorders that are seen in adult patients. The second part describes the two common connective tissue disorders—Marfan's and Ehlers–Danlos syndromes—and the more recently described Loeys–Dietz syndrome that shares some pathogenetic mechanisms with Marfan's. A number of other heritable diseases that affect the heart are listed in a table, without discussion in the text. Haemochromatosis (Chapter 12.7.1) and Friedreich's ataxia (Chapter 24.7.5) are discussed elsewhere; the others, though important to other organ systems, offer little opportunity to the cardiologist for diagnosis or management.

Syndromic congenital heart disease
Aneuploidy disorders

The two commonest chromosomal disorders in adult patients are Down's and Turner's syndromes, and each includes characteristic cardiac abnormalities. A third, Klinefelter's syndrome, does not.

Some 25 to 50% of patients with Down's syndrome (OMIM 190685) have congenital heart disease. The characteristic lesion, present in about one-half of the affected hearts, is atrioventricular canal defect. This ranges from the relatively simple primum atrial septal defect to the complete type, in which the defect involves both the atrial and ventricular septa, between which there lies a single atrioventricular valve ring. In other patients, ventricular septal defect, tetralogy of Fallot, and persistent ductus arteriosus are seen in roughly equal numbers. Patients with Down's syndrome undergo heart surgery most easily when they are infants, and the tendency has shifted from the nihilistic approach of past years to correcting serious cardiac malformations early in life.

Turner's syndrome causes coarctation of the aorta, and congenital abnormalities of the aortic valve, usually a bicuspid valve. These are lesions that commonly accompany one another, even in the absence of an identifiable genetic cause. Patients with either lesion frequently have aortic ectasia. In some patients with Turner's syndrome, the whole aorta is abnormal—either hypoplastic or weakened by the presence of cystic medial necrosis. Aortic dissection may occur, and aortic surgery, e.g. to repair coarctation, can sometimes be very difficult, owing to the fragile nature of the aortic wall. Other congenital heart abnormalities are not common in Turner's syndrome, except for anomalies of pulmonary venous return.

Mendelian syndromes that include congenital heart disease

Noonan's syndrome

Noonan's syndrome (OMIM 163950) is the most common heritable syndrome that characteristically causes congenital heart disease. The syndrome shares some features with the Turner phenotype, and the two were confused between 1930 and the 1960s. In 1963, Noonan described a small series of patients with pulmonary stenosis who shared a characteristic facial appearance. Since then, the expanded phenotype has been well described and shown to be associated with a normal karyotype and autosomal dominant inheritance. The condition is genetically heterogeneous, with causative mutations shown in eight proteins, all members of the RAS-MAPK growth-regulating pathway that links extracellular signalling proteins to gene transcription factors. Mutations in the intracellular signalling molecule protein tyrosine phosphatase SHP-2 (the gene is called *PTPN11*) are the most common, and account for 50% of cases. The pathogenetics are complicated by both clinical and genetic overlap.

Another syndrome—LEOPARD syndrome (OMIM 151100)—is also caused by *PTPN11* mutations, and the Noonan phenotype is closely related to disorders caused by mutations affecting other members of the RAS-ERK intracellular signalling cascade. Within Noonan's syndrome there is some suggestion that mutations of particular proteins within the signalling cascade may predict particular phenotypic features.

Patients with Noonan's syndrome are of short stature, with a facies that is variously described as elfin or triangular (Fig. 11.1.1), emphasized by ocular hypertelorism. The palpebral fissure may slope downwards and outwards, and display ptosis and an epicanthal fold. The ears are set low and rotated forwards so that the lobes are prominent, and there is characteristic webbing of the neck—the most obvious of the features that may lead to confusion with Turner's syndrome. Pectus deformities are common, as are other miscellaneous skeletal abnormalities, including cubitus valgus. Patients with Noonan's syndrome are prone to develop keloid scars. Cryptorchidism is common, as is delayed sexual maturation, but not infantilism as in Turner's syndrome. Unlike Turner's syndrome, many patients with Noonan's syndrome have a degree of mental handicap, but this is quite variable. Among the author's patients with Noonan's syndrome are a physician, an architect, a certified accountant, and a high-school mathematics teacher.

The frequency of cardiac involvement in Noonan's syndrome is high, estimated as more than 80%, but because the diagnosis is so easily missed in the absence of congenital heart disease the true frequency may be less. The most characteristic lesion is pulmonary stenosis, but in contrast to the almost stereotypical cardiovascular findings in Turner's syndrome, the range in Noonan's syndrome is broad. In many patients, the stenotic pulmonary valve leaflets are not simply fused, as in nonsyndromic pulmonary stenosis, but may be dysplastic, thickened, and immobile—unsuitable for simple

(a) (b) (c)

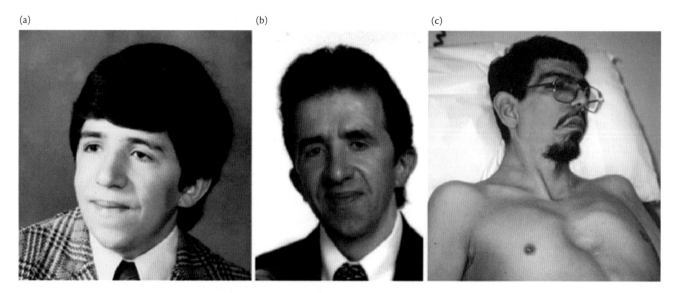

Fig. 11.1.1 Two patients with Noonan's syndrome: (a, b) patient 1 aged 18 and 40; (c) patient 2—note scars at site of plastic surgery for pterygium colli.

balloon or surgical valvotomy. Other congenital lesions found in Noonan's syndrome are ventricular and atrial septal defects, tricuspid atresia, single ventricle, and abnormalities of the left ventricle, including congenital mitral stenosis, subaortic stenosis, and a combination of these two lesions. The electrocardiogram often shows a superior axis (left-axis deviation), even when there is pulmonary stenosis and right ventricular hypertrophy.

The most ominous complication of Noonan's syndrome is cardiomyopathy, taking the form of myocardial hypertrophy complicated by progressive fibrosis. This leads, over the course of 5 to 15 years, to low cardiac output with very high ventricular diastolic pressures—the pathophysiology of restrictive cardiomyopathy. Since the valvular abnormalities are for the most part correctable, this hypertrophic restrictive cardiomyopathy is the main factor limiting life expectancy.

Familial supravalvar aortic stenosis and Williams' syndrome

Familial supravalvar aortic stenosis is caused by loss-of-function mutation or deletion affecting the gene for elastin located on chromosome 7. Affected patients develop a tight, fleshy constriction of the aorta, or sometimes the pulmonary artery, at the level of the sinotubular junction above the semilunar valve (Fig. 11.1.2). In some patients, both great arteries are affected. Supravalvar aortic stenosis can lead to severe left ventricular outflow obstruction, with left ventricular failure or even sudden death. This is not a setting for balloon dilation or stenting, but the results of surgery are good, for either lesion or for both.

Williams' syndrome (OMIM 194050) is one of the best-documented examples of a contiguous gene phenomenon seen in adult medicine. It is caused by macrodeletions of chromosome 7 that include the elastin gene. Hence, Williams' syndrome includes the cardiovascular features of familial supravalvar aortic stenosis described in the previous paragraph. In addition, more far-reaching effects caused by deletion of contiguous genes accompany these vascular abnormalities. The full syndrome includes a

characteristic facial appearance, with round, blue eyes, a distinctive stellate pattern of the irises, depression of the nasal bridge, outwards tilting of the nostrils, abnormal dentition, and big lips, together with small stature, mental retardation, and a history of infantile hypercalcaemia. Mental retardation in Williams' syndrome takes on very individual forms, the patients often being articulate and socially adept: several purported idiot savants have had Williams' syndrome. As in the purely cardiac syndrome, surgery may be required to relieve severe left (or right) ventricular outflow obstruction.

DiGeorge and velocardiofacial syndromes (chromosome 22 deletion syndrome)

DiGeorge syndrome (OMIM 188400), described in 1965, comprises abnormalities of the parathyroid glands, absence or hypoplasia of the thymus, and conotruncal abnormalities of the heart such as pulmonary atresia and severe forms of tetralogy of Fallot. A number of affected patients have learning disabilities or schizophrenia. It was recognized soon after the original description that the syndrome is generally caused by deletions in a region of chromosome 22.

Velocardiofacial syndrome (OMIM 192430), or Shprintzen's syndrome, described in 1981, comprises similar cardiac abnormalities along with cleft palate, a characteristic facies, and learning difficulty. It has since proved to be caused by deletions in the same region of chromosome 22, now often referred to as the DiGeorge critical region (DGCR). A third syndrome, known as 'conotruncal anomalies face', is also linked to this site.

With a broad spectrum of phenotypic variation, and deletions that are often quite large, it was suspected for some time that these syndromes are related manifestations of a contiguous gene phenomenon, just as in Williams' syndrome. However, it has emerged that the size of the deletion does not predict the extent of the phenotype, and that within a family the same (presumably stable) deletion can be the cause of a wide range of phenotypes. Two candidate genes lie within the DGCR—*TBX1* and *UFDIL*; it remains to be

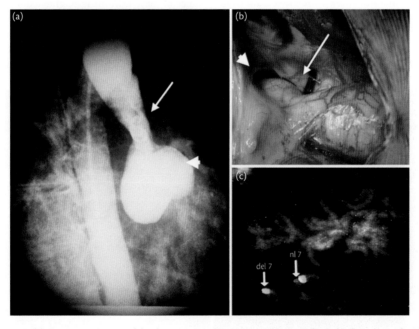

Fig. 11.1.2 Supravalvar aortic stenosis: (a) Contrast angiogram of the thoracic aorta showing normal sinuses of Valsalva (broad arrow) with constriction at the sino–tubular junction (narrow arrow). (b) Operative photograph. The patient's head is to the right. Arrows as in panel (a). (c) Fluorescence *in situ* hybridization (FISH) showing two markers for chromosome 7 (bright fluorescence), but only one for the elastin gene (orange fluorescence).

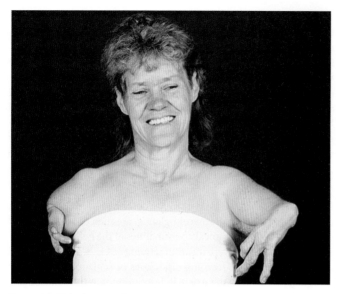

Fig. 11.1.3 Holt–Oram syndrome.

seen whether either can be implicated as the cause of the entire group of phenotypes.

Heart–hand syndromes

The two commonly recognized heart–hand syndromes are Holt–Oram syndrome and Ellis–van Creveld syndrome.

Holt–Oram syndrome

Holt–Oram syndrome (OMIM 142900), inherited as an autosomal dominant trait, was described in 1960. It includes a secundum atrial septal defect and skeletal abnormalities, principally affecting the upper limbs and shoulder girdle, never the legs, and usually more pronounced in the left arm (Fig. 11.1.3). Within a family, affected individuals may have skeletal abnormalities, congenital heart disease, or both. The limb abnormalities cover a wide spectrum from just a triphalangeal thumb to phocomelia. Abnormalities of the hand and forearm always involve the radial side and thumb (in contrast to Ellis–van Creveld syndrome). The characteristic cardiac abnormality is fossa ovalis (secundum) atrial septal defect, but

affected patients may have other relatively simple lesions, e.g. ventricular septal defect or pulmonary stenosis.

Holt–Oram syndrome is caused by mutation in a transcription factor, TBX5, a close homologue of a transcription factor seen as phylogenetically far away as the fruit fly, where mutations produce abnormalities of the wing.

Ellis–van Creveld syndrome

Ellis–van Creveld syndrome (OMIM 225500) is inherited as a recessive trait, hence the more complete clinical descriptions have come from studies in genetically circumscribed communities, notably the Old Order Amish of Pennsylvania where, thanks to a founder effect, the gene is common and homozygotes abound. The syndrome, described in 1940, includes dwarfism, caused mainly by shortening of the forearms and lower legs, and symmetrical polydactyly affecting the ulnar side with accessory sixth and even seventh digits attached to or beyond the little finger. Cardiac involvement is very common, present probably in three-quarters of homozygotes. The characteristic lesion is common atrium—a lesion that has the appearance, on echocardiography and to the surgeon, of a very large primum atrial septal defect. A few patients have more complete forms of atrioventricular canal defect, and—at least among the Amish—there is a high perinatal mortality rate among affected infants, suggesting the possibility of still more extensive cardiac involvement. The gene has been mapped to chromosome 4, sequenced, and named *EVC*. The protein has been identified as playing a role in the hedgehog signal transduction pathway.

Connective tissue disorders

Marfan's syndrome

Thanks principally to the work of McKusick and his collaborators, beginning in 1955, Marfan's syndrome (OMIM 154700) has become the paradigm for the clinical, genetic, and molecular investigation of the heritable disorders of connective tissue. The importance of the syndrome is heightened by the fact that its recognition and treatment have had a dramatic impact on survival among those affected. Untreated, patients had a median survival into the fourth decade before death from aortic dissection and rupture (Fig. 11.1.4). Today, affected patients have a near-normal lifespan,

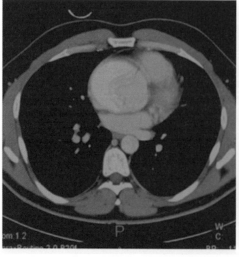
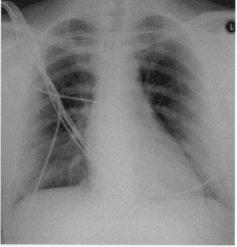

Fig. 11.1.4 Aortic ectasia and dissection in a patient with Marfan's syndrome. Note that the aortic root enlargement, to 7 cm, is not apparent from the chest radiograph.

and there are reasons to hope that recent advances in understanding the molecular pathogenesis may yet make this genetic disease, in a sense, 'curable'.

In 1896, Marfan described a weak, generally hypotonic child, with what he termed arachnodactyly. In the ensuing 100 years it was appreciated that the syndrome is Mendelian and pleiotropic, involving several apparently unrelated organs whose common feature seemed initially to be just the importance of elastic tissue to their structural integrity. Ocular involvement, with the lens subluxed because of failure of its suspensory ligament, was recognized early in the 20th century. Cardiovascular involvement was noted incidentally in the 1940s, and studied systematically from the 1950s onwards. Skeletal involvement includes—besides long limbs and arachnodactyly—scoliosis and other abnormalities of the thoracic cage. The sternum may be pushed outwards or inwards by the abnormally long ribs, hence pectus carinatum and/or excavatum, often asymmetrical. Skin involvement is identified by light-coloured striae, which should be looked for over the deltopectoral groove and the flanks. Less common findings are dural ectasia, which can sometimes be so marked as to cause radicular symptoms, and pulmonary involvement with emphysema, spontaneous pneumothorax or apical blebs. In severely affected children, like the one Marfan described, there may be generalized weakness and hypotonia. These last findings are hard to account for just on the basis of abnormal elastic tissue, and recognizing this led to an appreciation that the pathogenesis of Marfan's involves abnormal growth regulation, not simply a fixed physical abnormality of ground substance scaffolding.

The characteristic cardiovascular findings in Marfan's syndrome are aneurysmal dilatation of the aorta, and occasionally other large arteries, and floppy mitral valve. The former was recognized in the 1920s, but not really addressed until McKusick showed that it was the principal cause of early death in the disease. Shortly afterwards, echocardiography became available to identify and follow these abnormalities, and surgical techniques were developed by Bentall and Gott to repair the aneurysms. Until then, median life expectancy for men with Marfan's syndrome had been 45 years, for women a year or two longer.

Fibrillin-1 mutations

The syndrome (OMIM 134797) is caused by mutations of the fibrillin-1 gene (*FBN1*) on chromosome 15. It has recently emerged that besides a purely structural role, one that could hardly be replaced by any form of treatment, fibrillin-1 acts to modulate cell-to-cell signalling during development and, at least in a mouse model, after birth. The dominant negative hypothesis, in which the mutated fibrillin protein was believed to have its effect by interfering with polymerization of the product of the nonmutated allele, thus proves to have been an oversimplification. Rather, the pleiotropic effects of *FBN1* mutations prove to be mediated through up-regulation of the signalling pathway transforming growth factor-β1 (TGFβ1), which is modulated by fibrillin-1. Such findings have led to the likelihood of pharmacological treatment for the disease. Losartan, an angiotensin-II receptor blocker, which like the other members of its class also blocks TGFβ1 signalling, has been shown dramatically to prevent aortic dilation in a mouse model, also in a small clinical cohort study. Large randomized trials of treatment in children are in progress, and at least in one such there seems indeed to be a striking positive treatment effect.

The fibrillin molecule is large, and most of the disease-causing mutations have yet to be described, hence genetic diagnosis by screening for known mutations is often not possible and diagnosis usually depends on applying clinical criteria. There are many polymorphisms within the gene, so in some kindreds it is possible, by tracking particular haplotypes, to determine which is associated with the disease and therefore contains the pathogenetic mutation. This has allowed diagnosis of the syndrome in individual family members in whom the clinical findings were uncertain, and has been used for prenatal diagnosis. Furthermore, the technique makes it possible to infer the existence of a fibrillin-1 mutation in kindreds where the phenotype has not met clinical criteria for Marfan's syndrome; if aortic ectasia segregates with a particular fibrillin-1 haplotype, then the chances are high that a fibrillin mutation somewhere in that copy is the pathogenetic mechanism.

Diagnostic criteria

The clinical diagnosis of Marfan's syndrome rests on major and minor criteria. In an index case, involvement of three organ systems is required, with major criteria in two. Major criteria can be aortic aneurysm, lens subluxation, characteristic skeletal abnormalities, or dural ectasia. Minor criteria can be striae, mitral valve prolapse, joint laxity, the facies, or moderate pectus excavatum. Characteristic skeletal abnormalities can be arachnodactyly (encircling the wrist with the thumb and little finger, the 'wrist sign', and making a fist with a protruding thumb, the 'thumb sign'), marked pectus deformity, increased wingspan to 5% more than the height, and scoliosis. In the relative of an index case, the positive family history becomes another major criterion.

In clinical practice, determining whether a patient satisfies these criteria may be fairly subjective and requires experience with the syndrome. Often, it is enough to know whether or not there is cardiovascular involvement, and there are numerous families with aortic aneurysms or ectasia who do not satisfy clinical criteria for Marfan's syndrome, yet whose long-term management is identical. Indeed, in a busy cardiac surgery practice with expertise in aortic root replacement, such 'nonsyndromic' familial aortopathy represents a significant proportion of patients treated, and some of these families have yielded other loci as sites for the cause of their disease. On the other hand, a lanky patient who has a normal aorta needs only infrequent follow-up, even though there may be a suspicion that he has a mild case of the syndrome.

Clinical management

Patients with Marfan's syndrome should be followed up with annual or 6-monthly echocardiograms to examine the aortic root. If there is reason to suspect that the aorta may be dilated above the echo plane, then CT scanning or MRI is required at least once to validate the echo measurement. When the maximum measurement across the aorta reaches 5 cm, we generally recommend surgical replacement of the aortic root, to prevent aortic dissection (see Chapter 14.1), which becomes a real risk once the dimension reaches 6 cm. The traditional and very successful approach is with the composite graft, whereby a mechanical aortic valve prosthesis—to which is indissolubly attached a tubular vascular prosthesis—is used to replace the entire aortic root and annulus. The coronary artery ostia are excised from the native aorta and reattached to the prosthetic root. Recently, to avoid anticoagulation in certain patients, there has been interest in a valve-sparing technique of root replacement in which a vascular prosthesis is fitted snugly over the aortic valve commissures, with the native leaflets suspended in their normal anatomical arrangement. Long-term success with this approach will depend on the degree to which the valve leaflets themselves degenerate because of the connective tissue abnormality. The Ross (pulmonary autograft) procedure is not appropriate in Marfan's syndrome. After surgery, and especially in patients whose surgery was done as an emergency for dissection, follow-up is with periodic imaging by CT or MRI to keep the remaining aorta under surveillance. Management of mitral prolapse and regurgitation in Marfan's syndrome is the same as in other patients. Surgery is required for severe or symptomatic regurgitation; mitral valve repair has proved surprisingly successful.

It is usual to treat patients who have aortic involvement with β-adrenergic blockers to slow the progression to aneurysm, but the benefit is probably modest. In mice with fibrillin-1 mutations in which the Marfan phenotype is well reproduced, β-adrenergic blockade had only slight effect on aortic ectasia. This was in contrast to the dramatic effect of losartan, alluded to in a previous paragraph, and many clinicians now recommend use of this drug. We generally advise against excessively demanding sports, particularly competitive basketball, but in all affected children it is important to balance the risks of aortic disease against the importance of normal psychological development. Pregnancy is not contraindicated in all women with Marfan's syndrome, but genetic counselling should be offered, and it is advised that women not become pregnant if the aorta is enlarged to over 4 cm. Indeed, aortic dissection has been reported in a very few affected patients during pregnancy, even when they did not previously have aortic enlargement. In this autosomal dominant condition with high penetrance, the risk for the offspring of affected mothers or fathers is 50%. This can be mitigated, when the disease-causing mutation has been identified, by preimplantation genetic diagnosis.

Loeys–Dietz syndrome

If the pathogenesis of Marfan's syndrome lies with abnormal TGFβ signalling, then it should not come as a surprise that mutations in the TGFβ receptors also cause abnormalities of vascular and other tissues. Recently, this was confirmed in the description of Loeys–Dietz syndrome (OMIM 609192, 610380, 610168, 608967), a disease that shares some aspects of the Marfan's phenotype and is associated with mutations of either of the two TGFβ receptors. Patients with Loeys–Dietz syndrome have more diffuse vascular involvement than those with Marfan's, and may have dissection even in vessels that are only mildly dilated. In this, they resemble patients affected by the vascular form of Ehlers–Danlos syndrome, and the phenotypes may be very difficult to distinguish. Prominent nonvascular features include ocular hypertelorism with malar hypoplasia, bifid or broad uvula (Fig. 11.1.5), cleft palate, arachnodactyly, scoliosis, and pectus excavatum, yet excessive height is uncommon.

Ehlers–Danlos syndromes

In the early part of the 20th century, Ehlers and Danlos independently described an association between hyperextensibility of the skin, atrophic scarring, and hypermobility of the large joints. In

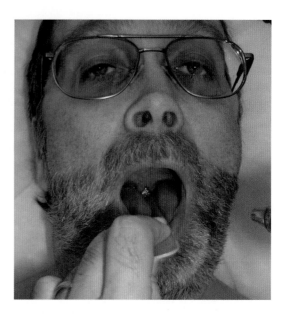

Fig. 11.1.5 Loeys–Dietz syndrome, illustrating the characteristic bifid uvula.

the following 75 years, numerous accounts were published of what we now recognize to be a group of related conditions, so that by 1988 a new classification of the Ehlers–Danlos syndrome included 10 separate phenotypes in an unwieldy classification. For practical purposes, clinicians distinguish 'classical' Ehlers–Danlos, formerly types I and II, from the potentially fatal 'vascular' form, previously type IV.

Classical Ehlers–Danlos

The classical Ehlers–Danlos syndrome (OMIM 130000, 130010) is characterized by skin elasticity, abnormal scars, and joint hypermobility, and is inherited as a dominant trait. Skin hyperextensibility is obvious, e.g. on tugging at the side of the neck or face. Joint laxity is much more marked than in Marfan's syndrome, and allows for tricks like placing the feet behind the head or other contortionist performances, besides permitting a remarkable span on the piano or violin. It also leads eventually to severe degenerative arthritis, often with considerable deformity of the hands. Ability to touch the nose with the tip of the tongue may also provide a clue to the diagnosis. The third aspect of the phenotype, atrophic scarring, if not immediately apparent, may be sought by inspecting the knees for the results of minor childhood injuries: there one may find characteristic wide, atrophic ('cigarette paper') scars still obvious from bygone years.

Cardiovascular findings in classical Ehlers–Danlos are for the most part benign. Affected patients frequently have mitral valve prolapse, as do many people with joint laxity who do not have diagnosable Ehlers–Danlos syndrome. Relatively few progress to develop severe mitral reflux or to the point of requiring surgery. Enlargement of the aortic sinuses of Valsalva may occur, but only rarely is this severe or progressive. Surgical replacement of the aortic root, as is performed in Marfan's syndrome, is unusual in Ehlers–Danlos syndrome.

Vascular Ehlers–Danlos

Unlike classical Ehlers–Danlos, vascular Ehlers–Danlos syndrome (OMIM 130050) is a potentially fatal condition, with a natural history worse than Marfan's syndrome. It is genetically and biochemically well characterized: patients have mutations in the *COL3A1* gene which encodes for type III procollagen, with inheritance as a dominant trait. The collagen defect leads to excessive fragility of blood vessels, bowel, and uterus, and the natural history of the condition is to present with spontaneous rupture of one of these three (in the case of the uterus, during pregnancy). Because of the intrinsic weakness of the affected tissues, surgical repair is challenging and these complications frequently prove fatal. Furthermore, in patients who have once undergone vascular or bowel rupture, the likelihood of a second event is high.

The joint and skin features of the vascular phenotype are less obvious than those of the classical form. Joint hypermobility is not seen, nor the resulting arthropathy. However, the skin feels soft and thin, and is abnormally translucent such that the veins are easily seen through it as one examines the shoulders and upper chest. The face is often thin and bony and the nose pinched.

Vascular complications are hard to anticipate. Aortic ectasia and aneurysm occur only in a few patients. Moreover, arterial rupture—as common as dissection—may occur in medium-sized vessels of the brain, thorax, or abdomen just as often as the aorta. In these regards, the vascular complications of this disease are comparable to those of the Loeys–Dietz syndrome. In affected patients and their families, detailed genetic evaluation is important and should include screening of *COL3A1* and biochemical analysis of type III collagen obtained from skin biopsy and cultured fibroblasts as well as screening the TGFβ receptor genes.

Table 11.1.1 Rare Mendelian disorders affecting the cardiovascular system

	Biochemical abnormality	Noncardiac features	Cardiovascular features
Osteogenesis imperfecta (OMIM 166200, and others)	Heterogeneous, abnormalities of type 1 procollagen	Bony fractures and deformity, blue scleras (four types described)	Mitral valve prolapse and regurgitation Aortic root enlargement and aortic regurgitation
Pseudoxanthoma elasticum (OMIM 264800)		Areas of thickened skin and pseudoxanthomas Vascular fragility and haemorrhage Fundus: angioid streaks	Extensive vascular narrowing and calcification with angina, claudication, and limb ischaemia
Hunter's syndrome (MPS II) (OMIM 309900)	Iduronate sulfate sulfatase	X-linked usually severe with dwarfing, mental retardation, gargoylism	Cardiomyopathy, coronary narrowing, valve lesions
Scheie's syndrome (MPS IS) (OMIM 607016)	α-Iduronidase (as in the much more severe, allelic, Hurler's syndrome, MPS IH)	Arthropathy, hepatosplenomegaly, corneal clouding	Aortic regurgitation Abnormal valve leaflets
Morquio's syndrome (MPS IV) (OMIM 253000 and others)	Galactosamine-6-sulfate sulfatase or α-galactosidase	Dwarfism, deafness, spinal cord compression and injury	Aortic regurgitation and stenosis
Homocystinuria (OMIM 236200)	Cystathionine-α-synthase	Osteoporosis, sternal deformity, lens subluxation, mental retardation	Vascular thrombosis, precocious coronary atherosclerosis
Fabry's disease (OMIM 301500)	α-Galactosidase A	Painful neuropathy, CNS disease, renal failure, corneal opacity	Coronary artery disease, myocardial infarction, mitral valve dysfunction
Friedreich's ataxia (OMIM 229300)	Frataxin	Spinocerebellar degeneration	Cardiomyopathy with increased wall thickness and restrictive physiology Ventricular arrhythmias
Duchenne's muscular dystrophy (OMIM 310200)	Dystrophin	X-linked muscular dystrophy with rapid progression during childhood and adolescence	Dilated cardiomyopathy, characteristic ECG
Becker's muscular dystrophy (OMIM 300376)	Dystrophin	X-linked muscular dystrophy, less severe than Duchenne's	Dilated cardiomyopathy, variable severity
Dystrophia myotonica (OMIM 160900)	Myotonin protein kinase	Weakness and myotonia, ptosis, cataracts, frontal balding, intellectual slowing	Bundle branch block, bradyarrhythmias, less frequently VT
Haemochromatosis (OMIM 235200 and others)	HFE protein	Diabetes, liver disease, pigmentation, arthritis, pituitary dysfunction	Dilated or restrictive cardiomyopathy
Arrhythmogenic right ventricular dysplasia (OMIM 107970 and others)	Desmosomes, Transforming growth factor-beta-3 (and others)	None	Palpitations, syncope, sudden death

CNS, central nervous system; MPS, mucopolysaccharidosis; VT, ventricular tachycardia.

Other heart-related connective tissue and metabolic disorders

Osteogenesis imperfecta causes aortic and mitral regurgitation, as do several of the mucopolysaccharidoses (Table 11.1.1). It is striking, particularly in the case of osteogenesis imperfecta, how healing is almost nonexistent where there is foreign material. If the opportunity arises, even years later, to inspect the operative result in a patient who has undergone valve replacement, the sutures look as though they had only just been placed, with minimal endothelial reaction and scar-tissue formation.

Further reading

Brooke BS, *et al.* (2008). Angiotensin II blockade and aortic-root dilation in Marfan's syndrome. *N Engl J Med*, **358**, 2787–95.

D'Asdia MC, *et al.* (2013). Novel and recurrent EVC and EVC2 mutations in Ellis-van Creveld syndrome and Weyers acrofacial dysostosis. *Eur J Med Genet*, **56**, 80–7.

Groenink M, *et al.* (2013). Losartan reduces aortic dilatation rate in adults with Marfan syndrome: a randomized controlled trial. *Eur Heart J*, **34**, 34913–500.

Habashi JP, *et al.* (2006). Losartan, an AT1 antagonist, prevents aortic aneurysm in a mouse model of Marfan syndrome. *Science*, **312**, 117–21.

Judge DP, Dietz HC (2005). Marfan's syndrome. *Lancet*, **366**, 1965–76.

Lowery MC, *et al.* (1995). Strong correlation of elastin deletions, detected by FISH, with Williams syndrome: evaluation of 235 patients. *Am J Hum Genet*, **57**, 49–53.

McKusick VA (2000). Ellis–van Creveld syndrome and the Amish. *Nat Genet*, **24**, 203–4.

Oderich GS, *et al.* (2005). The spectrum, management and clinical outcome of Ehlers–Danlos syndrome type IV: a 30-year experience. *J Vasc Surg*, **42**, 98–106.

Prendiville TW, *et al.* (2014). Cardiovascular disease in Noonan syndrome. *Arch Dis Child*, **99**, 629–34.

Pyeritz RE (1983). Cardiovascular manifestations of heritable disorders of connective tissue. *Progr Med Genet*, **5**, 191–302.

Roberts AE, *et al.* (2013). Noonan syndrome. *Lancet*, **381**, 333–42.

Congenital heart disease in the adult

CHAPTER 12.1

Congenital heart disease in the adult

S. A. Thorne

Essentials

Adults with congenital heart disease are a growing population, and now outnumber children with congenital heart disease in the United Kingdom. Many patients with repaired hearts can now, with specialist care, expect to live a normal or near normal lifespan. Other survivors have complex, surgically altered hearts and circulations that reflect the surgical and interventional practices of the preceding two decades. Their long-term outlook is unknown and they remain at lifelong risk of complications that may require further intervention. The organization of services to provide specialist care is key to their long-term survival.

The language of congenital heart disease

The classification and description of complex congenital heart disease can appear intimidating, but should be easily understood by using a simple physiological approach that takes into account whether a condition is cyanotic or acyanotic, whether there is a shunt, and the implications of the morphology for pulmonary blood flow.

The description of the congenitally malformed heart is aided by a sequential segmental analysis of the relationship of the three cardiac segments, which makes it possible to understand and describe how a complex heart is connected. The three segments to be considered are: (1) the atriums; (2) the ventricles; (3) the great vessels. The next step is to describe how each segment connects to the others.

Cyanosis and pulmonary hypertension

Cyanosis occurs as a result of a right-to-left shunt, with its natural history determined by the pulmonary blood flow. If pulmonary blood flow is limited (e.g. by pulmonary stenosis in the presence of a large ventricular septal defect), then pulmonary blood flow and arterial oxygen will be low, as will pulmonary artery pressure. Cyanotic patients with low or normal pulmonary artery pressure are usually amenable to surgical repair that abolishes the cyanosis. By contrast, if the pulmonary circulation is unprotected (e.g. if the defect includes a large ventricular septal defect and no pulmonary stenosis), then pulmonary blood flow will be high and at high pressure, pulmonary vascular remodelling will occur, and—without intervention—pulmonary vascular disease will eventually develop (pulmonary arterial hypertension; the Eisenmenger syndrome). Once pulmonary vascular disease is established, it is not possible to repair the defect and abolish the right-to-left shunt.

The right ventricle

Preservation of ventricular function is fundamental in allowing long-term survival with a good quality of life. The right ventricle is a key factor in the long-term outcome of many congenital cardiac conditions. It may fail as a result of either long-standing pressure or volume overload. (1) Pressure loading—this occurs in patients in whom the right ventricle supports the systemic circulation, such as those with congenitally corrected transposition of the great arteries, and in those who underwent interatrial repair (Mustard or Senning operation) of simple transposition of the great arteries. The right ventricle is hypertrophied, and ultimately fails, with tricuspid regurgitation secondary to annular dilatation hastening the decline. (2) Volume loading—this commonly occurs as a result of pulmonary regurgitation secondary to pulmonary valvotomy or repair of tetralogy of Fallot in early life. There may be no audible murmur because there are often only remnants of pulmonary valve tissue, such that the regurgitant flow is laminar. Partly because of the lack of physical signs, and partly because pulmonary regurgitation is usually tolerated for many years before the right ventricle begins to fail, patients may present very late with a very dilated and impaired ventricle. Long-standing large atrial septal defects produce similar right ventricular volume loading effects. The right ventricle may be inherently abnormal, as in Ebstein anomaly where a combination of a functionally small ventricle and volume loading from tricuspid regurgitation may cause the right ventricle to fail.

The Fontan circulation

Hearts which have only one functional ventricle present a particularly difficult challenge. Patients are cyanosed, and only a few will reach adulthood if left unoperated. The ultimate aim for patients with only one functional ventricle is a Fontan circulation: a palliative approach that reduces ventricular volume loading and abolishes cyanosis. It is critically dependent on a low pulmonary vascular resistance, hence early control of pulmonary blood flow is paramount. If pulmonary blood flow is too high, it is controlled by placing a pulmonary artery band: i.e. by the creation of iatrogenic, protective pulmonary stenosis. If pulmonary blood flow is too low, the infant will not thrive, and pulmonary blood supply is augmented by means of a systemic to pulmonary artery shunt. There are many variations of the Fontan operation, but all involve the separation of pulmonary and systemic circulations by using the single ventricle to support the systemic circulation and by connecting the systemic veins directly (or via the right atrium) to the pulmonary artery. There is thus no 'pump' in the pulmonary circulation, so although cyanosis is abolished, the Fontan circulation is one of a chronic low-output state. Thus, although the Fontan approach enables most patients with a single ventricle to reach adulthood, they have a fragile circulation and will develop a range of complications. They are particularly at risk if they have a tachyarrhythmia or acute noncardiac illness, since they tolerate such insults poorly and are dependent on their medical teams' understanding of their circulation to ensure good hydration, avoidance of vasodilatation, and rapid restoration of sinus rhythm.

Tachyarrhythmia

Tachyarrhythmias are a major cause of sudden death in patients with congenital heart disease, with scar-related atrial tachyarrhythmias being common in those who have had previous cardiac surgery, and probably a commoner cause of death than ventricular arrhythmias. Atrial tachyarrhymias are the reason that patients who underwent interatrial repair (Mustard or Senning operations) of transposition of the great arteries are the congenital cardiac group with the highest incidence of sudden death. Their surgically created atrial 'baffles' mean that atrial function is abnormal, and ventricular filling is impaired, particularly at high heart rates. Atrial flutter is common post Mustard or Senning, and patients are usually able to conduct 1:1 at a rate of 300 bpm, resulting in cardiovascular collapse. Correct management is rapid restoration of sinus rhythm, followed by flutter ablation. Patients with a Fontan circulation are similarly vulnerable to interatrial re-entry tachyarrhythmias. Ventricular and atrial tachycardias may both occur in most survivors of complex congenital heart disease, particularly after repair of tetralogy of Fallot. If ablation is not successful, consideration should be given to an internal cardioverter defibrillator.

Pregnancy and contraception

Many women with congenital heart disease wish to consider pregnancy. For most this can be undertaken with only a small increased risk, but for some pregnancy carries a significant risk of complication, long-term morbidity, and death. Outcomes can be optimized by preconception counselling and specialist joint cardiac and obstetric care. Access to safe and effective contraception is important to allow patients to avoid potentially high risk pregnancies. Oestrogen-containing preparations are not suitable for those at risk of intracardiac thrombus or who have a right-to-left shunt; long-acting progestogen-only methods offer safe and effective alternatives

Heart failure and end-of-life care

As the population of adults with congenital heart disease ages, so the number developing heart failure increases. Conventional heart failure drugs have not been shown to have much benefit in this situation, and there is a lack of clear guidance as to who will benefit from interventions such as cardiac resynchronization therapy. Cardiac transplantation is associated with a worse early mortality than acquired heart disease, but the long-term outcome is as good. Transplantation is limited both by suitability of the recipient with a complex, surgically modified heart, and by donor availability. Services caring for patients need to develop a robust end-of-life pathway that focuses on symptoms and quality of life, and runs in parallel with other therapies.

Introduction

The growing number of adult survivors of congenital heart disease will encounter medical staff from all areas of medicine and surgery. It is therefore important that all doctors have an understanding of the principles of congenital heart disease and enough knowledge to know when to refer such patients to a specialist centre.

As a result of advances in paediatric cardiac surgery and intervention, the outlook for the approximately 8 per 1000 babies born with congenital heart disease has changed dramatically in the last half-century. Fifty years ago, 70% of children born with congenital heart disease died before their 10th birthday; now more than 80% survive to adulthood and in the United Kingdom there are more adults than children living with congenital heart disease.

Despite such advances, only those with the simplest conditions, e.g. isolated secundum atrial septal defect or anomalous pulmonary venous drainage successfully repaired in childhood, may be considered cured of their heart disease. Most patients need continued specialist follow-up since they have residual lesions that may progress over many years and require timely intervention.

Surgical techniques evolve continually, creating new populations with different surgically modified conditions and long-term outcomes. Careful follow-up is therefore crucial, not only to provide high standards of clinical care, but also to provide feedback about late results in order to inform initial management in infancy. As a result of such long-term follow-up information, the operation of choice for transposition of the great arteries became the arterial switch from the late 1980s, because of the late problems encountered in patients who had undergone interatrial repair with the Senning or Mustard operations.

Surgical advances mean that patients with new surgically modified conditions are reaching adulthood. Their outlook and the complications they may face are not known, so lifelong specialist surveillance is important. Left unoperated, hypoplastic left heart syndrome is lethal; survivors of the three-stage surgical palliation are now reaching the adult clinics. They will form the largest new population over the next decade and face a more complex future than those with a 'standard' Fontan circulation.

Classification and nomenclature

The classification and description of complex congenital heart disease can appear intimidating. Nonetheless, a grasp of the basic principles is important to understand the anatomy and pathophysiology of congenital cardiac conditions. A simple physiological approach to classifying congenital heart disease takes into account whether a condition is cyanotic or acyanotic, whether there is a shunt, and the implications of the morphology for pulmonary blood flow (Table 12.1.1).

Sequential segmental analysis

The description of the congenitally malformed heart is aided by a segmental approach, which makes it possible to understand and describe how a complex heart is connected. Any heart can be described by considering it as three segments (the atrial chambers, the ventricular mass, and the great arteries) and describing in a sequential manner how each segment is arranged and connected to the next segment (Figs 12.1.1 and 12.1.2).

Table 12.1.1 Classification of congenital heart disease

| | Acyanotic | | | Cyanotic: obligatory right-to-left shunt | | | | | |
| | No shunt | Left-to-right shunt | | Eisenmenger syndrome | | High pulmonary blood flow | | Normal or low pulmonary blood flow | |
Level of lesion	Example of specific lesion	Level of shunt	Example of specific lesion	Level of shunt	Example of specific lesion (unoperated)	Level of shunt	Example of specific lesion	Level of shunt	Example of specific lesion
Right inflow	Ebstein anomaly	*Atrial*	PAPVD ASD AVSD	*Atrial*	Large ASD (uncommon cause)	*Atrial*	Large ASD	*Atrial, with obstruction to pulmonary blood flow*	Severe pulmonary stenosis with ASD Left SVC to LA connection
Left inflow	Parachute mitral valve Cor triatriatum	*Ventricular*	VSD	*Ventricular*	Large VSD	*Ventricular*	Large VSD: will develop Eisenmenger syndrome if left unoperated	*Ventricular, with obstruction to pulmonary blood flow*	Tetralogy of Fallot, Pulmonary atresia VSD, Univentricular heart with pulmonary stenosis
Right outflow	Infundibular stenosis Pulmonary stenosis	*Arterial*	PDA Aortopulmonary window	*Arterial*	Large PDA Aortopulmonery window	*Arterial*	Large PDA Aortopulmonery window : will develop Eisenmenger syndrome if left unoperated	*Extra cardiac*	Pulmonary AVM
Left outflow	Subaortic stenosis Bicuspid aortic valve	*Multiple*	AVSD	*Multiple*	Large AVSD	*Multiple*	Large AVSD: will develop Eisenmenger syndrome if left unoperated		
Arterial	Supravalvar stenosis Coarctation of the aorta								

ASD, atrial septal defect; AVSD, atriventricular septal defect; LA, left atrium; PAPVD, partial anomalous pulmonary venous drainage; SVC, superior vena cava; VSD, ventricular septal defect.

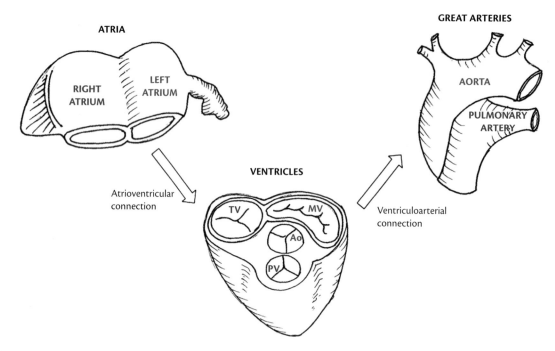

Fig. 12.1.1 The segments of the heart.

1. The arrangement of the atria (situs) is described

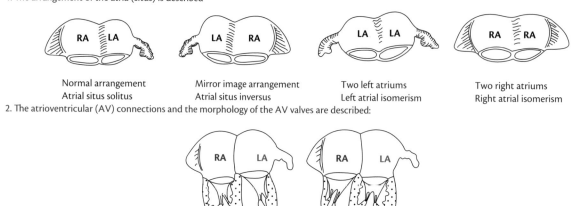

| Normal arrangement | Mirror image arrangement | Two left atriums | Two right atriums |
| Atrial situs solitus | Atrial situs inversus | Left atrial isomerism | Right atrial isomerism |

2. The atrioventricular (AV) connections and the morphology of the AV valves are described:

Atrioventricular concordance   Atrioventricular disccordance

3. The ventriculoarterial (VA) connections and the morphology of the great arteries are described:

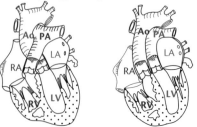

Ventriculoarterial concordance   Ventriculoarterial discordance

4. Associated malformations are then described

Fig. 12.1.2 Sequential segmental analysis.

Atrial arrangement

Situs solitus is the usual arrangement of asymmetrical structures, i.e. morphological left atrium on the left and right atrium on the right; morphological left main bronchus on the left and right main bronchus on the right; stomach on the left, liver on the right. Situs inversus is the mirror-image arrangement of these structures.

Isomerism describes abnormal symmetry of paired structures that usually show laterality, as shown in Table 12.1.2. The presence of isomerism of the atrial appendages should alert the physician to the coexistence of complex associated lesions, including a variety of abnormalities of venous connections that may cause technical difficulties at cardiac catheterization and permanent pacemaker insertion. Right isomerism is commoner in males and left isomerism in females. Survival to adulthood with right isomerism is uncommon because of associated asplenia and severe cyanotic heart disease,

including obstructed anomalous pulmonary venous drainage (the pulmonary venous confluence is a left atrial structure). The lesions associated with left isomerism tend to produce left-to-right shunts and little if any cyanosis.

Atrioventricular connections

In the normal heart, the atrioventricular connections are concordant (Fig. 12.1.2), i.e.

- the right atrium connects to the right ventricle via the tricuspid valve
- the left atrium connects to the left ventricle via a mitral valve.

If the atrioventricular connections are discordant:

- the right atrium connects to the left ventricle via a mitral valve
- the left atrium connects to the right ventricle via a tricuspid valve.

Table 12.1.2 Diagnosis of atrial arrangement

	Situs solitus (normal arrangement)	Situs inversus (mirror image arrangement)	Right atrial isomerism	Left atrial isomerism
Atrial & appendage[a] morphology	R-sided morphological RA & appendage L-sided morphological LA & appendage	R-sided morphological LA & appendage L-sided morphological RA & appendage	Bilateral morphological RA & appendages	Bilateral morphological LA & appendages
Pulmonary & bronchial morphology[b]	R lung trilobed L lung bilobed R-sided main bronchus: short, L-sided main bronchus: long	R lung bilobed L lung trilobed R-sided main bronchus: long, L-sided main bronchus: short	Bilateral trilobed lungs Bilateral short morphological R bronchi	Bilateral bilobed lungs Bilateral long morphological L bronchi
Abdominal arrangement[c]		Normal or mirror image		
Aorta	To L of spine		Aorta and IVC on same side	Aorta and azygos on same side
IVC	To R of spine		IVC anterior to aorta	Azygos posterior to aorta
Stomach	L-sided		Usually L-sided	Usually R-sided
Liver	R-sided		Midline	Midline
Spleen	R-sided		Usually absent	Often polysplenia

Ao, aorta, AV, azygos vein, IVC, inferior vena cava; L, left; LA, left atrium; R right; RA, right atrium; SVC, superior vena cava.

[a] Readily identified on transoesophageal echocardiography.

[b] Since bronchopulmonary situs nearly always follows atrial situs, atrial situs can be inferred from the chest radiograph.

[c] Echocardiography shows the intra-abdominal relations of the great vessels. In left isomerism, there is usually interruption of the IVC, and the abdominal venous return connects to the heart via a (right-sided) azygos or (left-sided) hemiazygos vein. The hepatic veins can be identified draining separately into the atriums.

Ventriculo-arterial connections

In the normal heart, the ventriculo-arterial connections are concordant (Fig. 12.1.2), i.e.

- the left ventricle connects to the aorta via the aortic valve
- the right ventricle connects to pulmonary artery via the pulmonary valve.

If the ventriculo-arterial connections are discordant (transposition of the great arteries), then:

- the left ventricle connects to the pulmonary artery via the pulmonary valve
- the right ventricle connects to the aorta via the aortic valve.

Cyanosis: a multisystem disorder

Cyanosis occurs as a result of a right-to-left shunt. Cyanotic heart disease is a multisystem disorder; its manifestations are listed in Table 12.1.3.

Secondary erythrocytosis

Chronic hypoxia is the stimulus to the increased red blood cell mass and high haematocrit found in cyanotic heart disease. This physiological response increases the oxygen-carrying capacity of the blood and improves tissue oxygenation sufficiently to reach a new equilibrium at a higher haematocrit. The secondary erythrocytosis of cyanotic heart disease is a physiological response, often associated with thrombocytopenia. It is fundamentally different from the pathological generalized increase in all haemopoietic stem cell lines found in the malignant disease polycythaemia rubra vera.

Venesection was advocated historically to reduce the haematocrit to less than 65% in patients with cyanotic heart disease because of concerns about the effects of hyperviscosity. However, although a raised haematocrit is associated with increased blood viscosity, it also correlates with improved exercise tolerance, and does not correlate well with symptoms classically regarded as those of hyperviscosity (Box 12.1.1). Conversely, iron deficiency brought about by venesection is associated with increased symptoms akin to those of hyperviscosity (but does not cause an actual increase in viscosity) as well as an increased risk of stroke. Restoration of iron stores improves exercise tolerance and symptoms. Cyanotic patients with iron deficiency should therefore have the cause of the deficiency treated and be given iron supplements sufficient to render them iron replete over a course of months. A prolonged course of low-dose iron should allow iron stores to be replenished without causing a rapid rise in haematocrit. There is no evidence that venesection improves symptoms beyond a few days, nor that it carries any prognostic benefit. Thus, venesection to reduce elevated haemoglobin and haematocrit is rarely, if ever, indicated for the physiological erythrocytosis of cyanotic heart disease.

Menorrhagia is common in women with cyanotic heart disease and may be sufficient to cause iron deficiency anaemia. It may be difficult to manage, the combined oral contraceptive pill being contraindicated because of the prothrombotic effects of the oestrogen it contains, and tranexamic acid may similarly be associated with thrombosis. Norethisterone may provide short-term relief. Progestogen-only contraceptives have unpredictable effects on menstruation: the subdermal implant (e.g. Nexplanon®) is safe and causes oligoamenorrhoea in some women. Mirena® IUS is a progestogen-eluting intrauterine device that causes oligoamenorrhoea in most women, but great care is needed for those with cyanotic heart disease or who have not undergone previous vaginal delivery because insertion may cause a vasovagal response and cardiovascular collapse. If menorrhagia is due to uterine fibroids, catheter embolization of the feeding uterine artery is safe and may be successful.

Table 12.1.3 Complications of cyanotic congenital heart disease

Haematological	Secondary erythrocytosis	→Hyperviscosity symptoms?
	Iron deficiency (venesection, menorrhagia)	↑ Risk of CVA
	Thrombocytopenia	
	Haemorrhage	
	Coagulopathy	
Neurological	CVA	2° to paradoxical embolism
	Cerebral abscess	
Hyperuricaemia	Impaired renal clearance of uric acid	→Gout
	Increased uric acid production?	
Renal abnormalities	↓ Uric acid clearance	→High risk of iatrogenic renal failure
	Glomerular proteinuria	
	Mesangial matrix thickening	
	Capillary and hilar arteriole dilatation	
Bilirubin kinetics	↑ Haem breakdown	→Pigment gallstones
Digits and long bones	Clubbing	
	Hypertrophic osteoarthropathy	
Dental	Gingival hypertrophy	→↑ Risk of endocarditis
Infection	Endocarditis	
	Cerebral abscess	
Skin	Acne	

CVA, cardiovascular accident.

Box 12.1.1 Symptoms of hyperviscosity

- Headache
- Faint, dizzy, light-headed
- Depressed mentation, sense of distance
- Blurred vision, amaurosis fugax
- Paraesthesiae
- Tinnitus
- Fatigue, lethargy
- Myalgia, muscle weakness
- Chest and abdominal pain
- Restless legs

Disorders of coagulation and blood vessels

It is poorly understood why patients with cyanotic disease are at increased risk of haemorrhage and thrombosis. There is often a mild thrombocytopenia that may be due partly to shortened platelet survival time, and the large multimeric forms of von Willebrand factor and other clotting factors may be depleted. Coagulation testing may yield spurious results in patients with haematocrit over 55% unless the amount of citrate anticoagulant is reduced.

Bleeding may be minor and mucocutaneous, but major haemorrhage may occur during surgery, or from the lungs. Pulmonary artery thrombosis is discussed below (see 'Eisenmenger syndrome: defects with secondary pulmonary vascular disease'). Interestingly, systemic arterial atherosclerosis is rare in the cyanotic population, perhaps because of a combination of thrombocytopenia, up-regulated nitric oxide, hyperbilirubinaemia, and hypocholesterolaemia.

Other complications of cyanotic heart disease

The risk of stroke is increased in cyanotic heart disease, with independent risk factors being intravenous lines, arterial hypertension, atrial fibrillation, iron deficiency, and prosthetic intravascular material such as endocardial pacing systems. The mechanism of stoke is often paradoxical embolism due to right-to-left shunting. Paradoxical air emboli are a cause of stroke in patients whose venous lines are not fitted with filters. Patients who require transvenous pacing should be anticoagulated with warfarin to prevent paradoxical thromboembolism from pacing leads.

Cerebral abscess is an uncommon but potentially devastating complication of cyanosis, with a mortality of around 13%. The right-to-left shunt allows systemic venous blood to avoid passing through the lungs, where bacteria are removed by phagocytosis. The diagnosis should be considered in all cyanotic patients who present with fever, headache and malaise, neurological signs, or altered consciousness. Similarly, patients who present with cerebral abscess of apparently unknown cause should have a right-to-left shunt excluded. The right-to-left shunt may be extracardiac: for example, pulmonary arteriovenous malformation, or a persistent left superior vena cava (SVC) draining to the left atrium. A bubble contrast echocardiogram without Valsalva manoeuvre, via the left brachial vein, will detect such right-to-left shunting. Empirical treatment is usually a third-generation cephalosporin and metronidazole; blood cultures, and if possible stereotactic aspiration of pus with narrow antibiotic therapy and surgical drainage may be necessary for large abscesses.

Despite the high incidence of hyperuricaemia, attacks of acute gout are uncommon and asymptomatic hyperuricaemia does not require treatment. Acute attacks should be treated with colchicine, avoiding nonsteroidal anti-inflammatory agents (NSAIDs) because of their detrimental effects on haemostasis and renal function. As in primary hyperuricaemia, allopurinol is useful in preventing recurrence.

The renal abnormalities outlined in Table 12.1.3 are frequently not associated with abnormal baseline renal function. However, renal failure may be precipitated by hypotension and dehydration, especially in combination with radiographic contrast media, NSAIDs, or aminoglycoside antibiotics. The mode of decline and eventual death is a combination of heart and renal failure in many patients with cyanotic heart disease, and care should be taken to titrate diuretic therapy cautiously to minimize worsening renal function. Renal dialysis or filtration is very poorly tolerated in this patient group and should be avoided: the failing cyanotic circulation does not cope with the haemodynamic demands of renal support, and deterioration and death is likely to occur rapidly.

Acne is a common complaint in adolescents and adults with cyanotic disease and may be widespread and psychologically debilitating. When severe it may also increase the risk of bacteraemia and endocarditis.

Digital clubbing is almost universal in cyanotic heart disease, and some degree of hypertrophic osteoarthropathy of the long bones may occur in up to one-third of patients. Symptoms include aching and tenderness of the long bones of the forearms and legs. There is oedema and cellular infiltration, causing lifting of the periosteum that is visible radiographically, with new bone formation and resorption. Localized activation of endothelial cells by an abnormal platelet population, with the ensuing release of fibroblast growth factors, may play a central role in the pathogenesis of both phenomena.

Cyanotic patients become more hypoxic during air travel, as the partial pressure of oxygen in a pressurized aircraft is lower than that at sea level. However, such travel seems to be well tolerated and supplemental oxygen should not normally be necessary. Travellers should be warned to avoid dehydration and to plan their journeys to avoid having to carry baggage for long distances within large airports.

Cyanotic patients are at risk of iatrogenic complications if they require surgery or intervention for noncardiac conditions. See Box 12.1.2.

Eisenmenger syndrome: defects with secondary pulmonary vascular disease

Eisenmenger syndrome is a cyanotic condition that occurs in patients with a large (nonrestrictive) communication between the systemic and pulmonary circulations that results in high pulmonary vascular resistance and pulmonary arterial hypertension, so that the shunt across the communication is reversed (right-to-left) or bidirectional. The communication may be at atrial, ventricular, or arterial levels.

In fetal life, pulmonary vascular resistance is high and there is muscularity of the pulmonary arterioles. In the normal circulation, pulmonary vascular resistance falls soon after birth and

---

Box 12.1.2 Checklist for patients at high risk[a] of iatrogenic complications during the perioperative period or during intercurrent illness

- Seek advice from the patient's congenital cardiology team
- Maintain hydration—intravenous fluids (via air filter if cyanotic to avoid the risk of paradoxical embolism) when nil by mouth
- Maintain haemoglobin commensurate with degree of cyanosis to optimize oxygen-carrying capacity
- Avoid vasodilator agents—especially at induction of anaesthesia
- Protect the kidneys—maintain hydration, avoid nephrotoxic agents (NSAIDs, aminoglycosides), use minimal volumes of contrast agents.

[a] Patients at high risk include those who are cyanotic and those with Eisenmenger syndrome or Fontan circulation.

remodelling of the pulmonary arterioles occurs. However, if there is a large communication, e.g. a ventricular septal defect, the effects of blood entering the pulmonary circulation at high volume and systemic pressure causes reverse remodelling, and instead of falling, the pulmonary vascular resistance rises. Endothelial dysfunction secondary to changes in shear stress and circumferential wall stress is thought to mediate these changes through altered expression of vasoactive mediators and growth factors such as endothelin-1, nitric oxide, prostacyclin, and vascular endothelial and fibroblast growth factors.

Corrective surgery in infancy usually prevents the development of this irreversible syndrome, so its incidence in the developed world is declining. However, when patients do present their management is dependent on a good understanding of their condition.

For patients with established right-to-left shunting and pulmonary arterial hypertension, the diagnosis is clear. However, some have intermediate pathologies, and European guidelines attempt to clarify these: it is important to understand that despite the absence of a right-to-left shunt and cyanosis, potentially life-threatening pulmonary artery hypertension is present (Table 12.1.4).

Clinical findings

Symptoms of breathlessness relate to the degree of hypoxia; many patients feel worse in hot weather or after a hot bath because the resulting systemic vasodilatation is not accompanied by a reduction in pulmonary vascular resistance, so the right-to-left shunt is enhanced and they become more hypoxic. Exercise-induced syncope may occur, and is exacerbated by hot weather and dehydration. Haemoptysis is common and may be fatal.

Whatever the underlying defect, some examination findings are shared. Patients are cyanosed and clubbed and may be plethoric. There is a right ventricular heave and the pulmonary component of the second heart sound is palpable and loud. A pulmonary ejection click and pulmonary regurgitation may be audible. A soft systolic flow murmur may be heard from the dilated pulmonary artery. No systolic murmur can be heard from the lesion responsible for the pulmonary vascular disease since the chambers on both sides of the lesion are at equal pressure.

It is frequently possible to distinguish between the common lesions associated with the Eisenmenger syndrome on clinical grounds. The patient with an Eisenmenger patent arterial duct has differential cyanosis and clubbing, since fully saturated blood from the left ventricle supplies the aortic arch and its branches before mixing occurs with desaturated pulmonary arterial blood via the patent duct. The right hand may therefore be pink with no clubbing, the left may be slightly more cyanosed because of the origin of the left subclavian artery opposite the duct, and the toes are more deeply cyanosed and clubbed. The second heart sound may be closely or normally split. In contrast, cyanosis and clubbing is uniform when the right-to-left shunt occurs at atrial, ventricular or ascending aortic (as in truncus arteriosus or aortopulmonary window) levels. The second sound is single in ventricular septal defect (VSD), atrioventricular septal defect (AVSD), and truncus, but may be split in an atrial septal defect (ASD).

Investigations

The chest radiograph shows a dilated pulmonary trunk because of high pulmonary blood flow in earlier life, but reduced blood flow as pulmonary vascular resistance rose means that the lung fields are oligaemic (Fig. 12.1.3). Unless cardiac failure intervenes, the heart size is usually normal, the effects of volume overload having regressed as pulmonary vascular resistance increased and the left-to-right shunt diminished and disappeared.

The electrocardiogram (ECG) shows P pulmonale and biventricular hypertrophy. The echocardiogram should establish the site of the shunt and allow an estimation of pulmonary arterial pressure and ventricular function.

Cardiopulmonary exercise testing may be used with caution: patients with Eisenmenger syndrome are among the most limited of those with congenital heart disease and maximal exercise testing may induce potentially fatal syncope. The less strenuous but still objective 6-min walk or shuttle tests are preferable measures of exercise capacity in these patients.

High-resolution CT scanning demonstrates the hypertensive pulmonary vasculature and any collateral vessels. It is also the investigation of choice to show *in situ* pulmonary thrombus and pulmonary artery aneurysms, and to demonstrate the site of any pulmonary haemorrhage. Care should be taken to avoid contrast-induced nephropathy by ensuring adequate hydration.

Cardiac catheterization is unnecessary and potentially dangerous for patients with established pulmonary vascular disease. The only

Table 12.1.4 Pulmonary arterial hypertension associated with congenital heart disease

A	Eisenmenger syndrome
	A large systemic to pulmonary artery shunt leads to a severe increase in pulmonary vascular resistance such that it exceeds systemic vascular resistance, and the shunt reverses (becomes right-to-left). The patient is cyanosed
B	Pulmonary artery hypertension associated with systemic to pulmonary shunt
	A moderate–large defect causes a rise in pulmonary vascular resistance, but it remains less than systemic vascular resistance and the shunt remains left-to-right
C	Pulmonary artery hypertension and a small systemic to pulmonary shunt
	A small defect (e.g. VSD <1 cm or ASD >2 cm) coexists with pulmonary arterial hypertension. If pulmonary vascular resistance exceeds systemic vascular resistance, the shunt reverses and the patient is cyanosed. The clinical course is akin to idiopathic pulmonary arterial hypertension. It is likely that two different diagnoses are present, i.e. a patient with idiopathic pulmonary artery hypertension coincidentally has a small septal defect
D	Pulmonary artery hypertension after surgery to correct systemic to pulmonary artery shunt
	A large systemic to pulmonary shunt is surgically repaired but pulmonary artery hypertension is still present

ASD, atrial septal defect; VSD, ventricular septal defect.

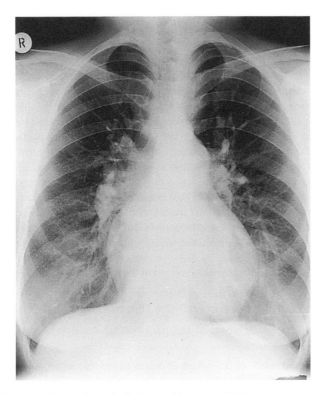

Fig. 12.1.3 Chest radiograph of a 35-year-old woman with Eisenmenger secundum atrial septal defect. The aortic knuckle is small and the central pulmonary arteries enlarged, indicating pulmonary arterial hypertension; the lung fields are clear. The cardiac silhouette is not enlarged.

indication is for those patients whose pulmonary vascular disease is suspected to be reversible and who would be considered for surgical repair if reversibility can be confirmed. This situation is rarely encountered in the adult population.

Histologically, pulmonary vascular disease progresses from medial hypertrophy through intimal proliferation with migration of smooth muscle cells, to progressive fibrosis and obliteration, dilatation, the development of angiomas and finally fibrinoid necrosis. Those who have developed fibrotic and obliterative changes are likely to have irreversible pulmonary vascular disease. Routine lung biopsy is not recommended; it carries a high risk in the pulmonary hypertensive adult and is unlikely to show reversible pathology. In addition, thoracotomy scars from open lung biopsy are a relative contraindication to heart–lung transplantation.

Outcome and complications

Survival into adulthood with Eisenmenger syndrome is common. Life expectancy may be around 20 years less than for the general population, but this is markedly better than for those with idiopathic pulmonary arterial hypertension. Markers of poorer prognosis include complex anatomy and physiology, decline in functional class, and the development of heart failure, renal dysfunction and clinical arrhythmia. Serum uric acid increases with disease progression and may also be used as a long-term predictor of mortality. The patient with Eisenmenger syndrome is prone to all the complications of cyanotic heart disease.

Haemoptysis is usually due to rupture of small hypertensive intrapulmonary vessels, or more rarely to thrombosis *in situ* and pulmonary infarction. Massive haemoptysis is a well-recognized cause of death. All patients should be admitted to hospital and the systemic pressure kept low by bed rest and β-blockade; the pulmonary artery pressure being the same as that measured in the brachial artery. NSAIDs should be stopped and vasodilators should not be given. If the haemoptysis is massive, diamorphine should be administered, fresh frozen plasma or cryoprecipitate may be given, and consideration should be given to selectively intubating the nonbleeding lung to allow an attempt to embolize a bleeding vessel. Bronchoscopy has no role and may worsen the haemorrhage.

In situ thrombosis in the dilated pulmonary arteries of adults with Eisenmenger syndrome is common (prevalence of 20–30%) and relates to the degree of cyanosis. It is best detected and quantified using high-resolution CT scanning. Anticoagulation of any sort has not been shown to resolve such thrombus, and patients are at risk of pulmonary embolic episodes. Warfarin may increase the risk of bleeding while failing to reduce the thrombus, and aspirin should be avoided as it may exacerbate haemorrhage associated with thrombocytopenia.

Right ventricular failure may be precipitated by atrial arrhythmia and usually occurs after the age of 30 years. Decline may be heralded by the onset of right ventricular failure, renal dysfunction, supraventricular arrhythmia, and haemoptysis. Death may be sudden and due to arrhythmia or massive haemoptysis. In some patients death follows progressive hypoxia terminating in bradycardia and asystole from which they cannot be resuscitated.

Intercurrent illness and noncardiac surgery may pose major risks. The latter is particularly dangerous when carried out without the benefit of expert cardiology, anaesthetic and perioperative care. A sound understanding of the pathophysiology is vital (Box 12.1.2).

Treatment options

Until recently, treatment of patients with Eisenmenger syndrome has been palliative and symptom led, directed at avoiding iatrogenic and natural complications. Gentle exercise should be encouraged, but strenuous exertion avoided, since it may result in syncope. Long-term oxygen therapy may improve symptoms in some patients, but has not been shown to have prognostic benefit.

Although this approach is still the mainstay of treatment, selective pulmonary vasodilators including phosphodiesterase inhibitors (e.g. sildenafil) and endothelin receptor antagonists (e.g. bosentan) may improve outcome and should be considered at least for patients with New York Heart Association (NYHA) class III symptoms. These drugs have been shown to improve outcome in other forms of pulmonary hypertension. Early data from small trials suggest that bosentan helps to maintain right ventricular function, quality of life, and exercise capacity. Sildenafil improves quality of life and exercise tolerance in many patients as they reach NYHA III.

Pregnancy and contraception

Pregnancy carries a particularly high risk (25–40% maternal mortality). Pregnancy and contraception in congenital heart disease are discussed below. All women with pulmonary hypertension of any cause should be counselled about the risks and given access to safe, effective contraception. If a woman with Eisenmenger syndrome becomes pregnant and chooses not to have a termination, she should be referred to a specialist pulmonary hypertension centre.

Valve and outflow tract lesions

Isolated pulmonary valve stenosis

Isolated pulmonary stenosis is common, occurring in up to 10% of patients with congenital heart disease. There is usually fusion of the valve cusps leading to a doming appearance. Syndromic associations are not unusual and include Noonan, Williams, and Alagille syndromes.

Significant pulmonary stenosis results in right ventricular hypertrophy and high right-sided pressures; right-to-left shunting causing cyanosis may occur if there is a coexistent ASD or patent foramen ovale (PFO).

Pulmonary stenosis is a better-tolerated lesion than aortic stenosis, with an excellent survival. Severe pulmonary stenosis usually presents in childhood, either as an asymptomatic murmur, or with failure to thrive, chest pain, dyspnoea, or cyanosis.

Physical signs

Patients are acyanotic unless there is an interatrial communication, in which case cyanosis can be severe. The venous pressure is raised only if the right ventricle has begun to fail and there is tricuspid regurgitation. There may be a right ventricular heave. The pulmonary component of the second heart sound is soft and there is a pulmonary ejection systolic murmur. An early diastolic murmur may also be present if there is coexistent pulmonary regurgitation.

Investigations

The ECG may demonstrate right ventricular hypertrophy. This regresses after relief of the stenosis. The chest radiograph reveals poststenotic dilation of the proximal pulmonary artery, and the lung fields may be oligaemic if the pulmonary stenosis is severe.

Transthoracic echocardiography confirms the diagnosis and allows functional assessment of the severity of pulmonary stenosis and regurgitation as well as right ventricular hypertrophy, dilatation, and function.

Management

Adults with trivial (<20 mmHg) pulmonary stenosis do not require regular follow-up, since progression is unlikely. Approximately 20% of adults with mild stenosis (<50 mmHg) may progress and ultimately require intervention, and most of those with a peak pulmonary valve gradient greater than 50 mmHg require intervention.

Balloon pulmonary valvotomy is the treatment of choice, unless the valve is thickened and dysplastic or regurgitant, or there are associated anomalies requiring a surgical approach. Valvotomy is usually successful and it is uncommon for stenosis to recur, however, the procedure invariably results in a degree of pulmonary regurgitation and so long-term follow-up is required.

Lone infundibular stenosis and double-chambered right ventricle

Abnormally placed muscle bands cause either infundibular obstruction or—if placed more inferiorly—subinfundibular obstruction and a double-chambered right ventricle. The degree of obstruction may be mild in childhood, but progresses in adult life and causes symptoms as the right ventricle hypertrophies and outflow obstruction becomes severe. A perimembranous VSD usually coexists and

may close spontaneously. Treatment is by surgical resection of the obstructing muscle bands.

Ebstein anomaly

This rare, complex defect of the tricuspid valve occurs in 1 in 20 000 live births and affects both sexes equally. The risk may be increased by maternal exposure to lithium during the first trimester.

In the normal heart, the tricuspid and mitral valves are formed from the endocardium of the right and left ventricles, respectively. The valve leaflets delaminate from the endocardium to form the atrioventricular valves. In Ebstein anomaly, there is failure of tricuspid valve leaflet delamination during fetal life, so that the leaflets adhere to the right ventricular myocardium, resulting in apical displacement of the functional tricuspid valve, tethering, redundancy, and fenestrations of the valve leaflets. There is a broad spectrum of severity of this condition, dependent upon the degree of failure of delamination.

Ebstein anomaly is characterized by a spectrum of features:

- Adherence of the tricuspid valve leaflets to the underlying myocardium due to failure of delamination in fetal life

- Apical displacement of the tricuspid valve hinge points and orifice:

  - As a result of the failure of delamination the septal and posterior (mural) leaflets insert further into the body of the right ventricle than in the normal heart (in which the mitral and tricuspid valves are offset so that the tricuspid valve is displaced up to 1.5 cm towards the right ventricular apex).

  - The 'atrialized' portion of the right ventricle is often thinner walled than the functional right ventricle due to congenital partial absence of the myocardium; as a result, the functional size of the right ventricle is reduced and that of the right atrium increased

- Dilation of the functional right atrium

- Dilatation of the true tricuspid valve annulus at the atrioventricular junction.

This combination of features usually results in tricuspid regurgitation (or very rarely stenosis) and right heart dilation, providing a substrate for atrial and ventricular arrhythmias.

Associated abnormalities

A PFO or ASD is present in most cases, and allows cyanosis to develop as the disease progresses and right-to-left shunting occurs. Left heart abnormalities occur as a consequence of alterations in left ventricular geometry due to leftwards displacement of the interventricular septum; e.g. mitral valve prolapse may occur as result of relatively long chordae in a left ventricle of reduced cavity size. Coexistent Wolfe–Parkinson–White syndrome, usually with single or multiple right-sided pathways, occurs in 20% of patients.

Ebstein anomaly may also form part of other complex congenital lesions, including pulmonary stenosis and atresia and tetralogy of Fallot. When it coexists with congenitally corrected transposition of the great arteries, the tricuspid valve is the systemic atrioventricular valve.

Clinical presentation and course

There is a broad spectrum of severity, ranging from intrauterine or neonatal death to presentation in late adulthood. Mortality, both with and without surgery, is influenced by age at presentation, the condition of the tricuspid valve, the cardiac rhythm, and the function and capacity of the right ventricle, including the severity of right ventricular outflow tract obstruction, and the size of the right atrium in relation to the other cardiac chambers.

Arrhythmia is the commonest mode of initial presentation in adult life; presentation earlier in life is usually associated with severe disease and additional cardiac lesions.

Cyanosis may develop in adulthood if there is an associated ASD or PFO; as the right ventricular filling pressure increases there is a parallel rise in right atrial pressure, and a right-to-left interatrial shunt is established. These patients are at risk of paradoxical embolism, but the risk of endocarditis is low because the tricuspid regurgitant jet is of low velocity.

Heart failure may intervene as a result of the combination of severe tricuspid regurgitation and the onset of atrial fibrillation or flutter. These atrial arrhythmias may be particularly troublesome if a coexistent accessory pathway allows a rapid ventricular response rate. The onset of atrial fibrillation is a predictor of death within 5 years, and may account for the increased death rate in the fifth decade.

Physical signs

The patient may be acyanotic or cyanosed and clubbed. Even when tricuspid regurgitation is severe the jugular venous pressure may not be particularly high or the 'v' wave prominent because of the capacity of the right atrium and thin-walled atrialized right ventricle to accommodate the low-pressure regurgitant volume. Once right ventricular failure develops the jugular venous pressure rises further and the 'a' and 'v' waves become more prominent. In the uncommon situation of tricuspid stenosis, the 'a' wave is increased and may be giant. The first heart sound is widely split with a delayed tricuspid component, due to the extra distance that the large anterior leaflet has to travel to reach the limit of its systolic excursion. The second heart sound may be single because low pressure in the right ventricular outflow tract renders the pulmonary component inaudible, or it may be widely split, reflecting right bundle branch block. Third or fourth ventricular filling sounds may be present. The systolic murmur of tricuspid regurgitation varies from inaudible to loud enough to generate a thrill, but is classically decrescendo and scratchy. Once the right ventricle begins to fail and the venous pressure rises, hepatomegaly, ascites, and peripheral oedema are common.

Investigations

The chest radiograph is characteristic (Fig. 12.1.4). The ECG typically shows a superior axis and right atrial enlargement, with or without right bundle branch block. The 'p' wave may be peaked and the PR interval prolonged, reflecting the prolonged conduction in the large right atrium, or there may be evidence of pre-excitation. Right bundle branch block may occur due to abnormal activation and conduction in the atrialized right ventricle.

Echocardiography establishes the diagnosis, severity, and associated abnormalities of Ebstein anomaly. The atrialized and functional portions of the right ventricle can be identified, as can the precise attachments and degree of tethering of the anterior leaflet of the tricuspid valve. Echocardiography is the investigation of choice in planning surgical intervention, tethering and restricted motion of the anterior leaflet and a small right ventricle being strong predictors of the need for tricuspid valve replacement rather than repair. Cardiac catheterization is only necessary if specific haemodynamic questions remain after noninvasive assessment.

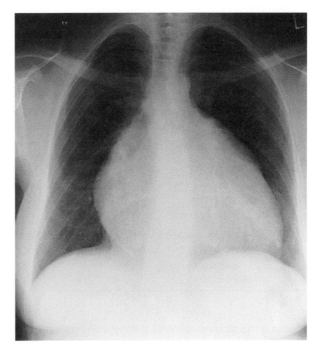

Fig. 12.1.4 Chest radiograph of a 43-year-old woman with classic cardiac silhouette of Ebstein anomaly due to right atrial enlargement. The aortic knuckle and pulmonary arteries are inconspicuous and the lung fields oligaemic.

Cardiopulmonary exercise testing is invaluable in assessing functional capacity when planning timing of surgery.

Treatment

Patients should be anticoagulated when atrial arrhythmias develop, particularly if there is an ASD. If re-entry tachycardias cannot be controlled with antiarrhythmic drugs, radiofrequency ablation of accessory pathways may be performed. However, ablation may be made difficult by the size and abnormal shape of the right atrium and abnormal position of the accessory pathway or pathways.

Symptomatic patients should be assessed for surgery. In addition, the asymptomatic patient with severe tricuspid regurgitation and normal cardiopulmonary exercise tolerance should be considered for repair if right ventricular function has begun to deteriorate. The timing of surgery may be difficult to decide in the adult patient, even in the few centres with reasonable experience. Once the patient has developed overt right heart failure with a raised venous pressure, hepatomegaly, ascites, and atrial fibrillation, ventricular function may have deteriorated such that repair of the valve is no longer possible and transplantation may need to be considered.

Successful repair of the ebsteinoid valve is difficult, as evidenced by the many techniques described. The aim is to achieve a competent native valve with its insertion at the true annulus and a reduction in right atrial size. Where possible, valve replacement should be avoided, since long-term outcomes are better with repair. A maze procedure should also be considered to reduce the long-term risk of atrial flutter and fibrillation.

For high-risk patients in whom the right ventricle is thought to be unable to support the pulmonary circulation with a competent tricuspid valve, techniques to reduce its workload may be considered. The '1½' ventricle repair combines tricuspid valve repair with

Table 12.1.5 Right ventricular cardiomyopathy and Uhl's anomaly

	Arrhythmogenic right ventricular cardiomyopathy	Uhl's anomaly 'Parchment heart'
Morphology	Patchy, localized fibro-fatty replacement of parietal myocardium mostly affecting outflow tract. Other parts of right and occasionally left ventricle may be involved	Congenital absence of parietal ventricular myocardium with direct apposition of endocardium and epicardium. Normal interventricular septum and left ventricle
Sex ratio	2:1 male:female	Equal
Typical presentation	As young adult Exercise-induced ventricular tachycardia: palpitation, syncope, sudden death	In infancy Congestive cardiac failure

a cavopulmonary anastomosis so that upper body systemic venous return is directly to the pulmonary arteries, thus offloading the right ventricle. A single-ventricle repair may also be used, resulting in a Fontan circulation (see 'Fontan operation').

Other right ventricular anomalies

Uhl's anomaly and arrhythmogenic right ventricular cardiomyopathy (see also Chapter 7.2) are rare sporadic or familial conditions affecting the right ventricle. Table 12.1.5 list the key distinguishing features.

Early diagnosis and the screening of family members of affected individuals is challenging and requires experience. MRI and high-resolution CT are useful tools, but early abnormalities are subtle and may be over interpreted.

Cor triatatrium and congenital mitral valve anomalies

Cor triatatrium

This is a very rare defect in which one of the atriums (nearly always the left) is partitioned by a fibromuscular membrane into an upper chamber that receives the pulmonary veins, and a lower chamber connecting with the atrial appendage and mitral valve. This is thought to occur due to a failure of the common pulmonary venous chamber to incorporate into the body of the left atrium early in fetal life. As a result, a persistent membrane inserts into the atrial septum at the fossa ovalis and into the posterolateral wall just above the mouth of the left atrial appendage. An ASD coexists in about 50% of cases, allowing communication between the right and left atriums. The membrane may be intact, or pierced by one or more holes that are usually restrictive, causing supramitral stenosis.

If the membrane obstructs pulmonary venous inflow, presentation is early in life, and adult survivors will have undergone surgical resection. First presentation in adulthood is unusual unless the membrane is nonrestrictive or coexists with a large ASD. Patients may have signs of an ASD or mitral stenosis. New symptoms in adulthood may be due to fibrosis or calcification of the membrane so that it becomes restrictive, or from progressive mitral regurgitation.

The diagnosis is made by echocardiography. The chest radiograph may also be characteristic, showing signs of pulmonary venous congestion, but not the left atrial appendage enlargement that accompanies valvar mitral stenosis, since the appendage lies in the low-pressure atrial chamber. The lateral chest radiograph may show enlargement of the pulmonary venous compartment of the left atrium.

Treatment is unnecessary if the membrane is unobstructive and there are no significant associated lesions. The results of surgical resection of obstructive membranes and the postoperative prognosis are good.

Congenital mitral valve anomalies

These are rare and frequently coexist with other lesions. A supramitral ring often coexists with congenital mitral stenosis. It differs from cor triatatrium in that the ring is sited inferiorly to the os of the appendage and lies immediately above the mitral valve.

Shone syndrome consists of four levels of left heart obstruction: supramitral ring, parachute mitral valve, subaortic stenosis (often with bicuspid aortic valve), and coarctation of the aorta. Parachute mitral valve occurs when the two papillary muscles are fused or there is hypoplasia or absence of one papillary muscle; the valve and its apparatus are often additionally dysplastic. Obstruction occurs at the level of the abnormal papillary muscles. The parachute mitral valve may also be regurgitant if the chordae are elongated and not significantly fused. Shone syndrome forms part of a spectrum of left heart obstruction that has bicuspid aortic valve at one end and hypoplastic left heart syndrome at the other. The recurrence risk is greater than for many forms of congenital heart disease at around 10%.

Isolated cleft mitral valve differs from the 'cleft' seen in an AVSD in being in the anterior (aortic) leaflet, directed towards the aortic outflow tract, rather than being in the space between the bridging leaflets and pointing towards the septum. The isolated cleft can be readily repaired to resemble a competent normal mitral valve.

Left ventricular outflow tract obstruction

Bicuspid aortic valve

This is the commonest congenital cardiac anomaly, occurring in 1 to 2% of the population. Bicuspid aortic valve is four times more common in males than in females. In 20% of cases it is associated with other lesions such as patent arterial duct and coarctation. There is also a familial association aortopathy, with aortic root dilatation and dissection—lifelong surveillance is necessary. Symptoms occur late in young people with aortic valve disease, hence regular follow-up is particularly important. Exercise testing is useful in planning the timing of surgery in those with asymptomatic aortic stenosis and left ventricular hypertrophy: ST segment changes and a failure of blood pressure to rise appropriately in response to stress indicate that intervention should be considered. Aortic stenosis and regurgitation are discussed in Chapter 6.1.

Supravalvar aortic stenosis

In this least common form of left ventricular outflow tract obstruction there is a localized narrowing of the aorta immediately above the aortic sinuses. Fibromuscular thickening of the aortic wall at the site of obstruction may encroach into the coronary ostia or onto the aortic valve leaflets and adversely influence prognosis. Unlike other forms of left ventricular outflow obstruction, the coronary arteries lie proximal to the obstruction and so are exposed to high left ventricular pressures, resulting in premature atherosclerosis. The condition may be associated with Williams' syndrome, when the prognosis may be worse since there is diffuse arterial involvement that may also involve the pulmonary and renal arteries (see Chapter 11.1).

Subaortic stenosis

Subaortic stenosis may be due to a discrete fibromuscular ridge or ring, or a long muscular tunnel. It may exist in isolation or as part of another lesion such as AVSD, where the 'unwedged' aorta; the elongated left ventricular outflow tract, and abnormal insertion of the left atrioventricular valve may all cause obstruction. Whether discrete or tunnel-like, subaortic stenosis tends to progress and may recur following surgical resection. It may result in functional disruption of the aortic valve and secondary aortic regurgitation, which can progress even after resection of subaortic stenosis.

Atrial septal defects

Interatrial communications are common both in congenital heart disease and in the general population. The different types of ASD are illustrated in Fig. 12.1.5. ASDs account for around 10% of congenital heart disease.

Patent foramen ovale

PFO is a normal variant that occurs in 20 to 30% of the population. There is no deficiency of atrial septal tissue, but after birth—when left atrial pressure exceeds right atrial pressure and closes the PFO—the valve of the foramen ovale fails to fuse with the septum.

Interest has risen in PFO in recent years because of its potential to be a route for paradoxical embolism or for thrombosis *in situ*, especially if associated with an aneurysmal interatrial septum. PFO is associated with cryptogenic embolic stroke in young adults, with neurological decompression sickness in divers, and with migraine with aura. Device closure of a PFO appears to protect against recurrent stroke due to paradoxical embolism and decompression sickness. Whether PFO closure should be considered for secondary provision following cryptogenic stroke is controversial.

Careful consideration should be given to all risk factors in assessing a patient with an embolic stroke and a PFO for suitability for device closure of the PFO. If there are multiple risk factors for arterial disease, such as advanced age, smoking history, diabetes, hyperlipidaemia, hypertension, or proven existing atherosclerotic disease, then device closure of a PFO is unlikely to reduce the risk of a further embolic event. The same is true for patients with risk factors for left-sided intracardiac thrombosis, such as atrial fibrillation, mitral valve disease with a dilated left atrium, or left ventricular aneurysm. In contrast, patients with a PFO and previous embolic stroke who have risk factors for venous thrombosis, such as a thrombophilia or previous venous thomboembolism—i.e. whose stroke was likely to be due to paradoxical embolism—may be protected against further events by device closure.

Ostium secundum atrial septal defect

Secundum ASD accounts for 40% of left-to-right shunts in adults aged over 40 years. It is commoner in females, with a sex ratio of 2:1, and may be familial. It may occur as an isolated abnormality with autosomal dominant inheritance, be associated with Holt–Oram syndrome (autosomal dominant skeletal abnormalities and atrioventricular conduction defects due to *TBX5* mutation), and is a common association with Down's syndrome.

ASD may be an incidental finding in an elderly patient at autopsy, and diagnosis in life may be delayed well into adulthood because of the absence of symptoms and subtlety of clinical signs. However, the natural history of this lesion is not benign: historically only 50% with unoperated nonrestrictive (large) ASD survived to the age of 40 years, and 10% beyond 60 years of age.

Presentation in adulthood may be with symptoms of exertional dyspnoea or palpitation, or as a result of incidental clinical or radiographic findings. However, 20% may have developed atrial fibrillation by 40 years, with the figure rising to around 60% by the age of 60 years. Similarly, the volume-loaded right ventricle is well tolerated for many years, but may ultimately fail, usually after the fifth decade.

Contributing factors to progression of symptoms with age may be increased left-to-right shunting due to an age-related reduction in left ventricular compliance causing an increase in left ventricular

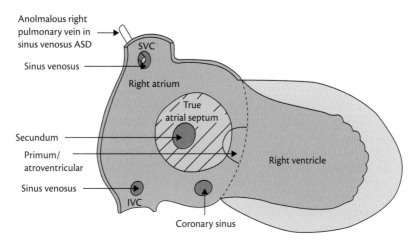

Fig. 12.1.5 Sites of atrial septal defects. The shaded area delineates the true atrial septum. Sinus venosus and coronary sinus defects are therefore not strictly atrial septal defects although they permit shunting at atrial level.

end-diastolic pressure and therefore left atrial pressure, and development of mitral regurgitation causing an increase in left atrial pressure. In addition, modest pulmonary arterial hypertension increases with age so the right ventricle is exposed to pressure as well as volume overload, precipitating right ventricular failure.

A left-to-right shunt at atrial level predisposes to paradoxical embolus since simple manoeuvres such as the Valsalva are sufficient to increase right atrial pressure and reverse the shunt. Patients with unoperated ASD are therefore at risk of embolic stroke, and should not dive because of the risk of paradoxical gas embolism.

Interactions with coexisting heart disease

Acquired disease may coexist and interact with congenital heart disease, especially in the ageing patient. Left ventricular dysfunction due to coronary artery disease and systemic hypertension may increase the left-to-right interatrial shunt, resulting in a more rapid clinical deterioration. Similarly, mitral regurgitation increases the effective interatrial shunt and mitral valve abnormalities may be acquired secondary to the effects of a secundum ASD. There may be distortion of the anterior mitral valve leaflet with fibrotic shortened chordae due to the abnormal position of the interventricular septum as a result of chronic right ventricular overload. Lutembacher's syndrome is the association of mitral stenosis with secundum ASD.

Mitral valve disease is underestimated in the presence of an ASD because the left atrium is able to decompress through the ASD. If significant mitral stenosis or regurgitation is overlooked at the time of ASD repair, left atrial pressure will rise and the patient may decompensate dramatically. It is therefore vital to ensure thorough assessment of the mitral valve in any patient in whom ASD closure is planned. Since left ventricular dysfunction may also be masked by an ASD, the defect serving to allow the left ventricle to offload, ventricular function must also be assessed carefully prior to ASD closure, particularly in elderly patients.

Coexisting pulmonary stenosis may be overestimated in the presence of an ASD, since Doppler velocities are increased in the presence of a left-to-right shunt.

Pulmonary vascular disease and atrial septal defect

Mild pulmonary hypertension with ASD is a common finding with advancing age, but pulmonary vascular resistance is rarely in excess of 6 Wood units and advanced pulmonary hypertension is rare. Few ASDs develop a right-to-left shunt secondary to pulmonary vascular disease, and a causal relationship between ASD and the Eisenmenger syndrome remains controversial. In ASD, unlike other lesions which may cause the Eisenmenger syndrome such as large VSD, the pulmonary vasculature is not exposed to increased flow at systemic pressure.

ASD with a right-to-left shunt due to pulmonary vascular disease and pulmonary hypertension occurs most commonly in young women, and in some cases may be due to idiopathic pulmonary arterial hypertension with an incidental ASD (see Table 12.1.4, pulmonary hypertension types A–D). In this combination, the prognosis may be better than for idiopathic pulmonary arterial hypertension with intact atrial septum, the septal defect protecting the right heart from pressure overload by allowing right-to-left shunting. Persistence of the fetal pulmonary vascular pattern may be implicated in the development of pulmonary hypertension in some young patients with ASD. Patients living or born at high altitude have a higher incidence of pulmonary vascular disease because of the effects of relative hypoxia on the pulmonary vasculature.

Clinical signs

If the defect is nonrestrictive the 'a' and 'v' waves of the jugular venous pulse tend to be equal. In older patients with reduced left ventricular compliance, the left and therefore right atrial pressure is raised, reflected by an elevated jugular venous pressure. A right ventricular heave may be felt at the left sternal border, and the dilated pulmonary artery may be palpable in the left second intercostal space. The first sound is loud because of increased diastolic flow across the tricuspid valve. If the left-to-right shunt is greater than approximately 2:1, the second heart sound is widely split and fixed, and there is loss of normal sinus arrhythmia. There may be a pulmonary flow murmur at the upper left sternal edge. Only if the ASD has a high gradient across it will it generate a murmur itself, usually a soft continuous murmur. This is the case if the defect is small and restrictive and the left atrial pressure high, e.g. if there is associated mitral stenosis. If the patient has pulmonary vascular disease, the signs will be the same as for pulmonary hypertension with right-to-left shunt.

Investigations

The ECG may show sinus node dysfunction, prolongation of the PR interval, right axis deviation, and QRS prolongation with rSr′ in lead V1—which does not represent incomplete right bundle branch block, but occurs since the last part of the myocardium to depolarize is the right ventricular outflow tract that is enlarged and thickened due to volume overload. Postoperatively the ECG may show sinus node dysfunction due to damage when the SVC is cannulated, and the PR interval returning to normal as right atrial size decreases. Macro re-entry circuits at the site of atrial surgery may result in postoperative ectopic atrial tachycardias.

The typical chest radiograph shows dilated proximal pulmonary arteries with a small aortic knuckle, plethoric lung fields, and cardiomegaly secondary to dilatation of the right atrium and ventricle.

Transthoracic echocardiography demonstrates the volume-loaded right atrium and ventricle. The size of the shunt can be estimated and colour-flow Doppler facilitates the detection of the site of the shunt. If transcatheter device closure is considered, a transoesophageal approach is necessary to define the site and size of the ASD precisely and to identify the pulmonary veins.

Cardiac catheterization is indicated only to calculate pulmonary vascular resistance if there is a suspicion of pulmonary hypertension, or to exclude coexisting congenital or acquired cardiac pathology such as coronary artery disease.

Indications for closure of atrial septal defect

Closure of an ASD is indicated if there is right heart volume overload, left-to-right shunt is 1.5:1 or more, and the ASD is 10 mm or more in diameter. Prevention of recurrent paradoxical embolism is an additional indication for closure. Contraindications to closure are significant pulmonary hypertension (which may be suggested by a right-to-left shunt on exercise or at rest) and severe left ventricular dysfunction. In addition, merely closing the ASD in the presence of significant mitral valve disease is contraindicated.

Irrespective of age, the benefits of device closure should be improved functional class, exercise capacity, and breathlessness. Repair of a large isolated secundum ASD by the third decade results in a normal life expectancy. Between the ages of 25 and 41 years it results in a good but shorter than normal life expectancy, but beyond the age of 41 years morbidity and mortality remain significantly higher than normal. Nonetheless, functional status and longevity are improved following repair over the age of 40 years, 5- and 10-year survival being estimated as 98% and 95% respectively for patients who underwent repair, and 93% and 84% for those treated medically. Repair in older patients does not reduce the risk of late atrial arrhythmia, particularly if there is right ventricular dysfunction, elevated pulmonary artery pressure or pre-existing atrial arrhythmia. Whether the incorporation of a modified maze procedure or cryoablation into the surgical repair of ASD will reduce the long-term incidence of existing or *de novo* atrial arrhythmia remains to be determined.

Secundum ASDs up to 4 cm stretched diameter may be closed by transcatheter devices so long as the surrounding rim of atrial septal tissue is sufficient. Criteria for device closure of secundum ASD are size less than 4 cm; a situation away from the atrioventricular valves and pulmonary and caval veins; and normal pulmonary venous drainage. The risk of major complication during device closure is 1 to 2%. Following closure, antiplatelet or anticoagulant therapy is recommended for 3 to 6 months. Surgical repair carries also carries a low mortality and morbidity, but perioperative atrial fibrillation is common and recovery time is longer.

Other forms of atrial septal defect

Sinus venosus atrial septal defect

Sinus venosus defects account for 2 to 3% of ASDs and have an equal sex incidence. They are not truly defects of the atrial septum, but since they allow shunting at atrial level, they are included in the classification of ASDs. The inferior border of the more common SVC type of sinus venosus defect is made by the superior limbus of the fossa ovalis, and the upper border comprises the junction of the SVC with the atrial mass. The superior caval vein overrides the atrial septum, connecting to both atriums, and the right upper pulmonary vein drains anomalously into the SVC. There may be an ectopic atrial pacemaker because the defect is located in the area of the sinoatrial node. This may be reflected by a leftwards 'p' wave axis and an inverted 'p' wave in lead III.

The sinus venosus defect may not be visualized with transthoracic echocardiography, and a transoesophageal approach is usually necessary to define the defect and is associated anomalous pulmonary venous drainage.

They are unsuitable for transcatheter device closure, both because there is no superior rim and because of anomalous drainage of one or more of the right pulmonary veins. The proximity of the sinus node to the SVC type of defect makes it vulnerable to damage during surgical repair; postoperative atrial pacing may be required.

Coronary sinus defect

The rarest form of ASD, this defect is at the site of entry of the coronary sinus to the right atrium. The unroofed coronary sinus is a variation of coronary sinus defect in which the partition between the coronary sinus and the left atrium is absent as the coronary sinus runs posteriorly along the floor of the left atrium. In this condition, a left SVC commonly connects directly to the left atrium, producing a right-to-left shunt and cyanosis.

Ostium primum atrial septal defect

This is a defect in the true atrial septum that exists as part of an AVSD and is discussed later in the chapter (see 'Atrioventricular septal defects').

Ventricular septal defects

With the exceptions of bicuspid aortic valve and mitral valve prolapse, VSD is the commonest congenital cardiac malformation, occurring in around 3 per 1000 live births. It occurs equally in both sexes. Defects may exist in isolation, in association with other lesions such as coarctation of the aorta, or as an integral part of lesions such as tetralogy of Fallot. This section deals with isolated VSDs.

Morphology and classification

An understanding of the basic anatomy of the ventricular septum is necessary to appreciate the various types of VSD. A VSD arises when there is failure of one of the components of the ventricular septum to develop correctly. The septum comprises four parts and is described as viewed from the right ventricle (Fig. 12.1.6):

- Inlet septum—separates the mitral and tricuspid valves

- Muscular trabeculated septum—extends from the tricuspid valve leaflet attachments to the muscle separating the tricuspid and pulmonary valves (the crista supraventricularis)

- Outlet septum—extends from the crista to the pulmonary valve

- Perimembranous septum—small fibrous area bordered by the aortic and tricuspid valves

VSDs are classified by their location within the septum and by their borders, again viewed from the right ventricle. There are three types: muscular, perimembranous and doubly committed subarterial (Figs. 12.1.6 and 12.1.7). The position of muscular and perimembranous VSDs may be inlet, trabecular, or outlet, depending on which part of the right ventricle they open into. Perimembranous VSD is the commonest type of defect. Only 5 to 7% of VSDs in Europe and North America are doubly committed subarterial defects, whereas they account for up to 30% of defects in Asian patients.

Clinical presentation and complications of unoperated ventricular septal defect

The presentation of an isolated VSD depends on its size and haemodynamic effects (Table 12.1.6). Perimembranous and doubly

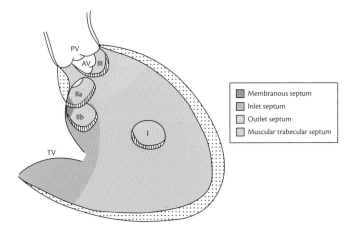

Fig. 12.1.6 Schematic representation to show the sites of different types of ventricular septal defects (VSDs). The heart is in cross-section, viewed from the right ventricular aspect. I, muscular VSD; IIa, perimembranous outlet VSD; IIb perimembranous inlet VSD; III doubly committed subarterial VSD. AV, aortic valve, seen through VSD; PV, pulmonary valve; TV, tricuspid valve.

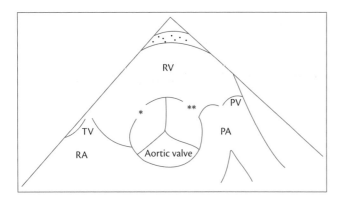

Fig. 12.1.7 Schematic representation of the transthoracic echocardiographic parasternal short-axis view, to demonstrate sites of ventricular septal defects (VSDs). **, site of doubly committed subarterial VSD—the aortic and pulmonary valves are in continuity and form the roof of the VSD. *, site of subaortic perimembranous VSD. PA, pulmonary artery; PV, pulmonary valve; RA, right atrium; RV, right ventricle; TV, tricuspid valve; VSD, ventricular septal defect.

committed subarterial VSDs may be associated with the development of aortic valve leaflet prolapse and aortic regurgitation, and the conduction tissue in these types of defects is vulnerable to damage at operation.

Adults with isolated unoperated restrictive VSDs are usually asymptomatic and acyanotic, with normal arterial and jugular venous pulses. There may be a thrill at the left sternal border, the left ventricular apex may be thrusting if the defect is large enough to cause volume overload, and a dilated pulmonary artery may be palpable. The second heart sound is usually normally split. There is a loud, harsh pansystolic murmur at the left sternal edge, which is softer and shorter (early systolic) in very small defects.

Late complications of unoperated small VSDs include significant risk of endocarditis due to the high-velocity jet from left to right ventricle, particularly if the jet is directed onto tricuspid valve tissue; aortic regurgitation if the aortic valve forms part of the border of the VSD; atrial arrhythmia if there is left heart volume overload; and small increased risk of sudden death and ventricular arrhythmia.

A moderate-sized restrictive VSD may cause left heart volume overload, and in the long term, atrial arrhythmias and left ventricular dysfunction. A VSD causes left, rather than right, ventricular dilatation because the left-to-right shunt reaches the right ventricle during ventricular systole: the right ventricle cannot dilate during contraction, so the additional blood is directed straight into the pulmonary circulation and back into the left heart during diastole. Thus the left heart is subject to volume overload.

Larger VSDs rarely present for repair in adulthood since the large left-to-right shunt is unlikely to allow unoperated survival unless pulmonary vascular disease has developed. Nonrestrictive defects are not associated with the classical VSD murmur since left and right ventricular pressures are equal.

Investigations

Investigation should determine the type and number of VSDs, the size of the defect (restrictive or nonrestrictive), an estimation of the size of the shunt (Qp:Qs), pulmonary artery pressure and resistance, and assessment of left and right ventricular function and volume and pressure overload. Associated lesions that may alter management should be identified, especially aortic regurgitation, subaortic stenosis, and right ventricular outflow tract obstruction.

The chest radiograph is normal if the defect has been small from birth. If the VSD is (or has been) larger, the left ventricle, left atrium, and pulmonary trunk may be dilated and there may be increased pulmonary vascularity. The ECG shows a normal QRS axis unless there are multiple defects, when there may be left axis deviation. In the presence of a large left-to-right shunt the 'p' wave may be broad and there may be evidence of left ventricular hypertrophy. Two-dimensional echocardiography identifies the number and site of defects as well as describing the morphology and associated defects. Doppler is used to estimate the size and direction of the shunt, and right ventricle to left ventricle pressure difference, but this may not be accurate if there is an obliquely lying muscular VSD. Cardiac catheterization is important to measure the size of shunt and pulmonary vascular resistance, with reversibility studies if baseline resistance is high.

Indications for repair and postoperative sequelae

Repair of a VSD is indicated in the presence of symptoms, if Qp:Qs is greater than 2:1, or if there is ventricular dysfunction with right ventricular pressure overload or left ventricular volume overload. Repair should also be undertaken if there are coexisting lesions such as significant right ventricular outflow tract obstruction, or more than mild aortic regurgitation or aortic valve prolapse in the presence of an outlet VSD. An episode of endocarditis may also be considered as an indication for VSD closure. If the pulmonary artery pressure is more than two-thirds systemic pressure, repair should only be considered if Qp:Qs exceeds 1.5:1 or if there is

Table 12.1.6 Grading of ventricular septal defects by size

	Small	Moderate	Large	Eisenmenger syndrome
Pulmonary artery pressure: systemic pressure ratio	<0.3	0.3–0.6	RV = LV pressure	RV ≥ LV pressure
Qp:Qs	<1.4:1	1.4–2.2:1	>2.2:1	<1.5:1
Clinical grading	Negligible haemodynamic changes, normal LV	LA and LV enlargement and reversible pulmonary hypertension	Pulmonary vascular disease (Eisenmenger syndrome) will develop unless there is RVOTO	
	Restrictive (RV pressure < LV pressure in absence of RVOTO)		Nonrestrictive (equal RV and LV pressures in absence of RVOTO)	

Qp, pulmonary blood flow; Qs, systemic blood flow; RVOTO, right ventricular outflow tract obstruction.

evidence of reversibility in response to pulmonary vasodilators such as oxygen and nitric oxide.

The surgical approach aims at avoiding damage to important structures such as the conducting tissues, which are especially vulnerable in perimembranous defects. Transatrial repair reduces the risk of postoperative ventricular arrhythmias by avoiding a right ventriculotomy. Transient postoperative complete heart block is associated with an increased risk of late high-degree block, and permanent pacemaker implantation is indicated in the 1 to 2% of patients in whom complete heart block persists, even if they are asymptomatic, because there is a significant risk of late sudden death.

The prognosis after VSD repair in the early years of life is good, but if repair is delayed into late childhood left ventricular dilatation may persist and systolic function be impaired. Long-term postoperative survival depends on the presence of pulmonary hypertension, left ventricular dysfunction, and complications such as aortic regurgitation and endocarditis.

Transcatheter device closure of VSDs is possible providing that valvar apparatus can be avoided. Both muscular and selected perimembranous VSDs may be device closed, the latter requiring experienced hands to avoid damage to the aortic valve and heart block. This approach is particularly useful for defects that are difficult to access or close surgically, and a hybrid surgical/interventional technique may be used.

Atrioventricular septal defects

The key feature of an AVSD (previously termed endocardial cushion defect or atrioventricular canal) is a common atrioventricular junction and atrioventricular valve ring (Fig. 12.1.8). The atrioventricular septum is absent and the atrioventricular valves share a common junction and fibrous ring, with a five-leaflet atrioventricular valve. Since they share common leaflets, the valves are not correctly called mitral and tricuspid valves, but left and right atrioventricular valves. As a consequence the normal offsetting of

the right atrioventricular valve towards the right ventricular apex is absent. In addition, the aorta is 'unwedged' from its normal position between the left and right atrioventricular valves. The left ventricular outflow tract is therefore elongated ('gooseneck') and has the propensity to develop obstruction, often due to septal attachments of the left atrioventricular valve. 'Cleft mitral valve' refers to the commissure between the anterior and posterior bridging leaflets that renders the left atrioventricular valve potentially regurgitant. The left ventricular papillary muscles are abnormally placed anteriorly and posteriorly instead of in the normal anterolateral and posteromedial positions. Ostium primum defect describes the atrial component of an AVSD.

There are two types of AVSD, partial and complete. Both have a common atrioventricular junction, but in a partial AVSD the right and left atrioventricular valves have separate orifices and the VSD is usually small or absent, and in a complete AVSD there is a common atrioventricular valve and valve orifice, and the VSD is usually large.

AVSD occurs with equal sex incidence. The complete form of the defect is most commonly associated with Down's syndrome. A single gene defect may be responsible for AVSD in nonsyndromic patients, when the recurrence risk is about 10% if the mother has an AVSD, less if the father is affected.

The physiological consequences of an AVSD are the same as for other conditions with left-to-right shunting at atrial or ventricular level, but may be complicated by left atrioventricular valve regurgitation or left ventricular outflow tract obstruction. Pulmonary vascular disease may develop if the VSD is large and nonrestrictive. Patients with Down's syndrome are at particular risk of this complication, and coexisting upper airway obstruction and sleep apnoea, and abnormal pulmonary parenchyma, may be contributory factors.

Investigations

The ECG is distinctive, with a left and superior QRS axis and notching of 'S' waves in the inferior leads. The chest radiograph

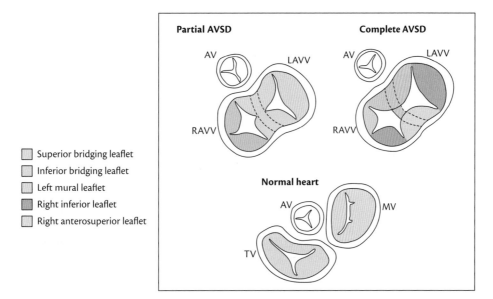

Fig. 12.1.8 Schematic representation of the atrioventricular junction in atrioventricular septal defect (AVSD). Short-axis view, seen from the atrial aspect. In both forms of AVSD, there is a common atrioventricular valve ring guarded by five valve leaflets. In the partial defect, the superior and inferior bridging leaflets fuse to create two separate valve orifices. This fusion does not occur in complete AVSD, so there is a common valve orifice. AV, aortic valve; LAVV, left atrioventricular valve; RAVV, right atrioventricular valve.

appearances depend on the degree of interatrial shunting and left atrioventricular valve regurgitation, the former producing cardiomegaly due to left heart dilatation and the latter left atrial enlargement. There may be increased pulmonary vascularity, particularly in young patients with complete AVSD and high pulmonary blood flow.

Transthoracic echocardiography reveals the detailed anatomy of the defect and establishes the site and degree of shunting, the presence and nature of left ventricular outflow tract obstruction, and the function and anatomy of the atrioventricular valves.

The indications for cardiac catheterization are the same as for secundum ASD, namely to exclude inoperable pulmonary vascular disease. In addition useful information may be obtained regarding the severity of left atrioventricular valve regurgitation and left ventricular outflow tract obstruction.

Clinical course

First presentation may occur in adulthood if the left-to-right shunt is small and the left atrioventricular valve is competent. Physical signs are the same as in other ASDs, and there may also be an apical pansystolic murmur. Paradoxical embolism is less common than in secundum ASD because the position of the primum defect low in the interatrial septum avoids the streaming of blood from the inferior vena cava that is most likely to carry emboli and is directed towards the midportion of the septum.

Most adult patients have undergone surgery to repair the defect and left atrioventricular valve: others have survived unoperated and may have developed pulmonary vascular disease.

Late complications after repair of AVSD include recurrent atrioventricular valve regurgitation, the severity of which may increase with age in response to changes in the left ventricle due to ageing, ischaemia, or systemic hypertension; residual ASD or VSD; residual or recurrent left ventricular outflow tract obstruction, which may be difficult to relieve surgically if it involves left atrioventricular valve tissue; complete heart block, related to the abnormally positioned atrioventricular node that is particularly vulnerable to intraoperative damage; endocarditis, relating largely to the left atrioventricular valve; and atrial arrhythmia. It is vital to read the original operation note when planning ablation, since the mouth of the coronary sinus is often left opening into the left atrium, making it inaccessible to the electrophysiologist.

Arterial disorders

Coarctation of the aorta

Aortic coarctation is a narrowing of the aorta, usually sited near the ligamentum arteriosum. It is one of the commonest congenital cardiac lesions, occurring in 1 in 12000 live births, with a male to female ratio of 3:1. Coarctation is part of a generalized arteriopathy with considerable variation in anatomy and severity, ranging from a mild obstruction to interruption of the aorta, and from a discrete fibromuscular shelf to hypoplasia of the arch. Coarctation is most strongly associated with bicuspid aortic valve, which coexists in up to 80% of cases. Ascending and descending aortopathy may be present, with medial changes and arterial wall stiffness; aneurysm formation, dissection, and the complications of hypertension require lifelong surveillance. Other associations are VSD, patent arterial duct, subaortic ridge, and mitral valve abnormalities. It is a frequent finding in Turner's

syndrome and is also associated with congenital aneurysm of the circle of Willis.

Presentation

Most patients present in infancy, but some survive into adulthood before being diagnosed at routine examination or during investigation for hypertension, leg claudication, angina, heart failure, or cerebral haemorrhage. Historically, more than 75% with unoperated coarctation died by age 50 years, from premature coronary disease, stroke, or aortic dissection.

Clinical findings include upper body hypertension: the leg blood pressure is lower, as is that in the left arm if the subclavian artery is involved in the coarctation. If there is a good collateral supply, femoral arteries may be easily palpable, but they are usually reduced, with radiofemoral delay. Intercostal collaterals may be both visible and palpable over the patient's back. There is an ejection systolic murmur from the site of coarctation, and systolic collateral murmurs may be heard. Fundoscopy shows a typical corkscrew appearance of the retinal vessels and there may be evidence of hypertensive retinopathy.

Investigations

There may be electrocardiographic evidence of left ventricular hypertrophy. The chest radiograph (Fig. 12.1.9) has a typical appearance.

Transthoracic echocardiography may show left ventricular hypertrophy, with the coarctation site visualized on two-dimensional imaging and its severity assessed using Doppler mode from the suprasternal notch. A peak gradient of over 20 mmHg is significant, especially if accompanied by a diastolic tail.

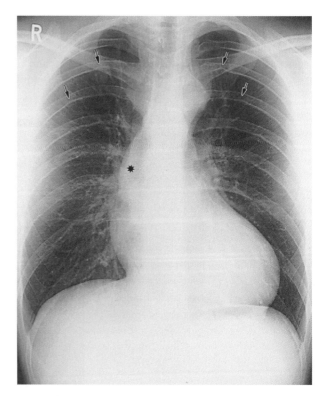

Fig. 12.1.9 Chest radiograph of an 18-year-old man with unoperated coarctation of the aorta and bicuspid aortic valve. There is bilateral rib notching (arrows) and a prominent deformed aortic knuckle. The dilated ascending aorta (*) indicates the associated aortopathy.

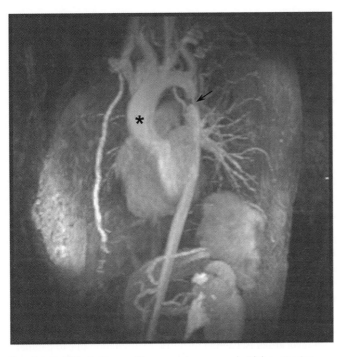

Fig. 12.1.10 MRI of a 20-year-old woman who presented with hypertension. There is a severe discrete coarctation (↓), multiple tortuous collaterals and a dilated ascending aorta (*) associated with a bicuspid aortic valve.

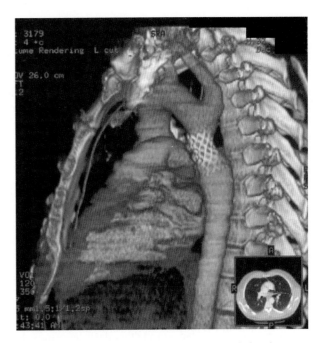

Fig. 12.1.11 High-resolution CT scan demonstrating stent deployed at native coarctation site.

MRI provides definitive noninvasive haemodynamic data and two- and three-dimensional images of the coarctation site, collaterals and related vessels (Fig. 12.1.10). It may obviate the need for angiography unless coronary disease is suspected. In the adult, diagnostic angiography is usually reserved for assessing coronary disease.

Repair of native coarctation

Surgical repair is the conventional approach in neonates and children, with a risk of less than 1% for those with simple coarctation. Extensive collateral vessels and nonelastic diseased aortic tissue make surgical repair of adult coarctation challenging, and this is associated with significant morbidity. The incidence of perioperative spinal cord ischaemia and paraplegia is up to 0.4%, those patients without an abundant collateral circulation probably being most at risk. Those with well-developed collaterals are at risk of significant intraoperative haemorrhage. Early postoperative hypertension is common and may be difficult to control, and postoperative intestinal ileus may persist for several days.

Transcatheter balloon dilatation and primary stenting of native coarctation in adults are usually the preferred alternatives to surgery. The use of primary stents, particularly covered stents, is likely to support the aorta following dilatation and to reduce the risk of aortic dissection or late aneurysm formation. However, this interventional approach is controversial and should only be done in specialist centres; careful follow-up is required.

Follow-up after coarctation repair

Follow-up after repair of coarctation should be lifelong, since late complications are frequent: residual or recoarctation, aneurysm formation, persistent hypertension despite adequate repair, premature atherosclerotic disease, and progression of associated lesions such as bicuspid aortic valve and aortopathy. Older age at repair is the main risk factor influencing longevity. Late survival is 92% for patients repaired in infancy, 25-year survival is 75% for those repaired between ages and 40 years, but 15-year survival is only 50% for those repaired at age more than 40 years.

Recoarctation may be diagnosed when the resting arm–leg systolic blood pressure gradient is 20 mmHg at rest and 50 mmHg after exercise. This occurs most commonly following neonatal repair by end-to-end anastomosis, and the diagnosis should be sought when there is new or persisting hypertension. Blood pressure should be recorded in both arms of all such patients; spuriously low readings may be obtained if one of the subclavian arteries (usually the left) is involved in the repair or recoarctation.

MRI is the investigation of choice for both recoarctation and aneurysm formation after coarctation repair. High-resolution CT is used following stent repair of coarctation (Fig. 12.1.11), since the artefact produced by the stent renders MRI unhelpful. Balloon angioplasty with or without stent insertion is used to relieve most recoarctations, but reoperation is required for some patients with complex anatomy.

The 14-year incidence of aneurysm formation at the site of repair is up to 27%; it occurs most commonly in adults and in those with Dacron patch repair. An aneurysm may rupture into the bronchial tree or oesophagus, hence any patient with a history of coarctation who presents with haemoptysis or haematemesis should undergo emergency noninvasive diagnostic imaging (MRI or CT) and surgical repair. Bronchoscopy and conventional angiography are contraindicated since they may cause further damage to the ruptured area.

Hypertension is a major risk factor for atherosclerotic disease and may persist despite an apparently good result from surgical repair. Continuing hypertension relates in part to older age at time of surgery. Nonetheless, late repair of coarctation or re-coarctation does render systolic hypertension easier to control.

Patent arterial duct

The pathophysiological consequences of a patent arterial duct in adulthood depend on the size of the shunt. Small ducts are of no haemodynamic significance and are associated with a low risk of infective endarteritis. Moderate-sized ducts may cause left heart volume overload and late atrial fibrillation and ventricular dysfunction. A large nonrestrictive duct may cause pulmonary vascular disease (see 'Eisenmenger syndrome', above).

Duct closure is usually recommended if a duct is clinically detectable, i.e. there is a systolic or continuous (machinery) murmur in the left subclavicular area, to avoid long-term haemodynamic complications. Ducts up to 14 mm in diameter are usually suitable for transcatheter device closure. Pulmonary vascular disease should be excluded before repair of large ducts is undertaken.

Aortopulmonary window

In this rare condition there is a direct communication between adjacent portions of the proximal ascending aorta and pulmonary artery. The communication is usually large and the physiological consequences are the same as for a large patent arterial duct. Rare patients surviving unoperated into adulthood will be cyanosed and have developed the Eisenmenger syndrome. If pulmonary vascular resistance is low at the time of childhood repair, long-term postoperative survival is good.

Truncus arteriosus/common arterial trunk

This condition accounts for 1 to 4% of all congenital heart disease. It may coexist with interrupted aortic arch, coarctation, coronary anomalies and DiGeorge syndrome. A single great artery arises from the heart and gives rise to the coronary arteries, aorta and pulmonary arteries. There is a single semilunar 'truncal' valve that has three or more leaflets, and a subtruncal VSD.

Most patients present in infancy with heart failure. If they are left unoperated, pulmonary vascular resistance rises, cyanosis becomes more marked, and the Eisenmenger syndrome becomes established. Repair before pulmonary vascular disease develops involves closure of the VSD, detachment of the pulmonary arteries from the common arterial trunk, and placement of a valved conduit from right ventricle to pulmonary artery. The truncal valve then functions as the aortic valve. Late complications following repair include truncal regurgitation, truncal (aortic root) dilation, ventricular dysfunction, and the need to replace stenotic conduits.

Sinus of Valsalva aneurysm

There is dilation of one of the aortic valve sinuses between the aortic valve annulus and sinotubular junction, and the aneurysm progressively dilates and may rupture. The right and noncoronary cusps are most often affected; rupture of a noncoronary sinus aneurysm is nearly always into the right atrium and of the right coronary sinus into the right ventricle or atrium. Involvement of the left coronary sinus is rare. Rupture usually occurs in early adulthood and may be precipitated by endocarditis. If sudden, it is accompanied by tearing chest pain, breathlessness, and sudden-onset symptoms suggesting heart failure, with a loud continuous murmur and good systolic ventricular function. Small perforations may remain asymptomatic for many years. The diagnosis and site of the rupture is confirmed echocardiographically and/or angiographically before surgical or transcatheter repair.

Coronary artery anomalies

The importance of congenital coronary anomalies lies in their potential to impair myocardial blood flow and cause ischaemia and sudden death. Evidence of ischaemia is the main indication for repair. The major types of coronary anomaly are summarized in Box 12.1.3.

Anomalous origin of the coronary arteries from an inappropriate aortic sinus

Ischaemia is particularly associated with an anomalous proximal coronary course between the aorta and pulmonary trunk, an intramural proximal segment of the coronary artery inside the aortic wall, and acute angulation between the origin of an anomalous coronary artery and the aortic wall.

Anomalous origin of the left coronary artery from the pulmonary artery

This rare condition, known as LCAPA, usually presents in infancy with myocardial ischaemia and left ventricular failure when pulmonary vascular resistance decreases. However, 10 to 15% survive into adulthood because an adequate intercoronary collateral circulation is established. Adults may be asymptomatic or present with myocardial ischaemia or mitral regurgitation due to papillary muscle dysfunction. Survival following surgical repair depends on the amount of ischaemic myocardial damage and degree of mitral regurgitation.

Congenital coronary arteriovenous fistulas

The coronary arteries arise normally from their aortic sinuses, but a fistulous branch communicates directly with the right ventricle in 40% of cases, the right atrium in 25%, pulmonary artery in 15%, or rarely the SVC or pulmonary vein. Survival to adulthood is usual, but lifespan may be reduced, depending on the size of the fistulous connection and the presence of myocardial ischaemia resulting from any coronary steal phenomenon. Symptoms increase with age and there is a risk of endocarditis, heart failure, arrhythmia, myocardial ischaemia and infarction, and sudden death. Surgical

---

Box 12.1.3 Major types of coronary anomaly

- ◆ Anomalous origin from inappropriate aortic sinus or coronary vessel
  - LAD from right aortic sinus or right coronary artery (RCA)
  - Absent LMS (separate origins of LAD and Cx)
  - Cx from right aortic sinus or RCA or absent Cx
  - RCA from left aortic sinus, posterior sinus or LAD
  - Single coronary artery from right or left aortic sinus
- ◆ Anomalous origin from other systemic artery (rare)
  - Innominate, subclavian, internal mammary, carotid, bronchial arteries, or descending aorta
- ◆ Anomalous origin from pulmonary artery
- ◆ Coronary arteriovenous fistulae

Cx, circumflex; LAD, left anterior descending; LMS, left main stem; RCA, right coronary artery.

repair is recommended unless there is a trivial isolated shunt. Some smaller fistulae are suitable for transcatheter device occlusion.

Systemic venous anomalies

These anomalies frequently form part a more complex lesion, particularly isomerism. Normal systemic venous drainage is illustrated in Fig. 12.1.12.

Superior caval vein anomalies

A persistent left-sided SVC occurs in 0.3% of the general population, approximately 3% of patients with congenital heart disease, and 15% of those with tetralogy of Fallot. The left SVC may be visible on the chest radiograph. It usually drains to the right atrium via the coronary sinus, which is seen to be dilated on two-dimensional echocardiography (Fig. 12.1.13). A right-sided SVC is usually also present, but the two caval veins do not usually communicate via the brachiocephalic vein. This common anomaly should be sought routinely at cardiac catheterization; although it does not have any haemodynamic significance, it may cause technical difficulties during transvenous pacemaker insertion and cardiac surgery (Fig. 12.1.14).

Other SVC anomalies are rare. An absent right SVC is associated with arrhythmias including atrioventricular block, sinus node dysfunction, and atrial fibrillation. The left, or rarely the right, SVC may connect directly to the left atrium, causing an obligatory right-to-left shunt and cyanosis. This may be associated with isomerism of the atrial appendages.

Inferior caval vein anomalies

Azygos continuation of the inferior vena cava (IVC) occurs in 0.6% of patients with congenital heart disease. The infrahepatic portion of the IVC is absent and continues to the SVC via an azygos vein; the hepatic veins drain directly into the right atrium. This is often

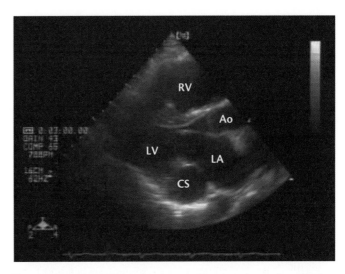

Fig. 12.1.13 Persistent left superior vena cava. Transthoracic two-dimensional echocardiogram, parasternal long-axis view. The coronary sinus, receiving the persistent left superior vena cava, is dilated. Ao, aorta; CS, coronary sinus; LA, left atrium; LV, left ventricle; RV, right ventricle.

associated with complex lesions, particularly left isomerism. The chest radiograph reveals an absence of the IVC at the junction of the diaphragm with the right heart border and a dilated azygos vein (Fig. 12.1.15). Direct connection of the IVC to the left atrium is rare: the patient is cyanosed, as in the SVC–left atrium connection.

Pulmonary venous anomalies

Total anomalous pulmonary venous drainage

Total anomalous pulmonary venous drainage occurs in 1 in 17 000 live births. All four pulmonary veins drain into the right atrium,

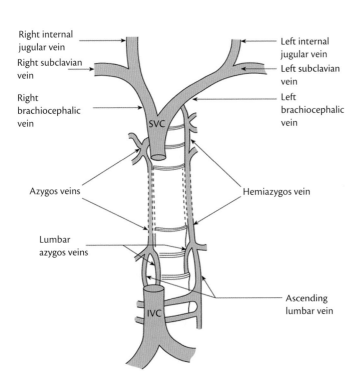

Fig. 12.1.12 Schematic diagram of normal systemic venous drainage.

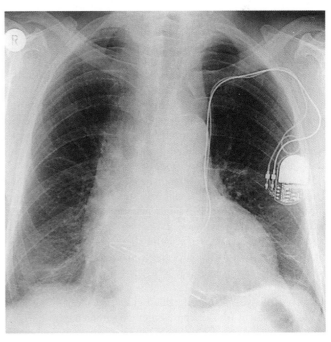

Fig. 12.1.14 Chest radiograph of a 56-year-old man with bicuspid aortic valve, aortic regurgitation, and coarctation. A left superior vena cava draining via the coronary sinus to the right atrium is marked by the path taken by the transvenous pacing leads, inserted for complete heart block.

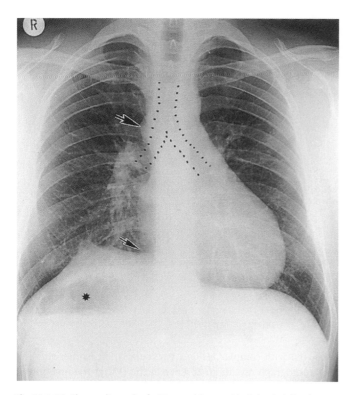

Fig. 12.1.15 Chest radiograph of a 50-year-old man with abdominal situs inversus (*) and laevocardia. Left atrial isomerism is inferred from the symmetrical long bronchi (bilateral morphological left lungs). The inferior vena cava is absent at the level of the diaphragm (small arrow), and the azygos vein receiving inferior caval venous blood is prominent (large arrow).

either directly or via a common vein into a systemic vein. The anomalous veins may follow (1) a supracardiac course draining to the SVC, azygos, or brachiocephalic veins; (2) a cardiac course, draining to the right atrium directly or to the coronary sinus directly or via a persistent left SVC connection; or (3) an infradiaphragmatic course, draining to the portal vein or IVC.

Since the pulmonary venous confluence is a left atrial structure, total anomalous venous drainage is obligatory in right isomerism: there are bilateral right atriums and no left atrium for the pulmonary veins to drain to. The presence of pulmonary venous obstruction is the most important predictor of a poor outcome. Associated anomalies include an obligatory right-to-left shunt, nearly always at atrial level.

The condition presents in infancy, hence 98% of patients reaching the adolescent or adult clinic will have survived corrective surgery in early life. Unless there is residual pulmonary hypertension most such adults should be asymptomatic, having a normal cardiovascular examination and an excellent prognosis. Patients who are still growing may develop obstruction of the redirected pulmonary venous pathway and present with dyspnoea, signs of pulmonary oedema, evidence of pulmonary venous congestion on the chest radiograph, and an obstructive echo Doppler flow signal at the site of the stenosis.

The rare patient who reaches adulthood unoperated is likely to have survived because of a large ASD and unobstructed pulmonary venous drainage. They will be cyanosed, have developed pulmonary vascular disease, and be at risk of atrial tachyarrhythmias and right heart failure. The chest radiograph has the appearance of a large ASD with a small aortic knuckle, cardiomegaly, and a dilated

main pulmonary artery. In addition, the anomalous veins may cause an abnormal vascular shadow.

Partial anomalous pulmonary venous drainage

There is anomalous drainage of some of the pulmonary veins to the right atrium. In 90% of cases the anomalous pulmonary venous connection is between the right upper or middle pulmonary vein to the SVC or right atrium, usually in association with an ASD, 10 to 15% of all ASDs and nearly all SVC-type sinus venosus ASDs being associated with partial anomalous pulmonary venous connection.

Partial anomalous pulmonary venous drainage may present in adult life with signs of a left-to-right shunt at atrial level; the pathophysiological consequences are the same as for an ASD with an equivalent shunt.

The chest radiograph may reveal the abnormally draining pulmonary vein. Transthoracic echocardiography may be indicative of a shunt at atrial level, but in adults it may not be possible to image the pulmonary veins and a transoesophageal approach is likely to be necessary. The identification of all the pulmonary veins is crucial in assessing the suitability of a secundum ASD for transcatheter device closure, this technique being contraindicated in the presence of anomalous pulmonary veins (see 'Atrial septal defects', above).

The indications for surgical repair are the same as those for repair of an ASD. In the most common variant of right pulmonary venous connection to the SVC in association with a sinus venosus defect, the patch closing the ASD is placed to direct the anomalous vein into the left atrium.

Scimitar syndrome

Partial anomalous pulmonary venous drainage also occurs as part of the rare familial 'scimitar syndrome' (OMIM 106700) in which part or all of the right pulmonary venous drainage is to the IVC below the diaphragm. The affected lung lobes are usually hypoplastic (Fig. 12.1.16) and are supplied with arterial blood from the descending aorta. Recurrent infection and bronchiectasis may develop in the hypoplastic lobes or lung. MRI demonstrates the abnormal arterial supply and venous drainage of the affected lung segment, and may obviate the need for diagnostic cardiac catheterization. Surgical repair may be complicated by difficulty in maintaining perfusion to the affected lung, and lobectomy may be required. In view of this it should be remembered that patients presenting with scimitar syndrome for the first time in adult life have a good unoperated prognosis, similar to that of a small ASD.

Transposition complexes

The nomenclature of the transposition complexes may cause confusion. There are two types:

- Complete transposition of the great arteries (TGA)—this condition is described as concordant atrioventricular connection and discordant ventriculo-arterial connection (Fig. 12.1.15), previously known as D-TGA (Fig 12.1.17). Without intervention it is not compatible with life, since once the arterial duct and foramen ovale have closed, there is complete separation of the systemic and pulmonary circulations such that deoxygenated blood from the systemic veins recirculates to the aorta, and oxygenated blood from the pulmonary veins recirculates to the pulmonary artery.

- Congenitally corrected transposition of the great arteries (cTGA)—this condition is described as discordant atrioventricular and ventriculo-arterial connections. (Fig. 12.1.18),

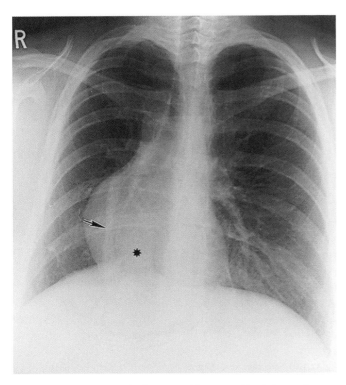

Fig. 12.1.16 Chest radiograph of a 25-year-old woman with scimitar syndrome. The heart is shifted into the right hemithorax because the right lung is small. The 'scimitar' shadow (arrow) is produced by the anomalous descending venous channel which drains into the dilated inferior vena cava (*).

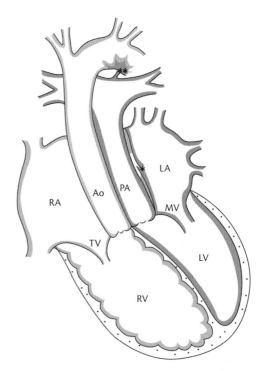

Fig. 12.1.17 Schematic representation of complete transposition of the great arteries (discordant ventriculo-arterial connections). The pulmonary and systemic circulations are completely separate once the arterial duct and foramen ovale close. Without intervention, the condition is not compatible with life. Ao, aorta; LA, left atrium; LV, left ventricle; MV, mitral valve; PA, pulmonary artery; RA right atrium; RV right ventricle; TV, tricuspid valve; **patent arterial duct; *patent foramen ovale.

previously known as L-TGA. cTGA is congenitally physiologically 'corrected': deoxygenated systemic venous blood reaches the pulmonary artery, albeit via the morphological left ventricle; oxygenated pulmonary venous blood reaches the aorta, but via the morphological right ventricle.

Complete transposition of the great arteries (discordant atrioventricular connection, concordant ventriculo-arterial connection)

TGA accounts for about 5% of congenital cardiac malformations and is four times more common in males than females. Associated anomalies such as VSD and pulmonary stenosis occur in approximately one-third of patients. As described above, unoperated survival after closure of the foramen ovale and arterial duct have closed is dependent upon the presence of other associated lesions, such as a VSD, which allow mixing of the two circulations. Without intervention, 30% die within the first week and only 10% survive their first year.

If the atrial and ventricular septums are intact, immediate neonatal management requires a prostaglandin infusion to maintain patency of the arterial duct until a balloon atrial septostomy is performed. Post septostomy, the neonate remains cyanosed, but there is usually adequate mixing to allow it to thrive until definitive surgery. There are survivors of four operative approaches in adult clinics: interatrial repair (Mustard or Senning), arterial switch, Rastelli and 'palliative' Mustard/Sennning or arterial switch operations. The indications and outcomes of each are described below.

Interatrial repair: Mustard or Senning operations

This approach was first described in 1957 and can be used for those with TGA or TGA with VSD. Interatrial repair involves excision of the atrial septum and placement of a saddle-shaped patch ('baffle') to direct pulmonary venous blood into the right atrium and right ventricle and thence to the aorta (Fig. 12.1.19). Systemic venous blood is directed into the left atrium, left ventricle, and pulmonary artery. The right ventricle and tricuspid valve therefore support the systemic circulation. The Senning operation uses the patient's own atrial septum to create the baffle, whereas the Mustard operation uses nonautologous material. The Mustard/Senning operations have been superseded by the arterial switch operation, apart from some uncommon situations in cTGA in which a Senning operation is part of a more complex procedure. However, there are still significant numbers of adult survivors of the interatrial repair.

Clinical signs and complications after interatrial repair

The systemic right ventricle causes a parasternal heave. The aortic component of the second heart sound may be palpable and loud, and the second sound single, due to the anterior-lying aorta. The presence of cyanosis suggests a baffle leak allowing right-to-left shunting between the systemic and pulmonary venous atriums. Systemic venous pathway obstruction may be associated with elevation of the jugular venous pressure and hepatomegaly.

Complications after interatrial repair include:

◆ Progressive bradycardias and sinus node disease, due to damage to the sinus node during repair.

◆ Atrial flutter and interatrial re-entry tachycardias, due to extensive atrial surgical scarring—these are often poorly tolerated, are associated with sudden death, and should be treated with urgent

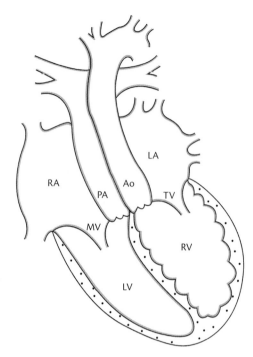

Fig. 12.1.18 Schematic representation of congenitally corrected transposition of the great arteries (discordant atrioventricular and ventriculo-arterial connections). The circulation is congenitally physiologically 'corrected' in that systemic venous blood reaches the pulmonary artery (via the left ventricle) and pulmonary venous blood reaches the aorta (via the right ventricle). Ao, aorta; LA, left atrium; LV, left ventricle; MV, mitral valve; PA, pulmonary artery; RA, right atrium; RV, right ventricle; TV, tricuspid valve.

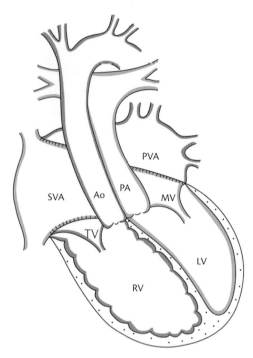

Fig. 12.1.19 Schematic representation of intra-atrial repair for complete transposition of the great arteries (Senning or Mustard operation). Ao, aorta; LV, left ventricle; MV, mitral valve; PA, pulmonary artery; PVA, pulmonary venous atrium; RV, right ventricle; SVA, systemic venous atrium; TV, tricuspid valve.

DC cardioversion rather than antiarrhythmic drugs, since the latter can precipitate cardiovascular collapse if there is underlying impaired ventricular function. After an episode of flutter, ablation should be performed.

◆ Systemic venous pathway obstruction, which usually only causes symptoms if both the IVC and SVC pathways are narrowed—if only one pathway is narrowed, the systemic venous blood flows along the azygos vein and drains to the heart via the unobstructed pathway; obstruction can usually be relieved by balloon dilation or stenting.

◆ Pulmonary venous pathway obstruction such that flow into the atrium and systemic ventricle is obstructed—the patient will be breathless, but clinical signs are few; it is demonstrated by echocardiography or MRI; surgical repair is usually necessary; transcatheter intervention is usually unsatisfactory.

◆ Baffle leak—holes along the baffle suture lines allow shunting which may be left-to-right, or right-to-left, causing cyanosis; an percutaneous approach sometimes allows successful closure of these interatrial communications.

◆ Systemic atrioventricular valve regurgitation—the tricuspid valve is poorly evolved to support systemic pressures and commonly becomes regurgitant; if right ventricular function is adequate, valve replacement should be performed because valve repair is rarely successful.

◆ Systemic ventricular failure—the right ventricle may fail because it is inherently unsuitable to support the systemic circulation in the long term, because of long-standing tricuspid regurgitation, and because of poor ventricular filling from the surgically constructed atrial pathways.

There has been much interest in whether placement of a pulmonary artery band to 'retrain' the left ventricle to enable it to support the systemic circulation will allow takedown of the Mustard operation and performance of an arterial switch operation. This approach only appears to be possible in young children, or in older patients with a degree of left ventricular outflow tract obstruction in whom the left ventricle has always retained near-systemic pressures.

Arterial switch operation

As a result of the late complications of interatrial repair, a different surgical approach was developed that restored the left ventricle to the systemic circulation and avoided extensive atrial surgery: the arterial switch.

Since the 1980s anatomical correction by the arterial switch operation has superseded interatrial repair as the operation of choice for most patients with TGA. Blood is redirected at arterial level by switching the aorta and pulmonary arteries so that the left ventricle becomes the subaortic ventricle supporting the systemic circulation. The coronary arteries are reimplanted into the neo-aortic root.

Late follow-up appears good for these patients, but vigilance is required to detect late problems including neo-aortic or pulmonary valve regurgitation, neo-aortic root dilation, and pulmonary arterial stenosis. Late myocardial ischaemia due to coronary anastomotic stenoses is a theoretical complication, but has not yet become apparent as a major problem.

Rastelli operation

This operation is performed for patients with TGA, VSD, and pulmonary stenosis (Fig. 12.1.20). The VSD is closed so that the left ventricle carrying oxygenated blood empties into the aorta. The stenotic pulmonary artery is ligated and a conduit is placed between the right ventricle and pulmonary artery. The main advantage of this operation is that the left ventricle supports the systemic

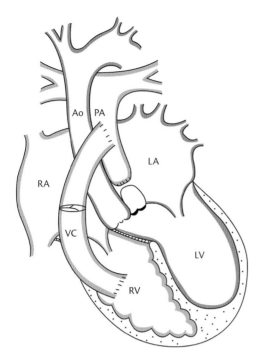

Fig. 12.1.20 Schematic representation of Rastelli operation for transposition of the great arteries with ventricular septal defect and pulmonary stenosis. Ao, aorta; LA, left atrium; LV, left ventricle; PA; pulmonary artery; RA, right atrium, RV, right ventricle, VC, valved conduit.

circulation, but it commits the patient to several further conduit replacements—some of which may now be carried out percutaneously rather than surgically.

'Palliative' Mustard/Senning or arterial switch operations

These procedures are performed for patients with TGA, VSD, and pulmonary vascular disease to improve mixing of blood and oxygenation. The VSD is left open. These patients should be treated in the same way as other patients with Eisenmenger syndrome.

Congenitally corrected transposition of the great arteries (discordant atrioventricular and ventriculo-arterial connections)

cTGA is a rare condition, accounting for less than 1% of all congenital heart disease. Both atrial and arterial connections to the ventricles are discordant, so pulmonary venous blood passes through the left atrium, through the right ventricle, and into an anteriorly lying aorta (Fig. 12.1.18). Similarly, systemic venous blood reaches the pulmonary trunk via the left ventricle. The circulation is therefore physiologically 'corrected', but the morphological right ventricle and tricuspid valve support the systemic circulation.

More than 95% of cases have associated anomalies, most commonly VSD and pulmonary stenosis, but also Ebstein anomaly of the systemic (tricuspid) atrioventricular valve, aortic stenosis, AVSD, abnormalities of situs, and coarctation. Congenital complete heart block occurs in around 5% of patients and may develop at any stage of life, particularly following surgery to the atrioventricular valve.

Presentation depends on associated lesions. Patients with isolated cTGA may remain asymptomatic and undiagnosed into old age, but failure of the systemic ventricle, systemic atrioventricular valve regurgitation, or the onset of complete heart block and atrial

arrhythmias usually results in presentation with symptoms from the fourth decade onwards. Those with VSD and pulmonary stenosis may be cyanosed, and those with VSD alone may present with pulmonary hypertension.

A parasternal heave is usually palpable from the pressure-loaded anteriorly lying systemic right ventricle; this may be especially prominent if it is also volume-loaded by systemic (tricuspid) atrioventricular valve regurgitation. There may be a prominent aortic pulsation in the suprasternal notch and the aortic component of the second heart sound may be palpable and loud. The pulmonary component is soft or inaudible due to the posterior position of the pulmonary artery.

The ECG may show varying degrees of atrioventricular block or evidence of pre-excitation due to accessory pathways (associated with Ebstein-like anomalies of the systemic atrioventricular valve). There may be left axis deviation. The right and left bundles are inverted, so the initial septal activation is right-to-left, resulting in Q waves in V1–2 and an absent Q in V5–6; this pattern may be wrongly interpreted as a previous anterior myocardial infarction. The chest radiograph has a typical appearance (Fig. 12.1.21). Echocardiography confirms the discordant relations and assesses ventricular and systemic (tricuspid) atrioventricular valve function as well as other associated lesions. Ebstein anomaly may be diagnosed if the tricuspid valve is apically displaced by more than 8 mm/m^2. Cardiac catheterization is indicated to assess the haemodynamic importance of associated lesions.

Angiotensin converting enzyme (ACE) inhibitors may be useful when there is systemic ventricular dysfunction or atrioventricular valve regurgitation, but there are no trial data to support their use.

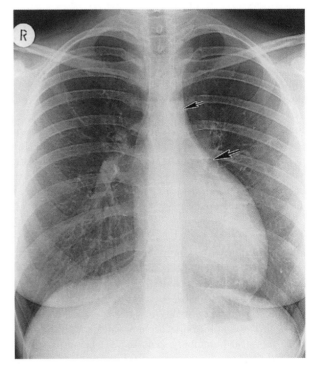

Fig. 12.1.21 Chest radiograph of a 23-year-old woman with congenitally corrected transposition of the great vessels. There is a narrow pedicle due to the abnormally related great arteries (small arrow) and the left heart border is straight (large arrow) due to the abnormal position of the left-lying anterior ascending aorta.

Transvenous atrioventricular sequential pacing is indicated for complete heart block; active fixation ventricular leads are required because of the absence of coarse apical trabeculations in the morphologically left subpulmonary ventricle. If there are associated intracardiac shunts, patients should be formally anticoagulated to reduce the risk of paradoxical embolism, or epicardial pacing should be considered.

The conventional surgical approach to systemic atrioventricular valve regurgitation is tricuspid valve replacement (repair is rarely successful), but if systemic ventricular function is poor (ejection fraction <40%) transplantation may be the only option. Replacement of the tricuspid valve before the systemic right ventricle fails improves prognosis. Where there is coexistent VSD and pulmonary stenosis, classical repair involved closure of the VSD and insertion of a valved conduit between the left ventricle and pulmonary artery, with the right ventricle continuing to support the systemic circulation.

Anatomical repair, so that the morphological left ventricle supports the systemic ventricle, has had success in children with systemic atrioventricular valve regurgitation and systemic ventricular dysfunction. For patients with an associated nonrestrictive VSD the left ventricle is at systemic pressure and therefore 'pretrained' to support the systemic circulation. If there is no pulmonary stenosis, a 'double switch' may be performed, combining an Senning operation with an arterial switch operation. If there is also pulmonary stenosis, the Senning operation is combined with a Rastelli-type repair. The regurgitant tricuspid valve and right ventricle are therefore placed in the pulmonary circulation. For children with corrected transposition whose left ventricle is at low pressure, a period of left ventricular 'training' is required before a double switch operation can be performed, which is achieved by placing a pulmonary artery band to increase left ventricular pressure and induce hypertrophy. Pulmonary artery banding *per se* may improve symptoms, since the increased left ventricular pressure causes the interventricular septum to move towards the systemic ventricle, reducing systemic atrioventricular regurgitation.

The long-term outcome of these anatomical approaches to corrected transposition is not yet known; complications relating to the dysfunction of the retrained left ventricular, conduit replacement, neo-aortic valve regurgitation, and arrhythmia may become significant. There are reports of adults with VSD and pulmonary stenosis having successfully undergone Senning–Rastelli repair, but it is probably not possible to adequately 'train' an adult left ventricle that has been at low pressure for many years.

Tetralogy of Fallot

Tetralogy of Fallot is the commonest cyanotic defect, occurring in 1 in 3600 live births; it affects males and females equally. Most patients reaching the adult clinics have undergone radical repair, but some natural and palliated survivors may present.

The fundamental abnormality in tetralogy of Fallot is anterocephalad deviation of the outlet septum which creates the four key features: subvalvar pulmonary stenosis, VSD, an aortic valve that overrides the VSD, and right ventricular hypertrophy (Fig. 12.1.22). There is great anatomical variation, ranging from minimal aortic override to double-outlet right ventricle (DORV), and from minimal pulmonary stenosis to pulmonary atresia. The VSD is perimembranous and there is usually additional pulmonary valvar stenosis.

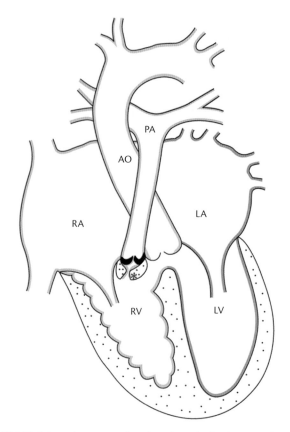

Fig. 12.1.22 Schematic representation of tetralogy of Fallot. *Anterocephalad deviation of outlet septum creates ventricular septal defect, subpulmonary stenosis, aorta overriding crest of interventricular septum, and secondary right ventricular hypertrophy. Ao, aorta, LA, left atrium, LV, left ventricle, PA, pulmonary artery, RA, right atrium, RV, right ventricle.

Associations

Microdeletions of chromosome 22q11 may occur in association with tetralogy of Fallot, especially in its most severe form with pulmonary atresia. 22q11 deletions are associated with a broad spectrum of phenotypic abnormalities that form the velocardiofacial syndrome (which includes DiGeorge syndrome; OMIM 601362): (1) other cardiac defects—Fallot with right aortic arch, truncus arteriosus, pulmonary atresia with VSD, interrupted aortic arch; (2) facial abnormalities—cleft palate, hare lip, hypertelorism, narrow eye fissures, puffy eyelids, a small mouth, deformed earlobes; (3) psychiatric disorders and learning difficulties; and (4) neonatal immune deficiency (thymic hypoplasia) and hypocalcaemia (parathyroid hypoplasia).

Cardiac defects associated with tetralogy of Fallot include a right-sided aortic arch in 16%, a left SVC in around 15%, additional VSDs in 5%, and a secundum ASD ('pentalogy' of Fallot) in 8%. The most important associated coronary anomaly is the crossing of the right ventricular outflow tract by a left anterior descending coronary artery arising anomalously from the right coronary sinus: this is vulnerable to damage during surgical repair.

Unoperated clinical course and management

Without surgical intervention, only 2% of patients survive to their fortieth year. Those that do survive may be a selected group in whom subpulmonary stenosis was not severe in early life, but progressed with advancing age. Unoperated patients are at risk of the complications of cyanosis, endocarditis, atrial and ventricular arrhythmias, progressive ascending aortic dilatation (without the high risk of dissection found in Marfan's syndrome), aortic regurgitation—causing volume overload of both ventricles and subsequent biventricular failure, and systemic hypertension—adding additional pressure overload to the work of both ventricles and further contributing to the onset of biventricular failure.

There is cyanosis and clubbing, a right ventricular heave, and sometimes a thrill over the right ventricular outflow tract. A right-sided aorta may be palpable to the right of the sternum. The second heart sound is usually single, and there is a loud pulmonary ejection murmur. There may be aortic regurgitation.

The ECG shows right axis deviation and right ventricular hypertrophy, and the QRS duration may be prolonged in older patients. The classical cardiac silhouette is a 'coeur en sabot', i.e. a clog-shaped heart, but this is more likely to be seen in tetralogy with pulmonary atresia (see 'Pulmonary atresia with VSD'). The heart size is usually normal and pulmonary vascularity reduced. There may be a right-sided aortic arch indenting the right of the trachea, and there may be a prominent dilated ascending aorta.

Two-dimensional echocardiography reveals infundibular stenosis with or without pulmonary valve stenosis, right ventricular hypertrophy, the typical VSD, and varying degrees of aortic override. There may be evidence of left ventricular volume overload, aortic root dilatation, and aortic regurgitation.

Cardiac catheterization should be performed prior to surgical repair in adults. The anatomy of the right ventricular outflow tract obstruction and pulmonary arteries is defined, and pulmonary vascular resistance assessed. Selective coronary angiography demonstrates any anomalous origin and course as well as acquired coronary disease. Aortography shows aortic root dilatation and any aortopulmonary collaterals. MRI may be performed instead of conventional cardiac catheterization, except that it does not provide pulmonary vascular resistance data.

Palliated history

Helen Taussig first suggested palliative surgery in 1943, and the first Blalock–Taussig shunt was performed in 1945 (Fig. 12.1.23 and Table 12.1.7). Nowadays, palliative shunts are usually performed as a staging procedure in small infants; however, occasional patients reach the adult clinic having had palliation without subsequent radical repair. They are cyanosed and clubbed and have a continuous murmur under the clavicle and over the scapula on the side of the shunt. In a classical Blalock–Taussig shunt the ipsilateral radial pulse is diminished or absent and the hand often small. Late complications of systemic to pulmonary artery shunts include infective endarteritis, acquired pulmonary atresia, aortic regurgitation, and biventricular failure, with increasing cyanosis and bronchopulmonary collateral development if the shunt blocks or is outgrown, and pulmonary vascular disease if the shunt is too big.

Radical repair, late follow-up, and reoperation

Radical repair involves patch closure of the VSD with infundibular resection with or without pulmonary valvotomy or replacement: 86% of patients who underwent such surgery in the 1980s survive to 32 years of age, and survival for those operated in the current era is further improved. However, patients remain at risk of late complications including pulmonary regurgitation and stenosis, aortic regurgitation, ventricular dysfunction, endocarditis,

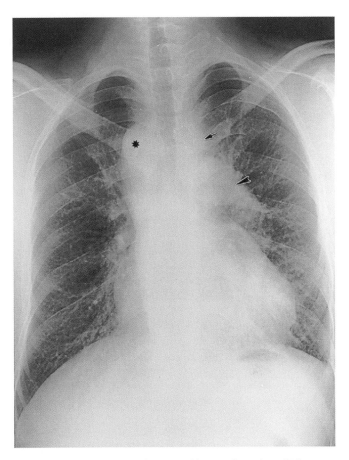

Fig. 12.1.23 Chest radiograph of a 36-year-old man with tetralogy of Fallot palliated by a classic left Blalock–Taussig shunt (small arrow). There is secondary dilatation of the left pulmonary artery (large arrow) and a right aortic arch (*).

arrhythmia, and sudden death. Those repaired in early childhood and by a transannular approach have a better long-term prognosis than those repaired later or by a transventricular approach.

In many patients repair involves placing a patch across the annulus of the pulmonary valve in order to create an unobstructed right ventricular outflow. As a result, the pulmonary valve is incompetent from the time of repair. The pulmonary regurgitant volume is relatively small early after repair, since the stiff hypertrophied right

Table 12.1.7 Systemic to pulmonary arterial shunts

Classical Blalock–Taussig shunt	Subclavian artery divided distally. Proximal subclavian artery anastomosed end-to-side to pulmonary artery
Modified Blalock–Taussig shunt	Prosthetic graft between subclavian and pulmonary arteries
Central shunts:	
Waterston shunt[a]	Side-to-side anastomosis between ascending aorta and (right) pulmonary artery
Potts shunt[a]	Side-to-side anastomosis between descending aorta and (left) pulmonary artery
Other	Prosthetic graft between aorta and pulmonary artery

[a] Now obsolete because not possible to adequately control the size of the shunt.

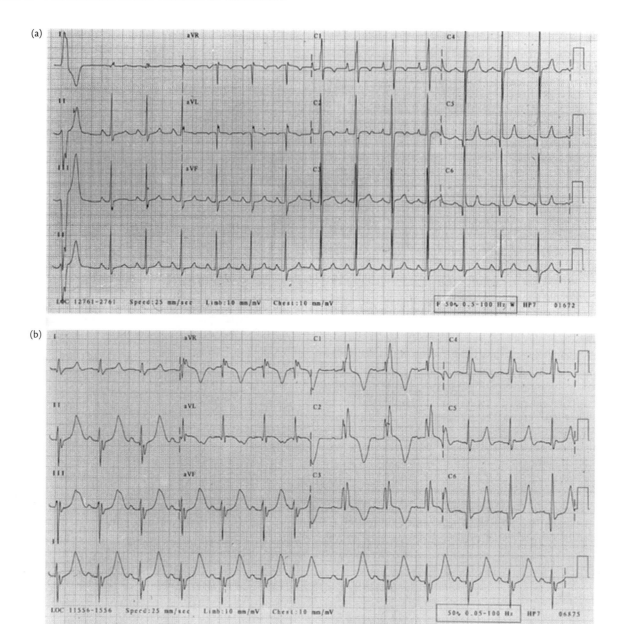

Fig. 12.1.24 Electrocardiograms of a 35-year-old woman who underwent radical repair of tetralogy of Fallot. Preoperatively (a) there is right ventricular hypertrophy; postoperatively (b) there is right bundle branch block, due to damage to the right bundle as it runs in the floor of the ventricular septal defect.

ventricle cannot accommodate the regurgitant blood, the fast heart rate of the small child reduces the time in which regurgitation can occur, and the capacitance of the child's pulmonary vasculature is low. However, the right ventricle remodels and by the time young adulthood is reached, pulmonary regurgitation is often severe and the right ventricle dilates. Although pulmonary regurgitation is well tolerated for many years, it results in progressive right ventricular dilation and dysfunction, impaired exercise tolerance, and increased risk of atrial and ventricular arrhythmias. A widening of the QRS complex beyond 180 ms may be a marker for right ventricular dilation and dysfunction, these being risk factors for developing worsening functional class, sustained ventricular tachycardia, and sudden death. Pulmonary valve replacement is indicated if there is impaired exercise tolerance, sustained arrhythmia, progressive right ventricular dilation, or any evidence of right ventricular dysfunction. Replacing the pulmonary valve before irreversible

right ventricular dysfunction occurs is likely to improve long-term outcome. MRI is a valuable tool for assessing right ventricular size and function, and any deterioration. The timing of redo surgery for pulmonary regurgitation remains controversial, although some centres consider that pulmonary valve replacement should be performed before the indexed right ventricular end diastolic volume reaches 150 ml/m^2.

Pulmonary regurgitation is worsened in the presence of pulmonary arterial stenosis that may occur at the site of a previous shunt. Right ventricular outflow tract obstruction may recur, especially if a valved right ventricular to pulmonary artery conduit was placed, this being due to excessive formation of neointima (peel) in the conduit or to calcification of the valve.

Most patients have right bundle branch block after repair (Fig. 12.1.24) due to surgical damage to the right bundle as it runs in the floor of the VSD. Bifasicular block and transient postoperative complete heart block carry a risk of developing late complete heart block. Atrial arrhythmias occur in 30% of long-term survivors and are a major cause of morbidity. Those with left-sided volume overload and left atrial dilatation secondary to residual VSD or previous shunts are at particular risk of atrial flutter and fibrillation. Rapidly conducted atrial flutter is particularly poorly tolerated and is likely to be responsible for a proportion of sudden deaths, as are the ventricular arrhythmias that occur in up to 45% of patients. Sustained monomorphic ventricular tachycardia is likely to be a significant risk factor for sudden death, as are atrial arrhythmias and heart block.

Adverse right ventricular risk factors include dilatation and dysfunction, outflow tract obstruction, hypertrophy, aneurysm, impaired myocardial blood flow, and pulmonary regurgitation. Surgical risk factors for late sudden death include transventricular versus transatrial repair, large ventriculotomy scar, residual VSD, previous complex or multiple operations, impaired left ventricular function, older age at operation, and length of follow-up.

Tetralogy of Fallot with absent pulmonary valve syndrome

This variation accounts for approximately 3% of cases of tetralogy of Fallot. There is a ring-like, usually stenotic malformation, with failure of development of the pulmonary valve cusps. The central pulmonary arteries are usually hugely dilated or aneurysmal.

Double-outlet right ventricle

In DORV more than one-half of the circumference of both great vessels arises from the morphological right ventricle. A complete or partial muscular infundibulum usually lies beneath each arterial valve. The anatomy and physiology are enormously varied, as are the surgical approaches to repair. The degree of pulmonary stenosis and the relation of the VSD to the great vessels determine the haemodynamics.

Most (80%) subaortic defects have pulmonary stenosis and Fallot-like physiology. The Taussig–Bing anomaly accounts for less than 10% of DORV and describes a subpulmonary defect without pulmonary stenosis. There is transposition-like physiology with cyanosis and high pulmonary blood flow. As the pulmonary vascular resistance rises, pulmonary blood flow falls and cyanosis increases. Unoperated survival to adulthood is uncommon, but occurs occasionally if the pulmonary vascular resistance establishes adequate but not excessive pulmonary blood flow. If such a survivor also has a patent arterial duct, there will be reversed differential cyanosis. Deoxygenated blood selectively enters the aorta to supply the arch vessels, whereas oxygenated blood enters the pulmonary artery and supplies the descending aorta via the duct; thus the fingers are more cyanosed and clubbed than the toes.

If the VSD is remote from the great vessels, a biventricular repair may not be possible and a single-ventricle repair (Fontan) may be necessary.

Pulmonary atresia with ventricular septal defect

This is a complex and heterogeneous cyanotic condition. The intracardiac anatomy is the same as tetralogy of Fallot, but the right ventricular outflow tract is blind-ended (atretic). The pulmonary blood supply is derived entirely from three different types of systemic vessels: (1) a large muscular duct that resembles a collateral; (2) a diffuse plexus of small 'bronchial' arteries arising from mediastinal and intercostal arteries; and (3) large tortuous systemic arterial

collaterals known as MAPCAs (major aortopulmonary collateral arteries), which arise directly from the descending aorta, from its major branches (usually the subclavian artery), or from bronchial arteries, and may connect with central pulmonary arteries or supply whole segments or lobes of lung independently.

Prognosis and management depends largely on the pulmonary vasculature, in which there is considerable anatomical variation. Confluent pulmonary arteries with pulmonary vessels having a near normal arborization pattern to all segments of the lungs are associated with the best prognosis. Here radical repair, with recruitment of MAPCAs to the native pulmonary arteries, a conduit from right ventricle to pulmonary artery, and closure of the VSD is likely to be possible, and the pulmonary vascular resistance is likely to be low. The 20-year survival after radical repair is about 75%. The outlook is worse if there are no native pulmonary arteries and multiple tortuous MAPCAs with poor arborization. Radical repair may be extremely challenging or impossible, and pulmonary vascular resistance likely to be high. Such patients may be suitable for no or only palliative surgery and will remain cyanosed. Following surgical palliation, 20-year survival is around 60%; unoperated survival is very poor, only about 8% reaching 10 years of age, and those that do reach adulthood have a mean age of death of 33 years.

Clinical findings

Examination findings in the unoperated or palliated patient are similar to those of the unoperated Fallot without pulmonary atresia, except that there are continuous collateral murmurs and often a collapsing pulse.

The chest radiograph shows a right aortic arch in 25% of cases and has a typical appearance (Fig. 12.1.25). The pulmonary collateral vessels may follow a bizarre pattern. Colour-flow Doppler may identify collateral vessels, but conventional angiography is required to precisely delineate their origin, degree of ostial stenosis, and intrapulmonary course. High-resolution CT and MRI are useful tools in imaging complex pulmonary vasculature.

Outcome

Late complications in unoperated or palliated survivors include increasing cyanosis due either to the development of pulmonary vascular disease in lung segments perfused at systemic pressure through nonstenosed collaterals, or to the progressive stenosis of collateral vessels. In the latter, good symptomatic relief may be obtained from stenting. The aortic root may become markedly dilated and aortic regurgitation may develop, resulting in biventricular volume overload and failure. Aortic valve endocarditis is a particular risk.

Late complications after radical repair include those that follow repair of tetralogy of Fallot. In addition, patients face inevitable repeated conduit replacements, and right ventricular failure secondary to high pulmonary vascular resistance.

Hearts with univentricular atrioventricular connection

Also known as univentricular or single-ventricle hearts, these hearts are defined by the connection of both atriums to one ventricle, or by the absence of one of the atrioventricular connections. There is only one functional ventricle, although there is nearly always a second rudimentary and incomplete ventricle. When the rudimentary ventricle is of right morphology, it nearly always lies

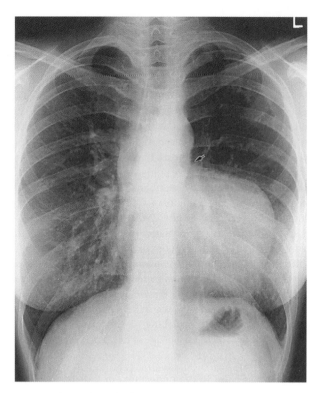

Fig. 12.1.25 Chest radiograph of a 21-year-old woman with tetralogy of Fallot and pulmonary atresia, no central pulmonary arteries, and multiple aortopulmonary collaterals which create an abnormal pulmonary vascular pattern. The typical 'coeur en sabot' silhouette is due to right ventricular hypertrophy and the pulmonary bay where the pulmonary artery should be (arrow).

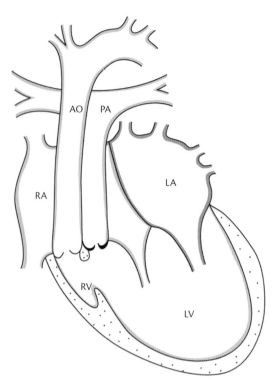

Fig. 12.1.26 Schematic representation of double-inlet left ventricle with discordant ventriculo-arterial connections. Both atriums connect to the left ventricle via the tricuspid and mitral valves, so that systemic and pulmonary venous blood mix in the left ventricle and the patient is cyanosed. The left ventricle supports both the systemic and pulmonary circulations. The aorta arises from the rudimentary right ventricle via the ventricular septal defect (VSD). If the VSD is restrictive, it creates obstruction to systemic blood flow. Ao, aorta; LA, left atrium; LV, left ventricle; PA, pulmonary artery; RA, right atrium; RV, right ventricle; VA, ventriculo-arterial; VSD, ventricular septal defect.

anteriorly. Less commonly, there is a posteriorly lying morphologically left rudimentary ventricle, and rarely, there is solitary ventricle of indeterminate morphology.

The two most common variants are double-inlet left ventricle (DILV) and tricuspid atresia (Figs. 12.1.26 and 12.1.27) which together account for around 4 to 5% of congenital heart disease. This section considers these two conditions, a discussion of more complex variants being beyond the scope of this text.

Clinical course: unoperated

Presentation depends largely on pulmonary blood flow, which in turn is dependent on the degree of pulmonary stenosis. Those with severe obstruction to pulmonary blood flow present as neonates with severe cyanosis. Neonates without pulmonary stenosis have excessively high pulmonary blood flow and present in congestive cardiac failure with breathlessness and only mild cyanosis. The presence of subaortic stenosis or other obstruction to systemic blood flow such as coarctation exacerbates heart failure and results in early decompensation.

The outcome is most favourable for patients with left ventricular morphology, moderate pulmonary stenosis, and no subaortic stenosis, and for those with 'balanced' pulmonary and systemic blood flow, i.e. moderately severe pulmonary stenosis and no obstruction to systemic blood flow. Unoperated survival into adulthood is uncommon: 50% of patients with DILV die before 14 years, 50% with DORV die by 4 years of age. Nonetheless, rare patients with balanced circulation reach their sixth decade without surgical intervention.

In the unoperated patient, there is cyanosis and clubbing. A giant 'a' wave may be present in the jugular venous pulse in tricuspid atresia. An absent right ventricular impulse and prominent left ventricular impulse are characteristic of DILV and tricuspid atresia. There may be a precordial thrill from pulmonary stenosis, particularly if the pulmonary artery lies anteriorly. If there are discordant ventriculo-arterial connections, the aortic pulsation of the anteriorly lying aorta may be prominent in the suprasternal notch. The second heart sound is usually single.

If pulmonary vascular disease has developed there will be additional signs of pulmonary hypertension. Signs of congestive heart failure may be present in the ageing patient, particularly with the onset of atrial arrhythmia, such that the venous pressure is raised, with hepatomegaly and peripheral oedema.

The chest radiograph shows cardiomegaly due to chronic ventricular volume overload. If ventriculo-arterial connections are discordant, there is a narrow pedicle and the ascending aorta forms a straight edge along the left heart border. Pulmonary vascularity reflects the pulmonary blood flow, the main pulmonary arteries being small where there is significant pulmonary stenosis, with large main pulmonary arteries indicating high pulmonary blood flow, either past or present.

In tricuspid atresia the ECG usually shows right atrial hypertrophy, normal PR interval, small or absent right ventricular forces, and left axis deviation. There are left axis deviation and large left

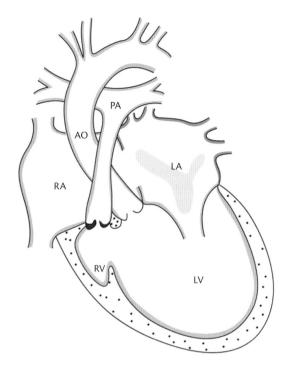

Fig. 12.1.27 Schematic representation of tricuspid atresia. Systemic venous blood leaves the right atrium via an atrial septal defect and mixes with pulmonary venous blood in the left atrium. The left ventricle thus supports both the systemic and pulmonary circulations and the patient is cyanosed. The rudimentary right ventricle does not play a functional role. Ao, aorta; LA, left atrium; LV, left ventricle; PA, pulmonary artery; RA, right atrium; RV, right ventricle.

ventricular forces in DILV. If the rudimentary chamber lies to the right the PR interval is usually normal, but if it lies to the left the PR interval may be prolonged or there may be complete heart block.

Two-dimensional echocardiography and colour-flow Doppler allow detailed assessment of the anatomy and physiology, including ventricular morphology and pulmonary and subaortic stenosis. Cardiac catheterization is required to assess pulmonary artery anatomy and resistance.

Surgical management of univentricular hearts: the Fontan operation

Management requires a staged approach, the ultimate aim of which is to achieve a pink patient in whom the functionally single ventricle supports only the systemic circulation: the Fontan operation.

The first stage, in early life, is to obtain control of pulmonary blood flow. In those with excessive flow a pulmonary artery band is placed to create supravalvar pulmonary artery stenosis and limit pulmonary flow. In neonates with severe pulmonary stenosis a systemic artery to pulmonary artery shunt is placed to augment pulmonary blood flow.

As the child 'grows out of the shunt' they become more cyanosed: the central shunt is replaced with a superior vena cava to pulmonary artery anastomosis (Glenn, or cavopulmonary anastomosis), as illustrated in Fig. 12.1.28. This reduces cyanosis, perfuses the pulmonary arteries at low pressure, and reduces the volume load on the single ventricle. However, as the child grows, the relative contribution of the SVC to the circulation diminishes, again resulting in progressive cyanosis.

The Fontan operation is usually completed by age 4 to 6 years. The principle of this approach is to separate the systemic and pulmonary circulations and abolish cyanosis. This is achieved by using the single functional ventricle to support the systemic circulation and leaving the pulmonary circulation without a ventricle, i.e. with phasic rather than pulsatile flow. Since its first description in 1972 the atriopulmonary Fontan operation has evolved, so that now several variations exist. The favoured approach nowadays is the total cavopulmonary connection (TCPC), which avoids some of the late complications of the original approach. Nonetheless, all the variations result in the same basic physiology, the 'Fontan circulation'.

The Fontan circulation is one of a chronic low cardiac output state, critically dependent upon adequate systemic venous filling pressure to drive forward flow across the pulmonary vascular bed. It is a fragile circulation in which small changes in haemodynamics can result in a serious, sometimes catastrophic, fall in cardiac output. Problems that can cause trouble include dehydration, stenosis at the site of connection of the right atrium or systemic veins to the pulmonary artery, pulmonary embolism from *in situ* right atrial thrombus, a rise in pulmonary vascular resistance, atrial flutter, mitral regurgitation, a rise in left ventricular end-diastolic pressure, aortic or subaortic stenosis, drug-induced vasodilatation (e.g. anaesthetic induction agents, nitrates), and positive pressure ventilation that reduces systemic venous return.

Clinical features after the Fontan operation

Most patients are acyanotic: new or worsening cyanosis is cause for concern. The jugular venous pulse is usually slightly raised and the second heart sound single. No murmur arises from the Fontan connection. There may be a murmur of mitral regurgitation. It patients with discordant venticuloarterial connections, a loud systolic murmur raises suspicion of subaortic stenosis (which may be at the level of the VSD). The liver edge is often palpable, but new or increasing hepatomegaly is a worrisome finding. Ascites often precedes peripheral oedema in young patients with complications subsequent to a Fontan procedure.

A combination of echocardiography and MRI provide anatomical and physiological data. Cardiac catheterization is needed to assess pulmonary vascular resistance. Cardiopulmonary exercise testing is a useful indicator of early signs of decompensation.

Complications after the Fontan operation

Patient selection is important in ensuring a good outcome of Fontan surgery. Survival ranges from 81% at 10 years for 'perfect candidates' to 60 to 70% for all patients. Preoperative risk factors for a poor outcome are pulmonary vascular resistance greater than 4 Wood units, mean pulmonary artery pressure more than 15 mmHg, ventricular hypertrophy, impaired systolic ventricular function, severe atrioventricular valve regurgitation, aortic outflow obstruction, and small or distorted pulmonary arteries. However, even patients with none of these risk factors are at risk of a great range of late complications which include intra-atrial re-entry tachycardia (IART)/atrial flutter, sinus node dysfunction, progressive ventricular dysfunction, atrioventricular valve regurgitation, development of subaortic stenosis, pathway obstruction, right lower pulmonary vein compression by dilated right atrium, thromboembolism (all adult patients should be anticoagulated), recurrent effusions, ascites, peripheral oedema, cyanosis (due to development of venous collaterals to the left atrium or pulmonary arteriovenous

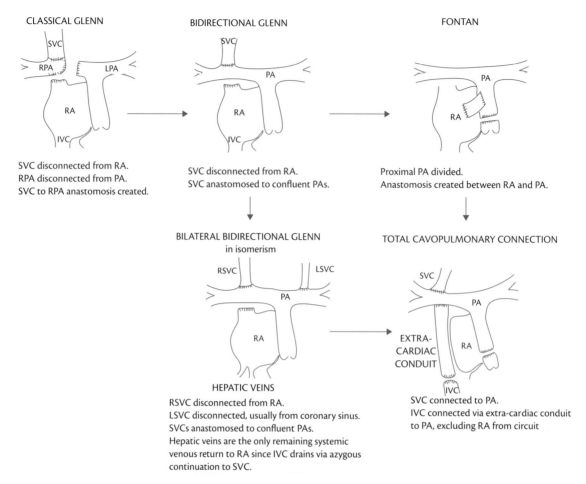

Fig. 12.1.28 Evolution of the Fontan and total cavopulmonary connection operations. IVC, inferior vena cava; PA, pulmonary artery; RPA, right pulmonary artery; SVC, superior vena cava.

fistulas), protein-losing enteropathy, and hepatic dysfunction including cirrhosis and hepatocellular carcinoma.

A detailed discussion of these many complications is beyond the scope of this book, but atrial flutter/IART merits further discussion because it is an acutely life-threatening complication (Fig. 12.1.29). Flutter is common after a Fontan procedure, and is poorly tolerated, causing a significant fall in cardiac output. Atrial transport is particularly important in the Fontan circulation to facilitate left ventricular filling, so simply controlling the rate of atrial flutter is inadequate: rapid restoration of sinus rhythm is required. Time may be wasted once the patient seeks medical attention, because the ECG appearances are often atypical and may be misinterpreted as sinus tachycardia. If in doubt, intravenous adenosine will reveal flutter waves and confirm the diagnosis, but will not terminate the arrhythmia. Other intravenous antiarrhythmics should be avoided since they may precipitate cardiovascular collapse. The safest approach is DC cardioversion. Intravenous fluids should be given while the patient is nil by mouth to maintain systemic venous filling pressure. Care must be taken to avoid excessive systemic vasodilation at induction of anaesthesia, and allowance must be made for the fall in cardiac output that accompanies ventilation.

Hypoplastic left heart syndrome

Until recently hypoplastic left heart syndrome (HLHS) was not discussed in adult texts, since there were no survivors to adulthood. With the introduction of the three-stage Norwood operation, resulting in a complex Fontan-type circulation, survivors are beginning to reach the adult clinic.

HLHS is a heterogeneous syndrome in which the left side of the heart is unable to support the systemic circulation because of hypoplasia, stenosis, or atresia at different levels of the left side of the circulation. The three-stage surgical approach to the condition is as follows:

◆ Stage I (Norwood operation)—performed in the first few days of life; the right ventricle and main pulmonary artery are used to reconstruct the systemic outflow tract; pulmonary blood flow is provided by a systemic–pulmonary artery shunt or right ventricle to pulmonary artery conduit.

◆ Stage II—this operation is performed at around 2 years; the systemic shunt or conduit to the pulmonary artery is taken down, and the superior vena cava anastomosed to the pulmonary artery (cavopulmonary or Glenn shunt).

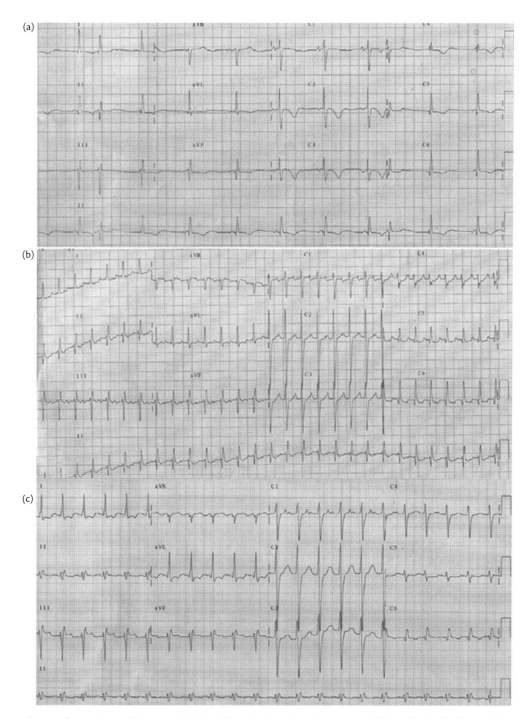

Fig. 12.1.29 Electrocardiograms from a 24-year-old woman with tricuspid atresia and previous Fontan surgery: (a) sinus rhythm; (b, c) interatrial re-entry tachycardias which were poorly tolerated and required urgent DC cardioversion.

♦ Stage III—Fontan completion is performed at around 5 years, usually with an extracardiac conduit.

Figure 12.1.30 shows a schematic representation of the Fontan circulation for HLHS. In early series only about 50% survived the three operations, but survival now approaches 70%. Those who reach the adult clinic will face the complications of any Fontan circulation, and in addition they are at risk of complications from ascending aorta and coarctation repair sites, coronary arteries arising from the hypoplastic remnant of ascending aorta, left pulmonary artery stenosis at site of arch repair, and failure of the right ventricle and tricuspid valve as they support the systemic circulation.

Pregnancy and contraception in congenital heart disease

Cardiac disease is the leading cause of pregnancy-related death in the United Kingdom. All patients with congenital heart disease should be counselled from adolescence on their risk of pregnancy

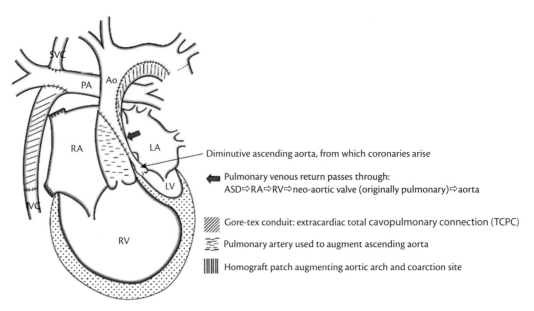

Diminutive ascending aorta, from which coronaries arise

Pulmonary venous return passes through:
ASD⇨RA⇨RV⇨neo-aortic valve (originally pulmonary)⇨aorta

Gore-tex conduit: extracardiac total cavopulmonary connection (TCPC)

Pulmonary artery used to augment ascending aorta

Homograft patch augmenting aortic arch and coarction site

Fig. 12.1.30 Hypoplastic left heart syndrome after the third stage Fontan completion. The right heart is used to support the systemic circulation and an ascending aorta is created from the pulmonary valve and pulmonary trunk. The aortic arch is enlarged with homograft tissue. An extracardiac conduit connects the IVC directly to the pulmonary arteries, and the SVC is also connected directly to the pulmonary arteries.

Ao, aorta; IVC, inferior vena cava; LA, left atrium; LV, left ventricle; PA, pulmonary artery; RA, right atrium; RV, right ventricle; SVC, superior vena cava.

and their contraceptive options. The risk of pregnancy in congenital heart disease ranges from being the same as that of the general population to a more than 25% risk of maternal death in pulmonary hypertension. Each patient requires specialist individual assessment before embarking on pregnancy. An outline of the risks associated with different conditions is shown in Table 12.1.8: it should be remembered that risks are additive, so a repaired septal defect with poor ventricular function moves from a low-risk to high-risk category.

Two principles should be remembered when considering contraceptive options: the efficacy of the method, and cardiovascular safety of the method. The risk of oestrogen-containing preparations (which include the combined oral contraceptive pill) relates to their thrombogenicity. Patients at risk of intracardiac or pulmonary thrombosis and those with right-to-left shunts should not use these preparations. Progestogen-only preparations are safe in cardiac disease, but the mode of delivery may carry risk. For example, insertion of a progestogen-eluting intrauterine device (Mirena®

IUS) carries a risk of vasovagal syncope in nulliparous women, a reaction that can provoke cardiovascular collapse in cyanotic, pulmonary hypertensive or post-Fontan patients. In addition, although the progestogen-only 'minipill' is safe, its efficacy is poor. The newer progestogen-only pill, desogestrel, combines cardiovascular safety with an efficacy equal to that of the combined pill. Other safe and effective methods useful for most women with cardiac disease are the subdermal implant Nexplanon® and the injectable DepoProvera®.

Bacterial endocarditis

Endocarditis is discussed in Chapter 9.2; the risks for specific congenital lesions are outlined in Table 12.1.9. However, it is noteworthy that United Kingdom guidelines on the use of antibiotic prophylaxis have been changed recently, such that this is no longer recommended for any procedure on an uninfected site. By contrast, North American guidelines recommend prophylaxis for those with

Table 12.1.8 Risk of maternal mortality in different cardiac conditions

Low risk (<1%)	Significant risk (1–10%)	High risk, pregnancy contraindicated (>10%)
Unoperated, small or mild: Pulmonary stenosis Septal defects Patent arterial duct	Mechanical valve	Pulmonary hypertension
Most repaired septal defects	Systemic right ventricle	Impaired systemic ventricular function
Successfully repaired coarctation	Cyanosis without pulmonary hypertension	Aortic aneurysm
Repaired tetralogy of Fallot	Fontan circulation	Severe left-sided obstruction, e.g. mitral and aortic stenosis
Most regurgitant valvar lesions		

Table 12.1.9 Risks of infective endocarditis or endarteritis in congenital heart disease

Unoperated	Operated
Low risk: lesions with no or low velocity turbulence and no prosthetic material	
Anomalous pulmonary venous drainage	Anomalous pulmonary venous drainage
Secundum ASD	Secundum ASD
Ebstein anomaly	Ebstein anomaly with repaired native valve
Mild pulmonary stenosis	VSD/tetralogy of Fallot without residual lesions
Isolated corrected transposition	Patent arterial duct
Eisenmenger syndrome without valvar regurgitation	Fontan-type procedures
	Arterial switch for transposition without residual lesions
Moderate risk	
Systemic AV valve regurgitation	Residual regurgitation of repaired native aortic or systemic AV valve
Subaortic stenosis	Nonvalved conduits
Moderate—severe pulmonary stenosis	
Tetralogy of Fallot	
Double-outlet right ventricle	
Univentricular heart with pulmonary stenosis	
Truncus arteriosus	
Coarctation	
Restrictive patent arterial duct	
High risk	
Bicuspid aortic valve	Prosthetic valves
Aortic regurgitation secondary to VSD or subaortic stenosis	Aortopulmonary shunts e.g. Gore-Tex, modified Blalock–Taussig
Restrictive VSD	Valved conduits

ASD, atrial septal defect; AV, atrioventricular; VSD, ventricular septal defect.

congenital heart disease that are unrepaired, have shunts or conduits, have prosthetic materials placed within 6 months, or have residual defects at the site of prosthetic material. It is likely that good oral hygiene and regular dental checks are more important in preventing endocarditis than whether or not antibiotic prophylaxis is given.

Further reading

Anderson RH, Shirali G (2009). Sequential segmental analysis. *Ann Pediatr Cardiol*, **2**, 24–35.

Broberg CS, *et al.* (2006). Blood viscosity and its relationship to iron deficiency, symptoms and exercise capacity in adults with cyanotic congenital heart disease. *J Am Coll Cardiol*, **48**, 256–65.

Cherian G, *et al.* (1983). Pulmonary hypertension in isolated atrial septal defect. *Am Heart J*, **105**, 952–7.

Clapp S, *et al.* (1990). Down syndrome, complete AV canal and pulmonary vascular obstructive disease. *J Thorac Cardiovasc Surg*, **100**, 115–21.

Del Sette M, *et al.* (1998). Migraine with aura and right-to-left shunt on trancranial Doppler: a case-control study. *Cerebrovasc Dis*, **8**, 327–30.

Diller GP, *et al.* (2006). Presentation, survival prospects and predictors of death in Eisenmenger syndrome: a combined retrospective and case-control study. *Eur Heart J*, **27**, 1737–42.

Driscoll DJ, *et al.* (1992). Five to fifteen year follow-up after Fontan operation. *Circulation*, **85**, 469–96.

Dupuis C, *et al.* (1992). The 'adult' form of the scimitar syndrome. *Am J Cardiol*, **70**, 502–7.

Fyfe A, *et al.* (2005). Cyanotic congenital heart disease and coronary artery atherogenesis. *Am J Cardiol*, **96**, 283–90.

Galiè N, et al. (2009). Guidelines for the diagnosis and treatment of pulmonary hypertension: the Task Force for the Diagnosis and Treatment of Pulmonary Hypertension of the European Society of Cardiology (ESC) and the European Respiratory Society (ERS), endorsed by the International Society of Heart and Lung Transplantation (ISHLT). *Eur Heart J*, **30**, 2493–537.

Geva T (2011). Repaired tetralogy of Fallot: the roles of cardiovascular magnetic resonance in evaluating pathophysiology and for pulmonary valve replacement decision support. *J Cardiovasc Magn Reson*, **13**, 9.

Hagen PT, Scholz DG, Edwards WD. (1984). Incidence and size of patent foramen ovale during the first 10 decades of life: an autopsy study of 965 normal hearts. *Mayo Clin Proc*, **59**, 17–20.

Ho SY, *et al.* (1995). *Colour atlas of congenital heart disease. Morphological and clinical correlations*. Mosby-Wolfe, London.

Kirklin JW, Barratt-Boyes BG (1993). *Cardiac surgery*, 2nd edition. Churchill Livingstone, New York.

Koller M, Rothlin M, Senning Å (1987). Coarctation of the aorta: review of 362 operated patients. Long term follow up and assessment of prognostic variables. *Eur Heart J*, **8**, 670–9.

Konstanides S, *et al.* (1995). A comparison of surgical and medical therapy for atrial septal defects in adults. *New Engl J Med*, **333**, 469–73.

Lumbiganon P, Chaitikpinyo A (2013). *Antibiotics for brain abscesses in people with cyanotic congenital heart disease*. Cochrane Collaboration/ John Wiley & Sons, London.

Mongeon FP, *et al.* (2008) Congenitally corrected transposition of the great arteries ventricular function at the time of systemic atrioventricular valve replacement predicts long-term ventricular function. *J Am Coll Cardiol*, **57**, 8–17.

Moodie DS, *et al.* (1984). Long term follow up in the unoperated univentricular heart. *Am J Cardiol*, **53**, 1124–8.

Moon RE, Camporesi EM, Kissolo JA (1989). Patent foramen ovale and decompression sickness in divers. *Lancet*, **i**, 513–14.

Murphy JG, *et al.* (1993). Long-term outcome in patients undergoing surgical repair of tetralogy of Fallot. *New Engl J Med*, **329**, 593–9.

Murtuza B, *et al.* (2011) Anatomic repair for congenitally corrected transposition of the great arteries: a single-institution 19-year experience. *J Thorac Cardiovasc Surg*, **142**, 1348–57.

NICE (2008). *Prophylaxis against infective endocarditis: antimicrobial prophylaxis against infective endocarditis in adults and children undergoing interventional procedures*. Clinical guideline 64. <http://guidance. nice.org.uk/CG64/Guidance/pdf/English>

Perloff JK, Child JS (1998). *Congenital heart disease in adults*. WB Saunders, Philadelphia, PA.

Redington AN, *et al.* (1998). *The right heart in congenital heart disease*. Greenwich Medical Media, London.

Roberts WC (1986). Major anomalies of coronary arterial origin seen in adulthood. *Am Heart J*, **111**, 941–62.

Sarris GE, *et al.* (2006). European Congenital Heart Surgeons Association. Results of surgery for Ebstein anomaly: a multicentre study from the European Congenital Heart Surgeons Association. *J Thorac Cardiovasc Surg*, **32**, 50–7.

Schamroth CL, *et al.* (1987). Pulmonary arterial thrombosis in secundum atrial septal defect. *Am J Cardiol*, **60**, 1152–6.

Stark J, de Leval MR (ed.) (1994). *Surgery for congenital heart defects.* W B Saunders, London.

Tay EL, *et al.* (2011). Replacement therapy for iron deficiency improves exercise capacity and quality of life in patients with cyanotic congenital heart disease and/or the Eisenmenger syndrome. *Int J Cardiol,* **151,** 307–12.

Thorne S, MacGregor A, Nelson-Piercy C (2006). Risks of contraception and pregnancy in heart disease. *Heart,* **92,** 1520–5.

Villafañe J, *et al.* (2013). Hot topics in tetralogy of Fallot. *J Am Coll Cardiol,* **62,** 2155–66.

Warnes CA (2006). Transposition of the great arteries. *Circulation,* **114,** 2699–709.

Warnes CA, *et al.* (2008). Guidelines for the management of adults with congenital heart disease: a report of the American College of Cardiology/American Heart Association Task Force on Practice Guidelines. *Circulation,* **118,** e714–833.

Wilson W, *et al.* (2007). Prevention of infective endocarditis: guidelines from the American Heart Association Rheumatic Fever, Endocarditis and Kawasaki Disease Committee, Council on Cardiovascular Disease in the Young, and the Council on Clinical Cardiology, Council on Cardiovascular Surgery and Anesthesia, and the Quality and Care Outcomes Research Interdisciplinary Working Group. *Circulation,* **116,** 1736–54.

Wood P (1958). Eisenmenger syndrome: or pulmonary hypertension with reversed central shunt. *Br Med J,* **ii,** 701–9, 755–62.

Coronary heart disease

CHAPTER 13.1

Biology and pathology of atherosclerosis

Robin P. Choudhury, Joshua T. Chai, and Edward A. Fisher

Essentials

Formation of an atheromatous plaque—this is an inflammatory process that involves the contribution of endothelial cells, monocytes, and smooth muscle cells in conjunction with the deposition of atherogenic lipoproteins in the intimal layer of the vascular wall. The initial stage involves activation of the endothelium at regions of nonlaminar flow in vessels resulting in increased permeability to Apo B-containing lipoproteins (LDL). Inflammatory cells, in particular monocytes, are recruited into the intimal layer of the vessel wall via the action of chemokines and adhesion molecules mobilized by activated endothelium.

Progression of atheroma—ingestion of LDL by monocytes, predominantly via scavenger receptors, generates lipid-rich foam cells. Atheroma progression is promoted by the failure to clear macrophages and foam cells that, on dying, release cholesterol-rich material promoting further inflammation. Leucocytes and endothelial cells also contribute through the release of growth factors that stimulate proliferation of vascular smooth muscle cells (VSMC). These cells migrate from the medial layer to the intima where they undergo transformation to both a synthetic phenotype (contributing to extracellular matrix formation), and 'macrophage-like' vascular smooth muscle cells capable of phagocytosis of LDL.

Further development of the atheromatous plaque—extracellular matrix formation by VSMC is stimulated by cytokines (e.g. TGFβ and platelet-derived growth factor) released from T cells, platelets, and macrophages. The extracellular matrix confers structural integrity to the atheromatous plaque and the overlying collagen-rich fibrous cap and promotes retention of lipoprotein molecules. Neovascularization of atheroma via the action of vascular endothelial growth factor (VGEF) results in susceptibility to plaque haemorrhage. Calcification is common although its pathogenic significance is uncertain. The progression of the atheromatous plaque is not always linear.

Clinical manifestations—stable angina may arise from progressive narrowing of the vessel lumen, but may also be contributed to by minor plaque rupture or haemorrhage resulting in stepwise progression. Acute coronary syndromes arise from more serious abrupt transformations of atheromatous plaques due to plaque haemorrhage, erosion, and rupture. Atheromatous lesions with a large lipid-rich core and thin fibrous cap are predisposed to plaque rupture, releasing lipid-containing prothrombotic material and giving rise to thrombosis and acute occlusion. Thrombotic occlusion due to plaque erosion arises in areas denuded of endothelium and is more common in women smokers.

Medical management—therapies to promote atheroma regression target plasma lipid profiles, plaque inflammation, and plaque remodelling. Dietary and pharmacological modification of plasma lipids are effective secondary prevention measures which have been shown to promote plaque regression, but their impact on clinical events appears to relate to complex mechanisms which modify inflammation, plaque stability, and thrombosis and are more difficult to assess using current techniques. Specific therapies targeting the inflammatory component of the atheromatous plaque, in particular monocyte recruitment, macrophage function, and apoptosis, are theoretically attractive and are currently under development.

Initiation of atheroma

Atherosclerotic plaques are not randomly distributed, but tend to form at the inner curvatures and branch points of arteries, where laminar flow is either disturbed or insufficient to support the normal, quiescent state of the endothelium (the lining of endothelial cells that separates the circulating blood from the arterial wall). The resulting activation of the endothelium leads to increased permeability to lipoproteins and an accumulation of extracellular matrix proteins that cause diffuse intimal thickening and the retention of the atherogenic apolipoprotein B (apoB)-containing lipoproteins.

Endothelial activation also promotes the recruitment of circulating monocytes that originate from either the bone marrow or spleen. Monocyte entry into the arterial intima depends on endothelial cell up-regulation of molecules that mediate their arrest on the luminal surface of the endothelium. The recruited monocytes transmigrate across the endothelium, where they differentiate into macrophages, some of which encounter the retained apoB-lipoproteins. The subsequent uptake of the retained apoB-lipoproteins by these macrophages is one of the earliest pathogenic events in the nascent plaque and results in the development of macrophage foam cells. The mechanisms of foam cell formation have been intensely studied. Although macrophages can take up apoB-containing lipoproteins through the low-density lipoprotein (LDL) receptor, expression of this receptor is down-regulated early during foam cell formation by the increased cellular cholesterol levels. These observations led to the hypothesis that lipoproteins must become modified in the artery wall and be taken up by other mechanisms, notably by scavenger receptors. Multiple means of LDL modification that facilitate cholesterol loading of macrophages *in vitro* have been identified, including oxidation. The physiologically relevant *in vivo* pathways of foam cell formation are still debated, though it is widely accepted that the appearance of foam cells in arterial sites represents the initiation of an atherosclerotic plaque.

Leucocyte recruitment

Though many cell types contribute to the formation of atherosclerotic plaques, including endothelial cells, monocytes, dendritic cells (DCs), lymphocytes, eosinophils, mast cells, and smooth muscle cells, macrophage foam cells are so central in the initiation and progression of atherosclerosis that emphasis has long been placed on understanding the mechanisms of monocyte recruitment into plaques. Circulating monocytes in mice consist of two major subsets, LY6C^{hi} and LY6C^{low}, with the corresponding subsets in humans being CD14$^+$CD16$^-$ and CD14^{low}CD16$^+$. In mice, and presumably in humans, the more inflammatory monocyte subsets (LY6C^{hi} and CD14$^+$CD16$^-$) make up the majority of cells recruited to progressing atherosclerotic plaques and are thought to be the source of the M1 (classically activated) macrophages found in both murine and human plaques that are responsible for maintaining a chronic inflammatory state.

Monocyte recruitment, as noted above, begins at the luminal surface of the endothelium. The capture and rolling phases of the recruitment cascade depend on the immobilization of chemokines, particularly CC-chemokine ligand 5 (CCL5) and CXC-chemokine ligand 1 (CXCL1), to endothelial cell glycosaminoglycans, and on P-selectin, which is expressed on the luminal side of endothelial cells. Vascular cell adhesion molecule 1 (VCAM1) and intercellular adhesion molecule 1 (ICAM1), which bind to the integrins VLA4 and lymphocyte function-associated antigen 1 (LFA1), respectively, are important for the firm adhesion of monocytes to the luminal surface of the endothelium.

The next phase is the transmigration of monocytes across the endothelium into the intimal (subendothelial) space. This is mediated by chemokines secreted by endothelial cells, intimal macrophages, and smooth muscle cells. Although several chemokines have been implicated in atherosclerosis, the three major chemokine receptor–chemokine pairs involved in monocyte transmigration are CCR2–CCL2, CX3CR1–CX3CRL1, and CCR5-CCL5. In addition to these chemokines, CD31 (also known von Willebrand factor; an endothelial cell surface immunoglobulin-like adhesion molecule) and VCAM1 may also have a role in monocyte transmigration into atherosclerotic plaques. See Fig. 13.1.1.

Although most studies of monocyte recruitment have been conducted in mice, the key players described above all have human homologues thought to function in similar ways.

Progression of atheroma

Beyond plaque initiation (see 'Initiation of atheroma' earlier), two factors conspire to promote the progression of atheroma. These are the ongoing entry and subsequent retention of the apoB-containing lipoproteins, and the continued recruitment of monoctyes, which follow the same path as their predecessors, namely to become macrophages, then foam cells that exhibit inflammatory changes. The

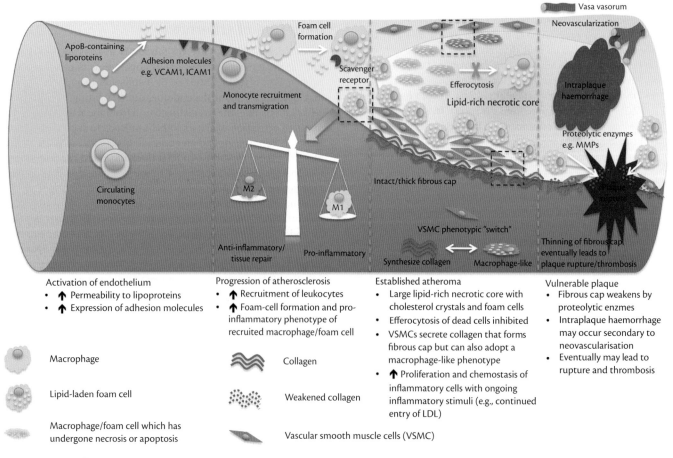

Fig. 13.1.1 Stages of atherosclerosis progression from activated endothelium, to leukocyte recruitment, established atheroma, to eventual development of vulnerable plaque features.

recruitment of these monocytes accelerates after plaque initiation because of increased expression on the endothelial surface of adhesion molecules (e.g. VCAM1 and ICAM1) and the robust secretion of attractant chemokines, particularly CCL2 (also termed MCP-1), by multiple cell types in the plaque, including the already established macrophages and foam cells.

Recruitment of monocytes to a site of inflammation is not abnormal; rather, it is the failure to remove macrophages and resolve the inflammation that leads to pathology. In part this is due to macrophage chemostasis (cellular paralysis) that is not typical in other settings (such as in pneumonia or wound healing) and which might reflect the expression of retention molecules that render the macrophages and foam cells relatively unresponsive to chemokines, as shown in mice. There is at least one other contributing factor: as in other tissues, a fraction of the macrophage population in plaques undergoes apoptosis, and is normally phagocytosed by healthy macrophages in a process called 'efferocytosis'. Even in an early plaque, in which the local environment is not fully toxic, clearance by efferocytosis cannot keep up with the influx of newly recruited monocytes, leading to plaque growth. As the disease advances, the plaque accumulates more inflammatory and injurious factors that can signal macrophages and other immune cells through Toll-like receptors (TLRs). Among other adverse effects, this reduces macrophage capacity to perform efferocytosis. This results in the disintegration of the dying macrophages, with the release into the extracellular plaque environment of inflammatory material, thrombotic factors, and the cholesterol-rich gruel found in the necrotic core.

In parallel with the macrophage 'itinerary' described above, as the atheroma advances, other immune cells—both innate (dendritic cells) and acquired (T and B lymphocytes)—also enter the plaque and modulate its inflammatory state. For example, T lymphocytes, depending on their stimuli, can either exacerbate macrophage activation by the secretion of Th1 cytokines (e.g. IL-1, IL-6, TNFα) or ameliorate it by secreting Th2 cytokines (e.g. IL-4, IL-10). Furthermore, B cells can elaborate antibodies to substances generated from the oxidation of LDL that resemble antigens derived from microorganisms, in an attempt to neutralize the harmful effects of these products, with levels of such antibodies considered by some as a marker of disease burden.

Smooth muscle cells

In normal arteries, vascular smooth muscle cells (VSMC) are confined to the medial layer, which is delimited from the intimal space, where plaques form and grow, and from the outer arterial wall by internal and external elastic laminae, respectively. The cells are in the 'contractile' state, meaning that they serve mainly to set the vascular tone in response to a variety of stimuli by either contracting or relaxing. Activated endothelial cells in coronary arteries not only up-regulate their leukocyte recruitment factors, they also down-regulate their production of nitric oxide, increasing arterial tone and adversely affecting blood flow to the myocardium. The loss of vasorelaxation is not the only change in VSMC in the progressing plaque. Both activated leucocytes and endothelium secrete growth factors that stimulate the proliferation of VSMC, which then migrate out of the medial layer into the intima. The migration of synthetic VSMC to the subendothelium and their elaboration of collagen forms the fibrous cap.

The historical view has been that the VSMC phenotype switches from 'contractile' to 'synthetic', in recognition of increased production of extracellular matrix (ECM) by these cells (see 'Extracellular matrix'). However, it is now appreciated that the phenotypic spectrum of VSMC in atheroma is more complex than originally realized. For example, VSMC can gain properties of inflammatory cells presumably because their TLRs become stimulated as they do in macrophages (see previous section). Another way in which the VSMC phenotype can be altered is by accumulating lipids. Relative to macrophages, whose transition to foam cells is enabled by their expression of scavenger receptors that take up large amounts of lipoprotein-derived lipids well after their LDL receptors are down-regulated, VSMC appear to become engorged more through a phagocytic process. Once it occurs to a significant degree, however, the cells in vitro and in vivo assume a macrophage foam cell-like state, both morphologically and phenotypically (in terms of cell-specific marker expression). In advanced plaques in patients, it has been estimated that as much as 40% of cells that would be traditionally classified as macrophage foam cells are actually of VSMC origin. Unlike the subendothelial VSMC that retain the synthetic phenotype, it is likely that the 'macrophage-like' VSMC have negative effects on plaque inflammation and stability.

Extracellular matrix

The ECM is made up of a mixture of macromolecules including collagen, elastin, glycoproteins, and proteoglycans, that confer tensile strength and viscoelasticity to the arterial wall. However, the ECM components function beyond furnishing a scaffold for the arterial wall and developing atherosclerotic plaque. Some constituents (notably proteoglycans) bind apoB-lipoproteins (described earlier), prolonging their residence in the intima. Retention of lipoprotein particles occurs due to steric hindrance and ionic interactions between positively charged amino acids in apoB-containing lipoproteins and negatively charged residues in the glycosaminoglycan chains. As a result, extravasated LDL are liable to retention and susceptible to the oxidative modification (and glycation) that drives atherogenesis.

In addition to lipoprotein retention, as atherosclerotic plaques develop, the ECM participates in other processes that are important in the context of atherosclerosis and its complications, including cell migration and proliferation, and thrombosis. Furthermore, the distribution of fibrous elements relative to other components, such as the lipid-rich necrotic core, can influence plaque behaviour. Elements of ECM can be found diffusely in a reticular distribution through the plaque but may also be found in a dense 'fibrous cap' overlying the lipid-rich necrotic core. Indeed, when considering pathogenicity, the deposition of ECM, comprised of fibrous and cellular components, confers structure and stability. Disruption of the fibrous cap (discussed later) is a precipitant of acute vascular syndromes.

The matrix also contains growth factors, and cleaving certain components such as laminin releases sequestered mediators that promote cellular migration. Cytokines such as TGFβ and platelet-derived growth factor (PDGF) from T cells, platelets, macrophages, and monocytes stimulate smooth muscle cells to produce ECM.

Atherosclerotic plaques

Cell death in atherosclerotic plaques

Intimal macrophages can undergo apoptosis, a type of programmed death that usually prevents necrosis. This process occurs throughout atherosclerotic lesion development, and in advanced atherosclerotic lesions, apoptotic macrophages necrose and coalesce to contribute to a lipid-rich necrotic core that harbours the tissue factor that contributes to the formation of the intraluminal clot after plaque rupture. As noted earlier, one mechanism underlying postapoptotic macrophage necrosis is the defective phagocytic clearance, or efferocytosis, of apoptotic cells. Studies in mouse models of advanced atherosclerosis have provided evidence that several molecules known to be involved in efferocytosis, including TG2, MFG-E8, complement C1q, Mertk, lysoPC, and Fas, play important roles in the clearance of apoptotic cells in advanced plaques.

Neovascularization in atherosclerotic plaques

Human arteries possess a microvasculature in their adventitial layers called the vasa vasorum. For the coronary arteries, normal vasa vasorum originate from branch points at regular intervals and run longitudinally along the vessel wall. A primary function of these vessels is to provide nutrients to the cells of the arterial wall. As plaques enlarge, angiogenic factors drive the formation of new blood vessels. For instance, oxidized phospholipids within the plaque can stimulate the production of vascular endothelial growth factor (VEGF) isoforms in both monocytes and endothelial cells. New endothelial cell sprouts can form immature, leaky microvessels within the plaque. These 'neo-vessels' also provide a site for entry of inflammatory monocytes that perpetuate the atherosclerotic process. Microvessels also present a potential site for intraplaque haemorrhage, which is associated with plaque progression.

Plaque calcification

Electron microscopy has shown that calcification can occur initially as microdeposits through mineralization of organelles in cells associated with the lipid-rich necrotic core. In some plaques, calcification progresses and can become diffuse and, particularly in older individuals, can become extensive.

The presence of calcification has been targeted for quantification using CT techniques. Electron beam CT sensitively detects arterial calcification and its level can enhance prediction of risk of vascular complications over and above that associated with conventional risk factors. Furthermore, the process of calcification can be identified using positron emission tomography for ^{18}F-sodium fluoride. In coronary arteries, tracer uptake can be demonstrated in 'culprit' plaques after acute coronary syndrome (ACS; see later), and in symptomatic carotid arteries uptake was associated with histological evidence of active calcification, macrophage infiltration, apoptosis, and necrosis. Yet to be determined, however, is the pathogenic significance of calcification. Although calcification may indicate the presence of atherosclerosis, it may at least in part reflect reparative processes.

While the level of calcification has found some acceptance as a stratifying factor for risk of cardiovascular disease, it does not seem well suited as a parameter to reflect treatment efficacy. Indeed, treatment with statins, which reduces the risk of complications of atherosclerosis, does not appear to alter plaque calcification.

Positive remodelling of the arterial wall

Atherosclerosis develops within the vessel wall and, as the lesion enlarges, its growth is often accommodated by positive remodelling of the artery. In other words, outward expansion of the artery can enable lesion growth without encroachment on the vessel lumen, at least initially. In the original description of this phenomenon in the left main stem coronary artery, the lumen area did not decrease in relation to the percentage of stenosis (i.e. the percentage of the vessel cross-sectional area occupied by the plaque) for values up to 40%, but did diminish markedly and in close relation to the percentage of stenosis for values beyond that. So, human coronary arteries can enlarge in response to plaque growth to maintain their patency, but eventually this protective mechanism reaches a limit, and if the plaque continues to expand, stenosis ensues. Importantly, the compensatory outward expansion of the artery's external elastic lamina can accommodate plaques with large lipid cores that do not appear on angiogram but may nonetheless rupture suddenly, causing thrombus formation and ACS.

Positive remodelling has important implications for identification of atheromatous lesions using arteriographic imaging techniques that, like angiography, focus on the lumen rather than the vessel wall. Intravascular ultrasound studies have shown that larger areas of plaque burden may exist in regions of the arteries with little or no luminal stenosis. Appreciation of this limitation has led to the emergence of imaging techniques that focus on quantification and characterization of lesions directly.

Patterns of disease progression

The course of pathological events associated with atheroma that are described above may suggest an ordered and formulaic progression of atherosclerosis. While atheroma may advance through gradual progression of these physical and cellular processes, the development of individual lesions can also be punctuated by abrupt events, for example intraplaque haemorrhage, plaque erosion, and cap rupture. These events may occur relatively frequently, with a majority remaining subclinical. The healing phase that follows may involve smooth muscle cell proliferation and matrix deposition, which may stabilize but also enlarge the plaque and promote stenosis by constrictive remodelling.

Acute coronary syndromes

An atherosclerotic plaque may develop over a period of several years and remain silent or subclinical throughout that time. Alternatively, encroachment of an enlarging but quiescent lesion may lead to symptoms of stable angina. Acute arterial syndromes typically occur due to the rupture or erosion of an atheromatous plaque. This exposes the contents of that plaque, including cellular debris, collagen and tissue factor, to the elements of circulating blood that can initiate blood coagulation, leading to partial or total thrombotic occlusion of the artery involved.

Plaque rupture and erosion

Post-mortem studies of human coronary artery have identified features that are associated with atherosclerotic plaque rupture. Atheromatous lesions with a large lipid-rich necrotic core and a thin fibrous cap with macrophage accumulation in the 'shoulder' regions seem to be susceptible to rupture. Propensity to rupture is further increased by the activity of proteolytic enzymes (matrix metalloproteinases) that digest and weaken elements of the fibrous cap. Plaque rupture exposes thrombogenic components of the plaque (including tissue factor and collagen) to the blood, leading to the generation of luminal thrombus, which may cause partial or total occlusion of the artery. As emphasized earlier, it is important to recognize that even lesions that do not cause a high degree of luminal stenosis can still behave in this way.

Plaque erosion, in which a patch of endothelium becomes denuded, thereby exposing the initma to the circulating blood, also causes acute thrombosis. Endothelial loss may occur due to apoptosis of endothelial cells or shedding of cells from the basement membrane due to the action of proteases such as gelatinases on type IV collagen, or other components of the basement membrane upon which endothelial cells rest. Sites of plaque erosion may not exhibit prominent macrophage or lymphocyte accumulation. The underlying plaque in erosions consists of a thickened intima or fibrous cap atheroma, and lesions may be eccentric or calcified. Fatal thrombosis due to plaque erosion is associated with smoking, especially in women. Compared with fibrous cap rupture, death due to plaque erosion occurs more often in younger individuals and may affect less severely narrowed arteries.

Vulnerable plaque and the vulnerable patient

While it is possible to identify individual lesions as the proximate cause of acute vascular events, these do not develop or behave in isolation. Numerous strands of evidence implicate systemic processes, especially in relation to inflammation, as drivers for atherosclerosis and or potential importance in affecting plaque behaviours acutely. Specifically, systemic inflammatory disease, such as rheumatoid arthritis, promotes atherosclerosis and its complications. In an experimental model, acute myocardial infarction itself led to increased atherosclerotic plaque macrophage content and atherosclerosis progression. Appreciation of the role of systemic factors in the pathogenesis of atherosclerosis has implications for diagnosis, risk prediction, and treatments and is an emerging area of great clinical interest with a number of relevant patient intervention trials in progress and planned.

Atherosclerosis regression

While delayed progression of atherosclerosis is a worthy clinical goal, the disease process starts early in life and by the time most patients begin risk factor treatments, they have considerable plaque burden, making regression a more desirable goal. Indeed, in multiple studies a number of interventions, including dietary approaches, genetic manipulations, infusion therapies, and pharmacological treatments in multiple animal species (rabbits, pigs, mice), including nonhuman primates, have demonstrated favourable effects on established atherosclerotic plaques. Most of these interventions have been 'lipid/lipoprotein centric' and involved either lowering plasma levels of the apoB-containing lipoproteins to reduce the formation and ongoing engorgement of the foam cells, or raising levels of cholesterol-efflux agents (e.g. high-density lipoproteins, HDL) to unload cholesterol from these cells and return it to the liver for elimination through the bile as part of the process dubbed 'reverse cholesterol transport'. See Fig. 13.1.2.

A general finding has been that during atherosclerosis regression, the plaque content of foam cells decreases. From recent studies in mouse models, evidence has accumulated to identify kinetic contributions to this decrease to include changes in monocyte recruitment, macrophage emigration, macrophage apoptosis and efferocytosis, and local macrophage proliferation. Knowledge of the critical role that the chronic inflammatory state of the plaque

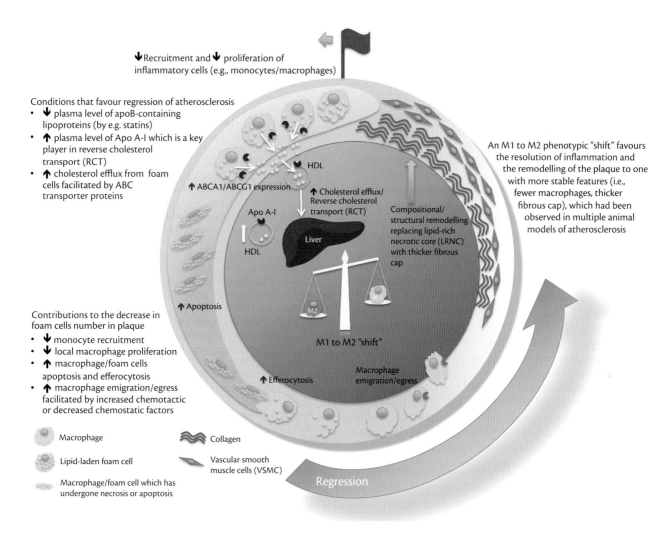

Fig. 13.1.2 Mechanisms involved in atherosclerosis regression in experimental models.

plays in the clinical disease process, especially the erosion and eventual rupture of a vulnerable plaque, has focused attention on therapies that would dampen or even resolve the inflammatory state in plaques. Preclinical findings give cause for optimism that this approach will join the lipid-centric approaches to realize plaque regression. For example, in mouse models it has been shown that the inflammatory state of the plaque foam cells is dynamic. Most are in the M1 activated state (which encourages inflammation) during disease progression, but under experimental regression conditions, there is enrichment of cells in the M2 state, which are sometimes referred to as anti-inflammatory or tissue repair macrophages. It is tempting to envision that this change is instrumental in the resolution of the inflammation and remodelling of the plaque to one with more stable features (i.e. fewer macrophages, thicker fibrous cap) that have been observed in multiple mouse models of atherosclerosis.

That this shift from M1 to M2 macrophages can be manipulated pharmacologically is supported by recent preclinical studies in which the administration of agents that are strong polarizers of macrophages *in vitro* to the M2 state (such as IL-13) has consistently led to delayed progression of atherosclerosis. One challenge for anti-inflammatory therapies, of course, is targeting agents to the plaque for those having adverse systemic effects, but improvements in nanoparticle-based therapies to achieve such specificity are rapidly advancing.

There are limited clinical studies that have also shown that significantly lowering plasma apoB-containing lipoprotein levels or increasing the levels of functional HDL particles resulted in plaque regression, as judged by quantitative angiography or intravascular ultrasound. Patients in most of these trials had evidence of ACS, and the imaging techniques used were not only invasive (and therefore not appropriate in primary prevention studies), but also primarily sensitive to changes in plaque size, rather than composition or inflammatory state. These 'qualitative' changes are likely to be exceedingly important clinically as they are key components of plaque regression in preclinical models. Evidence of plaque regression in the much larger primary prevention group is limited and largely restricted to noninvasive measurement of carotid intima-media thickness. Improved noninvasive techniques that assess plaque composition and activity are under development to assess the ability of current and future candidate therapies to favourably affect plaque characteristics.

There are a number of agents in clinical trials, or contemplated for such testing, to cause plaque regression, or less ideally, stop their progression. These include even more aggressive LDL-lowering using antibodies to PCSK9, infusions of HDL or artificial cholesterol acceptors (e.g. apoA1 Milano), anti-inflammatory treatments such as an antibody against the potent inflammatory cytokine IL-1β, or the use of methotrexate to reduce systemic inflammation. Finally, therapeutics can be envisioned that will manipulate the content of plaque macrophages by regulating monocyte recruitment or macrophage emigration, macrophage apoptosis and efferocytosis, and the proliferation of macrophages in plaques. Advances in genetic, immunological, and nanoparticle therapies will further enhance the likelihood of successful implementation of these and other, yet to be discovered, promising approaches.

Further reading

Allahverdian S, *et al.* (2014). Contribution of intimal smooth muscle cells to cholesterol accumulation and macrophage-like cells in human atherosclerosis. *Circulation*, **129**, 1551–9.

Arad Y, *et al.* (2005). Treatment of asymptomatic adults with elevated coronary calcium scores with atorvastatin, vitamin C, and vitamin E: The St. Francis Heart Study randomized clinical trial. *J Am Coll Cardiol*, **46**, 166–72.

Burke AP, *et al.* (1997). Coronary risk factors and plaque morphology in men with coronary disease who died suddenly. *N Engl J Med*, **336**, 1276–82.

Cardilo-Reis L, *et al.* (2012). Interleukin-13 protects from atherosclerosis and modulates plaque composition by skewing the macrophage phenotype. *EMBO Mol Med*, **4**, 1072–86.

Detrano R, *et al.* (2008). Coronary calcium as a predictor of coronary events in four racial or ethnic groups. *N Engl J Med*, **358**, 1336–45.

Dutta P, *et al.* (2012). Myocardial infarction accelerates atherosclerosis. *Nature*, **487**, 325–9.

Galis ZS, *et al.* (1994). Increased expression of matrix metalloproteinases and matrix degrading activity in vulnerable regions of human atherosclerotic plaques. *J Clin Invest*, **94**, 2493–503.

Glagov S, *et al.* (1987). Compensatory enlargement of human atherosclerotic coronary arteries. *N Engl J Med*, **316**, 1371–5.

Hansson GK, Hermansson A. (2011). The immune system in atherosclerosis. *Nat Immunol*, **12**, 204–12.

Joshi NV, *et al.* (2014). ^{18}F-fluoride positron emission tomography for identification of ruptured and high-risk coronary atherosclerotic plaques: A prospective clinical trial. *Lancet*, **383**, 705–13.

Leibundgut G, *et al.* (2013). Oxidation-specific epitopes and immunological responses: Translational biotheranostic implications for atherosclerosis. *Curr Opin Pharmacol*, **13**, 168–79.

McGill HC Jr, *et al.* (2000). Effects of coronary heart disease risk factors on atherosclerosis of selected regions of the aorta and right coronary artery. PDAY Research Group. Pathobiological Determinants of Atherosclerosis in Youth. *Arterioscler Thromb Vasc Biol*, **20**, 836–45.

Moore KJ, Freeman MW (2006). Scavenger receptors in atherosclerosis: Beyond lipid uptake. *Arterioscler Thromb Vasc Biol*, **26**, 1702–1711.

Moore KJ, *et al.* (2013). Macrophages in atherosclerosis: A dynamic balance. *Nat Rev Immunol*, **13**, 709–21.

Moreno PR, *et al.* (1996). Macrophages, smooth muscle cells, and tissue factor in unstable angina. Implications for cell-mediated thrombogenicity in acute coronary syndromes. *Circulation*, **94**, 3090–7.

Naghavi M, *et al.* (2003). From vulnerable plaque to vulnerable patient: A call for new definitions and risk assessment strategies: Part I. *Circulation*, **108**, 1664–72.

Naghavi M, *et al.* (2003). From vulnerable plaque to vulnerable patient: A call for new definitions and risk assessment strategies: Part II. *Circulation*, **108**, 1772–8.

Owen DR, *et al.* (2011). Imaging of atherosclerosis. *Annu Rev Med*, **62**, 25–40.

Rong JX, *et al.* (2003). Transdifferentiation of mouse aortic smooth muscle cells to a macrophage-like state after cholesterol loading. *Proc Natl Acad Sci U S A*, **100**, 13531–6.

Rumberger JA, *et al.* (1995). Coronary artery calcium area by electron-beam computed tomography and coronary atherosclerotic plaque area. A histopathologic correlative study. *Circulation*, **92**, 2157–62.

Tabas I, Glass CK (2013). Anti-inflammatory therapy in chronic disease: Challenges and opportunities. *Science*, **339**, 166–72.

Tacke F, *et al.* (2007). Monocyte subsets differentially employ CCR2, CCR5, and CX3CR1 to accumulate within atherosclerotic plaques. *J Clin Invest*, **117**, 185–94.

Thorp E, *et al.* (2008). Mertk receptor mutation reduces efferocytosis efficiency and promotes apoptotic cell accumulation and plaque necrosis in atherosclerotic lesions of apoe-/- mice. *Arterioscler Thromb Vasc Biol*, **28**, 1421–8.

Weber C, Noels H (2011). Atherosclerosis: Current pathogenesis and therapeutic options. *Nat Med*, **17**, 1410–22.

Williams KJ, *et al.* (2008). Rapid regression of atherosclerosis: Insights from the clinical and experimental literature. *Nat Clin Pract Cardiovasc Med*, **5**, 91–102.

Williams KJ, Tabas I (1995). The response-to-retention hypothesis of early atherogenesis. *Arterioscler Thromb Vasc Biol*, **15**, 551–61.

Wolfbauer G, *et al.* (1986). Development of the smooth muscle foam cell: Uptake of macrophage lipid inclusions. *Proc Natl Acad Sci U S A*, **83**, 7760–4.

Coronary heart disease: epidemiology and prevention

Goodarz Danaei and Kazem Rahimi

Essentials

Coronary heart disease (CHD) is now the leading cause of death and disability globally. Despite recent declines in age-standardized death rates from CHD globally, the number of CHD deaths have been increasing due to a combination of growth in population numbers and their longevity. In addition, manifestation and outcome of CHD varies substantially between and within countries.

Unlike many medical conditions that are common, disable, and kill, CHD is to a large extent preventable. There are strong, unconfounded relationships between several risk factors and CHD mortality and nonfatal myocardial infarction. The most important risk factors for CHD are smoking, high blood pressure, dyslipidaemia, diabetes, physical inactivity, unhealthy diet, and obesity. Controlling these risk factors, even in middle-aged individuals, through medical treatment as well as population-level interventions, may reduce CHD incidence by almost one-half.

Despite the apparent triumph in risk prediction and control, the search for new biomarkers, both phenotypic and genotypic, remains a major focus of cardiovascular research. Several novel markers of risk have already been identified and many more are likely to emerge during the next few years. However, the causal significance of these biomarkers, or their contribution to risk prediction, awaits further clarification.

Introduction

CHD is a group of diseases characterized by insufficient circulation in coronary arteries potentially leading to angina pectoris, myocardial infarction, heart failure and (sudden) coronary death. The underlying pathophysiology is most often coronary atherosclerosis, which is discussed in detail in Chapter 13.1. The process of atherosclerosis may begin in utero and is largely preventable by controlling the common risk factors of atherosclerosis discussed below. In this chapter we present the current evidence on the global distribution of CHD and its determinants, focusing on risk factors for atherosclerosis. Other, less common and nonatherosclerotic variants of CHD include those caused by vasoconstriction such as Prinzmetal's angina, paradoxical embolism, Kawasaki syndrome

leading to coronary aneurysms and stenosis, chest trauma, irradiation, spontaneous coronary dissection, and cardiac syndrome X. They collectively constitute a relatively minor proportion of the global CHD disease burden. Therefore, in this chapter we use CHD and ischaemic heart disease (IHD) interchangeably.

Global perspective

Coronary disease was a rare condition at the beginning of the twentieth century—a time when deaths from CHD were greatly outnumbered by those due to infectious diseases. CHD is now the leading cause of death and disability in almost all regions of the world, causing 7 million deaths in 2010 compared with 5.2 million in 1990. This 35% global increase in the number of CHD deaths has occurred despite a 20% decline in the age-standardized mortality rates over the same period and can be solely accounted for by the growth in population numbers and their longevity. CHD mortality rates have declined since 1980 in most high-income and many middle-income countries in the world with the notable exception of the countries of the former Soviet Union and South Asia in the 1990s where there was an increase in CHD deaths that only started to decline in the mid 2000s. There are also substantial regional differences. In 2010, countries in eastern Europe and Central Asia had the highest CHD mortality rates whereas those in eastern sub-Saharan Africa had the lowest. The rates in the former groups of countries were 10 times that in the latter group (see Fig. 13.2.1).

There are vast disparities in age at death from CHD, deaths occurring at much younger ages in Central Asia, North Africa, the Middle East, and sub-Saharan Africa. The differences in death rates and age at presentation across nations point to the largely preventable nature of CHD. Half the decline in CHD mortality in high-income countries in the recent decades is thought to be due to improvements in treatment, the remainder due to modification of CHD risk factors.

Substantial disparities in CHD within countries and across social and racial/ethnic subgroups have been identified. The increased risk compared to the white population in African Americans in the United States of America and the Asian population in the United Kingdom is largely explained by higher levels of well-known risk factors such as blood pressure, smoking, and diabetes. The importance of modifiable risk factors is emphasized by the fact that

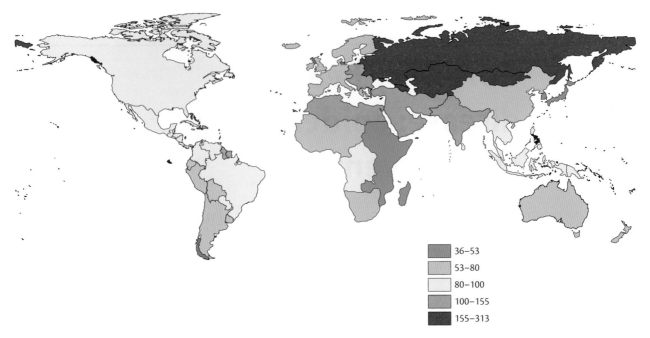

Fig. 13.2.1 Map of age-standardized ischaemic heart disease mortality rate per 100 000 persons in 21 world regions in 2010: the Global Burden of Disease 2010 Study. From Moran AE, Forouzanfar MH, Roth GA, Mensah GA, Ezzati M, Murray CJ, *et al.* Temporal trends in ischemic heart disease mortality in 21 world regions, 1980 to 2010: the Global Burden of Disease 2010 study. *Circulation.* 2014;129(14):1483–92.

individuals from low-risk ethnic groups tend to adopt the cardiovascular risk of their adopted country. Individuals with lower education, social status, or in lower income groups in Europe and America also exhibit higher rates of CHD due to a combination of worse risk factor profiles and lower access to, and quality of, health care.

A substantial body of epidemiological knowledge has been generated in the past seven decades and the collective evidence from cross-country comparison studies, prospective epidemiological studies, and randomized clinical trials has helped us understand the determinants of CHD and design clinical and public health interventions to reduce CHD burden worldwide. Next we summarize the key risk factors and the corresponding evidence that substantiates their effect on CHD.

Modifiable and nonmodifiable risk factors

Overview of risk factors

The most important risk factors for CHD are smoking, high blood pressure, dyslipidaemia, diabetes, physical inactivity, unhealthy diet, and obesity. Globally in 2010, 53% of the CHD burden (as measured by disability-adjusted life years) was attributable to non-optimal blood pressure, 40% to diet low in nuts and seeds, and about 30% separately to each of the following risk factors: alcohol use, smoking, physical inactivity, and high serum cholesterol (see Table 13.2.1). The sum of these proportions far exceeds 100% because one CHD case can be attributable to more than one risk factor. Lifelong exposure to these risk factors collectively explains about 70–80% of the incidence of CHD and over 75% of patients presenting with CHD will have at least one traditional risk factor. Controlling these risk factors, even in middle-aged individuals, may reduce CHD incidence by almost one-half.

Tobacco smoking, second-hand smoke, and other forms of tobacco use

Tobacco smoking is a major driver of CHD worldwide. Strong evidence from many prospective epidemiological studies and laboratory experiments clearly indicate the harmful effects of tobacco on CHD through its impact on reducing oxygen-carrying capacity, increasing blood pressure, damaging the endothelial cells, increasing inflammation, thrombosis, and oxidation of low-density lipoprotein (LDL) particles among many other pathways. There is a strong dose–response relationship between the duration and intensity of smoking and risk of CHD and heavy smokers may have up to five times higher risk of CHD than never smokers. The relative risks of tobacco smoking and CHD decline with age and are at least as large among women as among men. The twentieth century has aptly been named the 'tobacco century' to signify the substantial rise in tobacco consumption initially in the high-income nations and subsequently its export into developing countries. After the publication of the first report of the Royal College of Physicians in the United Kingdom in 1962 and the Surgeon General's report of 1964 in the United States of America, various public health interventions and policies including educational campaigns and raising taxes and banning advertising have led to lower tobacco smoking in many high-income countries which may have contributed substantially to reductions in CHD rates. For example, in the United States 12% of the decline in the CHD rates between 1980 and 2000 has been attributed to reductions in smoking prevalence. Smoking cessation is the most effective preventive measure for CHD. The harmful impact of smoking on CHD takes up to 10 years to revert to normal after quitting smoking; however, the impact is large, with a risk reduction of over 30% (Fig. 13.2.2).

Table 13.2.1 Proportion of ischaemic heart disease burden (measured in disability-adjusted life years) attributable to individual risk factors, worldwide, Global Burden of Disease Study results 2010

Risk factors	Proportion of CHD burden attributable
Physiological risk factors	
High blood pressure	53%
High total cholesterol	29%
High body mass index	23%
High fasting plasma glucose	16%
Alcohol use	33%
Tobacco smoking, including second-hand smoke	31%
Physical inactivity and low physical activity	31%
Dietary risk factors	
Diet low in nuts and seeds	40%
Diet low in fruits	30%
Diet low in seafood omega-3 fatty acids	22%
Diet low in whole grains	17%
Diet high in sodium	17%
Diet high in processed meat	13%
Diet low in vegetables	12%
Diet low in fibre	11%
Diet low in polyunsaturated fatty acids	9%
Diet high in trans fatty acids	9%
Diet high in sugar-sweetened beverages	2%
Air pollution	
Ambient particulate matter pollution	22%
Household air pollution from solid fuels	18%
Other environmental risks	
Lead exposure	4%

Reprinted from *The Lancet* Vol. 380 (9859), Lim SS, Vos T, Flaxman AD, Danaei G, Shibuya K, Adair-Rohani H, *et al*. A comparative risk assessment of burden of disease and injury attributable to 67 risk factors and risk factor clusters in 21 regions, 1990-2010: a systematic analysis for the Global Burden of Disease Study 2010:2224–60 © (2012), with permission from Elsevier.

Cessation programs including nicotine patches and gums, behavioural counselling and group therapy programmes, and the use of antidepressants, in particular buproprion and nortriptyline, may increase quitting success rates but prevention of uptake remains the key challenge. Population-level interventions to prevent smoking including bans on sales of tobacco products to minors, bans on advertising, and increasing taxes are among the most cost-effective ways to reduce CHD burden and 179 countries have signed a global treaty, the Framework Convention on Tobacco Control, adopted in 2003, to implement these policies.

Other forms of tobacco smoking (cigar, pipe, hookah) increase risk for CHD, chronic respiratory diseases, and mortality to a similar extent to cigarettes.

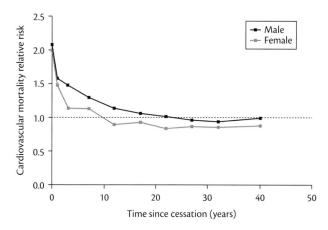

Fig. 13.2.2 Relative risk of cardiovascular mortality by time since cessation of smoking.
From Ezzati M, Lopez AD, Rodgers A, Murray CJL. Smoking and oral tobacco use. *Comparative quantification of health risks: Global and regional burden of disease attributable to selected major risk factors*. Geneva: World Health Organization; 2004. pp. 883–957.

Passive smoking

A significant component of the global impact of smoking on the incidence of CHD is related to passive smoking. Although the *relative* risk of CHD due to passive smoking is much lower than for active smoking, a substantially larger number of individuals are exposed to this harmful effect, raising the importance of banning smoking in public places.

E-cigarettes

Since 2004, electronic cigarettes (or e-cigarettes) have been launched as a smoke-free and implicitly harm-free nicotine delivery device to aid quitting. Although a recent review of chemical and toxicological studies did not find severe contamination of the aerosols by other substances, the amount of nicotine delivered by e-cigarettes easily surpasses the threshold limit values used in occupational health investigations for nicotine. There is some evidence that e-cigarettes may increase success rates for smoking cessation but uptake of e-cigarettes among non-smokers may lead to taking up smoking later in life.

Blood pressure

As early as the first or second decade of the twentieth century, the relationship between very high blood pressure and mortality was known and had led to the designation of 'malignant hypertension'. The invention of the sphygmomanometer in the last decade of the nineteenth century made the measurement of blood pressure at the bedside possible and the landmark description of the sounds and their relationship with pulse waves by Korotkoff in 1905 made the measurements more precise and standardized. However, the view in these early decades was that blood pressure lower than 210/110 mmHg was 'benign' and did not need to be treated. A vivid example of such views can be seen in the last years of the life of American president Franklin Delano Roosevelt, who died from a stroke in 1945 and had a systolic blood pressure of 300/190 mmHg on the day of his death. He had a recorded blood pressure of 186/108 one year earlier, but his personal physicians had considered it 'normal for a man of his age'. Despite a correct diagnosis of hypertension, hypertensive heart disease, and heart failure made by his cardiologist several months later, the understanding of blood pressure as a risk factor and options for treatment at that time were rather limited. Three years after Roosevelt's death, his successor Harry Truman signed the National Heart Act which stated that 'the Nation's health is seriously threatened by diseases of the heart and circulation, including high blood pressure. . .'.

Early evidence from analyses of life insurance records indicated that even 'normal' levels of blood pressure are associated with higher mortality. This view was further strengthened with large prospective studies in the United States and other high-income countries conducted in the 1950s and onwards. It is now clear, based on evidence from more than 100 prospective cohort studies and many randomized trials, that both systolic and diastolic blood pressure act as a continuous variable for CHD risk and that blood pressure levels even within the clinically 'normal' range may lead to higher risk of CHD (see Fig. 13.2.2). These studies collectively indicate that in people without any known vascular disease the 'optimal' level of systolic blood pressure may be as low as 115 mmHg. However, the debate on the exact 'optimal' level continues as evidence is still insufficient for individuals with very low blood pressure levels and those with known cardiovascular disease.

Among various measures of blood pressure, systolic blood pressure measured via the brachial artery has been shown to be most strongly associated with CHD risk. Other measures such as diastolic blood pressure, pulse pressure, ankle–brachial blood pressure index, and blood pressure measured at the wrist have also been used in epidemiological studies but are weaker determinants of CHD risk. Mean systolic blood pressure levels have been declining in high-income countries by as much as 4 mmHg per decade, possibly due to better diagnosis and treatment of cases as well as reduced smoking prevalence and intensity.

By contrast, during the past three decades blood pressure levels have increased in some developing countries, especially in eastern sub-Saharan Africa, and have remained stable elsewhere. Figure 13.2.4 shows the mean systolic blood pressure by country in 2008.

Analyses of data from more than 100 prospective observational studies show similar relative risks from different cohorts in Western and Asian populations as well as similar relative risks by gender. However, it is clear that relative risks decline by age, possibly due to higher competing risks by other causes of death as well as higher baseline CHD risks. Nonetheless, because of high absolute risk of CHD in elderly people, lowering blood pressure levels in the elderly is expected to have preventive effects similar to those in younger age groups. Pooled analysis of many large prospective studies indicate a 45% higher risk of CHD for each 20 mmHg higher systolic blood pressure level among individuals 55 to 64 years old.

Evidence from these observational prospective studies is corroborated by a large number of randomized clinical trials of antihypertensive treatment, starting from trials of the Veteran's Affairs healthcare system in the United States in the 1960s. Clinical trials of antihypertensive drugs have also shown that proportional effects are rather similar in different patient groups and using different classes of drug. See Chapter 17.2 for more details on diagnosis and management of hypertension.

Serum lipids

Dyslipidaemias are a major risk factor for CHD and are themselves affected by unhealthy diet as well as alcohol use, physical inactivity, and genetic factors. Early studies of familial hypercholesterolemia and studies by Ansel Keys and others on cross-country comparison

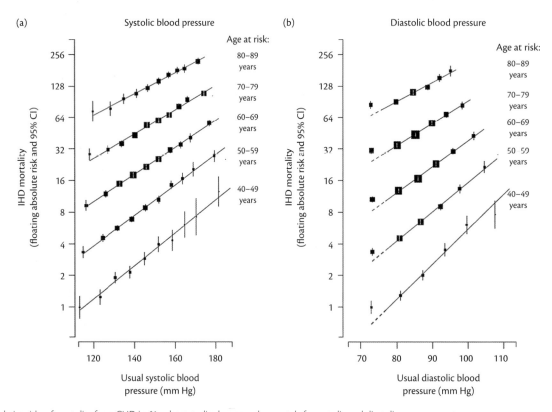

Fig. 13.2.3 Relative risks of mortality from CHD in 61 cohort studies by age and separately for systolic and diastolic measurements.
Reprinted from *The Lancet* Vol. 360, Prospective Studies Collaboration, Age-specific relevance of usual blood pressure to vascular mortality: a meta-analysis of individual data for one million adults in 61 prospective studies, 1903–13, 2002, with permission from Elsevier.

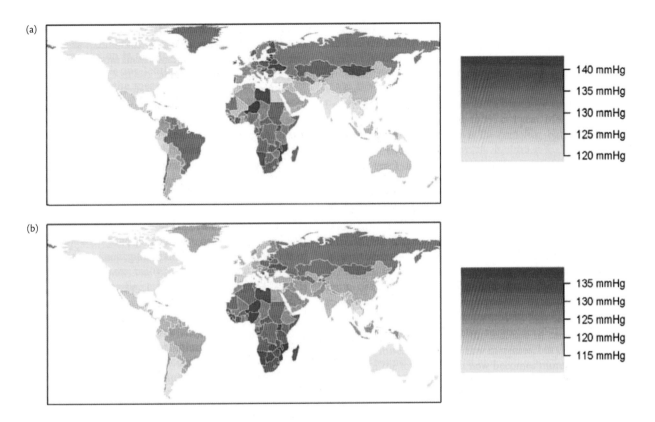

Fig. 13.2.4 Mean systolic blood pressure by country and gender in 2008 in men (a) and women (b).

Reprinted from *The Lancet* Vol. 377, Danaei G, Finucane MM, Lin JK, Singh GM, Paciorek CJ, Cowan MJ *et al.* National, regional, and global trends in systolic blood pressure since 1980: systematic analysis of health examination surveys and epidemiological studies with 786 country-years and 5.4 million participants. 569–77, 2011 with permission from Elsevier.

of CHD rates pointed to the potential role of cholesterol in CHD. Subsequently, analysis of data from the Framingham Heart Study and other prospective epidemiological studies indicated that high serum cholesterol was indeed positively associated with CHD risk. Separation of subfractions of serum lipids based on their density led to the identification of LDL and high-density lipoprotein (HDL) particles with opposite impacts on CHD risk.

In the past three decades, serum total cholesterol levels have declined in high-income countries, which back in the 1980s had some of the highest levels observed worldwide. In contrast, serum cholesterol levels have increased in many developing countries, especially in southeast Asia, therefore showing a 'global convergence' in serum total cholesterol levels.

As with high blood pressure, evidence from observational studies indicates a continuous increase in CHD risk with serum total cholesterol levels with no threshold at the commonly used clinical cut-off of 200 or 240 mg/dl (5–6 mmol/litre) and CHD risk continues to decline to very low levels of LDL cholesterol (about 80 mg/dl or 2 mmol/litre). Pooled analysis of multinational studies shows similar *relative risks* for dyslipidaemia across different populations and even in very low-risk populations such as the Chinese an association has been found between serum cholesterol and coronary mortality. Although the relationship between cholesterol and risk is not strong in elderly people it remains a major contributor because of their higher absolute risk of CHD.

Many randomized primary and secondary prevention clinical trials of cholesterol lowering, initially with fibrates and then with HMG coenzyme A reductase inhibitors (statins), support the

important role of serum cholesterol in CHD. The results clearly demonstrate the beneficial effects of these drugs with an estimated 20 to 40% reduction in coronary events that is largely independent of the starting cholesterol level. Initial fears that these statins were associated with an increased risk of cancer are unfounded; however, there appears to be a slightly increased risk of diabetes.

Although beneficial effects of having a higher HDL-cholesterol are well documented in epidemiological studies, clinical trials that aimed at increasing HDL using niacin, fibrates, or cholesteryl ester transfer protein (CETP) inhibitors have not been successful in reducing CHD risk. A few large-scale studies are still under way.

Observational studies have also found an association between apolipoproteins (i.e. apoAI and apoB) and lipoprotein-associated phospholipase A2 with CHD risk. There is also some evidence that levels of nonfasting serum total cholesterol are as predictive as fasting levels for CHD risk. The current evidence on the role of serum triglycerides on CHD is mixed, with some large pooling projects reporting no association between triglycerides and CHD after adjusting for other dyslipidaemias.

Obesity

Excess body fat (adiposity) has been linked to higher mortality since the first decades of the twentieth century. Since then, various measures of adiposity have been used in clinical and epidemiological studies including body weight, body mass index (BMI), waist circumference, waist-to-hip ratio, weight in water, and measurements of body fat using imaging modalities such as CT scans.

Among these measures, BMI, which 'standardizes' body weight to height (by dividing weight in kilograms by the square of height in metres) is most commonly used in epidemiological studies because of its ease of measurement and strong relationship with CHD and other health outcomes. However, it is well known that BMI does not measure fat mass and is a poor measure of adiposity in athletes and in elderly people. Furthermore, BMI does not reflect the distribution of fat in the body, which is a main determinant of the biological impact of adiposity. For example, there is a large body of evidence that abdominal fat is much more biologically active and therefore harmful than subcutaneous fat, and measures of abdominal obesity such as waist circumference and waist-to-hip ratio appear to be better predictors of cardiovascular outcomes.

The main determinants of adiposity are increased caloric intake and lower physical activity, as well as changes in body metabolism and genetic factors. The impact of obesity on CHD is partly mediated by hypertension, dyslipidaemia, and diabetes which collectively explain about 50% of the impact of adiposity on CHD. Other factors including low-grade chronic inflammation and increased coagulability are less important mediators.

Globally, the number of obese adults has doubled in the past 30 years and obesity is on the rise in almost all regions of the world. About one-third of the adult population in the United States of America are obese and another one-third are overweight by current World Health Organization (WHO) standards. Furthermore, childhood obesity is also on the rise in the United States and many other developed countries.

Observational epidemiological studies clearly indicate a continuous relationship between BMI and CHD at levels above 25 kg/m^2 and, in a similar manner to blood pressure and serum cholesterol,l there seems to be no threshold value to define obesity. The optimal levels of adiposity are the current focus of interest in many studies: some studies have shown risk reduction for CHD to levels as low as 21 kg/m^2; others have shown that the nadir may be higher, at around 23–25 kg/m^2. Epidemiological evidence on the impact of weight change on CHD (especially weight loss) is mixed. This is partly because it is hard to separate any beneficial effect of weight loss from the harmful impact of undiagnosed diseases in which weight loss is a feature. Nonrandomized studies of bariatric surgery in morbidly obese patients show rapid reversal of physiological changes, especially diabetes after surgery, but these observations may be due to hormonal changes rather than weight loss per se.

There is little evidence, if any, from randomized clinical trials on the beneficial effect of weight loss in CHD. Clinical trials of diet have often managed to induce weight loss in the first year but the weight loss has not been maintained for a sufficient period to detect a benefit. However, weight loss trials do show improvements in metabolic profiles such as reduced blood pressure and serum cholesterol and improved glucose tolerance, which should in principle lead to future reductions in CHD risk. Such lack of evidence for benefits of weight loss increases the importance of preventing weight gain, starting in early adolescence.

Diabetes mellitus

Diabetes is a major risk factor for CHD. There has been a substantial increase in the number of diabetic patients in almost all regions of the world, with a global prevalence of about 10% in adults. This rise has been partly fuelled by increases in obesity and therefore is expected to continue in the coming decades if current trends in unhealthy diet, urbanization, and physical inactivity continue.

Earlier studies of diabetes patients mostly focused on microvascular complications and the threshold levels above which the risk of these complications sharply increased. These thresholds were then used to set clinical cut-offs to diagnose diabetes.

Recent studies indicate that similar to blood pressure and serum cholesterol, the relative risks for different cardiovascular outcomes (when shown on a doubling scale) are linearly associated with various measures of blood glucose such as fasting plasma glucose, even down to levels below the conventional thresholds used to define diabetes (up to 4.9–5.3 mmol/L); see Fig. 13.2.5.

The landmark UKPDS study identified a quintet of modifiable risk factors for CHD in non-insulin-dependent diabetes mellitus comprising HDL and LDL cholesterol, haemoglobin A$_{1C}$, systolic blood pressure, and smoking. Of these the relative risks were highest for LDL cholesterol and blood pressure. CHD risk in diabetic patients may be further refined by the detection of microalbuminuria as a reflection of early endothelial and microvascular damage.

The optimal levels of blood glucose for CHD risk are still under debate, partly because several large randomized clinical trials of intensive glucose control among diabetic patients failed to show

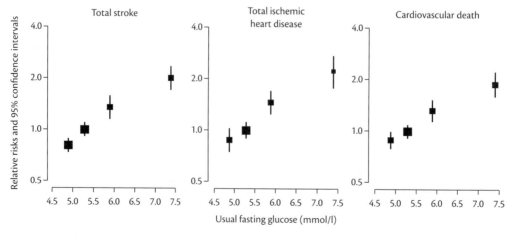

Fig. 13.2.5 Relative risk of stroke and CHD by fasting glucose levels.
From Lawes CM, Parag V, Bennett DA, Suh I, Lam TH, Whitlock G, *et al.* Blood glucose and risk of cardiovascular disease in the Asia Pacific region. *Diabetes Care* 2004;**27**(12):2836–42.

consistent reduction in risk. Early trials of intensive treatment were not powered to detect a small reduction in CHD risk and more recent trials showed mixed results: some studies indicated increased risk possibly due to higher age at enrolment or side effects of drugs, including hypoglycaemia, and others did not detect an effect, possibly due to use of other preventive drugs in the control groups that reduced the power to detect any change in the outcomes.

Several large randomized trials have shown that modification of lifestyle (such as quitting smoking, weight loss, and a healthy diet) and medical intervention may substantially reduce the risk of diabetes among high-risk patients (i.e. obese individuals or those who have borderline high blood glucose). A particular focus of interest in diabetes prevention and control is improving the quality of dietary carbohydrates to include less processed carbohydrates and more whole grains. Another potential preventive intervention is reducing sugar-sweetened beverage intake, which is associated with higher risk of obesity.

Diet quality

The evidence on the link between diet quality and CHD has grown substantially in the last few decades and the focus of this line of research has changed from analysis of specific macro- and micro-nutrients to foods and dietary patterns. Early epidemiological data identified the Mediterranean diet which is high in olive oil, cereals, nuts, and vegetables and low in animal fat as protective against cardiovascular disease, and a recent large randomized trial has corroborated this finding. Below, we summarize the main evidence on CHD prevention by improving diet quality.

Fat composition

The relationship between dietary fat composition and CHD has been one of the major sources of controversy in the field of nutritional epidemiology. The recommendation for a low-fat diet in the 1970s was based mostly on ecological studies in the 1960s that had shown a positive correlation between average saturated fat intake and CHD mortality across countries and short-term feeding studies and animal studies that had shown a rise in serum total cholesterol with higher saturated fat intake. However, more recent reanalyses of the feeding studies and results of prospective studies of diet and CHD showed no increased risk of CHD if saturated fat was substituted by carbohydrates, which could partly be explained by increases in both LDL- and HDL-cholesterol.

The importance of polyunsaturated fats (in particular those high in n-3 and n-6 fatty acids) was proposed following observational studies in the 1970s suggesting a low incidence of coronary disease in Greenland and Alaskan Eskimos consuming a diet based on oily cold-water fish. The beneficial effects could be mediated by the impact of polyunsaturated fats on coagulation, platelet and endothelial function, and serum LDL and HDL composition and levels. The effect of higher intake of polyunsaturated fatty acids in reducing CHD risk is consistent with recent evidence from a large randomized trial which showed lower CHD risk among individuals who received a serving (about 30 g) of nuts every day for 5 years. The impact of n-3 fatty acids on CHD prevention has also been widely studied. Meta-analysis of observational studies show a protective effect of higher omega-3 intake with beneficial effects for an intake of up to 250 mg/day. However, the most recent meta-analysis of randomized trials of omega-3 supplementation did not find any reduction in mortality or risk of myocardial infarction. There is now a general consensus that *trans* fats from hydrogenated oils increase the risk of CHD by increasing LDL- and lowering HDL-cholesterol, and there is strong evidence that substituting saturated fats with polyunsaturated fats reduces CHD risk.

The current trends toward higher intake of animal meet and processed foods as developing countries progress economically may well increase the harmful impact of fat composition on CHD. However, a recent global analysis of nutritional surveys indicated that between 1990 and 2010 intakes of *trans* and saturated fatty acids remained fairly stable while those of n-6 and n-3 fatty acids increased.

Salt

Our perception of salt has changed from being a useful food preservative to becoming one of the main causes of high blood pressure which is itself the leading risk factor for CHD worldwide. The levels of salt intake in many countries have been fairly stable in the past 20 years. However, the current global intake (c.10 g/day) is almost double the recommended level. Salt intake is highest in East and Central Asia, and eastern Europe.

Many observational studies have reported a positive association between salt intake and risk of CHD but some studies have also reported a lower intake of salt to be associated with higher risk of mortality in particular groups of patients, such as those with chronic renal failure or congestive heart failure, which is most likely due to 'reverse causation' where the underlying disease leads to both reduction in salt intake and higher cardiovascular mortality.

Several dozen randomized clinical trials of sodium reduction have shown reduction in blood pressure following short-term feeding interventions that reduce sodium intake. In meta-analyses of these trials, each 100 mmol/litre reduction in sodium intake (equivalent to 2.3 g salt) has been associated with 4–7 mmHg reduction in systolic blood pressure and the effects are larger in older or hypertensive individuals. Although a reduction in blood pressure is expected to reduce the risk of CHD and stroke, only the long-term follow-up of one of the larger sodium reduction trials has shown some reduction in CHD risk.

The optimal level of salt intake is still highly debated and the most recent recommendations from national guidelines in the United States of America and the United Kingdom suggest 5.8 g/day. There is some evidence that current efforts to reduce salt intake in the United Kingdom may have been responsible for further reductions in CHD risk at the population level, and WHO recommends salt reduction programmes as one of the most cost-effective ways to prevent CHD.

Other dietary components

Fruit and vegetables

Low intake of fruits and vegetables has been linked to higher CHD risk in several prospective observational studies, leading to recommendations of at least five daily servings of fruits and vegetables to prevent CHD and other noncommunicable diseases. In the absence of randomized trials that directly evaluate this effect, there is still potential for such associations to be due to confounding by other lifestyle factors. The mechanisms and pathways for such potential effects are not quite clear and could include the effects of fruits on increasing potassium intake and therefore lowering blood pressure.

Red and processed meat

The controversy about the effect of fresh red meat intake on CHD continues but there is ample evidence from several observational studies on the harmful effects of processed meat on CHD which could partly be due to the increased risk of diabetes: each 50 g per day higher intake of processed meat is associated with 42% higher risk of CHD.

Folate, B$_{12}$, and homocysteine

There is fairly strong evidence from observational studies that higher serum homocysteine levels are associated with CHD risk. However, randomized clinical trials of folate and vitamin B$_{12}$ supplementation have found mixed results for benefits of homocysteine reduction. A large 'Mendelian randomization study' that used the *MTHFR* gene as the instrument to examine the effect of lower homocysteine on cardiovascular disease did not find any benefits.

Dietary cholesterol

Despite the strong epidemiological data relating serum cholesterol to the incidence of cardiovascular disease, studies based on the lowering of dietary cholesterol alone have not been conclusive and there is currently insufficient evidence on the impact of dietary cholesterol on serum cholesterol levels and risk of CHD.

Dairy products

There is no evidence that higher dairy intake is associated with CHD risk, possibly due to beneficial effects through blood pressure reduction which are balanced by harmful effects through increased risk of arterial calcification. Similarly, there is no evidence that intake of whole-fat dairy would increase the risk of CHD.

Exercise, fitness, and sedentary lifestyle

Physical inactivity is associated with higher risk of CHD and increased urbanization and mechanization has the potential to reduce activity levels in many developed and developing countries worldwide. Early studies in the 1960s on London bus conductors and longshoremen in San Francisco (California) and more recent research on various types and durations of activity has shown a dose–response relationship with 30 to 35% risk reduction for CHD in the most active individuals compared with the least active. The current prevention guidelines recommend at least half an hour of moderate or vigorous activity at least 5 days a week.

More than a dozen observational studies have found a beneficial effect on CHD, which is partly mediated through weight loss as well as reductions in blood pressure. Vigorous physical activity can also be a trigger for acute myocardial infarction and the overall risk should be balanced when encouraging patients to increase their physical activity.

Cardiorespiratory fitness can be considered the consequence of physical activity and is often measured by exercise tolerance testing. A recent meta-analysis of observational studies reported that each 1 km/h higher speed of running or jogging is associated with a 15% reduction in risk of CHD.

Finally, a new line of research has identified sedentary lifestyle as a risk factor for CHD (and mortality) above and beyond physical inactivity. Each additional 2 h of screen time is linked to 5% higher risk of cardiovascular events. The associations were weaker but still significant for overall sitting time. Reducing television watching time in children is one of the few interventions that have proved beneficial in controlling childhood obesity.

In summary, higher physical activity levels are associated with reduced risk of CHD even if the achieved levels do not quite reach the recommended frequencies and intensities.

Alcohol

More than 30 observational studies have found beneficial effects of regular and moderate alcohol drinking on CHD risk and all types of alcohol beverages seem to confer this benefit similarly. Heavy and binge drinking will offset these beneficial effects. The potential mechanism of benefits may include reducing platelet adhesion. However, there is also evidence of harmful effects through increasing blood pressure, higher risk of cardiac arrhythmias, and myocardial damage at higher levels of intake.

In 2005, just over 40% of adults worldwide drank alcohol. Massive and rapid changes in alcohol intake were responsible for the largest observed increase CHD mortality in modern times, which happened in Russia in the 1990s.

Illicit drugs

Among various illicit drugs, cocaine abuse has been clearly identified as a trigger for acute myocardial events. Intake of marijuana also has the biological potential to increase the risk of atherosclerosis and act as a trigger of acute events, but trials of cannabinoid receptor antagonists failed to reduce CHD risk. There is recent evidence from a large observational study in Iran that opium use may increase CHD mortality.

Sleep duration and quality

Insufficient sleep is associated with higher risk of CHD, possibly through its effect on blood pressure as well as systemic inflammation, oxidative stress, and endothelial dysfunction. An extreme example is obstructive sleep apnoea which is linked to a potential doubling of CHD risk.

Psychosocial factors

Major depression has been associated with higher CHD risk in observational studies with the risk increasing by 80% in patients with a history of major depression episode. However, randomized trials of antidepressant treatment among CHD patients have provided mixed results.

The role of stress in CHD was initially investigated by identifying 'character types' in early prospective studies such as the Framingham Heart Study. Chronic stress is a clear cause of high blood pressure and acute stress can act as a trigger for myocardial events. Evidence is also emerging from studies of relaxation response which seem to indicate a beneficial response on blood pressure levels.

Various types of psychosocial stress are associated with higher CHD risk. These include acute and chronic stressors and anxiety as well as a sense of deprivation and inequality, social isolation, and poor social support. The opposite may also be true: positive emotions are associated with a lower risk of CHD in observational studies. Stronger evidence on the causal relationship between these factors and CHD is required. The few trials that have so far been conducted failed to show a protective effect for psychosocial interventions, possibly due to simultaneous improvements occurring in the usual care group.

Environmental factors

The harmful effect of outdoor and indoor air pollution on CHD has been shown in observational studies. Higher concentrations of smaller particles (PM 2.5) is more strongly associated with risk of CHD than larger particles (PM 10). Globally in 2010, 22% of the burden of disease from CHD was attributed to ambient air pollution. In rural areas and developing countries, similar harmful effects have been observed due to burning solid fuels indoors for cooking or heating which causes 18% of the burden of disease due to CHD.

Recent evidence has also linked high road traffic noise levels to risk of CHD, possibly through increasing blood pressure. Chronic lead exposure has been associated with higher blood pressure, which could itself lead to higher CHD risk. Harmful effects have also been reported for cadmium exposure and high doses of arsenic.

HIV and other infections

With more successful and accessible HIV treatments, the interaction between HIV and its treatment with CHD and other cardiovascular diseases has become a novel area of research. It is well known that some antiretroviral drugs increase serum cholesterol levels and the pathophysiology of HIV infection may itself lead to dyslipidaemia, and there is some evidence that effective HIV treatment may lead to weight gain. However, the overall impact of long-term HIV infection and antiretroviral treatment on CHD remains unknown. Other viral or bacterial infections have also been associated with CHD risk. However, there is currently no strong evidence that such associations are independent of other well-known risk factors.

Chronic renal insufficiency

There is now fairly strong evidence from observational studies that chronic renal disease increases the risk of CHD and cardiac disease is the leading cause of death among endstage renal disease patients. Even smaller rises in serum creatinine have been linked to slightly higher risk of CHD and point to the need for more aggressive management of classic risk factors in these patients. The potential mechanisms are through higher blood pressure levels, dyslipidaemia, anaemia, and increased systemic inflammation.

Novel biomarkers

A number of inflammatory, haemostatic and coagulation markers have been associated with higher CHD risk. Among these C-reactive protein, fibrinogen, and interleukin-6 are the most well known. However, there is still insufficient evidence on the exact role of these biomarkers and therefore it is not clear how they may be used to design preventive interventions. Of particular interest is their use in improving risk prediction models and discovery of new therapeutic targets.

Gender and genetic influences

Despite a lower incidence of myocardial infarction in women compared to men, CHD is the most common cause of death in women in most developed countries. The rate of decline in death from coronary disease has also been less for women than for men.

The difference in incidence of coronary disease between men and women is not explained by conventional risk factors alone. Although there is no distinct inflection in the incidence of coronary disease in women around the menopause, the difference in incidence of CHD has been attributed to the impact of hormonal changes. This concept was supported by theoretical considerations on the impact of oestrogens and progesterone on the vasculature and thrombogenesis and a meta-analysis of observational studies suggesting that hormone replacement therapy (HRT) might be protective. The Women's Health Initiative trial of HRT strongly refuted this hypothesis, finding an increased risk of events (OR 1.29) among women randomized to HRT.

Several studies have demonstrated the independent association of family history with the risk of cardiovascular disease. However, the observed associations tend to add very little to risk discrimination when risk prediction models include other traditional risk factors. Nonetheless, based on twin and family studies, there is little doubt that a large proportion of susceptibility to CHD is heritable. This knowledge has sparked numerous genetic studies, which have the advantage of not being confounded by environmental exposures, in an effort to establish causality of known risk factors and risk markers and to identify novel pathways and therapeutic targets.

To date, multiple genome-wide association studies (GWAS) investigating tens of thousands of single nucleotide polymorphisms (SNPs) have been reported. These studies have convincingly identified multiple loci that are associated with CHD risk. The largest meta-analysis of these studies, involving 63 746 CHD cases and 130 681 controls of European and South Asian ancestry, reported 45 SNPs across the genome which were significantly associated with an increased risk of CHD. However, associations were relatively weak (odds ratios between 1.031 and 1.126 per risk allele) and, taken together, they explained no more than 10.6% of the genetic variance of CHD. Many of the variants appeared to contribute to risk through traditional risk factors. More specifically, 5 were associated with blood pressure and 12 with lipid concentrations. By contrast, there was no significant association of any of the loci tested with type 2 diabetes. In the same study, the investigators employed a network analysis with 233 candidate genes to reveal potential pathways of gene disease interaction. The four most significant pathways mapping to these networks were linked to lipid metabolism and inflammation, underscoring the causal role of these activities in the genetic aetiology of CHD.

Although genetic markers, in particular those that show potential new causal pathways, are highly valuable for identification of new molecular targets for prevention and management of CHD, so far their incremental value on risk prediction has not been established. For example, a genetic risk score created from 101 SNPs associated with cardiovascular disease (CVD) did not improve discriminatory ability of a risk score based on traditional risk factors.

It has been argued that more precise classification of subtypes of CHD is needed in order to better understand the impact of different mutations on the biology and pathophysiology of CHD. Supporting evidence for this line of thinking comes from a study that showed different SNPs to be associated with different manifestations of CHD, with some increasing the risk of coronary atherosclerosis while others are associated with the risk of plaque rupture and acute myocardial infarction. In addition to pathophysiological pathways, the impact of genetic variants may differ by presence or absence of comorbid conditions. In one large-scale study, the same

SNP was associated with a significantly higher risk of CHD among patients with diabetes but no significant difference in risk of CHD among patients without diabetes was observed.

Clusters of risk factors: the metabolic syndrome

The concept of metabolic syndrome (syndrome X or insulin resistance syndrome) was proposed in the late 1980s to designate a constellation of risk factors for CVD. The idea was that co-occurrence of several risk factors may be due to common underlying pathophysiological processes and may confer a level of risk that is larger than the sum of the effect of each risk factor alone. The components of metabolic syndrome include hyperglycaemia, hypertriglyceridaemia and low HDL levels, high blood pressure, and abdominal obesity. Some studies have found that the patients with metabolic syndrome have twice as high a CHD risk compared with individuals with no risk factor. However, others have argued based on similar analyses in different settings that the 'syndrome' may just be a co-occurrence of a subset of cardiovascular risk factors and not an entity by itself. Irrespective of these debates, many clinicians

continue to use this term to alert others of the presence of the cluster of risk factors in an individual.

Combining risk factors to predict and manage risk in individuals

Successful and cost-effective prevention of CHD requires identification of high-risk individuals who would benefit more from risk reduction. One way of identifying high-risk individuals is to measure their risk factor levels and use clinical thresholds for each risk factor separately to designate a high-risk status (e.g. hypertensive or diabetic). This approach has been used in the past 50 years and is still the method commonly used by many clinicians and clinical practice guidelines. However, as summarized above, CHD is a multifactorial disease and most risk factors increase CHD even at levels well below the conventional thresholds used to define high-risk status. Generally, single risk factors are rarely accurate enough in predicting future risk for individuals. For example, for a binary risk marker to provide good discrimination between those who will suffer an event from those who will not,

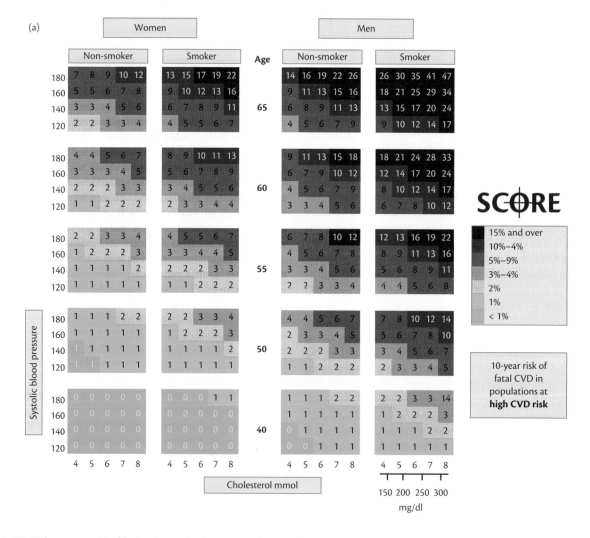

Fig. 13.2.6 SCORE chart: 10 year risk of fatal cardiovascular disease in populations at high (a) and low CVD (b) risk calculating using the following risk factors: age, gender, smoking, systolic blood pressure (SBP), and total cholesterol.

From Conroy, R. M., Pyörälä, K., Fitzgerald, A. E., Sans, S., Menotti, A., De Backer, G. et al. (2003). Estimation of ten-year risk of fatal cardiovascular disease in Europe: the SCORE project. *European Heart Journal*, 24(11), 987–1003.

the odds ratio of that marker with the outcome would need to be greater than about 9, which is not the case for any single risk factor described here. Therefore, to predict an individual's risk one has to combine the information on levels of the most important risk factors. A common way of doing this is to use a 'risk prediction score'. Most risk prediction scores combine CHD and stroke to provide a predicted risk for overall CVD.

The most well-known risk score is the Framingham Risk Score, which is based on the analysis of the Framingham Heart Study cohort in Massachusetts (USA). Each risk score is a combination of a 'baseline' or average risk and a set of coefficients for different risk factors that predict how each individual deviates from that average risk based on how much his/her risk factor levels deviate from mean risk factor levels in the target population. To apply a risk score to a new population, the average risk and mean risk factor levels have to be recalibrated to correspond to the target population; otherwise the risk score will be biased. Most risk scores use information on the major CVD risk factors such as smoking, blood pressure, serum cholesterol, and diabetes. Others include socioeconomic factors and family history of heart disease as well.

Although risk prediction scores, even when based on a few simple risk factors, are usually more accurate in estimating risk than individual risk factors or a qualitative summary of several risk factors

by clinicians, their performance is still far from ideal. In particular, for those individuals classified as having an intermediate level of risk, application of risk scores is often inadequate and inconsistent. Therefore, many researchers are focusing on identifying new risk factors or risk markers that can help improve the performance of prevailing models that are based on traditional risk factors. Several potentially useful novel risk factors are summarized earlier in the chapter, of which so far inflammatory markers have had the greatest potential in improving the predictive value of risk scores. In addition to the risk factors mentioned above, several other biomarkers have been evaluated. For instance, blood BNP levels or different types of vascular imaging (carotid intima-media thickness and coronary calcium scoring) have shown some promising results. However, further research is under way to establish the value of such markers to subgroups of patients and healthcare systems.

Most risk scores provide an approximate 10-year risk of CHD or CVD risk and the clinicians can then use this information along with current clinical guidelines to propose a prevention strategy for each patient. Primary intervention (i.e. for patients without pre-existing vascular disease) is based on a threshold of risk. One example, the SCORE chart (Fig. 13.2.6) is based on fatal CVD risk. All individuals with a fatal CVD risk greater than 5% (corresponding to a Framingham risk of CHD of approximately 20%) should

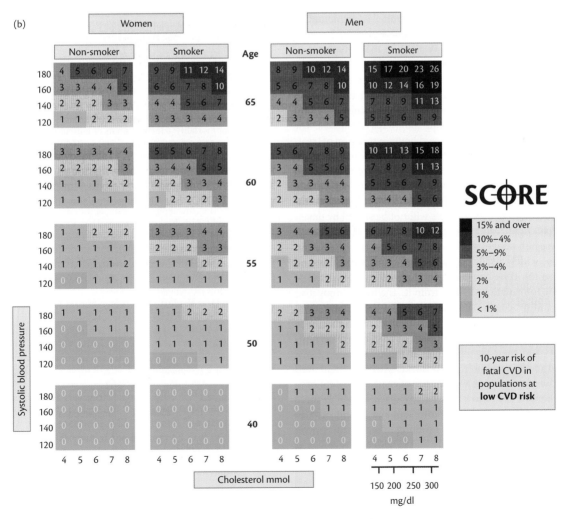

Fig. 13.2.6 Continued

be offered lifestyle advice and specific treatment for individual risk factors. Use of the SCORE chart in conjunction with guidelines for treatment of hypertension (see Chapter 17.2) will guide priorities in drug therapy. Very high levels of individual risk factors (blood pressure >160/110 mmHg or a total cholesterol of >8 mmol/litre) should be treated in their own right.

Risk prediction scores have also been used to assign antithrombotic treatment to patients without a prior vascular event. However, the use of aspirin for primary prevention is controversial because, despite the clear evidence for its beneficial effects on the risk of vascular events, it is also known to cause gastrointestinal bleeding and haemorrhagic stroke. Because the risk of vascular events as well as bleeding events both increase with age, it is hard to justify the use of aspirin in people beyond a certain age. However, more recent evidence suggests that aspirin may also reduce the risk of gastrointestinal cancer. If this effect is confirmed, it is likely that aspirin use in the primary prevention setting will lead to net clinical benefits.

Likely future developments

Several risk factors have been shown to be significantly associated with future risk of CHD and a few of these, largely through randomized trials, are known to cause CHD.

Although new research into new CHD risk factors is likely to help identify new molecular targets for its management, the shorter-term advantage that such new markers may offer is an increasing accuracy in the estimation of CHD risk and treatment benefits. Large-scale observational studies investigating the utility of new biomarkers, both phenotypic and genotypic, will help improve the accuracy of existing risk scores. This, combined with randomized evidence (e.g. from large individual patient data meta-analyses), will provide more granular information about the safety and efficacy of specific interventions in specific subgroups of patients. The combination of better risk prediction and better estimation of treatment effects in subgroups of patients is expected to lead to personalized or precision medicine, where those with the greatest risk and greatest opportunity for treatment will be offered an intervention. However, the challenge of maximizing benefits of preventive therapies for individuals as well as societies will not be solved by developing better risk engines and risk management algorithms alone.

Previous research suggests that cardiovascular risk prediction models are not widely used, partly because many clinicians find risk calculation too time consuming and remain unconvinced of the value of the information derived from it. The use of innovative technologies and processes, such as automated data capture systems and better techniques for risk visualization, could minimize user burden and facilitate communication of risks and uncertainties to patients and their families. Similar tools could also make information directly accessible to consumers, which might well increase their engagement, as well as that of their healthcare providers. Ultimately, a scenario could be envisaged in which there is seamless linkage between data capture, risk and benefit estimation, and clinical practice guidelines, resulting in the routine provision of personalized guidance for care that is both evidence-based and cost-effective. However, given that the introduction of such innovative models in complex healthcare environments can have multiple intended and unintended effects, appropriately designed studies are needed to evaluate the actual effects of such system changes before more general recommendations are made.

Further reading

American College of Sports Medicine; American Heart Association (2007). Exercise and acute cardiovascular events: placing the risks into perspective. *Med Sci Sports Exerc*, **39**, 886–97.

Armitage JM, *et al.* (2012). Effects of homocysteine-lowering with folic acid plus vitamin B12 vs placebo on mortality and major morbidity in myocardial infarction survivors: A randomized trial. *JAMA*, **303**, 2486–94.

Boussageon R, *et al.* (2011). Effect of intensive glucose lowering treatment on all cause mortality, cardiovascular death, and microvascular events in type 2 diabetes: meta-analysis of randomised controlled trials. *BMJ*, **343**, d4169.

Conroy RM, *et al.* (2003). Estimation of ten-year risk of fatal cardiovascular disease in Europe: the SCORE project. *Eur Heart J*, **24**, 987–1003. Epub 2003/06/06.

Danaei G, *et al.* (2010). The promise of prevention: the effects of four preventable risk factors on national life expectancy and life expectancy disparities by race and county in the United States. *PLoS Med*, **7**, e1000248.

Deloukas P, *et al.* (2013). Large-scale association analysis identifies new risk loci for coronary artery disease. *Nat Genet*, **45**, 25–33.

Ezzati M, *et al.* (2005). Role of smoking in global and regional cardiovascular mortality. *Circulation*, **112**, 489–97.

Ezzati M, *et al.* (2004). Smoking and oral tobacco use. In: Comparative quantification of health risks: Global and regional burden of disease attributable to selected major risk factors. Geneva: World Health Organization, pp. 883–957.

Ford ES, Caspersen CJ. (2012). Sedentary behaviour and cardiovascular disease: a review of prospective studies. *Int J Epidemiol*, **41**, 1338–53.

Lewington S, *et al.* (2002). Age-specific relevance of usual blood pressure to vascular mortality: a meta-analysis of individual data for one million adults in 61 prospective studies. *Lancet*, **360**(9349), 1903–13.

Lewington S, *et al.* (2007). Blood cholesterol and vascular mortality by age, sex, and blood pressure: a meta-analysis of individual data from 61 prospective studies with 55,000 vascular deaths. *Lancet*, **370**(9602), 1829–39.

Lu Y, *et al.* (2014). Metabolic mediators of the effects of body-mass index, overweight, and obesity on coronary heart disease and stroke: a pooled analysis of 97 prospective cohorts with 1.8 million participants. *Lancet*, **383**(9921), 970–83.

Moran AE, *et al.* (2014). Temporal trends in ischemic heart disease mortality in 21 world regions, 1980 to 2010: the Global Burden of Disease 2010 study. *Circulation*, **129**, 1483–92.

Mozaffarian D, *et al.* (2010). Effects on coronary heart disease of increasing polyunsaturated fat in place of saturated fat: a systematic review and meta-analysis of randomized controlled trials. *PLoS Med*, **7**, e1000252.

Powles J, *et al.* (2013). Global, regional, and national sodium intakes in 1990 and 2010: a systematic analysis of 24 h urinary sodium excretion and dietary surveys worldwide. *BMJ Open*, **3**: e003733.

Turner RC, *et al.* (1998). Risk factors for coronary artery disease in non-insulin dependent diabetes mellitus: United Kingdom Prospective Diabetes Study (UKPDS: 23). *BMJ*, **316**(7134), 823–8.

Yusuf S, *et al.* (2004). Effect of potentially modifiable risk factors associated with myocardial infarction in 52 countries (the INTERHEART study): case-control study. *Lancet*, **364**(9438), 937–52.

CHAPTER 13.3

Management of stable angina

Adam D. Timmis

Essentials

Angina—the pain provoked by myocardial ischaemia—is usually caused by obstructive coronary artery disease that is sufficiently severe to restrict oxygen delivery to the cardiac myocytes. Quality of life is impaired in direct proportion to the severity of symptoms.

Clinical history remains the most useful basis for diagnosis and referral decisions to specialist services, the commonest indications being (1) new-onset angina, (2) exclusion of angina in high-risk individuals with atypical symptoms, (3) worsening angina in a patient with previously stable symptoms, (4) new or recurrent angina in a patient with history of myocardial infarction or coronary revascularization, (5) assessment of occupational fitness (e.g. airline pilots).

Investigation—noninvasive testing is used primarily for diagnosis, but whatever test is employed—exercise ECG, myocardial perfusion imaging, stress echocardiography, or multidetector CT—the incremental diagnostic value is greatest for patients with an intermediate pretest probability of coronary artery disease in whom uncertainty is greatest. Such tests also have a role in risk assessment to inform decisions about the urgency and aggressiveness of treatment in individual cases.

Medical treatment of angina involves (1) dealing with exacerbating comorbidities, (2) secondary prevention by lifestyle modification (smoking cessation, exercise training, Mediterranean-style diet, etc.) and drugs (aspirin, statins, etc.), (3) antianginal drugs (most commonly β-blockers, calcium channel blockers, and short-acting nitrates).

Patients with continuing moderate or severe stable angina despite optimal medical treatment should undergo coronary angiography, particularly if they are identified as being at high risk on noninvasive testing. In symptomatic patients, revascularization is generally indicated if one or more of the major coronary arteries—or their large branches—have flow-limiting stenoses (>70% luminal narrowing) or occlusions. Percutaneous coronary intervention (PCI) and coronary artery bypass grafting (CABG) produce comparable symptomatic benefit. With regard to life expectancy, PCI does not produce survival benefit in patients with stable angina. By contrast, studies more than 40 years ago showed that CABG produced small gains in life expectancy in some patients.

With current management strategies, patients with angina are living longer, but a few remain symptomatic with poor quality of life despite optimal medical treatment and having exhausted revascularization options. Psychological support is important to treat anxiety and depression and improve confidence, but other treatment options such as neuromodulatory techniques are not evidence-based and do not have guideline recommendations.

Introduction

Angina—the pain provoked by myocardial ischaemia—is usually caused by obstructive coronary artery disease that is sufficiently severe to restrict oxygen delivery to the cardiac myocytes (Box 13.3.1). It is one of the most common initial manifestations of coronary artery disease, occurs almost as commonly in women as in men, and is not showing the steep decline in incidence seen for acute myocardial infarction. When angina occurs in patients without coronary artery disease it may be attributable to other ischaemic mechanisms such as severe anaemia resulting in inadequate oxygen delivery to the cardiac myocytes, or left ventricular hypertrophy secondary to hypertension or aortic stenosis resulting in increased oxygen demand. The appropriately named syndrome X is a diagnosis of exclusion in patients with angina and unobstructed coronary arteries for which there is no clear cause despite full cardiac investigation: abnormal microvascular function is one proposed mechanism, but although symptoms are often resistant to treatment, prognosis is usually good in terms of life expectancy.

In most patients with angina caused by coronary artery disease, quality of life is impaired in direct proportion to the severity of symptoms (Fig. 13.3.1). Prognosis is often good, particularly in patients with chronic stable symptoms receiving contemporary secondary prevention therapy, but in those with recently diagnosed angina risk is greater, with a 2 to 3% incidence of death or nonfatal myocardial infarction in the first year. Recognition of the need for early investigation has led to the widespread implementation of chest pain clinics in the United Kingdom and elsewhere to provide patients with suspected angina prompt treatment to relieve symptoms and reduce risk.

Referral for specialist assessment

Referral for specialist assessment (Box 13.3.2) is indicated in all patients with known coronary artery disease—particularly those with previous myocardial infarction or coronary revascularization—who experience abrupt worsening of symptoms, often indicating plaque rupture and risk of impending infarction.

However, referral decisions may be more difficult in patients presenting for the first time with chest pain. A noncardiac diagnosis accounts for most cases, but it is the task of the primary care or general physician to ensure that all those with suspected

Box 13.3.1 Causes of angina

Reduced myocardial oxygen supply

◆ Coronary artery disease

• Atherosclerosis

• Spasm

• Vasculitic disorders

• Post radiation therapy

◆ Severe anaemia

Increased myocardial oxygen demand

◆ Left ventricular hypertrophy

• Hypertension

• Aortic stenosis

• Aortic regurgitation

• Hypertrophic cardiomyopathy

◆ Right ventricular hypertrophy

• Pulmonary hypertension

• Pulmonary stenosis

◆ Rapid tachyarrhythmias

Indeterminate mechanism

◆ Syndrome X

Box 13.3.2 Angina—indications for specialist cardiological referral

◆ New-onset angina

◆ Exclusion of angina in high-risk individuals with atypical symptoms

◆ Worsening angina in a patient with previously stable symptoms

◆ New or recurrent angina in a patient with history of:

◆ Myocardial infarction

• Coronary revascularization

◆ Assessment of occupational fitness (e.g. airline pilots)

In primary care, screening is based largely on the character of the symptoms and the age and gender of the patient, other risk factors further helping to identify those with a high probability of coronary artery disease (see below). Access to noninvasive diagnostic tests can be helpful in primary care or the nonspecialist clinic, but there is often insufficient recognition of their limitations, the exercise ECG (for example) having a diagnostic sensitivity of only about 68%, which means that up to one-third of all cases with coronary disease are missed. For this reason, the clinical history remains the most useful basis for diagnosis and referral decisions. Thresholds for referral should be lowered in high-risk patients, including those with previous myocardial infarction and diabetes, and also in airline pilots and public service drivers whose occupations might put others at risk in the event of myocardial infarction or sudden death.

The recommendation that all patients with suspected angina be referred for specialist assessment leaves little room for prevarication. Yet studies repeatedly show inequitable management of patients with chest pain, those with the greatest need often being the very patients who receive the least intensive treatment. Thus elderly patients with chest pain are at heightened risk, but are less likely than their younger counterparts to receive referral to chest pain clinics. Women are also disadvantaged and are less likely than men to be referred, even though it is increasingly recognized that angina in women is almost as common as in men and prognosis little better (Fig. 13.3.2). The reasons for this inequity are complex and poorly understood, but the consequences for health care are important.

Diagnosis of angina

Angina varies considerably in its clinical presentation and its overlap with other entities can make the differential diagnosis of chest pain difficult. A detailed description of the symptom complex is the most important step in the diagnostic process and in the context of other factors, particularly age and gender, allows the clinician to estimate the probability of coronary artery disease. The extent of work-up required to exclude a noncardiac cause needs to be individually determined. The diagnosis is informed by the clinician's intuition, experience, and interviewing skills, supported by investigations such as resting ECG, stress testing, and coronary angiography.

Clinical evaluation

A careful history of the character, location, radiation, provocation, and duration of the chest pain provides the most useful

angina receive specialist assessment for confirmation of the diagnosis and risk stratification to identify those at greatest risk who need more intensive treatment. As in any screening process, false-negative diagnoses in which patients receive inappropriate reassurance must be avoided. By contrast, a proportion of false-positive diagnoses and referrals is acceptable, and among patients referred from primary care to chest pain clinics 75% have a non-cardiac diagnosis.

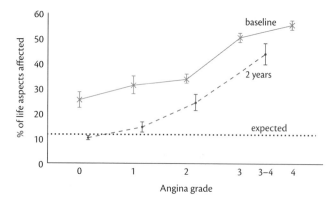

Fig. 13.3.1 Effect of angina on quality of life. Data are at baseline and 2 years after randomization in the RITA trial, showing impact of angina on life aspects encoded in part 2 of the Nottingham Health Profile. Note how quality of life deteriorates rapidly with worsening angina.

Pocock SJ, Henderson RA, Seed P, Treasure T, Hampton JR. Quality of life, employment status, and anginal symptoms after coronary angioplasty or bypass surgery.3-year follow-up in the Randomized Intervention Treatment of Angina (RITA) Trial. *Circulation* 1996;**94**:135–42.

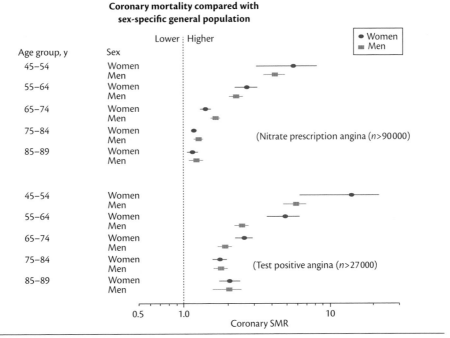

Coronary mortality compared with sex-specific general population

CI indicates confidence interval.

Fig. 13.3.2 Prognosis of angina in women and men. Primary care electronic records for Finland linked with mortality data have permitted estimation of the prognosis of angina for men and women, presented here as standardized mortality ratios. Two mutually exclusive case definitions of angina were used based on nitrate prescription and test positivity, yielding respectively over 90 000 and over 27 000 cases. The data show that the contemporary prognosis of angina is not always good and at all ages is similar for men and for women. SMR, standardized mortality ratio.

Hemingway H, McCallum A, Shipley M, Manderbacks K, Martikainen P, Keskimaki I. Incidence and prognostic implications of stable angina pectoris among women and men. *JAMA*, 2006;**295**:1404–11.

diagnostic information. Typically angina is experienced as a constricting, centrally located chest discomfort, radiating to the arms, throat, or jaw, provoked by exertion, less commonly by stress, and relieved by rest usually within 5–10 min. Symptoms are often worse in the morning, shortly after getting up, probably because catecholamine levels and blood pressure peak at this time of day. For similar reasons angina tends to be worse in cold weather and also after a heavy meal. In addition to age and gender, diagnostic probability is also influenced by a family history of premature coronary artery disease and also by other risk factors—particularly diabetes, smoking, hypertension, and dyslipidaemia. Thus, in the patient with chest pain, the probability of coronary disease is very low in men and women under 30, almost regardless of the typicality of the symptoms, while in men and women over 60 with multiple risk factors the probability of coronary disease is high even when the history has atypical features. The experienced clinician makes these probability judgements intuitively in the consulting room and they provide the main basis for the diagnosis of angina. For further discussion see Chapter 2.1.

Despite the reliance on clinical history in making a diagnosis of angina, it can be misleading, with atypical features, such as exertional dyspnoea in the absence of chest pain. Atypical presentations are said to be more common in patients with diabetes but, contrary to popular belief, there is little evidence that this also applies in women and South Asian people.

The physical examination is often normal in the patient with angina but may contribute to diagnosis if signs of major risk factors

are identified, particularly hypertension, cutaneous manifestations of dyslipidaemia, and complications of diabetes such as retinopathy and neuropathy. Patients with signs of peripheral vascular disease (e.g. absent pulses, arterial bruits) have associated coronary involvement in most cases.

Simple laboratory investigations may also contribute to diagnosis by identifying groups at heightened risk of coronary disease due to renal dysfunction, dyslipidaemia, or diabetes. Anaemia is also important to document because it may cause or—more commonly—exacerbate myocardial ischaemia.

Noninvasive investigation

Noninvasive testing is used primarily for diagnosis of coronary artery disease, but also has a role in risk assessment (see below). By tradition, nearly all patients presenting with chest pain have an ECG, although it is of limited diagnostic value. Many patients with angina have a normal recording and, although regional ST-segment or T-wave changes are commonly associated with coronary disease, only pathological Q waves, reflecting previous myocardial infarction, are diagnostic. Other features of the ECG of potential relevance include tachycardia—particularly in patients with atrial fibrillation—and evidence of left ventricular hypertrophy, either of which may cause or exacerbate myocardial ischaemia.

Diagnostic indications for noninvasive testing depend largely on the level of uncertainty following the clinical assessment. Thus, a 60-year-old man with multiple risk factors who experiences constricting chest pain relieved by rest when he walks up stairs does

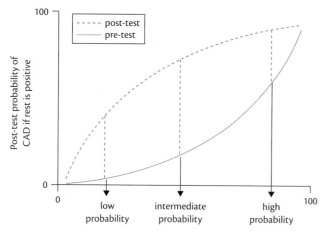

Fig. 13.3.3 Diagnosis of coronary artery disease (CAD)—probability analysis. If the pretest probability of CAD is very low (e.g. a young patient with very atypical chest pain) or very high (e.g. an elderly patient with typical angina), stress testing is generally unhelpful for diagnostic purposes because a positive test does not increase the probability of CAD very much. By contrast, in patients with an intermediate probability of disease, where there is real uncertainty about the diagnosis, a positive test produces a much larger increase in the probability of disease.

not need noninvasive testing for diagnostic purposes—he clearly has angina and a negative test would do nothing to change that diagnosis. Similarly, a 25-year-old with transient stabbing pains in the left side of the chest unrelated to exertion does not have angina and a positive test would not modify that diagnostic judgement. These Bayesian considerations apply to all noninvasive tests that commonly provide false-positive or false-negative results with little incremental value when the probability of coronary disease based on clinical assessment is respectively very low or very high. Incremental diagnostic value is greatest for patients with an intermediate pretest probability of coronary artery disease (say 10–90%) in whom uncertainty is greatest (Fig. 13.3.3). In these

patients the results of noninvasive testing, positive or negative, can help resolve the uncertainty and contribute to the appropriate further management (Fig. 13.3.4). The choice of noninvasive test is driven in part by the probability of coronary disease, a low probability (say 10–30%) favouring a test with very high sensitivity such as CT calcium scoring and angiography, which allows confident rule-out of coronary artery disease if the test is normal. By contrast, when the probability of coronary artery disease is higher, perfusion imaging or stress echo are favoured over the exercise ECG because the specificity of these imaging techniques is higher and an abnormal result strongly suggestive of coronary artery disease. When the probability of coronary disease is very high (>60%) the United Kingdom NICE guidance is for coronary angiography without prior noninvasive testing. However, other contemporary guidelines consider noninvasive ischaemia testing a necessary prerequisite to coronary angiography in the diagnostic work-up of these patients.

Exercise ECG

Once widely used for diagnosis of coronary artery disease, it is now giving way to the newer generation of noninvasive diagnostic tests described below. Details are described in Chapter 3.1. The sensitivity and specificity of the exercise ECG is 68% and 77% respectively, with diagnostic value tending to be lower in women than in men. The regional development of planar or down-sloping ST-segment depression, with gradual recovery when exercise stops, is usually diagnostic, particularly when associated with typical chest pain (Fig. 13.3.5a). The exercise ECG may also provide prognostic information: low exercise tolerance, ST depression early during exercise, an exertional fall in blood pressure, or exercise-induced ventricular arrhythmias all point to an increased risk of myocardial infarction or sudden death. The Duke treadmill score, which takes into account duration of exercise, degree of ST-segment deviation, and angina provides a quantitative prognostic assessment and a useful basis for determining the urgency of coronary arteriography.

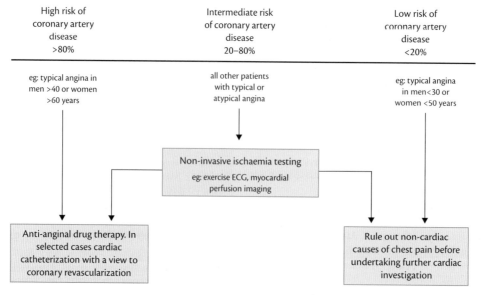

Fig. 13.3.4 Risk-based management strategy in chronic stable angina.

Timmis AD, Nathan AW, Sullivan ID. *Essentials of cardiology*, 3rd edition. Oxford, Blackwell Scientific Publications, 1997.

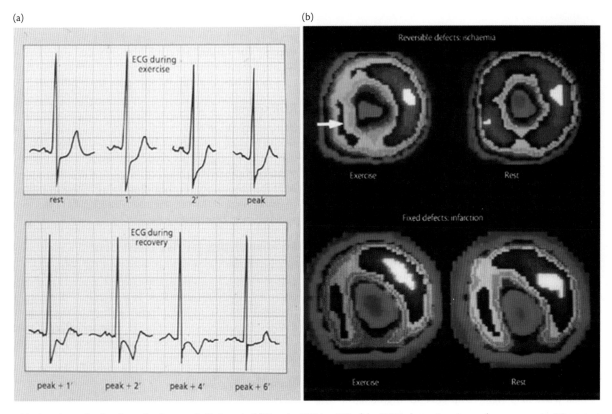

Fig. 13.3.5 Noninvasive testing for diagnosis of myocardial ischaemia. (a) Exercise ECG: lead V2 of the ECG is shown. Exercise produces progressive ST-segment depression with gradual resolution during the recovery period. (b) Isotope perfusion imaging. These are colour-coded perfusion images obtained during exercise stress. The upper panels shows reversible ischaemia with an exertional perfusion defect (arrowed) affecting the lateral left ventricular wall with resolution at rest. The lower panels show fixed perfusion defects denoting prior infarction.

Isotope perfusion imaging

This is also widely used for diagnostic purposes in patients with an intermediate probability of coronary artery disease and, although more costly and time-consuming than the exercise ECG, has enhanced diagnostic accuracy (sensitivity and specificity about 90%). Details are described in Chapter 3.3. Fixed defects, present at rest and during stress, indicate areas of myocardial infarction but reversible defects are indicative of ischaemia in patients with angina (Fig. 13.3.5b). Isotope perfusion imaging also provides useful prognostic information, the extent and severity of perfusion defects (fixed or reversible), the degree of lung uptake of radioisotope (reflecting level of pulmonary capillary pressure), and the calculated ventricular volume and ejection fraction all predicting risk of future events.

Cardiac magnetic resonance (CMR) perfusion imaging

This has now found an important role in the investigation of patients with an intermediate probability of coronary artery disease. First-pass perfusion imaging with gadolinium offers high levels of diagnostic accuracy (sensitivity *c.*90%, specificity 80%) for detection of myocardial ischaemia. Although currently unable to provide the same coronary anatomical definition as CT or conventional angiography, it also provides additional prognostic information about ventricular volumes, ejection fraction, and the extent of myocardial infarction which combine to predict risk of future events. The identification of viable and hibernating myocardium with CMR may be used to guide revascularization strategies.

Stress echocardiography

This too is used increasingly for diagnostic purposes in patients with an intermediate probability of coronary artery disease, but is more dependent than other noninvasive tests on the technical and interpretive skills of the operator. Details are described in Chapter 3.2. In expert hands it has similar sensitivity to exercise ECG but higher specificity for diagnosing coronary artery disease in patients with suspected angina. Left ventricular imaging during dobutamine infusion permits assessment of regional wall motion in response to adrenergic stress, with decreasing systolic wall motion or wall thickening indicating ischaemia and the likelihood of coronary artery disease.

Multidetector CT (MDCT)

The current generation of multidetector (or multislice) CT scanners have sufficient image acquisition speed and spatial resolution to provide noninvasive coronary arteriograms that are finding increasing clinical application particularly for exclusion of coronary artery disease based on high levels of diagnostic sensitivity that exceed 95%. (Fig. 13.3.6). Details are described in Chapter 3.3. Unlike conventional coronary arteriography information is also provided about the arterial wall, particularly the severity and distribution of coronary calcification which relates to the severity of coronary atherosclerosis. MDCT provides real promise for delivery of noninvasive coronary arteriography which is already having a significant impact on the outpatient assessment of patients with chest pain, particularly as a rule-out test in those with a low probability of coronary disease.

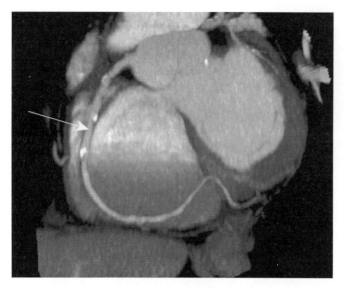

Fig. 13.3.6 Noninvasive coronary angiography by MDCT. The right coronary artery (arrowed) is patent but has localized areas of dense calcification in its proximal and mid segments denoting atherosclerosis.

Risk assessment of angina

Recent clinical trials of patients with chronic angina show that aggressive treatment under cardiological supervision reduces risk considerably such that long-term prognosis is good, with all-cause mortality rates of about 1.5% per year. However, prognosis is worse in cohorts attending chest pain clinics in the early weeks or months after symptom onset, with mortality rates in excess of 3% in the first year. Identification of high-risk patients is therefore an important part of the initial assessment to inform decisions about the urgency and aggressiveness of treatment in individual cases.

Clinical indicators of risk

As with diagnosis, it is the clinical assessment that provides the most useful prognostic information in angina. Risk is greatest in patients who are old, those with typical symptoms and—contrary to conventional wisdom—those with more severe symptoms. Women and South Asians with angina do not appear to be at greater risk. Risk increases with the number of 'reversible' risk factors, particularly diabetes, smoking, hypertension, and dyslipidaemia, all of which are important targets for treatment. Risk is also increased in patients with a history of myocardial infarction or stroke. Tachycardia is associated with increased risk, although treatment to slow the heart rate is directed primarily at preventing exertional ischaemia. Heart failure increases risk substantially. The most useful laboratory markers of risk are blood concentrations of lipids (particularly LDL cholesterol and apolipoproteins), glycated haemoglobin, and creatinine, but the search is on for novel biomarkers to identify high-risk stable angina patients with greater precision.

Noninvasive testing for risk assessment

Abnormalities of the resting ECG, particularly pathological Q waves and left bundle branch block, are associated with heightened risk in the patient with angina. Other noninvasive tests, including the exercise ECG and perfusion imaging, are also used for risk

assessment (see 'Diagnosis of angina' earlier). Generally speaking, negative test results indicate a good prognosis and a low level of urgency for further invasive investigation. However, when test results suggest severe and extensive ischaemia, risk is often high with important implications for future management.

Risk scores

Many scores have been developed for determining cardiovascular risk in healthy populations and in patients with acute myocardial infarction. Scores are also available for risk assessment in chronic stable angina based on many of the clinical and laboratory variables described above, plus echocardiographic measurement of left ventricular function. As yet, angina risk scores have not found major application in clinical practice.

Invasive testing for risk assessment

In patients with angina, risk of myocardial infarction and cardiovascular death is related to the extent and severity of angiographic coronary artery disease. Risk is particularly high when disease (luminal stenosis >50%) affects all three of the major coronary arteries. In patients with left main coronary artery disease death is inevitable in the event of left main occlusion and urgent revascularization is usually recommended.

Novel biomarkers

A range of inflammatory markers, including C-reactive protein, have been assessed in stable patients with coronary artery disease, but their incremental predictive value for future coronary events is very low once conventional risk factors have been taken into account. Brain natriuretic peptide may be more useful in this group of patients, although currently its main clinical application is in the diagnosis of heart failure (see Chapter 2.1). Recent data suggest a role for high-sensitivity proponin as a risk marker in stable coronary disease.

Treatment of angina

The purpose of treatment is to correct symptoms and reduce risk, thereby improving both the quality of life and its duration (Fig. 13.3.7).

General measures

Comorbidities that exacerbate angina include anaemia, obesity, and thyrotoxicosis, all of which need treating. Most important, however, is hypertension, which increases myocardial oxygen demand in proportion to its severity. Simple lowering of blood pressure will often correct angina without the need for additional symptomatic treatment. Atrial fibrillation is also important because it is common, particularly in elderly patients, and increases myocardial oxygen demand due to tachycardia. Symptom relief can often be achieved by heart rate control or cardioversion. Aortic stenosis is another cause of angina that can be corrected by valve replacement.

Secondary prevention

The risk of myocardial infarction, stroke, and cardiovascular death can be reduced by lifestyle modification and specific drug therapy. Logic also requires that major atherogenic risk factors—particularly diabetes, smoking, hypertension, and dyslipidaemia—are treated vigorously in patients with angina, evidence for risk reduction being best for blood pressure control, smoking cessation, and

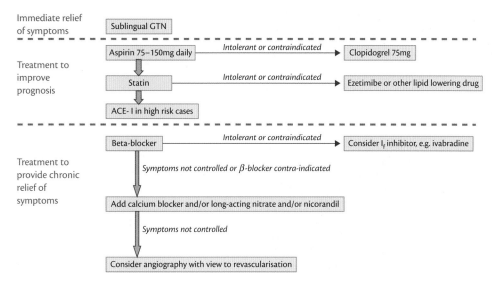

Fig. 13.3.7 Medical management of stable angina.
European Society of Cardiology guidelines. *Eur Heart J* 2006;**27**:1341–81. With permission of Oxford University Press (UK) © European Society of Cardiology, www.escardio.org/guidelines.

LDL cholesterol reduction. Strict glycaemic control in type 2 diabetes, on the other hand, provides little demonstrable protection against cardiovascular endpoints although microvascular complications (renal failure and retinopathy) are effectively diminished.

Lifestyle modification
Evidence-based recommendations are for smoking cessation, exercise training, and a Mediterranean-style diet characterized by low intake of total and saturated fats and increased intake of fresh fruits and vegetables, and cereals rich in fibre, antioxidants, minerals, vegetable proteins, and B-group vitamins. Weight reduction in obese patients is also recommended, particularly those with hypertension, dyslipidaemia, or diabetes.

Secondary prevention drugs
All patients with angina should receive aspirin 75–150 mg daily, its antiplatelet activity reducing the thrombotic response to plaque rupture and protecting against myocardial infarction and stroke. Patients intolerant of aspirin despite proton pump inhibition should be treated with clopidogrel, which offers equivalent protection.

Patients with angina should also receive statin therapy to lower LDL cholesterol, thereby reducing lipid accumulation in the arterial wall and stabilizing the atherosclerotic plaque against rupture. Risk reduction is independent of baseline LDL cholesterol concentration, but the more it is lowered the greater the protection against cardiovascular events. At present, therefore, recommendations are to treat to a target of 4 mmol/litre for total cholesterol and 2 mmol/litre for LDL cholesterol. This often requires treatment with a potent statin such as atorvastatin or rosuvastatin. In patients who cannot be treated to target or who are unable to tolerate statins, ezetimibe is usually added (or substituted) to reduce cholesterol absorption from the bowel, although there is no current evidence of prognostic benefit. The cardiovascular risk associated with low HDL is well established, but treatment to increase HDL with nicotinic acid derivatives or the more potent cholesteryl ester transfer protein (CETP) inhibitors that are currently under investigation, does nothing to reduce risk in patients with coronary artery disease.

Angiotensin converting enzyme (ACE) inhibition provides some additional protection against cardiovascular endpoints in patients with angina, but this probably relates to their blood pressure lowering effect and current recommendations are for their use only in patients with angina who have additional indications for ACE inhibition such as hypertension, heart failure, or diabetes.

β-Blockers, though widely used for symptomatic treatment, have no clear evidence-based indication for secondary prevention in patients with angina unless there is associated left ventricular dysfunction, when prognostic benefit is well established. Antioxidant vitamins C and E and omega-3 fatty acids have failed the test of clinical trials for secondary prevention in coronary artery disease. Similarly, there appears to be no role for hormone replacement therapy for protecting against coronary events in postmenopausal women.

Antianginal drugs
Drugs used to treat angina reduce ischaemia by improving the balance between myocardial oxygen supply and demand (Fig. 13.3.8). Guideline recommendations are that medical therapy with antianginal drugs should be tried before angioplasty or surgery is considered, except in those patients with stable angina with left main stem or multivessel coronary disease in whom there is evidence that surgical revascularization might improve prognosis.

The antianginal drugs recommended for initial treatment are β-blockers and calcium channel blocker, together with a short-acting nitrate for prompt alleviation of angina attacks. If these drugs are not tolerated, are contraindicated, or fail to correct symptoms, alternative antianginals may be considered.

β-Blockers
These drugs reduce myocardial oxygen demand, principally by slowing the heart rate, although reductions in left ventricular wall tension (blood pressure) and contractility also contribute. Choice of β-blocker is largely determined by patient acceptability, with preference given to once-daily cardioselective agents such as bisoprolol. Effective relief of exertional angina can often be obtained without recourse to other drugs if the heart rate response to exercise can be

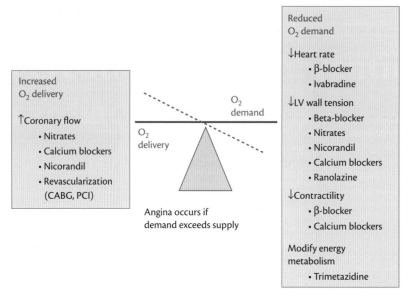

Fig. 13.3.8 Symptom relief with drugs.

reduced sufficiently. There is a clear indication for β-blockers when angina occurs in patients with heart failure or asymptomatic left ventricular dysfunction. They are usually well tolerated, but non-cardiac side effects, particularly fatigue and erectile dysfunction, may be troublesome even with cardioselective agents. β-Blockers are contraindicated in patients with bronchial asthma.

Calcium blockers

Like nitrates, these are vasodilators and improve myocardial oxygen balance by their effect on coronary flow and peripheral resistance. Angina complicated by hypertension provides a clear indication for drugs of this class, and amlodipine is usually the preferred agent. Diltiazem and verapamil are also useful because, in addition to vasodilator activity, they often produce minor reductions in heart rate, although combination therapy with β-blockers is best avoided. Nifedipine, which tends to increase heart rate, is not recommended for treatment of angina. Side effects of calcium blockers are related to vasodilatation and include facial flushing, postural dizziness, and mild ankle oedema.

Nitrates

These drugs improve myocardial oxygen delivery and reduce demand by direct coronary and peripheral vascular dilatation. Sublingual glyceryl trinitrate by tablet or spray should be given to all patients with angina, rapid absorption through the buccal mucosa providing symptomatic relief within 3 min. It can also be used prophylactically to prevent angina during exertion. Long-acting isosorbide mononitrate for regular oral administration is widely used, although variable tolerance to its therapeutic action may occur. Side effects are rarely troublesome apart from headache during the first few days of treatment.

Potassium channel openers

Nicorandil is the only drug in this group licensed to treat angina. It is a vasodilator with effects comparable to those of long-acting nitrates. The principal side effect is headache.

Trimetazidine

This interesting compound is licensed for treatment of angina in a number of European countries (not the United Kingdom). Its pharmacological effects are metabolic, not haemodynamic, with coupling between glycolysis and carbohydrate oxygenation restored by shifting cardiac energy metabolism from oxygenation of fatty acids (the preferred myocardial substrate) to glucose, thus preserving intracellular ATP levels. Antianginal effects are comparable to other agents. Side effects, including gastrointestinal disturbance, are rarely troublesome.

Ivabradine

Ivabradine inhibits the I_f channel in the sinus node, reducing the slope of diastolic depolarization and slowing the heart rate. The effect of ivabradine on heart rate is comparable to that of β-blockers, but it is only effective in patients with normal sinus rhythm (rate reduction does not occur in atrial fibrillation). Based on the results of a recent trial, however, the indication for ivabradine is restricted to patients with continuing symptoms in whom β-blockers fail to reduce the heart rate below 70 beats per minute. In such patients the addition of ivabradine may be helpful but heart rate should not be allowed to fall excessively. There is an additional indication for ivabradine in patients who have a contraindication to or intolerance of β-blockers and in whom calcium channel blockers such as amlodipine have failed to control symptoms. Ivabradine is generally well tolerated and mild visual side effects tend to resolve during treatment.

Ranolazine

Ranolazine's mechanism of action appears to involve inhibition of the late inward sodium channel which indirectly prevents calcium overload of ischaemic myocytes and reduces diastolic wall tension and oxygen demand. Heart rate or blood pressure are unaffected. Antianginal effects are additive to those of β-blockers and calcium blockers. Side effects including constipation and dizziness are rarely troublesome.

Revascularization

In the patient with angina, revascularization provides a nonpharmacological means of improving myocardial oxygen delivery by restoring coronary flow to the ischaemic myocardium. More than 60% of all revascularization procedures in stable angina are now by percutaneous intervention (PCI) using balloon angioplasty and stenting (Fig. 13.3.9). The remainder are by coronary artery bypass surgery (CABG), the choice depending largely on the extent and severity of coronary artery disease. At present, this can only be determined by coronary angiography which is an essential prerequisite of revascularization in the management of angina. See Chapters 13.5 and 13.6 for further discussion.

Which patients with stable angina should undergo coronary angiography?

Guideline recommendations are for angiography in patients with continuing moderate or severe angina despite optimal medical treatment. Other groups for whom angiography is recommended include those who have been successfully resuscitated from sudden cardiac death or who have life-threatening ventricular arrhythmias and those with suspected or known coronary artery disease whose jobs (e.g. piloting aircraft, driving public service vehicles) are dependent on a normal or fully revascularized coronary circulation. It may also be indicated in patients unwilling or unable to take antianginal drugs, or those in whom there is important diagnostic uncertainty despite noninvasive investigation. In patients whose angina has responded satisfactorily to medical treatment there is no absolute requirement for angiography but the potential for small gains in life expectancy with CABG for high-risk coronary anatomy (left main or three-vessel disease) should be discussed, and angiography offered to those who wish to have the coronary anatomy defined.

Choice of revascularization procedure—CABG vs PCI

In symptomatic patients who have undergone cardiac catheterization, revascularization is generally indicated if one or more of the major coronary arteries—or their large branches—have flow-limiting stenoses (>70% luminal narrowing) or occlusions. The choice of revascularization procedure is dependent on a range of factors and should be discussed in a multidisciplinary group that includes cardiologists and cardiac surgeons:

- Coronary anatomy—historically, PCI has been preferred for single-vessel and two-vessel coronary artery disease and CABG for more extensive disease. This preference, based largely on presumed prognostic benefit for CABG in patients with three-vessel or left main stem disease (see below), has now given way to procedure selection based on coronary scoring systems. Most widely used is the SYNTAX score designed to quantify the complexity of left main or three-vessel disease according to simple lesion criteria readily accessible from the coronary arteriogram. If the SYNTAX score is <22, signifying low lesion complexity, 5-year outcomes favour revascularization by PCI, regardless of the number of diseased vessels. If, on the other hand, the SYNTAX score is higher CABG should be considered and for scores >33, signifying severe lesion complexity, CABG produces unequivocally better 5-year outcomes compared with PCI. In making revascularization decisions however other factors are also important, particularly patient preference.

- Patient preference—PCI is often preferred because it avoids surgery, requires no more than 48 h hospitalization (day-case PCI is now feasible) and permits early return to normal activities within a few days of the procedure. In expressing a preference, however, it is important that the patient is properly informed of the relative risks and benefits of PCI and CABG in his or her particular case.

- Procedural risk— mortality is lower for PCI than CABG (0.9% vs 2.2%). Stroke risk may also lower but rates of nonfatal myocardial infarction are comparable.

- Symptomatic benefit—this is comparable for PCI and CABG, but recurrence of symptoms and need for repeat revascularization is higher for PCI because of coronary restenosis in the months following a successful procedure. Indeed restenosis has been the Achilles heel of PCI, and until the introduction of coronary stents affected 30% or more of all patients. Since then stenting has become widespread, producing more effective coronary patency although reductions in rates of restenosis to less than 10% had to await the introduction of drug-eluting stents that

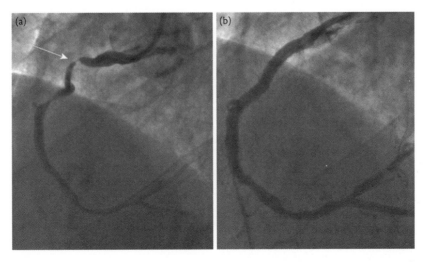

Fig. 13.3.9 Coronary stenting. Right coronary arteriogram (a) before stenting and (b) after deployment of a drug-eluting stent across the diseased segment (arrowed) in the proximal part of the vessel. The patient had stable angina and experienced complete relief of symptoms after the procedure.

deliver antiproliferative drugs (e.g. sirolimus, paclitaxel) locally within the coronary artery. The prospect of providing long-term relief of symptoms without the need for repeat procedures has considerably enhanced the clinical value of PCI.

◆ Prognostic benefit—There have been no studies showing survival benefit for PCI in patients with stable angina. For CABG, small gains in life expectancy have been reported in patients with left main stem coronary disease and three-vessel disease but are from studies nearly 40 years ago and their contemporary relevance may have changed with advances both in surgical techniques and in medical therapy. Indeed it is generally accepted that improvements in the prognosis of coronary artery disease in the last 25 years have little to do with revascularization, but much to do with lifestyle changes and advances in secondary prevention therapy.

Management of refractory angina

With current management strategies patients with angina are living longer, but a proportion, perhaps 5 to 10%, remain symptomatic on optimal medical treatment, having exhausted revascularization options. These patients commonly have extensively collateralized coronary circulations and well-preserved left ventricular function such that prognosis is not worse than other patients with angina, but the quality of life is poor because of refractory symptoms. Psychological support is important to treat anxiety and depression and improve confidence. Other options for further antianginal therapy are not evidence-based and are not recommended in international guidelines. They include neuromodulatory techniques (stellate ganglion block, transcutaneous electrical nerve stimulation, spinal cord stimulation) and enhanced counterpulsation therapy using pressure cuffs applied to the lower limbs that are inflated sequentially during diastole.

Further reading

Sekhri N, *et al.* (2007). How effective are rapid access chest pain clinics? Prognosis of incident angina and non-cardiac chest pain in 8762 consecutive patients. *Heart,* **93**, 458–63.

Cooper A, *et al.* (2010). Assessment of recent onset chest pain or discomfort of suspected cardiac origin: summary of NICE guidance. *BMJ,* **340**, c1118. http://guidance.nice.org.uk/CG95/NICEGuidance.

Timmis A, *et al.* (2011). Management of stable angina. http://guidance.nice.org.uk/CG126/NICEGuidance.

Head SJ, *et al.* (2014). The SYNTAX score and its clinical implications. *Heart,* **100**, 169–77.

Rapsomaniki E, *et al.* (2014). Prognostic models for stable coronary artery disease based on electronic health record cohort of 102,023 patients. *Eur Heart J,* **35**, 844–52.

Boden WE, *et al.* (2007). Optimal medical therapy with or without PCI in stable coronary disease. *N Engl J Med,* **35**, 1503–16.

NICE Guideline 2010: Chest Pain of Recent Onset (CG 95). http://www.nice.org.uk/guidance/cg95.

NICE Guideline 2011: Management of Stable Angina (CG126). http://publications.nice.org.uk/management-of-stable-angina-cg126.

Montalescot G, *et al.* (2013). 2013 ESC guidelines on the management of stable coronary artery disease: the Task Force on the management of stable coronary artery disease of the European Society of Cardiology. *Eur Heart J,* **34**. 2949-3003

Fihn SD, *et al.* (2012). ACCF/AHA/ACP/AATS/PCNA/SCAI/STS Guideline for the diagnosis and management of patients with stable ischemic heart disease: a report of the American College of Cardiology Foundation/American Heart Association Task Force on Practice Guidelines, and the American College of Physicians, American Association for Thoracic Surgery, Preventive Cardiovascular Nurses Association, Society for Cardiovascular Angiography and Interventions, and Society of Thoracic Surgeons. *J Am Coll Cardiol,* **60**, e44-e164.

CHAPTER 13.4

Management of acute coronary syndrome

Keith A. A. Fox and Rajesh K. Kharbanda

Essentials

The acute coronary syndrome (ACS) is precipitated by an abrupt change in an atheromatous plaque, resulting in increased obstruction to perfusion and ischaemia or infarction in the territory supplied by the affected vessel. The clinical consequences of plaque rupture can range from an entirely silent episode, through to unstable symptoms of ischaemia without infarction, to profound ischaemia complicated by progressive infarction, heart failure, and risk of sudden death. Clinical presentation with an ACS identifies a patient at high risk of further cardiovascular events requiring a defined acute and long-term management strategy.

The choice and timing of acute management strategy is critically dependent on the extent and severity of myocardial ischaemia, with the spectrum of ACS broken down into three elements: (1) Unstable angina: typical ischaemic symptoms without ST elevation on ECG and without elevated biomarkers of necrosis. (2) Non-ST-elevation myocardial infarction (NSTEMI): typical ischaemic symptoms without ST elevation on ECG but with biomarkers of necrosis above the diagnostic threshold. (3) ST-elevation MI (STEMI): typical ischaemic symptoms with ST elevation on ECG and with biomarkers of necrosis above the diagnostic threshold.

An acute reperfusion strategy (primary percutaneous coronary intervention (PCI) or thrombolysis) is of proven benefit only in ST-segment elevation infarction (or MI with new bundle branch block).

Prompt relief of pain is important, not only for humanitarian reasons, but also because pain is associated with sympathetic activation, vasoconstriction, and increased myocardial work. Effective analgesia is best achieved by the titration of intravenous opioids, with concurrent administration of an antiemetic. High-flow oxygen is recommended in those patients with evidence of desaturation, particularly in those who are breathless or who have features of heart failure or shock.

The management of prehospital cardiac arrest requires special attention: at least as many lives can be saved by prompt resuscitation and defibrillation as by reperfusion. Patients may also require management of arrhythmic and haemodynamic complications, including heart failure.

Acute coronary syndromes without ST elevation (unstable angina/non-ST elevation MI)
Risk stratification and initial management

Patients without ST elevation or left bundle branch block can be triaged into low, intermediate, and high-risk categories. (1) High-risk—patients with typical clinical features of ischaemia and ST-segment depression or transient ST-segment elevation, or with troponin elevation and a high-risk score (risk calculator downloadable from <http://www.outcomes.org/grace> or <http://www.timi.org/>). Patients are also at high risk when ischaemia provokes arrhythmias or haemodynamic compromise. (2) Intermediate or low risk—patients with clinical features of ACS and nonspecific ECG changes (T-wave inversion, T-wave flattening, minor conduction abnormalities, etc.). (3) Low risk or an alternative diagnosis—patients with a normal ECG, normal biomarkers, normal cardiac examination, and normal echo.

Patients at high risk—(1) High-risk patients with acute ischaemia at initial presentation, or those who develop such features after hospital admission, and especially those with haemodynamic compromise, require emergency assessment for revascularization and potentially benefit from glycoprotein IIb/IIIa inhibition. (2) Those proceeding to emergency revascularization should receive (a) aspirin; (b) $P2Y_{12}$ receptor inhibitor; (c) unfractionated or low molecular weight heparin (LMWH), or a direct thrombin inhibitor, and in selected cases (d) glycoprotein IIb/IIIa inhibition. (3) Some patients should receive anti-ischaemic therapy, antiarrhythmic management, or haemodynamic support (e.g. intra-aortic balloon pump to reduce ischaemia and stabilize the patient for revascularization).

Where the clinical features support a diagnosis of a primary ACS, patients developing ST elevation require emergency assessment with coronary angiography and where appropriate reperfusion by primary PCI, or—when a primary angioplasty service is not available—by thrombolysis (see below).

Patients at intermediate or low risk—patients with non-ST-elevation ACS and an intermediate risk score require dual antiplatelet therapy (aspirin plus $P2Y_{12}$ receptor inhibitor, e.g. ticagrelor, prasugrel, or clopidogrel) plus anticoagulation. They are candidates for an early elective revascularization strategy (within c.72h).

Clinically stable patients with minor or nonspecific ECG abnormalities and a low risk score (including negative repeat troponin) are at very low risk for in-hospital, major cardiac events. Such patients may, nevertheless, have significant underlying coronary artery disease. They require assessment of the cardiovascular risk and stress testing or perfusion scanning to identify the presence and extent of inducible ischaemia, ideally prior to discharge.

Specific pharmacological therapies

Anti-ischaemic therapies—(1) nitrates—effective in reducing ischaemia in the in-hospital management of non-ST-elevation ACS, but there is no evidence that they improve mortality; (2) β-blockers—patients with suspected acute coronary syndromes should be initiated on β-blocker therapy unless contraindicated; (3) dihydropyridine calcium entry blockers—should only be employed with β-blockers in ACS to avoid reflex tachycardia. In patients unable to tolerate β-blockers, a heart-rate-slowing calcium antagonist, e.g. diltiazem or verapamil, may be appropriate. Short-acting dihydropyridines should not be used in isolation in ACS.

Antiplatelet therapies—(1) aspirin 75–325 mg daily—indicated in all patients with ACS unless there is good evidence of aspirin allergy or evidence of active bleeding; (2) $P2Y_{12}$ receptor inhibitor —patients with non-ST-elevation ACS should be given a loading dose of either ticagrelor 180 mg, prasugrel 60 mg, or clopidogrel 300–600 mg, followed by continued treatment, in combination with aspirin. Dual antiplatelet therapy (DAPT) should be maintained for 12 months, unless the risks of bleeding exceed potential benefits. (3) GPIIb/IIIa inhibitors—e.g. abciximab, eptifibatide, tirofiban—result in improved outcome in patients requiring urgent percutaneous intervention for non-ST-segment-elevation ACS and in those at intermediate to high risk. Current indications for treatment with GPIIb/IIIa inhibitors are mainly as a bailout at PCI.

Anticoagulation—this is required in addition to antiplatelet therapy. Indirect thrombin inhibitors: LMWH is better than unfractionated heparin (UFH) and is most commonly used. In the absence of an urgent/early invasive strategy, fondaparinux (a synthetic pentasaccharide that selectively binds antithrombin and causes inhibition of factor Xa) has the most favourable efficacy/safety profile. Bilvalirudin is the only direct thrombin inhibitor currently used in ACS management.

ST-segment-elevation myocardial infarction

Patients with clear-cut evidence of ST-elevation infarction (STEMI) require immediate triage to reperfusion therapy. 'Fast-track' systems have been developed to minimize in-hospital delay to reperfusion: these aim to achieve clinical assessment and electrocardiography within 15 min of arrival and rapid transfer for PCI or the institution of thrombolytic therapy within 30 min. Audit programmes and continuous training are necessary for centres to achieve this 30-min median 'door-to-needle' time.

PCI—Randomized clinical trials of primary PCI vs thrombolysis have shown consistent findings: primary PCI is better, providing more effective restoration of vessel patency, achieving better ventricular function, and improving important clinical outcomes with lower rates of death, reinfarction, stroke, major bleeding, and recurrent ischaemia. Particular gains are seen in haemodynamically compromised patients. In consequence, primary PCI is the preferred therapeutic option in national and international guidelines.

Thrombolysis—prehospital thrombolysis is the next best option if a primary PCI programme is not available, or if transfer times are sufficiently prolonged that reperfusion may not be achieved within 120 min of patient call.

The current reference standard for the comparison of fibrinolytic agents is the accelerated infusion regimen of alteplase (tPA), or—for simplicity—the single-bolus administration of tenecteplase (TNK), which does not require an infusion pump or refrigeration and hence is particularly suited for prehospital administration. Internationally, streptokinase remains the most widely used fibrinolytic agent, principally because it is relatively inexpensive.

Antiplatelet agents and anticoagulants—(1) Aspirin 75–325 mg daily—indicated in all patients with ACS unless there is good evidence of aspirin allergy or evidence of active bleeding. (2) $P2Y_{12}$ receptor inhibitors should be given to all patients, continuing for at least 1 month in patients managed with fibrinolysis (or as determined by the type of stents implanted). (3) Anticoagulants—bivalirudin is indicated in patients managed with primary PCI. Patients treated with fibrinolytic therapy should receive LMWH or fondaparinux. (4) GPIIb/IIIa inhibitors are indicated in patients managed with primary PCI, but not in those managed with fibrinolysis.

Secondary prevention measures in patients with ACS

Patients require advice and help regarding cessation of smoking (including the avoidance of passive smoking), dietary modification, exercise, rehabilitation, and management of obesity.

The following therapies have been shown to reduce the risk of subsequent cardiovascular events: (1) antiplatelet therapy—aspirin in a dose of 75 mg/day, clopidogrel 75 mg/day; (2) β-blockers in those without contraindications; (3) lipid lowering with 3-hydroxy-3-methylglutaryl coenzyme A (HMG CoA) reductase inhibitors (statins); (4) angiotensin converting enzyme (ACE) inhibitors/angiotensin receptor blockers (ARB), especially in those with left ventricular dysfunction and heart failure, and benefit is also possible in other patients with vascular disease. (5) Aldostrone blockade (e.g. eplerenone) in those with left vntricular ejection fraction (LVEF) <35% and diabetes or clinical features of heart failure.

Introduction

The term 'acute coronary syndrome' (ACS) describes the clinical manifestations of a heterogeneous spectrum of conditions that share key pathophysiological features: disruption or erosion of coronary atheromatous plaque, changes in vascular tone, and a

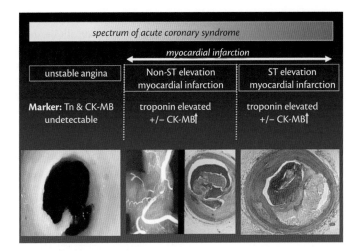

Fig. 13.4.1 The spectrum of acute coronary syndromes.

variable extent of thrombotic occlusion. The clinical presentations are determined by the extent of coronary obstruction, the volume of ischaemic myocardium, and temporal pattern of the atherothrombotic disease process. ACS occurs in patients with underlying, symptomatic or occult coronary artery disease and flow-limiting or non-flow-limiting atheromatous plaques in the coronary arterial wall (Fig. 13.4.1).

The ACS is precipitated by an abrupt change in an atheromatous plaque, resulting in increased obstruction to perfusion and ischaemia or infarction in the territory supplied by the affected vessel. For discussion of the mechanisms involved, see Chapter 13.1. The pattern and severity of clinical manifestations are dependent not only on the degree of obstruction to perfusion, but also on the presence or absence of collateral perfusion, the extent and distribution of fragmented microthrombi, and myocardial oxygen demand in the perfused territory. Thus, the clinical consequences of plaque rupture can range from an entirely silent episode, through to unstable symptoms of ischaemia without infarction, to profound ischaemia complicated by progressive infarction, heart failure, and risk of sudden death.

The goals of early management of ACS are to relieve ischaemia (by reducing myocardial oxygen demand, inhibiting thrombotic occlusion, and reducing coronary obstruction), to prevent further thrombotic occlusion, and to prevent or manage complications. The choice and timing of management strategy, including pharmacological treatment and percutaneous or surgical revascularization, is critically dependent on the extent and severity of myocardial ischaemia. Despite sharing key pathophysiological mechanisms across the spectrum of ACS, ST-segment-elevation acute myocardial infarction (STEMI) and non-ST-elevation ACS (unstable angina and non-STEMI) need to be considered separately because an acute reperfusion strategy (primary percutaneous coronary intervention (PCI) or thrombolysis) is of proven benefit in STEMI (or MI with new bundle branch block), but not in the remainder of the syndrome. Thus, although the management of STEMI differs, the remainder of the ACS should be managed as a continuous spectrum, but influenced by risk stratification.

Clinical presentation and definition of ACS

The ACS may present *de novo* (as new-onset angina), with typical ischaemic discomfort at rest (rest angina) or on minimal exertion. Alternatively, a previously stable pattern of angina may change, resulting in episodes of typical rest angina or angina provoked by minor exertion (crescendo angina). New-onset exertional angina has not previously been recognized as part of 'acute coronary syndrome', but the outcomes are similar—c.7% develop nonfatal MI and 4% die, and a further 19% require revascularization within 15 months—and such patients may fulfill the clinical and ECG/biomarker characteristics of the syndrome (Euroheart survey, GRACE, and CRUSADE registries).

There are three components to the clinical diagnosis of ACS: the symptom description, the ECG, and biomarker evidence of myocyte necrosis. The symptoms must be distinguished from noncardiac pain, and from stable angina. To improve the specificity of diagnosis, clinical trials use a more restricted definition, requiring at least 15 to 20 min of typical ischaemic discomfort or two 5-min episodes at rest. The specificity is further improved when the definition requires objective evidence of ischaemia or evidence of underlying coronary artery disease. ST-segment depression on the ECG, especially in association with typical pain, is highly predictive, whereas the less specific ECG abnormalities, including T-wave inversion, are less strong predictors. Markers of myocardial damage (troponins or cardiac enzymes) are powerfully predictive, in the presence of a typical clinical syndrome. ST elevation or depression on the ECG and elevated biomarkers of necrosis are markers of higher risk and adverse outcome (Table 13.4.1). In the absence of such markers, documented evidence of underlying coronary artery disease (prior infarction or angiographically demonstrated coronary disease) helps to confirm the diagnosis.

In brief, the three components of ACS are:

* unstable angina—typical ischaemic symptoms without ST elevation on ECG and without elevated biomarkers of necrosis

* non-STEMI—typical ischaemic symptoms without ST elevation on ECG but with biomarkers of necrosis above the diagnostic threshold

Table 13.4.1 Prognostic value of admission ECG for early risk stratification in 12 142 patients with an acute coronary syndrome

Outcome	ST elevation + ST depression(n = 15)	ST elevation(n = 28)	ST depression(n = 35)	T-wave inversion (n = 23)	p
Acute infarction on admission (%)	87	81	47	31	<0.0001
Death (%)	6.8	5.0	5.0	1.8	<0.001
(Re)infarction (%)	6.9	5.1	6.7	4.3	<0.001

Death and reinfarction at 30 days follow-up.

Data from the GUSTO IIb trial.

Box 13.4.1 Universal classification of myocardial infarction

◆ Type 1—spontaneous MI related to ischaemia due to a primary coronary event such as plaque fissuring, erosion or rupture, or dissection

◆ Type 2—MI secondary to ischaemia due either to increased oxygen demand or to decreased supply (e.g. coronary spasm or embolism, anaemia, arrhythmias, hypertension, or hypotension)

◆ Type 3—sudden unexpected cardiac death, including cardiac arrest, with symptoms suggestive of myocardial ischaemia, accompanied by new ST elevation, or new left bundle branch block, or definite new thrombus by coronary angiography (death before blood samples obtained) or in the lag phase of cardiac biomarkers

◆ Type 4— (a) MI associated with PCI; (b) MI related to stent thrombosis

◆ Type 5—MI associated with CABG

◆ STEMI—typical ischaemic symptoms with ST elevation on ECG and with biomarkers of necrosis above the diagnostic threshold.

The definition of MI has recently been revised by a global task force of the European Society of Cardiology, the American College of Cardiology, the American Heart Association (AHA), and others and has identified five subtypes of MI (Box 13.4.1).

Outcome of acute coronary syndrome

Trial data and large-scale observational registry studies

Overall, based upon large-scale registries with consistent disease definitions, there are approximately two patients with non-STEMI ACS for each patient with STEMI. Previously, inclusion of patients with chest pain, but without diagnostic features of acute ischaemia, under the term 'unstable angina' may have masked the true hazards of the syndrome. Comparisons between studies may be confounded by different disease definitions and varying use of more sensitive markers of myocyte necrosis (troponins), but on the basis of data from randomized trials and prospective registry studies there is no doubt that patients with ACS (with or without persistent ST elevation) are at substantial risk of subsequent cardiac events despite current therapy. About 9 to 11% suffer death or MI in the first 6 months following presentation, and almost half of this risk is within the first 7 days (GUSTO IIb, OASIS registry, and GRACE registry). Whereas patients with STEMI are most at risk of death, especially in the first hours of symptom onset, those with non-STEMI ACS are at higher risk after discharge (Fig. 13.4.2 and Table 13.4.2). These observations highlight the need for treatment of both the acute and longer-term phases of ACS.

The clinical syndrome and outcome

The Braunwald classification categorizes unstable angina according to the mode of onset and time course (Table 13.4.3). It was empirically based, but has been validated by prospective studies. Patients with unstable ischaemic pain at rest and those with ST depression have the highest risk of an adverse cardiac event. Similarly, those with unstable angina following acute MI are at an increased risk. Although the classification is useful, many of the patients that present with ACS are in Braunwald class 3B and additional methods of risk characterization are required to optimize management.

A diagnostic triage system can be developed for patients with suspected ACS (see 'Emergency Department—triage and establishing a working diagnosis'). This is based on ECG changes, biomarker release, and stress or perfusion testing. Patients with evolving STEMI are identified, and those with higher risk separated from those with lower risk. The respective categories of patients require different management strategies.

The ECG and outcome

The 12-lead ECG (performed on admission) provides direct prognostic information (Table 13.4.1). The greatest risk of death and

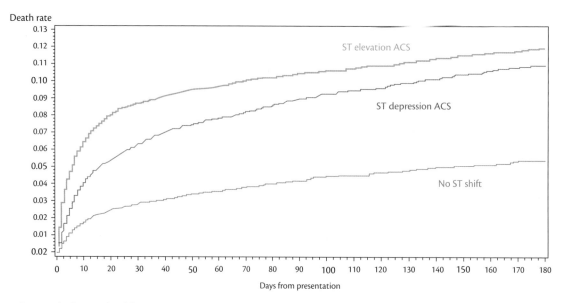

Fig. 13.4.2 Mortality over the first 180 days following presentation with ACS: patients stratified according to ST shift on presentation to hospital.
Reproduced with permission from Bassand J-P *et al.* (2007) Guidelines for the diagnosis and treatment of non-ST-segment elevation acute coronary syndromes. *Eur Heart J*, **28**, 1598–660.

Table 13.4.2 Mortality in hospital and at 6 months in low-, intermediate-, and high-risk categories in registry populations according to the GRACE) risk score

Risk category (tertiles)	GRACE risk score	In-hospital deaths (%)
Low	≤108	<1
Intermediate	109–140	1–3
High	>140	>3
Risk category (tertiles)	**GRACE risk score**	**Post-discharge to 6 months deaths (%)**
Low	≤88	<3
Intermediate	89–118	3–8
High	>118	>8

The Global Registry of Acute Coronary Events (GRACE) risk score, assigns risk on the basis of the following patient characteristics on admission: age, heart rate, systolic blood pressure, serum creatinine, evidence of congestive heart failure, also the presence/absence of cardiac arrest, ST-segment deviation, and elevated cardiac enzymes/markers. For calculations, see <http://www.outcomes.org/grace>

Reproduced from *BMJ*, Fox KA, *et al.* **333**, 1091–4 (2006) with permission from BMJ Publishing Group.

subsequent MI is seen in patients with simultaneous ST elevation and depression; the next highest risk is seen in those with transient ST-segment elevation or ST-segment depression (defined as being >0.5 mm in TIMI score); isolated T-wave inversion carries a lower risk. The number of leads demonstrating ST deviation also yields prognostic information: among those with ST deviation in the anterior leads a rate of death or MI of 12.4% was seen at 1 year—higher than seen with similar changes in other locations (TIMI III trial). Patients with a left main and three-vessel coronary artery disease may show a combination of ST-segment elevation and depression.

Ambulatory ST-segment recording can identify patients with unstable angina and either silent or symptomatic myocardial ischaemia with an increased risk for major subsequent cardiac events. However, conventional ambulatory monitoring usually requires offline analysis and is not suitable for the prediction of imminent events. Computer-assisted, continuous, multilead, ECG monitoring techniques have become available for real-time ECG and ST-segment monitoring. The occurrence and extent of ischaemic territory identified by such continuous recordings can provide additional prognostic information over and above the admission ECG. The information can be combined with biomarkers and, together, they provide additional prognostic information (FRISC study).

Biochemical markers and outcome
Markers of myocardial damage
Enzymes and biomarkers of necrosis are gradually released into the systemic circulation following complete or transient occlusion of

the coronary artery, or fragmentation of a thrombus and embolization. Following total occlusion of the vessel, troponins and creatine kinase (or more specifically CK-MB) are released and are detectable at clearly abnormal levels about 6 to 8 h after the event unless there is extensive collateral perfusion.

The cardiac isoforms of troponin I and troponin T are exclusively expressed in cardiac myocytes and provide specific evidence of myocardial damage. Following infarction, troponins are released from the cytosolic pool and first appear in the circulation in detectable concentrations between 3 and 4 h after the ischaemic event, and reach diagnostic concentrations at 6 to 8 h. Troponin release is evidence of myocardial injury and carries prognostic significance: the greater the troponin release, the greater the risk of subsequent MI and death. Recently, high-sensitivity or ultrasensitive assays have been introduced that have a 10-to 100-fold lower limit of detection than current assays. MI is detected more frequently and earlier using these assays. However, it is important to recognize that other causes of myocyte necrosis (including myocarditis, pulmonary embolism, and severe heart failure, see Fig. 13.4.3) can give rise to detectable troponin concentrations in the circulation; so the diagnosis of ACS requires the presence of an appropriate clinical syndrome. A clinical assessment of the reasons for troponin detection in the circulation is necessary so that patients can be treated according to the correct diagnosis (see Fig. 13.4.3).

When should the cardiac enzymes be measured? The time course of the release of troponins (or enzymes) from myocardium is such that diagnostic concentrations may not be achieved until between 6 and 8 h after an ischaemic event, depending on the assays employed.

Table 13.4.3 Classification of unstable angina (Braunwald)

Class		A Secondary unstable angina	B Primary unstable angina	C Postinfarction (<2 weeks) unstable angina
I	New-onset, severe or accelerated angina	IA	IB	IC
II	Subacute rest angina (<48 h ago)	IIA	IIB	IIC
III	Acute rest angina (within 48 h)	IIIA	IIIB	IIIC

Braunwald E. Unstable angina. A classification. *Circulation*, 1989;**80**, 410–14.

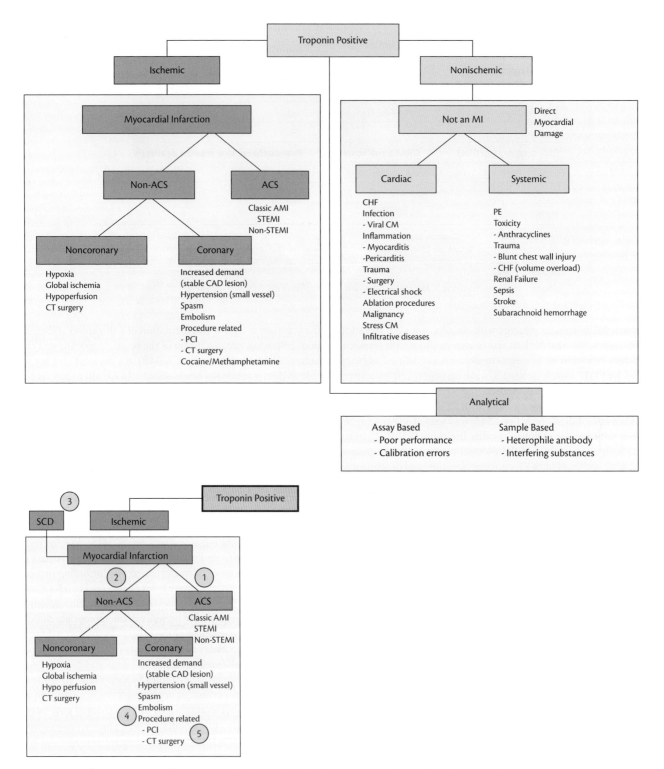

Fig. 13.4.3 Troponin elevation can occur due to a range of conditions. Clinical judgement is required to establish the correct. diagnosis CT = cardiothoracic.
Newby LK, *et al.* (2012). ACCF 2012 expert consensus document on practical clinical considerations in the interpretation of troponin elevations: a report of the American College of Cardiology Foundation task force on Clinical Expert Consensus Documents. *J Am Coll Cardiol*, **60**, 2427–63.

Thus, a normal value for a patient on arrival does not exclude infarction or unstable angina, but an elevated value is highly predictive of subsequent infarction. Troponins should be measured on arrival and at approximately 8 to 12 h: these provide the highest predictive accuracy. The latest generation of sensitive troponin assays increase diagnostic performance and improve the early diagnosis of MI regardless of the time of chest-pain onset and retest within 3 hours maybe feasible. Implementation of a sensitive troponin assay, and lowering the diagnostic threshold for MI, reduces recurrent MI and death in patients with suspected ACS.

Among those with persistently negative troponins and without significant ECG changes, there is a very low risk of subsequent infarction and death (provided that severe underlying coronary artery disease is excluded). Such patients should undergo predischarge risk assessment and stress testing. The best tests are myocardial perfusion scanning or stress echocardiography, but treadmill ECGs on exercise are more widely available (see Chapter 3.1).

Markers of left ventricular wall stress

Natruiretic peptides such as brain natriuretic peptide (BNP) or its N-terminal prohormone fragment (NT-proBNP) are associated with left ventricular dysfunction and elevated levels are associated with adverse prognosis; however, current management protocols are not determined by BNP levels.

Markers of inflammation

Inflammatory changes in the vessel wall promote plaque fissuring or erosion, and inflammatory changes also follow episodes of minor myocardial damage. In ACS there is evidence that inflammatory markers, such as C-reactive protein (CRP) and interleukins IL-6 and IL-1, are independently associated with adverse outcome. After the acute phase, continuing inflammation—e.g. with elevated CRP—occurs in one-half of those whose levels are acutely elevated and identifies a category of patients at increased risk. However, although inflammatory mechanisms are implicated in plaque growth and plaque destabilization, specific anti-inflammatory therapies have not yet been demonstrated to improve outcome, and measurement of CRP or other inflammatory markers is not part of routine clinical practice.

Risk characterization in ACS

The timing and the nature of key management decisions in ACS are dependent upon risk estimation. For example, the choice of reperfusion therapy in ST elevation may be influenced by the presence of comorbidity, bleeding risk, and time delay from symptom onset. Similarly, in non-STEMI ACS, ongoing ischaemia with ST depression or the presence of hypotension or a high-risk score may initiate very early revascularization. Specific pharmacological (e.g. glycoprotein IIb/IIIa inhibitors) or interventional therapies (PCI) have demonstrated benefit in high- or moderate-risk patients but not in low-risk patients (5-year outcome: RITA 3, FRISC-II).

In patients with ACS, risk can be separated into two components: 'prior risk' and 'acute ischaemic risk'. Prior risk is determined by patient characteristics (age and gender), prior ischaemic heart disease (MI, heart failure, prior angina, etc.), and systemic factors that influence risk (hypertension, diabetes, renal dysfunction, and other life-threatening systemic disorders). These can be considered as the background level of risk that the patients bring with them to the point of presentation. Although several of the individual risk components may not be modifiable, the combined impact of prior risk influences the balance between benefit and risk for each of the therapeutic strategies in ACS. Thus, prior risk sets the baseline for risk–benefit decisions.

By contrast, 'acute ischaemic risk' is potentially modifiable and determined by the severity of coronary obstruction and the extent of the territory affected. Collateral perfusion, embolization, myocardial oxygen demand, and cytoprotection mechanisms all influence the extent of ischaemia. Patients with similar clinical features may have experienced transient complete occlusion, or severe subtotal occlusion complicated by distal embolization of fragments

> **Box 13.4.2** Practical steps to assess risk (in addition to clinical symptoms)
>
> - 12-lead ECG—obtained directly after first medical contact, repeated after recurrent symptoms
> - Troponin estimation (cTnT or cTnI)—repeated after 6–12 h, if the initial test is negative
> - Apply a risk score (such as GRACE, TIMI—see Table 13.4.2)
> - An echocardiogram may be required to rule in/out alternative diagnoses and assess left ventricular function
> - In patients with no recurrence of pain, normal ECG and no troponin elevation, a noninvasive stress test may be required

of a platelet-rich thrombus, and altered vascular tone in the distal territory. Clinical markers of acute ischaemic risk include ECG changes, release of biomarkers of necrosis into the systemic circulation, and mechanical and arrhythmic complications of the ischaemic episode.

Simplistically, prior risk can be regarded as the 'baggage' that the patient carries with them, and acute ischaemic risk as an 'acquired hazard' arising from the new ischaemic event. The distinction is important because management strategies for prior risk aim to treat heart failure, underlying coronary and systemic disease, and risk factors. The management of acute ischaemic risk aims to reverse the impact of acute coronary obstruction and thrombosis and is the first priority in the management of patients with ACS. Assessment of the extent and impact of underlying coronary artery disease (e.g. with stress testing) and assessment of left ventricular function can take place later in the management of these patients (Box 13.4.2), and are important determinants of the longer-term outcomes.

In summary: (1) A diagnosis of ACS is a clinical diagnosis based on the suspicion that coronary ischaemia due to atherothrombosis is responsible for the patients presentation (2) clinical examination and ECG provide early and rapid assessment tools (3) patients with STEMI require consideration of emergency reperfusion therapy, and those without require further risk assessment to guide the ongoing management (Table 13.4.4).

Management of ACS without ST elevation (unstable angina/non-STEMI)

Anti-ischaemic therapy

Anti-ischaemic therapy can decrease myocardial oxygen consumption by reducing heart rate, lowering blood pressure, or depressing left ventricular contractility, and may also act by inducing vasodilatation. In consequence, anti-ischaemic therapy can limit the progression of occlusion and improve perfusion and improve the supply–demand imbalance. Mechanical revascularization (PCI and coronary bypass surgery) also aims to relieve obstruction and reduce a patient's susceptibility to ischaemia and its complications—these interventions will be considered separately (see later section of this chapter and Chapter 13.5).

Nitrates

Nitrates act by venodilatation and—in higher dose—by arteriolar dilatation, and hence reduce preload and afterload, thereby

Table 13.4.4 Recommendations for diagnosis and risk stratification for patients without persistent ST-segment elevation

Recommendations	Class[a]	Level[b]
In patients with a suspected NSTE-ACS, diagnosis and short-term ischaemic/bleeding risk stratification should be based on a combination of clinical history, symptoms, physical findings, ECG (repeated or continuous ST monitoring), and biomarkers	I	A
ACS patients should be admitted preferably to dedicated chest pain units or coronary care units	I	C
It is recommended to use established risk scores for prognosis and bleeding (e.g. GRACE, CRUSADE)	I	B
A 12-lead ECG should be obtained within 10 min after first medical contact and immediately read by an experienced physician. This should be repeated in the case of recurrence of symptoms, and after 6–9 and 24 h and before hospital discharge	I	B
Additional ECG leads (V_{3R}, V_{4R}, V_7–V_9) are recommended when routine leads are inconclusive	I	C
Blood has to be drawn promptly for troponin (cardiac troponin T or I) measurement. The result should be available within 60 min. The test should be repeated 6–9 h after initial assessment if the first measurement is not conclusive. Repeat testing after 12–24 h is advised if the clinical| condition is still suggestive of ACS	I	A
A rapid rule-out protocol (0 and 3 h) is recommended when highly sensitive troponin tests are available	I	B
An echocardiogram is recommended for all patients to evaluate regional and global LV function and to rule in or rule out differential diagnoses	I	C
Coronary angiography is indicated in patients in whom the extent of CAD or the culprit lesion has to be determined	I	C
Coronary CT angiography should be considered as an alternative to invasive angiography to exclude ACS when there is a low to intermediate likelihood of CAD and when troponin and ECG are inconclusive	IIa	B
In patients without recurrence of pain, normal ECG findings, negative troponin tests, and a low risk score, a noninvasive stress test for inducible ischaemia is recommended before deciding on an invasive strategy	I	A

[a]Class of recommendation.

[b]Level of evidence.

ACS, acute coronary syndromes; CAD, coronary artery disease; CRUSADE, Can Rapid risk stratification of Unstable angina patients Suppress ADverse outcomes with Early implementation of the ACC/AHA guidelines; ECG, electrocardiogram; GRACE, Global Registry of Acute Coronary Events; LV, left ventricular; NSTE-ACS, non-ST-segment elevation acute coronary syndrome.

Reproduced from Hamm CW, et al. (2011). ESC guidelines for the management of acute coronary syndromes in patients presenting without persistent ST-segment elevation. *European Heart Journal*, **32**, 2999–3054. With permission of Oxford University Press (UK) © European Society of Cardiology, <www.escardio.org/guidelines>.

decreasing oxygen demand. In addition, nitrates can also induce coronary vasodilatation. They are effective in relieving symptoms of ischaemia. In the acute phase of the syndrome, where dose titration is required, they are most conveniently administered intravenously. Once dose titration is no longer required, oral administration is feasible.

Continuous nitrate administration can induce tolerance; so when symptoms are controlled, oral nitrates should be prescribed with appropriate nitrate-free intervals. An alternative is to use drugs with nitrate-like properties but without the same problems of tolerance, such as a potassium channel activator (see 'Potassium channel activators and other antianginals').

Large outcome trials have been conducted with nitrates in acute MI but not in other ACS. However, patients without ST-segment elevation or bundle branch block were randomized within the ISIS-4 trial: their mortality was 5.3% for nitrate treatment and 5.5% for placebo treatment, a nonsignificant difference.

Nitrates are effective in reducing ischaemia in the in-hospital management of non-ST-elevation ACS, but there is no evidence that they improve mortality.

β-Blockers

β-Adrenoceptor antagonists reduce heart rate and blood pressure and myocardial contractility and hence decrease myocardial oxygen consumption. They are primarily employed to reduce ischaemia in ACS. Large-scale trials have not been conducted in patients with non-ST-elevation ACS. However, in the context of acute MI, β-blockers reduce mortality by approximately 10 to 15% (ISIS-1 study). They may act by reducing ventricular arrhythmias, reinfarction, and myocardial rupture. However, this trial was conducted before the widespread use of reperfusion therapy and the findings may not be relevant to contemporary practice. More recently the large COMMIT/CCS study demonstrated that immediate intravenous (metoprolol 5–15 mg) followed by oral metoprolol 200 mg daily had no effect on mortality, with reductions in recurrent MI and cardiac arrest offset by increased cardiogenic shock. A meta-analysis of five trials involving 4700 patients with threatened MI (treated with intravenous β-blockers followed by oral therapy for c.1 week) resulted in a 13% reduction in the risk of MI. Patients with significantly impaired atrioventricular conduction or asthma or acute left ventricular dysfunction should not receive β-blockers. Although β-blockers may exacerbate acute heart failure, extensive trials have produced strong evidence of a benefit for the gradual introduction of β-blockers in ambulant patients with heart failure (see Chapter 5.3).

In the absence of bradycardia or hypotension, patients with suspected ACS should be initiated on β-blocker therapy unless contraindicated.

Calcium entry blockers

These agents inhibit the slow inward current induced by the entry of extracellular calcium through the cell membrane, especially in cardiac and arteriolar smooth muscle. They act by lowering myocardial oxygen demand, reducing arterial pressure, and reducing contractility. Calcium channel blockers can provide symptom relief in patients already receiving nitrates and β-blockers, and may be useful in patients with contraindications to β-blockade. Some agents induce a reflex tachycardia (e.g. nifedipine, nicardipine, amlodipine) and are best administered in combination with a β-adrenoceptor antagonist. By contrast, diltiazem and verapamil are suitable for patients who cannot tolerate a β-blocker because they inhibit conduction through the atrioventricular node and tend to cause bradycardia. All calcium antagonists reduce myocardial contractility and may aggravate heart failure. Calcium entry blockers have been demonstrated to reduce the frequency of angina in patients with variant angina.

A meta-analysis of calcium entry blockers in ACS indicates a nonsignificant trend towards a higher mortality in treated vs control patients (5.9% vs 5.2%, in 7551 patients). In individual trials, diltiazem has been compared with propranolol, and both agents produced a similar reduction in anginal episodes.

Dihydropyridine calcium entry blockers should be employed with β-blockers in ACS to avoid reflex tachycardia. In patients unable to tolerate β-blockers, a heart-rate-slowing calcium antagonist may be appropriate. Short-acting dihydropyridines should not be used in isolation in ACSs.

Potassium channel activators and other antianginals

These agents (e.g. nicorandil) have arterial and venous dilating properties, but do not exhibit the tolerance seen with nitrates. They have been shown to be better than placebo in relieving the symptoms of angina. A randomized trial of nicorandil (a combined nitrate-like and potassium channel activator) suggested benefit on a composite clinical endpoint (IONA study), and this drug may be considered as an alternative to nitrate administration.

> ### Box 13.4.3 Recommendations for anti-ischaemic therapy
>
> - Anti-ischaemic therapy should be administered in conjunction with antithrombotic and interventional therapy (see below), with the overall strategy guided by risk evaluation of the patient (see risk stratification)
>
> - Patients with suspected ACS should be initiated on nitrate and β-blocker therapy, unless there are contraindications to the use of β-blockers
>
> - In patients with contraindications to β-blockers, heart-rate-slowing calcium antagonists should be employed
>
> - The combination of a calcium antagonist and β-blocker is superior to either agent alone
>
> - Angiography and revascularization should be considered in patients with recurrent or persistent ischaemia, or patients with troponin elevation (including non-STEMI). The timing of angiography should be guided by the risk status of the patient

Ivabridine selectively inhibits the primary pacemaker current in the sinus node and maybe used in selective patients with contraindications to β-blockers. Ranolozine inhibits the late sodium current, and can reduce recurrant ischaemia in non-ST-elevation ACS.

The recommendations in Box 13.4.3 are based on current clinical and trial evidence.

Antiplatelet therapy

Aspirin

Exposure of the contents of atheromatous plaque to circulating blood triggers platelet activation by several different pathways. Aspirin is a potent and irreversible inhibitor of platelet cyclooxygenase, blocking the formation of thromboxane A_2 and inhibiting platelet aggregation. Although the effects of aspirin can be overcome in the presence of potent thrombogenic stimuli, nevertheless the benefits of aspirin treatment in unstable angina are clearly defined and substantial. The Antiplatelet Trialists Collaboration demonstrated a reduction of 36% in death or MI with antiplatelet treatment (predominantly aspirin) vs placebo in unstable angina trials. Aspirin treatment significantly reduces subsequent MI, stroke, and vascular death, with the largest reductions seen among patients at highest risk. In patients with unstable angina, four key studies have demonstrated that aspirin significantly reduces the risk of cardiac death or nonfatal MI by approximately 50%.

The efficacy of lower-dose aspirin (75 mg/day) therapy has been demonstrated in several studies, including those of Wallentin and colleagues where long-term effects were evaluated in men under 70 years of age with unstable coronary artery disease. After 6 and 12 months of aspirin treatment, the risk of MI or death was reduced by 54% and 48%, respectively (risk ratio 0.52 with 95% confidence intervals 0.37–0.72). The strength of evidence and magnitude of benefit demonstrated with aspirin treatment in non-ST-segment-elevation ACS is such that aspirin is indicated in all patients with ACS, unless there is a clear contraindication. Nevertheless, patients with ACS remain at significant risk despite aspirin therapy. In prospective registry studies of unstable angina/non-STEMI, and in spite of aspirin treatment in more than 80% of patients, the risk of death or MI is approximately 10% at 6 months and the risk of death/MI or refractory angina is approximately 22 to 33% over the same period (OASIS registry, PRAIS registry).

Aspirin treatment (75–325 mg daily) is indicated in all patients with ACS unless there is good evidence of aspirin allergy or evidence of active bleeding.

P2Y$_{12}$ receptor inhibitors

Ticlopidine and clopidogrel are ADP receptor antagonists, and they block the ADP-induced pathway of platelet activation by inhibiting the P2Y$_{12}$ ADP receptor.

Clopidogrel replaced ticlopidine on account of a superior safety profile and has been tested in a large-scale trial of patients with unstable angina/non-STEMI ($n = 12\,562$, CURE trial). The agent was used on top of existing therapy, and in addition to aspirin. It reduced death, nonfatal MI, and stroke from 11.4 to 9.3% (95% confidence interval 0.72–0.90, $p < 0.001$). For every 1000 patients treated, there were 28 fewer major cardiovascular complications but 6 more transfusions. Importantly, benefits were seen across risk groups (diabetics, hypertensives, biomarker elevation or not, revascularization or not). In a substudy (PCI-CURE), clopidogrel also reduced death and MI in those undergoing percutaneous revascularization (2.9% clopidogrel vs 4.4% for placebo). Thus, with the combination of clopidogrel and aspirin, there is evidence of early and sustained reductions in the risks of death and MI in patients that present with ACS.

A number of smaller studies have used higher loading doses of clopidogrel (usually 600 mg), and these show more rapid inhibition of platelet aggregation than that achieved with 300 mg. The CURRENT-OASIS 7 trial assessed the effects of double-dose (600 mg loading, 150 mg for 1 week, then 75 mg daily) vs standard dose (300 mg loading, then 75 mg daily) clopidogrel in patients with ACS and intended early revascularization. The double-dose clopidogrel regimen was associated with a reduction in cardiovascular events and stent thrombosis compared with the standard dose in patients who underwent PCI.

Long-term clopidogrel administration was tested in the CHARISMA study of 15 603 patients with documented vascular disease or risk factors for vascular disease. Overall, there was no difference in the primary endpoint of cardiovascular death, MI, or stroke. However, in the subgroup of patients with documented cardiovascular disease, the same endpoint was significantly reduced with dual antiplatelet therapy (DAPT), when compared with aspirin (6.9 vs 7.9%, relative risk 0.88, 95% confidence interval 0.77–0.99). Thus, longer-term treatment with DAPT should only be considered in those in whom the risk of ischaemic events exceeds the risk of bleeding complications.

Prasugrel is a more potent thienopyridine with faster onset than clopidogrel. Similar to clopidogrel, prasugrel is a prodrug that requires metabolism by enzymatic hydrolysis in the liver for activation. In moderate–high-risk patients with ACS scheduled to undergo PCI, prasugrel (60 mg loading dose, 10 mg maintenance) compared to clopidogrel (300 mg loading dose, 75 mg maintenance), reduced MI and stent thrombosis particularly in diabetic patients, but with an increased risk of major bleeding, including fatal bleeding. Prasugrel should therefore be avoided in patients older than 75 years, with previous intracerebral bleeding or transient ischaemic attack, or who weigh less than 60 kg. Prasugrel is approved for use in patients with ACS undergoing PCI.

Ticagrelor is a reversible inhibitor of the platelet $P2Y_{12}$ receptor and belongs to a new class of antiplatelet agents, the cyclopentyl-triazolopyrimidines. It does not require hepatic metabolism to an active form and therefore has a rapid onset with more predictable platelet inhibition. The PLATO study demonstrated that ticagrelor (180 mg loading dose, 90 mg twice daily thereafter) as compared to clopidogrel (300–600 mg loading dose, 75 mg daily thereafter) reduced cardiovascular death, MI, and stent thrombosis without increasing the rate of major bleeding in patients with ACS. This was the first study to demonstrate a mortality benefit with the addition of an antiplatelet agent to aspirin in patients with ACS.

Guidelines for antiplatelet therapy are listed in Table 13.4.5.

Glycoprotein IIb/IIIa inhibitors

Platelet adhesion is the initial step in haemostasis after disruption of an atheromatous plaque. It is triggered by damage to the vessel wall and exposure of the subendothelium, and is followed by platelet activation and aggregation. Regardless of the agonist, the final common pathway leading to the formation of a platelet aggregate is mediated by the glycoprotein (GP) IIb/IIIa receptor. GPIIb/IIIa receptor antagonists inhibit platelet aggregation irrespective of the

agonist, and they prevent binding of fibrinogen to its receptor on the platelet surface.

Three GPIIb/IIIa receptor antagonists have been approved for clinical use: abciximab, eptifibatide, and tirofiban. They all require intravenous administration. Abciximab is a chimeric human–murine monoclonal antibody that binds with high affinity to the receptor: it has a long biological half-life of 6 to 12 h, and low levels of receptor occupancy are detected even 2 weeks after treatment. Eptifibatide is a synthetic cyclic heptapeptide with high affinity for the arginine–glycine–aspartic acid ligand-adhesion site of the IIb/IIIa receptor. It inhibits platelet aggregation in a dose-dependent manner and is readily reversible due to competitive binding and a short half-life of approximately 2.5 h. Tirofiban is a nonpeptide tyrosine derivative which also binds to the arginine–glycine–aspartic acid site with high specificity. It inhibits platelet aggregation in a dose- and concentration-dependent manner and is rapidly reversible, with platelet function approaching normal levels in 90% of patients within 4 to 8 h.

Although it is convenient to group glycoprotein IIb/IIIa receptor antagonists together, and undoubtedly there is evidence of a class effect, there are biological and pharmacological differences between the agents. It is also important to note that there are limited data about the use of combination GPIIb/IIIa and the newer $P2Y_{12}$ receptor inhibitors.

Trials of GPIIb/IIIa inhibitors

More than 32 000 patients have been randomized in clinical trials involving GPIIb/IIIa inhibitors (16 trials). A highly significant ($p < 0.001$) benefit is observed for the combined endpoint of death or MI at 48 to 96 h, 30 days, and 6 months. At 30 days the odds ratio is 0.76, or 20 fewer events per 1000 patients treated, and a highly significant benefit is observed for the combined endpoint of death/MI or revascularization at all time points. By contrast, mortality benefits are seen only at 48 to 96 h, with no significant benefit at 30 days or 6 months. A pooled analysis of abciximab trials has revealed a net mortality benefit, but there is no evidence of benefit for abciximab in medically treated patients (GUSTO-4-ACS). The impact of GPIIb/IIIa inhibitors is influenced by the risk status of the patient and whether administered in the context of percutaneous coronary intervention (PCI). In a meta-analysis of 29 570 patients, there was a 9% reduction in relative risk overall, but with no significant benefit in those who were medically managed (death and MI at 30 days of 9.3% for IIb/IIIa vs 9.7% placebo, OR 0.95, 95% confidence interval 0.86–1.04). Significant benefit was observed when GP IIb/IIIa inhibitors were maintained during PCI (10.5 vs 13.6%, OR 0.74, 95% confidence interval 0.57–0.96). The EARLY-ACS study demonstrated that the use of eptifibatide 12 h or more before coronary angiography was not superior to provisional use after angiography, and early use was associated with more nonfatal bleeding. Similarly, there is no convincing evidence of benefit in low-risk patients, irrespective of interventional strategy. However, there are limited data on the use of GPIIb/IIIa in the context of newer DAPT regimens, and the value of upstream GPIIb/IIIa inhibition is uncertain.

Current indications for treatment with GPIIb/IIIa inhibitors are mainly as a bailout at PCI when there is large thrombus burden or evidence of no-reflow, since reecent trials suggest similar clinical efficacy with reduced bleeding using novel DAPT and bivalirudin.

Anticoagulant therapy for for non-ST-elevation ACS is summarized in Box 13.4.4.

Table 13.4.5 Guidelines for the use of oral antiplatelet agents in non-ST-elevation ACS

Recommendations	Class[a]	Level[b]
Aspirin should be given to all patients without contraindications at an initial loading dose of 150–300 mg, and at a maintenance dose of 75–100 mg daily long-term regardless of treatment strategy	I	A
A P2Y$_{12}$ inhibitor should be added to aspirin as soon as possible and maintained over 12 months, unless there are contraindications such as excessive risk of bleeding	I	A
A proton pump inhibitor (preferably not omeprazole) in combination with DAPT is recommended in patients with a history of gastrointestinal haemorrhage or peptic ulcer, and appropriate for patients with multiple other risk factors (*Helicobacter pylori* infection, age ≥65 years, concurrent use of anticoagulants or steroids)	I	A
Prolonged or permanent withdrawal of P2Y$_{12}$ inhibitors within 12 months after the index event is discouraged unless clinically indicated	I	C
Ticagrelor (180 mg loading dose, 90 mg twice daily) is recommended for all patients at moderate-to-high risk of ischaemic events (e.g. elevated troponins), regardless of initial treatment strategy and including those pre-treated with clopidogrel (which should be discontinued when ticagrelor is commenced)	I	B
Prasugrel (60 mg loading dose, 10 mg daily dose) is recommended for P2Y$_{12}$-inhibitor-naive patients (especially diabetics) in whom coronary anatomy is known and who are proceeding to PCI unless there is a high risk of life-threatening bleeding or other contraindications	I	B
Clopidogrel (300 mg loading dose, 75 mg daily does) is recommended for patients who cannot receive ticagrelor or prasugrel	I	A
A 600-mg loading dose of clopidogrel (or a supplementary 300 mg dose at PCI following an initial 300 mg loading dose) is recommended for patients scheduled for an invasive strategy when ticagrelor or prasugrel is not an option	I	B
A higher maintenance dose of clopidogrel 150 mg daily should be considered for the first 7 days in patients managed with PCI and without increased risk of bleeding	IIa	B
Increasing the maintenance dose of clopidogrel based on platelet function testing is not advised as routine, but may be considered in selected cases	IIb	B
Genotyping and/or platelet function testing may be considered in selected cases when clopidogrel is used	IIb	B
In patients pre-treated with P2Y$_{12}$ inhibitors who need to undergo non-emergent major surgery (including CABG), postponing surgery at least for 5 days after cessation of ticagrelor or clopidogrel, and 7 days for prasugrel should be considered, if clinically feasible and unless the patients is at high risk of ischaemic events	IIa	C
Ticagrelor or clopidogrel should be considered to be (re-)started after CABG surgery as soon as considered safe	IIa	B
The combination of aspirin with an NSAID (selective COX-2 inhibitors and non-selective NSAID) is not recommended	III	C

[a] Class of recommendation.

[b] Level of evidence.

[c] Prasugrel is given a IIa recommendation in the ESC guidelines (Wijns W, et al. (2010). Guidelines on myocardial revascularization: the Task Force on Myocardial Revascularization of the European Society of Cardiology (ESC) and the European Association for Cardio-Thoracic Surgery (EACTS). *Eur Heart J*, **31**, 2501–2555) as the overall indication including clopidogrel-pre-treated patients and/or unknown coronary anatomy. The class I recommendation here refers to the specifically defined subgroup.

CABG, coronary artery bypass graft; COX, cyclo-oxygenase; DAPT, dual (oral) antiplatelet therapy; NSAID, non-steroidal anti-inflammatory drug; PCI, percutaneous coronary intervention.

Reproduced from Hamm CW, et al. (2011). ESC guidelines for the management of acute coronary syndromes in patients presenting without persistent ST-segment elevation. *European Heart Journal*, **32**,2999–3054. With permission of Oxford University Press (UK) © European Society of Cardiology, <www.escardio.org/guidelines>.

Anticoagulant therapy

Unfractionated heparin

Unfractionated heparin is widely used for the treatment of non-ST-elevation ACS, but the evidence on which this is based is less robust than for other widely adopted treatment strategies. In practice, unfractionated heparin is difficult to control because of its unpredictable levels of binding to plasma proteins, and this may be amplified by the acute-phase response. In addition, heparin has reduced effectiveness against platelet-rich and clot-bound thrombin.

Oler and colleagues conducted a meta-analysis of the influence of adding heparin to aspirin in the treatment of patients with unstable angina. Only 6 randomized trials were available, with 1353 patients included: there were 55 deaths or MIs in the aspirin plus heparin arm and 68 in the aspirin-alone arm, giving a risk reduction of 0.67

and a 95% confidence interval of 0.44 to 1.02. These results do not produce conclusive evidence of benefit from adding heparin to aspirin, but it must be stressed that appropriately powered, larger-scale trials have not been conducted. Nevertheless, clinical practice has adopted unfractionated heparin treatment with aspirin as a pragmatic extrapolation of the available evidence.

LMWH

Trials vs placebo

The FRISC trial tested dalteparin against placebo in aspirin-treated patients with unstable angina/non-STEMI. Some 1506 patients were randomized to receive dalteparin (twice daily for the first 6 days and then once daily at a lower dose for approximately 6 weeks), and the trial showed a highly significant reduction in the frequency of death or new MI at 6 days (1.8% vs 4.8%, with a risk

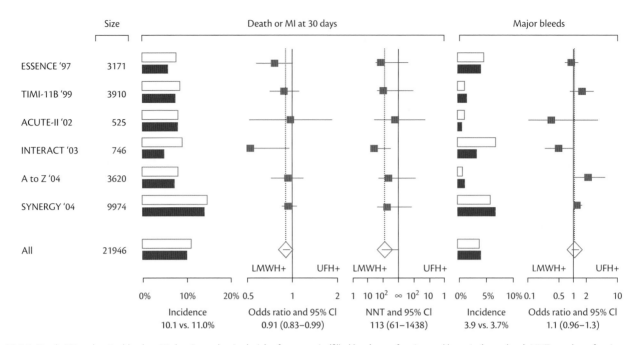

Fig. 13.4.4 Death, MI, and major bleeds at 30 days in randomized trials of enoxaparin (filled bars) vs unfractionated heparin (open bars). NNT, number of patients who needed to be treated to avoid one event.

Reproduced with permission from Bassand J-P, *et al.*, (2007). Guidelines for the diagnosis and treatment of non-ST-segment elevation acute coronary syndromes. *Eur Heart J*, **28**, 1598–1660.

ratio of 0.37). The effects were sustained to 42 days, but were attenuated at 6 months, the differences no longer maintaining significance. Nevertheless, this trial clearly showed the benefit of LMWH over placebo in the presence of aspirin.

Trials vs unfractionated heparin

LMWH possesses enhanced anti-Xa activity in relation to anti-IIa (antithrombin) activity, compared with unfractionated heparin. It also exhibits decreased sensitivity to platelet factor 4 (PF4), more predictable anticoagulant effect, and lower rates of thrombocytopenia. In view of its enhanced bioavailability, it offers the substantial practical advantage of subcutaneous administration based on a dose per kilogram of body weight and without the need for laboratory monitoring.

Acute-phase treatment (c.2–8 days)

In the FRIC trial, dalteparin was tested against unfractionated heparin in 1400 patients with unstable angina: it had limited power to show a difference, and no significant difference was seen between unfractionated heparin and dalteparin.

The ESSENCE trial was double-blinded and placebo-controlled and tested enoxaparin against unfractionated heparin. The treatments were given for 2 to 8 days (median 2.6 days) and the primary endpoints were death, MI, or recurrent angina. Enoxaparin reduced the primary endpoint from 19.6% to 16.6% at 14 days (odds ratio 0.80 and confidence intervals 0.67–0.98; see Fig. 13.4.4). A similar and significant odds ratio was maintained at 30 days and 1 year. At 1 year, there were 3.7 fewer events/100 patients (p = 0.022). The study was not powered for death/MI alone, but demonstrated corresponding trends for these endpoints.

The TIMI 11b trial was also double-blinded and tested enoxaparin vs unfractionated heparin, but additionally it examined 72 h of treatment vs 43 days of treatment. The results up to 14 days mirrored those seen in the ESSENCE trial: at 14 days the primary outcome

occurred was 16.6% (heparin) vs 14.2% (enoxaparin), risk ratio 0.85 (p = 0.03). A combined analysis of ESSENCE and TIMI 11b indicated an absolute reduction of 3.1 per 100 for death/MI/refractory angina, and showed a similar risk ratio of 0.79 (confidence interval 0.65–0.96) for death and MI. Taken together, these findings indicate that short-term treatment with enoxaparin results in about 3 per 100 fewer major cardiac endpoints compared to unfractionated heparin treatment, and this is achieved without additional major bleeding.

Prolonged outpatient treatment

The FRAXIS trial tested fraxaparin, for 6 or 14 days, against unfractionated heparin in 3468 patients; no difference was seen in efficacy, but there was a significant excess of major bleeds with longer-term outpatient treatment. In TIMI 11b, the curves remained separated over the succeeding treatment interval: at 43 days there were 19.6% events (heparin) vs 17.3% (enoxaparin) (p = 0.049), with no evidence of a further separation of the curves. There was 1.4% absolute excess in major bleeds over the chronic phase.

Conclusions from the LMWH studies

There is convincing evidence in aspirin-treated patients (heparin or LMWH is not indicated in the absence of antiplatelet therapy) that LMWH is better than placebo (FRISC trial). The two trials using enoxaparin have provided consistent data in favour of LMWH over unfractionated heparin when administered as an acute regimen. The other trials have produced a similar outcome for the acute phase of treatment and it can be concluded that acute treatment is at least as effective as unfractionated heparin There is no convincing evidence to support longer-term treatment with LMWH. The use of the Xa antagonist fondaparinux is now preferred to LMWH in high risk ACS (see below).

Anti-Xa inhibitors

Fondaparinux is a synthetic pentasaccharide that selectively binds antithrombin and causes inhibition of factor Xa. In the OASIS-5 study, 20,078 patients with non-ST-elevation ACS were randomized (double-blind design) to receive 2.5 mg subcutaneous fondaparinux once daily vs subcutaneous enoxaparin 1 mg/kg twice daily for up to 8 days. Fondaparinux was noninferior at 9 days (the primary endpoint), but subsequently those randomized to fondaparinux had reduced mortality and approximately half the rate of major bleeding. In those undergoing PCI, there was an excess of catheter-related thrombi, and administration of this agent requires additional antithrombin therapy (the excess thrombi were not seen when combined with unfractionated heparin and there was no evidence of excess bleeding with this combination).

Direct thrombin inhibitors

Direct thrombin inhibitors (e.g. hirudin, bivalirudin) bind directly to thrombin (factor IIa) and inhibit thrombin-induced conversion of fibrinogen to fibrin. They bind to and inactivate fibrin-bound thrombin as well as thrombin in the circulation. They do not bind to plasma proteins nor interact with PF4, and hence their anticoagulant effect is predictable.

Hirudin has been tested in large-scale trials (e.g. OASIS-1, OASIS-2, TIMI 9b, GUSTO IIb) against heparin and a combined analysis suggests a 22% relative risk reduction in cardiovascular death or MI at 72 h, 17% at 7 days, and 10% at 35 days. This combined analysis is significant at 72 h and 7 days but not beyond. Hirudin is licensed for heparin-induced thrombocytopenia but not for ACS.

Bivalirudin was tested in the open-label randomized ACUITY trial in 13 819 patients with moderate- to high-risk non-ST-elevation ACS with a planned invasive strategy. The composite endpoints included death, MI, or unplanned revascularization for ischaemia, major bleeding (noncoronary artery bypass graft (CABG)-related), and net clinical outcome (composite ischaemia or major bleeding). Bivalirudin plus GPIIb/IIIa had similar outcomes (noninferior) to heparin/LMWH plus GPIIb/IIIa and similar rates of bleeding. Bivalirudin alone had similar outcome (noninferior composite) to heparin/LMWH plus GPIIb/IIIa, but had superior safety (less bleeding). An interaction with the effects of clopidogrel was evident; benefits were seen with clopidogrel but not without. The HORIZON-AMI trial tested a bivalirudin strategy in PPCI for ST-elevation ACS and showed superiority over GPIIb/IIIa/UFH, primarily driven by a reduction in bleeding. A reduction in cardiovascular mortality was found at 30 days and 3 years. The recent Euromax study studied the use of bivalirudin in the prehospital phase and demonstrated a reduction in the 30-day combined primary endpoint of death, MI, and bleeding, but an increase in acute stent thrombosis. Further studies are needed to define the uses of adjuvant antithrombotics in the context of the newer antiplatelet agents.

Oral antithrombotics:

A number of oral factor Xa inhibitors (e.g. rivaroxaban, apixaban, and otamixaban) are available and have been assessed in dose-ranging and safety phase II trails of patients with ACS. An efficacy study of apixaban in patients with ACS (APPRAISE 2) was stopped due to excess bleeding. The ATLAS 2 study assessed the effect of rivaroxaban in addition to DAPT. A recent metanalysis concluded that the addition of new oral anticoagulants to antiplatelet therapy

---

Box 13.4.4 Anticoagulation for non-ST-elevation ACS

- Anticoagulation is required in addition to antiplatelet therapy

- Anticoagulant options include unfractionated heparin, LMWH, fondaparinux, and bivalirudin, with choice dependent on the initial strategy (early invasive, or not) and the bleeding risk

- With an urgent invasive strategy, unfractionated heparin, enoxaparin, or bivalirudin are treatment options

- In the absence of an urgent/early invasive strategy, fondaparinux (2.5 mg SC) has the most favourable efficacy/safety profile

- If fondaparinux is not available enoxaparin (1 mg/kg twice daily) is recommended

- Bivalirudin with bailout GPIIb/IIIa are recommended as an alternative to UFH/ GPIIb/IIIa in patients with intended invasive management and high bleeding risk

---

was associated with a modest reduction in cardiovascular events but a substantial increase in bleeding. Further studies using single agents or shorter duration of therapy are underway. Oral platelet thrombin receptor antagonists (TRA) are currently under evaluation in a phase III clinical trial programme (TRA 2 degrees P-TIMI 50). SCH 530348 selectively inhibits the cellular actions of thrombin via the protease-activated receptor 1 (PAR-1) on the surface of platelets. Given that the generation of fibrin by thrombin is not affected by PAR-1 inhibition, it is anticipated that this molecule will have potent antithrombotic effects with less bleeding than other novel antiplatelet agents.

Revascularization

The aim of revascularization in non-ST-elevation ACS is to relieve angina, to alleviate myocardial ischaemia, and to prevent progression to MI or death. The indications for myocardial revascularization are dependent on the risk status of the patients and the presence or absence of evidence of ongoing myocardial ischaemia and/or evidence that the ischaemia has resulted in mechanical or electrical complications. Following angiography, the choice of PCI or coronary artery bypass grafting (CABG) is dependent on the extent and severity of angiographic stenoses and the comorbidity of the patient. Angiographic analyses from the TIMI-3B and FRISC-2 studies demonstrates that about 30 to 38% of patients with non-ST-elevation ACS have single-vessel disease and 44 to 60% have multivessel disease (>50% diameter stenosis).

Observational studies

Large-scale observational studies have demonstrated wide variations between countries in the use of cardiac catheterization and revascularization for patients with acute ischaemic syndromes, and a paradox whereby lower-risk patients are less likely to receive aggressive antithrombotic and interventional treatment than moderate- or higher-risk patients. Similar findings have been observed in the United States of America in the CRUSADE registry. Nevertheless, there is clear evidence over time of increasing use of guideline-indicated therapies (especially class 1 indicated treatments) in non-ST-elevation ACS, including angiography and interventional procedures. Overall, the changing pharmacological and interventional therapies have been associated with striking improvements in outcome, including a halving of new heart failure and a reduced risk of death. Higher rates of revascularization have been associated with an increased frequency of procedural complications, including stroke and major bleeding. Definitive assessment of the impact of revascularization on outcomes requires randomized trials and longer-term follow-up.

Randomized trial data

Several smaller and older trials (including TIMI 3B and VANQWISH) tested the impact of a routine invasive strategy in ACS. These largely predated modern antithrombotic therapy, interventional technology (including PCI and stents), and the use of radial access.

The FRISC-II trial compared an invasive strategy with a conservative strategy in patients who were initially stabilized with approximately 6 days of treatment with LMWH. Coronary angiography was performed within the first 7 days and revascularization performed in 71% of those in the invasive arm and 9% of those in the noninvasive arm within 10 days. This was, therefore, the first trial to achieve substantial separations in strategy and to include an appropriately powered population. After 6 months, death or MI occurred in 9.4% of the invasive group compared with 12.1% of the noninvasive group (a risk ratio of 0.78, $p = 0.031$) and the results remained significant at 1 year, but the mortality and the death or MI outcomes were no longer significant at 5 years. However, the results at 5 years clearly demonstrate that most benefit was seen in higher-risk patients, with no evidence of benefit in low-risk patients. A similar relationship between patient risk status and long-term outcome had been demonstrated in the RITA-3 trial.

The FRISC-II and the RITA-3 trials demonstrated that invasive therapy was associated with an excess early (within 30 days) rate of death or MI due to periprocedure complications. Overall, there

was a consistency of benefit (for the efficacy endpoints) across the FRISC-II, TACTICS, and RITA-3 trials. RITA-3 demonstrated that most benefit in the first year was in preventing refractory angina, but over 5 years there was a significant benefit in death or MI, and in preventing cardiovascular death, in those randomized to intervention. The more recent ICTUS trial was smaller and had a high rate of intervention in the 'selective invasive' arm of the trial, about as high as the intervention arm in RITA-3 and only modestly lower than in the intervention arm of FRISC-II. ICTUS employed a high rate of adjunctive therapies (including GPIIb/IIIa inhibitors), and the trial did not show an overall benefit for intervention. Differences in trial design, in the risk status of the trial populations, and in the definitions of MI in the respective trials must be taken into consideration. Nevertheless, a pooled analysis of all the trials is likely to represent the most reliable interpretation of all of the randomized trial data.

A number of meta-analyses have been published recently. In a meta-analysis of 8 trials, there was clear evidence for overall benefit on the outcomes of death, MI, or ACS in men and biomarker-positive women. A meta-analysis of FRISC-II, ICTUS, and RITA-3 confirmed that a routine invasive strategy reduced 5-year cardiovascular death and MI (17.9% vs 14.7%, OR 0.83 (CI 0.710–.93), $p = 0.002$), with most benefit in the highest risk group (Fig. 13.4.5).

Risk stratification of patients with non-ST-elevation ACS

Risk stratification is required to guide management and therapeutic decisions in patients with non-ST-elevation ACS. Some patients are clearly at high risk at the time of initial presentation, e.g. those with typical ongoing ischaemic pain and ST depression on the ECG and elevated biomarkers. However, for the remainder it may not be possible to identify higher-risk patients on the basis of biomarkers and ECG findings alone. Additional clinical criteria

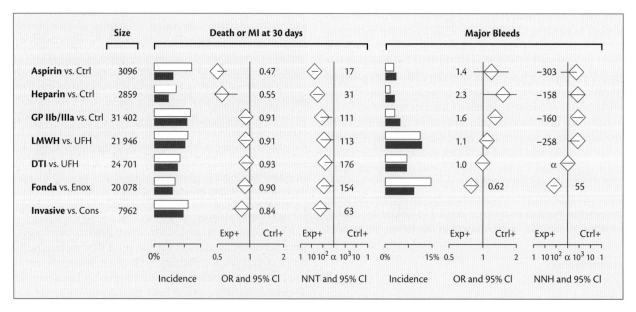

Fig. 13.4.5 Summary of the effects of antiplatelet and anticoagulant regimens in NSTEMI. CI, confidence interval; Cons, conservative; Ctrl, control; DTI, direct thrombin inhibitor; Enox, enoxaparin; Exp +, experimental therapy; Fonda, fondaparinux; GP, glycoprotein; LMWH, low molecular weight heparin; MI, myocardial infarction; NNH, numbers needed to harm; NNT, numbers needed to treat; OR, odds ratio; UFH, unfractionated heparin.

Reproduced from Hamm CW, et al. (2011). ESC guidelines for the management of acute coronary syndromes in patients presenting without persistent ST-segment elevation. *European Heart Journal*, **32**, 2999–3054. With permission of Oxford University Press (UK) © European Society of Cardiology, <www.escardio.org/guidelines>.

such as diabetes, renal insufficiency, impaired LV function, early post-MI angina, recent PCI, prior CABG are important high risk factors. Several studies have demonstrated that simple risk scores can accurately predict short- and longer-term outcome, not only in those with defined characteristics of ACS, but also in patients with suspected cardiac chest pain (GRACE and TIMI risk scores). Using a handheld device, a computer, or a scorecard, risk status can be calculated in less that a minute (risk calculator downloadable from <http://www.outcomes.org/grace> or <http://www.timi.org/>, Table 13.4.2). International comparisons have demonstrated superior predictive accuracy for the GRACE score and the European Society of Cardiology (ESC) guidelines for non-ST-elevation ACS recommend this score. The ESC guidelines also recommend that risk status be re-evaluated, especially if clinical or biochemical features change.

Troponin (cTnT or cTnI) measurement should be performed at presentation (on the basis that those with elevated markers of necrosis on arrival are at increased risk) and repeated after 6 to 12 h if the initial test is negative. Echocardiography may be required to demonstrate the presence or absence of contractile dysfunction or to rule out alternative diagnoses.

There is a substantial late mortality in non-STEMI that is currently under-recognized with 5-year death rates equivalent to patients with STEMI. Although the GRACE risk score was derived and validated for in-hospital and 6-month outcomes, this analysis demonstrates that it has similarly high predictive accuracy for long-term outcomes. The late consequences of presentation with ACS, in terms of death, MI, and stroke, are substantially greater than those seen during the initial in-hospital phase and novel approaches to diminish long-term risk are required.

An integrated approach to the patient with non-ST-elevation ACS

Patients with ACS may present to primary care physicians or directly to emergency hospital services. In addition, 15 to 20% of those presenting directly to chest pain clinics have ACS. Among patients presenting with an ACS, approximately 40% have evidence of prior coronary artery disease (e.g. MI, angiographically demonstrated disease, documented angina with a positive stress test).

The evaluation of patients with suspected ACS needs to be considered in a stepwise approach, proceeding from initial assessment and formulation of a working diagnosis (on the basis of clinical evaluation and the results of immediately available diagnostic tests) to confirmation of the diagnosis and stratification of the patients for emergency, urgent, and elective management.

Emergency Department—triage and establishing a working diagnosis

For the patient with chest pain, two issues must be resolved urgently. First, is the chest pain/discomfort thought to be of cardiac origin? This is a clinical judgement and requires prompt and skilled assessment. Secondly, in those with suspected cardiac pain, is there evidence of evolving infarction?

Patients with evolving infarction (ST-segment elevation or bundle branch block and clinical features of infarction) require emergency reperfusion with primary angioplasty, or if unavailable, thrombolysis (see below).

Patients without ST elevation or left bundle branch block can be triaged into low, intermediate, and high-risk categories (Fig. 13.4.6):

- High-risk ACS—patients with typical clinical features of ischaemia and ST-segment depression or transient ST-segment-elevation, or with troponin elevation and a high risk score (e.g. GRACE >140 and/or 1 high risk feature—see Table 13.4.2). Patients are also at high risk when ischaemia provokes arrhythmias or haemodynamic compromise. These patients should have early invasive assessment (i.e.within 24 h).

- Intermediate or low-risk ACS—patients with clinical features of ACS and nonspecific ECG changes (e.g. T-wave inversion, T-wave flattening, minor conduction abnormalities).

- Patients with a normal ECG, normal biomarkers, normal cardiac examination, and normal echo are potentially low-risk ACS; however, an alternative diagnosis should be actively sought in this group.

Management of patients with non-ST-elevation and high-risk status

High-risk patients with acute ischaemia at initial presentation, and especially those with haemodynamic compromise, require emergency assessment for revascularization (Fig. 13.4.6). Those proceeding to emergency revascularization should receive (1) aspirin, (2) $P2Y_{12}$ receptor inhibitors, (3) Fondaparinux, LMWH, or bivalirudin, and consideration of GPIIb/IIIa inhibition, depending on the timing of planned invasive assessment. In addition, patients should receive anti-ischaemic therapy (see above) and some patients require antiarrhythmic management or haemodymamic

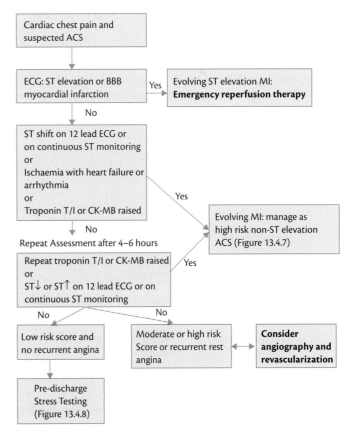

Fig. 13.4.6 Diagnostic triage for suspected acute coronary syndromes. Flowchart to illustrate the key diagnostic features for evolving MI, for higher-risk unstable angina, and for low-risk patients.

support (e.g. intra-aortic balloon pump to reduce ischaemia and stabilize the patient for revascularization).

Management of patients with non-ST-elevation ACS at intermediate or low risk

Patients without high-risk features on initial presentation require further assessment to guide management (Fig. 13.4.7). Application of a risk score will reveal that a significant proportion have unsuspected higher risk (approximately one-third based on registry studies). Such patients require monitoring and repeat ECGs (ideally ST-segment continuous analysis) and evaluation in a dedicated chest pain, cardiac, or combined assessment unit (while awaiting the results of biomarker and other investigations).

- Patients who develop high-risk features after initial presentation should be considered for urgent angiography and revascularization (within 24–72 h). See Table 13.4.5. Those developing ST elevation require emergency reperfusion (by primary PCI or—if PCI not available—by thrombolysis).

- Patients with non-ST-elevation ACS and an intermediate risk score require DAPT plus anticoagulation (heparin, LMWH, fondaparinux, or bivalirudin). All patients at intermediate and high risk are candidates for an early elective revascularization strategy (within c.72 h).

- Clinically stable patients without further chest pain, heart failure, no evolving ECG changes, and biomarker negative are at very low risk for in-hospital major cardiac events. Such patients may, nevertheless, may have significant underlying coronary artery disease. They require further assessment of cardiovascular risk and stress testing or perfusion scanning, ideally prior to discharge.

Other considerations

Coronary artery bypass surgery

As demonstrated by the FRISC-II study, those with three-vessel or left main coronary artery disease and an ACS can be stabilized in the acute phase with antiplatelet and anticoagulant therapy and can proceed to coronary artery bypass surgery with a low perioperative and postoperative morbidity and mortality in experienced centres (c.2%, 30-day mortality). Based on the findings of the CURE study, bleeding risk is minimized if the thienopyridine (clopidogrel) is stopped for 5 or more days prior to surgery. Patients at high risk for thrombotic events in the pre-surgery phase may require an intravenous small molecule GP IIb/IIIa inhibitor (to provide more potent but reversible platelet inhibition up until the time of surgery). See Chapter 13.6 for further discussion.

Antiplatelet and LMWH therapy in patients on warfarin.

There is continuing debate concerning the use of dual antiplatelet therapy in patients undergoing stent implantation for ACS who are on warfarin. Bleeding risk is increased in patients on triple therapy and this has to be balanced against the risk of stent thrombosis with a single antiplatelet agent. Dual antiplatelet thereapy is generally recommended for at least 4 weeks for bare metal stents and for 6 months in patients with drug eluting stents. Where the indication for warfarin is atrial fibrillation alone, oral anticoagulation is often discontinued for this period if the embolic risk is low. Evidence is currently lacking to provide firm recommendations regarding patients on NOAC's.

Secondary prevention

All patients with ACS require cardiovascular secondary prevention measures (Table 13.4.6) including lifestyle modification (smoking cessation, diet, exercise), oral pharmacological therapy (antiplatelet, cholesterol-lowering, ACE inhibitor/ARB) and the management of established and newly detected comorbidities (e.g. diabetes, hypertension, renal dysfunction, heart failure). These are the same in patients with non-ST-elevation ACS as they are for those with STEMI (Table 13.4.6).

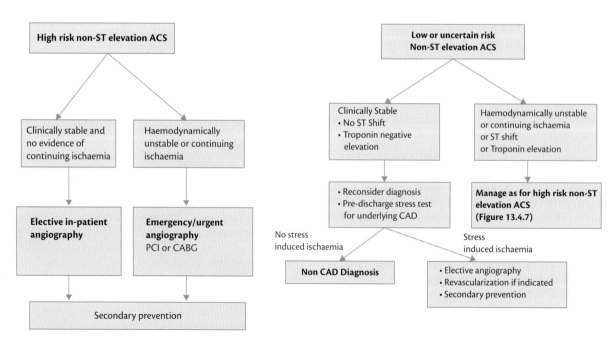

Fig. 13.4.7 Flow chart to indicate the key management steps for patients with non-ST elevation acute coronary syndromes.

Table 13.4.6 Recommendations for secondary prevention for patients with proven ACS

Therapy	Regime
Aspirin	Continue lifelong
P2Y$_{12}$ inhibitor	Continue for 12 months (unless at high risk of bleeding)
β-Blocker	If LV function depressed
ACE inhibitor/ARB	If LV function depressed
	Consider for patients devoid of depressed LV function
Aldosterone antagonist/eplerenone	If depressed LV function (LVEF ≤35%) and either diabetes or heart failure, without significant renal dysfunction
Statin	Titrate to achieve target LDL-C levels <1.8 mmol/litre (<70 mg/dl)
Lifestyle	Risk-factor counselling, referral to cardiac rehabilitation/secondary prevention programme

ACE, angiotensin converting enzyme; ARB, angiotensin receptor blocker; LDL-C, low-density lipoprotein cholesterol; LV, left ventricular; LVEF, left ventricular ejection fraction.

ST-segment elevation myocardial infarction (STEMI)

Outcome in STEMI is critically determined by the extent and severity of myocardial ischaemia. In addition, the eventual extent of irreversibly injured myocardium is influenced by residual myocardial perfusion (via collaterals or subtotal coronary occlusion), the duration of myocardial ischaemia, and cytoprotective mechanisms including preconditioning. As a result, the clinical consequences of abrupt coronary occlusion can range from an entirely silent episode, to profound ischaemia with major cardiac rhythm disturbances (ventricular fibrillation or asystole), to acute mechanical decompensation with heart failure or cardiogenic shock. The outcome is influenced by the extent to which ischaemia is modified by prompt and effective reperfusion and the presence or absence of significant complications, especially arrhythmias (ventricular tachycardia, ventricular fibrillation, and asystole) and acute heart failure. Prompt and successful reperfusion, e.g. within the first hour of symptom onset, may 'abort' or greatly attenuate the eventual extent of MI. Importantly, prompt and effective resuscitation for early ventricular arrhythmias (especially ventricular fibrillation) may have a big impact on survival and freedom from cardiac complications.

The priorities in the management of STEMI are to manage acute life-threatening complications (resuscitation), relieve acute distress, limit the extent of infarction, and treat complications. Beyond the acute phase, attention focuses on secondary prevention and rehabilitation.

Outcome in STEMI

Historically, community-based studies in various populations demonstrated that the case fatality from acute MI, prior to the advent of resuscitation and reperfusion and other modern therapies, was approximately 50% by 1 month after the onset (MONICA studies). About one-half of those deaths were within the first 2 h of symptom onset. However, the risk of death, prior to hospitalization, varies with age: 80% of those above 85 years die before reaching hospital but only 40% of those below 55 years. Before the introduction of cardiac care units in the 1960s, in-patient mortality was in the range of 25 to 30%, and in the 1980s—before the introduction of reperfusion—in-patient mortality averaged about 18%. More recently, the MONICA study from five cities has indicated that the 28-day mortality for patients admitted to hospital with a MI

ranged from 13 to 27%, and other studies have provided figures of 10 to 20%.

There is a marked discrepancy between mortality figures from randomized clinical trials and those from observational studies. Publications reporting the outcome for individuals ineligible for inclusion in trials have demonstrated substantially higher death rates than seen in those entered into contemporary trials in the same centres. Clinical trials can provide accurate information on what is possible in defined populations (often excluding patients with important comorbidity), and carefully conducted registries can provide an accurate reflection of 'real-world' clinical practice. Both approaches are required.

The multinational GRACE registry has demonstrated a decline in in-hospital mortality from 8.4 to 4.6% and new heart failure from 19.5 to 11.0% between 1999 and 2006. The more widespread application of evidence-based pharmacological and reperfusion therapy is closely linked with the improved outcome (with no change in the risk status of patients at presentation), highlighting the importance of 'closing the gap' between evidence from guidelines and clinical trials and application in clinical practice. International organizations including the American College of Cardiology and the ESC have stressed this. Special attention needs to be drawn to the more comprehensive provision of acute resuscitation and defibrillation in the community and to the provision of early effective reperfusion.

Prehospital care

The priorities in prehospital care are to establish a prompt diagnosis of suspected acute infarction, to provide effective resuscitation (especially for ventricular fibrillation), and to initiate prehospital thrombolysis if primary PCI is not available. In addition, patients require effective analgesia and the management of acute complications. Where available, telemetry of the ECG can confirm the diagnosis, expedite emergency transfer for primary PCI, and prepare the cardiac team for receiving the patient in the cardiac catheter laboratory. The aim is to provide reperfusion within 90 min of symptom onset. Although this has been demonstrated to be feasible in many centres and various countries, there are major logistic challenges. 'Door-to-balloon' times exclude the prehospital phase and, in many instances, 'door-to-balloon' times are longer than 90 min, just for this phase of treatment. In rural and other communities with prolonged transfer times to a hospital with PCI facilities, appropriate equipment and training needs to be established to allow prehospital thrombolysis to be administered safely and effectively.

Making a diagnosis of suspected infarction and initiating treatment

A working diagnosis of suspected infarction is based upon typical severe chest discomfort of more than 15 min duration which is unresponsive to glyceryl trinitrate. Characteristically, the pain may radiate to the neck, lower jaw, and arms, and is often accompanied by autonomic features including sweating and pallor. Unless complications are present, physical examination may reveal no significant abnormalities, other than those associated with autonomic disturbance, but signs can include tachycardia or bradycardia, the presence of a third or fourth heart sound, and features of heart failure (see Chapter 2.1).

The initial ECG is seldom normal, but may not show the classical features of ST-segment elevation or evidence of Q waves (unless prior MI had occurred). Hyperacute T-wave changes can be present within minutes of the onset of ischaemia due to coronary occlusion, and this may be followed by the evolution of characteristic ST-segment elevation. However, minor or nonspecific ECG abnormalities in conjunction with a characteristic history may signal the early stages of infarction. The working diagnosis relies heavily on the clinical history, and when this suggests MI, repeat ECG within 30 to 60 min (or continuous ST analysis) will frequently reveal the evolution of recognizable ECG changes. It is critically important

that infarction that evolves after initial presentation should be detected promptly.

In the prehospital setting, a paramedic or primary care physician may have to rely on the clinical findings to establish the working diagnosis and to initiate immediate treatment. Prompt relief of pain is important, not only for humanitarian reasons, but because pain is associated with sympathetic activation, vasoconstriction, and increased myocardial work. Effective analgesia is best achieved by the titration of intravenous opioids, although some paramedic crews only have access to nonopioid analgesia. Side effects of analgesia include nausea and vomiting, hypotension, and respiratory depression. Antiemetics can be administered concurrently; hypotension and bradycardia will usually respond to atropine and respiratory depression to naloxone. Oxygen should be administered, especially to those who are breathless or those with any features of heart failure or shock (see Chapter 4.2 for information on basic and advanced life support in the management of cardiac arrest or ventricular fibrillation).

The logistics of providing acute care for patients with MI depend upon the locally available facilities. Guidelines recommend an integrated service involving prehospital emergency care (ambulance and paramedic personnel, primary care physicians, etc.) and hospital-based specialists, including cardiologists and emergency care physicians. Within an urban setting, with relatively short transfer times, the shortest delays and the most prompt initiation

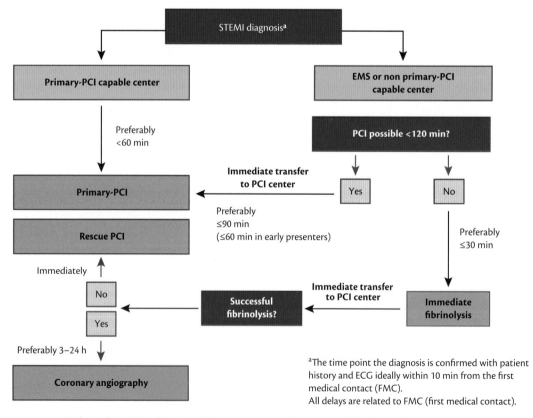

Cath = catheterization laboratory; EMS = emergency medical system; FMC = first medical contact; PCI = percutaneous coronary intervention; STEMI = ST-segment elevation myocardia l infarction.

Fig. 13.4.8 Prehospital and in- hospital management and reperfusion strategies for STEMI within 24 h of first medical contact. Cath, catheterization laboratory; EMS, emergency medical system; FMC, first medical contact; PCI, percutaneous coronary intervention; STEMI, ST-segment elevation mycocardial infarction.
Adapted from Wijns W, *et al.* (2010). Guidelines on myocardial revascularization. *Eur Heart J*, **31**, 2501–2555.

of reperfusion occurs when the patient seeks an emergency medical ambulance and achieves direct transfer to a hospital with available primary PCI facilities. Studies have shown that once the diagnosis is confirmed (e.g. by telemetry of the ECG) substantial time can be saved by direct transfer of the patient to the catheterization laboratory for PCI rather than transfer via an Emergency Department (Fig. 13.4.8).

Prehospital thrombolysis

If a primary PCI programme is not available, or if transfer times are sufficiently prolonged that reperfusion may not be achieved within 120 min of patient call, then prehospital thrombolysis is the next best option. The combined analysis of primary PCI vs thrombolysis trials clearly shows superior outcome (deaths, recurrent MI, stroke, etc.) and less bleeding complications (especially intracerebral bleeds) for primary PCI. However, whether primary PCI—with the inherent transfer delays—is superior to very early thrombolysis (administered within the first hour of symptom onset) remains untested in trials of sufficient power.

To date, eight trials have been conducted comparing prehospital with in-hospital administration of thrombolytic therapy. Depending upon the clinical setting, between 30 and 130 min are saved by prehospital thrombolysis (fibrinolytic drug plus aspirin). Overall, for the complete study population of 6607 patients, the 30-day mortality was 10.7% for those receiving in-hospital administration of thrombolysis, and 9.1% for those where it was administered prior to hospital admission. This amounts to a 17% relative reduction in early mortality with a *p* value of 0.02 (1.6% absolute reduction). Complication rates were similar for community-treated and hospital-initiated thrombolysis, although ventricular fibrillation occurred more frequently with community administration and necessitated well-trained staff and the availability of defibrillators. The greatest benefit is seen when prehospital treatment is applied in remote settings where transport delays are more than 1 h. Several studies have indicated that about 20 patients with chest pain require evaluation for each patient found to be eligible for thrombolytic therapy in the community. Nevertheless, with appropriate training and facilities, prehospital care can provide a gain of approximately 20 lives per 1000 treated among eligible patients.

Prehospital cardiac arrest

The management of prehospital cardiac arrest requires special attention. At least as many lives can be saved by prompt resuscitation and defibrillation as by reperfusion. For these reasons, emergency assessment of the patient with suspected infarction necessitates that the clinician or paramedic has access to a defibrillator and the skills to manage cardiac arrest promptly and effectively. The provision of basic or advanced life support training to paramedic ambulance crews, together with semiautomatic defibrillators, has resulted in a substantial increase in the number of patients surviving out-of-hospital cardiac arrest. Before the institution of such programmes, successful resuscitations were opportunistic and often relied on the availability of a bystander with medical or nursing training. Nationwide figures indicate that resuscitation now achieves survival in 7 to 10% of those patients found with cardiac arrest and in whom the initial rhythm is thought to be ventricular fibrillation. With effective integrated programmes, higher success rates have been achieved: for instance, in the south-eastern region of Scotland, about 14% survive to reach hospital alive, and in Seattle, with a well-established community training and resuscitation programme, the figure exceeds 20%. About one-half of those reaching hospital alive survive to be discharged home.

Emergency Department triage and management

Ideally, in those with typical clinical features and ST elevation on the ECG, a working diagnosis has been made in the prehospital setting (by paramedics with ECG telemetry or by a primary care physician) and early management initiated prior to hospital arrival. Where facilities are available, the patient should be transferred directly to the catheterization laboratory (with the team alerted while the patient is in transit), or if the decision is made for thrombolysis, then this is administered before arrival in hospital.

In-hospital evaluation is required in the remainder, where the symptoms are unclear, the ECG not diagnostic, or if significant comorbidity is present (e.g. bleeding risks). The priority immediately after arrival at the hospital is to identify those patients with ST elevation infarction for prompt reperfusion therapy (Fig. 13.4.9). Triage is usually performed in the Emergency Department, or, in some institutions, patients with a high probability of infarction gain direct access to a cardiac care assessment area. An integrated strategy involving the paramedic or ambulance system, the emergency physicians, and the cardiologists is required. 'Fast-track' systems have been developed to minimize in-hospital delay to reperfusion: these are facilitated by specifically trained medical and nursing staff, with the aim of ensuring clinical assessment and ECG within 15 min of arrival and rapid transfer for PCI or the institution of thrombolytic therapy within 30 min. Audit programmes and continuous training are necessary for centres to achieve this 30-min median 'door-to-needle' time.

Definite vs suspected infarction

Rapid triage systems allow the identification of patients with clearly defined clinical and ECG features of infarction, i.e. characteristic symptoms of infarction which persist at rest and are not relieved by glyceryl trinitrate, in the presence of at least 1 mm ST-segment

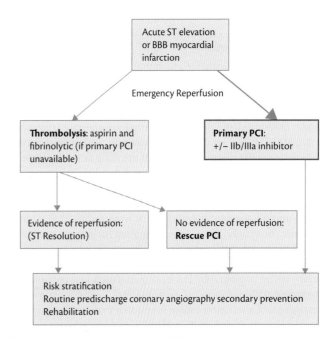

Fig. 13.4.9 Management of ST elevation MI.

elevation in two or more contiguous leads, or the development of bundle branch block. Clinical trials have employed ECG criteria of 1 mm ST elevation for limb leads and 2 mm for chest leads, a definition that improves specificity, but is associated with reduced sensitivity.

Among those without diagnostic ECG changes, a working diagnosis of suspected MI or non-ST-elevation ACS can be established. Such patients require repeat clinical and ECG assessments or continuous ST analysis to detect those with evolving infarction and separate them from those with unstable angina or non-ST-elevation infarction.

The rationale for minimizing delays to reperfusion

Experimental and clinical data demonstrate that the duration of ischaemia prior to reperfusion is a critical determinant of the eventual extent of myocardial damage. These data are supported by the improved outcome seen with prehospital vs in-hospital thrombolysis, also observational data from large clinical trials in which survival gain diminishes with each additional hour of ischaemia. The Fibrinolytic Trials Overview suggests about 1.6 additional deaths per hour of delay per 1000 treated, and a more recent meta-analysis suggests that early time delay is especially important.

The relationship between the duration of ischaemia and the extent of infarction is nonlinear: the greatest potential for salvage occurs when reperfusion is initiated within 60 min of the onset of infarction. Under such circumstances, a proportion of patients (5–7%) will have the infarction aborted and will not develop Q waves or significant enzyme elevation despite characteristic ST elevation on the initial ECG. Minimizing the time delay is, therefore, critical in salvaging myocardium. Based on data from individual trials, and from the Fibrinolytic Trials Overview, most benefit occurs within the first 3 h of the onset of infarction, and highly significant benefits still occur at up to 6 h. Statistically significant gains are still present at 12 h, but beyond 12 h the benefits are marginal. However, some patients present with a stuttering pattern and in the presence of persistent or intermittent ST-segment elevation and continuing symptoms of ischaemia, reperfusion beyond 12 h may salvage significant ischaemic myocardium.

Differential diagnosis

Critically, thrombolytic therapy or angiography for anticipated primary angioplasty will be of no benefit to those who do not have MI and may convey significant hazards. Such patients suffer the dual hazards of thrombolysis or angiography in the acute phase of their illness and the delay in initiating appropriate treatment. Furthermore, those treated inappropriately with thrombolysis will experience the bleeding hazards of the drug (a net increase in intracerebral haemorrhage of c.0.5%) and the disrupted coagulation system will render other emergency surgery (e.g. for perforated peptic ulceration) more hazardous. Alternative cardiac diagnoses include non-ST-segment-elevation ACS, myocarditis, pericarditis, and aortic dissection. Noncardiac diagnoses include gastrointestinal pain of oesophageal, peptic, or biliary origin; pancreatitis; pulmonary embolism; and respiratory and musculoskeletal disorders. Equally, where angiography has been performed in a patient with a suspected ACS and is found to be normal a careful review and investigation of alternative causes is essential prior to discharge.

Aortic dissection presents a particular problem when it extends proximally to the origin of the right coronary artery and produces inferior infarction. CT, MRI, or transoesophageal echocardiography may be required to establish the diagnosis (see Chapter 14.1).

Transthoracic echocardiography can be valuable when infarction is suspected, but characteristic ECG features are absent: normal left ventricular function excludes significant infarction, and conversely a regional contraction abnormality helps to confirm the diagnosis of ischaemia or possible infarction. However, in those with prior myocardial damage, the differentiation of new from old mechanical dysfunction is complex and requires specialist assistance.

Cardiac enzymes are helpful when abnormal, but most patients present within 3 h of the onset of symptoms and insufficient time has elapsed to produce a diagnostic release of biomarkers of necrosis—troponins, creatine kinase (CK), or CK-MB. Patients with suspected infarction but normal ECGs require further clinical ECG and biomarker estimations 4 to 6 h after the suspected event.

Among elderly and very elderly patients (>90 years of age), the presentation of infarction is often atypical. They may not experience a typical pattern of symptoms and concomitant multisystem disorders may obscure the diagnosis. MI must be considered in the differential diagnosis of abrupt collapse, haemodynamic disturbance of sudden onset, or severe nonspecific symptoms in elderly patients.

Continuing management in the Cardiac Department

Administration of analgesia, management of rhythm and haemodynamic compromise, and initiation of pharmaocological therapy (heparin, LMWH, aspirin, $P2Y_{12}$ receptor inhibitors, etc.) should have been initiated shortly after the diagnosis of ST-elevation MI is made (in the Emergency Department or Cardiac Assessment Area or prehospital). The first priority is for emergency reperfusion (primary PCI, or if unavailable thrombolysis). Patients may require management of heart failure and arrhythmias and pain relief while in transit to reperfusion therapy, but every effort should be made to avoid delays to reperfusion.

Percutaneous coronary intervention
Primary PCI

Primary angioplasty is defined as PCI without concomitant fibrinolytic therapy. It requires prompt availability of a highly skilled interventional cardiology team with substantial experience of the procedure.

Randomized clinical trials of primary PCI vs thrombolysis have shown consistent findings: primary PCI has superior outcomes. In experienced centres it is more effective in restoring patency, achieves better ventricular function, and improves important clinical outcomes, with lower rates of death, reinfarction, stroke, major bleeding, and recurrent ischaemia (Table 13.4.7). Particular gains are seen in haemodynamically compromised patients and those with cardiogenic shock. In consequence, primary PCI is the preferred therapeutic option in national and international guidelines (SIGN, ESC PCI Guidelines, American College of Cardiology, and AHA).

Patients are transferred as an emergency to the cardiac catheterization laboratory and angiography undertaken (radial artery or femoral artery access) to establish coronary anatomy and the nature of the vessel occlusion. A flexible guide wire is then passed across the occluded lesion and balloon angioplasty (usually accompanied by stent implantation) performed ('primary PCI'), thereby restoring patency to the previously occluded coronary artery.

Table 13.4.7 Advantages of primary percutaneous coronary intervention over thrombolysis

Clinical indices	Event rate (%)		Absolute risk (%)	Relative risk (%)	NNT
	Thrombolysis	PCI			
Short-term mortality (4–6 weeks)	8	5	3	36	33
Long-term mortality (6–18 months)	8	5	3	38	33
Stroke	2	<1	2	64	50
Reinfarction	8	3	5	59	20
Recurrent ischaemia	18	7	11	59	9
Death or nonfatal reinfarction	12	7	5	44	20
Need for CABG	13	8	5	36	20

CABG, coronary artery bypass graft; NNT, number needed to treat; PCI, percutaneous coronary intervention.

Data from Hartwell D, *et al.* (2005). Clinical effectiveness and cost-effectiveness of immediate angioplasty for acute myocardial infarction: systematic review and economic evaluation. *Health Technol Assess*, **9**(17).

• Primary percutaneous coronary angioplasty (PCI) is the treatment of choice in patients with STEMI.

• Primary PCI requires a highly experienced interventional team with 24-h availability and an integrated approach to management to achieve reperfusion with the minimum of delay—ideally within 120 min of symptom onset.

• Where primary PCI is unavailable, the patient should undergo prompt thrombolytic therapy, provided no contraindications are present.

• The limit in treating all potentially eligible patients with reperfusion therapy has not been reached. Internationally, at least one-third of all MIs (without a major bleeding risk) receive neither thrombolysis nor primary PCI.

Rescue PCI

Thrombolytic therapy may fail to achieve effective reperfusion in 30% or more of those in whom it is administered for STEMI. Patients experience continuing symptoms of ischaemia and failure of resolution of ST elevation on the ECG (<50% resolution of the ST elevation within 1 h of administration). Rescue PCI is more effective than repeat thrombolysis or conservative treatment in improving outcome (REACT trial). Thus, in centres where primary PCI is not available, logistics need to be established for prompt transfer for rescue percutaneous coronary intervention of patients in whom thrombolysis does not result in signs of reperfusion.

Facilitated PCI

The combination of full-dose or reduced-dose fibrinolysis followed by emergency PCI has been tested in large-scale trials and shown worse outcomes and greater bleeding risks (ASSENT 4 trial). Hence, planned emergency PCI after thrombolysis is not recommended. although later PCI—after the impact of thrombolysis has resolved—may be of benefit (GRACIA 2 study). The latter approach should be considered as part of the strategy to deal with residual stenoses after PCI (prior to hospital discharge), rather than as 'facilitated' PCI.

Thrombolytic treatment

Thrombolytic treatment refers to the combination of antiplatelet therapy (aspirin and clopidogrel) with fibrinolytic treatment. The fibrinolytic agent, directly or indirectly, converts plasminogen to plasmin and plasmin lyses fibrin in the clot. Cross-linked fibrin is more resistant to fibrinolytic drugs than a newly formed fibrin clot.

The combination of aspirin and a fibrinolytic agent has undergone extensive clinical testing in trials involving more than 100 000 patients. Additional trials have been conducted comparing one fibrinolytic agent with another. For patients presenting within 6 h of symptom onset, and with ST elevation or bundle branch block, approximately 30 deaths are prevented per 1000 patients treated. For those presenting between 7 and 12 h, approximately 20 deaths are prevented per 1000 patients treated, and beyond 12 h the benefits are inconclusive. Thrombolysis is a very cost-effective treatment for acute MI. A sustained benefit on survival has been demonstrated 14 years after thrombolysis.

The ISIS-2 trial demonstrated that the benefits of aspirin treatment were additional to those of fibrinolytic treatment, each achieving about 25 lives saved per 1000 patients treated (for the whole of the study population). Thus, in combination, about 50 lives are saved per 1000 patients treated, but the benefits are larger than this among those presenting within 3 h of infarction with ST-segment elevation or bundle branch block.

Overall, the largest absolute benefit is seen in patients at highest risk, although the proportional benefit may be similar for all. High-risk patients include those over 65 years of age, those with a systolic blood pressure below 100 mmHg, and those with anterior infarction or more extensive ischaemia (see 'Primary PCI'). The absolute benefit in lives saved per 1000 treated is 11 ± 3 for those under 55 years of age; 18 ± 4 for those between 55 and 64; 27 ± 5 for those 65 to 74; and 10 ± 13 for those over 75. However, for ST depression there is a net hazard of 14 lives lost per 1000 treated, and for those with a normal ECG 7 lives lost per 1000 treated (Fibrinolytic Trials Overview). Thus, evidence supports thrombolysis treatment only for those patients with ST elevation or bundle branch block.

Hazards of thrombolysis

Thrombolytic therapy is associated with a significant excess of haemorrhagic complications, including cerebral haemorrhage. Overall, about 2 nonfatal strokes occur per 1000 patients treated, and of these half are moderately or severely disabling. An additional 2 strokes per 1000 patients are fatal, and the net impact on mortality includes such patients. The risk of stroke increases with age, especially for those over 75 years of age, and for those with systolic hypertension. There is also an excess of noncerebral bleeds of about 7 per 1000 treated. Bleeding occurs at arterial and venous puncture sites, hence blood sampling or cannulation of vessels should be limited to sites where external compression can achieve haemostasis.

Streptokinase and other streptokinase-containing agents can produce hypotension and, rarely, allergic reactions. Routine administration of hydrocortisone is not indicated. When hypotension occurs, it can be managed by interrupting the streptokinase infusion, lying the patient flat or head down, and by the administration of atropine or intravascular volume expansion.

Comparison of thrombolytic agents

The most widely used thrombolytic agents are streptokinase, alteplase (tissue plasminogen activator, tPA), tenecteplase (TNK), and reteplase (rPA). The GISSI International Trial and ISIS-3 international trial both failed to find a difference in outcome between streptokinase and tPA. However, the GUSTO trial (Global Utilization of Streptokinase and Tissue plasminogen active for Occluded coronary arteries) employed an accelerated administration of alteplase over 90 min and intravenous heparin adjusted using the activated partial thromboplastin time, finding 10 fewer deaths per 1000 patients treated with alteplase compared with the streptokinase group. Meta-analysis confirms the superiority of clot-specific agents (e.g. alteplase, tenecteplase) over streptokinase.

The current reference standard for the comparison of fibrinolytic agents is the accelerated infusion regimen of alteplase (tPA), or for simplicity the single-bolus administration of tenecteplase (TNK). Tenecteplase does not require an infusion pump or refrigeration and hence is particularly suited for prehospital administration, but internationally streptokinase remains the most widely used fibrinolytic agent, principally because it is relatively inexpensive.

Invasive assessment after fibrinolysis

Following lytic therapy a strategy of routine early angiography (3–24 h) is recommended. This approach reduces the risk of recurrent infarction and ischaemia, without an increased risk of stroke or bleeding. Patients should have DAPT, and antithrombin therapy as indicated in PPCI. Revascularization by PCI or CABG depends upon the extent and location of underlying coronary disease.

Coronary artery bypass surgery (CABG)

In the acute phase of MI, the role of CABG is limited to those patients with acute mechanical complications, such as ventricular septal defect or mitral regurgitation due to papillary muscle rupture. Unless such mechanical complications are present, the hazards of acute bypass surgery are significantly increased compared to delayed revascularization in a stabilized patient. The Danish DANAMI study investigated the role of revascularization in those with ischaemia during the recovery phase of MI. It suggested that, following infarction, individuals with symptomatic or electrocardiographic ischaemia on stress testing experience significant long-term benefit from surgical revascularization.

Further in-hospital management

The period of hospitalization for reperfused and uncomplicated patients following STEMI has progressively shortened, and is now in the range of 2 to 5 days. Thus there are time pressures to initiate lifestyle modifications, drug therapy for secondary prevention, and rehabilitation measures. It is essential to initiate these management steps before hospital discharge to minimize the risk that they are not carried out afterwards.

The main aims of further in-hospital management are the identification and treatment of acute complications of infarction, identification of patients at increased risk for subsequent cardiac events, and initiation of secondary prevention and rehabilitation.

Major complications may be apparent at the time of presentation and haemodynamic, arrhythmic, or ischaemic complications may be evident shortly thereafter. Nevertheless, in the period beyond the first 12 to 24 h, it is appropriate to focus attention on the points listed above.

Identification and treatment of complications of infarction
Failure of reperfusion

Electrocardiographic markers of failed thrombolysis reperfusion are the persistence of ST-segment elevation together with clinical and haemodynamic features of continuing ischaemia. Continuous computed ST analysis allows the most accurate definition of ECG changes, but an approximation can be obtained with repeated 12-lead ECGs and measurement of ST-segment elevation. In those with successful reperfusion, ST segments decrease to less than 50% of peak elevation within 60 min.

In addition, some patients exhibit reperfusion arrhythmias (ventricular tachycardia, idioventricular rhythm, and—rarely—ventricular fibrillation). Such arrhythmias are more common in the presence of marked ischaemia and prompt reperfusion within 60 to 90 min of occlusion.

Rescue angioplasty is the appropriate management for failed reperfusion, and consists of mechanical recanalization of the occluded vessel with percutaneous intervention, including stent implantation. This strategy achieves an 'open artery', and randomized trial data (REACT trial) shows superior outcome compared with repeat thrombolysis or conservative management.

Cardiogenic shock

In cardiogenic shock, mechanical contractile abnormalities of the left ventricle or acute haemodynamic complications (papillary muscle rupture or ventricular septal defect) lead to reduced blood pressure and impaired tissue perfusion. Clinically, the condition is recognized by a systolic blood pressure of less than 90 mmHg together with impaired tissue flow, as reflected by oliguria, impaired cerebral function, and peripheral vasoconstriction. Between 5 and 20% of those patients admitted to hospital with acute MI demonstrate cardiogenic shock, although the frequency has been reduced by thrombolytic therapy and primary PCI. The mortality rate when cardiogenic shock complicates an acute coronary event is in excess of 70%, if acute revascularization is not possible.

Time delay is critically important in the management of cardiogenic shock: mortality rises progressively if more than 2 h have elapsed since its onset. Treatment aims to improve the recovery of acutely ischaemic myocardium (mechanical and surgical revascularization) and to support the circulation with a combination of inotropes, vasodilators, and loop diuretics. Evidence suggests that the most important treatment may be to reopen the infarct-related artery.

In addition to achieving reperfusion, management of the patient with cardiogenic shock after MI may require inotropic support. Dopamine is commonly used, initially at a low 'renal dose' (1–5 micrograms/kg per min) that activates dopaminergic receptors (but also has an effect on the circulation), but if necessary at higher doses of 5 to 20 micrograms/kg per min that have positive inotropic and chronotropic effects. In doses above 20 micrograms/kg per min, there is activation of α-adrenoceptors with undesirable peripheral vasoconstriction and a decline in renal perfusion. Dobutamine acts mainly as a β_1-adrenoceptor agonist and is used in the range of 2 to 40 micrograms/kg per min. Phosphodiesterase inhibitors have both inotropic and vasodilator effects and, although they have produced favourable haemodynamic responses, the studies conducted have not shown an improvement in outcome.

The management of pulmonary oedema consists of opiates (to relieve distress and to reduce vascular resistance), oxygen, vasodilators, and diuretics. If it is severe, patients may require positive end-expiratory ventilation or even full mechanical ventilation. Vasodilators (including nitrates, salbutamol, and sodium nitroprusside) reduce venous and pulmonary arterial pressure, but tachycardia may be a limiting feature and their use is limited in those who are profoundly hypotensive. Loop diuretics are employed in bolus intravenous doses or by infusion.

In all instances, decisions to proceed to mechanical external support of the circulation or mechanical ventilation need to take account of the extent to which the cardiac dysfunction may be reversible, the presence of comorbidity, and the wishes of the patient and their family.

Left ventricular dysfunction and heart failure

Large-scale trials of angiotensin converting enzyme (ACE) inhibitors and angiotensin receptor blockers (ARBs) have been conducted in patients with left ventricular dysfunction and those with clinical and radiological features of heart failure (see Chapter 5.1). Clear evidence demonstrates improved short- and long-term outcome with ACE inhibitors/ARBs in patients with heart failure and those with asymptomatic left ventricular dysfunction.

Caution must be exercised with the introduction of ACE inhibitors in patients with intravascular volume depletion, when they can cause hypotension, and in patients with low arterial pressure or renal impairment. ACE inhibition should commence with a very small dose (e.g. 6.25 mg of captopril), with dosages increased progressively in conjunction with clinical monitoring. They can provoke deterioration in renal function in patients with renal artery stenosis and in those with significant pre-existing renal impairment, hence it is important to check serum electrolytes and creatinine during early treatment and follow-up.

Arrhythmias

A wide variety of arrhythmias can be seen in the context of acute MI and its treatment. The most serious, including ventricular fibrillation, ventricular tachycardia, and heart block, can lead to cardiac arrest. However, routine administration of antiarrhythmic agents is not indicated. They are almost invariably negatively inotropic, and they may also be proarrhythmic in the context of acute coronary ischaemia. An overview of randomized trials into the use of prophylactic lidocaine (lignocaine) showed that it increased mortality. Ventricular fibrillation should be treated with direct current (DC) cardioversion, and recurrent ventricular arrhythmias require antiarrhythmics (e.g. amiodarone). Importantly, attention should be paid to electrolyte imbalance and the correction of reversible

ischaemia or other factors provoking arrhythmias. (see Chapter 4.1 for details of the diagnosis and treatment of arrhythmias).

Heart block of any degree can occur after acute MI. It is more common with inferior than anterior infarction because the right coronary artery supplies the atrioventricular node, and also because vagal reflexes are more likely from this area. It is often transient, and does not necessarily imply a large infarct, except when it occurs with anterior infarction, in which case the prognosis is grave. Temporary transvenous pacing is justified when bradycardia compromises the circulation, but is not advocated 'prophylactically'.

Ventricular septal defect, papillary muscle rupture, and myocardial rupture

Rupture of the interventricular septum occurs in up to 3% of acute infarctions and is responsible for about 5% of deaths due to MI. Rupture in the apical area may complicate anterior infarction and in the basal inferior area may complicate inferior infarction. Clinically, the condition is associated with the development of a new pansystolic murmur and clinical features of a left-to-right shunt with increased pulmonary congestion. The findings are confirmed on echocardiography or cardiac catheterization. Surgery should be undertaken as soon as possible: the outlook for those who are not operated upon is very bleak, with few surviving. However, some patients with small shunts survive the acute phase, in which case they may suffer the later consequences of the shunt.

Papillary muscle rupture occurs as a result of acute ischaemic damage due to obstruction of either the left anterior descending or circumflex coronary arteries. It causes the abrupt onset of severe mitral regurgitation and accounts for 5% of deaths after acute MI. The complication generally occurs within the first week after infarction, and may be recognized as the abrupt onset of acute pulmonary oedema. It is often accompanied by a new systolic murmur, but when the left atrial pressure rises acutely the murmur may be insignificant. The findings are confirmed with echocardiography. The management is acute surgical repair with or without revascularization.

In the patient who deteriorates haemodynamically after MI—with hypotension, pulmonary oedema, or both—it is important to consider the possibility of a ventricular septal defect or acute mitral regurgitation. However, it can be impossible to distinguish between the two on clinical grounds. Both classically produce a new pansystolic murmur, and although differences between the murmurs have been described, these are not robust enough to discriminate with certainty in the individual case. Acute mitral regurgitation is best diagnosed by echocardiography, but transthoracic echocardiography may be unable to detect a ventricular septal defect in a reliable manner. Transoesophageal echocardiography is better, as is the use of a contrast-enhanced technique. If this is unavailable, an alternative approach is to pass a flow-directed pulmonary catheter and take blood samples from the pulmonary artery, right ventricle, and right atrium. A step-up in oxygen tension between the right atrium and the pulmonary artery indicates the presence of a left-to-right shunt and confirms the diagnosis of a ventricular septal defect.

Myocardial rupture may follow acute infarction, usually involving the free wall of the left ventricle. It is responsible for approximately 10% of all deaths in acute MI. Half of the ruptures occur within the first week, and 90% within 2 weeks. The location of rupture is usually within the infarcted area, but may be at the junction with adjacent normal myocardium. In most cases, death is immediate and due to electromechanical dissociation. The patient is unresponsive to resuscitation measures but, rarely—with subacute rupture—patients can be supported until surgical repair is performed. The diagnosis is made on clinical and echocardiographic criteria with assessment for possible cardiac tamponade (see Chapter 8.1). In some patients, partial rupture of the free wall can result in the late development of a false aneurysm.

Left ventricular thrombus

A left ventricular thrombus can be detected using echocardiography in up to 40% of patients with acute anterior MI. The thrombus is usually located at the apex in association with a dyskinetic or aneurysmal section of myocardium with impaired contractile function. The thrombus may be large, and is associated with risks of embolization (in 15–20% of cases). Anticoagulation with heparin followed by warfarin is advised in patients with extensive infarction and those in whom apical aneurysms or mural thrombi are detected for up to 6 months. Both, thrombolysis and surgical repair, have been successfully conducted. However, there is no clear evidence that either strategy is superior (provided there is no evidence of embolization). Combining oral anticoagulation with DAPT increases bleeding risk. The duration of therapy is unknown but should reflect the relative risk of bleeding and stent thrombosis. Repeat imaging may help to confirm thrombus resolution and/or improvement of LV function to guide a decision about long-term therapy.

Right ventricular infarction

Right ventricular infarction may occur in isolation, or associated with inferior STEMI. The triad of hypotension, clear lung fields, and raised central venous pressure should prompt its diagnosis. ECG may show ST elevation in V1 and V4R. The chest radiograph is characteristically clear despite the presence of shock. Echocardiography conforms right ventricular (RV) dilatation, low pulmonary artery (PA) pressure, dilated hepatic veins. Fluid loading to maintain RV filling is the key therapeutic intervention, and PA catheter insertion maybe necessary for accurate monitoring. Maintaining sinus rhythm and atrioventricular synchrony is important.

Pericarditis

Pericarditis may complicate an extensive MI, and may be manifest clinically as a pericardial friction rub accompanied by pleuritic chest pain. A small pericardial effusion may be detected using echocardiography. Dressler's syndrome is a rare late complication and is associated with pericarditis between 2 weeks and 3 months after acute infarction. It has an autoimmune basis, often accompanied by pleural and pericardial effusions. It is managed with salicylates, paracetamol, or colchicine. The frequency of both pericarditis and Dressler's syndrome is reduced with acute reperfusion.

An integrated approach to the management of STEMI

Prehospital management

In a patient with suspected acute infarction, the priorities are to establish whether typical clinical features and ST elevation (or left bundle branch block) are present, and if so to initiate reperfusion with the absolute minimum of delay. Where possible, the diagnosis is confirmed and the transfer of the patient arranged by telemetry of the ECG. The phrase 'time is muscle' has been coined for acute STEMI. Acute resuscitation may be required for cardiac arrest or

major arrhythmic complications, especially ventricular fibrillation. Additional priorities are to provide analgesia and oxygen. Prehospital thrombolysis may be given by appropriately trained paramedic crews, when transfer times to a PCI hospital are such that more than 120 min will elapse from diagnosis to PCI.

In-hospital management

Initial triage and management

Initial assessment involves the identification of those with clear-cut evidence of STEMI (based on clinical and diagnostic ECG criteria). Such patients require immediate triage to reperfusion therapy (primary PCI, or if unavailable thrombolysis with a fibrinolytic agent plus an antiplatelet agents). In transit to primary PCI or while preparing pharmacological reperfusion, patients may require further analgesia and management of arrhythmic and haemodynamic complications, including heart failure.

Patients in whom the diagnosis of MI is suspected, but the ECG criteria are not diagnostic, should be managed in an intensive care setting (in the Emergency Department or Cardiac Care Unit with repeat ECG evaluation at 30-min intervals (or ST-segment analysis). Cardiac biomarkers (troponins) may be elevated at presentation, if sufficient time has lapsed from onset of ischaemia (4–6h), or they may become elevated following arrival (repeat measurement at 8–12h). Such patients may be divided into those with evidence of non-STEMI (ECG and troponin elevation) and those with unstable angina (T-wave inversion, ST-segment depression, or transient ST-segment elevation, without elevated cardiac troponins). Among those with minor or nonspecific ECG changes and no enzyme elevation, re-evaluation should take place for alternative diagnoses, and stress testing performed subsequently to detect underlying coronary artery disease (Fig. 13.4.8). A key component of initial evaluation of those without ST elevation or left bundle branch block involves risk stratification (see Table 13.4.2). Echocardiography may be valuable to detect signs of ischaemia/infarction or to demonstrate normal contractile function in those with an alternative diagnosis.

Later in-hospital management

During this phase the management of complications, initiation of secondary prevention, and early cardiac rehabilitation should take place. In high-risk patients (those with recurrent acute ischaemia or those with failure of ST-segment resolution and continuing pain), emergency PCI or surgical revascularization can be performed in appropriately equipped centres (Fig. 13.4.8).

Regular clinical and electrocardiographic assessments are required during the recovery phase to detect acute mechanical and arrhythmic complications, and to identify impaired contractile function in patients who will benefit from ACE inhibitor/ARB treatment. This treatment is indicated in those with overt heart failure in the acute phase and also indicated for secondary prevention in patients with established vascular disease (HOPE trial). Thus, ACE inhibitors or ARBs are indicated for those with vascular disease, irrespective of whether there is evidence of overt heart failure or impaired left ventricular function in acute phase. Patients also require lipid-lowering therapy: robust evidence demonstrates that all patients with MI or non-ST-elevation ACS will benefit (MRC/BHF Heart Protection Study). There is evidence to support management of diabetes with glucose and insulin during the in-hospital and early posthospital phase.

All patients will benefit from smoking cessation, the management of hypertension (systolic pressure to <140 mmHg), and dietary and lifestyle modification, including exercise (SIGN Guideline 2007). After STEMI, patients benefit from participation in a rehabilitation programme, with improved quality of life, symptom relief, and return to an active lifestyle or occupation.

Secondary prevention measures in those with STEMI or non-STEMI ACS

Following an ACS, patients require dietary and lifestyle advice including the support necessary to discontinue smoking with the introduction of nicotine replacement therapy. (SIGN Guideline 2007). Lipids should be measured within the first 24 h of admission, with evidence supporting the use of lipid-lowering therapy. Individuals with documented coronary artery disease, and especially those with left ventricular contractile dysfunction or heart failure, have reduced long-term risks of death and MI if maintained on an ACE inhibitor or ARB. In addition, patients may require antianginal therapy if revascariztion is incomplete and all should receive long-term, low-dose aspirin. DAPT should be given for at least 1 month in STEMI (the limits of the evidence) and a year for non-ST-elevation ACS (or as determined by the type of stents implanted).

Nonpharmacological interventions

Evidence supports the following nonpharmacological interventions in secondary prevention: cessation of smoking (including the avoidance of passive smoking), dietary modification, exercise, rehabilitation, and management of obesity.

Patients with impaired LV function and or later symptomatic heart failure may need to considered for defibrillator or resynchronization therapy (see chapter 16.05.01.03 adapt for stand alone volume).

Pharmacological interventions

Trial evidence supports therapeutic interventions to modify the following conditions: hyperlipidaemia, left ventricular dysfunction and heart failure, diabetes mellitus, and hypertension.

Table 13.4.8 Estimated benefits of long-term secondary prophylactic treatment/intervention after MI

Treatment/intervention	Problems prevented per 1000 patient-years of treatment	
All post-MI patients (unless specific contraindications exist)		
Aspirin (meta-analysis)	7	vascular deaths
	9	nonfatal reinfarctions
	3	nonfatal strokes
Oral β-blocker	21	deaths
	21	reinfarctions
Statin (hyperlipidaemia, post-MI)	7	deaths
	11	revascularizations
	12	nonfatal MIs
	3	strokes
	4	congestive heart failure
	13	angina
Statin (average cholesterol, post-MI, CARE)	2	deaths
	9	re-vascularizations
	4	nonfatal MIs
	2	strokes
	4	unstable angina
Smoking cessation (observational studies)	15	deaths
	46	reinfarctions
Post-MI patients with LVD or heart failure (additional treatment unless specific contraindications exist)		
ACE inhibitor (left ventricular ejection fraction ≤ 40%)	12	deaths
	9	MIs
	10	congestive heart failure (requiring hospital admission)
ACE inhibitor (heart failure)	45	deaths
	26	congestive heart failure (severe)

LVD, left ventricular dysfunction.

Sivers, F. (1999). Evidence-based strategies for secondary prevention of coronary heart disease, 2nd edn. A&M Publishing, Guildford, Surrey.

Table 13.4.9 Comparison of the treatment benefits from interventions to prevent cardiovascular events

Problems/therapy	Events prevented	NNT*
Severe hypertension (DBP 115–129 mmHg)	Death or stroke or MI	3
Coronary artery bypass surgery for left main stem stenosis	Death	6
Aspirin for transient ischaemic attack	Death or stroke	6
Statin for hyperlipidaemia, post-MI/angina (4S)	Death or nonfatal MI or CABG/PTCA or cerebrovascular event	6
Warfarin for atrial fibrillation	Stroke	7
ACE inhibitor for LV dysfunction post-MI	CV death or hospitalization for CHF	10
Statin for average cholesterol post-MI (CARE trial) or stroke	Death or nonfatal MI or CABG/PTCA	11
Aspirin post-MI	CV death or stroke or MI	12
Statin for average/elevated cholesterol, post-MI/unstable angina (LIPID trial)	Death or nonfatal MI or CABG/PTCA or stroke	15
Beta-blocker post-MI	Death	20
ACE inhibitor for LV dysfunction	CV death or hospitalization for CHF	21
ACE inhibitor for vascular disease (HOPE)	Deaths	50
	MI	42
	Stroke	67
Statin for hypercholesterolaemia in primary prevention	Death or nonfatal MI or CABG/PTCA or stroke	26
Mild hypertension (DBP 90–109 mmHg)	Death or stroke or MI	141

ACE, angiotensin converting enzyme; CABG, coronary artery bypass grafting; CARE, Cholesterol and Recurrent Events Trial; CHF, congestive heart failure; CV, cardiovascular; DBP, diastolic blood pressure; HOPE, Heart Outcomes Prevention Evaluation Trial; LIPID, Long-term Intervention with Pravastatin in Ischaemic Disease Trial; LV, left ventricle; MI, myocardial infarction; NNT, estimated number of patients that need to be treated for 5 years to prevent one event; PTCA, percutaneous transluminal coronary angioplasty.

Sivers, F. (1999). Evidence-based strategies for secondary prevention of coronary heart disease, 2nd edn. A&M Publishing, Guildford, Surrey.

Reduction of cardiovascular risk

Evidence (summarized in Tables 13.4.8 and 13.4.9) supports the following therapies to reduce the risk of subsequent cardiovascular events: antiplatelet therapy (aspirin in a dose of 75 mg/day, clopidogrel 75 mg day); β-blockers in those without contraindications; lipid lowering with 3-hydroxy-3-methylglutaryl coenzyme A (HMG CoA) reductase inhibitors (statins); ACE inhibitor or ARB, especially in those with left ventricular dysfunction and heart failure, although benefit is also possible in other patients with vascular disease (Table 13.4.9).

Anticoagulants

These are indicated in those with high risks of embolism due to left ventricular or atrial thrombus. There is evidence to support the use of anticoagulants in post-MI patients but no definitive evidence that such treatment is superior to aspirin therapy. Current trials are evaluating the role or oral antithrombins and oral anti-Xa inhibitors following ACS.

Hormone replacement therapy (HRT)

HRT is not indicated for risk reduction after ACS. When used to relieve menopausal symptoms, HRT is associated with a small, but increased, risk of thrombotic events.

Calcium channel blockers

An overview of data from 19 000 patients, based on all randomized trials of acute infarction and unstable angina, suggests that the available calcium channel blockers are unlikely to reduce the rate of subsequent infarct development, infarct size, or subsequent infarction. They may, however, have indications for the relief of angina (especially heart-rate-lowering calcium antagonists).

Antiarrhythmic agents

A review of the effects of antiarrhythmic agents (with the exception of β-blockers) does not demonstrate a beneficial impact on mortality. Many have significant proarrhythmic complications and negative inotropic effects.

Further reading

Antithrombotic Trialists Collaboration (2002). Collaborative meta-analysis of randomised trials of antiplatelet therapy for prevention of death, myocardial infarction, and stroke in high risk patients. *BMJ*, **324**, 71–86.

Antman EM, *et al.* (1996). Cardiac-specific troponin I levels to predict the risk of mortality in patients with acute coronary syndromes. *N Engl J Med*, **335**, 1342–9.

Antman EM, *et al.* (1999). Abciximab facilitates the rate and extent of thrombolysis: results of the thrombolysis in myocardial infarction (TIMI) 14 trial. *Circulation*, **99**, 2720–32.

Antman EM, *et al.* (1999). Assessment of the treatment effect of enoxaparin for unstable angina/non-Q-wave myocardial infarction. TIMI IIB–ESSENCE meta-analysis. *Circulation*, **100**, 1602–8.

Antman EM, *et al.* (2006). Enoxaparin versus unfractionated heparin with fibrinolysis for ST elevation myocardial infarction. *N Engl J Med*, **354**, 1477–88.

Armstrong PW, *et al.* (1998). Acute coronary syndromes in the GUSTO-IIb trial: prognostic insights and impact of recurrent ischemia. *Circulation*, **98**, 1860–8.

ASSENT-2 Investigators (1999). Single-bolus tenecteplase compared with front-loaded alteplase in acute myocardial infarction: the ASSENT-2 double-blind randomised trial. *Lancet*, **354**, 716–22.

ASSENT-3 Investigators (2001). Efficacy and safety of tenecteplase in combination with enoxaparin, abciximab, or unfractionated heparin: the ASSENT-3 randomised trial in acute myocardial infarction. *Lancet*, **358**, 605–13.

Bassand J-P, *et al.* (2007). Guidelines for the diagnosis and treatment of non-ST-segment elevation acute coronary syndromes. *Eur Heart J*, **28**, 1598–660.

Bhatt DL, *et al.* (2004). Utilization of early invasive management strategies for high-risk patients with non-ST-segment elevation acute coronary syndromes: results from the CRUSADE Quality Improvement Initiative. *JAMA*, **292**, 2096–104.

Bhatt DL, *et al.* (2006). Clopidogrel and aspirin versus aspirin alone for the prevention of atherothrombotic events. *N Engl J Med*, **354**, 1706–17.

Bode C, *et al.* (1999). Randomised comparison of coronary thrombolysis achieved with double-bolus reteplase (recombinant plasminogen activator) and front-loaded, accelerated alteplase (recombinant tissue plasminogen activator) in patients with acute mycocardial infarction. *Circulation*, **94**, 891–8.

Boden WE, *et al.* (1998). Outcomes in patients with acute non-Q-wave mycocardial infarction randomly assigned to an invasive as compared with a conservative management strategy. Veterans Affairs Non-Q-Wave Infarction Strategies in Hospital (VANQWISH) Trial Investigators. *N Engl J Med*, **38**, 1785–92.

Boersma E, *et al.* (2002). Platelet glycoprotein IIb/IIIa inhibitors in acute coronary syndromes: a meta-analysis of all major randomized clinical trials. *Lancet*, **359**, 189–98.

Boersma E (2006). Does time matter? A pooled analysis of randomized clinical trials comparing primary percutaneous coronary intervention and inhospital fibrinolysis in acute mycocardial infarction patients. *Eur Heart J*, **27**, 779–88.

Bradley EH, *et al.* (2006). Strategies for reducing the door-to-balloon time in acute myocardial infarction. *N Engl J Med*, **355**, 2308–20.

Braunwald E (1989). Unstable angina: a classification. *Circulation*, **80**, 410–14.

Braunwald E, *et al.* (1994). Effects of tissue plasminogen activator and a comparison of early invasive and conservative strategies in unstable angina and non-Q-wave mycocardial infarction, results of the TIMI III trial. *Circulation*, **89**, 1545–56.

Briel M, *et al.* (2006). Effects of early treatment with statins on short-term clinical outcomes in acute coronary syndromes: a meta-analysis of randomized controlled trials. *JAMA*, **295**, 2046–56.

Cannon CP, *et al.* (1995). Prospective validation of the Braunwald classification of unstable angina: results from the Thrombolysis in Myocardial Ischemia (TIMI) III Registry. *Circulation*, **92**, 1–19.

Cannon CP, *et al.* (2001). Comparison of early invasive and conservative strategies in patients with unstable coronary syndromes treated with the glycoprotein IIb/IIIa inhibitor tirofiban. *N Engl J Med*, **344**, 1879–87.

CAPTURE Investigators (1997). Randomised placebo-controlled trial of abciximab before and during coronary intervention in refractory unstable angina: the CAPTURE study. *Lancet*, **349**, 1429–35.

Chen ZM, *et al.* (2005). Addition of clopidogrel to aspirin in 45,852 patients with acute mycocardial infarction: randomised placebo-controlled trial. *Lancet*, **366**, 1607–21.

Chen ZM, *et al.* (2005). Early intravenous then oral metoprolol in 45,852 patients with acute myocardial infarction: randomised placebo-controlled trial. *Lancet*, **366**, 1622–32.

Cohen MD, *et al.* (1997). A comparison of low-molecular-weight heparin with unfractionated heparin for unstable coronary artery disease. *N Engl J Med*, **337**, 447–52.

Collinson J, *et al.* (2000). Clinical outcomes, risk stratification and practice patterns of unstable angina and myocardial infarction without ST elevation: Prospective Registry of Acute Ischaemic Syndromes in the UK (PRAIS-UK). *Eur Heart J*, **21**, 1450–7.

Cox J, Naylor CD (1992). The Canadian Cardiovascular Society grading scale for angina pectoris: is it time for refinements? *Ann Int Med*, **117**, 677–83.

de Araujo Goncalves P, *et al.* (2005). TIMI, PURSUIT, and GRACE risk scores: sustained prognostic value and interaction with revascularization in NSTE-ACS. *Eur Heart J*, **26**, 865–872.

de Lemos JA, Braunwald E (2001). ST segment resolution as a tool for assessing the efficacy of reperfusion therapy. *J Am Coll Cardiol*, **38**, 1283–94.

De Luca G, *et al.* Abciximab as adjunctive therapy to reperfusion in acute ST-segment elevation myocardial infarction: a meta-analysis of randomized trials. *JAMA*, **293**, 1759–65.

de Winter RJ, *et al.* (2005). Early invasive versus selectively invasive management for acute coronary syndromes. *N Engl J Med*, **353**, 1095–104.

Eikelboom JW, *et al.* (2000). Unfractionated heparin and low-molecular-weight heparin in acute coronary syndrome without ST elevation: a meta-analysis. *Lancet*, **355**, 1936–42.

Eikelboom JW, *et al.* (2006). Adverse impact of bleeding on prognosis in patients with acute coronary syndromes. *Circulation*, **114**, 774–82.

Fibrinolytic Therapy Trialists' (FTT) Collaborative group (1994). Indications for fibrinolytic therapy in suspected acute myocardial infarction: collaborative overview of early mortality and major morbidity results from all randomised trials of more than 1000 patients. *Lancet*, **343**, 311–22.

Fox KA, *et al.* (2002). Management of acute coronary syndromes. Variations in practice and outcomes: findings of the Global Registry of Acute Coronary Events (GRACE). *Eur Heart J*, **23**, 1177–89.

Fox KA, *et al.* (2004). Benefits and risks of the combination of clopidogrel and aspirin in patients undergoing surgical revascularization for non-ST-elevation acute coronary syndrome: the Clopidogrel in Unstable angina to prevent Recurrent ischemic Events (CURE) Trial. *Circulation*, **110**, 1202–8.

Fox KA, *et al.* (2005). 5-year outcome of an interventional strategy in non-ST-elevation acute coronary syndrome: the British Heart Foundation RITA 3 randomised trial. *Lancet*, **366**, 914–20.

Fox KA, *et al.* (2006). Prediction of risk of death and myocardial infarction in the six months after presentation with acute coronary syndrome: prospective multinational observational study (GRACE). *BMJ*, **333**, 1091–4.

Fox KA, *et al.* (2007). Intervention in acute coronary syndromes: do patients undergo intervention on the basis of their risk characteristics? The global registry of acute coronary events (GRACE). *Heart*, **93**, 177–82.

Fox KA, *et al.* (2010). Underestimated and under-recognized: the late consequences of acute coronary syndrome (GRACE UK-Belgian Study). *Eur Heart J*, **31**, 2755–64.

Fox KA, *et al.* (2010). Long-term outcome of a routine versus selective invasive strategy in patients with non-ST-segment elevation acute coronary syndrome a meta-analysis of individual patient data. *J Am Coll Cardiol*, **55**, 2435–45.

Fox KA, *et al.* (2007). Decline in rates of death and heart failure in acute coronary syndromes, 1999–2006. *JAMA*, **297**, 1892–900.

FRAX.I.S. Study Group (1999). Comparison of two treatment durations (6 days and 14 days) of a low molecular weight heparin with a 6-day treatment of unfractionated heparin in the initial management of unstable angina or non-Q wave myocardial infarction: FRAX.I.S. (FRAxiparine in Ischaemic Syndrome). *Eur Heart J*, **20**, 1553–62.

FRISC-II Investigators (1999). Invasive compared with non-invasive treatment in unstable coronary artery disease: FRISC-II prospective randomised multicentre study. *Lancet*, **354**, 708–15.

Gandhi MM, Lampe FC, Wood DA (1995). Incidence, clinical characteristics, and short-term prognosis of angina pectoris. *Br Heart J*, **73**, 193–8.

Gershlick AH, *et al.* (2005). Rescue angioplasty after failed thrombolytic therapy for acute myocardial infarction (REACT Trial). *N Engl J Med*, **353**, 2758–68.

GISSI (Gruppo Italiano per lo Studio Della Streptochinasi Nell'Infart Miocardico) (1988). Effectiveness of intravenous thrombolytic treatment in acute myocardial infarction. *Lancet*, **i**, 397–402.

Giugliano RP, *et al.* (2009). Early versus delayed, provisional eptifibatide in acute coronary syndromes. *N Engl J Med*, **360**, 2176–90.

Grines CL, *et al.* (2007). Prevention of premature discontinuation of dual antiplatelet therapy in patients with coronary artery stents. A Science Advisory from the American Heart Association, American College of Cardiology, Society for Cardiovascular Angiography and Interventions, American College of Surgeons, and American Dental Association, with Representation from the American College of Physicians. *Circulation*, **115**, 813–8.

GUSTO Investigators (1993). An international randomised trial comparing four thrombolytic strategies for acute mycocardial infarction. *N Engl J Med*, **329**, 673–82.

GUSTO-V Investigators (2001). Reperfusion therapy for acute mycocardial infarction with fibrinolytic therapy or combination reduced fibrinolytic therapy and platelet IIb/IIIa inhibition: the GUSTO V trial. *Lancet*, **357**, 1905–14.

Hamm CW, *et al.* (1992). The prognostic value of serum troponin T in unstable angina. *N Engl J Med*, **327**, 146–50.

Hamm CW, *et al.* (1997). Emergency room triage of patients with acute chest pain by means of rapid testing for cardiac troponin T or troponin I. *N Engl J Med*, **337**, 1648–53.

Hamm CW, *et al.* (2011). ESC guidelines for the management of acute coronary syndromes in patients presenting without persistent ST-segment elevation. *Eur Heart J*, **32**, 29993–30054.

Hartwell D, *et al.* (2005). Clinical effectiveness and cost-effectiveness of immediate angioplasty for acute myocardial infarction: systematic review and economic evaluation. *Health Technol Assess*, **9**(17). http://www.hta.ac.uk/fullmono/mon917.pdf

Hasdai D, *et al.* (2002). A prospective survey of the characteristics, treatments and outcomes of patients with acute coronary syndromes in Europe and the Mediterranean basin. The Euro Heart Survey of Acute Coronary Syndromes. *Eur Heart J*, **23**, 1190–201.

Held PH, et al. (1989). Calcium channel blockers in acute myocardial infarction and unstable angina: an overview of randomized trials. *BMJ*, **299**, 1187–92.

Herrington DM (1999). Erratum, Comparison of the Heart and Estrogen/Progestin Replacement Study (HERS) cohort with women with coronary disease from the National Health and Nutrition Examination Survey III (NHANES). *Am Heart J*, **138**, 800. [First published in *Am Heart J* 1998, **136**, 115–24].

HOPE Study Investigators (The Heart Outcomes Prevention Evaluation) (2000). Effects of an angiotensin-converting-enzyme inhibitor, ramipril, on death from cardiovascular causes, myocardial infarction, and stroke in high-risk patients. *N Engl J Med*, **342**, 145–53.

IONA Study Group (2002). Effect of nicorandil on coronary events in patients with stable angina: the Impact Of Nicorandil in Angina (IONA) randomized trial. *Lancet*, **359**, 1269–75.

ISIS-2 (Second International Study of Infarct Survival) Collaborative Group (1988). Randomised trial of intravenous streptokinase, oral aspirin, both, or neither among 17,187 cases of suspected acute myocardial infarction. *Lancet*, **ii**, 349–60.

ISIS-3 (Third International Study of Infarct Survival) Collaborative Group (1992). A randomised comparison of streptokinase vs tissue plasminogen activator vs anistreplase and of aspirin plus heparin vs aspirin alone among 41,299 cases of suspected acute myocardial infarction. *Lancet*, **339**, 153–70.

ISIS-4 (Fourth International Study of Infarct Survival Collaborative Group) (1995). A randomised factorial trial assessing early oral captopril, oral mononitrate, and intravenous magnesium sulphate in 58,050 patients with suspected acute myocardial infarction. *Lancet*, **345**, 669–85.

Kastrati A, *et al.* (2006). Abciximab in patients with acute coronary syndromes undergoing percutaneous coronary intervention after clopidogrel pretreatment: the ISAR-REACT 2 randomized trial. *JAMA*, **295**, 1531–8.

Keeley EC, Boura JA, Grines CL (2003). Primary angioplasty versus intravenous thrombolytic therapy for acute myocardial infarction: a quantitative review of 23 randomized trials. *Lancet*, **361**, 13–20.

Keller T, *et al.* (2009). Sensitive troponin I assay in early diagnosis of acute myocardial infarction. *N Engl J Med*, **361**, 868–77.

Kong DF, *et al.* (1998). Clinical outcomes of therapeutic agents that block the platelet glycoprotein IIb/IIIa integrin in ischemic heart disease. *Circulation*, **98**, 2829–35.

Lagerqvist B, *et al.* (2002). A long-term perspective on the protective effects of an early invasive strategy in unstable coronary artery disease: two-year follow-up of the FRISC-II invasive study. *J Am Coll Cardiol*, **40**, 1902–14.

Lewis WR, Amsterdam EA (1994). Utility and safety of immediate exercise testing of low-risk patients admitted to the hospital for suspected acute myocardial infarction. *Am J Cardiol*, **74**, 987–90.

Lindhal B, Venge P, Wallentin L (1996). Relation between troponin T and the risk of subsequent cardiac events in unstable coronary artery disease. *Circulation*, **93**, 1651–7.

Luescher MS, *et al.* (1997). Applicability of cardiac troponin T and I for early risk stratification in unstable coronary disease. *Circulation*, **96**, 2578–85.

Maas ACP, *et al.* (1999). Sustained benefit at 10–14 years follow-up after thrombolytic therapy in myocardial infarction. *Eur Heart J*, **20**, 819–26.

Madsen JK, *et al.* (1997). Danish multicentre randomised study of invasive versus conservative treatment in patients with inducible ischaemia after thrombolysis in acute myocardial infarction (DANAMI). *Circulation*, **96**, 748–55.

Mehta SR, *et al.* (2001). Effects of pretreatment with clopidogrel and aspirin followed by long-term therapy in patients undergoing percutaneous coronary intervention: the PCI-CURE study. *Lancet*, **358**, 528–33.

Mehta SR, *et al.* (2005). Routine vs selective invasive strategies in patients with acute coronary syndromes: a collaborative meta-analysis of randomized trials. *JAMA*, **293**, 2908–17.

Mehta RH, *et al.* (2006). Recent trends in the care of patients with non-ST-segment elevation acute coronary syndromes: insights from the CRUSADE initiative. *Arch Intern Med*, **166**, 2027–34.

Mehta SR, *et al.* (2010). Double-dose versus standard-dose clopidogrel and high-dose versus low-dose aspirin in individuals undergoing percutaneous coronary intervention for acute coronary syndromes (CURRENT-OASIS 7): a randomised factorial trial. *Lancet*, **376**, 1233–43.

Mills NL, *et al.* (2011). Implementation of a sensitive troponin I assay and risk of recurrent myocardial infarction and death in patients with suspected acute coronary syndrome. *JAMA*, **305**, 1210–16.

Montalescot G, *et al.* (2006). Enoxaparin versus unfractionated heparin in elective percutaneous coronary intervention. *N Engl J Med*, **355**, 1006–17.

Montalescot G, *et al.* (2009). Prasugrel compared with clopidogrel in patients undergoing percutaneous coronary intervention for ST-elevation myocardial infarction (TRITON-TIMI 38): double-blind, randomised controlled trial. *Lancet*, **373**, 723–31.

MRC/BHF Heart Protection Study (HPS Study) of cholesterol lowering with simvastatin in 20,536 high-risk individuals: a randomised placebocontrolled trial. *Lancet*, **360**, 7–22.

Nunn CM, *et al.* (1999). Long-term outcome after primary angioplasty. Report from the primary angioplasty in myocardial infarction (PAMI-I) trial. *J Am Coll Cardiol*, **33**, 640–6.

Oler A, *et al.* (1996). Adding heparin to aspirin reduces the incidence of myocardial infarction and death in patients with unstable angina. A meta-analysis. *JAMA*, **276**, 811–15.

Petersen JL, *et al.* (2004). Efficacy and bleeding complications among patients randomized to enoxaparin or unfractionated heparin for antithrombin therapy in non-ST-segment elevation acute coronary syndromes: a systematic overview. *JAMA*, **292**, 89–96.

Pitt B, *et al.* (1999). Effects of losartan versus captopril on mortality in patients with symptomatic heart failure: rationale, design, and baseline characteristics of patients in the Losartan Heart Failure Survival Study—ELITE II. *J Cardiac Fail*, **5**, 146–54.

Pocock SJ, *et al.* (1995). Meta-analysis of randomised trials comparing coronary angioplasty with bypass surgery. *Lancet*, **346**, 1184–9.

PRISM. The Platelet Receptor Inhibition in Ischemic Syndrome Study Investigators (1998). A comparison of aspirin plus tirofiban with aspirin plus heparin for unstable angina. *N Engl J Med*, **338**, 1498–505.

PRISM-PLUS. The Platelet Receptor Inhibition in Ischemic Syndrome Management in Patients Limited by Unstable Signs and Symptoms Study Investigators (1998). Inhibition of the platelet glycoprotein IIb/IIIa receptor with tirofiban in unstable angina and non-Q-wave myocardial infarction. *N Engl J Med*, **338**, 1488–97.

Ravkilde J, *et al.* (1995). Independent prognostic value of serum creatine kinase isoenzyme MB mass, cardiac troponin T and myosin light chain levels in suspected acute myocardial infarction. Analysis of 28 months of follow-up in 196 patients. *J Am Coll Cardiol*, **25**, 574–81.

Rawles J, *et al.* (1994). Halving of mortality at 1 year by domiciliary thrombolysis in the Grampian Region Early Anistreplase Trial (GREAT). *J Am Coll Cardiol*, **23**, 1–5.

Ryan TJ (1999). Early revascularisation in cardiogenic shock—a positive view of a negative trial. *N Engl J Med*, **341**, 687–8.

Sabatine MS, *et al.* (2005). Addition of clopidogrel to aspirin and fibrinolytic therapy for myocardial infarction with ST-segment elevation. *N Engl J Med*, **352**, 1179–89.

Savonitto S, *et al.* (1997). Prognostic value of the admission electrocardiogram in acute coronary syndromes. Results from the GUSTO-IIb trial. *Eur Heart J*, **18** (Suppl), **335**, 5–82.

SIGN (2007). *Risk estimation and the prevention of cardiovascular disease.* SIGN Publication no. 97, Scottish Intercollegiate Guidelines Network, Edinburgh. http://www.sign.ac.uk.

Sivers F (1999). *Evidence-based strategies for secondary prevention of coronary heart disease*, 2nd edition. A&M Publishing, Guildford.

Stone GW, *et al.* for the ACUITY Investigators (2006). Bivalirudin for patients with acute coronary syndromes. *N Engl J Med*, **355**, 2203–16.

Tunstall-Pedoe H, *et al.* (1996). Sex differences in myocardial infarction and coronary deaths in the Scottish MONICA population of Glasgow 1985–1991. *Circulation*, **93**, 1981–92.

Van de Werf F, *et al.* (2005). Access to catheterization facilities in patients admitted with acute coronary syndrome: multinational registry study. *BMJ*, **330**, 441.

Wallentin L, *et al.* (2009). Ticagrelor versus clopidogrel in patients with acute coronary syndromes. *N Engl J Med*, **361**, 1045–57.

Wiviott SD, *et al.* (2007). Prasugrel versus clopidogrel in patients with acute coronary syndromes. *N Engl J Med*, **357**, 2001–15.

Yusuf S, *et al.* (1985). B-blockade during and after myocardial infarction: an overview of the randomized trials. *Progr Cardiovasc Dis*, **27**, 335–71.

Yusuf S, *et al.* (1998). Variations between countries in invasive cardiac procedures and outcomes in patients with suspected unstable angina or myocardial infarction without initial ST elevation. *Lancet*, **352**, 507–14.

Yusuf S, *et al.* (2001). Effects of clopidogrel in addition to aspirin in patients with acute coronary syndromes without ST-segment elevation. *N Engl J Med*, **345**, 494–502.

Yusuf S, *et al.* (2004). Effect of potentially modifiable risk factors associated with myocardial infarction in 52 countries (the INTERHEART study): case–control study. *Lancet*, **364**, 937–52.

Yusuf S, *et al.* (2006). Effects of Fondaparinux, a factor Xa inhibitor, on mortality and reinfarction in patients with acute myocardial infarction presenting with ST-segment elevation. Organization to Assess Strategies for Ischemic Syndromes (OASIS)-6 Investigators. *JAMA*, **295**, 1519–30.

Yusuf S, *et al.* (2006). Efficacy and safety of fondaparinux compared to enoxaparin in 20,078 patients with acute coronary syndromes without ST segment elevation. The OASIS (Organization to Assess Strategies in Acute Ischemic Syndromes)-5 Investigators. *N Engl J Med*, **354**, 1464–76.

CHAPTER 13.5

Percutaneous interventional cardiac procedures

Edward D. Folland

Essentials

Percutaneous coronary intervention (PCI) is the term applied to a variety of percutaneous, catheter-based procedures that accomplish revascularization by angioplasty (enlargement of a vessel lumen by modification of plaque structure), stenting (deployment of an internal armature or stent), atherectomy (removal or ablation of plaque), or thrombectomy (removal of thrombus).

The most common single indication for PCI is acute coronary syndrome. Randomized trials have shown that direct intervention for ST-elevation myocardial infarction (STEMI) is superior to initial thrombolytic therapy when performed in appropriate centres, and it can be used as a salvage procedure after failed thrombolytic therapy.

Balloon angioplasty is the traditional, basic technique of coronary intervention, but it is now uncommonly employed as a stand-alone treatment and finds its chief application in deployment of balloon-expandable stents, which have become the intervention of choice in about 90% of cases undergoing PCI. A variety of percutaneous techniques can be used to remove atheroma or thrombus from coronary arteries as a prelude to angioplasty/stenting.

There are two main types of coronary stent—'bare metal' and 'drug-eluting'. The latter contain a drug (e.g. sirolimus, paclitaxel, etc.) that inhibits smooth muscle proliferation and thereby considerably reduces the risk of restenosis, which is the most common complication of stenting. Restenosis typically presents as exertional angina at 1 to 6 months following intervention: if it is not present at 6 months, it is unlikely to occur.

Percutaneous techniques can also be used to treat some forms of valvular disease and close cardiac defects in (highly) selected cases. Balloon valvuloplasty is the preferred treatment, when feasible, for patients with stenosis of mitral and pulmonic valves. Transcatheter aortic valve implantation has proven safe and effective as an alternative to surgical valve replacement in patients for whom surgical risk is very high or prohibitive. Atrial septal defect can be successfully closed with a clamshell device in many cases. Patent foramen ovale likewise can be closed with a percutaneously delivered device, although the indications for this procedure remain controversial. Percutaneous clipping of mitral valve leaflets in some patients with mitral regurgitation has been accomplished with safety equivalent to that of surgical treatment. Nevertheless, the benefit of this procedure is less than that of surgery.

Introduction

The birth of interventional vascular medicine is generally credited to Charles Dotter, a radiologist from Portland, Oregon, who in 1964 first dared to relieve atherosclerotic stenosis of a patient's femoral artery by passage of a percutaneously introduced dilator. Although Dr Dotter had a few notable successes, which were widely publicized in the lay press, the scientific community scorned him. His radical concept lay dormant until a decade later when Andreas Gruentzig, a young German radiologist studying in Zurich, revived it. Dr Gruentzig was convinced that percutaneous dilatation of atherosclerotic stenosis was a sound concept and proposed that Dotter's solid dilator be replaced by a catheter with an inflatable cylindrical balloon at its tip. Using catheters he created in his own kitchen, he proceeded carefully and logically in applying his technique first to animal models, then to human peripheral vessels, and finally in 1977 to his ultimate goal, the human coronary artery. News of Gruentzig's percutaneous transluminal coronary angioplasty (PTCA) was quickly embraced by the medical community, and the era of percutaneous coronary intervention (PCI) was born. This chapter deals with percutaneous approaches to treating coronary, valvular, and congenital heart disease.

Percutaneous coronary intervention

PCI is the current general term applied to a variety of percutaneous catheter-based procedures that accomplish revascularization by either angioplasty (enlargement of a vessel lumen by modification of plaque structure), stenting (deployment of an internal armature or stent), atherectomy (removal or ablation of plaque), or thrombectomy (removal of thrombus). Several different devices have been developed to perform these procedures. The interventional cardiologist chooses among these approaches to best suit the particular requirements of each individual patient.

Indications

The indications for percutaneous revascularization have expanded dramatically during the past 35 years. In the early days of PTCA it was indicated for subtotal proximal occlusions of single vessels in patients with chronic stable angina pectoris who had failed medical therapy. As experience grew and equipment improved, patients with unstable angina, total occlusions, bypass grafts, multivessel disease, and acute myocardial infarction were added to the list. Currently, the most common single indication for PCI is acute coronary syndrome (see Chapter 13.4).

PCI has traditionally been performed only in hospitals having cardiac surgical backup. However, as the procedure has become safer and the need for emergency bypass surgery less common (currently <1% of all cases), it has become more common, particularly in Europe, for these procedures to be performed in facilities where surgical backup is not on site. Likewise, all patients undergoing PCI were once required to be potential candidates for bypass surgery in case of failure of the percutaneous procedure. Now some patients who are poor surgical candidates may undergo salvage intervention as their best or only avenue for revascularization. The choice of initial treatment (pharmacological, interventional, or surgical) for patients with each of the above coronary syndromes has been guided by evidence from a number of randomized clinical trials and is treated in more detail in the later section headed 'Outcomes'.

Devices and techniques

Balloon angioplasty

Balloon angioplasty is the traditional, basic technique of coronary intervention, although it is now uncommonly employed as a stand-alone treatment. Nevertheless, it is fundamental to the deployment of coronary stents, which are currently the most widely utilized of the interventional devices. The equipment for angioplasty is shown in Fig. 13.5.1 and consists of a coaxial array of guiding catheter, balloon catheter, and steerable guide wire. The procedure is accomplished by first engaging the left or right coronary orifice with the tip of the guiding catheter to access the vessel containing the target lesion and to provide backup support during advancement of the guide wire and balloon across the lesion (Fig. 13.5.2a). Next, the guide wire is advanced through the guide catheter into the appropriate vessel and across the lesion to be treated. Typical guide wires are 0.014 of an inch in diameter (*c.*0.36 mm) and have a flexible spiral coil tip that can be directed by rotating their proximal end outside the body. The balloon catheter is then advanced over the guide wire until the deflated balloon lies across the target lesion. Finally, the balloon is inflated with a solution of dilute contrast medium to a pressure sufficient to expand the cylindrical balloon to its nominal manufactured diameter (Fig. 13.5.2b). The balloon size is selected to match the estimated diameter of the nearest segment of normal vessel and the length of the target lesion. Sometimes intravascular ultrasound is used to assist in this choice. The balloon is then withdrawn and the result assessed by angiography and, occasionally, by ultrasound (Fig. 13.5.2c).

Traditional angioplasty now finds its chief application in deployment of balloon-expandable stents. However, angioplasty may serve as a stand-alone interventional technique for the treatment of lesions of small vessels (<2.5 mm in diameter) and lesions located far distally or beyond tortuous segments where more rigid devices such as stents cannot reach. In experienced hands, with appropriate case selection, the initial success rate of balloon angioplasty should exceed 95%. Abrupt closure of the vessel might be expected in about 3% of cases (usually due to dissection), but most of these can be corrected by deployment of a stent, resulting in a need for emergency bypass surgery in less than 1% of cases. The clinical consequence of vessel closure is often insufficient to justify surgery in vessels too small or distal for grafting.

The technology of guide, balloon, and guide wire systems has advanced to the point where few locations in the coronary anatomy are inaccessible. Totally occluded vessels can usually be successfully crossed with appropriate manipulation of the right guide wire, enabling successful angioplasty. The success rate for angioplasty of totally occluded vessels depends upon the age, length, and composition (thrombus vs plaque) of the occlusion; it is well over 90% in cases of acute thrombotic occlusion, and over 50% in cases of chronic occlusion (>3 months). The chief disadvantage of balloon angioplasty is the phenomenon of restenosis, which is discussed in

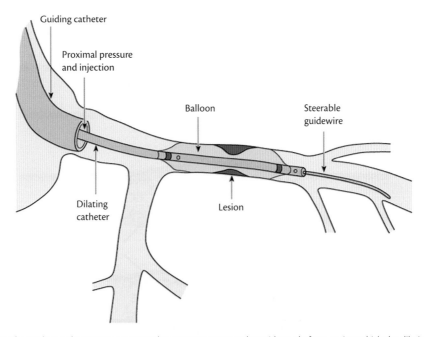

Fig. 13.5.1 Balloon angioplasty. The guiding catheter gives access to the coronary artery and provides a platform against which the dilating apparatus can be advanced. The steerable guide wire is passed down the vessel being treated and provides a rail over which the balloon catheter can be advanced. Once centred on the atherosclerotic lesion, the balloon is inflated under pressure to dilate the narrowed segment of artery.

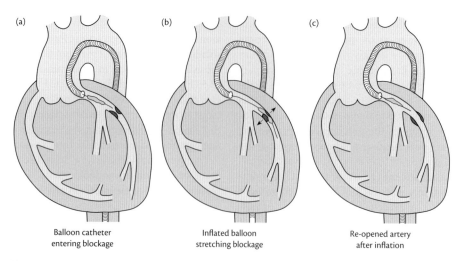

| Balloon catheter entering blockage | Inflated balloon stretching blockage | Re-opened artery after inflation |

Fig. 13.5.2 A typical lesion (a) before, (b) during, and (c) after balloon angioplasty.

more detail later in this chapter, and which spurred the development of newer devices in the hope of preventing restenosis.

Stenting

Bare metal stents

Stenting has become the intervention of choice in about 90% of cases undergoing PCI. A modern-day vascular stent is actually an armature, or internal skeleton, for restoring and maintaining the cylindrical structure of the diseased vessel. Most stents are made from a thin-walled stainless steel or cobalt–chromium steel tube in which slots have been carved. The slotted tube is then mounted securely on a deflated angioplasty balloon and deployed at the target lesion of the coronary artery by inflating the balloon at high pressure with dilute contrast medium. When the balloon is deflated the stent remains expanded against the vessel wall, its slots stretched into diamond-shaped apertures (Fig. 13.5.3). Approximately 20% of the vessel wall is covered by metal, the remainder being an intrastrut aperture. This accounts for the surprisingly high patency of side branches following stent deployment, and the ability to access these side branches when necessary for further intervention.

A variation of the slotted-tube stent is a balloon-deployed coiled wire (Wallstent and others). A coiled wire made from nitinol, or another alloy with shape-retaining characteristics, is compressed into a tubular delivery sheath, which is advanced over a guide wire across the target lesion. Once in its proper position the sheath is drawn back, allowing the stent to expand to its original size and shape (Fig. 13.5.4). As with slotted-tube stents, pre- or post-deployment dilation with a balloon may be necessary, depending upon the nature of the lesion treated and the device used. Although one of the original stent designs, the self-expanding stent is now used less commonly for coronary artery applications, but it still finds use in many peripheral vascular cases. Most current stent

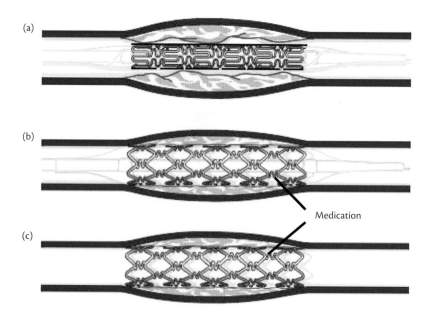

Medication

Fig. 13.5.3 A balloon-deployed coronary artery stent before (a), during (b), and after (c) deployment.
With permission from Maisel WH, Laskey WK. (2007). Drug eluting stents. *Circulation,* **115**, e426–7.

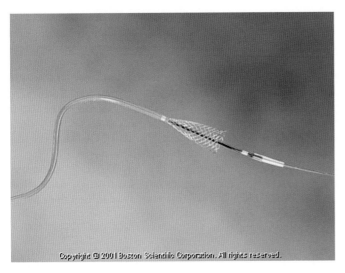

Fig. 13.5.4 A self-deploying coil stent. The stent unfurls as its delivery (containment) sheath is pulled back.
Copyright 2001. Boston Scientific Corporation.

designs are hybrids, which incorporate desirable properties of both the slotted-tube and coiled-wire designs.

Stents have gained remarkable popularity, mainly for three reasons. (1) Immediate complications are reduced because abrupt closure of the vessel due to dissection is less likely, emphasized by the fact that a stent is the best treatment for a balloon-induced dissection. (2) The immediate result is better in terms of the diameter and smoothness of the lumen, which turns out to be of more than cosmetic value because the early gain in lumen size relates directly to the late outcome. (3) Stents have been demonstrated in randomized clinical trials to be effective in reducing the likelihood of late restenosis.

However, stents do have some disadvantages, which include the fact that they cannot be deployed under some circumstances, their propensity to subacute thrombosis, and the persistence of some degree of restenosis (depending upon the size of the vessel and length of the lesion). Subacute thrombosis, a complication unique to stents, usually occurs within a few weeks after stent deployment. By contrast to restenosis, which is a gradual phenomenon, stent thrombosis is usually sudden, presenting as acute myocardial infarction and requiring emergency revascularization, usually by balloon angioplasty. The likelihood of subacute thrombosis has been reduced to less than 1% by dual antiplatelet therapy with a combination of aspirin plus a thienopyridine (clopidogrel, prasugrel, ticagrelor, or ticlopidine).

Drug-eluting stents

The development of stents that gradually elute a drug into the surrounding vessel wall has reduced the need for repeat intervention due to restenosis from approximately 15% for bare metal stents to less than 5%. This technology is largely responsible for the rapid and sustained growth in popularity of stent procedures, such that most patients requiring coronary revascularization are now treated by percutaneous rather than surgical techniques. The design of the drug-eluting stent incorporates a polymer matrix coating that contains a drug which inhibits the proliferation of smooth muscle cells in the surrounding vessel wall. The active drug slowly elutes from this coating into the underlying tissue while the vascular response

to injury caused by vessel dilation is most active. Drug elution is usually complete by 2 months after stent deployment, but by modulating the proliferation of smooth muscle cells the growth of neointima covering the stent struts is limited, reducing the likelihood of restenosis of the treated vessel.

The first two types of drug-eluting stents to be commercially available use sirolimus and paclitaxel as the active drug. These drugs inhibit cell proliferation through different mechanisms, but have proven to be equally effective. Other drugs currently available include everolimus and zotarolimus. Although excessive neointimal growth is undesirable, some is needed in order to cover the stent struts and prevent thrombosis. Dual antiplatelet drug therapy is necessary to minimize this risk as long as the struts are exposed. Bare metal stents are usually fully covered by 2 months, but drug-eluting stents may remain uncovered for 6 months or longer. For this reason, most cardiologists recommend that dual antiplatelet therapy be continued along with aspirin for at least 1 year following deployment of drug-eluting stents.

Cutting balloon

The cutting balloon has several tiny longitudinally mounted blades that become erect when the balloon is inflated and create linear cuts along the vessel wall. This was conceived as a method to dilate a vessel less traumatically and thereby reduce the likelihood of restenosis. This goal was never realized for *de novo* lesions, but the device has been advantageous for treatment of recurrent stenosis within previously deployed stents (in-stent restenosis) and for dilating lesions located at the ostium of a vessel, which are otherwise often subject to elastic recoil when dilated.

Atherectomy
Rotational ablation

Rotational ablation (Rotablator) is a method of pulverizing plaque into particles smaller than the size of a capillary, which wash away with the circulating blood. This process is accomplished by means of a diamond-studded burr, which rotates at approximately 150 000 rev/min (Fig. 13.5.5) and is advanced along a guide wire into the plaque. The diamond studs on the forward face of the olive-shaped burr selectively cut into hard substances such as plaque and calcium, sparing the soft surface of normal tissue. During rotational atherectomy a vasodilating solution is infused into the artery proximal to the burr to prevent spasm and to maintain maximal coronary flow, which carries away particulate debris. Burrs are manufactured in sizes ranging from 1.5 mm to 2.5 mm in diameter. Atherectomy often requires the use of two or three burrs of progressively larger size until an adequate lumen size is achieved. Although occasionally used as a stand-alone procedure, rotational ablation is usually employed to 'debulk' lesions prior to final dilation with a balloon or stent.

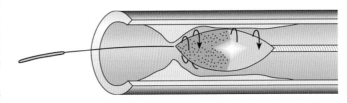

Fig. 13.5.5 Rotational atherectomy. The rotating burr pulverizes plaque as it is advanced over the guide wire into the lesion.

Rotational ablation was originally conceived as a potential solution to the problem of postintervention restenosis. Unfortunately, it has failed to outperform balloon angioplasty in this regard and has assumed the role of a 'niche' device for special situations. It is most commonly used in the treatment of heavily calcified lesions that do not respond well to balloons and stents. It is also useful in treating diffuse, osteal, and bifurcating lesions. The frequency with which rotational ablation is employed varies by operator, but averages less than 5% of most centres' cases. It has the disadvantages of being an expensive addition to other interventional modalities, is unable to adequately increase the lumen of large vessels, and is contraindicated in lesions containing thrombus. Due to its tendency to transiently decrease contractility during the ablation process, it is also relatively contraindicated in patients whose left ventricular function is severely impaired.

Directional coronary atherectomy

Directional coronary atherectomy (DCA) is achieved with a device illustrated in Fig. 13.5.6 that utilizes a rotating cylindrical blade which is advanced across an open aperture near the tip of a cone-shaped catheter directed by a guide wire. Opposite the aperture is an eccentric balloon, which when inflated compresses plaque of the opposite vessel wall into the aperture, where it is cut away by the rotating blade and pushed into the nose cone. The direction of the aperture can be rotated so that slices of plaque are removed in a radial fashion by multiple cuts taken at different locations around the circumference of the vessel. The catheter can then be withdrawn and the excised plaque removed from the nose cone. The catheter may be reintroduced, if necessary, for more atherectomy.

Although DCA was originally devised with the hope of reducing the incidence of restenosis, it has failed to outperform balloon angioplasty in most circumstances. It has therefore assumed the role of a 'niche' technology, which is useful in particular situations such as very eccentric proximal lesions, and lesions involving the ostia of major side branches. Removal of plaque at branch points seems to reduce the likelihood of plaque shifting from one branch to another as the respective lesions are dilated with balloons or stents. However, DCA has the disadvantage of requiring a rather large, stiff device, limiting its application to proximal lesions of large vessels. Furthermore, the removal of plaque seems to have surprisingly little effect on restenosis. DCA is currently employed in less than 5% of interventional cases.

Other devices

The transcutaneous excision catheter (TEC) device was developed at about the same time as DCA. It employs a rotating conical blade that cuts away plaque and clot as it is advanced over a guide wire. The resulting debris is sucked back through the catheter into a reservoir outside the body. Although originally developed as an atherectomy device, it has found its chief application in treating clot-laden lesions, but it has not gained wide usage.

Excimer laser coronary atherectomy (ELCA) employs a fibre-optic catheter directed by a guide wire to deliver bursts of excimer laser energy to the plaque. Disintegrated plaque washes away in the circulation. However, ELCA has also failed to solve the restenosis problem and is used uncommonly in most

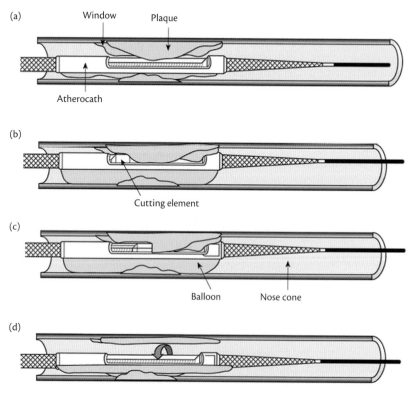

Fig. 13.5.6 Directional coronary atherectomy: (a) The catheter is inserted such that the blade housing is adjacent to the plaque to be removed. (b) The balloon on the opposite side of the blade housing is inflated, pushing the aperture over the plaque. (c) The rotating cylindrical blade is advanced across the window of the housing and cuts away plaque, packing it into the nose cone. (d) The catheter can be rotated to remove plaque elsewhere on the circumference of the vessel.

centres, but remains the sole surviving member of a number of laser applications that have been tried and failed over the past 35 years. It finds its most frequent application in treatment of osteal lesions, stent restenosis, and diffuse calcified disease. Because of the limitations of fibre size it is usually followed by balloon or stent treatment.

Thrombectomy

Thrombectomy is an adjunct to angioplasty and stent procedures in patients with acute myocardial infarction and thrombus-laden lesions. Its purpose is to prevent distal embolization by removing the thrombus prior to balloon dilation and stent deployment. The devices for achieving this have become simpler over time. The simplest and least expensive is called a Pronto, which is a catheter, delivered over a guide wire, that has a relatively large inner lumen attached to a suction syringe. As blood is withdrawn through the catheter, its tip is moved back and forth through the thrombus, picking it up and removing it. A more complex device called AngioJet uses the Venturi effect from a high-velocity jet of water, which draws thrombus into a window near the tip of a catheter directed by a guide wire and propels it into a reservoir. Another device called the Excisor employs a helical screw at the end of a catheter, which breaks up the clot so that it can be withdrawn through the catheter. Both these devices currently find their chief application in the treatment of degenerated and clot-laden vein-graft lesions.

Distal protection

Distal protection devices are methods of capturing and collecting thrombus and other debris that may embolize distally from the target lesion during the use of many of the interventional tools mentioned above. They may be particularly beneficial during the treatment of old, degenerated vein grafts in which distal embolization is especially common. Two general approaches are employed. The simplest is a guide wire with a filter on its end (Filterwire, Fig. 13.5.7). The filter looks like a windsock and catches debris released proximal to it. The other approach (PercuSurge) is to use a guide wire with a balloon near its tip which is progressively inflated until it occludes the distal portion of the vessel being treated. Intervention is then performed over the guide wire proximal to the occlusion balloon. Once the intervention is complete an export catheter is advanced over the guide wire and any debris removed by

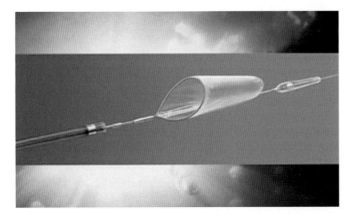

Fig. 13.5.7 Distal protection device: FilterWire.
Copyright 2001. Boston Scientific Corporation.

suction. Finally, the distal balloon is deflated, restoring flow and the guide wire removed.

Brachytherapy

The local, catheter-based delivery of β- or γ-radiation has been demonstrated to reduce the incidence of recurrent stent restenosis. Radiation is delivered with the assistance of a radiation therapist after initial treatment of stent restenosis with a cutting balloon, Rotablator, or conventional balloon. The benefit of brachytherapy appears to be limited to treatment of stent restenosis and it is not recommended following initial deployment of a stent. Brachytherapy also prolongs the period of risk for subacute thrombosis, making it necessary to treat patients with both aspirin and clopidogrel for at least 6 months after treatment. However, the need for brachytherapy has been virtually eliminated by drug-eluting stents. Not only is restenosis less likely after initial deployment of a drug-eluting stent, but restenosis—when it does occur—is most effectively treated by concentric deployment of a second drug-eluting stent.

Selection and evaluation of treatment targets

Fractional flow reserve

In cases of acute myocardial infarction or single-vessel disease the identification of the treatment target (so-called 'culprit lesion') is usually straightforward. However, in patients having lesions of multiple vessels it is often unclear which vessels require treatment. Treating a lesion that is not responsible for causing ischaemia can create a problem where previously none existed. An unnecessary stent can still lead to restenosis and other complications, not to mention needless additional cost. On the other hand, failure to treat a vessel having borderline stenosis may overlook a source of ischaemia. Measurement of fractional flow reserve has proven to be a useful method of identifying the physiological significance of coronary artery lesions, especially in vessels having lesions with borderline percentage stenosis (50–70%). It is performed using a pressure wire to cross an area of disease in a coronary artery; the pressure drop across a lesion is measured at rest and during maximal dilatation with an adenosine infusion. Fractional flow reserve (FFR) is the quotient of the mean pressure on either side of a coronary stenosis during maximum vasodilation. An FFR quotient of less than 0.75 correlates with stress-induced defects in myocardial perfusion imaging studies. Such a lesion is capable of causing ischaemia and merits treatment. The FFR therefore facilitates clinical decisions in the catheterization laboratory. Well-designed studies have shown that use of this method to guide treatment results in improved clinical outcomes.

Intravascular ultrasound

Intravascular ultrasound (IVUS) is a useful adjunct to interventional coronary procedures. It is performed by passing a small catheter having a rotating ultrasound crystal at its tip down a guide wire positioned in a coronary artery. Tomographic cross-sectional images of the artery are produced as the crystal is withdrawn. These images enable precise measurement of the dimensions of the arterial lumen plus visualization of the arterial wall and any plaque that might be present. Minimum cross-sectional area of coronary artery stenosis measuring less than $4.0\,mm^2$ indicates that the stenosis is severe enough to cause ischaemia and likely to need treatment. The most common application of IVUS is in measuring the diameter of normal artery adjacent to a lesion in order to choose a stent of appropriate size. IVUS is also very useful for assessing whether a stent has been adequately deployed.

Optical coherence tomography

Optical coherence tomography (OCT) is a method of creating cross-sectional images of the artery similar to those produced by IVUS. The difference is that reflected light, rather than ultrasound, is used to create the images. The advantage of OCT is that its spatial resolution is 10 times greater than that of IVUS. However, the use of light requires that the artery be flushed with saline in order to clear blood from the imaging field. Although this can be achieved safely, it is cumbersome enough that OCT has not yet gained widespread use in clinical practice.

Complications

PCI exposes the patient to all the potential complications of cardiac catheterization presented in Chapter 3.4. In addition, it carries the risk of other complications unique to interventional procedures. Most of these stem from four general processes that cause adverse outcomes in coronary artery intervention: abrupt closure, distal embolization, stent thrombosis, and restenosis. Patient characteristics such as age, acute coronary syndrome, previous bypass surgery, and renal insufficiency are major determinants of risk. When considering PCI for a patient, it is important to weigh the likelihood of these adverse outcomes against the expected chance of adverse events without intervention. The approximate frequencies of various specific complications from PCI are listed in Table 13.5.1. As in diagnostic catheterization, the likelihood of these complications also depends upon operator skill.

Abrupt closure and distal embolization

Abrupt closure and distal embolization account for most of the immediate complications of PCI, especially acute myocardial infarction and emergency coronary artery bypass surgery. Dissection, spasm, and thrombosis are the leading causes of abrupt closure. The availability of stents has reduced the need for emergency bypass surgery to less than 1% because these are an effective treatment for acute dissection in most cases. Nevertheless, dissection sometimes extends with the addition of each stent, and occasionally the stent itself can be the cause of dissection at one of its edges. Acute thrombosis may occur in spite of routine prophylactic treatment with anticoagulants (heparin, low molecular weight heparin, or bivalirudin) and aspirin: glycoprotein IIb/IIIa inhibitors may stop this process and are sometimes given prophylactically, especially in high-risk cases. Incomplete stent deployment seems to be a leading cause of thrombotic occlusion. Distal embolization is surprisingly uncommon, except when patients have acute coronary syndromes or visible thrombus. It is especially troublesome for patients with degenerated or thrombus-laden vein grafts. Embolization may result in discrete occlusion of branch vessels or the phenomenon called 'no reflow', which is manifest by reduced flow without identifiable occlusion and thought to be due to capillary plugging from showers of microemboli. Distal protection devices (Fig. 13.5.7) may help prevent these problems. Both abrupt closure and no reflow usually cause some degree of myocardial infarction, the likelihood of infarction being a matter of how it is defined: non-ST-elevation infarction indicated only by a rise of troponin or creatine kinase enzymes is more common than ST-elevation (Q wave) infarction.

Stent thrombosis

Thrombosis is a serious complication of particular concern for stents. It rarely occurs after the first 24 h following isolated balloon angioplasty or atherectomy. However, when a stent is deployed it may occur at a later time and is manifest by acute myocardial infarction. It is a medical emergency that must be managed in a fashion similar to spontaneous acute infarction. Emergency reperfusion by balloon angioplasty is usually preferred, unless a catheterization laboratory is unavailable, in which case thrombolytic therapy is recommended. In the early days of stenting this complication occurred in over 3% of cases in spite of vigorous anticoagulation including intravenous heparin and warfarin, a treatment that required several days of hospital stay for the initiation of warfarin therapy and delayed the widespread acceptance of stenting. However, once the current treatment using oral antiplatelet agents was proven to be superior, the length of hospital stay and local bleeding complications were reduced, and the use of stents grew rapidly. Stent thrombosis now occurs in less than 1% of cases. Thrombosis is defined as subacute when it occurs between 1 day and 1 month following stent deployment. Subacute thrombosis is equally likely for bare metal and drug-eluting stents. Thrombosis occurring more than 1 month after stent deployment is called late stent thrombosis and is particularly associated with drug-eluting stents. To minimize the risk of late stent thrombosis, dual antiplatelet therapy with aspirin and thienopyridine should be continued without interruption for at least 6–12 months following implantation of drug-eluting stents.

Restenosis

Restenosis was once the Achilles heel of coronary intervention. In patients undergoing isolated balloon angioplasty the likelihood of restenosis at 6 months following intervention lies between 30 and 50% if defined by angiographic criteria, and approximately 25% if defined by the clinical recurrence of symptoms. The use of bare metal stents reduced the angiographic rate of restenosis to about 25% and the clinical rate to as little as 10%. Drug-eluting stents have further reduced the rate to 5% or less, depending upon clinical and anatomic circumstances. The risk of restenosis varies according to individual factors such as vessel diameter and lesion length. Restenosis typically presents clinically as exertional angina at 1 to 6 months following intervention: if it is not present at 6 months, it is unlikely to occur. As described above, it is caused by the

Table 13.5.1 Complications of percutaneous coronary intervention

Complication	Frequency (%)[a]
Death	0.5–2
Acute myocardial infarction	2–5
Emergency bypass surgery	0.5–2
Abrupt closure	1–2
Subacute stent thrombosis	<1
Peripheral arterial complications	5
Restenosis (clinical)	5–30

[a] These rates are approximate and vary widely with the clinical setting and patient characteristics. These are in addition to the usual complications of cardiac catheterization presented in Chapter 3.4.

proliferation and migration of smooth muscle cells into the lumen of the treated vessel, a process that can be significantly modulated by use of drug-eluting stents.

Outcomes

Chronic stable angina

Randomized clinical trials have shown that patients with single- and double-vessel disease experience a more rapid and complete resolution of symptoms, and a greater improvement in treadmill exercise performance, when treated by balloon angioplasty rather than by pharmacological therapy for chronic stable angina pectoris. However, this comes at the price of a greater likelihood of repeat intervention or bypass surgery at 6 months, largely due to the need to treat restenosis. Nevertheless, the rate of bypass surgery becomes equal in both groups by 3 years. More recent studies employing drug-eluting and bare metal stents continue to support these findings. Therefore medical therapy is an acceptable initial strategy for low-risk patients. Intervention is recommended for higher-risk patients and those not responding to medical therapy. When compared to coronary bypass surgery, PCI provides similar relief of symptoms and similar rates of mortality and myocardial infarction at 5-year follow-up, with the exception of diabetic patients who have somewhat better 5-year survival rates when treated surgically. Otherwise, the main difference between patient groups randomly assigned to surgery or percutaneous intervention is that repeat catheterization or revascularization is less frequent for those having surgery. Again, this difference is largely due to the effect of restenosis and less complete revascularization in the interventional group. See Chapter 13.4 for further discussion.

Unstable angina

The choice between initial aggressive treatment (catheterization and revascularization) and initial conservative treatment (medical therapy with catheterization and revascularization only for those who have continued evidence of ischaemia) for patients with unstable angina has been controversial. However, recent studies favour an aggressive approach to these patients, especially those having high clinical risk or evidence of non-STEMI. See Chapter 13.4 for further discussion.

Acute myocardial infarction

Percutaneous intervention has been shown to be an effective treatment for acute myocardial infarction with ST-segment elevation (STEMI), both as a salvage procedure after failed thrombolytic therapy and as a direct initial approach to reperfusion. Randomized trials have shown that direct intervention for STEMI is superior to initial thrombolytic therapy when performed in centres with expert interventionists and catheterization facilities that are available around the clock. Direct PCI is also an option for patients presenting outside these centres provided that they can be transferred and effectively treated in less than 90 min. In any case, direct PCI is the treatment of choice for patients in whom thrombolytic therapy is contraindicated and for patients who are haemodynamically unstable. See Chapter 13.4 for further discussion.

Economic considerations

The cost of equipment and supplies for percutaneous coronary procedures may become a limiting factor, particularly in developing countries and in healthcare systems with stringent budgets. Most catheters, guide wires, and other supplies are intended for one-time use. Expendable supplies alone cost approximately £750 ($US 1200) for a simple balloon angioplasty procedure. That cost may be multiplied several-fold when drug-eluting stents are used—these are two to three times more costly than bare metal stents, although the added cost is offset somewhat by the reduced likelihood of repeat procedures necessitated by restenosis. The coverage of this additional cost varies considerably throughout the world, depending on insurance and government policies. Nevertheless, the cost of a single percutaneous revascularization procedure usually remains less than that of a comparable coronary bypass operation. However, when the added cost of repeat percutaneous revascularizations necessitated by restenosis is considered, the price difference between the two therapeutic approaches narrows.

Noncardiac surgery in patients following coronary intervention

An estimated 5–10% of patients undergo noncardiac surgery within 1 year following coronary stent implantation. When surgery is performed within 6 weeks of intervention there is a high risk of death or myocardial infarction usually secondary to stent thrombosis, this risk is highest in patients with drug-eluting stents. The risk continues to be significant for at least 6 months. In individual cases the risk is higher, for example where a major coronary artery is stented (left main stem or proximal left anterior descending artery. For this reason it is reasonable try to defer elective surgery for at least 6 months following stent implantation. Where urgent surgery is required then a delay of 6 weeks is advisable. Where possible dual antiplatelet therapy should be continued in those operated on within 6 months except where the risks of perioperative bleeding are unacceptable.

Percutaneous treatment of valvular disease

Allain Cribier in France developed the treatment of valvular stenosis by means of balloon catheters in the 1980s. The clinical utility of the procedure depends on the valve treated and the age of the patient. Percutaneous aortic valve replacement is now an effective alternative to surgery in patients having very high surgical risk. Catheter-deployed clips can reduce the severity of mitral regurgitation.

Mitral stenosis

Balloon valvuloplasty of the mitral valve has become the treatment of choice for selected patients with rheumatic mitral stenosis. The most common approach to the mitral valve is via trans-septal puncture of the left atrium from percutaneous access of the right femoral vein. After passing a stiff guide wire with a curved soft tip across the mitral valve, an appropriately sized balloon is centred on the valve and inflated with dilute contrast medium, tearing open the fused commissures and allowing the valve to open more normally. A dumbbell-shaped balloon, named after Dr Inoue, is often utilized, preventing the balloon from slipping off the valve during inflation (see Fig. 13.5.8). Clinical improvement, complications, and durability of the outcome from balloon mitral valvuloplasty have been shown to be comparable to surgical commissurotomy in appropriately selected patients. To be a candidate for balloon mitral valvuloplasty a patient must have no evidence of thrombus in the left atrium. Other features which auger poorly include immobility

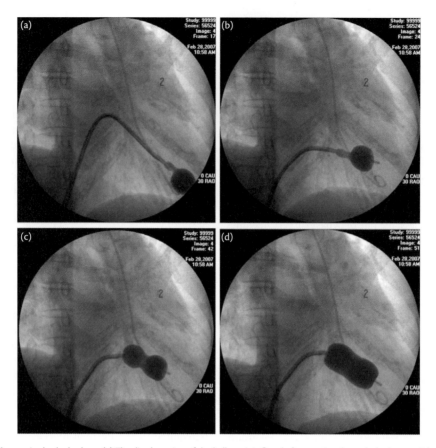

Fig. 13.5.8 Percutaneous balloon mitral valvuloplasty. (a) The distal portion of the balloon is inflated after passing through the intra-atrial septum and mitral valve. (b) The distal balloon is pulled back against the stenotic valve. (c) The proximal portion of the balloon is inflated, locking it across the valve. (d) The waist of the balloon is inflated, dilating the valve orifice.

Nobuyoshi M, *et al*. Percutaneous balloon mitral valvuloplasty: A review. *Circulation* **119**, e211–e219.

of the valve leaflets, severe calcification, thickening of the chordae tendineae, and more than mild regurgitation. Balloon mitral valvuloplasty is generally recommended as the procedure of first choice for patients with favourable anatomy.

Mitral regurgitation

Percutaneous treatment of mitral regurgitation is being approached by two different strategies. The first involves applying a clip to the mitral valve commissures, effectively creating a dual orifice valve. The second approach is to pass a ring into the coronary sinus which constricts the mitral valve annulus, enabling better coaptation of the valve leaflets. Experience is greatest with the clip device (MitraClip). The EVEREST II trial indicates that the severity of mitral regurgitation can be safely reduced in two-thirds of cases. An attractive aspect of this procedure is that its performance does not preclude surgical repair if subsequently needed. Survival in this randomized trial is similar at 4 years follow-up, but the likelihood of requiring surgery or repeat clipping is nearly 25% in the clip-treated group.

Aortic stenosis

Experience with balloon valvuloplasty for patients with aortic stenosis has been disappointing, largely due to an almost universal tendency for the stenosis to recur within 1 year. Consequently, it is performed as a stand-alone procedure only under unusual

circumstances. It has a role for children with congenital aortic stenosis, where temporary treatment by valvuloplasty may allow the child to complete growth before requiring surgical valve replacement. It is now used to prepare the aortic valve in advance of transcatheter aortic valve implantation (TAVI). These valves are fashioned from bovine pericardium inside a cylindrical cage that is either balloon expandable (Edwards SAPIEN) or self-expanding (Medtronic CoreValve) (see Fig. 13.5.9). TAVI has been studied in a randomized trial comparing the SAPIEN percutaneous valve with medical therapy in patients whose surgical risk for valve replacement is prohibitively high (PARTNER Study, cohort B). Patients randomized to TAVI showed improved outcome at one year compared to patients assigned to medical therapy (mortality 30.7% vs 50.7%). Cohort A of this study randomized patients whose surgical risk was considered high, but not prohibitive. Mortality for patients receiving TAVI was less than surgically assigned patients at 1 month (3.45 vs 6.5%), but similar at 1 year (24.3% vs 26.8%) and 2 years (33.9 vs 35.0). Symptom improvement was similar for both treatments. Risk of stroke was greater for TAVI at 1 month (5.5% vs 2.4%) but not different by 1 and 2 years. As a result of this study TAVI is now clinically available throughout the world.

Pulmonary stenosis

Balloon valvuloplasty is the treatment of choice for patients with pulmonary stenosis. Most are children whose valves respond well

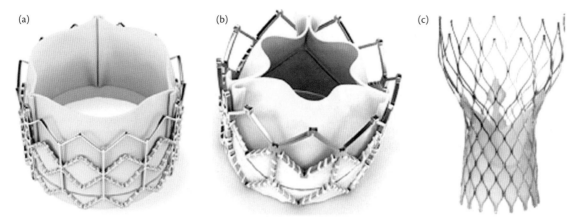

Fig. 13.5.9 Current widely available transcatheter valves. (a) The Edwards SAPIEN THV balloon-expandable valve (Edwards Lifesciences, Irving California, USA) incorporates a stainless steel frame, bovine pericardial leaflets and a fabric sealing cuff. (b) The SAPIEN XT THV (Edwards Lifesciences) utilizes a cobalt chromium alloy frame and is compatible with lower profile delivery catheters. (c) The Medtronic CoreValve (Medtronic, Minneapolis, Minnesota, USA) incorporates a self-expandable frame, porcine pericardial leaflets and a pericardial seal.
With permission from Webb JG, Wood DA (2012). Current status of transcatheter aortic valve replacement. *J Am Coll Cardiol*, 60, 483–92.

to this treatment, the advantage of avoiding surgery outweighing the moderate tendency for restenosis of these valves.

Percutaneous closure of cardiac defects

Atrial septal defects and patent ductus arteriosus can be closed percutaneously with catheter-delivered devices. One such device, called a clamshell (brand names include Amplatzer, Helex, and STARFlex), has been used for this purpose for a

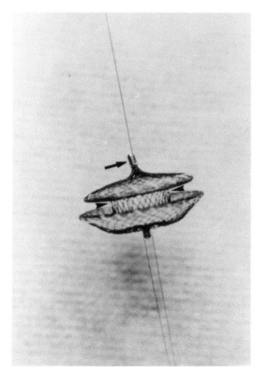

Fig. 13.5.10 Amplatzer septal occluder made of 0.005 inch (0.127 mm) Nitinol wire tightly woven into two round disks with a 4 mm connecting waist (arrowheads). Arrow indicates the negative microscrew adaptor mounted on the right atrial disk.
J Am Coll Cardiol (1998), **31**, 1110–16. Reproduced with permission of Elsevier.

number of years (Figure 13.5.10). It is now available throughout the world and is useful for closing smaller defects, although larger defects still require surgical closure. A concurrent non-randomized trial comparing outcome for percutaneous versus surgical closure of atrial septal defect suggests shorter hospital stay and fewer complications for the percutaneous approach, which is now often preferred for patients with smaller ostium secundum type defects.

Closure of patent foramen ovale can be accomplished by devices similar to the clamshell used for atrial septal defect. However, no study has yet proven that percutaneous closure reduces the likelihood of recurrent stroke due to paradoxical embolism. Patent foramen ovale closure has also been advocated for migraine sufferers, but the MIST trial did not show significant reduction of the primary study endpoint, although the overall burden of migraine was reduced. Consequently, the closure of these defects remains controversial.

Further reading

De Bruyne B, Pijls NH, *et al.* (2012). Fractional flow reserve guided-PCI versus medical therapy in stable coronary disease. *N Engl J Med*, **367**, 991–1001.

Dowson A, *et al.* (2008) Migraine Intervention With STARFlex Technology (MIST) Trial. A prospective, multicenter, double-blind, sham-controlled trial to evaluate the effectiveness of patent foramen ovale closure with STARFlex septal repair implant to resolve refractory migraine headache. *Circulation*, **117**, 1397–1404.

Du Z-D, *et al.* (2002) Comparison between transcatheter and surgical closure of secundum atrial septal defect in children and adults. *J Am Coll Cardiol*, **39**, 1836–1844.

Leon MB, *et al.* (2010) Transcatheter aortic-valve implantation for aortic stenosis in patients who cannot undergo surgery. *N Engl J Med*, **363**, 1597–1607.

Meier B, Kalesan B, *et al.* (2013) Percutaneous closure of patent foramen ovale in cryptogenic embolism. *N Engl J Med* **368**, 1083–1100.

Messe SR, Kent DM. (2013) Still no closure on the question of PFO closure. *N Engl J Med*, **368**, 1152–53.

Sharma SK, Chen V. (2006). Coronary interventional devices: balloon, atherectomy, thrombectomy and distal protection devices. *Cardiol Clin*, **24**, 201–15.

Smith CR, Leon MB, Mack MJ, *et al.* (2011) Transcatheter versus surgical aortic-valve replacement in high-risk patients. *N Engl J Med*, **364**, 2187–98.

Stefanini GG, Holmes DR. (2013). Drug-eluting coronary-artery stents. *N Engl J Med*, **368,** 254–65.

Stettler C, *et al.* (2007). Outcomes associated with drug-eluting and bare-metal stents: a collaborative network meta-analysis. *Lancet*, **370**, 937–48.

The Task Force on the management of ST-segment elevation acute myocardial infarction of the European Society of Cardiology (ESC) (2012). ESC guidelines for the management of acute myocardial infarction in patients presenting with ST-segment elevation. *Eur Heart J*, **33**, 2569–619.

Tonino PA, De Bruyne B, *et al.* (2009). Fractional flow reserve versus angiography for guiding percutaneous coronary intervention. *N Engl J Med*, **360**, 213–24.

Topol EJ, Teirstein PS (ed) (2011). *Textbook of interventional cardiology*, 6th edition. Elsevier, Philadelphia.

Webb JG, Wood MD (2012). Current status of transcatheter aortic valve replacement. *J Am Coll Cardiol*, **60**, 483–92.

Wijeysundera HC, Ko DT, *et al.* (2013). Coronary artery bypass graft surgery vs percutaneous interventions in coronary revascularization: a systematic review. *JAMA*, **310**, 2086–95.

Coronary artery bypass and valve surgery

Rana Sayeed and David Taggart

Essentials

Coronary artery bypass grafting (CABG)—the two main indications are for relief of symptoms, usually angina and/or breathlessness, that persist even with optimal medical therapy (OMT), and/or prognosis. There is a prognostic benefit for CABG in patients with large volumes of ischaemia (i.e. affecting >12% of the ventricular mass), and the benefit of revascularization increases with increasing volumes of ischaemia. The overall mortality for elective CABG in the United Kingdom is around 1% and has continued to fall over the last decade despite an increasingly adverse risk profile of patients undergoing surgery. In randomized trials and large propensity-matched cohort registries CABG, in comparison to percutaneous coronary intervention (PCI) even with drug-eluting stents, has been shown to improve survival and to reduce the subsequent risk of myocardial infarction and recurrent angina. Approximately 80% of patients are alive a decade after surgery of whom around 70% are still free from angina.

Valve surgery—this is primarily performed for patients with severe valvular disease and symptoms. Indications also include deteriorating ventricular function and the requirement for coronary artery surgery in patients with coexistent valve disease. Mitral valve repair is a highly successful procedure in patients with nonrheumatic valvular regurgitation and is associated with an excellent long-term survival. Aortic valve disease is usually treated with aortic valve replacement. A range of biological and mechanical valves are available for valve surgery, with no difference in outcomes between mechanical and biological valves in respect of mortality, prosthetic valve endocarditis, or thromboembolism, but biological valves have a higher rate of reoperation, and the haemodynamic profiles of biological and newer mechanical valves are similar. Biological valves are particularly attractive for elderly patients in whom anticoagulation is deemed high risk, and are now the commonest type of valve implanted worldwide. Patients with aortic stenosis may also be considered for transcatheter valve intervention (TAVI) when the risks of conventional surgery are high. The indications for TAVI for aortic stenosis are likely to expand significantly as the technique develops.

Introduction

Valve surgery first developed in the 1920s for the treatment of congenital heart disease and mitral stenosis. The development of durable valve prostheses in the 1950s allowed surgery for a wider range of acquired valvular heart disease. Currently, degenerative disease causing aortic stenosis, aortic regurgitation, and mitral regurgitation is prevalent in North America and Europe; rheumatic heart disease remains a significant cause of valvular stenosis and/or regurgitation elsewhere. Every year, over 13 000 valve procedures are performed in the United Kingdom and almost 100 000 in the United States of America.

Coronary artery bypass grafting (CABG) has now been performed for almost half a century and it is estimated that approximately three-quarters of a million such operations are performed worldwide annually. Over the last decade the numbers of CABG operations have fallen in most developed countries because of improved medical therapy and advances in percutaneous coronary intervention (PCI), while the numbers of CABG operations continue to increase in the developing world.

Attempts to improve the blood supply to the heart through indirect means were first attempted over a century ago. However, it was technological advances in the 1960s that allowed direct suturing of either the internal mammary artery (IMA) or saphenous grafts to the native coronary artery that led to dramatic improvements in the relief of angina and the explosive growth in CABG surgery. The publication of randomized trials comparing CABG to medical therapy in the 1970s demonstrated the superior efficacy of CABG in relieving angina and a subsequent meta-analysis of these trials also reported that CABG resulted in a survival benefit over a 10 year follow-up period. This led to further dramatic increases in the number of CABG operations in developed countries over the following two decades. Initially most CABG operations were performed using only saphenous vein grafts conduits but the demonstration of superior patency and clinical outcomes with an IMA graft eventually resulted in the vast majority of patients receiving an IMA graft to the anatomically and functionally most important coronary artery, the left anterior descending artery. The superior angiographic patency of the IMA in comparison to vein grafts is largely explained by the tendency to develop intimal hyperplasia and atherosclerosis in vein grafts, a pathological process from which the IMA remains largely immune. Over the last decade there have been attempts to promote the use of more arterial grafts during multivessel CABG surgery, and particularly the use of both IMAs. Over the last two decades there has also been considerable enthusiasm for the use of off-pump CABG to avoid the deleterious effects of cardiopulmonary bypass, but recent large trials have shown no difference in clinical outcome for the majority of patients whether CABG surgery is performed on or off pump.

General considerations in assessing patients for cardiac surgery

The decision to proceed to cardiac surgery involves a careful assessment of the operative risk. In an ageing population with multiple comorbidities these considerations become increasingly important and significantly influence the decision to intervene with surgery and the choice between surgery and percutaneous or trans-catheter intervention. The presence of significant comorbidity exerts a greater influence when surgery is being performed for prognostic rather than symptomatic grounds. In some patients long-term prognosis is determined to a greater degree by their comorbidity than by their coronary or valvular disease, and in those who have asymptomatic disease the benefits of intervention have to be carefully weighed against the risks.

All patients will have routine haematological and biochemical assessment, coronary angiography, and echocardiography. Patients undergoing valve surgery should have a dental assessment including a panoramic radiograph. Angiographic assessment can be refined by the use of pressure wire studies, particularly in those cases where the presence of a given coronary stenosis will determine the choice between PCI and surgery. In patients in whom coronary bypass surgery is being performed for prognostic benefit, in particular those with significant left ventricular impairment, assessment with myocardial perfusion imaging or MRI will guide the decision to revascularize based on the extent of viable myocardium and reversible ischaemia. Right heart catheterization may be required in the assessment of mitral valve disease or where significant pulmonary hypertension has been identified on echocardiography.

Antiplatelet therapy with the exception of aspirin should be withdrawn in patients undergoing elective surgery (see Box 13.6.1).

A number of scoring systems have been developed to estimate the risks of cardiac surgery. In the EuroSCORE II a number of parameters have been identified on univariate analysis to influence the outcome of surgery, as shown in Table 13.6.1.

The operative mortality in elderly patients has fallen substantially over the past 30 years and it is no longer unusual to consider surgery in patients over the age of 80 if their overall risk is acceptable. The risk of coronary artery bypass surgery in patients over the age of 85 is approximately 9% compared to less than 1% in those aged 60 or under; the corresponding figures for isolated valve surgery are 7% and 2.6% respectively. The risks are substantially affected by

> **Box 13.6.1** Management of antiplatelet therapy before coronary artery bypass grafting surgery
>
> ◆ Assessment of the risk of bleeding and ischaemia is recommended when making the decision for CABG surgery
>
> ◆ Low-dose aspirin (75–160 mg daily) should be maintained in patients undergoing CABG surgery
>
> ◆ In patients with increased bleeding risk and in those who refuse blood transfusion, cessation of aspirin 3–5 days before surgery is recommended based on individualized assessment of ischaemic and bleeding risks
>
> ◆ In patients on $P2Y_{12}$ inhibitors it is recommended to postpone surgery for 5 days after interruption of ticagrelor or clopidogrel, and 7 days for prasugrel, unless the patient is at high risk of ischaemic events
>
> Adapted from Sousa-Uva M, Storey R, Huber K, et al., on behalf of ESC Working Group on Cardiovascular Surgery and ESC Working Group on Thrombosis (2013). Expert position paper on the management of antiplatelet therapy in patients undergoing coronary artery bypass graft surgery. *Eur Heart J*, **10**, 1093.

comorbidities such as chronic obstructive airways disease, cerebrovascular disease, and renal disease, which are more common in this age group. Frailty in elderly people, though increasingly important, is difficult to define and is probably best assessed by an experienced physician reviewing the patient, although attempts have been made to develop a frailty index to assist in decision-making.

Moderate to severe chronic obstructive airways disease (i.e. $FEV_1/FVC <0.7$ and $FEV_1 <80\%$ predicted) increases surgical mortality threefold and if combined with a D_{LCO} of less than 50% the mortality increases tenfold. Many patients with chronic obstructive pulmonary disease (COPD) are wrongly classified prior to cardiac surgery and routine pulmonary function testing in patients with a smoking history or history of COPD is advised.

Carotid artery disease is associated with an increased risk of stroke during cardiac surgery; however, there is no evidence that routine screening of all patients is required. Screening of patients aged over 70 with an additional risk factor (carotid bruit, history of cerebrovascular disease, diabetes mellitus, or peripheral vascular disease) is

Table 13.6.1 Variables associated with mortality for cardiac surgery (EuroSCORE II)

Patient-related factors	Cardiac-related factors	Operation-related factors
Age	CCS angina class 4	Urgent operation
Female	NYHA class (>II)	Emergency operation
Extracardiac arteriopathy	Left ventricular ejection fraction	Salvage operation
Neurological/musculoskeletal dysfunction	Recent myocardial infarction	Additional surgical procedures
Previous cardiac surgery	Pulmonary artery pressure	Postinfarct VSD
Serum creatinine		Thoracic surgery
Acitve endocarditis		Aortic arch surgery
Critical preoperative state[a]		

[a] Critical preoperative state is defined as ventricular tachycardia or fibrillation, aborted sudden death or cardiac massage, ventilation prior to surgery, inotropic support, ventricular assist device/balloon pump pre-operatively or acute renal failure (anuria or oliguria <10 ml/h).

Adapted from Nashef SAM, et al. (2012). Euroscore II. *Eur J Cardiothorac Surg*, **41**, 734–45.

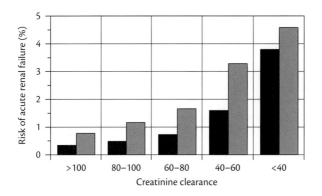

Fig. 13.6.1 Risk of acute renal failure according to baseline creatinine clearance. Adapted from Chertow GM, Lazarus JM, Christiansen CL, Cook EF, Hammermeister KE, Grover F, & Daley J (1997). Preoperative renal risk stratification. *Circulation*, **95**(4), 878–884.

probably justified. Intervention for carotid disease should be considered at or before surgery in patients with a history of cerebrovascular disease and a carotid stenosis (50–99% in men and 70–99% in women). The role of carotid surgery in asymptomatic patients is controversial but it should be considered in men with bilateral severe carotid stenosis or contralateral occlusion if the operative complication rate for carotid surgery is low and life expectancy is good.

The 30 day mortality of patients with acute renal failure in the postoperative period approaches 60% in some series. The risk is largely dependent on the baseline creatinine clearance (see Fig. 13.6.1). Cardiac surgery in patients on dialysis carries a threefold greater mortality and patients are more likely to suffer a stroke, pneumonia, or sepsis in the postoperative period. There is some evidence that off-pump bypass surgery reduces the risks of surgery in this group of patients.

The decision to proceed to cardiac surgery involves a multidisciplinary team of cardiologists, surgeons, and physicians and detailed preoperative assessment is required for an informed decision to be made.

Coronary artery bypass surgery

Indications

Indications for revascularization by either PCI or CABG are shown in Table 13.6.2. The major indications for CABG are the relief of angina

or breathlessness in patients who remain symptomatic despite optimal medical therapy and for prognosis in patients with substantial volumes of ischaemia (classified as involving >12% of the ventricle mass).

Recent guidelines published in Europe and North America broadly agree that there is a prognostic advantage of CABG in patients with the most severe coronary artery disease and particularly in the presence of complex three-vessel disease and/or left main disease. Revascularization is also indicated in patients with impaired left ventricular function and severe coronary artery disease and especially with the demonstration of significant ischaemia and viable myocardium.

Non-ST-elevation myocardial infarction

Patients with non-ST-elevation myocardial infarction (NSTEMI) often require urgent revascularization by either PCI or CABG. For isolated one- or two-vessel disease, and particularly where the culprit lesions are not complex, PCI is an appropriate strategy. In contrast, for those patients with complex multivessel coronary artery disease CABG is still the preferred treatment option soon after medical stabilization of the patient using optimal medical therapy.

ST-elevation myocardial infarction

There is universal agreement that the primary treatment of ST-elevation myocardial infarction (STEMI) is immediate PCI, preferably within 90 min. There is a prohibitively high risk for CABG surgery in patients with acute myocardial infarction. CABG is therefore reserved for patients who exhibit persistent symptoms or evidence of ischaemia despite PCI or who become haemodynamically unstable, and those who develop mechanical complications of myocardial infarction such as papillary muscle rupture or ventricular septal defect.

The CABG operation

The vast majority of CABG operations are performed through a median sternotomy which allows excellent access to all anatomical regions of the heart. In certain situations CABG can be performed through a minithoracotomy with or without the aid of robotic instruments.

After median sternotomy one or both IMAs are harvested while vein from the lower limb and/or the radial artery from the forearm may also be harvested simultaneously as additional conduits. The

Table 13.6.2 Indications for revascularization in stable angina or silent ischaemia

	Subset of coronary disease by anatomy	Evidence class
For prognosis	Left main stem stenosis >50%	IA
	Any proximal LAD >50%	IA
	Two-vessel or three-vessel disease with impaired LV function	IB
	Proven large area of ischaemia (>10%)	IB
	Single remaining patent vessel >50% stenosis	IC
	Single-vessel disease without proximal LAD and without >10% ischaemia	IIIA
For symptoms	Any stenosis >50% with limiting angina or angina equivalent unresponsive to optimal medical treatment	IA
	Dyspnoea/CHF and >10% LV ischaemia/viability supplied by >50% stenotic artery	IIA
	No limiting symptoms with optimal medical therapy	IIIC

CHF, chronic heart failure; LAD, left anterior descending artery; LV, left ventricle.

The Task Force on Myocardial Revascularization of the European Society of Cardiology (ESC) and the European Association for Cardio-Thoracic Surgery (EACTS) (2010). Guidelines on myocardial revascularization. *Eur Heart J*, **31**, 2501–55.

left IMA remains attached proximally to the subclavian artery and the right IMA can either be left *in situ* or anastomosed as a composite graft to the left IMA.

Around 80% of all CABG operations are completed using cardiopulmonary bypass by draining venous blood from the right atrium into the extracorporeal perfusion circuit, where it is oxygenated and cooled, and then returning it to the ascending aorta so that the heart and lungs are effectively bypassed. A large clamp is then placed across the ascending aorta and a cardioplegia solution—usually either crystalloid or blood containing a high concentration of potassium—is used to arrest the heart to provide the surgeon with a motionless, bloodless operating field. After completion of the distal anastomoses the aortic clamp is removed so that the heart is reperfused while the proximal end of the radial artery or vein graft is sewn to the ascending aorta after isolating part of the ascending aorta with a side-biting clamp.

If the operation is performed off pump (without the use of cardiopulmonary bypass) a stabilizing device is used to immobilize a small area of the heart to allow the anastomosis to be performed to the coronary artery.

Outcomes

The 10-year survival for a standard CABG operation using an IMA and saphenous vein grafts is expected to be in the region of 80%. Half of late deaths are due to vein graft failure and this has been a driving force for increasing the use of two IMAs. At 10 years the patency of the IMA is around 95% in comparison to 25 to 50% for vein grafts. Recent studies have shown that the patency of the IMA remains at over 90% two decades after follow-up.

In younger patients there is general agreement to try to maximize the use of mammary arteries and radial arteries because of their improved patency over the longer term. There is evidence that two IMAs improve survival and freedom from further interventions in comparison to a single IMA. Similarly, there is increasing evidence that the more frequent use of arterial grafts also reduces rates of myocardial infarction and recurrent angina.

Secondary prevention

The use of secondary prevention is mandatory in patients who have undergone any revascularization whether by PCI or CABG. Minimum therapy should be at least one antiplatelet medication, β-blockers, statins, and angiotensin converting enzyme (ACE) inhibitors in the presence of impaired left ventricular function.

The choice between CABG and PCI

There is strong evidence from randomized trials such as SYNTAX and FREEDOM (in diabetic patients), and from several large-scale propensity-matched registries with tens of thousands of patients, of a persistent survival advantage of CABG by around 5%, 3 to 5 years after intervention (see also Chapter 13.4). In patients with the most severe disease the difference in survival in favour of CABG is around 10%. These survival curves continue to diverge with further duration of follow-up, suggesting that over the longer term the benefits of CABG may be even greater. This difference between CABG and PCI has persisted despite advances in PCI technology from balloon angioplasty to bare metal stents to drug-eluting stents and to the newer generation of drug-eluting stents. The likely reason for the persistent survival advantage of CABG is that placing bypass grafts to the mid-coronary vessels makes the complexity of proximal coronary artery disease irrelevant and protects against the development of new proximal disease, which is still common despite optimal medical therapy. In contrast, PCI can only deal with localized proximal culprit lesions and has no prophylactic benefit against the development of new disease.

Heart valve surgery

Indications

The indications for valve surgery are covered in more detail elsewhere (see Chapter 6.1). In brief, surgery is indicated for symptomatic (breathlessness, angina, syncope) severe valvular disease or for asymptomatic severe valvular disease with evidence of pathophysiological changes, e.g. abnormal exercise test for asymptomatic severe aortic stenosis, left ventricular dysfunction, pulmonary hypertension, or atrial fibrillation for asymptomatic severe mitral regurgitation.

Repair or replacement

The suitability and success of valve repair rather than replacement depends on valve pathology, the pathophysiological consequences, and surgical expertise. The advantages of valve repair are the avoidance of anticoagulation, prosthetic valve dysfunction, and paravalvular leak, with lower procedural risks and better long-term outcome.

Techniques for mitral valve repair for degenerative disease are well established with excellent long-term outcomes with respect to reoperation. More than 90% of degenerative mitral valves are suitable for repair using a combination of techniques: resection or plication of prolapsing or redundant leaflet tissue; chordal replacement with expanded polytetrafluoroethylene neochords; or annuloplasty, usually with implantation of a prosthetic ring or band to support the repair and prevent further annular dilatation. The cumulative reoperation rate is less than 1%/year, better for isolated posterior leaflet repair (0.5%), and worse for bileaflet (0.9%) or anterior leaflet (1.6%) repairs. Current guidelines support early mitral valve repair for asymptomatic severe mitral regurgitation when there is a high expectation of successful durable repair and low procedural mortality.

Surgical repair for rheumatic mitral valve disease is more limited, depending on the extent and chronicity of rheumatic changes: closed and open commissurotomy may be performed to palliate mitral stenosis. Several techniques for aortic valve repair for aortic regurgitation in bicuspid and trileaflet valves have been described to treat cusp, commissural, and annular pathology in selected cases, but long-term outcomes are uncertain.

Surgical approaches

The majority of valve procedures are performed through a median sternotomy on cardiopulmonary bypass, as described for CABG. Several minimal-access approaches have been described that allow better cosmesis compared with median sternotomy. Aortic valve replacement may be undertaken through a partial upper sternotomy with a J-shaped or inverted T sternal incision through the third or fourth intercostal space, or through a right anterior thoracotomy. The mitral valve may be approached through a lower partial sternotomy, right thoracotomy, or a port access approach through the right chest using a thoracoscopic camera for guidance and specialized instruments; robotic mitral valve surgical techniques have also been developed, but these are limited to specialized centres owing to the high costs of a surgical robot. Depending on the exposure, these minimal-access approaches may require peripheral cannulation for cardiopulmonary bypass, with specialized surgical equipment for venting and arresting the heart, and clamping the aorta. There is a recognized learning curve for these newer surgical approaches, and, although a shorter in-hospital stay and faster early recovery have been reported, the medium-term outcomes remain equivalent to standard open approaches.

Transcatheter valve intervention

Percutaneous valve intervention techniques have been developed that have replaced surgery in cases with prohibitive surgical risk. Transcatheter aortic valve implantation (TAVI) for aortic stenosis uses standard pericardial bioprosthetic valves mounted in balloon-expandable or self-expanding alloy frames, implanted through the femoral or subclavian artery, ascending aorta, or left ventricular apex, depending on the type of device, presence of vascular disease, and institutional expertise. The procedural success rate is 95% with a 90% or lower 30-day mortality and lower than 2% stroke rate. TAVI is recommended for inoperable patients (logistic EuroSCORE ≥ 20, STS PROM ≥ 8) following the PARTNER B study that found a significant reduction in 2-year all-cause mortality with TAVI compared with optimal medical therapy in inoperable severe aortic stenosis (43.3% vs 68%). The PARTNER A study found TAVI to be noninferior to surgical aortic valve replacement with respect to 2-year all-cause mortality (33.9% vs 35%) in a high-risk surgical cohort (STS predicted mortality ≥10). TAVI devices for aortic regurgitation have not yet been widely introduced. Further improved devices are under development to facilitate intraprocedural positioning and to reduce the risks of acute coronary ostial occlusion and paravalvular leak.

Types of valve prosthesis

Biological valves

Biological or bioprosthetic valves may be xenografts, homografts (allografts), or autografts. Xenograft valves are made from glutaraldehyde-fixed animal leaflet tissue with a proprietary anticalcification treatment, most commonly bovine pericardium or porcine aortic valve mounted in an alloy frame for a stented valve, or a whole porcine aortic root for a stentless prosthesis. The advantages of stented xenograft valves are the ease of implantation, the avoidance of long-term anticoagulation, and the ease of reoperation; the development of transcatheter valve-in-valve implantation offers an additional less invasive option. Porcine stentless valves became popular in the 1990s because of their excellent haemodynamics and avoidance of long-term anticoagulation; however, these valves are more challenging to implant reliably, either as a subcoronary implant or as a mini-root replacement, and the rate of structural valve deterioration is higher than for stented valves.

Homografts (allografts) are antibiotic-treated cryopreserved cadaveric grafts including the aortic root and valve. Homografts are resistant to infection and are used for aortic root replacement, particularly for aortic valve endocarditis, in younger patients to avoid the need for anticoagulation, and where there is extensive periannular infection and tissue destruction to allow left ventricular outflow tract reconstruction. However, although the durability at 10 years is similar to pericardial bioprosthetic valves, the reoperation rate for structural valve deterioration at 15 years is as high as 20% in patients aged 41 to 60 years, and reoperation is challenging owing to homograft calcification.

Finally, the Ross procedure described in 1962 uses a pulmonary autograft for aortic root replacement with the pulmonary outflow tract replaced with an aortic homograft. The pulmonary autograft is viable tissue and is able to grow in young patients, has excellent haemodynamics with a low thromboembolic risk, and is resistant to infection. The complexity of the Ross procedure limits its use to specialist centres for selected cases, e.g. women of childbearing age keen to avoid anticoagulation. The Ross procedure is complicated by homograft stenosis in 10 to 20% and aneurysmal dilatation of the autograft causing aortic regurgitation; the 10 year structural valve deterioration rate is up to 30%.

'Sutureless' or rapid-deployment valves are bioprosthetic aortic valves incorporating many features of transcatheter valves, to allow faster implantation in the debrided aortic annulus after open surgical resection of the diseased valve. Cardiopulmonary bypass and cardioplegic arrest are still required, but these valves facilitate minimally invasive approaches and allow shorter procedural times, although the longer-term benefits have yet to be confirmed.

Mechanical valves

Mechanical valves offer the advantage of excellent durability but the disadvantages of long-term anticoagulation and the risks of bleeding; modern low-profile valves have better haemodynamic properties and lower thromboembolic risk than earlier generations. The PROACT study is comparing standard anticoagulation against lower intensity anticoagulation for high thromboembolic risk cases and dual antiplatelet therapy for low-risk cases with the On-X bileaflet valve: early results are encouraging, with a 0.6%/year thromboembolic event rate and 0.4%/year significant bleeding rate.

Meta-analyses of the randomized studies comparing mechanical with biological valves have found no difference in outcomes between mechanical and biological valves with respect to mortality, prosthetic valve endocarditis, or thromboembolism; biological valves have a higher rate of reoperation, mechanical valves a higher risk of significant bleeding complications. The Veterans Administration study found a better 15 year survival for mechanical valves, but the Edinburgh Heart Valve trial found no difference in survival at 20 years. The choice of valve prosthesis for an individual patient depends on several factors including, most importantly, the wishes of the patient, age and life expectancy, metabolic factors predisposing to calcification and early structural valve deterioration (e.g. chronic kidney disease), any contraindication to anticoagulation, expectation of pregnancy, previous infection, and risk of reoperation. There has been a steady increase in the proportion of biological valves implanted over the last decade with these valves now making up more than 80% of valves implanted.

Anticoagulation

Anticoagulation for prosthetic valves

Anticoagulation is required for all currently available mechanical valves. The intensity of anticoagulation depends on valve characteristics and its position, and patient factors such as a history of thromboembolism, atrial fibrillation, left atrial enlargement, and left ventricular dysfunction. Current recommendations for anticoagulation are summarized in Box 13.6.2.

Management of anticoagulation for noncardiac surgery

Anticoagulation is usually stopped for noncardiac surgery depending on the prosthesis type and bleeding risk of surgery. Patients with modern bileaflet or tilting disk mechanical aortic valves at low risk of thromboembolism and with no risk factors such as atrial fibrillation,

Box 13.6.2 Guidelines for choice of prosthetic heart valve

Guidelines favouring bioprosthetic valves

	ECS/EACTS 2012 guidelines
Anticoagulation contraindicated, unavailable, or unable to be managed appropriately	Class IC
Patient preference	Class IC
Re-operation for mechanical valve thrombosis despite good long-term anticoagulation	Class IC
Women of childbearing age contemplating pregnancy	Class IIaC
Low risk for future redo valve replacement	Class IIaC
A bioprosthesis should be considered in those aged >70 years (>65 years for aortic valve replacement in European guidelines)	Class IIaC

Guidelines favouring mechanical valves

	ECS/EACTS 2012 guidelines
Patient already on anticoagulation for a mechanical valve in another position	Class IC
Patient preference	Class IC
Accelerated risk of structural valve deterioration (age <40 years, hyperparathyroidism)	Class IC
Reasonable life expectancy (>10 years) and high risk for future repeat valve replacement	Class IIaC
A mechanical prosthesis is reasonable for those aged <60 years (<65 years for mitral valve replacement in European guidelines)	Class IIaC
Patient already on anticoagulation due to high risk of thromboembolism (AF, venous thromboembolism, thrombophilia, severe LV dysfunction)	Class IIbC

history of thromboembolism or hypercoagulability, or left ventricular dysfunction, may stop warfarin 3 to 5 days before surgery, with no need for bridging therapy with low molecular weight or unfractionated heparin. In all other cases, bridging therapy is indicated before and after surgery for an INR of 2.0 or less; heparin should be resumed after surgery as soon as the immediate risk of bleeding has passed.

Excessive anticoagulation

Anticoagulation may need to be reversed because of an excessive INR, for bleeding, or for emergency surgery. Prothrombin complex concentrate is recommended for rapid reversal for bleeding. A mildly elevated INR with no signs of bleeding may be managed by the omission and/or adjustment of warfarin doses. Oral vitamin K and omission of warfarin are recommended for the correction of a higher INR with no bleeding.

Complications of cardiac surgery

Operative mortality

The overall mortality for all CABG in the United Kingdom is around 1.8%, being just under 1% for elective CABG and approximately 2% for all urgent CABG. Overall mortality has remained low despite an increasing risk profile in patients who are ever more elderly with significant comorbidities. Valve surgery caries a slightly higher risk: the mortality rates for uncomplicated mitral valve repair and aortic valve replacement are approximately 2%. A consistently low mortality almost certainly reflects improvements in medical management of patients as well improvements in anaesthetic, surgical, and perfusion techniques.

Neurological injury

Significant neurological injury is arguably the most feared complication of cardiac surgery and occurs with an incidence of around 1 to 2% during surgery or in the perioperative period. Of patients with neurological injury approximately one-third will die, one-third will remain severely disabled, and one-third will make a good recovery. The incidence of stroke is statistically higher in patients with left main disease than those with isolated three-vessel disease and this may reflect a concomitant higher burden of carotid artery disease in patients with left main disease. The major risk factors for stroke are advanced age, significant disease of the ascending aorta, carotid artery disease, previous neurological injury, and the development of postoperative atrial fibrillation. There is strong evidence that CABG performed off pump using a no-touch aortic technique is the best surgical methodology for reducing incidence of stroke.

Sternal wound complications

Sternal wound dehiscence is another particularly troublesome complication of median sternotomy. The overall incidence is around 0.6% and the major risk factors are insulin-dependent diabetes and especially in combination with obesity. In such patients the use of two IMAs leads to a small but significant increase in this risk of sternal dehiscence and is therefore generally avoided. The treatment of sternal dehiscence is prolonged and complex and usually requires a period of vacuum-assisted dressings followed by plastic surgical reconstruction with muscle flaps.

Pleural effusion

Pleural effusions are usually small and self-limiting and easily treated by chest drainage. They may also develop after patient discharge as a late event.

Pericardial effusion

All patients develop pericardial effusions after cardiac surgery and in the vast majority these are self-limiting and require no specific therapy. A small percentage of patients may develop significant pericardial effusions which can usually be drained by a small incision under the xiphisternum or by using a thoracoscope through the pleural cavity and the pericardium. Pericardial effusions can also appear after patient discharge and can usually be drained without having to reopen the full sternotomy.

Atrial fibrillation

Atrial fibrillation occurs temporarily in around 30% of patients after CABG and the incidence may be reduced by peri- and postoperative β-blockade. It is now standard practice to anticoagulate these patients as well as treat with amiodarone for 6 weeks. If the patient remains in atrial fibrillation after this period then cardioversion is indicated.

Conduction defects

Cardiac conduction defects are common after valve surgery, particularly aortic valve replacement owing to the proximity of the atrioventricular node and bundle of His to the right coronary–noncoronary commissure: conduction pathways may be damaged during valve debridement, by direct injury from a suture, or by postoperative oedema. First-degree or higher degrees of heart block are common after aortic valve surgery and most surgeons routinely place epicardial atrial and ventricular pacing wires for temporary postoperative pacing. Complete heart block requiring implantation of a permanent pacemaker is needed in 3 to 8% of aortic valve replacement cases, being more common in the elderly, with pre-existing conduction defects, and in valve surgery.

Structural valve deterioration

Acute primary valve failure is rare in current mechanical or biological valves, but emergent or urgent reoperation is indicated. Structural valve deterioration is a complication of biological valves owing to leaflet fibrosis and calcification causing progressive valvular stenosis, and perforation and leaflet tearing leading to regurgitation. Structural valve deterioration develops at a predictable rate related to younger patient age, valve position, mitral more affected than aortic, altered calcium metabolism (e.g. chronic kidney disease), and pregnancy. Pericardial valves deteriorate more slowly than porcine bioprostheses. The indications for reoperation for structural valve deterioration are the same as for native valve disease, based on symptoms, ventricular size and function, and pulmonary hypertension.

Thromboembolism

The incidence of clinical thromboembolic events is up to 2.3 cases per 100 patient-years. The risk is similar for biological and anticoagulated mechanical valves. Risk factors for thromboembolism include prosthesis type and position, a history of thromboembolism or hypercoaguability, atrial fibrillation and left atrial size, and left ventricular dysfunction. Thromboembolism with a mechanical valve is managed by ensuring that the INR is in the therapeutic range, or if the INR is already therapeutic, by increasing the target INR or adding low-dose aspirin.

Prosthetic valve thrombosis

Thrombosis of a mechanical valve may be a life-threatening complication. The diagnosis is suggested by heart failure, signs of a low cardiac output, or thromboembolism with reduced or absent prosthetic valve sounds, new murmurs, or documented inadequate anticoagulation. Mitral and tricuspid valves are more commonly involved. Echocardiography or fluoroscopy usually confirm reduced leaflet or disk motion caused by an occluding thrombus. Emergency reoperation is recommended for left-sided valve thrombosis with shock or New York Heart Association (NYHA) III or IV symptoms or cases with large thrombi (>0.8 cm^2 on transoesophageal echocardiography (TOE)) but the operative mortality is up to 30%. Fibrinolysis with tPA or streptokinase may be used for left-sided valves with less severe symptoms (NYHA I and II) or smaller thrombus burdens and for patients unsuitable for reoperation;

fibrinolysis is recommended for right-sided valve thrombosis. Fibrinolysis for left-sided valve thrombosis is associated with a 15 to 20% risk of systemic embolism or death.

Prosthetic valve endocarditis

Prosthetic valve endocarditis (PVE) is more common early after surgery, with an incidence up to 3% at 1 year. Mechanical valves are more commonly involved over the first year, but the incidence for mechanical and biological valves is similar thereafter. Early PVE (within 1 year) in most commonly due to nosocomial coagulase-negative staphylococci; late PVE (after 1 year) is caused by a similar range of organisms as native valve endocarditis. PVE follows a more aggressive course than native valve endocarditis with early perivalvular tissue destruction and abscess formation. TOE is important to establish the diagnosis and identify complications indicating early surgery. Medical therapy is usually ineffective in PVE. Early surgery is recommended for heart failure, abscess formation, valve dehiscence or other dysfunction, or infection with a resistant organism; surgery is also indicated for a persistent bacteraemia despite adequate antibiotic therapy or recurrent embolism from vegetations. The operative mortality for early surgery for PVE is up to 35%.

Paravalvular leak

A paravalvular leak may develop because of poor surgical technique, suture dehiscence, poor native tissue strength, and infection: PVE must always be excluded in the setting of a new paravalvular leak. A small leak may cause a haemolytic anaemia due to mechanical red cell damage; iron and folic acid supplements may be beneficial. Reoperation is indicated for heart failure, a persistent need for transfusion, or an impaired quality of life. Large leaks, particularly mitral, may cause volume overload: the development of intractable heart failure is an indication for reoperation. Catheter-based approaches may be helpful to avoid redo surgery.

Further reading

Iqbal J, *et al.* (2013). Optimal revascularization for complex coronary artery disease. *Nat Rev Cardiol*, **10**, 635–47.

Mohr FW, *et al.* (2013). Coronary artery bypass graft surgery versus percutaneous coronary intervention in patients with three-vessel disease and left main coronary disease: 5-year follow-up of the randomised, clinical SYNTAX trial. *Lancet*, **381**(9867), 629–38.

Partridge JS, *et al.* (2012). Frailty in the older surgical patient: a review. *Age Ageing*, **41**, 142–7.

Taggart DP (2013). Current status of arterial grafts for coronary artery bypass grafting. *Ann Cardiothorac Surg*, **2**, 427–30.

Taggart DP, *et al.* (2001). Effect of arterial revascularisation on survival: a systematic review of studies comparing bilateral and single internal mammary arteries. *Lancet*, **358**(9285), 870–5.

Vahanian A, *et al.* (2012). Guidelines on the management of valvular heart disease (version 2012) The Joint Task Force on the Management of Valvular Heart Disease of the European Society of Cardiology (ESC) and the European Association for Cardio-Thoracic Surgery (EACTS). *Eur Heart J*, **33**, 2451–96.

Vohra HA, *et al.* (2013). Outcomes following cardiac surgery in patients with preoperative renal dialysis. *Interact Cardiovasc Thorac Surg*, **18**, 103–11.

Windecker S, *et al.* (2014). 2014 ESC/EACTS Guidelines on myocardial revascularization. Task Force on Myocardial Revascularization of the European Society of Cardiology (ESC) and the European Association for Cardio-Thoracic Surgery (EACTS); European Association of Percutaneous Cardiovascular Interventions (EAPCI). *Eur Heart J*, **35**, 2541–619.

SECTION 14

Diseases of the arteries

CHAPTER 14.1

Acute aortic syndromes

Andrew R. J. Mitchell, James D. Newton, and Adrian P. Banning

Essentials

The acute aortic syndromes are acute dissection, intramural haematoma, and penetrating ulcer, and all involve disruption of the wall of the aorta with potentially devastating consequences. Although relatively uncommon, left unrecognized and untreated they can carry a mortality rate of up to 2% per hour and 50% within the first few weeks.

Clinical presentation—the pain of an acute aortic syndrome is typically of instantaneous onset, cataclysmic in severity, pulsatile and tearing in quality, located either in the anterior thorax or back, and migrating if a dissection extends through the thorax. Patients usually appear shocked, but blood pressure may be normal or raised and heart rate relatively slow. Physical signs typically reflect the region of the aorta involved and effects of pressure on adjacent structures: evidence of new aortic regurgitation or development of pulse deficits should be actively sought.

Diagnosis—abnormalities on the chest radiograph and ECG are common, but neither investigation is diagnostic and further imaging is always necessary by MRI, contrast-enhanced CT, or transoesophageal echocardiography, depending on local availability and the clinical condition of the patient.

Management—every patient with a clinical suspicion of an acute aortic syndrome should receive effective pain relief and antihypertensive medication (intravenous labetalol or esmolol), aiming to maintain systolic blood pressure <120 mmHg. For confirmed intramural haematoma or dissection of the ascending aorta (type A), emergency surgery is indicated. Penetrating ulcers can be treated with endovascular stenting. When the ascending aorta is spared (type B), aggressive control of blood pressure is the usual initial management, with surgery being considered if there is evidence of further progression of dissection or ischaemic complications. In the long term, strenuous efforts to control blood pressure are indicated for all patients who have survived aortic dissection, with repeat imaging at least once a year.

Introduction

An acute aortic syndrome should be considered, even if only briefly, in the differential diagnosis of any patient complaining of acute chest pain and other symptoms (Box 14.1.1). A careful history and physical examination will often secure the diagnosis, which is then confirmed by appropriate noninvasive investigations.

The consequences of missing an acute aortic syndrome can be disastrous: when managing a patient with acute chest pain it is always prudent for clinicians to ask themselves 'could this be an acute aortic syndrome?' to ensure it features in the differential diagnosis before any antiplatelet or anticoagulant agents are administered.

The three mechanisms of acute aortic syndromes are acute aortic dissection, acute intramural haematoma, and penetrating ulcer of the aortic wall (Fig. 14.1.1)

Pathogenesis

The aortic wall is composed of three layers: a thin intimal lining, a thicker medial layer (largely composed of elastin fibres that provide strength), and a thinner adventitial outer layer from which small blood vessels (the vasa vasorum) arise to nourish the outer layers of the media.

Acute aortic dissection occurs when a breach in the integrity of the intima allows blood at high pressure to penetrate through and into the media. Through this tear, pulsatile blood flow can then propagate distally, parallel to the lumen, often spiralling and splitting the arterial wall into an inner (intima–medial) and outer layer (media–adventitial). This process of tearing within the wall results in the formation of a false lumen, parallel to the original true lumen, and commonly of a similar or larger size (Fig. 14.1.2).

Further communication between the lumens (or re-entry tears) can occur and may reduce the pressure within the false lumen, thus limiting propagation of the dissection. However, the process often extends along the entire length of the aorta to the common iliac arteries, threatening the origins of branch vessels that may be avulsed or narrowed by the mass effect of the false lumen, and leading to ischaemia in the dependent vascular territories. When dissection extends retrogradely towards the heart it can cause occlusion of a coronary artery and distortion of the aortic valve, resulting in

---

Box 14.1.1 Symptoms that warrant consideration of an acute aortic syndrome

◆ Chest pain

◆ Syncope

◆ Thoracic back pain

◆ Neurological, mesenteric, or limb ischaemia

◆ Abdominal pain

◆ Symptoms of pericardial tamponade

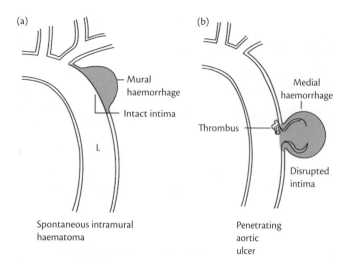

Fig. 14.1.1 *Mechanism of acute thoracic aortic syndromes: (a) acute aortic dissection; (b) spontaneous intramural haematoma; (c) penetrating atherosclerotic ulcer.*

acute aortic regurgitation. Dissection may also rupture into the pericardial space, causing cardiac tamponade. The weakened aortic wall can rupture at any point along its length; this is usually fatal.

Acute intramural haematoma was described by pathologists in 1920. It usually occurs when the small arterioles that run in the outer media of the aorta (the vasa vasorum) rupture and bleed, rarely it can occur following trauma. It is a medial/adventitial event, with the intima remaining intact, and there is no false lumen (Fig. 14.1.3). The clinical presentation is very similar to that of acute aortic dissection, with thoracic pain being the commonest presenting symptom. The diagnosis can only be made by exclusion of an intimal tear or a penetrating atherosclerotic ulcer. The intramural haematoma is not readily identifiable by aortography, but using noninvasive imaging, a circular or crescentic thickening of the aortic wall of more than 7 mm in depth associated with central displacement of any intimal calcification supports the diagnosis. There is increasing evidence that spontaneous intramural haematoma may be a precursor of aortic dissection. Clinical studies have

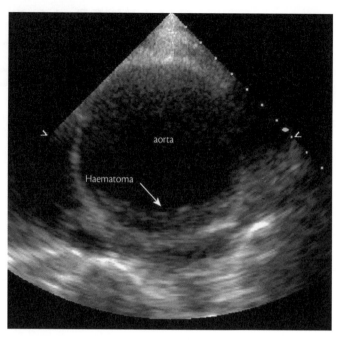

Fig. 14.1.3 *Transthoracic echocardiography of the ascending aorta. The aorta is dilated and there is a posterior intramural haematoma.*

supported this assertion: despite aggressive blood pressure control, up to 50% of patients with an intramural haematoma develop dissection or aortic rupture. Surgery is generally indicated when the ascending aorta is involved.

Penetrating atherosclerotic ulcer presents with similar symptoms to aortic dissection, usually in elderly patients with disseminated atheroma. Intimal disruption caused by atheroma results in perforation and secondary haemorrhage into the media. Imaging demonstrates an out-pouching from the lumen into the aortic wall with localized haemorrhage and evidence of diffuse atheroma. Rarely, this can cause a localized dissection, but the main threat is the high incidence of rupture. Pseudoaneurysm formation can occur (Fig. 14.1.4). Treatment is usually with endovascular stenting to cover the ulcer, or with high-risk surgery.

Classification

The commonest sites for thoracic aortic dissection to originate are in the ascending aorta, just above the sinuses of the aortic valve, and in the upper descending aorta just beyond the origin of the left subclavian artery. The Stanford group proposed a classification that is directly linked to patient management (Fig. 14.1.5). Aortic dissection that involves the ascending thoracic aorta is classified as type A and demands consideration of immediate surgery, whereas dissection that spares the ascending aorta is classified as type B and initial management is usually medical.

Aetiology

The most common predisposing risk factor (70% of patients) for aortic dissection is hypertension. Although the processes involved in the initiation of dissection remain incompletely understood, medial haemorrhage from rupture of vasa vasorum appears to be important. When this process is self-limiting and there is no expansion of the resultant haematoma by recurrent bleeding, healing may occur

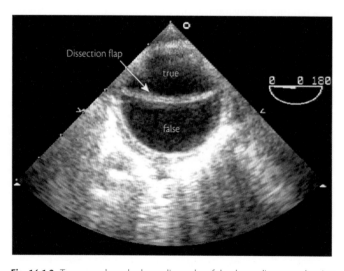

Fig. 14.1.2 *Transoesophageal echocardiography of the descending aorta showing a dissection flap separating the true and false lumens.*

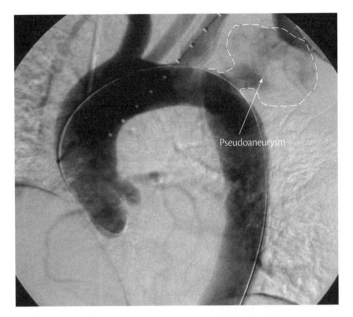

Fig. 14.1.4 Emergency aortography during endovascular closure of a pseudoaneurysm occurring due to a penetrating atherosclerotic ulcer.

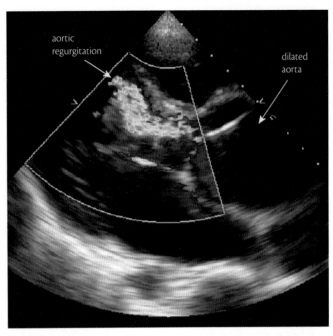

Fig. 14.1.6 Transthoracic echocardiography in a patient with Marfan's syndrome. The aortic root is significantly dilated with a central jet of aortic regurgitation.

with reabsorption of the haemorrhage. Alternatively, and particularly when the bleeding is extensive or recurrent, a large intramural haematoma may form around the circumference of the aorta. This alters the distribution of tensile stresses within the aorta, with much of the redistributed stress affecting the intima/endothelium overlying the mass. An intimal tear may then result in splitting and separation of the media, propagation of a false lumen, and dissection.

Specific risk factors

Patients with Marfan's syndrome (see Chapter 11) may present with aortic dissection or aortic root dilatation and aortic regurgitation (Fig. 14.1.6). Abnormal fibrillin within the aortic media results in intimal instability, particularly when aortic dilation leads

to increased wall stress. Although the absolute risk of dissection rises with increasing size of the ascending aorta, it is important to remember that all patients with Marfan's syndrome are at risk, particularly when there is a family history of aortic dissection (Box 14.1.2). Patients with Ehlers–Danlos syndrome are also at risk of spontaneous dissection, not only of the aorta but of its principal branches, including the coronary arteries.

Patients with coarctation of the aorta and those with bicuspid aortic valves also appear to be at increased risk of dissection, possibly related to defects in aortic wall composition. Dissection may also occur in patients with Turner's syndrome, Noonan's syndrome, and in the later stages of pregnancy, particularly in patients with Marfan's syndrome. In high-risk patients with Marfan's syndrome with dilated aortas or a family history of dissection, deferring pregnancy until after elective aortic root replacement may be advisable.

Clinical features

Most patients present with characteristic symptoms and clinical findings, in which case the diagnosis of dissection can be made

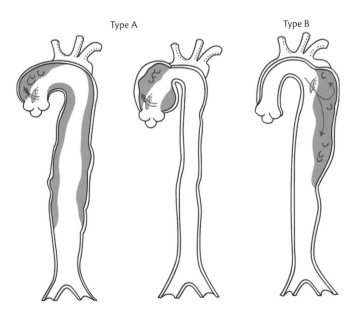

Fig. 14.1.5 The Stanford classification of aortic dissection. Type A dissection involves the ascending aorta, irrespective of the distal extent of dissection.

Box 14.1.2 High-risk conditions for acute aortic syndromes
◆ Marfan's syndrome
◆ Loeys–Dietz syndrome
◆ Bicuspid aortic valve
◆ Recent aortic manipulation
◆ Prior aortic dissection
◆ Known thoracic aortic aneurysm
◆ Family history of aortic dissection or thoracic aneurysm
◆ Hypertension

with reasonable assurance. However, a few present atypically and it is worth considering the possibility of aortic dissection in any patient who is haemodynamically unstable without satisfactory explanation.

The pain of acute dissection of the aorta can be described in terms of its (1) instantaneous onset, (2) cataclysmic severity, (3) pulsatile and tearing quality, (4) location either in the anterior thorax or back, and (5) migration as it follows the course of the dissection through the thorax. Careful interrogation about the presence of these five features will usually allow differentiation from other causes of chest pain. The instant onset, tearing/pulsatile quality, and migratory pattern contrast with the pain of cardiac ischaemia, which is usually gradual in onset (over minutes), tight or crushing, and more unchanging in its distribution in the anterior chest. Syncope shortly after the onset of typical pain is not common, but is another characteristic presentation of dissection, often caused by rupture of the false lumen into the pericardial cavity. Other uncommon modes of presentation include stroke and limb ischaemia, with or without pain, and very occasionally congestive heart failure resulting from severe aortic regurgitation.

Although patients with dissection usually appear shocked, their blood pressure may be normal or raised and their heart rate relatively slow. The distribution of the abnormalities detected by physical examination usually reflect the region of the aorta involved in the dissection and pressure on adjacent structures. Signs of aortic regurgitation or tamponade are likely to be found in a patient with dissection involving the ascending aorta, whereas absent upper limb pulses and cerebral abnormalities suggest involvement of the aortic arch. Expansion of the arch may compress venous return and cause engorgement of one or both jugular veins. Similarly, hoarseness and Horner's syndrome can follow pressure on the left recurrent laryngeal nerve and superior cervical ganglion, respectively. Tenderness over a carotid artery may be due to dissection extending up the artery from the arch. Involvement of the descending aorta can result in visceral and lower limb ischaemia.

Although traditional teaching emphasizes the relevance of blood pressure discrepancy between the arms, this is not a particularly sensitive sign, particularly when dissection spares the ascending aorta and arch. However, evidence of new aortic regurgitation or development of pulse deficits are specific signs of dissection and should be actively sought by the examining physician.

Clinical investigation

Abnormalities of the chest radiograph and electrocardiogram (ECG) are common in patients with dissection, but neither investigation is diagnostic and further imaging is always necessary.

Chest radiograph

Potential abnormalities on the chest radiograph include a widened aortic contour, aortic kinking, tracheal deviation, left pleural effusion, and a widened mediastinum (Fig. 14.1.7). The 'calcium sign' is medial displacement of the calcium in the aortic knuckle by more than 6 mm and occurs in 20% of cases. The chest radiograph is normal in 10% of patients with acute aortic dissection. Urgent portable anterior–posterior chest radiographs are often of insufficient quality to comment on the mediastinal contours and cannot be relied upon.

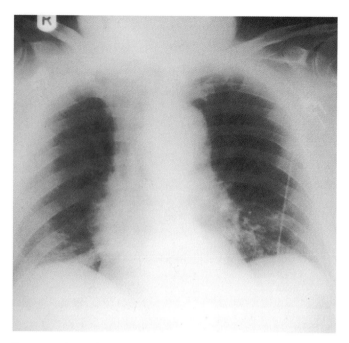

Fig. 14.1.7 Chest radiograph in aortic dissection showing mediastinal enlargement.

ECG

Nonspecific ST-segment and T-wave changes on the ECG are often found, as are changes of left ventricular hypertrophy related to previous hypertension. The ECG is normal in one-third of patients. Actual involvement of a coronary artery is relatively uncommon, presentation is usually with features of right coronary occlusion since involvement of the left main stem is usually rapidly fatal. An atypical distribution of ST-elevation changes (i.e. generalized acute changes, affecting the anterior and inferior leads) is well recognized and should always alert the physician to the possibility of a diagnosis other than acute myocardial infarction and thereby reduce the possibility of inadvertent administration of thrombolytic treatment.

Blood tests

The diagnosis of aortic dissection should not be delayed while the results of blood tests are awaited. Nevertheless, immunoassays of monoclonal antibodies to smooth muscle myosin heavy chains have a high sensitivity and specificity for the diagnosis of aortic dissection. Cardiac enzymes are usually normal, but an elevated cardiac troponin on admission is a marker for a worse in-hospital outcome. If there is haemolysis of blood in the false lumen, lactate dehydrogenase may be elevated. Haemoglobin may be reduced if there has been significant leakage of blood from the aorta. A mildly raised leucocyte count, and raised C-reactive protein (CRP) are common. D-dimer is often elevated in dissection but is a nonspecific finding. A normal D-dimer test has been used to identify patients unlikely to benefit from further aortic imaging.

Key imaging studies

The priorities when imaging a patient with suspected dissection are to confirm the diagnosis and to decide if the ascending aorta is involved (Stanford type A), as this will determine whether or

Table 14.1.1 Sensitivity and specificity of investigations for the diagnosis of aortic dissection

Investigation	Sensitivity (%)	Specificity (%)
MRI	99–100	99–100
CT	96–100	96–100
Transoesophageal echocardiography	98	95
Transthoracic echocardiography	59–85	63–96
Aortography	77–88	94

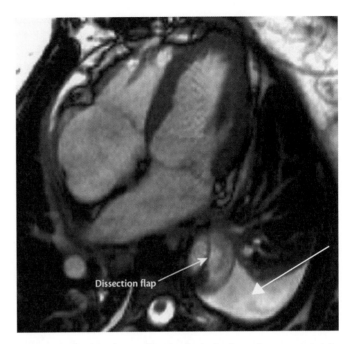

Fig. 14.1.8 MRI of the chest. A dissection flap in the descending aorta and a left-sided pleural effusion (large arrow) are visible.

not surgery is required. The surgeon wants to know the entry site of the dissection, if the aortic valve is competent, if there is a pericardial effusion or tamponade, and if there is involvement of the coronary arteries. Several diagnostic techniques are available (Table 14.1.1).

Historically, aortography was the investigation of choice, but it has several disadvantages. These include delay during the assembly of the catheter laboratory team, the risk of aortic rupture during catheter manipulation, and the nephrotoxicity of radiological contrast media when renal function may already be compromised by hypotension or renal artery involvement. CT, MRI, and echocardiography all have proven advantages over aortography. However, with the advent of primary percutaneous coronary intervention (PCI) some patients do present to the angiography suite with a diagnosis of acute coronary syndrome (ACS). Aortic dissection should always be considered in those in whom coronary angiography is normal and further imaging performed if appropriate.

Contrast-enhanced CT is noninvasive, but requires the use of radiological contrast medium. In sensitivity and specificity it is at least equivalent to aortography, but its accuracy is inferior to MRI, although this has been improved by the use of newer multislice CT scanners. MRI is noninvasive and provides excellent images of the whole aorta. Its sensitivity and specificity for dissection are up to 100% in some series, and the addition of cardiac gated and cine techniques can give information on luminal blood flow and valvular regurgitation (Fig. 14.1.8). MRI is therefore the investigation of choice for most diseases affecting the aorta, but it has several limitations in patients with suspected acute dissection of the aorta. These include the requirement for patient transfer to the scanner,

with attendant delays, restricted access to the patient during scanning, and the high degree of patient cooperation required to obtain artefact-free images.

The limited sensitivity and specificity of transthoracic echocardiography mean that it cannot be used to exclude aortic dissection. However, in some patients dissection of the ascending aorta can be confidently diagnosed using parasternal and suprasternal imaging, mandating urgent transfer to a surgical centre where additional information can be obtained by transoesophageal echocardiography in the anaesthetic room. Transoesophageal echocardiography provides detailed anatomical information about the morphology of a dissection and can also demonstrate the consequences of proximal extension, including the presence of aortic regurgitation, pericardial effusion, and involvement of the coronary artery ostia, thus making complementary investigations such as angiography unnecessary (Fig. 14.1.9).

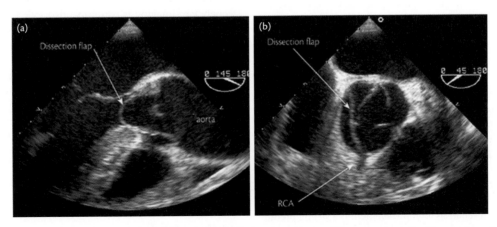

Fig. 14.1.9 Transoesophageal echocardiography at the level of the aortic valve: (a) view along the aorta; (b) cross-sectional view. There is a large dissection flap in the ascending aorta (type A) that nearly involves the ostium of the right coronary artery (RCA).

Management

Emergency management

Lowering systolic blood pressure and limiting shear stress reduces the likelihood of progression of dissection. Every patient with a clinical suspicion of dissection should therefore receive effective pain relief (intravenous morphine is usually required) and antihypertensive medication pending a definitive diagnosis by imaging. Patients should be cared for in a high-dependency area with continuous monitoring of the ECG and regular blood pressure and urine output measurement. Ideally, systolic blood pressure should be maintained below 110 mmHg and heart rate to less than 60 bpm, using intravenous labetalol (initial dose 50 mg bolus followed by 1–2 mg/min) or intravenous esmolol. Both of these agents produce a rapid and titratable reduction in blood pressure, with β-blockade particularly appropriate in this context because it reduces the force of cardiac contraction and the rate of rise of the arterial pressure (dP/dt). If blood pressure control remains suboptimal, an additional infusion of sodium nitroprusside may be used (0.5–8 micrograms/kg per min). Intravenous nitrates and oral calcium antagonist are alternatives in patients who are intolerant of β-blockers.

Patients presenting with or developing cardiogenic shock should undergo immediate echocardiography for investigation of pericardial tamponade. Emergency surgery is the treatment of choice, as percardiocentesis can accelerate bleeding and is usually ineffective.

The optimal management of patients with aortic dissection requires close liaison between those who admit patients as medical emergencies and cardiac surgical centres, using local guidelines for investigation that should reflect the available expertise and surgical opinion. Patients with a low clinical index of suspicion of dissection who are in a stable cardiovascular state should undergo prompt investigation in their local hospital, using a nominated noninvasive technique—usually CT scanning. Unless noninvasive imaging is available immediately, unstable patients with a high clinical index of suspicion should receive medical treatment and be transferred immediately to a surgical centre for both diagnostic imaging and management. This approach minimizes delay, a critical aspect of the management of acute aortic dissection.

Surgery

When the dissection involves the ascending aorta (type A), immediate surgery is required as there is a high risk of proximal extension causing dissection of the coronary arteries, incompetence of the aortic valve, and rupture into the pericardium. Surgery usually involves excision of the intimal tear in the ascending aorta and interposition of a Dacron graft. This procedure protects the lower ascending aorta and valve from progressive dissection and prevents distal extension by reducing pressure within the false lumen. The false lumen may subsequently thrombose, or—in cases with multiple intimal tears—may remain patent but decompressed.

Replacement of the aortic valve is usually performed only when resuspension of the valve is not possible. However, in patients with Marfan's syndrome the ascending aorta and valve are usually replaced with a composite graft to prevent subsequent annular dilatation. In cases where dissection extends into the aortic arch, some surgeons advocate that the arch and great vessels should be included in the initial repair as arch involvement is a strong predictor of a requirement for repeat surgery. However, extended surgery can increase the duration of the operation and the risk of damage to the central nervous system, hence inclusion of the arch in dissection repair is generally restricted to centres with particular expertise.

Spinal cord damage and paraplegia is a common complication of aortic dissection repair, resulting from cross-clamping of the aorta. Techniques to improve distal aortic perfusion can reduce the incidence of this complication to less than 5%. The overall operative mortality for surgical repair is between 10 and 20%.

Further management of descending aortic dissection

Proximal extension towards the heart is less likely when the dissection begins distal to the left subclavian artery (type B). These patients tend to be older than those with ascending aortic involvement and are more likely to have comorbidity. Diligent blood pressure management is the usual initial treatment, as surgery on the descending thoracic aorta carries significant mortality and morbidity, including impaired blood supply to the spinal cord and paraplegia. However, some centres recommend elective surgery (after several weeks) in selected patients with Marfan's syndrome, in younger patients with dissection associated with large aneurysms, and if thrombosis of the false lumen fails to occur.

Surgery for type B dissection should be considered if there is evidence of proximal extension of the dissection, progressive aortic enlargement threatening external rupture, or ischaemic complications from involvement of major arteries. For example, the prognosis is extremely poor when ischaemia occurs in the territory of a major abdominal artery, in which case emergency surgical fenestration of the intimal flap can be life-saving.

Encouraging results have recently been achieved using endovascular stenting for patients with complicated dissection starting distal to the left subclavian artery. Using vascular access from a groin incision, a covered stent can be delivered to cover the intimal tear. In suitable cases this obliterates flow into the false lumen, relieving branch ischaemia and preventing further aneurysmal dilatation.

Follow-up and prognosis

Strenuous efforts to control blood pressure are indicated for all patients who have survived aortic dissection. β-Blockers are the agents of choice for most, with other agents added as required. Most patients will require a combination of antihypertensive agents to achieve satisfactory blood pressure control (systolic <120–130 mmHg). Imaging at least once a year is recommended, using the modality with which there is most local expertise. Increased frequency of imaging is recommended following any acute event, for example severe chest pain, and for some patients with Marfan's syndrome.

The long-term survival of patients with type A aortic dissection who have surgery and survive to discharge is encouraging: 90% are still alive at 3 years. Although patients who are treated medically have extremely high in-hospital mortality (50%), two-thirds of patients who survive to hospital discharge are alive 3 years later. The mortality is often not related to dissection but from other cardiovascular conditions. Patients with a history of atherosclerosis or prior cardiac surgery are at increased risk of death. In-hospital mortality for patients treated medically with type B dissection is 10%, and 3-year survival is approximately 70%.

Further reading

Dake MD, *et al.* (1999). Endovascular stent graft placement for the treatment of acute aortic dissection. *N Engl J Med*, **340**, 1546–52.

Estrera AL, *et al.* (2006). Outcomes of medical management of acute type B aortic dissection. *Circulation*, **114**, 384–9.

Evangelista A, *et al.* (2005). Acute intramural hematoma of the aorta. A mystery in evolution. *Circulation*, **111**, 1063–70.

Klompas M (2002). Does this patient have an acute thoracic aortic dissection? *JAMA*, **287**, 2262–2272.

Kodolitsch Y, *et al.* (2004). Chest radiography for the diagnosis of acute aortic syndrome. *Am J Med*, **116**, 73–7.

Macura KJ, *et al.* (2003). Pathogenesis in acute aortic syndromes: aortic dissection, intramural hematoma, and penetrating atherosclerotic aortic ulcer. *Am J Roentgenol*, **181**, 309–16.

Nienaber CA, Eagle KA (2003). Aortic dissection: new frontiers in diagnosis and management. Part I: from etiology to diagnostic strategies. Circulation 108, 628–35; Part II: Therapeutic management and follow-up. *Circulation*, **108**, 772–8.

Nienaber CA, *et al.* (1993). The diagnosis of thoracic aortic dissection by noninvasive imaging procedures. *N Engl J Med*, **328**, 1–9.

Trimarchi S, *et al.* (2006). Role and results of surgery in acute type B aortic dissection: insights from the international registry of acute aortic dissection (IRAD). *Circulation*, **114**, 357–64.

Tsai TT (2005). Acute aortic syndromes. *Circulation*, **112**, 3802–13.

Tsai TT, *et al.* (2006). Long-term survival in patients presenting with type A acute aortic dissection: insights from the international registry of acute aortic dissection (IRAD). *Circulation*, **114**, 350–356.

Vilacosta I, *et al.* (1998). Penetrating atherosclerotic ulcer: documentation by transoesophageal echocardiography. *J Am Coll Cardiol*, **32**, 83–9.

CHAPTER 14.2

Peripheral arterial disease

Janet Powell and Alun Davies

Essentials

The most common presentations of peripheral arterial disease are intermittent claudication and abdominal aortic aneurysm. In patients under 50 years of age the cause of disease is most likely to be genetic, congenital, immunological, infectious, or traumatic; over 50 years of age the principal risk factor is smoking.

Diagnosis—the main diagnostic method used to confirm the diagnosis of peripheral arterial disease is Doppler ultrasonography, in particular to estimate the ratio of systolic blood pressure at the ankle and in the arm, the ankle–brachial pressure index (ABPI; normal value 1.0–1.4, <0.9 abnormal). Ultrasonography is the standard technique for demonstrating abdominal aortic aneurysms, usually defined as being when the maximum aortic diameter exceeds 3 cm.

Critical leg ischaemia is defined as gangrenous change, ulceration, tissue loss, or rest pain lasting for 2 weeks, with an absolute ankle pressure of less than 50 mmHg.

Acute leg ischaemia

Presents as a painful, pale and pulseless limb, and is usually caused by thrombosis at the site of an atherosclerotic stenosis. Requires administration of analgesia and, if appropriate, rapid surgical intervention: (1) for irreversible ischaemia the options are amputation or palliative care; (2) for severe but potentially reversible ischaemia (white leg), surgery is usually the treatment of choice; and (3) for moderate limb ischaemia (no paralysis and only mild sensory loss), arteriography with consideration of thrombolysis, endovascular angioplasty/stenting, or surgical embolectomy/endarterectomy/bypass.

Chronic leg ischaemia

Most commonly presents with claudication affecting the calf and thigh. This is associated with high cardiovascular risk, but only 5% will go on to lose a limb, and surgical or endovascular intervention is not usually required. Key elements in management are smoking cessation, aspirin, and statins.

Abdominal aortic aneurysm

Ruptured abdominal aortic aneurysm typically causes collapse and severe back or abdominal pain: less than 20% reach hospital alive, and almost one-half of those undergoing emergency surgical die within 30 days.

By standard definition, more than 5% of men older than 55 years have an abdominal aortic aneurysm, but most of these are small (3–5.5 cm). These should be managed by ultrasound surveillance, with attention to modification of cardiovascular risk factors.

Repair is generally recommended for asymptomatic aneurysms larger than 5.5 cm (perhaps >5 cm in women), or symptomatic aneurysms of any size. Minimally invasive endovascular aneurysm repair has an operative mortality of about 2%, which is only one-third of that associated with traditional open repair, but within 2 years the mortality advantage of endovascular repair has been lost and long-term outlook is unknown.

Introduction

Peripheral arterial disease, defined for the purpose of this chapter as diseases of the abdominal aorta and its branches, has risk factors and features that overlap with, but can be distinguished from, those of coronary artery disease. The two conditions often coexist, but patients with coronary disease are almost always referred directly to physicians, whereas those with peripheral arterial disease are referred directly to vascular surgeons, particularly in regions where angiology is a poorly developed specialty, since medical therapies are limited. Vascular surgeons also manage patients with arterial disease in the carotid vessels and upper limbs. These aspects receive only passing mention in this chapter: for discussion regarding the clinical features and management of carotid artery disease, see Chapter 24.10.1.

The most common presentations of peripheral arterial disease are intermittent claudication and abdominal aortic aneurysm. Most peripheral arterial disease remains asymptomatic. It is not a new disease that results from a modern Westernized lifestyle. Atherosclerotic disease, partially occluding the peripheral arteries, has been described in the mummies of ancient Egypt. Life as a cavalry officer was associated with an increased risk of popliteal aneurysm, a condition treated by ligation by John Hunter, the pioneering 18th-century surgeon. Albert Einstein died of a ruptured abdominal aortic aneurysm.

Techniques for repairing abdominal aortic aneurysms were not developed until the middle of the 20th century. This was the golden era for the development of vascular surgery as a specialty, with the increasing use of bypass surgery that reduced the need for amputation. Today newer, less invasive approaches are being employed—angioplasty and endovascular stenting—but few specific medical therapies are on the horizon.

Aetiology and epidemiology

Peripheral arterial disease may occur in young people, but the prevalence increases sharply with age. Both young and old may suffer from occlusive (stenosing) disease of the peripheral arteries or dilating (aneurysmal) disease, while vasospastic disease is uncommon.

However, the underlying causes of peripheral arterial disease in those below and above 50 years of age tend to be very different.

Peripheral arterial disease in patients less than 50 years old

In younger patients, the cause of disease is most likely to be genetic, congenital, immunological, infectious, or traumatic. Patients with familial hypercholesterolaemia and related inherited disorders of lipid metabolism may present with peripheral limb ischaemia. There are also congenital causes of early-onset leg ischaemia. These include aortic hypoplasia, which occurs during the embryonic fusion of the distal aortas, and popliteal entrapment, where the popliteal artery takes an unusual course through the head of the gastrocnemius muscle, with exercise involving knee flexion causing intermittent occlusion of the artery and calf pain that resembles intermittent claudication. A fierce immunological inflammatory response to smoking causes Buerger's syndrome, which involves the artery, vein, and associated nerves in both the legs and the arms. This disease, seen principally in men, is particularly prevalent in the Indian subcontinent, and may resolve if the patient stops smoking. Sudden thrombotic occlusion of the iliac and distal arteries may occur in those below 50 years of age, suggesting the presence of an inherited thrombotic disorder. Embolic occlusion from a proximal source is also possible.

Marfan's syndrome may sometimes be confirmed only after a patient has presented with a ruptured abdominal aortic aneurysm. In some variants of Ehlers–Danlos syndrome, patients with mutations in type III collagen present with visceral artery aneurysms. In South Africa (and elsewhere), aneurysms of the abdominal, femoral, or popliteal arteries in those under 50 years have been attributed to infectious causes, from HIV to tuberculosis. Syphilitic aneurysms, which used to affect principally the thoracic aorta, are now rare.

Peripheral arterial disease in patients over 50 years old

For patients over 50 years of age, the principal risk factor for peripheral arterial disease—stenosing, aneurysmal, or vasospastic—is smoking. The pathology is atherosclerotic change with superimposed thrombosis. Of patients who present with peripheral arterial disease, less than 5% have never smoked. For this reason, more men than women presented with peripheral arterial disease in the past, but recently more women are affected, perhaps a reflection of the increasing number who smoke. Nevertheless, unlike Buerger's disease, cessation of smoking is not associated with an immediate dramatic improvement in symptoms and it may take several years without smoking to improve prognosis.

Diabetes is another important risk factor for stenosing peripheral arterial disease. Other risk factors include hypertension, raised levels of plasma fibrinogen, and hyperlipidaemia, with elevated plasma triglycerides being a common finding. The risk factors for dilating arterial disease are similar, with the exception of diabetes, which is rare.

For aortic aneurysms, strong familial clustering has been observed, and a recent genome-wide study has confirmed association with a variant low-density lipoprotein receptor related protein-1, which acts as a receptor for proteases and antiproteases. White and northern European populations appear to be at higher risk of aneurysmal disease than black populations. Stenosing and aneurysmal disease are associated with degenerative changes of the

Table 14.2.1 The increasing prevalence of peripheral arterial disease with age in the populations of northern Europe

Age	Population	Asymptomatic peripheral arterial disease (ABPI <0.9)	Intermittent claudication	Abdominal aortic aneurysm (>3 cm)
(years)		(%)	(%)	(%)
55–64	Men	8	1.2	5
55–64	Women	7	0.8	0.7
65–74	Men	16	2.5	7.5
65–74	Women	11	1.2	1.3
75+	Men	>30	4.0	9
75+	Women	>30	1.5	1.5

ABPI, ankle–brachial pressure index.

Most peripheral arterial disease, both stenosing and dilating, is asymptomatic. The data have been derived from several studies and geographical variation may occur.

artery wall, the prevalence of both diseases increasing sharply with age (Table 14.2.1). Epidemiological studies also indicate a difference between stenosing and aneurysmal disease, with death from aneurysmal disease (aortic aneurysm) being more common among those of higher social classes and in affluent geographical areas.

Leg ischaemia

Clinical features

The terms acute and chronic relate purely to the length of time that symptoms have been present and must not be confused with terms related to severity, such as critical limb ischaemia.

Critical leg ischaemia

Critical leg ischaemia is defined as gangrenous change, ulceration, tissue loss, or rest pain lasting for 2 weeks, with an absolute ankle pressure of less than 50 mmHg, although patients with diabetes are difficult to include in this classification because ankle pressures in such patients may be unreliable due to arterial calcification.

Acute leg ischaemia

The incidence of acute leg ischaemia, which presents as a painful, pale, and pulseless limb, is 1 in 12 000 patients per year. It can be due either to an embolic event or to thrombosis of an atherosclerotic stenosis. The commonest cause of a peripheral embolus used to be rheumatic heart disease in a patient with atrial fibrillation, but this is now uncommon, and other sources of emboli, such as an aortic aneurysm, must be considered. The development of a thrombosis at the site of an atherosclerotic stenosis, in either the superficial femoral artery or the popliteal artery, is undoubtedly now the commonest cause of acute leg ischaemia. However, it should be stressed that, whatever the cause, there is no difference on clinical examination of the acutely ischaemic limb.

Arterial trauma due to road traffic accidents and knife or gunshot wounds is becoming commoner, as is iatrogenic trauma following the insertion of intra-arterial catheters for diagnosis or therapy. A rare but dramatic cause of acute leg ischaemia is phlegmasia cerulea dolens, in which massive thrombosis of all the major veins of the limb occurs with gross swelling that obstructs the arterial supply.

Patients with a thrombosis of a popliteal aneurysm may present with classic symptoms of pain, paralysis, loss of power, paraesthesia, pallor, lack of pulse, and perishing cold. If the blood supply is not restored, fixed blue staining of the skin is a further sign of irreversible ischaemia, as is a tense calf with plantar flexion. However, most patients presenting with acute ischaemia have symptoms that are less severe.

Chronic leg ischaemia

Chronic leg ischaemia is much more common than acute ischaemia (Table 14.2.1), and its main cause is atherosclerosis. In the young patient, one should also consider cystic adventitial disease, entrapment of the popliteal artery, and occasionally fibromuscular hyperplasia of the iliac arteries, particularly in women.

Symptoms are pain on walking, claudication affecting the calf and thigh, rest pain, ulceration, and gangrenous change. Less commonly, patients may present with buttock claudication and impotence (Leriche's syndrome). Although the differential diagnoses of the acutely ischaemic limb are few, in the chronically ischaemic limb pain may be due to spinal stenosis or nerve-root compression (spinal claudication) or arthritis of the hip or knee. Classically the patient with claudication will complain of cramp-like pain in the calf, appearing after walking a particular distance, relieved by a few minute's rest, and recurring again at the same distance if the patient resumes walking. Failure of the pain to disappear on resting, or its reappearance after a shorter distance after each rest, suggests a possible musculoskeletal cause, particularly if distal pulses are present on examination. However, it should also be remembered that distal pulses may be felt at rest in the limbs of patients with claudication due to peripheral vascular disease, but disappear on exercise to the point of pain.

Investigations

The main diagnostic method used to confirm the diagnosis of peripheral arterial disease is Doppler ultrasonography (duplex scanning), an example of which is shown in Fig. 14.2.1. The ratio of systolic blood pressure at the ankle and in the arm, the ankle–brachial pressure index (ABPI), provides a physiological measure of blood flow at the level of the ankle. At rest, in a normal leg, the ABPI lies between 1.0 and 1.4. As the blood flow in the leg is compromised, the ABPI falls sharply and values below 0.9 are considered abnormal and likely to confirm the diagnosis of peripheral vascular disease. To emphasize the important overlap between this condition and coronary artery disease, a reduction in ABPI nearly always signals the presence of coronary artery disease, which is the cause of death in most patients with peripheral arterial disease.

Exercise testing provides an objective method of assessing walking distance and helps with the identification of disease processes, such as angina, that may be limiting. It only needs to be used in those people who have a history of claudication but have normal resting ABPI, and can be used as a way of eliminating or suggesting other diagnoses.

In addition to establishing the diagnosis of peripheral arterial disease, duplex ultrasonography is able to determine the site of disease and indicate the degree of stenosis or length of an occlusion and hence aid in the planning of interventional treatment. Other imaging modalities such as CT scanning and magnetic resonance (MR) angiography can provide three-dimensional reconstructions

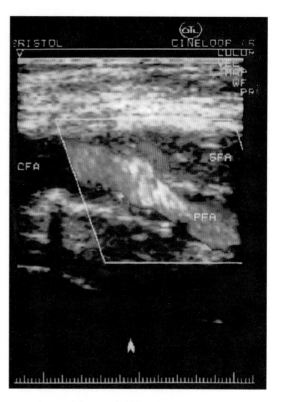

Fig. 14.2.1 Occlusion of the superficial femoral artery demonstrated by colour-coded duplex ultrasonography. On the left, the common femoral artery (CFA) lies outside the colour box. In the colour box antegrade flow through the profunda femoris artery (PFA) is shown in blue. The red flash represents rebound flow against the occluded origin of the superficial femoral artery (SFA).

of the diseased vessels and may be used for planning surgical treatment. Angiography is only required as an adjuvant to endovascular treatment, for surgical planning in some circumstances, or in the management of the acutely ischaemic limb.

Attention to risk factors, in particular smoking, blood pressure, and exercise, are important issues.

Management

Critical and acute leg ischaemia

Critical limb ischaemia requires administration of analgesia and rapid surgical intervention. The severity of ischaemia will determine the treatment options considered. However, all patients with a severely ischaemic limb should be given adequate analgesia and 5000 units of heparin intravenously. Many will be old and frail, with significant medical comorbidities. These issues must be considered in deciding whether or not surgical intervention is appropriate for any individual case, with action taken to improve those aspects of the patient's medical condition that can be improved before surgery, or as part of continuing medical management.

For a patient with irreversible ischaemia (fixed skin staining and tense muscles), the main decision is whether a primary amputation or palliative care should be offered. If severe but potentially reversible ischaemia is present (white leg), surgery is usually the treatment of choice. Delay while thrombolytic therapy is tried is not advisable in this group. For patients with moderate limb ischaemia, where there is no paralysis and only mild sensory loss, arteriography with consideration of the potential use of thrombolysis should

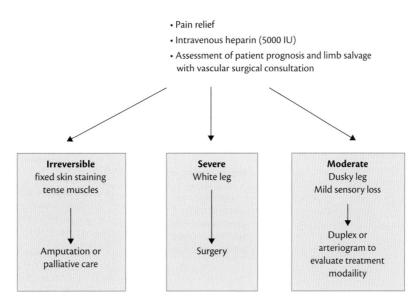

Fig. 14.2.2 Management of the patient with an acutely ischaemic leg.

be performed. However, it should be remembered that thrombolysis is associated with numerous potential complications, most notably gastrointestinal haemorrhage and stroke, and is contraindicated in the early postoperative period. If the limb is salvageable, it may be possible to offer the patient an endovascular procedure, such as an angioplasty (with or without stenting). Surgical treatment can involve simple embolectomy, but may require a bypass procedure or endarterectomy, and in the severely ischaemic limb fasciotomies may be needed to treat or prevent a compartment syndrome. For at least 10% of patients, it will not be possible to offer revascularization: a few of these may benefit from the use of a prostacyclin analogue (iloprost), which might diminish amputation rates and alleviate pain. Any benefits of gene therapy on avoidance of amputation, with vascular endothelial growth factor (VEGF), fibroblast growth factor (FGF), or other molecular mediators, are far from established and the only large randomized trial was disappointing. Limb salvage rates for patients presenting with critical limb ischaemia are variable, probably 50 to 60% at 2 years, dependent on the severity of disease.

In a patient presenting with acute leg ischaemia the outlook is poor, with only about 60% leaving hospital with an intact limb. The 30-day mortality for this group of patients can be as high as 30%, the main cause of death being cardiac disease. The strategy for management is described in Fig. 14.2.2. Controversial areas in the treatment of acute leg ischaemia include the role of arteriography, which technique of thrombolysis is the safest and most cost-effective, and whether initial treatment with thrombolysis is beneficial or harmful as compared to surgery. A recently updated Cochrane review, which included five randomized trials comparing thrombolysis and surgery for the initial treatment of acute limb ischaemia, found no overall difference in outcomes (limb salvage or death) at 1 year. Initial thrombolysis was associated with higher risk of major haemorrhage, stroke, and distal embolization, but also less severe degree of intervention overall.

In the patient who has had an embolic event, long-term anticoagulation should not be forgotten, and nor should a search for the source of embolus. If the patient is not in atrial fibrillation, and has normal cardiac enzymes and 12-lead electrocardiogram (ECG),

then they should have an echocardiogram to exclude any valvular lesion, a 24-h electrocardiogram (ECG) to look for arrhythmia, an ultrasound scan to exclude abdominal aortic aneurysm, and a screen for thrombophilia.

Chronic leg ischaemia

In chronic limb ischaemia, management depends upon the severity of the disease. Most patients present with claudication, which is relatively benign: symptoms of intermittent claudication will progress to critical limb ischaemia in less than one in five patients and only about 5% will go on to lose a limb. However, claudication identifies patients with a threefold increased risk of death from either heart disease or cerebrovascular disease compared with age- and sex-matched controls. It is important when planning treatment that all the potential risk factors are covered. In the past surgical intervention was usually considered unnecessary: at least one-third will have improvement of symptoms with simple medical treatment and exercise. However recent trials have suggested that either angioplasty with adjunct and stents or coated balloons or angioplasty combined with exercise therapy may offer early benefits (to 2 years) and longer term results are awaited eagerly. The current treatment of patients with chronic lower leg pain is shown in Fig. 14.2.3.

General management

Careful attention must be paid to the cleanliness of ischaemic feet to avoid infection, and particular care should be given to the cutting of toenails. In many patients this is best done by a careful relative or chiropodist, since apparently minor lacerations can lead to ulcers, infection, and gangrene. Patients are recommended to exercise. Walking to the point of claudication is not harmful, and may improve collateral circulation with beneficial results. Supervised exercise therapy appears to be more effective than merely providing advice to exercise more.

Smoking is by far the most significant risk factor for occlusive arterial disease and every effort should be made to encourage smokers to stop. If patients undergo surgical treatment, then the long-term patency rate following arterial reconstruction is four times greater in smokers who stop than in those who persist.

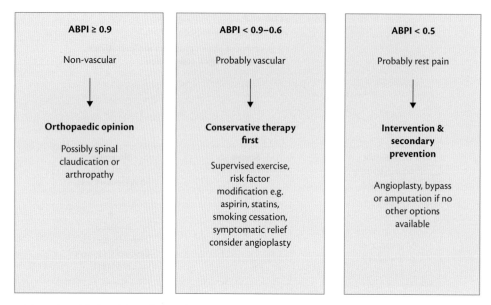

ABPI ≥ 0.9	ABPI < 0.9–0.6	ABPI < 0.5
Non-vascular	Probably vascular	Probably rest pain
↓	↓	↓
Orthopaedic opinion	**Conservative therapy first**	**Intervention & secondary prevention**
Possibly spinal claudication or arthropathy	Supervised exercise, risk factor modification e.g. aspirin, statins, smoking cessation, symptomatic relief consider angioplasty	Angioplasty, bypass or amputation if no other options available

Fig. 14.2.3 Management of the patient with chronic lower leg pain, but no tissue loss, stratified by ankle–brachial pressure index (ABPI).

Pharmacological treatment

Since coronary artery disease is the main cause of death in those with peripheral arterial disease, patients with the latter condition should receive similar cardiovascular risk reduction therapy to patients with coronary heart disease. Low-dose aspirin therapy (75–325 mg/day) should be recommended for all. If aspirin cannot be tolerated, ADP receptor antagonists, such as clopidogrel, are equally effective in reducing the risk of cardiovascular events (stroke, myocardial infarction, and vascular deaths).

Secondary prevention trials have demonstrated the benefits of statin therapy in reducing cardiovascular morbidity and mortality in those with stenosing atherosclerotic disease of the peripheral arteries. Statins also may improve operative cardiovascular morbidity and mortality, but neither fibrates nor chelation therapy offer benefits.

The options for facilitating smoking cessation are increasing and nicotine replacement therapy or e-cigarettes can be used with either bupropion or varenicline if necessary, although many will not stop smoking until surgery threatens.

Vasodilators may be used where supervised exercise does not bring symptomatic improvement and further endovascular or surgical intervention is decided against, or as a bridge to future angioplasty or surgery. There is good evidence that cilostazol (a selective cAMP phosphodiesterase inhibitor) improves walking distance in those with intermittent claudication, although the mechanism of action is not clear, side effects are frequent, and the drug is contraindicated in patients with congestive heart failure.

Surgical treatment

In general, surgeons are conservative with respect to interventional treatment for patients with claudication, despite a possible early benefit for those having an endovascular procedure. However, in the patient who has severe claudication, with symptoms that significantly affect their quality of life, it is certainly possible and appropriate to offer interventional treatment.

Both endovascular techniques (angioplasty with or without stent) and bypass surgery are effective treatments, with little to choose between the two. For infrainguinal bypass, good-quality autologous vein is the conduit of choice. However, reasonable results can be obtained with synthetic grafts, particularly where the distal anastomosis is above the knee. Below the knee, an adjuvant vein interposition in the form of either a Miller cuff or Taylor patch is used. Stenting is used widely, but its use is contentious, and, at least in the infrainguinal arteries, it may not be of value. The role of exercise therapy compared with angioplasty in the treatment of mild to moderate claudication continues to be debated, but it might be prudent to consider the conjoint treatment of angioplasty with exercise therapy.

Ischaemia of the arm

Ischaemia of the arm is usually a result of embolism from the heart. Occasionally the subclavian artery is diseased or has suffered traumatic injury or radiation damage following radiotherapy. The basic principles of investigation and management are the same as for the leg. However, it should be noted that the upper limb has multiple interconnection of collateral vessels, hence occlusion of the major arterial supply may still leave a viable limb. The other disease process that needs to be considered in differential diagnosis is the thoracic outlet syndrome, which gives rise to symptoms in the arm as a result of arterial, venous, or neurological compression caused by an additional cervical rib or by scalene bands. Management may require surgical intervention, either cervical rib excision or thoracic outlet decompression with the removal of the first rib.

Mesenteric ischaemia

Mesenteric ischaemia is uncommon. Over one-third of cases of acute mesenteric ischaemia are due to arterial embolism, with emboli lodging at the ostium of the superior mesenteric artery in many cases. Patients with acute mesenteric artery thrombosis have often had symptoms of mesenteric ischaemia prior to the acute episode. Chronic mesenteric ischaemia typically presents with weight loss and abdominal pain on ingestion of food, the classic story being that the patient is constantly hungry, but frightened to eat. Other causes of acute mesenteric ischaemia include venous thrombosis and nonocclusive ischaemia secondary to hypoperfusion.

Patients with acute mesenteric ischaemia will usually present with abdominal pain, but the abdominal physical signs may be much less dramatic than would be anticipated from the subsequent clinical course. Suspicion of the diagnosis should be heightened in the presence of atrial fibrillation or widespread atheromatous vascular disease. Patients may deteriorate suddenly and present in shock.

The diagnosis of acute mesenteric ischaemia is difficult to make. In the acute situation, clues to look for include leucocytosis, hyperamylasaemia, and unexplained acidosis. Liver function tests are usually normal. Radiological imaging is rarely able to make a positive diagnosis, although it can be very useful in excluding other possibilities. Angiography is not always accurate. CT scanning can be helpful in the diagnosis of mesenteric venous thrombosis.

Intensive resuscitation to replace fluids is essential. Surgery is usually necessary for the patient to survive, and the possibility of acute mesenteric ischaemia remains one of the dwindling number of reasons for requiring an emergency diagnostic laparotomy. Depending on the findings, resection of small bowel may suffice, but formal arterial surgery may be necessary, and in some unfortunate instances the extent of irreversible ischaemia can preclude any attempt at resection or revascularization. In cases where the surgeon is unsure of the viability of bowel remaining after resection, a second laparotomy may be planned to assess the situation a few days later. Repeat laparotomy may also be required to examine, and if necessary resect, more bowel in the patient who is not 'doing well' postoperatively. The prognosis for patients who present with acute mesenteric ischaemia is poor.

For patients who present with chronic mesenteric ischaemia, the aim of treatment is to improve blood flow and to act as a prophylactic procedure to prevent the catastrophic disaster of arterial occlusion. The potential options, having identified the site of the disease process by duplex scanning and angiography, include angioplasty, endarterectomy, reimplantation, or a surgical bypass procedure.

Abdominal aortic aneurysm

Definition

There is no fixed definition of an abdominal aortic aneurysm beyond agreement that it is a localized dilatation of the abdominal aorta, usually fusiform, with dilation starting distal to the renal arteries. Some would apply the term when the maximum aortic diameter is more than 1.5 times the diameter of the undilated proximal aorta.

Manual palpation to detect abdominal aortic aneurysms is unreliable, unless undertaken by a specialist on a nonobese patient. The most convenient method of screening for the presence of these aneurysms is ultrasonography, measuring the anterior–posterior diameter. Since the reproducibility of ultrasound measurements of the suprarenal aorta is poor, a convenient working definition of an abdominal aortic aneurysm is when the maximum diameter exceeds 3 cm, which in most people is more than 1.5 times the diameter of the undilated proximal aorta. In practice, it is only aneurysms of 4 cm or greater in diameter that have been of clinical concern.

Epidemiology

Population screening studies in northern Europe have shown that the disease is usually without symptoms, much more common in men than in women (Table 14.2.1), and strongly associated with smoking. The associations with hypertension and hyperlipidaemia are inconsistent. The prevalence of large aneurysms (>5 cm in diameter) detected by screening is only about 1% in men and the large majority of screen-detected aneurysms are 3 to 5 cm in diameter. The natural history of abdominal aortic aneurysms is progressive enlargement (with the diameter increasing by 2–5 mm each year) without symptoms, until the aortic wall is so weakened that it ruptures, which is a catastrophic event.

The infrarenal aorta is by far the most common site of aneurysmal dilatation, and usually the abdominal aorta is the only site of dilatation. When patients present with aneurysms of the iliac, femoral, or popliteal arteries, abdominal aortic aneurysm is often present and screening for this is mandatory. This emphasizes the tendency of some patients to have a more generalized form of dilating arterial disease.

Most patients (60%) with abdominal aortic aneurysm die from cardiovascular causes, and up to 25% of other male family members may develop occult aneurysms.

Ruptured aneurysms

The symptoms of a ruptured abdominal aortic aneurysm are collapse (shock) and severe back or abdominal pain. Rarely a ruptured aneurysm will present with gastrointestinal bleeding from an aortoduodenal fistula or high-output cardiac failure from an aortocaval fistula.

Less than 20% of patients with a ruptured abdominal aortic aneurysm reach hospital alive, and even among those that undergo emergency surgical repair almost one-third will die within 30 days. New evidence indicates that mortality may be reduced considerably if the rupture is repaired using endovascular repair under local anaesthesia. With this bleak prognosis and the very significant costs associated with emergency repair following rupture, evidence has accumulated that screening of men over 65 years of age to detect those with the largest aneurysms, at highest risk of rupture, is cost-effective. Accordingly, national screening programmes for abdominal aortic aneurysm in men have been implemented in the United Kingdom, Sweden, and other countries.

Management of ruptured aneurysms requires:

◆ Access lines, cross-matched blood, and resuscitation—maintaining moderate hypotension at $c.70$ mmHg may be beneficial

◆ Confirmation of diagnosis—ultrasound (to show aneurysm); CT scan or experienced vascular surgeon (to confirm diagnosis of rupture)

◆ Rapid assessment of whether patient would benefit from emergency repair—if yes, immediate surgical or endovascular repair.

Aneurysms detected before rupture

Abdominal aortic aneurysms are commonly symptomless, but rupture—as explained above—is catastrophic. However, elective repair of an abdominal aortic aneurysm, a major surgical procedure, is not without risk. Traditionally, larger aneurysms have been repaired by cross-clamping of the aorta and insertion of a Dacron

3.0–3.9 cm	4.0–5.5 cm	5.6 + cm or symptomatic
Ultrasound surveillance at 1–2 yearly intervals Stop smoking Control hypertension Check lipids	**Ultrasound surveillance** at 6 monthly intervals **Cardiovascular risk reduction** With statin, smoking cessation, aspirin, etc	**Consider intervention** **Cardiovascular risk reduction** With statin, smoking cessation, aspirin, etc.

Fig. 14.2.4 Management of men with asymptomatic, unruptured abdominal aortic aneurysm stratified by aneurysm diameter.

inlay graft at open surgery. This is a durable procedure and effectively 'cures' the patient. However, although some specialized surgical centres report an operative mortality of less than 2% associated with this elective procedure, on a population basis the mortality is more likely to be 5 to 8%, which is an important reason for avoiding surgery in those with small aneurysms.

Minimally invasive endovascular aneurysm repair, via femoral access vessels, has developed rapidly. Only about one-half of patients have an aneurysm that is anatomically suitable for this mode of repair, but randomized trials have shown that the operative mortality associated with endovascular repair is less than 2%, which is only one-third of the mortality associated with traditional open repair. However, within 2 years the mortality advantage of endovascular repair has been lost and a significant proportion of patients with endovascular repair require further interventions to ensure continued exclusion of the aneurysm. Hence patients with endovascular repair are likely to require lifelong surveillance. The long-term durability and cost-effectiveness for this newer technique has not been established. In the United Kingdom endovascular repair is considered cost-effective for elective procedures (<http://www.nice.org.uk/TA167>), and most patients would prefer this approach, although some still prefer open repair principally because there is no requirement for long-term follow-up. For endovascular repair, late secondary rupture is a greater problem than for open repair. Although the endovascular approach was initially developed for patients not considered fit for open surgery because of numerous comorbidities, the operative mortality rises to 9% in this cohort and there is no evidence that endovascular aneurysm repair prolongs patient survival.

Two large randomized trials have shown that for aneurysms of 4.0 to 5.5 cm in diameter a policy of early elective open surgery confers no long-term survival benefit, and hence early surgery should not be recommended. Later, two small trials comparing early endovascular repair versus surveillance also showed that early intervention conferred no survival benefit. The data of all four trials are summarized in a Cochrane review. For such patients surveillance, with measurement of ultrasound diameter every 6 months, is a safe policy that engenders little patient anxiety, and the risk of aneurysm rupture is very low—1% per year. By contrast, for patients with aneurysms greater than 6 cm in diameter the risk of rupture may be as high as 25% per year, and in most such cases elective repair is recommended. Over 90% of the patients enrolled in the

trials were men, and it is possible that the diameter threshold for considering surgery should be 5 cm in women.

Repair is also recommended when symptoms are attributed to the aneurysm, whatever its size, the commonest being back or abdominal pain, or tenderness to palpation. It is assumed that such aneurysms are at high risk of rupture and need early repair. As the aneurysm dilates, onion-skin layers of laminated thrombus deposit in the lumen, to leave a blood-flow channel of approximately normal aortic diameter. These layers of thrombus are very stable and only in rare circumstances are the sources of emboli to the legs. The aneurysms which most often provoke symptoms have very thick, inflamed, fibrotic walls, which entrap nerves and may become adherent to other tissues. These are known as inflammatory aneurysms and the thickened wall can often be detected by CT or MRI. They are technically demanding to repair. There is no convincing evidence that a course of preoperative corticosteroids is beneficial. In the Japanese population, inflammatory aneurysms have been associated with active cytomegalovirus infection.

A strategy for the management of abdominal aortic aneurysms detected before rupture is shown in Fig. 14.2.4. Patients with small aneurysms should stop smoking and have their blood pressure controlled. Since screening detects mainly small aneurysms, it would clearly be beneficial if a treatment to limit aneurysm growth were available. Although β-blockers have proved effective in limiting the dilation of the proximal aorta in patients with Marfan's syndrome, there is no evidence that they are effective for abdominal aortic aneurysms. Furthermore, many patients with abdominal aortic aneurysm have impaired lung function, perhaps through smoking, and β-blockers are often poorly tolerated. However, effective control of blood pressure and cessation of smoking are both likely to minimize the rate of aneurysm growth and the risk of rupture, and statins may also be helpful. Intervention to exclude the aneurysm remains the only available treatment for aneurysms larger than 5.5 cm in diameter.

Medical management

Just as for patients with limb ischaemia, patients with abdominal aortic aneurysm are at high risk of cardiovascular events. All patients with abdominal aortic aneurysm should be offered statin therapy to reduce the risk of morbidity and mortality from other forms of coexistent cardiovascular disease. Antiplatelet therapy should be considered, and there is some evidence that, for hypertensive patients, angiotensin converting enzyme (ACE) inhibitors minimize the chance of aneurysm rupture.

Conventional surgical management

Preoperative evaluation requires CT or MRI to define the anatomy and extent of the aneurysm. Cardiac, pulmonary, and renal function should always be assessed and optimal treatment instituted before surgery: poor renal and lung function are associated with an increased risk of postoperative morbidity and mortality.

The most common surgical approach to an abdominal aortic aneurysm is through a transperitoneal incision under general anaesthesia. The retroperitoneal approach, which avoids bowel manipulation and permits a more rapid return to oral diet, has similar cross-clamp, operating, and recovery times. The transperitoneal approach offers the advantage of exploring the abdominal cavity for other pathology. In this approach, after the bowel has been removed from the operative field, the aorta is exposed anteriorly from the left renal vein to the bifurcation. The infrarenal neck of the aneurysm is exposed anteriorly and laterally so that an occluding clamp may be applied. Both common iliac arteries are exposed for the placement of the distal occluding clamps. The aneurysm is opened longitudinally on the anterior surface and the remainder of the procedure performed from inside the aneurysm cavity. Usually following a small dose of intravenous heparin, arterial clamps are applied. Clot and debris are evacuated and any back-bleeding lumbar or mesenteric arteries ligated. A Dacron prosthesis is then sutured, end-to-end, to the normal-diameter aorta above the aneurysm. This anastomosis is tested for leaks before the graft is trimmed to appropriate length and sutured in place above the aortic bifurcation. The aneurysmal sac is closed over the prosthesis, before replacement of abdominal contents. Such tube grafts are the most common type, but when the iliac arteries are dilated or diseased a bifurcated prosthesis is used. The cross-clamp time should be less than 1 h and the whole procedure completed within 2 to 4 h. The longest procedures involve inflammatory aneurysms and cases where the proximal aneurysm neck lies above the renal arteries. The patient should be ready to leave hospital 7 to 12 days after the operation, with a durable repair.

Endovascular aneurysm repair

The technique of endovascular repair was introduced in the early 1990s and the technology has now stabilized. The procedure may be performed under general, regional, or even local anaesthesia. This flexibility allows endovascular repair in patients where general anaesthesia is risky, and the avoidance of aortic cross-clamping is an additional benefit for those with limited cardiac reserve.

Preoperative investigation to evaluate the extent and size of the aneurysm (spiral CT or MRI) is of critical importance. The length of the aneurysm neck below the renal arteries, angulation of the aorta, and tortuosity of the iliac arteries must be evaluated precisely so that the correct size of graft can be placed via the femoral artery.

The insertion of the graft is performed under fluoroscopic control. This requires the use of significant amounts of contrast material, which may underlie the unfavourable results reported in patients with pre-existing renal impairment. The proximal end of the graft is held in place by hooks and barbs, balloon, or self-expandable stents.

The length of the procedure is similar to that for open repair but the transfusion requirements are similar to those for open repair but the transfusion requirements are less and the patient recovers more rapidly and is ready to leave hospital within 2 to 5 days. The long-term success of the procedure depends on the successful exclusion of the aneurysmal sac and the security of the proximal attachment to prevent graft migration. Endoleaks may develop when the aneurysm is not completely excluded, the graft migrates or fatigues, or there is back-bleeding from lumbar vessels or the inferior mesenteric artery into the aneurysm sac. These are associated with an important risk of continued aneurysm expansion and rupture. For these reasons, continued vigilance and repeated evaluation of the aneurysm with duplex or CT scanning is necessary at annual intervals.

The endovascular revolution has affected the management of all categories of peripheral arterial disease, although in many instances the advantages and indications for the use of the (often more expensive) endovascular approach are not based on evidence from randomized trials.

Further reading

ACC/AHA (2006). 2005 guidelines for the management of peripheral arterial disease. *J Am Coll Cardiol*, **47**, 123–312.

BASIL Trial Participants (2005). Bypass versus angioplasty in severe ischaemia of the leg (BASIL): multicentre, randomized controlled trial. *Lancet*, **366**, 1925–34.

Belch J, et al. (2011). Effect of fibroblast growth factor NV1FGF on amputation and death: a randomised placebo-controlled trial of gene therapy in critical limb ischaemia. *Lancet*, **377**, 1929–37.

Berridge DC, Kessel DO, Robertson I (2013). Surgery versus thrombolysis for initial management of acute limb ischaemia. *Cochrane Database Syst Rev*, **6**(6), CD002784.

Filardo G, Powell JT, Martinez MA, Ballard DJ (2012). Surgery for small asymptomatic abdominal aortic aneurysms. *Cochrane Database Syst Rev*, **14**(3), CD001835.

Moll FL, et al.; European Society for Vascular Surgery (2011). Management of abdominal aortic aneurysms: clinical practice guidelines of the European Society for Vascular Surgery. *Eur J Vasc Endovasc Surg*, **41**(Suppl 1), S1–58.

RESCAN Collaborators (2013) Surveillance intervals for small abdominal aortic aneurysms: a meta-analysis. *JAMA*, **309**, 806–13.

Setacci C, Ricco JB; European Society for Vascular Surgery (2011). Guidelines for critical limb ischaemia and diabetic foot—introduction. *Eur J Vasc Endovasc Surg*, **42**(Suppl 2), S1–3.

Thompson PD, et al. (2002). Meta-analysis of results from eight randomized, placebo-controlled trials on the effect of cilostazol on patients with intermittent claudication. *Am J Cardiol*, **90**, 1314–19.

CHAPTER 14.3

Cholesterol embolism

Christopher Dudley

Essentials

Cholesterol embolism occurring after vascular surgery or intra-arterial angiographic procedures is not uncommon, but is often unrecognized. The clinical features mimic a number of conditions, including contrast nephropathy and systemic vasculitis, and—if misdiagnosed—can result in the inappropriate use of powerful immunosuppressive drugs. A high index of suspicion is required when an elderly patient with widespread vascular disease develops a nonspecific systemic illness with progressive renal impairment, particularly after vascular surgery or arteriography. Biopsy of affected tissue, especially skin or kidney, is diagnostic—showing biconvex, needle-shaped cholesterol clefts within the lumen of arteries or arterioles. Treatment is supportive and the prognosis is often poor.

Introduction

When atheromatous plaques ulcerate and become denuded of their endothelial covering, the underlying cholesterol-rich extracellular matrix can become detached and embolize. If the dislodged plaque and superimposed thrombi are sufficiently large, occlusion of a major systemic artery results in infarction of the organ or ischaemia of the limb supplied. This has been termed 'thromboembolism'. By contrast, 'atheroembolism' or cholesterol-crystal embolism occurs when much smaller and more numerous particles, composed principally of cholesterol crystals, lodge in a number of small arteries or arterioles simultaneously. The presence of a collateral circulation usually prevents infarction, and the event frequently passes unrecognized by the patient or their physician. However, tissue damage in a number of organs can result from multiple showers of emboli. Because severe ulcerative atherosclerosis is most frequently present in the abdominal aorta, cholesterol embolism commonly affects the legs, gastrointestinal tract, and kidneys. The condition usually presents as a complication of vascular surgery or angiographic procedures, when mechanical dislodgement of crystals from ulcerated plaques occurs. Anticoagulant and thrombolytic use has also been implicated as a predisposing factor. The clinical features are those of a systemic disorder with renal failure that can mimic vasculitis, although more indolent cases with stable renal failure have been observed.

Epidemiology

The incidence of cholesterol-crystal embolism found at post-mortem is high: 77% after aortic surgery, 30% after aortography, and 25.5% after cardiac catheterization. By contrast, the clinical syndrome of cholesterol-crystal embolism is rare, complicating less than 2% of cardiac catheterizations. In two large renal biopsy series, an incidence of 1% was reported, and it has been suggested that cholesterol-crystal embolism could account for 5–10% of cases of acute kidney injury, although most nephrologists would regard this as an overestimate.

Since the condition occurs in patients with severe atheromatous disease, it is most often seen in older male patients with obvious risk factors (e.g. hypertension, diabetes mellitus, smoking) and overt vascular disease (e.g. ischaemic heart disease, abdominal aortic aneurysm, cerebrovascular disease). Although spontaneous cholesterol embolism can occur, it is much more common after vascular surgery or invasive radiology including aortography, angiography, and angioplasty. Under these circumstances, direct trauma to the vessel may result in detachment of atheromatous material from a ruptured plaque, or denude the endothelial lining of the vessel exposing the underlying atheroma for subsequent embolization. Angiography is the most common cause of cholesterol-crystal embolization, accounting for approximately 80% of cases in some series. Anticoagulant use has been associated with cholesterol embolism, and it has been proposed that by preventing thrombosis of ulcerating atheromatous plaques, anticoagulants favour the dissemination of atheromatous material. However, a causal relationship is unproven and many patients with widespread atherosclerosis coincidentally receive anticoagulants for a variety of reasons. Cholesterol embolism following the use of thrombolytic agents has been rarely reported.

Prevention

Prevention is important, particularly with the increasing number of older patients submitted to invasive angiography. Noninvasive methods of arterial imaging such as CT or magnetic resonance (MR) angiography are to be preferred in patients with diffuse atherosclerosis. When invasive angiography is unavoidable, careful attention must be paid to the angiographic technique, including the arterial approach (brachial, or radial instead of femoral, for cardiac catheterization), use of softer, more flexible catheters, and reduced catheter manipulation.

Clinical features

Symptoms are often nonspecific with fever, weight loss, and myalgia. The clinical features are, otherwise, determined by the pattern of organ involvement and are usually referable to the gastrointestinal tract, kidneys, and legs. Bilateral skin changes over the lower extremities are the commonest physical finding and include livedo reticularis, a purpuric rash, 'trash feet', blue toes (acral cyanosis),

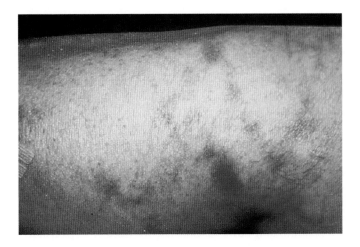

Fig. 14.3.1 Livedo reticularis and vasculitic-like erythematous nodules on the leg of a patient in whom cholesterol-crystal embolization occurred after coronary angiography.

and focal digital necrosis (Figs 14.3.1 and 14.3.2). Ulceration, nodules, and petechiae have also been described. Despite these skin changes and the presence of calf claudication (or frank myositis), pedal pulses may be felt easily, emphasizing that small vessels are occluded in this disorder. Carotid and femoral bruits are frequently heard, reflecting widespread and generalized atherosclerosis.

Abdominal pain, gastrointestinal bleeding, and pancreatitis may occur, and embolism to the stomach, small bowel, colon, gallbladder, and spleen have all been reported. The most frequently involved of these sites is the colon.

Because of their large blood supply and proximity to the abdominal aorta, the kidneys are commonly affected. This usually manifests as a subacute stepwise deterioration in renal function over 2 to 6 weeks, invariably accompanied by a worsening of pre-existing hypertension that can be labile and difficult to control. Cardiac failure with pulmonary oedema is a common accompaniment. Thus, a typical case is an elderly man presenting after angiography with progressive renal failure accompanied by a low-grade fever,

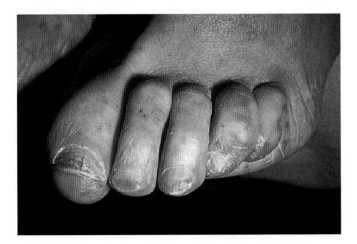

Fig. 14.3.2 Purpuric spots and acral cyanosis of the toes from cholesterol embolism after aortic aneurysm repair.

abdominal pain, livedo reticularis of the lower body, and purpura over the feet with focal digital ischaemia of the toes. Acute kidney injury with necrotizing glomerulonephritis and crescent formation on renal biopsy has been described, but is rare. A further presentation is with slowly progressive chronic kidney disease. This form is underdiagnosed because extrarenal manifestations are absent and renal biopsy rarely undertaken.

Transient ischaemic attacks, amaurosis fugax, and strokes can occur when embolism is from the carotid arteries or aortic arch. Retinal cholesterol-crystal emboli may be observed on ophthalmoscopy as bright refractile plaques within the retinal arterioles, especially at their bifurcation. Spinal cord infarction has also been reported.

Differential diagnosis

The diagnosis is frequently missed during life, or confused with that of acute renal failure induced by radiocontrast media (contrast nephropathy) when renal failure occurs after arteriography. A high index of clinical suspicion is therefore required, particularly in elderly patients with evidence of atherosclerotic disease who develop renal failure after arteriography or following aortic or cardiac surgery; cholesterol embolism should also be considered in the differential diagnosis of a multisystem disease in elderly patients. Spontaneous cholesterol-crystal embolism associated with renal failure, fever, rash, and eosinophilia may, not surprisingly, be misdiagnosed as a vasculitic illness such as granulomatosis with polyangiitis (Wegener's granulomatosis), microscopic polyangiitis, Churg–Strauss syndrome, polyarteritis nodosa, or bacterial endocarditis (see Chapter 21.10.2). A false-positive antineutrophil cytoplasmic antibody (ANCA) test (not uncommonly by immunofluorescence, rarely to specific antigen) may further compound the diagnostic difficulty. Under these circumstances, renal biopsy is mandatory to make the correct diagnosis.

Clinical investigation

Laboratory findings are nonspecific, but frequently include a raised erythrocyte sedimentation rate (ESR), plasma viscosity, and C-reactive protein (CRP). Leucocytosis and a transient eosinophilia are common and may be pronounced. Depending on the tissue involvement, an elevation in creatine phosphokinase, amylase, lactate dehydrogenase (LDH), serum aspartate aminotransferase (AST), and alkaline phosphatase may all be seen. Hypocomplementaemia is rare and usually mild. As stated above, ANCA have been reported, and their presence may further confuse the diagnosis with a multisystem vasculitic process. Mild proteinuria is generally present, and nephrotic-range proteinuria has been reported. Urine microscopy may be bland or reveal red cells, white cells (particularly eosinophils), and hyaline and granular casts. Renal failure is frequently nonoliguric.

Histology

The definitive histological diagnosis of cholesterol-crystal embolism can usually be made from biopsies of kidney, skin, or muscle (including clinically uninvolved areas), although sampling error may miss the lesion due to its patchy distribution. Ante-mortem histological diagnoses have also been made from other tissues, including a gastric biopsy, prostatic currettings, and a bone marrow biopsy. The diagnostic feature is of biconvex, needle-shaped

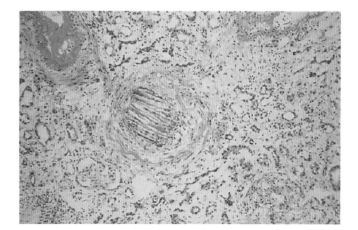

Fig. 14.3.3 Renal biopsy demonstrating the characteristic needle-shaped cholesterol clefts occluding a medium-sized renal arteriole with surrounding inflammatory cell infiltration, intimal proliferation, thickening, and concentric fibrosis. There is extensive autolysis (post-mortem sample).

cholesterol clefts within the lumen of arteries or arterioles that remain after the crystals have dissolved during routine histological preparation (Fig. 14.3.3). In fresh samples, the crystals can be identified by birefringence under polarized light or by specific histochemical staining of cholesterol. In the kidneys, the typical finding is occlusion of small arteries and arterioles of between 150 and 200 μm in diameter, such as the arcuate and interlobular arteries, resulting in patchy areas of ischaemia and small areas of infarction. Crystals can also be seen within the glomeruli. In chronic cases, ischaemia produces a wedge-shaped lesion involving all components of the renal cortex radiating towards the capsule. The glomeruli appear ischaemic and sclerosed and the tubules become atrophic and separated by interstitial fibrosis. Grossly, the kidneys may be reduced in size with a rough granular surface and wedge-shaped scars.

Based on animal studies involving the injection of atheromatous material, the presence of cholesterol crystals in the vascular lumen is thought to trigger a localized inflammatory and endothelial vascular reaction. Inflammatory cells (mainly macrophages and eosinophils) infiltrate, and multinucleated giant cells engulf the cholesterol crystals, but these are resistant to the scavenger effects of macrophages and may persist for many months. The inflammatory phase is followed by marked intimal thickening with concentric fibrosis and occlusion of the vessel. Depending on the extent of organ involvement, these pathological changes result in ischaemia, infarction, or—rarely—necrosis of the distal tissue.

Management

There is no effective therapy and no clinical trials of treatment in this condition have been done. Steroids, aspirin, dipyridamole, and low molecular weight dextran have all been tried, but without any clear effect. There are anecdotal reports of a response to hydroxyl methyl glutaryl coenzyme A (HMG CoA) reductase inhibitors (statins), theoretically inducing plaque stabilization, but recovery may have been spontaneous. Nevertheless, statin use is recommended, even when started after the condition has been diagnosed. Anticoagulants are of no proven benefit and should be avoided given their potential role in the pathogenesis of the disorder. Encouraging results with iloprost and low-density lipoprotein (LDL) apheresis have been reported, but these observations require replication.

CT scanning of the aorta has been used to identify the precise source (e.g. aortic aneurysm, localized aortic plaque) of cholesterol emboli, and surgical replacement of the diseased vessel with a graft has been advocated. However, major surgery in elderly patients with widespread vascular disease and renal impairment carries significant risks and is generally avoided.

Supportive therapy is directed at stopping anticoagulation unless essential, avoiding further angiographic or vascular surgical procedures, controlling hypertension, and appropriate management of renal failure. Use of angiotensin converting enzyme (ACE) inhibitors or angiotensin receptor blockers (ARB) has been advocated, but careful monitoring of renal function is required.

Prognosis

Mortality is high, due to the coexistence of cardiac and vascular disease with renal failure in elderly patients. Renal impairment may remain stable, but frequently progresses such that dialysis is required, although partial recovery has been reported, even after several months of dialysis. The mechanism of this recovery is uncertain.

Further reading

Belenfant X, Meyrier A, Jacquot C (1999). Supportive treatment improves survival in multivisceral cholesterol crystal embolism. *Am J Kidney Dis*, **33**, 840–50.

Elinav E, Chajek-Shaul T, Stern M (2002). Improvement in cholesterol emboli syndrome after iloprost therapy. *BMJ*, **324**, 268–9.

Fine MJ, Kapoor W, Falanga V (1987). Cholesterol crystal embolization: a review of 221 cases in the English literature. *Angiology*, **38**, 769–84.

Hasegawa M, Sugiyama S (2003). Apheresis in the treatment of cholesterol embolic disease. *Ther Apher Dial*, **7**, 435–8.

Hyman BT, et al. (1987). Warfarin-related purple toes syndrome and cholesterol microembolization. *Am J Med*, **82**, 1233–7.

Mannesse CK (1991). Renal failure and cholesterol crystal embolization: a report of 4 surviving cases and a review of the literature. *Clin Nephrol*, **36**, 240–5.

Meyrier A (2006). Cholesterol crystal embolism: diagnosis and treatment. *Kidney Int*, **69**, 1308–12.

Mulay SR, Evan A, Anders HJ (2014). Molecular mechanisms of crystal-related kidney inflammation and injury. Implications for cholesterol embolism, crystalline nephropathies and kidney stone disease. *Nephrol Dial Transplant*, **29**, 507–14.

Saric M, Kronzon I. (2011). Cholesterol embolization syndrome. *Current Opin Cardiol*, **26**, 472–9.

Scolari F, et al. (2000). Cholesterol crystal embolism: a recognizable cause of renal disease. *Am J Kidney Dis*, **36**, 1089–90.

Scolari F, et al. (2007). The challenge of diagnosing atheroembolic renal disease: clinical features and prognostic factors. *Circulation*, **116**, 298–304.

Scolari F, et al. (2010). Atheroembolic renal disease. *Lancet*, **375**, 1650–60.

CHAPTER 14.4

Takayasu's arteritis

Yasushi Kobayashi

Essentials

Takayasu's arteritis is a chronic granulomatous vasculitis of unknown cause characterized by stenosis, occlusion, and aneurysm of large elastic arteries, mainly the aorta and its branches. It mainly affects young women, predominantly in Asian, Middle Eastern, and South American countries.

Clinical presentation—symptoms in the acute stage are nonspecific, such as general fatigue and fever, which can persist for months to years. Symptoms in the chronic stage depend on the anatomical location of the vascular lesions, with typical complaints relating to ischaemia of the brain, eyes, or arms. The commonest finding on physical examination is a weak or absent pulse in one or both brachial, radial, and/or ulnar arteries. Bruits can often be heard over affected arteries. Hypertension and aortic insufficiency are strongly associated with poor prognosis.

Diagnosis—comprehensive angiographic imaging is required for diagnosis, evaluation of the extent of disease, and to guide therapy. American College of Rheumatology diagnostic criteria require the presence of three out of the following six to diagnose Takayasu's arteritis: (1) age of onset less than 40 years; (2) claudication of a limb; (3) decreased brachial artery pulse; (4) systolic pressure difference between two limbs greater than 10 mmHg; (5) bruit over aorta or subclavian arteries; and (6) angiographic narrowing/occlusion of aorta, its primary branches, or large arteries in proximal arms or legs.

Treatment—is with prednisolone and antiplatelet agents, with other immunosuppressants added if necessary. Surgical bypass graft procedures are often required.

Introduction

Takayasu's arteritis is a chronic granulomatous vasculitis characterized by stenosis, occlusion, and aneurysm of large elastic arteries, mainly the aorta and its branches, including the coronary arteries (Fig. 14.4.1). The pulmonary arteries can also be affected. Pathologically the condition is defined as vasa vasoritis of the aorta, which generally affects young women during their reproductive period.

Acute severe inflammation sometimes causes dilatation of vessel walls and/or aneurysm formation. Chronic inflammation causes arterial stenosis and occlusion due to thrombus. In the early stages patients often have nonspecific inflammatory symptoms such as intermittent fever, fatigue, and malaise, which may exist for months to years prior to the onset of full-blown vasculitis, when clinical manifestations then depend on the arteries involved.

Historical perspective

Takayasu's arteritis was described by Mikito Takayasu at the 12th Annual Meeting of the Japanese Ophthalmology Society in 1908. He reported a case of a 21-year-old woman who had a peculiar wreath-like arteriovenous anastomosis, termed a 'coronary anastomosis', around the optic papilla (Fig. 14.4.2). As is often the case for eponymous diseases, the condition had almost certainly been observed before. In 1761 Morgagni reported a 40-year-old woman in Italy whose radial pulses were impalpable for many years. In 1856 Savoy described a young woman in whom the main arteries of both arms and of the left side of the neck were completely obliterated.

Takayasu's arteritis has also been called pulseless disease, aortitis syndrome, aortic arch syndrome, long-segment atypical coarctation of the aorta, Martorell's syndrome, and occlusive thrombo-aortopathy.

Aetiology and pathology

The aetiology of Takayasu's arteritis remains unknown. For a long time tuberculosis was suspected to be the cause in India and

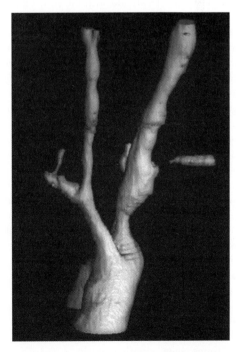

Fig. 14.4.1 Three-dimensional CT image showing narrowing and aneurysmal dilatation in the aorta and vessels arising from the aorta in Takayasu's arteritis.

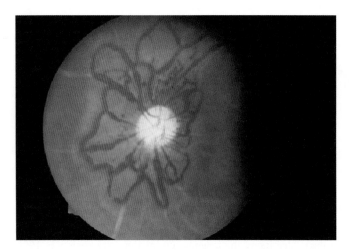

Fig. 14.4.2 Typical coronary anastomosis of retinal vessels in Takayasu's arteritis.

Mexico, but the incidence of proven tuberculosis in patients with Takayasu's arteritis was not higher than that in the general population and it is not now considered to be a causative agent. Takayasu's arteritis after hepatitis B vaccination has also been reported, but so far no clear bacterial or viral organism has been incriminated as the cause, although it may be that aberrant host response to infection is a trigger.

The observations that there is a strong predilection for women, higher incidence in Asian, Middle Eastern, and South American populations, and that cases have been described in monozygotic twins, are all consistent with a role for genetic factors in causing Takayasu's arteritis (OMIM 207600). But balanced against this must be the fact that only 1% of Japanese patients with Takayasu's arteritis have affected relatives.

Human leucocyte antigen (HLA) studies in Japan revealed positive associations of Takayasu's arteritis with the class II alleles HLA DRB1*1502 and DPB1* 0901, and with the class I alleles B*5201 and B*3902, with the two class II alleles mentioned in strong linkage disequilibrium with HLA B*5201 in the Japanese population. An association of HLA with Takayasu's arteritis has also been reported in Mexico and Colombia. Recently, the *IL12B* gene was reported to be significantly associated with Takayasu's arteritis among Japanese and Turkish populations. Such HLA and *IL12B* associations suggest that genetic factors may play a role in the pathogenesis of this condition.

Pathologically Takayasu's arteritis is defined as an inflammatory vasculopathy that involves mainly large and mid-sized vessels. The aorta is thick and often rigid secondary to fibrosis of all three arterial layers, particularly the adventitia and intima. It is characteristic that narrowings of the aortic lumen may alternate with aneurysmal dilatations of the aortic wall ('skipped lesions'). The gross appearance of the intima may be of cobblestones, with smooth, round, white, gelatinous, well-circumscribed plaques of variable size alternating with intervening normal intima. When thickened the intima may reveal longitudinal wrinkling and ridges that give the gross appearance of tree bark. In endstage Takayasu's arteritis the aorta may have a 'lead pipe' appearance.

Takayasu's arteritis may be divided into an acute florid inflammatory phase and a chronic healed fibrotic phase, with both types sometimes seen simultaneously, suggesting recurrent

inflammation. In the acute phase the inflammatory lesions originate in the vasa vasorum and are characterized by perivascular cuffing, mainly composed of γδ T lymphocytes, cytotoxic T cells, and helper T cells. Luminal stenosis of small adventitial arteries due to intimal thickening is relatively common, and an increase in the adventitial thickness due to fibrosis is a histopathological feature found in the chronic phase. Inflammatory infiltrates in the arterial wall are typically arranged in granulomas that are dependent on T cells regulating the activity and integrity of macrophages. The media has neovascularization often accompanied by infiltrates of lymphocytes, plasma cells and occasional Langerhans-type giant cells. Patches of medial coagulation necrosis surrounded by a fence-like arrangement of epithelioid cells are occasionally seen at the periphery. In the chronic stage of Takayasu's arteritis, intimal fibrosis is often accompanied by well-formed fibrous atherosclerotic plaques and calcification. Extension of the adventitial fibrosis and round cell infiltration to adjacent structures may result in retroperitoneal fibrosis.

Epidemiology

Although Takayasu's arteritis has been reported from all over the world, there is a wide variation in its prevalence in different geographical regions. It is predominantly found in Asian, Middle Eastern, and South American countries, although recently patients with the condition have been increasingly recognized in Africa, Europe, and North America. The incidence rate of Takayasu's arteritis in Japan in 2005 was 4.2 persons per 100 000 population; by contrast, in Sweden and the United States of America the prevalence was reported to be between 0.26 and 0.64 persons per 100 000 population.

Takayasu's arteritis affects healthy young women, the average age of onset in Japanese and Indian patients being 15–35 years.

Clinical features

Some patients are asymptomatic and diagnosed as having Takayasu's arteritis incidentally when they are found to lack pulses, to have a significant difference in blood pressure between their arms, or to have raised inflammatory markers on blood testing. When they occur, clinical symptoms may be divided into those of acute and chronic stages.

In the acute stage the symptoms of Takayasu's arteritis are usually nonspecific and generalized, including fever, easy fatigability, general malaise, neck pain, weight loss, and arthralgia. Faintness and/or dizziness are sometimes reported, perhaps due to hypersensitivity of the baroreceptors in the aortic arch leading to hypotension. The vague and nonspecific nature of these symptoms means that the diagnosis is often missed for a long time. Stroke and sudden blindness may be caused by thrombosis of cerebral arteries.

In the chronic stage most patients with Takayasu's arteritis present with features related to specific vascular lesions, although they may also have the constitutional symptoms described above. In East Asian countries the condition affects the aortic arch most frequently, hence typical complaints relate to ischaemia of the brain, eyes, or arms; namely, dizziness, syncope, visual disturbance, and easy fatigability of the arms, with pain due to intermittent claudication. By contrast, in south Asian countries Takayasu's arteritis tends to affect the abdominal arteries such that hypertension may

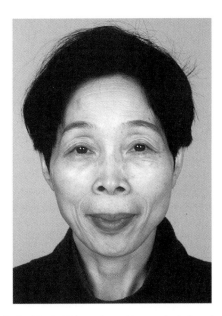

Fig. 14.4.3 The 'bird face' of Takayasu's arteritis: note the hollow cheeks and eye sockets.

be the first clue. This may be caused by atypical coarctation of the aorta, loss of vascular compliance of the aorta, aortic insufficiency, or renal artery stenosis.

The commonest finding on physical examination is a weak or absent pulse in one or both brachial, radial, and/or ulnar arteries (usually on the left side), which is noted in about 80% of Japanese patients. Reduced blood pressure in one or both arms is often observed. Bruits can often be heard over affected arteries. A 'bird face' due to atrophy of facial muscles (Fig. 14.4.3), intermittent claudication of the jaw muscles, and perforation of the nasal septum— all due to ischaemia—are helpful diagnostic clues.

Cardiac manifestations of Takayasu's arteritis are associated with poor prognosis and are the commonest cause of death in Japanese patients. Aortic insufficiency is present in almost one-third in Japanese series, typically caused by annulo-aortic ectasia, and left ventricular hypertrophy is often observed, presumed related to hypertension. The combination of aortic insufficiency and left ventricular hypertrophy may eventually result in heart failure. The inflammation of Takayasu's arteritis may involve the ostia of the coronary arteries and thus lead to exertional angina or acute myocardial infarction.

Pulmonary lesions are frequently found with imaging techniques, but clinical symptoms such as haemoptysis and dyspnoea are uncommon. Isolated pulmonary arteritis has rarely been reported.

Renal artery involvement in Takayasu's arteritis causes hypertension and renal dysfunction. In India almost one-half of all patients with Takayasu's arteritis exhibit ostial and/or proximal renal arterial involvement. Hypertension, nephritic/nephrotic syndrome and renal failure are reported consequences or associations.

Acute gastrointestinal bleeding may be the first symptom in Takayasu's arteritis, and Crohn's disease, ulcerative colitis, and nonspecific inflammatory colitis are rarely associated with the condition.

The ocular complications of Takayasu's arteritis are decreasing due to advances in early diagnosis and therapy. Emboli may cause sudden blindness in the acute stage. Hypertensive retinopathy is commonly reported, with other ocular complications including cataracts, optic atrophy, loss of eye reflexes, iris atrophy, and rubeosis iris.

Erythema nodosum is the most common skin lesion associated with Takayasu's arteritis in white populations, and ulcerative subacute nodular lesions have been described in Mexico and Japan.

Differential diagnosis

The nonspecific symptoms of the acute stage of Takayasu's arteritis are most commonly misdiagnosed as being due to viral infection, tuberculosis, rheumatoid arthritis, or other causes of a 'fever of unknown origin'. The differential diagnosis of the chronic stage includes atherosclerosis, inflammatory abdominal aortic aneurysm, Behçet's disease, syphilitic aortitis, temporal arteritis, and congenital vascular abnormality.

Investigation

The most frequent laboratory abnormalities are elevation of erythrocyte sedimentation rate (ESR; 70–90% of cases) and C-reactive protein (CRP; 50–70%), which are good indices of acute disease activity. The white blood cell count (40%) and gammaglobulin level are often elevated, and mild anaemia (50%) and elevation of complement factors are also observed. Coagulopathies and platelet activation are seen in the acute stage. HLA typing may help with prognosis of Takayasu's arteritis in some countries.

On the chest radiograph, segmental, fine dystrophic calcification with abrupt termination is very suggestive of Takayasu's arteritis in a young patient (Fig. 14.4.4). Rib notching due to aortic aneurysm or dilatation of ascending aorta may also be found.

A comprehensive angiogram is performed to diagnose Takayasu's arteritis and evaluate the extent of disease and guide therapy (Fig. 14.4.5). Digital subtraction angiography (DSA), CT,

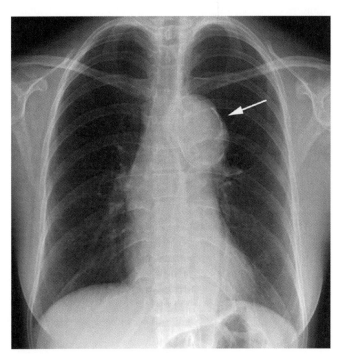

Fig. 14.4.4 Chest radiograph showing calcification along the aorta (arrow) in Takayasu's arteritis.

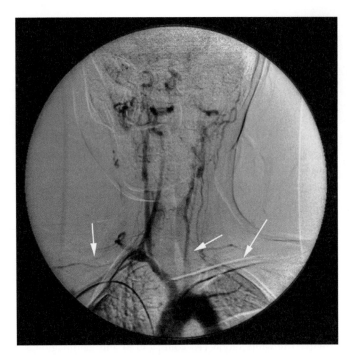

Fig. 14.4.5 Angiogram showed marked narrowing of the left common carotid artery and both subclavian arteries (arrows) in Takayasu's arteritis.

and magnetic resonance angiography (MRA) may also provide valuable information. Localized narrowing or irregularities of the aortic wall are early changes on arteriography. Obliterative vascular lesions range from narrowing and stenosis to complete occlusion. The vessel may be dilated or aneurysmal, and there may be a combination of obstruction and aneurysmal dilatation. The classification proposed by the international cooperative study on Takayasu's arteritis is used to standardize description of disease based on location of vascular lesion (Table 14.4.1); involvement of coronary or pulmonary arteries is designated as C(+) or P(+), along with any of the types.

Aortic insufficiency and cardiac function should be assessed by echocardiography. The measurement of intracardiac pressure may be necessary for correct assessment of blood pressure in some patients. Doppler ultrasonography can demonstrate lesions of the carotid artery and estimate intimal thickness, which may reflect disease activity, as can the use of MRI to detect vessel wall oedema. ^{18}F-fluorodeoxyglucose positron emission tomography (^{18}F-FDG-PET) can show inflammatory activity and—in conjunction with CT or MRI—define its anatomical location,

Table 14.4.1 Classification of Takayasu's arteritis

Type	Site of involvement
I	Branches from aortic arch
IIa	Ascending aorta, aortic arch and its branches
IIb	Ascending aorta, aortic arch, its branches, and thoracic descending aorta
III	Thoracic descending aorta, abdominal aorta and/or renal arteries
IV	Only abdominal aorta and/or renal arteries
V	Combination of types IIb and IV

potentially enabling early prestenotic diagnosis of Takayasu's arteritis with estimation of the inflammatory burden (Fig. 14.4.6). However, ^{18}F-FDG can also be accumulated in atherosclerotic lesions and other vascular diseases, hence FDG-PET data must be interpreted carefully in conjunction with other clinical and laboratory findings.

Criteria for diagnosis

The diagnosis of Takayasu's arteritis is based on the finding of vascular lesions in large and middle size vessels by angiogram, CT, or MRI. Age of onset should also be considered in making the diagnosis. The American College of Rheumatology has proposed the following diagnostic criteria, which are generally accepted, with presence of three out of the six required for diagnosis:

1. Age of onset under 40 years

2. Claudication of an extremity

3. Decreased brachial artery pulse

4. Difference of more than 10 mmHg systolic pressure between two limbs

5. Bruit over subclavian arteries or the aorta

6. Angiographic evidence of narrowing or occlusion of the aorta, its primary branches, or large arteries in the proximal upper or lower extremities.

Treatment

The goal of treating Takayasu's arteritis in the acute stage is to terminate vascular wall inflammation. Corticosteroids are now used as a first-line therapy. The use of low-dose aspirin or other antiplatelet drugs in addition reduces the likelihood of ischaemic complication. A typical initial regimen would be oral prednisolone at a dose of 0.5–1 mg/kg per day, depending on the clinical symptoms and general inflammatory markers, ESR and CRP levels. However, these inflammatory markers are suboptimal for evaluating disease activity during treatment because both pathological and ^{18}F FDG CT-PET analyses have shown that vascular wall inflammation can exist even when inflammatory marker levels are normal. Evaluation of patient symptoms and imaging studies may therefore be helpful in assessing ongoing vascular inflammation. About 60 to 80% of patients will go into remission, but relapse during corticosteroid taper occurs in more than 50%. Low-dose corticosteroids are usually used to maintain remission, but if patients cannot then be tapered to an alternate-day regimen without disease exacerbation, a cytotoxic agent such as ciclosporin, cyclophosphamide, azathioprine, or methotrexate can be used, ciclosporin typically being administered as a daily oral dose of 1 to 3 mg/kg per day in conjunction with prednisolone 10 to 20 mg daily. Tumour necrosis factor (TNF) antagonists may be considered in refractory cases. Recently, anti-TNF-α therapy and anti-IL-6 receptor therapy have been introduced for refractory Takayasu's arteritis because of the roles that TNF and interleukin (IL)-6 appear to play in the development of lesions.

Established vascular lesions are usually not reversible with medical treatment alone, hence surgical intervention may be needed if

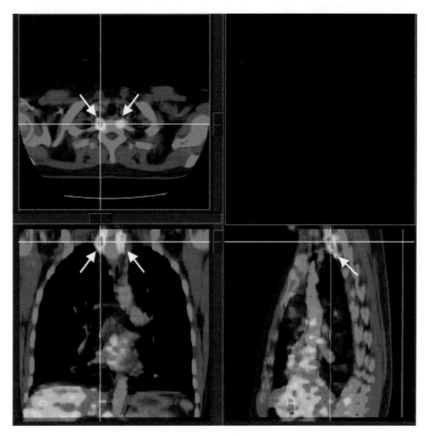

Fig. 14.4.6 ^{18}F-FDG PET showing inflammation in both vertebral arteries (arrows) in Takayasu's arteritis.

severe ischaemic organ dysfunction is present. This is commonly required in patients with severe complications of Takayasu's arteritis, particularly for cerebrovascular disease due to cervicocranial vessel stenosis, coronary artery disease, severe to moderate aortic regurgitation, severe coarctation of the aorta, renovascular hypertension, limb claudication and progressive aneurysm enlargement. Bypass graft procedures are often performed, with good long-term outcomes reported.

Takayasu's arteritis is a disease that affects women of childbearing age, but it does not alter fertility, hence it sometimes presents during pregnancy and around the time of delivery, and recurrences may also occur at these times. Inflammation during pregnancy may be managed with prednisolone, with dose based on the activity of inflammation. Management of labour and/or the decision to proceed to caesarean section are based on standard assessment of maternal and fetal risk factors.

Prognosis

Earlier diagnosis of Takayasu's arteritis, attributable to increased clinical awareness of the condition and advances in imaging techniques, means that the reported prognosis of the condition has improved. In recent series most patients are well controlled, with no or minimal symptoms, and many are on no treatment. However, 25 to 30% have a poor prognosis, the major factors contributing to this being cardiovascular complications, particularly aortic insufficiency and hypertension causing congestive heart failure. Cerebrovascular events, myocardial infarction, and pulmonary infarction may be fatal.

Further reading

Arend WP, *et al.* (1990). The American College of Rheumatology criteria for the determination of Takayasu arteritis. *Arthritis Rheum*, **33**, 1129–34.

Andrews J, Mason JC (2006). Takayasu's arteritis—recent advances in imaging offer promise. *Rheumatology*, **46**, 6–15.

Gravanis MB (2000). Giant cell arteritis and Takayasu aortitis: morphologic, pathogenetic and etiologic factors. *Int J Cardiol*, **75** Suppl 1, S21–33.

Hashimoto Y, *et al.* (1992). Aortic regurgitation in patients with Takayasu arteritis: assessment by color Doppler echocardiography. *Heart Vessels*, **7** Suppl, 111–15.

Hata A, *et al.* (1996). Angiographic findings of Takayasu arteritis: new classification. *Int J Cardiol*, **54** Suppl, S155–63.

Hoffman GS, *et al.* (1994). Treatment of glucocorticoid-resistant or relapsing Takayasu arteritis with methotrexate. *Arthritis Rheum*, **37**, 578–82.

Jennette JC, *et al.* (1994). Nomenclature of systemic vasculitides. Proposal of an international consensus conference. *Arthritis Rheum*, **37**, 187–92.

Kerr GS, *et al.* (1994). Takayasu arteritis. *Ann Intern Med*, **120**, 919–29.

Kimura A, *et al.* (2000). Mapping of the HLA-linked genes controlling the susceptibility to Takayasu's arteritis. *Int J Cardiol*, **75** Suppl 1, S105–10.

Kobayashi Y, *et al.* (2005). Aortic wall inflammation due to Takayasu arteritis imaged with ^{18}F-FDG PET coregistered with enhanced CT. *J Nuclear Med*, **46**, 917–22.

Mason JC (2010). Takayasu arteritis—advances in diagnosis and management. *Nat Rev Rheum*, **6**, 406–15.

Miyata T, *et al.* (2003). Long-term survival after surgical treatment of patients with Takayasu's arteritis. *Circulation*, **108**, 1474–80.

Molloy ES, *et al.* (2008). Anti-tumour necrosis factor therapy in patients with refractory Takayasu arteritis: long-term follow-up. *Ann Rheum Dis*, **67**, 1567–9.

Numano F (2000). Vasa vasoritis, vasculitis and atherosclerosis. *Int J Cardiol*, **75** Suppl, 1–8.

Numano F, *et al.* (2000). Takayasu's arteritis. *Lancet*, **356**, 1023–5.

The pulmonary circulation

CHAPTER 15.1

Structure and function of the pulmonary circulation

Nicholas W. Morrell

Essentials

The normal pulmonary circulation distributes deoxygenated blood at low pressure and high flow to the pulmonary capillaries for the purposes of gas exchange. The structure of pulmonary blood vessels varies with their function—from large elastic conductance arteries, to small muscular arteries, to thin-walled vessels involved in gas exchange.

Pulmonary vascular resistance (PVR) is about one-tenth of systemic vascular resistance, with the small muscular and partially muscular arteries of 50 to 150 μm diameter being the site of the greatest contribution to resistance. The gas-exchanging capillary surface area (c.125 m^2) contains a blood volume of about 150 ml at any one time, with the blood–gas barrier being only 0.2 to 0.3 μm thick at its thinnest part. In the normal pulmonary circulation, a large increase in cardiac output causes only a small rise in mean pulmonary arterial pressure because PVR falls on exercise: this is accomplished by a combination of vascular distensibility and recruitment. Pulmonary blood flow is heterogeneous: gravity causes increased blood flow in the more dependent parts of the lung; within a horizontal region—or within an acinus—blood-flow heterogeneity is imposed by the branching pattern of the vessels.

Many neural and humoral mediators can influence pulmonary vascular tone, including nitric oxide and prostacyclin. Alveolar hypoxia causes constriction of the small pulmonary arteries, whereas systemic arteries dilate when hypoxic: this hypoxic pulmonary vasoconstriction can reduce venous admixture and improve arterial oxygenation in the presence of bronchial obstruction. Despite large regional differences in the matching of ventilation and perfusion within the normal lung, the overall lung ventilation–perfusion ratio is maintained remarkably steady at around 0.85.

Introduction

The main function of the pulmonary circulation is respiratory gas exchange, a vital function that the lungs take over from the placenta at birth. The structure of the pulmonary circulation is highly adapted to fulfil this role. It receives the entire cardiac output from the right ventricle during each cardiac cycle, and this mixed venous blood is delivered at high flow but low pressure to the delicate alveolar structures where gas exchange occurs. Blood flow is matched closely to the regional ventilation within the lung to optimize and maintain systemic arterial oxygenation. This chapter discusses the anatomy and physiology of the pulmonary circulation.

Structure of the pulmonary circulation

The pulmonary arteries and bronchi, together with lymphatics, run in a single connective tissue sheath in the centre of pulmonary segments and lobules, the so-called bronchovascular bundle. The 'conventional' pulmonary arteries branch dichotomously and symmetrically, along with the airways, and they also give off extra branches between the conventional branching points, called 'supernumerary' or short branches. The intrapulmonary veins pursue a different course along the edges of lobules and segments, in the interlobular septa. The branching pattern of veins is similar to that of the pulmonary arteries.

The branching pattern of the pulmonary arteries can be described by a 'divergent' approach, where the main pulmonary artery is called generation 1, with each division giving rise to generation 2, 3, etc. An alternative is the 'convergent' approach where the most peripheral branch is numbered 'order 1', and the orders increase until the main pulmonary artery (order 17) is reached. Figure 15.1.1 shows this arrangement going from the precapillary arteriole of order 1, whose diameter is about 13 μm, to the main pulmonary artery (order 17) with a diameter of 30 000 μm. Note the ninefold expansion in cross-sectional area of the pulmonary vascular bed from order 2 to order 1: it is these precapillary vessels that are often involved in disease processes that affect the pulmonary circulation. In the normal lung, the site of the greatest pulmonary vascular resistance (PVR) is in the small partially muscular and muscular pulmonary arteries (orders 4 to 6; 50–150 μm diameter).

The wall structure of the pulmonary arteries changes along their length depending on the function of the vessel (Fig. 15.1.2). All preacinar arteries have a complete muscular coat, but the muscle layer may be incomplete or absent in smaller intra-acinar vessels.

- Elastic arteries (orders 17–13)—these larger arteries have adventitial, muscular, and intimal layers. The media, or muscular layer, is bounded by internal and external elastic laminae, with three or more elastic laminae within the muscle coat. Medial thickness is about 1 to 2% of external diameter.

- Muscular arteries (orders 13–3)—these small arteries have a thicker muscle layer in relation to their external diameter (2–5%),

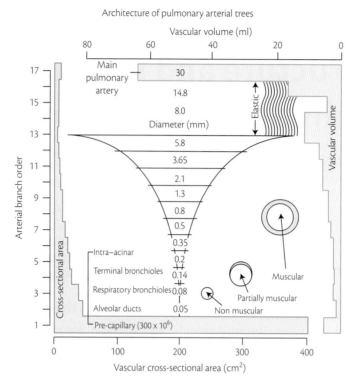

Fig. 15.1.1 Map of the pulmonary arterial tree showing how vascular volumes, cross-sectional areas, diameters, and wall structure vary with branch order number.

and they possess only internal and external elastic laminae; in the smallest arteries, the internal elastic lamina disappears.

- Partially muscular arteries (orders 5–3)—the smooth muscle fibres investing the smallest pulmonary arteries taper off in a spiral, leading to an incomplete muscular coat (Fig. 15.1.2). Most arteries of 50 to 100 μm external diameter are partially muscular.

- Nonmuscular arteries (orders 5–1)—these arteries have no elastic laminae. The smooth muscle cell is replaced by pericytes whose basement membrane fuses with that of the endothelial cell lining the vascular lumen.

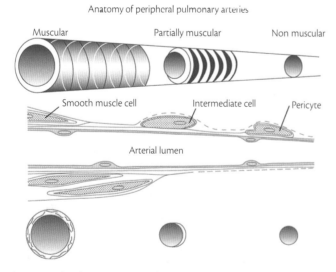

Anatomy of peripheral pulmonary arteries

Fig. 15.1.2 The changing structure of pulmonary arteries.

- Supernumerary arteries—these are small, relatively thin-walled arteries that branch sharply from the parent vessel between bifurcations of the conventional branching system, starting from orders 11 to 12. They provide a short cut for blood supplying the alveoli adjacent to the conduit arteries and bronchi, which would otherwise require a long and circuitous supply by the axial route.

- Pulmonary veins—the branching pattern and organization of the pulmonary veins is similar to that of the arteries, but with only 15 orders, because the 4 pulmonary veins converge on the left atrium without joining up to form an additional 2 orders. Veins do not have an internal elastic lamina. Their walls contain more elastic tissue and less muscle than arteries of the same size. There are supernumerary veins like the supernumerary arteries.

- Capillary network—the 300 million precapillary vessels lead into a network of alveolar septal capillaries with a blood volume (150 ml) equal to that in the pulmonary arterial or venous systems. The capillary surface area is about 125 m^2 (c.86% of the alveolar surface area). Individual capillaries are not much wider than a single erythrocyte, hence the microvascular bed at normal vascular pressures is essentially a sheet of blood one red cell thick, exposed to alveolar gas on both sides. Alveolar capillaries have a thick side and a thin side. The thin side consists of the cytoplasmic extensions of the luminal endothelial cell and the alveolar epithelial cell with their fused basement membrane (0.2–0.3 μm across). The thick side, up to 2 μm across, contains collagen, elastin, and fibroblast processes to give structural support to the alveolus.

Pulmonary vascular resistance

The pulmonary circulation is a high-flow, low-pressure system whose vascular resistance is one-tenth of systemic vascular resistance. PVR is the ratio of the mean pulmonary arterial–venous pressure difference ($Ppa - Ppv$) to mean pulmonary blood flow (Qp):

$$(Ppa - Ppv) / Qp = PVR\,(\mathrm{mmHg} / \mathrm{litre\ per\ min})$$

The normal PVR is less than 2 mmHg/litre per min at rest.

The main determinants of PVR are captured in the equation for Poiseuille flow (steady flow of a Newtonian fluid through long, straight, unbranched tubes):

$$PVR \sim 8\mu L / \pi D^4$$

where L is vascular path length, μ is the viscosity of blood, and D is vessel diameter. L/D^4 is known as the geometric factor, the importance of which can be seen by considering that a 16% decrease in D leads to a twofold increase in PVR. In reality, the situation is more complicated because blood flow in the lungs is not of uniform velocity, but is, of course, pulsatile.

PVR normally falls on exercise despite the increase in cardiac output, hence Ppa rises only modestly, perhaps from 15 mmHg at rest to 23 mmHg. The fall in PVR during exercise is accomplished by a combination of vascular 'distensibility' (vascular compliance) and 'recruitment' (number of parallel pathways with flow). Vascular recruitment means that a vessel goes from a state of zero flow to one of finite flow. An increase in pulmonary arterial pressure during exercise can distend pulmonary arteries. The total compliance of the pulmonary circulation is about 20 ml/mmHg, hence on heavy exercise, if all vascular pressures rose by 10 mmHg, pulmonary vascular volume would increase by 200 ml, provided vessels had not reached their limiting size.

The distribution of PVR can be partitioned into a three-segment model, which can be described as having (1) arterial, (2) 'middle', and (3) venous segments. In isolated lungs, about 20% of the total PVR lies in the distensible 'middle' segment (capillaries and small arteries and veins), with 40% each in the arterial and venous segments. This distribution can be altered by factors, e.g. hypoxia, that increase resistance predominantly in the 'middle' segment. Blood viscosity is a further factor that affects PVR, e.g. when polycythaemia increases PVR.

Distribution of pulmonary blood flow

Blood flow within the lung is heterogeneous in distribution. For example, between lung regions of secondary lobule size ($c.10\,\mathrm{cm}^3$) there is a modest amount of gravity-dependent heterogeneity, with flow increasing with vertical distance (more to the lower zones than the upper zones). Within these lung regions and within the respiratory acinus there is a greater degree of heterogeneity, which is independent of gravity.

Gravity-dependent flow

The effects of gravity are best illustrated by considering that, in the human erect posture at rest, mean pulmonary artery pressure (Ppa) at the level of the hilum is about 18 cmH$_2$O, whereas the apex of

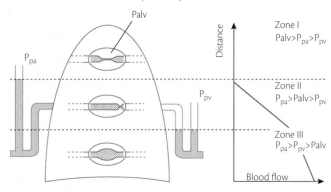

Three zone model of pulmonary blood flow distribution

Fig. 15.1.3 The three-zone model of pulmonary blood flow distribution.

the lung is 20 cmH$_2$O above the hilum. Consequently, the apex of the lung will be perfused only during the systolic pressure peak. In the supine position, the apical blood flow increases, with the result that the distribution from apex to base becomes more uniform. During exercise, with the increase in cardiac output, both upper and lower zone blood flow increases, but the upper increases more than the lower, so that flow becomes more even. The role of gravity in determining pulmonary blood flow was extended by West and encompassed in the three-zone model of pulmonary circulation (Fig. 15.1.3). This model relies on the assumption that the site of major flow resistance is in the small vessels whose extravascular pressure is the alveolar pressure ($Palv$). There is no flow in zone I because $Palv$ is greater than Ppa. Flow increases down zone II because the driving pressure increases by 1 cm of H$_2$O for each 1 cm distance down the lung. Flow increases with distance down zone III, although ΔP ($Ppa - Ppv$) remains constant, because local PVR decreases due to capillary distension and recruitment. The driving pressure for blood flow is determined by the relationship between $Palv$, Ppa, and pulmonary venous pressure (Ppv) down the upright lung. A further zone (zone IV) is found at the lung base: in this zone, blood flow is observed to decrease with distance down the lung due to increased perivascular pressure in extra-alveolar vessels.

Gravity-independent flow

The branching pattern of pulmonary arteries imposes changes in perfusion that are independent of gravity. Within any given horizontal level of the upright lung, there is a decrease in blood flow in peripheral lung regions compared to central hilar regions. This is thought to be due to the reduction in Ppa in small acinar arteries with increasing distance from the hilum. This pattern is also seen at the level of the secondary lobule (the group of acini supplied by one terminal bronchiole), with a decreasing gradient of blood flow from the centre to the periphery.

Regulation of pulmonary vasomotor tone

The pulmonary circulation differs from the systemic in that it is under minimal resting tone and is almost fully dilated under normal conditions. Circulating and local production of vasodilators and vasoconstrictors contribute to the resting tone, with the balance tipped in favour of vasodilators. Nitric oxide, produced locally by endothelial cells, and the arachidonic acid metabolite prostacyclin are important vasodilators that contribute to this low pulmonary vascular tone.

The autonomic nervous system interacts with humoral mediators and haemodynamic forces in the control of pulmonary vascular tone, autonomic innervation of the lung being via parasympathetic (cholinergic: predominantly vasodilator) and sympathetic (adrenergic: predominantly vasoconstrictor) nerves in the periarterial plexus.

Hypoxic pulmonary vasoconstriction

The pulmonary circulation responds to a reduction in the partial pressure of alveolar oxygen by vasoconstriction. This is opposite to the response to hypoxia in the systemic circulation, where tissue hypoxia leads to vasodilatation, hence improving tissue oxygen delivery. Hypoxic pulmonary vasoconstriction (HPV) probably plays little role in the normal distribution of pulmonary blood flow or regulation of ventilation–perfusion relationships in humans. However, in diseases characterized by airway obstruction, such as acute asthma or chronic obstructive lung disease, HPV can divert blood flow away from poorly ventilated lung regions, reducing venous admixture (shunt through poorly ventilated lung regions) and preserving arterial oxygenation. The magnitude of the response varies widely between individuals and is, at best, 50% efficient. It is noteworthy that populations indigenous to high-altitude regions, e.g. Tibetans, lack HPV with no obviously detrimental effect. At high altitude, with low atmospheric partial pressures of oxygen, HPV would lead to generalized vasoconstriction and pulmonary hypertension, which is presumably more detrimental than the lack of HPV.

Ventilation–perfusion relationships

In the normal lung, it is remarkable that pulmonary blood flow and ventilation are, in general, well matched given the heterogeneity of blood flow described above. Of course, regional ventilation is also under similar constraints and forces as the blood flow. In terms of the structure and function of the airways and alveoli in brief, the airways run with the arteries in the bronchovascular bundle and the branching patterns are similar. Regional ventilation is under the influence of gravity: the lung sits in the thorax under its own weight, which leads to a gradient of intrapleural pressure, with more negative pressures at the top of the lung than at the bottom in the upright position. This means that the lung is more expanded at the apex than at the base at the end of a normal breath (functional residual capacity). Thus, the upper and lower parts of the lung are operating on different portions of their pressure–volume curves. The result is that, during normal breathing, greater ventilation is delivered to the bottom than to the top of the lung. This gradient of regional ventilation down the lung is reminiscent of the gradient of blood flow described above. In fact, with increasing distance up the lung, the rate of change of ventilation per unit of alveolar volume is somewhat less than the rate of change of perfusion (about one-third). This leads to large regional differences in the ventilation–perfusion ratio up the lung (Fig. 15.1.4): alveoli at the bottom of the lung are relatively overperfused, leading to a low ventilation–perfusion ratio (c.0.6); by contrast, alveoli at the apex of the lung are relatively under-perfused, leading to ventilation–perfusion ratios over 3.0. Nevertheless, the overall ventilation–perfusion ratio for the whole lung is approximately 0.85. The regional ventilation–perfusion ratio will determine the partial pressures of oxygen and

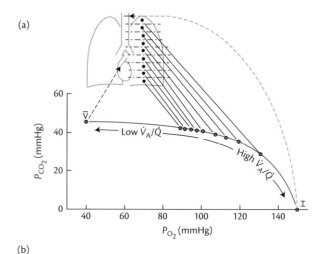

(a)

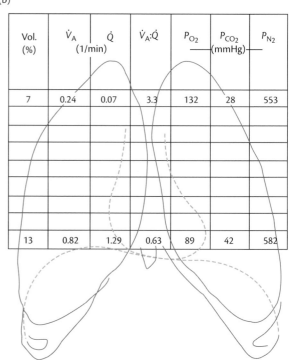

(b)

Vol. (%)	$\dot{V}_A$ (1/min)	$\dot{Q}$ (1/min)	$\dot{V}_A:\dot{Q}$	P_{O_2}	P_{CO_2} (mmHg)	P_{N_2}
7	0.24	0.07	3.3	132	28	553
13	0.82	1.29	0.63	89	42	582

Fig. 15.1.4 (a) O_2–CO_2 diagram showing how the change in ventilation–perfusion ratio up the lung determines the regional composition of alveolar gas. Dashed lines show the composition of mixed venous (pulmonary arterial) blood and inspired (tracheal) gas. (b) Effects of change in ventilation–perfusion ratio up the lung on the regional composition of alveolar gas, with volumes of lung slices, ventilations, and blood flows also shown.

CO_2 found in the alveoli at a given level of the lung, and this will be reflected in the gas tensions found in pulmonary venous blood draining those alveoli. The result is that the P_{O_2} is higher, and the P_{CO_2} lower, in blood draining from the top of the lung, compared with the bottom. The matching of ventilation and perfusion in the normal lung ensures that the overall ventilation–perfusion ratio remains fairly constant with changes in posture or exercise.

Acknowledgement

Much of the chapter written for the third edition of the *Oxford Textbook of Medicine* by the late J. S. Prichard has been retained here.

Further reading

De Mello DE, Reid LM (1997). Arteries and veins. In: Crystal RG, *et al.* (eds.) *The lung: scientific foundations*, 2nd edition, pp. 1117–27. Lippincott-Raven, Philadelphia.

Hughes JMB (1997). Distribution of pulmonary blood flow. In: Crystal RG, *et al.* (eds.) *The lung: scientific foundations*, 2nd edition, pp. 1523–36. Lippincott-Raven, Philadelphia.

Hughes JMB, Morrell NW (2001). *Pulmonary circulation: from basic mechanisms to clinical practice*. Imperial College Press, London.

Singhal S, *et al.* (1973). Morphometry of the human pulmonary arterial tree. *Circ Res*, **33**, 190–7.

West JB, Dollery CT, Naimark A. (1964). Distribution of blood flow in isolated lung: relation to vascular and alveolar pressures. *J Appl Physiol*, **19**, 713–24.

West JB (1985). *Ventilation/blood flow and gas exchange*, 4th edition. Blackwell Scientific Publications, Oxford.

CHAPTER 15.2

Pulmonary hypertension

Nicholas W. Morrell

Essentials

Symptoms of unexplained exertional breathlessness or symptoms out of proportion to coexistent heart or lung disease should alert the clinician to the possibility of pulmonary hypertension, and the condition should be actively sought in patients with known associated conditions, such as scleroderma, hypoxic lung disease, liver disease, or congenital heart disease. Heterozygous germ-line mutations in the gene encoding the bone morphogenetic protein type II receptor (BMPR2) are found in over 70% of families with pulmonary arterial hypertension (PAH).

Pulmonary hypertension is defined as a mean pulmonary arterial pressure greater than 25 mmHg at rest, or 30 mmHg on exercise, and may be due to increased pulmonary vascular resistance (e.g. PAH), increased transpulmonary blood flow (e.g. congenital heart disease), or increased pulmonary venous pressures (e.g. mitral stenosis). Exercise tolerance and survival in pulmonary hypertension is ultimately related to indices of right heart function, such as cardiac output.

Investigation—echocardiography is a good screening tool for the presence of pulmonary hypertension, but right heart catheterization is needed to confirm the diagnosis and guide treatment. CT pulmonary angiography and high-resolution CT are important to exclude underlying parenchymal lung disease and chronic thromboembolic pulmonary hypertension. In idiopathic PAH a vasodilator study should be undertaken at the time of right heart catheterization to detect the few (5–10%) patients who will have good long-term survival on calcium channel blockers.

Management—treatments for PAH include prostanoids, endothelin receptor antagonists, and phosphodiesterase inhibitors, which improve symptoms of breathlessness, exercise tolerance, quality of life, and probably survival. Chronic thromboembolic pulmonary hypertension (CTEPH) is an important diagnosis to make because selected patients with predominantly proximal disease can be cured by pulmonary endarterectomy.

Introduction

The normal pulmonary circulation, as described in Chapter 15.1, is a low-pressure, high-flow system that delivers the output of the right ventricle to the alveolar capillary network during each cardiac cycle for the purposes of gas exchange. Pulmonary hypertension is defined as a sustained elevation of mean pulmonary arterial pressure to more than 25 mmHg at rest.

Many diseases can lead to an elevation of pulmonary arterial pressure. Therefore, the term 'pulmonary hypertension' is not a final diagnosis, but a starting point for further investigation. In general terms, the main causes of pulmonary hypertension are (1) a narrowing or obstruction of the precapillary pulmonary arteries, (2) an increase in pulmonary venous pressure, (3) a persistent elevation of pulmonary blood flow, (4) chronic thromboembolic disease, or (5) miscellaneous causes. This simplified approach is worth keeping in mind during the assessment of patients found to have pulmonary hypertension, because it has major consequences for prognosis and management.

Classification of pulmonary hypertension

Table 15.2.1 shows the 5th World Symposium on Pulmonary Hypertension (2013) classification of pulmonary hypertension as determined by an international panel of experts. The grouping of causes in this classification takes into account similarities in aetiology, pathology, and haemodynamic assessment at right heart catheterization. The classification helps to understand the underlying cause of pulmonary hypertension in a given patient and to plan management, hence it is a useful framework to consider the various causes of pulmonary hypertension, described in more detail below.

Pulmonary arterial hypertension

The term pulmonary 'arterial' hypertension (PAH) refers to conditions characterized predominantly by a precapillary obstruction to blood flow through the pulmonary vascular bed, characterized hemodynamically by a mean pulmonary arterial pressure of greater than 25 mmHg, an end-expiratory pulmonary artery wedge pressure (PAWP) ≤15 mmHg, and a pulmonary vascular resistance >3 Wood units. This elevation of pulmonary vascular resistance increases the driving pressure required to maintain blood flow through the lungs: pulmonary arterial pressure rises to maintain adequate left ventricular filling. The normal mean pulmonary arterial pressure (c.17 mmHg) is about one-fifth of the systemic mean blood pressure. In PAH, mean pulmonary arterial pressure may approach systemic levels. The normally thin-walled right ventricle struggles to cope with the increasing pressure. At first it undergoes a degree of hypertrophy, which increases its ability to generate higher pressures, but ultimately it begins to fail and cardiac output declines. It is the reduction in cardiac output that generates most of the clinical symptoms in patients, with dyspnoea and fatigue being the most common (Fig. 15.2.1). The function of the right heart is the main determinant of prognosis in patients with PAH.

Epidemiology and aetiology

PAH is broadly divided into idiopathic PAH (previously known as primary pulmonary hypertension), and PAH found with other

Table 15.2.1 Clinical classification of pulmonary hypertension (NICE 2013)

1 Pulmonary arterial hypertension
1.1 Idiopathic PAH
1.2 Heritable PAH
1.2.1 BMPR2
1.2.2 ALK-1, ENG, SMAD9, CAV1, KCNK3
1.2.3 Unknown
1.3 Drug and toxin induced
1.4 Associated with:
1.4.1 Connective tissue disease
1.4.2 HIV infection
1.4.3 Portal hypertension
1.4.4 Congenital heart diseases
1.4.5 Schistosomiasis
1' Pulmonary veno-occlusive disease and/or pulmonary capillary hemangiomatosis
1'' **Persistent pulmonary hypertension of the newborn (PPHN)**
2 Pulmonary hypertension due to left heart disease
2.1 Left ventricular systolic dysfunction
2.2 Left ventricular diastolic dysfunction
2.3 Valvular disease
2.4 **Congenital/acquired left heart inflow/outflow tract obstruction and congenital cardiomyopathies**
3 Pulmonary hypertension due to lung diseases and/or hypoxia
3.1 Chronic obstructive pulmonary disease
3.2 Interstitial lung disease
3.3 Other pulmonary diseases with mixed restrictive and obstructive pattern
3.4 Sleep-disordered breathing
3.5 Alveolar hypoventilation disorders
3.6 Chronic exposure to high altitude
3.7 Developmental lung diseases
4 Chronic thromboembolic pulmonary hypertension (CTEPH)
5 Pulmonary hypertension with unclear multifactorial mechanisms
5.1 Haematologic disorders: **chronic haemolytic anaemia**, myeloproliferative disorders, splenectomy
5.2 Systemic disorders: sarcoidosis, pulmonary histiocytosis, lymphangioleiomyomatosis
5.3 Metabolic disorders: glycogen storage disease, Gaucher disease, thyroid disorders
5.4 Others: tumoral obstruction, fibrosing mediastinitis, chronic renal failure, **segmental PH**

Main modifications to the previous Dana Point classification are in **bold**.

BMPR, bone morphogenic protein receptor type II; CAV1, caveolin-1; ENG, endoglin; PAH, pulmonary arterial hypertension.

NICE (2013). Reproduced from Simonneau G, *et al. Journal of the American College of Cardiology* Volume 62, Issue 25, Supplement, 2013, pages D34–D41

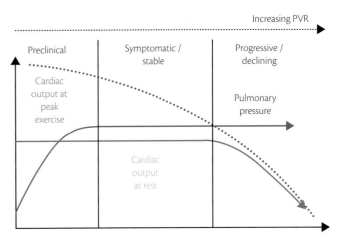

Fig. 15.2.1 Relationship between pulmonary hypertension, right ventricular function, and symptoms in pulmonary hypertension. Pulmonary arterial hypertension (PAH) is characterized by progressively increasing pulmonary vascular resistance. In the early stages, the disease is asymptomatic and only manifests during exercise or during unusually demanding activities, but over time there is a progressive reduction in cardiac output and increasing pulmonary vascular resistance (PVR), eventually progressing to cardiac failure and death.

known associated conditions or triggers. Idiopathic PAH is further divided into familial or sporadic disease, with about 10% of patients with idiopathic PAH having an affected relative. Idiopathic PAH is a rare disorder with an estimated incidence of 1 to 2 per million per year. It is more common in women (female:male sex ratio = 2.3:1), can occur at any age, but most commonly occurs between the ages of 40 and 50 years.

PAH that is pathologically indistinguishable from the idiopathic form can occur in a range of associated conditions (Table 15.2.1). Of the autoimmune rheumatic diseases, the most common association is with systemic sclerosis, where PAH can complicate the clinical course in 15 to 20% of patients in the absence of interstitial lung disease. Other associated conditions include mixed connective tissue disease and systemic lupus erythematosus, and more rarely rheumatoid arthritis, dermatopolymyositis, and primary Sjögren's syndrome.

There is a well-recognized association of PAH with congenital heart disease leading to left-to-right shunts. Overall, the prevalence of PAH is 15 to 30%, but varies depending on the nature of the underlying cardiac defect. Portal hypertension, usually associated with cirrhosis, is associated with PAH in less than 5% of patients. There is an unusually high prevalence of PAH (c.0.5%) in patients with HIV infection. Epidemiological studies have confirmed the association of PAH with amphetamine-like diet pills: in the 1970s, increased numbers of patients with PAH were found to have been exposed to Aminorex, and in the 1990s further studies confirmed an association of PAH with appetite-suppressant drugs of the fenfluramine and dexfenfluramine group. An epidemic of PAH also occurred in Spain in the 1980s, following the ingestion of contaminated rapeseed oil. Other more rarely associated conditions are listed in Table 15.2.1.

The classification of PAH includes two other rare pulmonary vascular diseases—pulmonary veno-occlusive disease (PVOD) and pulmonary capillary haemangiomatosis (PCH). Both are rarer than idiopathic PAH, but their true prevalence is unknown. Persistent pulmonary hypertension of the newborn is a disorder characterized by a failure of vascular transition from fetal to a neonatal circulation and estimated to affect 0.2% of liveborn term infants.

Genetics

Familial or heritable PAH is a rare autosomal dominant condition, with reduced penetrance. It is indistinguishable on clinical or pathological grounds from idiopathic PAH. Linkage studies localized the gene to the long arm of chromosome 2 (2q33). In 2000, heterozygous germ-line mutations were identified in the *BMPR2* gene encoding the bone morphogenetic protein type II receptor, which is a constitutively active serine-threonine kinase that acts as a receptor for bone morphogenetic proteins (BMPs), these being members of the transforming growth factor β (TGFβ) superfamily. Mutations in BMPR-II have now been identified in over 70% of cases of familial PAH, and similar mutations are also found in 15 to 26% of patients thought to have sporadic or idiopathic disease. Many of these are unexpected examples of familial disease with low penetrance, although *de novo* mutations have also been reported. BMPR-II mutations have been identified in most of the 13 exons of the *BMPR2* gene, most (*c*.70%) being nonsense or frameshift mutations predicted to cause haploinsufficiency due to nonsense-mediated mRNA decay of the mutant transcript: only the wild-type allele is expressed in these cases, reducing the amount of BMPR-II protein to about 50% of normal. About 30% of the mutations are mis-sense mutations, which cause retention of mutant protein within the endoplasmic reticulum or affect important functional domains of the receptor, such as the ligand-binding domain or the kinase domain. Mutations in BMPR-II have also been found in a small proportion (*c*.10%) of patients with PAH associated with appetite suppressants, and in children with complicated PAH associated with congenital heart disease.

Mutations in another TGFβ receptor, ALK-1, have also been reported in association with PAH. These are usually found in families with hereditary haemorrhagic telangiectasia, but occasionally some family members develop severe PAH. These findings have highlighted the central role of the TGFβ signalling pathway in the pathogenesis of PAH. The BMPR-II/ALK-1 receptor complex on endothelial cells has been found to be the major signalling complex for BMPs 9 and 10, providing major mechanistic insights into the pathobiology of PAH. Mutations in other TGFβ-related genes have also been identified in rare cases of heritable PAH, including endoglin, BMPR-1B, Smad1, Smad4, and Smad9. In addition, mutations in caveolin-1 and the potassium channel KCNK3 have been reported in rare cases of heritable PAH. Mutations in the eukaryotic translation initiation factor 2-alpha kinase 4 were recently identified in families with autosomal recessive PVOD.

Pathology

Typical morphological appearances include increased muscularization of small (<200 μm diameter) arteries and thickening or fibrosis of the intima, referred to as concentric intimal fibrosis (Fig. 15.2.2). In severe cases, dilatation of small pulmonary arterioles is seen and, sometimes, fibrinoid necrosis. In the larger elastic arteries, aneurysmal dilatation and atherosclerotic change may occur, the latter being otherwise extremely unusual in the normotensive pulmonary artery. The term plexogenic arteriopathy is used to describe the presence of plexiform lesions (200–400 μm), which are tangles of capillary-like channels adjacent to small pulmonary arteries. Plexiform changes are found in some 50% of cases of idiopathic

PAH, but also in other causes of severe pulmonary hypertension, such as that due to congenital heart disease.

In some cases of idiopathic PAH, there are pathological changes in the pulmonary venous circulation as well as in the arterial. If the venous changes dominate the pathology, the diagnosis is PVOD, which has some distinct clinical features. The pathological hallmark of PVOD is the extensive and diffuse occlusion of pulmonary veins by intimal fibrous tissue, which may be loose and oedematous or dense and sclerotic. The intimal thickening is confined usually to the smaller veins. Accompanying arterial changes, particularly muscular hypertrophy, often coexist. Pulmonary and pleural lymphatics are dilated, and longstanding venous hypertension may lead to oedema and fibrosis.

A further distinct pathological entity is PCH, characterized by the presence of numerous foci of proliferating, congested, thin-walled capillaries, which invade alveolar tissue, as well as the pleural, bronchial, and vascular tissue.

Pathogenesis

The process of pulmonary vascular remodelling described above involves proliferation of smooth muscle cells, fibroblasts, and endothelial cells in the vessel wall (Fig. 15.2.3). Endothelial dysfunction contributes to the pathogenesis of PAH, manifesting as an increase in the release of vasoconstrictors and a deficiency of endogenous vasodilators. Initially, there is an increased tendency towards endothelial cell apoptosis, though clonal survival of endothelial cells may lead to the plexiform lesions seen in severe PAH. The increase in medial and adventitial thickness and cell number may result from increased proliferation, but also from migration of precursor cells from within the vessel wall, the surrounding interstitium, and from circulating progenitor cells. At least in some forms of PAH, increased vasoreactivity may precede the structural changes in the vessels.

A number of mediators and growth factors have been shown to be involved in driving the cellular changes (Fig. 15.2.4). Increased circulating and local pulmonary vascular expression of endothelin-1 is observed in patients with PAH. As well as being a potent vasoconstrictor, endothelin stimulates smooth muscle and fibroblast proliferation via the endothelin A (ET_A) and/or endothelin B (ET_B) receptors, the expression of which is increased in small hypertensive pulmonary arteries—ET_B receptors on the endothelium mediating endothelin-1 clearance as well as release of nitric oxide and prostacyclin. Circulating levels of serotonin (5HT) are also elevated in PAH, and the known association of severe PAH with appetite-suppressant drugs of the fenfluramine/dexfenfluramine group is thought to be partly due to increased serotonergic signalling by metabolites of these drugs. Serotonin stimulates mitogenesis of vascular cells via serotonin receptors, including the $5HT_{2A}$, $5HT_{2B}$, and $5HT_{1B}$ receptors. In human pulmonary artery smooth muscle cells, a major proliferative pathway involves activation of mitogen-activated protein kinases via the serotonin transporter, increased expression of which is found in hypertensive arteries.

A relative deficiency of vasodilator pathways is observed in severe PAH, leading to an imbalance that enhances the activity of mitogenic and vasoconstrictor pathways. Patients with PAH produce less endothelial-derived prostacyclin. They also exhibit reduced expression of nitric oxide synthase in their small pulmonary arteries, and consequently less nitric oxide release. More recent studies have also shown a deficiency of the neuropeptide vasodilator

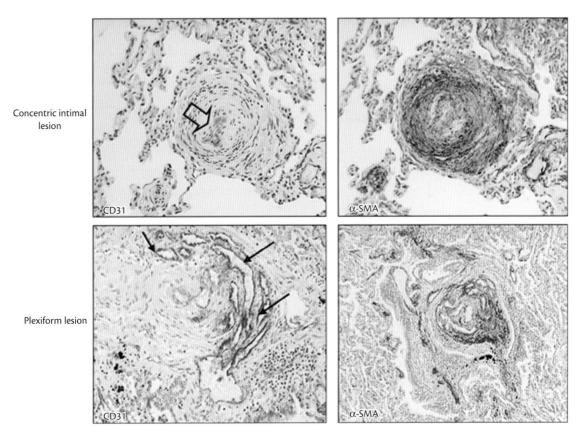

Fig. 15.2.2 Representative images of vascular lesions in idiopathic PAH immunostained for the endothelial marker CD31, or the smooth muscle cell marker α-smooth muscle specific actin (α-SMA). In concentric intimal lesions, a single layer of cells adjacent to the vascular lumen stains for CD31 (upper left panel, open arrow), with concentric layers of cells comprising the vascular wall staining for α-SMA (upper right panel). In plexiform lesions, CD31 stains a single layer of cells lining endothelial channels (lower left panel, arrows), with the supporting stroma staining for α-SMA (lower right panel).

From Atkinson C, *et al.* Primary pulmonary hypertension is associated with reduced pulmonary vascular expression of type II bone morphogenetic protein receptor. *Circulation,* **105**, 1672–8.

vasoactive intestinal polypeptide (VIP) in the lungs of patients with PAH. Many of these important vasodilator pathways also exert antiproliferative effects on smooth muscle cells and fibroblasts via production of the cyclic nucleotides cAMP and cGMP. Deficiency of these key vasodilator pathways has provided the rationale for

many of the new therapies that have emerged over the past two decades (see 'Newer agents').

Another important pathway involved in the process of pulmonary vascular remodelling includes loss of potassium channel (Kv1.5 and Kv2.1) expression and function, promoting smooth muscle cell

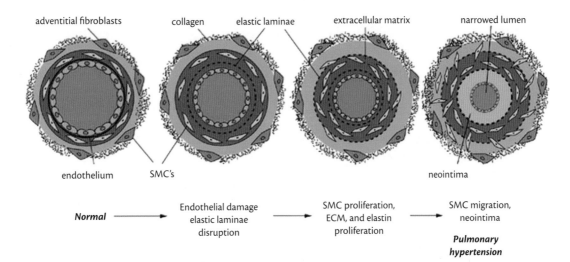

Fig. 15.2.3 Cellular mechanisms of pulmonary vascular remodelling. ECM, extracellular matrix; SMC, smooth muscle cell.

By Hughes, J.B.M. From *Pulmonary circulation: Basic mechanisms to clinical practice* (2001). With permission of Imperial College Press.

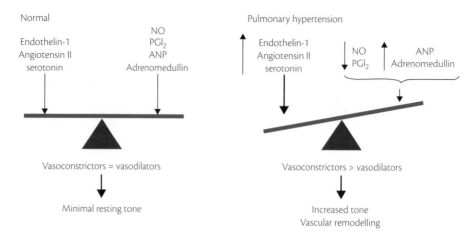

Fig. 15.2.4 An imbalance of pulmonary vascular vasodilators and vasoconstrictors contributes to the vascular constriction and remodelling in pulmonary hypertension. ANP, atrial natriuretic peptide; NO, nitric oxide; PGI$_2$, prostacyclin.

contraction and survival. Activation of vascular elastases within the vessel media and disruption of the elastic laminae is also a key step in disease pathogenesis. Inflammatory cells may also contribute, especially in PAH associated with autoimmune conditions, accompanied by increased expression of inflammatory cytokines and chemokines in small pulmonary arteries.

Pathological studies have identified the presence of thrombosis in small pulmonary arteries of patients with PAH. It is not clear whether this represents *in situ* thrombosis as a consequence of the reduced blood flow, or embolic phenomena. Platelet dysfunction has also been recognized in PAH, and an increased frequency of antiphospholipid antibodies associated with an increased thrombotic risk.

The identification of mutations in the BMPR-II receptor has highlighted the important role of the TGFβ superfamily in the pathogenesis of familial PAH. Most mutations lead to a reduction in a critical signalling pathway, the Smad pathway, downstream of BMP receptors. This, in turn, leads to the failure of BMPs to activate transcription of important target genes. In smooth muscle cells, BMPR-II mutation leads to a failure of the normal growth suppressive and proapoptotic effects of bone morphogenetic proteins, favouring excessive pulmonary artery smooth muscle cell proliferation and survival (Fig. 15.2.5). In endothelial cells, by contrast, BMPR-II mutation promotes endothelial dysfunction and endothelial cell apoptosis. The combination of endothelial cell dysfunction and smooth muscle cell proliferation within the pulmonary circulation favours the development of vascular obliterative lesions and pulmonary hypertension. Clonal expansion of apoptosis-resistant endothelial cells may contribute to the formation of plexiform lesions. However, this simple model does not

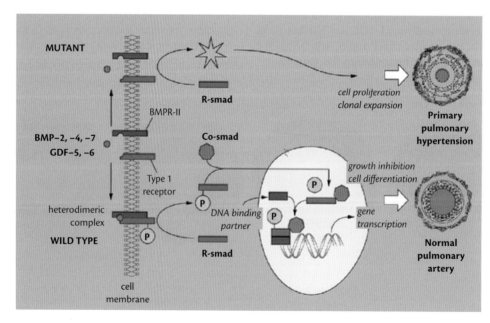

Fig. 15.2.5 The potential role of mutations in the bone morphogenetic protein type II receptor (BMPR-II) in familial PAH. The wild-type receptor signals in response to ligands by activating receptor-regulated Smad proteins (R-Smads), which dimerize with common partner Smads (Co-Smads) to regulate gene expression in the vascular cell. Mutation in BMPR-II disrupts Smad signalling and leads to abnormal vascular cell proliferation. BMP, bone morphogenetic protein; GDF, growth differentiation factors.
By Hughes, J.B.M. From *Pulmonary circulation: Basic mechanisms to clinical practice* (2001). With permission of Imperial College Press.

explain all of the features of heritable PAH. In particular, it does not explain why disease is confined to the lung circulation, while BMPR-II is widely expressed in many tissues. In addition, it does not explain why the presence of the mutation is not sufficient on its own to cause disease, with gene penetrance as low as 20% in some families. These observations indicate that additional environmental and/or genetic factors are necessary for disease manifestation. This putative 'second hit' may further impact on BMP signalling pathways, leading to a critical reduction in bone morphogenetic signalling via Smad proteins and initiation of the process of pulmonary vascular remodelling.

Although mutations in BMPR-II are not generally found in most secondary forms of PAH, it is now becoming clear that dysfunction of the BMPR-II pathway is involved in their pathogenesis. Further research is likely to reveal further clues to the involvement of this important pathway in vascular disease.

Clinical features

Symptoms

The three main presenting symptoms are dyspnoea, chest pain, and syncope. The severity of symptoms is related to prognosis. A modified New York Heart Association (NYHA) score is a useful way to assess symptom severity and follow response to treatment (Box 15.2.1).

Unexplained breathlessness on exertion should always raise the possibility of PAH, particularly in the setting of conditions known to be associated with pulmonary hypertension (Table 15.2.1). The condition may have an insidious onset: frequently, there is a delay of up to 3 years between the onset of first symptoms and diagnosis. Syncope is an ominous sign, usually reflecting severe right ventricular dysfunction. Other symptoms include lassitude, abdominal swelling from ascites, and ankle swelling. Small haemoptyses may occur at later stages.

Clinical signs

Tachypnoea may be present, even at rest. Peripheral cyanosis is common due to a low cardiac output. Central cyanosis occurs later

---

Box 15.2.1 Modified New York Heart Association functional classification of pulmonary hypertension

- Class I—pulmonary hypertension without resultant limitation of physical activity. Ordinary physical activity does not cause undue dyspnoea or fatigue, chest pain, or near syncope

- Class II—pulmonary hypertension resulting in slight limitation of physical activity. The patient is comfortable at rest. Ordinary physical activity causes undue dyspnoea or fatigue, chest pain, or near syncope

- Class III—pulmonary hypertension resulting in marked limitation of physical activity. The patient is comfortable at rest. Less than ordinary activity causes undue dyspnoea or fatigue, chest pain, or near syncope

- Class IV—Pulmonary hypertension with inability to carry out any physical activity without symptoms. These patients manifest signs of right heart failure. Dyspnoea and/or fatigue may be present at rest. Discomfort is increased by any physical activity

---

as pulmonary gas exchange deteriorates or right-to-left shunting occurs through a patent foramen ovale. The jugular venous pulse may be elevated with a prominent 'a' wave, reflecting the increased force of atrial contraction, or—if tricuspid regurgitation is present—there may be a large 'V' wave. There may be a right ventricular heave and a pulsatile liver. On auscultation, forceful closure of the pulmonary valve leads to an accentuated pulmonary arterial component of the second heart sound. There are often a third and fourth right heart sound. The murmurs of tricuspid regurgitation (systolic) or pulmonary regurgitation (diastolic) may be heard. Jaundice, ascites, and peripheral oedema may be present at advanced stages of the disease.

Differential diagnosis

If the symptoms and clinical signs suggest pulmonary hypertension, the differential diagnosis should be considered with reference to the classification in Table 15.2.1. Most importantly, the presence of left heart disease, parenchymal lung disease, or congenital heart disease should be excluded. Pulmonary hypertension due to chronic thromboembolic disease is important to detect because specific surgical treatment is available. Idiopathic PAH remains a diagnosis of exclusion.

Clinical investigation

The investigation of a patient with suspected pulmonary hypertension involves (1) the exclusion of other underlying causes and (2) an assessment of severity of pulmonary hypertension and right heart failure for prognosis and treatment. The investigations that are useful in identifying the aetiology of newly diagnosed, unexplained pulmonary hypertension are listed in Box 15.2.2.

Blood tests

A thrombophilia screen, including antithrombin III, proteins C and S, factor V Leiden, anticardiolipin antibodies, and lupus anticoagulant should be performed, and may reveal clotting abnormalities predisposing to chronic thromboembolic pulmonary hypertension (CTEPH). Thyroid function should be checked since both hypo- and especially hyperthyroidism are commonly reported associations. An autoantibody screen should be performed to exclude underlying autoimmune rheumatic or vasculitic disease: positive antinuclear antibodies (ANA) can be found in 30 to 40% of patients with idiopathic PAH, but a positive test for antineutrophil cytoplasmic antibodies (ANCA) would be uncommon. Since there is an increased incidence of unexplained pulmonary hypertension in HIV-positive patients, this diagnosis should always be considered.

Imaging

The plain chest radiograph shows enlargement of the proximal pulmonary arteries, which may be dramatic, with peripheral pruning of the pulmonary vascular pattern, giving rise to increased peripheral radiolucency. If heart failure is present the heart may be enlarged, with particular enlargement of the right atrium (Fig. 15.2.6). The chest radiograph may also give clues to underlying diagnoses such as interstitial lung disease.

Spiral contrast-enhanced CT will detect proximal pulmonary arterial obstruction suggestive of acute or chronic thromboembolic disease (Fig. 15.2.7). A pattern of mosaic perfusion of the lung parenchyma is also a feature of CTEPH, and may be the only sign

Box 15.2.2 Investigation of the patient with suspected idiopathic pulmonary hypertension

Blood tests

- Full blood count/film/differential
- Hb electrophoresis
- Urea and electrolytes
- Liver function including gamma GT
- Thyroid function
- Thrombophilia screen:
  - Antithrombin III
  - Protein C
  - Protein S
  - Factor V Leiden
  - Anti-cardiolipin antibody
  - Lupus anticoagulant
- CMV deaff
- Autoantibodies:
  - RhF
  - ANA
  - ENAs
  - AntidsDNA
  - Anticardiolipin IgG and IgM
  - Antism/anti-SCL/anti-SS
  - Complement C3, C4, CH50
  - ANCA
- Serum angiotensin converting enzyme
- Hepatitis screen
- HIV test

Imaging

- Chest radiograph
- Ventilation-perfusion lung scan
- High-resolution and spiral CT
- Pulmonary artery angiography

Lung function

- Pulmonary function tests
- Exercise tests with saturation monitoring
- Arterial blood gases on air

Cardiac function

- ECG
- Echocardiogram
- Diagnostic cardiac catheterization

Miscellaneous

- Urine microscopy
- Abdominal ultrasound—?cirrhosis

in predominantly distal disease (Fig. 15.2.8). A high-resolution CT scan will pick up unsuspected parenchymal abnormalities, such as fibrosis. CT scanning is also useful to indicate more uncommon forms of PAH, such as PVOD, when there may be a degree of mediastinal lymphadenopathy and septal lines in the lung periphery, presumably indicating lymphatic and venous obstruction (Fig. 15.2.9).

On ventilation–perfusion lung scanning, the pattern of ventilation is usually normal in idiopathic PAH, and uneven ventilation should suggest underlying lung disease. The pattern of perfusion is also virtually normal, although small patchy perfusion defects may be present. This is in contrast to the appearance in CTEPH when segmental or larger perfusion defects persist, often indistinguishable from the pattern of acute pulmonary embolism (Fig. 15.2.10).

Pulmonary artery angiography is really only required if the diagnosis is likely to be CTEPH, in which situation angiography will provide precise anatomical information regarding the location of vascular obstruction, indicated by abrupt cut-off of vessels or intravascular webs, that may be of great use if surgical endarterectomy is being contemplated. However, CT pulmonary angiography or MR angiography may be employed in place of conventional angiography.

The main contribution of MRI is in the assessment of patients with suspected intracardiac shunts or with anomalous vascular anatomy, e.g. if a shunt is suspected on the basis of right heart catheterization but cannot be demonstrated by echocardiography. MRI can also provide further pulmonary angiographic images.

Pulmonary function tests

The typical pattern for standard pulmonary function test for disease confined to the pulmonary circulation is to find normal lung

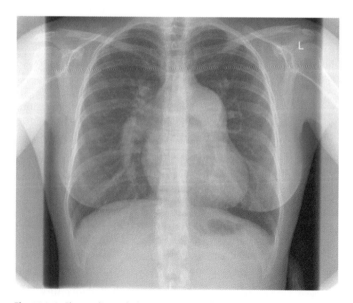

Fig. 15.2.6 Chest radiograph demonstrating cardiomegaly with dilated right heart chambers and dilatation of the proximal pulmonary arteries in a patient with PAH secondary to an atrial septal defect.

Courtesy of Dr Nick Screaton, Addenbrooke's Hospital.

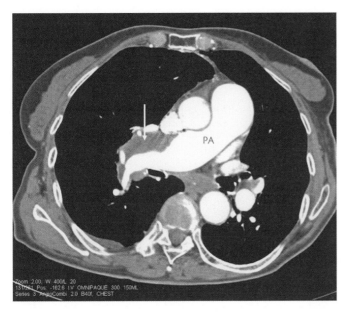

Fig. 15.2.7 Image from a CT pulmonary angiogram at the level of the right main pulmonary artery demonstrating dilatation of the main pulmonary artery (PA) with laminated thrombus in the distal right pulmonary artery (arrow) in keeping with proximal CTEPH.

Courtesy of Dr Nick Screaton, Addenbrooke's Hospital.

volumes; normal forced expiratory volume in 1 s (FEV_1)/vital capacity (VC) ratio (>0.75), indicating no airflow obstruction; and low transfer factor (diffusing capacity, TLco), and low transfer coefficient (Kco).

The low diffusing capacity probably results from a combination of a reduced cardiac output and disease affecting the small arterioles, thereby reducing local perfusion. Additional findings in the pulmonary function tests—such as marked airflow obstruction (e.g. severe chronic obstructive pulmonary disease) or a restrictive

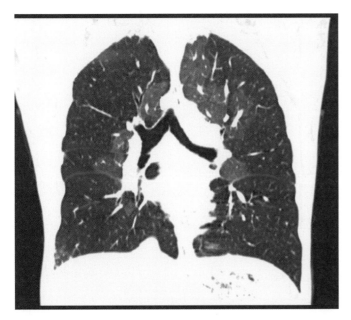

Fig. 15.2.8 Coronal multiplanar reconstruction demonstrating extensive mosaic perfusion in both lungs in a patient with CTEPH.

Courtesy of Dr Nick Screaton, Addenbrooke's Hospital.

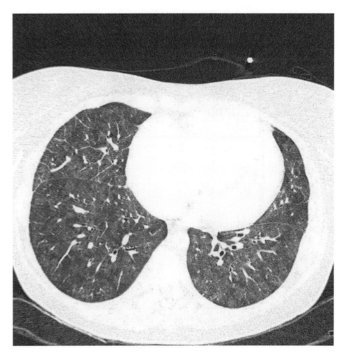

Fig. 15.2.9 Transverse CT image through the lower zones demonstrating heterogeneous attenuation of the lung parenchyma, centrilobular ground-glass opacities, and smooth thickening of the interlobular septa in a patient with pathologically proven veno-occlusive disease.

Courtesy of Dr Nick Screaton, Addenbrooke's Hospital.

defect (e.g. pulmonary fibrosis)—would indicate the presence of an underlying cause for the pulmonary hypertension. However, subtle changes in lung volumes and mild airflow obstruction have been reported in a few patients with PAH. In some groups of patients at high risk of developing PAH, e.g. in scleroderma, the low transfer coefficient can be monitored at intervals, with breathlessness accompanied by a fall in the low transfer coefficient sometimes being the first sign of this complication.

Exercise testing

Significant PAH is always associated with a reduced exercise capacity, one of the most useful tests of this being the 6 min walk test, with monitoring of heart rate and oxygen saturation. This can readily be repeated to assess patients over time and as a measure of response to treatment. A normal distance is more than 500 m, with a low 6 min walk predictive of a poor survival.

Full cardiopulmonary exercise testing is technically more demanding to perform and is only recommended if the diagnosis is in doubt, e.g. if there was a need to document cardiovascular limitation on exercise. Peak oxygen uptake on exercise is low and the anaerobic threshold is reduced to about 40% of normal. There is excessive ventilation for a given degree of oxygen consumption or CO_2 output, even at rest. There is no ventilatory impairment when underlying lung disease is absent. There is often a pronounced tachycardia at submaximal exercise, and usually arterial oxygen desaturation.

ECG

In symptomatic PAH, the ECG is abnormal in 80 to 90% of cases, but it has inadequate sensitivity (55%) and specificity (70%) as a screening tool for detecting pulmonary hypertension. The typical appearances are right-axis deviation (more than + 120°) in

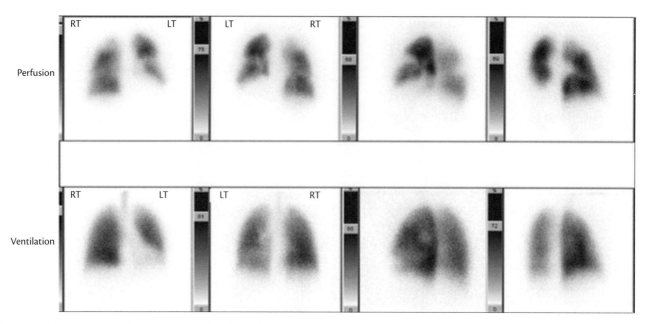

Fig. 15.2.10 Perfusion scintigram demonstrates multiple perfusion defects in a patient with CTEPH.
Courtesy of Dr Nick Screaton, Addenbrooke's Hospital.

the limb leads, and a dominant R wave and T wave inversion in the right precordial leads, accompanied by a dominant S wave in the left precordial leads, suggesting right ventricular hypertrophy (Fig. 15.2.11). Tall, peaked P waves in the right precordial and inferior leads denote right atrial enlargement. Right bundle branch block is common.

Echocardiography

Echocardiography remains the best screening test for significant pulmonary hypertension. It detects the presence, and direction,

of intracardiac shunts. Usually this is possible using conventional transthoracic techniques, but if visualization is poor or a small shunt is still suspected, then transoesophageal echocardiography may be necessary. In addition, the left ventricle can be assessed to determine whether there is a contribution from left ventricular systolic or diastolic dysfunction to elevated pulmonary arterial pressure. The function of the right side of the heart can also be assessed qualitatively and quantitatively. Atrial and ventricular dimensions and wall thickness can be measured, and paradoxical bowing of the intraventricular septum into the left ventricular

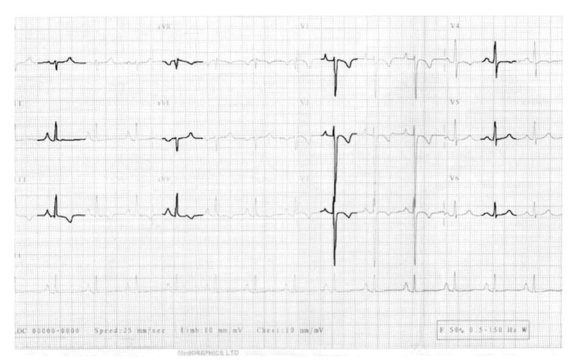

Fig. 15.2.11 12-lead ECG from a patient with idiopathic PAH showing a rightward axis, p pulmonale, poor R wave progression and ST segment changes indicative of right ventricular strain in the anterior chest leads.

cavity may be seen during systole as a consequence of greatly elevated right-sided pressures. Continuous-wave Doppler echocardiography is used to measure high-flow velocities across cardiac valves, one of the most commonly derived indices in the right heart being the pulmonary artery systolic pressure estimated by Doppler echocardiography from measurement of the velocity of the tricuspid regurgitant jet (c.80% of patients with PAH and 60% of normal subjects, have measurable tricuspid regurgitation). The maximum flow velocity (v) of the regurgitant jet is measured and inserted into the modified Bernoulli equation for convective acceleration pressure change, giving an estimate of right ventricular systolic pressure (RVSP):

$$RVSP = 4v^2 + RAP$$

where RAP is right atrial pressure, which can be estimated clinically from the height of the jugular venous pressure. In the absence of pulmonary valve stenosis, the right ventricular systolic pressure is equal to the pulmonary artery systolic pressure (PASP). There is a reasonable correlation between Doppler estimates of PASP and catheter measurements. Newer echocardiographic techniques such as three-dimensional echo and tissue Doppler are being evaluated.

Right heart catheterization

Right heart catheterization remains the best technique for confirming the diagnosis of pulmonary hypertension and for providing important prognostic information. An elevated mean pulmonary arterial pressure of greater than 25 mmHg at rest, or 30 mmHg on exercise, is the accepted definition. In patients with idiopathic PAH the mean pulmonary arterial pressure may exceed 60 mmHg. The pulmonary capillary wedge pressure (PCWP) can also be determined at catheterization, which is an approximation of left atrial pressure. An elevated PCWP (>15 mmHg) generally indicates left heart disease, but can also be elevated in PVOD. Measurement of PCWP is often unreliable in the presence of CTEPH. Sampling of venous blood oxygen saturation as the catheter passes down from the right atrium to right ventricle may detect a sudden 'step-up' in oxygenation, which would indicate the presence of a left-to-right shunt. Cardiac output can be determined by thermodilution or the Fick method.

Indicators of right heart failure, and hence poorer prognosis, include (1) an elevated right atrial pressure (>10 mmHg), (2) an elevated right ventricular end-diastolic pressure (>10 mmHg), (3) a reduced mixed venous oxygen saturation (Svo_2 <63%), and (4) reduced cardiac output (<2.5 litre/min).

Vasoreactivity studies

A subgroup (5–10%) of patients with idiopathic and anorexigen-associated PAH demonstrate a marked reduction in pulmonary vascular resistance following the administration of a vasodilator. These patients are the only group that respond favourably to long-term treatment with vasodilator therapy in the form of calcium channel blockers (see 'Disease-targeted therapies'), and are thus an important group to identify. Vasodilator studies are undertaken at the time of right heart catheterization, the preferred agent being inhaled nitric oxide, or an intravenous infusion of prostacyclin or adenosine. A positive response is defined as a fall in mean pulmonary arterial pressure of at least 10 mmHg to below 40 mmHg, accompanied by an increase or no change in cardiac output.

Conventional treatments

All patients with suspected severe PAH are best referred to a specialist centre for initial assessment and treatment. A multidisciplinary team approach to planning treatment is preferred, with input from respiratory physicians and cardiologists, transplant physicians and cardiothoracic surgeons, radiologists, specialist nurses, and palliative care specialists. Assisting patients to adapt to the uncertainty associated with chronic, life-shortening disease is essential if they are to successfully adjust to the demands of their illness and its treatment. The overall aims are to improve symptoms and quality of life, increase exercise capacity, and improve prognosis.

Supportive medical therapy

Patients with right heart failure and fluid retention may require diuretics. Decreasing cardiac preload with diuretics is often enough to alleviate episodes of right heart failure. However, caution should be exercised because faced with a reduction in vascular filling pressures, patients with severe PAH will not be able to increase cardiac output effectively, which may result in systemic hypotension and syncope.

Antiarrhythmics may be required for sustained or paroxysmal atrial fibrillation. Patients with severe PAH are prone to this complication because of stretching of the overloaded right atrium, and atrial fibrillation can significantly compromise the already reduced cardiac output in patients with PAH, hence it should be treated aggressively. Rate control with digoxin is possible, but if not contraindicated, pharmacological cardioversion with amiodarone is preferable. Electrophysiological mapping of arrhythmias and ablation of arrhythmogenic pathways may be indicated in selected patients.

Anticoagulation

Warfarin therapy to maintain the international normalized ratio (INR) between 2 and 3 is recommended in all patients with idiopathic and familial PAH. Two retrospective studies and one small prospective study have demonstrated a survival benefit of anticoagulation, almost doubling survival rate in idiopathic PAH over a 3 year period. The consensus is that patients with PAH associated with autoimmune rheumatic tissue disease should also receive warfarin, unless contraindicated. The risk–benefit ratio of anticoagulation in other forms of PAH is undetermined.

Oxygen therapy

Oxygen therapy is indicated for symptomatic relief of breathlessness. There are no published trials of the benefit of long-term oxygen therapy in hypoxaemic patients with PAH. Nocturnal oxygen has been shown to be of no benefit in Eisenmenger's syndrome. Ambulatory oxygen may be beneficial if there is evidence of correctable desaturation of 4% and to less than 90% during a 6 min walk test. Consideration should be given to in-flight supplemental oxygen for air travel.

Disease-targeted therapies

Calcium channel blockers

Patients with idiopathic PAH and a documented acute vasodilator response at cardiac catheterization, as defined above, should be offered long-term treatment with a calcium channel blocker. This is associated with very significant improvement in symptoms and prognosis in this subset of patients, although only 50% of those who respond in the cardiac catheterization laboratory will maintain a long-term response. Long-term responders account for less than 5% of idiopathic PAH patients.

Calcium channel blockers should be avoided in any patient with significant signs of right ventricular failure, or until this is controlled, because of their negative inotropic effects. For this reason, and the risk of systemic hypotension, calcium channel blockers should not be prescribed without confirmation of a vasodilator response at cardiac catheterization: indiscriminate prescribing will lead to increased mortality in the PAH population. Treatment should be started in hospital, using diltiazem, amlodipine, or nifedipine, and carefully titrated against systemic blood pressure. The aim is to increase the dose to the maximum tolerated.

Newer agents

In recent years, remarkable advances have been made in the availability of therapeutic agents for PAH. In the early 1980s, carefully timed heart–lung transplantation was the only option known to improve prognosis. We now have a range of pharmacological agents available and licensed for treatment in this condition, based on data from clinical trials that have almost exclusively recruited patients with idiopathic and anorexigen-associated PAH, although often including a subset of patients with PAH associated with systemic sclerosis. The drugs are used to reduce pulmonary vascular resistance and improve cardiac output: they all improve exercise performance and some prolong life. Figure 15.2.12 presents an algorithm summarizing the pharmacological approach to treating PAH, based on current recommendations.

Prostanoids

Epoprostenol was the first treatment to be developed for the treatment of PAH during the 1980s. This has minimal oral bioavailability, has a half-life in the circulation of less than 2 min, and thus must be given by continuous intravenous infusion. It produces acute haemodynamic effects in some patients; most experience a fall in pulmonary vascular resistance with long-term use even in the absence of acute improvements. These observations support the view that long-term administration of these agents may reverse some of the vascular remodelling, as well as having a vasodilator effect. Epoprostenol has been shown to improve haemodynamics, exercise tolerance, quality of life, and survival in patients in NYHA class III and IV. The dose may have to be increased on a regular basis because of tachyphylaxis, and side effects are usually experienced when starting epoprostenol or when escalating the dose, including jaw pain, cutaneous flushing, nausea, and diarrhoea, as well as myalgias. Acute withdrawal of epoprostenol, e.g. if the infusion pump fails, can causes severe rebound pulmonary hypertension that can be fatal. Recurrent sepsis due to line infection can also be problematic.

Although epoprostenol remains a proven therapy in PAH, the complexity of its administration and the availability of newer oral agents mean that its use tends to be reserved for patients with severe haemodynamic compromise. Stable analogues of prostacyclin have been developed with longer half-lives and improved bioavailability: iloprost can be given by the intravenous or inhalation route; treprostinil can be given subcutaneously or intravenously and is approved for use in patients in NYHA class II, III, and IV.

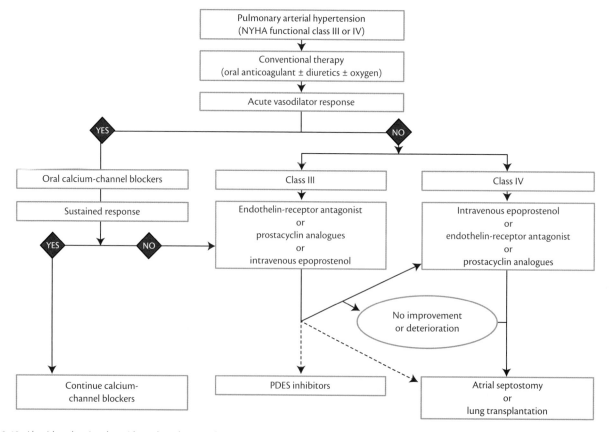

Fig. 15.2.12 Algorithm showing the evidence-based approach to treatment in patients with PAH.

Beraprost is an orally available prostacyclin analogue, although the dose may be limited by gastrointestinal side effects and it is presently only available in Japan.

Endothelin receptor antagonists

Bosentan, an orally active dual-selective ET_A/ET_B receptor antagonist, has been shown to improve exercise capacity, functional class, haemodynamics, echocardiographic, and Doppler variables, and time to clinical worsening in idiopathic PAH. Its most significant side effect is elevation of the hepatic transaminases, which is usually reversible on stopping the drug. Sitaxsentan and ambrisentan are newer ET_A selective agents with similar efficacy to bosentan, though sitaxsentan was recently withdrawn due to reports of irreversible hepatotoxicity. All patients on these agents require monthly monitoring of liver function tests. The United States Food and Drug Authority (FDA) recently approved a new dual-selective ET receptor antagonist, macitentan, for PAH.

Phosphodiesterase inhibitors

Sildenafil is an orally active selective inhibitor of cGMP-phosphodiesterase type 5. It acts by inhibiting the breakdown of cGMP, with vasorelaxant and antiproliferative effects in pulmonary vascular smooth muscle. Sildenafil improves exercise tolerance and pulmonary haemodynamics in short-term studies in PAH. Longer-acting phosphodiesterase (PDE5) inhibitors such as tadalafil also show promise. Tadalafil is a once daily PDE5 antagonist licensed for use in PAH.

Stimulators of soluble guanylate cyclase

Riociguat, a novel stimulator of soluble guanylate cyclase, was recently approved by the FDA for use in patients with PAH and in patients with chronic thromboembolic pulmonary hypertension. Hypotension may limit dosing and the drug should be avoided in combination with a PDE5 inhibitor.

Combination therapy

There is considerable theoretical and experimental evidence to support the use of combinations of the above disease-targeted therapies in PAH, which is a progressive disease. Most patients eventually deteriorate on monotherapy, and the addition of further agents has been shown to provide clinical benefit, although the evidence for precise recommendations is lacking at present.

Other strategies

Atrial septostomy

Atrial septostomy involves creating a right-to-left shunt between the atria, the preferred technique being percutaneous graded balloon dilatation. The rationale for this procedure is that patients with PAH and a patent foramen ovale have improved survival. Creating the shunt reduces right ventricular preload, which relieves the failing right ventricle and can increase cardiac output and improve exercise capacity. The increase in cardiac output is at the expense of a reduction in systemic arterial oxygen saturation, but systemic oxygen delivery is usually improved. The procedure is usually reserved for patients who are failing on maximal medical therapy or as a bridge to transplantation for PAH patients in NYHA class IV. Patient selection is vital. A high right atrial pressure (>20 mmHg) and low arterial oxygen saturation (<80% on air) prior to septostomy are associated with a high mortality related to the procedure, although impact on survival has not been formally assessed.

Transplantation

Transplantation of the lungs or heart and lungs developed as a treatment for endstage PAH during the 1980s. The advent of modern, targeted therapies has reduced the number of patients referred for transplantation, but the long-term outcome of patients who remain in NYHA functional class III or IV remains poor. Lung or heart–lung transplantation therefore remains an important mode of treatment for patients failing medical therapy. Patients with PVOD and PCH have a particularly poor outlook; they respond poorly to available medical therapies and should be referred early for transplantation assessment.

In general, patients presenting with NHYA class IV symptoms should be referred for transplantation assessment at the time of presentation, because their prognosis is poor. Additional indicators of poor prognosis include (1) a 6 min walking distance less than 332 m, (2) peak oxygen consumption less than 10.4 ml/min per kg, (3) cardiac index less than 2 litre/min per m², (4) right atrial pressure greater than 20 mmHg, (5) mean pulmonary arterial pressure greater than 55 mmHg, (6) mixed venous oxygen saturation of less than 63%. Those with significant improvement after 3 months of medical therapy can be removed or suspended from listing for transplant. The choice of procedure varies between centres, but single lung, bilateral lung, and heart–lung transplantation are used in patients with PAH. International registry figures show that the 1 year mortality post-transplantation is highest in patients with idiopathic PAH, compared with any other indication, with median survival post-transplantation between 4 and 5 years.

Prognosis

The prognosis of PAH varies depending on the underlying association or cause. Prognosis is most closely linked to indices of cardiac function, especially cardiac index. Historical data in the period prior to the availability of modern, targeted therapies suggest an expected median survival for idiopathic pulmonary arterial hyper tension between 2.5 and 4 years, and a 3 year survival of about 60%. The prognosis is worse for patients with underlying systemic sclerosis, autoimmune rheumatic disease, HIV disease, and anorexigen-associated PAH, and that for patients surviving to adulthood with PAH associated with a congenital intracardiac defect is substantially better than patients with idiopathic disease. At least in patients with idiopathic PAH, targeted therapies seem to improve survival to some extent, though definitive studies are awaited. Women with severe PAH should be advised that pregnancy carries a very high mortality because of the associated increased burden on the right heart.

Other conditions associated with pulmonary hypertension

One of the commonest causes of pulmonary hypertension is that occurring as a complication of chronic lung disease including interstitial lung disease and chronic obstructive pulmonary disease (COPD). In COPD, pulmonary hypertension is due to a combination of hypoxic pulmonary vasoconstriction, hypoxia-driven pulmonary vascular remodelling, and a reduction in capillary cross-sectional area in emphysema. Lung hyperinflation and polycythaemia may also contribute. The prevalence of pulmonary hypertension in patients with severe COPD may be as high as 50%, but the average mean pulmonary arterial pressure is of the order of 25 mmHg and progresses slowly (<1 mmHg/year). It is likely that ventilatory impairment due to obstructed airways contributes most to the exercise limitation in these patients. Nevertheless, there are relatively unusual cases of COPD in which the pulmonary hypertension dominates. Patients with combined pulmonary fibrosis and emphysema (CPFE) are particularly prone to develop severe pulmonary hypertension. These patients are often profoundly hypoxic, have emphysema with variable degrees of fibrosis on CT scanning, and demonstrate a low DL_{CO}. Severe pulmonary hypertension in the setting of chronic lung disease is defined as a mean pulmonary arterial pressure of 35 mmHg or more, or 25 mmHg or more with low cardiac index (<2.0 litres min^{-1} m^{-2}). In these patients targeted therapy for PAH may be indicated in addition to optimization of their lung disease medication.

Pulmonary hypertension is detectable in some 5% of patients with sarcoidosis. This may develop in the context of endstage pulmonary fibrosis, but may also present as an isolated sarcoid vasculopathy in patients with relatively little parenchymal lung involvement. A falling DL_{CO} in the face of preserved lung volumes may be the first clue to this in a sarcoid patient with worsening dyspnoea. In patients with vasculopathy, there may be a marked response to immunosuppression with prednisolone, which is worth trying before embarking on targeted PAH therapy.

It is often stated that the commonest worldwide cause of pulmonary hypertension is schistosomiasis. When one considers how many patients are infected with schistosomiasis, this may be true, but true prevalence figures are hard to come by. The clinical picture in schistosomiasis is usually dominated by the effect on the urinary tract (*Schistosoma haematobium*) or liver (*S. mansoni* and *S. japonica*). Pulmonary hypertension is thought to be due to granulomata in or adjacent to pulmonary arterioles caused by the reaction to the presence of schistosome eggs.

Likely future developments

The next few years will see further important advances in our understanding of the pathobiology of PAH. Intensive research into the TGFβ/BMP signalling pathway in pulmonary vascular cells and tissues should elucidate the mechanisms by which mutation in the *BMPR2* gene leads to PAH. This knowledge will allow the development of new therapies aimed at prevention, arrest, or reversal of the process of pulmonary vascular remodelling in PAH. Already trials are under way to explore the impact of growth factor inhibition in PAH, and the next few years is likely to see more of these experimental studies using drugs initially developed for use in oncology. Cell-based therapy using circulating progenitor cells is also being evaluated. New pathways are being targeted which impact on ion channels, cell survival, and endothelial function, including drugs such as statins and activators of the peroxisome proliferator-activated receptors. Novel biomarkers of disease activity and progression are being identified. Imaging modalities using the latest advances in echocardiography, CT scanning, and MRI are being developed to maximize the information derived from these techniques, which may then replace invasive right heart catheterization.

Chronic thromboembolic pulmonary hypertension (CTEPH)

Pathogenesis

CTEPH occurs when a clot fails to resolve completely after an acute pulmonary embolic event. The rate of resolution of clots after acute pulmonary embolism varies and is longer in patients with pre-existing cardiopulmonary disease, but normal perfusion should be restored by 4 to 6 weeks after an acute event. To some extent, the rate of resolution depends on the initial clot burden or the size of the acute pulmonary embolism. If the clot fails to resolve, it becomes organized before it can be completely fibrinolysed, and this organized thrombus is incorporated into the wall of the pulmonary artery, becomes covered by endothelial cells, and forms a false intima. The organized material occludes the vascular lumen, which increases pulmonary vascular resistance and leads to pulmonary hypertension.

The true prevalence of CTEPH is hard to ascertain, because it is not usually sought in patients who are recovering from acute pulmonary embolism, but it is almost certainly underdiagnosed. One well-designed study found that 4% of patients with a history of acute pulmonary embolism had a persistent elevation of pulmonary arterial pressure after 2 years. Those with a higher initial clot burden (massive pulmonary embolism) are more likely to develop CTEPH than those with minor pulmonary embolism. The more widespread use of thrombolysis for acute pulmonary embolism is often assumed to reduce the prevalence of CTEPH, but no data at present support this view.

It is of note that some of the classic risk factors for acute deep vein thrombosis (DVT)/pulmonary embolism are not found with increased frequency in the population that develops CTEPH. For example, the factor V Leiden polymorphism, which leads to activated protein C resistance and is found with high prevalence in the population of patients with acute DVT, is not overrepresented in patients with CTEPH. By contrast, the prevalence of protein C and S deficiency is increased in patients with CTEPH, but these conditions account for only a small minority of patients. In addition, some 10% of patients with CTEPH may have circulating antiphospholipid antibodies. Recent research points to a deficiency in the ability to fibrinolyse established clots as a predisposing factor. Other important predisposing factors include previous splenectomy and inflammatory bowel disease.

Clinical presentation

Patients often present with persistent symptoms of dyspnoea after an acute embolic event despite the recommended period of anticoagulation, up to 60% having a prior documented episode of previous venous thromboembolism, although some patients may present with gradually worsening dyspnoea in the absence of acute events. On physical examination, there may be pulmonary flow murmurs resulting from turbulent flow across partially obstructed large pulmonary arteries: these are audible on chest auscultation in up to 30% of patients with CTEPH. Otherwise, the clinical presentation is similar to that described above for PAH.

Investigation

The work-up of patients referred with a suspected diagnosis of CTEPH requires a multidisciplinary approach involving surgeons, physicians, and radiologists. Imaging plays a key role in determining whether a patient is suitable for the surgical procedure of choice, pulmonary endarterectomy. CT pulmonary angiography with modern multislice scanners is a rapid and noninvasive technique that can provide several important pieces of information in the assessment of patients with suspected CTEPH, both assessing the presence of any associated lung disease or tumours, and most importantly giving an accurate assessment of the extent of proximal organized clots (Fig. 15.2.7). Although occlusion of very small arteries cannot be visualized directly in the case of predominantly distal disease, the characteristic appearance of 'mosaic perfusion' suggests the presence of peripheral disease (Fig. 15.2.8), and ventilation–perfusion lung scans also usually show multiple segmental perfusion defects not matched by defects in ventilation in this circumstance (Fig. 15.2.10). CT can also reveal the extent of right ventricular hypertrophy and dilatation, although this is probably best seen by MRI. Three-dimensional reconstruction of the two-dimensional CT and MR images can help decide whether the distribution of disease is suitable for pulmonary endarterectomy. The use of a combination of these techniques means that the more invasive traditional pulmonary angiogram can be avoided in most patients.

Treatment

About 60% of cases of CTEPH is potentially suitable for surgery. Of the patients who are not suitable for surgical management, many may be suitable for targeted therapy with the new pharmacological agents described previously for PAH.

Pulmonary endarterectomy involves removal of organized thrombi from the proximal pulmonary arteries. The procedure is a major operation that usually requires the patient to undergo repeated cycles of cardiopulmonary bypass with cerebral cooling, which ensures a bloodless field of view for the surgeon, who can then enter the left and right main pulmonary arteries via an arteriotomy. The aim is to identify a dissection plane along the base of the false intima and to dissect distally as far as possible, when it is often possible to remove organized material down to the level of segmental pulmonary arteries (Fig. 15.2.13). With successful clearance of proximal clots the pulmonary vascular resistance can fall dramatically postoperatively, and near normalization of resistance can be achieved in the long term.

There are two main aspects to patient selection for this procedure. Comorbidities are important predictors of perioperative mortality and require careful assessment. A further important consideration is the distribution of the disease, as organized clots need to be anatomically accessible to the surgeon. If the organized material is predominantly of a distal distribution within the pulmonary arteries, i.e. involves subsegmental vessels, there is a high risk that pulmonary vascular resistance will not decrease after the procedure and that the patient will be left with significant pulmonary hypertension.

Despite careful patient selection, the operation is high risk, with perioperative mortality varying between 7% and 20% depending on the experience of the centre. However, in those who survive surgery, the long-term outlook is often excellent after a successful procedure, with marked improvements in exercise capacity, NYHA functional status, and quality of life. To prevent further thromboembolism, patients have an inferior vena cava filter sited prior to the operation and are maintained on lifelong warfarin.

Likely future developments

Much remains unknown about the natural history of CTEPH and the risk factors for failure of resolution of an acute embolic event. Large studies designed to prospectively follow up patients with acute embolism over many years will be necessary to get a clearer picture of the underlying causes. Whether chronic thromboembolic pulmonary embolism always results from embolic phenomena or whether in situ thrombosis also contributes remains uncertain. The distinction between CTEPH leading to occlusion of small peripheral pulmonary arteries and idiopathic PAH can be difficult in some cases, and indeed they may be part of the same spectrum of disease.

Selection of patients likely to respond favourably to surgery can be difficult, and improved imaging or physiological assessments are needed. These, along with advances in anaesthetic technology and surgery, are likely to improve further the already impressive results of surgery. The use of angioplasty for the dilatation of proximal partially occlusive chronic thromboembolic disease is currently being evaluated. The response of inoperable CTEPH to targeted pharmacological therapy has been evaluated recently and has led to the recent approval of riociguat, a stimulator of soluble guanylate cyclase, in CTEPH. We are also likely to see further medical interventions aimed at reducing the incidence of CTEPH after acute pulmonary embolism.

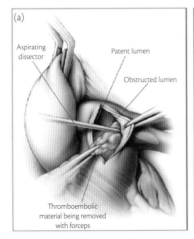
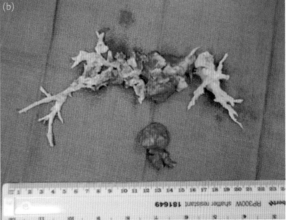

Fig. 15.2.13 The surgical technique of pulmonary endarterectomy (a) and the surgical specimen obtained from a patient undergoing surgery for CTEPH (b).

Further reading

Abenhaim L, *et al.* (1996). Appetite-suppressant drugs and the risk of primary pulmonary hypertension. *N Engl J Med*, **335**, 609–16.

Archibald CJ, *et al.* (1999). Long-term outcome after pulmonary thromboendarterectomy. *Am J Respir Crit Care Med*, **160**, 523–8.

Barst RJ, *et al.* (1994). Survival in primary pulmonary hypertension with long-term continuous intravenous prostacyclin. *Ann Intern Med*, **121**, 409–15.

Barst RJ, *et al.* (1996). A comparison of continuous intravenous epoprostenol (prostacyclin) with conventional therapy for primary pulmonary hypertension. *N Engl J Med*, **334**, 296–301.

Bonderman D, *et al.* (2007). Predictors of outcome in chronic thromboembolic pulmonary hypertension. *Circulation*, **115**, 2153–8.

Deng Z, *et al.* (2000). Familial primary pulmonary hypertension (gene PPH1) is caused by mutations in the bone morphogenetic protein receptor-II gene. *Am J Hum Genet*, **67**, 737–44.

Fedullo PF, *et al.* (2011). Chronic thromboembolic pulmonary hypertension. *Am J Respir Crit Care Med*, **183**, 1605–13.

Fuster V, *et al.* (1984). Primary pulmonary hypertension: natural history and the importance of thrombosis. *Circulation*, **70**, 580–7.

Galie N, *et al.* (2005). Sildenafil citrate therapy for pulmonary arterial hypertension. *N Engl J Med*, **353**, 2148–57.

Galie N, *et al.* (2013). Updated treatment algorithm of pulmonary arterial hypertension. *J Am Coll Cardiol*, **62**, Suppl, D60–D72.

Heath D, Segel N, Bishop J (1966). Pulmonary veno-occlusive disease. *Circulation*, **34**, 242–8.

Heath D (1996). Pulmonary vascular disease. In: Hasleton PS (ed.) *Spencer's pathology of the lung*, pp. 649–93. London: McGraw-Hill.

Higenbottam T, *et al.* (1984). Long-term treatment of primary pulmonary hypertension with continuous intravenous epoprostenol (prostacyclin). *Lancet*, **i**, 1046–7.

Hoeper MM, *et al.* (2002). New treatments for pulmonary arterial hypertension. *Am J Respir Crit Care Med*, **165**, 1209–16.

Hoeper MM, *et al.* (2013). Definitions and diagnosis of pulmonary hypertension. *J Am Coll Cardiol*, 62, Suppl, D42–D50.

Humbert M, *et al.* (2004). Cellular and molecular pathobiology of pulmonary arterial hypertension. *J Am Coll Cardiol*, **43**, Suppl 1, S13–24.

Humbert M, Sitbon O, Simonneau G (2004). Treatment of pulmonary arterial hypertension. *N Engl J Med*, **351**, 1425–36.

International PPH Consortium, *et al.* (2000). Heterozygous germ-line mutations in *BMPR2*, encoding a TGF-β receptor, cause familial primary pulmonary hypertension. *Nat Genet*, **26**, 81–4.

Kay JM, Smith P, Heath D (1971). Aminorex and the pulmonary circulation. *Thorax*, **26**, 262–70.

Loyd JE, Primm RK, Newman JH (1984). Familial primary pulmonary hypertension: clinical patterns. *Am Rev Respir Dis*, 129, 194–7.

Kim NH, *et al.* (2013). Chronic thromboembolic pulmonary hypertension. *J Am Coll Cardiol*, **62**, Suppl, D92–D99.

McGoon MD, *et al.* (2013). Pulmonary arterial hypertension : epidemiology and registries. *J Am Coll Cardiol*, **62**, Suppl, D51–D59.

Moser KM, *et al.* (1983). Chronic thrombotic obstruction of major pulmonary arteries. Results of thromboendarterectomy in 15 patients. *Ann Intern Med*, **99**, 299–304.

Newman JH, *et al.* (2004). Genetic basis of pulmonary arterial hypertension: current understanding and future directions. *J Am Coll Cardiol*, **43**, Suppl 1, S33–39.

Olschewski H, *et al.* (2002). Inhaled iloprost for severe pulmonary hypertension. *N Engl J Med*, **347**, 322–9.

Palevsky HI, *et al.* (1989). Primary pulmonary hypertension: vascular structure, morphometry, and responsiveness to vasodilator agents. *Circulation*, **80**, 1207–21.

Pengo V, *et al.* (2004). Incidence of chronic thromboembolic pulmonary hypertension after pulmonary embolism. *N Engl J Med*, **350**, 2257–64.

Pepke-Zaba J, *et al.* (1991). Inhaled nitric oxide as a cause of selective pulmonary vasodilatation in pulmonary hypertension. *Lancet*, **338**, 1173–4.

Piazza G, Goldhaber SZ (2011). Chronic thromboembolic pulmonary hypertension. *N Engl J Med*, **364**, 351–60.

Rich S, Kaufmann E, Levy PS (1992). The effect of high doses of calcium-channel blockers on survival in primary pulmonary hypertension. *N Engl J Med*, **327**, 76–81.

Rich S, *et al.* (1987). Primary pulmonary hypertension. A national prospective study. *Ann Intern Med*, **107**, 216–23.

Rubin LJ, *et al.* (2002). Bosentan therapy for pulmonary arterial hypertension. *N Engl J Med*, **346**, 896–903.

Rudarakanchana N, *et al.* (2002). Functional analysis of bone morphogenetic protein type II receptor mutations underlying primary pulmonary hypertension. *Hum Mol Genet*, **11**, 1517–25.

Seeger W, *et al.* (2013). Pulmonary hypertension in chronic lung diseases. *J Am Coll Cardiol*, **62**, Suppl, D109–D116.

Simonneau G, *et al.* (2013). Updated clinical classification of pulmonary hypertension. *J Am Coll Cardiol*, **62**, Suppl, D34–D41.

Soubrier F, *et al.* (2013). Genetics and genomics of pulmonary arterial hypertension. *J Am Coll Cardiol*, **62**, Suppl, D13–D21.

Tuder RM, *et al.* (2013). Relevant issues in the pathology and pathobiology of pulmonary hypertension *J Am Coll Cardiol*, **62**, Suppl, D4–D12.

Wagenvoort C, Wagenvoort N (1970). Primary pulmonary hypertension: a pathological study of vessels in 156 clinically diagnosed cases. *Circulation*, **42**, 1163–84.

Venous thromboembolism

CHAPTER 16.1

Deep venous thrombosis and pulmonary embolism

Paul D. Stein, Fadi Matta, and John D. Firth

Essentials

Deep venous thrombosis

Deep venous thrombosis (DVT) is diagnosed in 1 to 2% of hospitalized patients, but is often silent and is found much more frequently at autopsy. Patients typically complain of pain and/or swelling of the leg, but often the diagnosis will be considered only when the physician detects unilateral leg swelling.

Investigation—given the sinister nature of untreated DVT, it is important to confirm or refute the diagnosis with appropriate investigations whenever clinical suspicion is aroused, unless the general condition of the patient makes this inappropriate. Management algorithms have been developed to guide strategy for investigation. These typically use scoring systems to stratify the clinical probability that the particular patient has a DVT (or pulmonary embolism). Those with a low clinical probability proceed to D-dimer testing, with further investigation not pursued if this is negative. Patients with either a high clinical probability, or a low clinical probability but elevated D-dimer, proceed to tests for the presence of thrombus in the leg veins, typically by ultrasonography.

Management—a first episode of proximal DVT, diagnosed by noninvasive testing, should be treated with anticoagulation for 3 months. Longer duration of treatment may be recommended for those whose thrombosis occurred in the absence of a reversible risk factor or in those with a thrombophilic condition or cancer. Treatment is initiated with heparin (low molecular weight or unfractionated) or fondaparinux for ≥5 days and warfarin (or other vitamin K antagonist), with the heparin or fondaparinux stopped when the international normalized ratio (INR) is greater than 2.0 for ≥24 h. There is increasing experience and use of extended therapy with an oral factor Xa inhibitor (rivaroxaban, apixaban, edoxaban) or direct thrombin inhibitor (dabigatran) as alternatives to heparin/warfarin (see Chapter 16.2).

DVT carries extensive morbidity irrespective of pulmonary embolism: severe postphlebitic syndrome occurs in 9% of patients by 5 years.

Pulmonary embolism

Acute pulmonary embolism (PE) is the third most common cardiovascular problem after coronary heart disease and stroke. It is a complication of DVT, with emboli originating in the legs in 80% or more of cases. Immobilization, irrespective of the cause, is the most frequent predisposing factor.

Common symptoms are dyspnoea (c.75%), pleuritic chest pain (c.50%), cough (c.35%), and calf or thigh pain or swelling (c.40%). Circulatory collapse (systolic blood pressure <80 mmHg or loss of consciousness) is an uncommon (8–15%) mode of presentation in patients entered into clinical trials, but likely to be more frequent in routine clinical practice. Tachypnoea (respiratory rate ≥20 cycles/min or greater) is the most common physical sign (50–70%), and abnormalities may be found on respiratory (30–50%) or cardiac (20–30%) examination.

Investigation—algorithms similar to those used to guide management of patients with suspected DVT are used when PE is suspected or needs to be excluded. Patients with a low, 'unlikely', or moderate clinical probability and negative D-dimer are not investigated further. Patients with a high clinical probability, and those with an elevated D-dimer, proceed to tests for the presence of pulmonary emboli, typically by contrast-enhanced spiral CT, perhaps in combination with CT venous phase imaging.

Management—treatment with anticoagulants while awaiting the outcome of diagnostic tests may be appropriate, particularly if the tests cannot be obtained immediately. All patients who are hypoxic should be given supplementary oxygen at high concentration. Anticoagulation is as described for DVT. Thrombolytic therapy is not indicated for routine treatment, but is advised for those who are hypotensive or require ventilatory support.

Inferior vena cava filter—this is recommended for patients with proximal DVT or PE if anticoagulants are contraindicated, PE has recurred while on adequate anticoagulant therapy, or PE is severe and any recurrent PE may be fatal. Administrative data show a lower in-hospital all-cause mortality with vena cava filters in patients with PE if they are haemodynamically unstable (in shock or on ventilatory support), require thrombolytic therapy or pulmonary embolectomy, have solid malignant tumours or chronic obstructive pulmonary disease.

A very few survivors of acute PE develop chronic pulmonary thromboembolic hypertension. Treatment is pulmonary thromboendarterectomy, but only at experienced centres.

Introduction

Deep venous thrombosis (DVT) and pulmonary embolism (PE) are sometimes described together using the term 'thromboembolism'. PE is a complication of DVT, with thrombi in 80% or more of cases originating in the legs. Management strategies of PE have been developed that are based on the diagnosis of either PE or DVT, provided the patient has good respiratory reserve. Treatment with anticoagulants is the same for both. Some physicians believe that patients can be managed better if it is known whether acute PE is present, even if a diagnosis of DVT is already established.

Prognosis of untreated disease

The frequency of fatal PE in patients with untreated DVT has diminished as diagnostic tests have made it possible to diagnose DVT before it becomes extensive. In 1955, prior to the use of sensitive noninvasive tests for the early detection of DVT, the risk of fatal PE in untreated patients with clinically apparent DVT was 37%. Based on a diagnosis by radioactive fibrinogen scintiscans, the risk of fatal PE in patients with untreated DVT, most of which were subclinical, was about 5%.

Early diagnosis has also reduced the risk of death from PE. In the early 1960s the mortality in untreated patients with acute PE, diagnosed on the basis of clinical features, was 26 to 37%, and an additional 36% died of recurrent PE. In 2008, the estimated case fatality rate from acute PE was 6.2%. Among patients in the Prospective Investigation of Pulmonary Embolism Diagnosis (PIOPED) with mild PE who inadvertently escaped treatment, the mortality was 4% to 5%.

Deep venous thrombosis

Incidence and pathology

In 2008, DVT was diagnosed in 1.7% of hospitalized patients aged 18 years or more in the United States of America. This represented 250 patients per 100 000 adult population. The condition is often silent: among patients with DVT detected by screening with ^{125}I-fibrinogen scans, clinical evidence was present in 49%. Proximal DVT was found at autopsy in 22% of patients who died of various causes in a tertiary care hospital.

Thrombosis of the leg veins usually occurs without inflammation. Inflammation of the walls of the veins, when it occurs, is usually secondary to the thrombosis. No clear evidence indicates that inflammation of the veins prevents embolization, or that embolization is more frequent in those patients with thrombi not associated with venous inflammation. The valve pockets are a frequent site of origin of thrombi.

Clinical features

Patients may complain of pain or swelling of the leg, but physical examination remains the means by which attention is usually drawn to the potential diagnosis of DVT. DVT sometimes, but not always, leads to swelling of the leg. If restricted to the popliteal and calf veins, swelling is confined to below the knee, but if thrombosis involves the femoral and pelvic veins (or inferior vena cava), then swelling of the thigh is also expected. A difference of circumference of the calves of 1.0 cm or more, measured 10 cm below the tibial tuberosity, is abnormal. It is important to repeat the measurement of circumference of the calves and thighs at frequent intervals: proximal extension of a thrombus is likely to cause increased swelling, and to allow repeated measurements to be made from a fixed point it is good practice for the position of the first measurement to be marked indelibly on the patient's skin.

Homans' sign is positive when active and/or passive dorsiflexion of the foot associated with any of the following: (1) pain, (2) incomplete dorsiflexion (with equal pressure applied) to prevent pain, or (3) flexion of the knee to release tension in the posterior muscles with dorsiflexion. This sign was present in 44% of patients with DVT of the lower leg, and in 60% of patients with femoral venous thrombosis.

The elicitation of pain with inflation of a blood pressure cuff around the calf to 60 to 150 mm Hg has been recommended as a test for DVT. However, this test has not been shown to be more helpful than the assessment of direct tenderness or leg circumference.

In one study, the sensitivity of oedema, erythema, calf tenderness, palpable cord, or Homans' sign alone, or 1 cm or more calf asymmetry alone was 55 to 80%, but the specificity was only 49%. The combination of one of these signs plus 1 cm or more ipsilateral calf asymmetry increased the specificity to 87%, but decreased the sensitivity to 15 to 33%. The specificity increased to 91% with one of these signs in combination with 2 cm or more calf asymmetry. Only 3 to 10% of patients had one or more qualitative signs plus 3 cm or more ipsilateral calf asymmetry: in these the specificity for DVT was 96%.

Other clinical features of DVT, whose sensitivity and specificity have not been tested, include increased temperature on the affected side, cyanotic discoloration of the limb, and persistent engorgement of superficial veins. Superficial varicose veins almost always empty when the patient lies down: if they remain engorged, this suggests problems with drainage through the deep veins. In very rare cases, tense venous oedema can cause arterial compression and venous gangrene.

Differential diagnosis

The clinical diagnosis of DVT is not always straightforward. Many of the findings described above can also be found in those with muscular strains and bruising, ruptured Baker's cyst or plantaris tendon, superficial thrombophlebitis, cellulitis, and other traumatic conditions. The presence of bruising near either malleolus suggests ruptured Baker's cyst or other cause of calf haematoma.

Given the sinister nature of untreated DVT it is important to confirm or refute (so far as is possible) the diagnosis with appropriate investigations whenever clinical suspicion is aroused, unless the general condition of the patient makes this inappropriate.

Investigation

Detection of evidence of thrombus within the circulation: D-dimer

D-dimer is a specific degradation product released into the circulation by endogenous fibrinolysis of a cross-linked fibrin clot. A D-dimer measured by enzyme-linked immunosorbent assay (ELISA) below a cut-off of 300 to 540 ng/ml (the values differ slightly from one study to another) make the diagnosis of DVT (or PE) unlikely. However, a concentration of D-dimer above the cut-off level is not useful for making a positive diagnosis because of the large number of false-positive tests.

Conventional ELISA assays are cumbersome and not suited for emergency use, which limited the practical utility of D-dimer measurements until the development of rapid ELISA assays. These provide the best balance of sensitivity and specificity among the various assays for the safe diagnostic handling of patients with suspected DVT and PE.

Detection of the physical presence of thrombus in leg veins

The 'gold standard' is contrast venography, but this can be unpleasant for patients, time consuming for radiology departments, and expensive. This has driven the search for acceptable noninvasive methods of diagnosis, and contrast venography is now rarely performed except as part of research protocols.

Contrast venography has been replaced by B-mode ultrasonography as the preferred first-line diagnostic technique. Among patients with DVT proven by contrast venography, B-mode ultrasonography using compression showed a 95% sensitivity in symptomatic patients. In asymptomatic patients who were evaluated because of a high risk of DVT, venous compression ultrasound showed a sensitivity of only 67%. Regarding veins of the calves, venous compression ultrasound was 93% sensitive in symptomatic patients, but only 26% sensitive in asymptomatic high-risk patients subsequently found to have DVT. In all instances, specificity was 97 to 99%.

Venous-phase contrast-enhanced spiral CT is useful for imaging the veins of the pelvis and thighs, particularly in combination with spiral CT pulmonary angiograms. This offers a comprehensive study for thromboembolism, but increases exposure to ionizing radiation. Whether CT pulmonary angiography should routinely be accompanied by CT venography is a matter of controversy. Among patients with suspected PE who were evaluated by 64-detector CT, 10.8% were shown to have PE by CT angiography and an additional 1.3% had venous thromboembolism based on a positive CT venogram with a negative CT angiogram. A 1.3% yield would seem poorly cost effective; however, among the patients shown to have venous thromboembolism, 11% were diagnosed only by CT venography—a proportion that some would consider sufficiently high to merit consideration of its use.

Gadolinium-enhanced magnetic resonance (MR) venography following an intravenous injection was sensitive for DVT in the veins of the thighs and pelvis but often technically inadequate. Specificity in all regions was 95 to 100%. Usage is restricted by cost, availability, and risk of nephrogenic systemic fibrosis/nephrogenic fibrosing dermopathy in patients with poor renal function.

Fibrinogen-uptake radionuclide scanning was used extensively in the 1960s. It is more sensitive for DVT in the calves than in the thighs, meaning that its value is limited because of the greater risk of PE with DVT in the thighs than in the calves.

Strategy for diagnosis

Management algorithms have been developed to identify patients at low risk of DVT who can be spared extensive testing. These algorithms typically use scoring systems to stratify the clinical probability that the particular patient has a DVT and then proceed to D-dimer testing of those with low probability. Patients with a low clinical probability and a negative D-dimer test should not be investigated further for thromboembolic disease. Patients with a high or moderately high clinical probability, or a low clinical probability but elevated D-dimer, proceed to tests for the presence of thrombus in the leg veins, typically by ultrasonography. An example of a pretest scoring system and management algorithm is shown in Table 16.1.1.

Prevention

The prevention of DVT is critical in the prevention of PE. Risk factors for DVT are almost certainly the same as those for PE (see later section in this chapter). Recommendations for the prevention of DVT are shown in Tables 16.1.2–16.1.7. Despite recommendations for the prevention of DVT in hospitalized patients, an increase in secondary DVT in patients hospitalized in the United States of America from 1991 through 2006 suggests that efforts to prevent DVT in high-risk patients are inadequate (Figure 16.1.1). In the

United Kingdom, recognition of such inadequacy has led commissioners of health care to mandate use of a risk scoring tool for venous thromboembolism in all patients admitted to hospital, with the possibility of financial penalties for those that do not achieve a very high rate of compliance.

Treatment

Proximal DVT leads to PE more frequently than DVT confined to the calf. Patients with acute isolated calf vein DVT without severe symptoms or risk for extension can be followed with serial noninvasive testing for 2 weeks without treatment with anticoagulants unless there is extension. Recommendations for treatment are shown in Table 16.1.8, with further details discussed in Chapter 16.2. With generally increasing pressure to avoid hospital admission, or to keep admissions as short as possible, some patients with a primary diagnosis of PE or DVT are being discharged from hospital before adequate heparin can be administered and before vitamin K antagonists can become antithrombotic. An increased mortality has been observed among patients with PE discharged in ≤4 days if inadequately treated. If patients are to be discharged before adequate heparin can be administered, outpatient treatment with low molecular weight heparin (LMWH) for at least 5 days and until the international normalized ratio (INR) is ≥2.0 for 24 hours is recommended, or extended outpatient treatment with LMWH may be considered. Treatment with novel oral anticoagulants (factor Xa or factor IIa inhibitors) is another option.

Complications

DVT itself carries extensive morbidity irrespective of PE. Severe postphlebitic syndrome (venous ulcer or combinations of pain, cramps, heaviness, pruritus, paraesthesia, pretibial oedema, induration, hyperpigmentation, venous ectasia, redness or pain with calf compression) occurs in 9% of patients by 5 years after a 3-month course of treatment with anticoagulants. Randomized controlled trials have shown that elastic compression stockings applied directly after an episode of DVT can reduce the chances of the patient developing postphlebitic syndrome by about 70%, but there is no clear evidence on which to recommend how long such stockings should be worn after an acute episode.

Acute pulmonary embolism

Incidence

Acute PE is the third most common cardiovascular problem after coronary heart disease and stroke. In 2008, 0.9% of patients aged 18 years or more hospitalized in short-stay hospitals in the United States of America had PE. This represented 135 patients per 100 000 adult population. Age-adjusted rates were similar in men and women. Silent PE, on average, was diagnosed in 36% of patients with proximal DVT and 13% with distal DVT. The incidence of acute PE increases exponentially with age and is much more frequent in adults than in children, but it is not rare in children.

In autopsy studies encompassing university as well as nonuniversity hospitals, when the pathologist judged that PE contributed to death or caused death, the diagnosis was unsuspected ante-mortem in over one-half of cases. Some of these were in patients who died of malignancy, in whom a diagnosis of PE may (appropriately) not have been actively pursued. However, the time-honoured point remains as valid today as ever: a high index of suspicion is necessary to reduce the number of patients with unsuspected PE.

Table 16.1.1 Pretest clinical probability scoring system and care pathway for the patient with suspected deep venous thrombosis

(a) Pretest probability score

Criteria	Score
Active cancer	+1
Paralysis, plaster cast	+1
Bed rest >3 days, surgery within 4 weeks	+1
Tenderness along veins	+1
Entire leg swollen	+1
Calf swollen >3 cm	+1
Pitting oedema	+1
Collateral veins	+1
Alternative diagnosis likely	−2

(b) Pretest probability

Low	0
Moderate	1 or 2
High	3 or more

(c) Management algorithm

Pretest probability score	Action	Result	Further action
0 or 1	Perform D-dimer	Negative	No further investigation
		Positive	Perform ultrasonography
2 or more	Do not perform D-dimer		
	Perform ultrasonography	Negative	Withhold treatment and repeat ultrasonography in 10–14 days. If serial ultrasonography is negative, PE rarely occurs
		Positive	Diagnosis of venous thrombosis established

Notes

1. Pretest probability score from Wells *et al.* (1997).

2. This management algorithm is typical of many used, but further prospective evaluation is warranted.

3. If the physician's judgement is that DVT is very likely in a particular case, then they should proceed to investigations directed at detecting thrombus in leg veins whatever the scoring algorithm would suggest. If the result of ultrasonography is negative, and repeat ultrasonography in 10–14 days is also negative, PE rarely occurs.

4. All patients who are discharged with 'DVT excluded' should be given written information describing how they can be reassessed if symptoms worsen or fail to settle over the next few days.

Thromboembolic events have been linked to oestrogen-containing oral contraceptives, but the absolute risk is low and their frequency has been reduced with the use of preparations that contain less than 50 μg of oestrogen. Oral contraceptives may increase the risk of venous thromboembolism after surgery even if their oestrogen content is low.

Predisposing factors

Immobilization, irrespective of the cause, is the most frequent predisposing factor (Table 16.1.9). Immobilization of even 1 or 2 days may predispose to PE and most patients with PE are immobilized less than 2 weeks. Obesity is also a risk factor.

Pregnancy-associated DVT has increased in recent years, the rate being over twice that in nonpregnant women. The rate of DVT following caesarean section is twice the rate following vaginal delivery. By contrast, higher rates of PE have not been shown in pregnancy, but this may be because of reluctance to perform imaging studies in pregnant women.

There has been much interest in the subject of genetic predisposition to thromboembolism. Heterozygosity for the factor V Leiden mutation increases susceptibility three- to eight-fold in a variety of circumstances. Other genetic and acquired thrombophilic factors include protein C deficiency, protein S deficiency, antithrombin deficiency, prothrombin 20 201A, high concentration of factor VIII, hyperhomocystinaemia, heparin cofactor II deficiency, dysfibrinogenaemia, decreased levels of plasminogen, decreased levels

Table 16.1.2 Recommendations for prevention of venous thromboembolism in patients undergoing general, abdominal–pelvic, cardiac, and thoracic surgery

Indication	Recommendation
General and abdominal–pelvic surgery	
Very low risk patients VTE	Early ambulation
Low risk VTE	Mechanical prophylaxis, preferably intermittent pneumatic compression
Moderate-risk VTE, not high risk major bleeding	LMWH or low-dose unfractionated heparin or mechanical prophylaxis, preferably with intermittent pneumatic compression
Moderate-risk VTE, high risk major bleeding	Mechanical prophylaxis, preferably with intermittent pneumatic compression
High-risk VTE, not high risk major bleeding	LMWH or low-dose unfractionated heparin and elastic stockings or intermittent pneumatic compression
High-risk VTE, cancer surgery, not high risk major bleeding	LMWH, 4 weeks
High-risk VTE, high risk major bleeding	Mechanical prophylaxis, preferably with intermittent pneumatic compression. Start LMWH or low-dose unfractionated heparin when risk of bleeding diminishes
Cardiac surgery	
Uncomplicated	Mechanical prophylaxis, preferably with intermittent pneumatic compression
Complicated	LMWH or low-dose unfractionated heparin and mechanical prophylaxis, preferably with intermittent pneumatic compression
Thoracic surgery	
Moderate risk VTE, not high risk bleeding	Low-dose unfractionated heparin or LMWH or intermittent pneumatic compression
High risk VTE, not high risk bleeding	LMWH or low-dose unfractionated heparin and intermittent pneumatic compression or elastic stockings
High risk VTE, high risk bleeding	Mechanical prophylaxis, preferably with intermittent pneumatic compression. Start LMWH or low-dose unfractionated heparin when risk of bleeding diminishes

LMWH, low molecular weight heparin; VTE, venous thromboembolism.

Adapted from Guyatt GH *et al.* (2012). Antithrombotic therapy and prevention of thrombosis, 9th ed. American College of Chest Physicians Evidence-Based Clinical Practice Guidelines. *Chest* **141**(suppl), 7S–47S.

of plasminogen activators, antiphospholipid antibodies, heparin-induced thrombocytopenia, and myeloproliferative disorders. For full discussion of these and related issues, see Chapter 22.6.4.

Clinical features

The clinical characteristics of acute PE have been derived from prospectively acquired data of patients recruited in trials of diagnostic investigations or therapies such as the PIOPED studies. Such trials clearly only include those in whom there was sufficient clinical

suspicion to lead physicians to obtain diagnostic tests: whether subtle PE was overlooked is undetermined. The specificity of signs, symptoms, and ordinary clinical tests was low among patients with suspected PE in whom the diagnosis was eventually excluded.

Symptoms

In patients in whom the diagnosis is not confused by pre-existing cardiac or pulmonary disease, dyspnoea is the most common symptom, occurring in 73% of cases both in PIOPED and PIOPED II (Table 16.1.10), with dyspnoea only on exertion in 16%. Dyspnoea

Table 16.1.3 Recommendations for prevention of venous thromboembolism in patients undergoing orthopaedic surgery

Surgical procedure	Recommendation
Total hip arthroplasty or total knee arthroplasty	LMWH, fondaparinux, apixaban, dabigatran, rivaroxaban, low-dose unfractionated heparin, adjusted-dose vitamin K antagonist, aspirin, or intermittent pneumatic compression for minimum of 10–14 days, preferably up to 35 days. LMWH is the preferred antithrombotic agent. Antithrombotic agent and intermittent pneumatic compression recommended in hospital. Intermittent pneumatic compression only if high risk of bleeding. Suggest against inferior vena cava filter even if contraindication to both pharmacological and mechanical thromboprophylaxis
Hip fracture surgery	LMWH, fondaparinux, low-dose unfractionated heparin, adjusted-dose vitamin K antagonist, aspirin, or intermittent pneumatic compression for minimum of 10–14 days and preferably up to 35 days. LMWH is the preferred antithrombotic agent
Knee arthroscopy, no history of prior venous thromboembolism	No thromboprophylaxis

INR, international normalized ratio; LMWH, low molecular weight heparin; VTE, venous thromboembolism.

Adapted from Guyatt GH *et al.* (2012). Antithrombotic therapy and prevention of thrombosis, 9th ed. American College of Chest Physicians Evidence-Based Clinical Practice Guidelines. *Chest* **141**(suppl), 7S–47S.

Table 16.1.4 Recommendations for prevention of venous thromboembolism in patients undergoing neurosurgery

Surgical procedure	Recommendation
Spinal surgery or craniotomy	
Not high risk VTE	Mechanical prophylaxis, preferably with intermittent pneumatic compression
High risk VTE	Mechanical prophylaxis, preferably with intermittent pneumatic compression and pharmacological prophylaxis after risk of bleeding decreases

LMWH, low molecular weight heparin; VTE, venous thromboembolism.

Adapted from Guyatt GH *et al.* (2012). Antithrombotic therapy and prevention of thrombosis, 9th ed. American College of Chest Physicians Evidence-Based Clinical Practice Guidelines. *Chest* **141**(suppl), 7S–47S.

(at rest or during exertion) and orthopnoea were more frequent in patients with PE in main or lobar pulmonary arteries than in patients in whom the largest vessel with PE was a segmental pulmonary artery. The onset of dyspnoea occurred within seconds or minutes in 72% of cases, and within seconds, minutes, or hours in 83%. In some, however, the onset of dyspnoea occurred over days.

Pleuritic chest pain (66% of patients with PE and no pre-existing cardiopulmonary disease in PIOPED and 44% in PIOPED II) occurred much more often than haemoptysis (13% in PIOPED and 5% in PIOPED II).

Cough was common (37% and 34% in PIOPED and PIOPED II) among patients with PE and no pre-existing cardiopulmonary disease. This was nonproductive or productive of bloody (typically blood-streaked, but it can be pure blood or blood-tinged) or purulent (5% of cases) sputum.

Signs

Tachypnoea (respiratory rate ≥20/min) was the most common sign of acute PE among patients with no prior cardiac or pulmonary disease (70% of patients in PIOPED and 54% in PIOPED II) (Table 16.1.11). Tachycardia (heart rate >100/min) occurred in 30% and 24% of patients with PE in PIOPED and PIOPED II, and

Table 16.1.5 Recommendations for prevention of venous thromboembolism in patients following major trauma, traumatic brain injury, acute spinal cord injury

Indication	Recommendation
Major trauma	LMWH or low-dose unfractionated heparin or mechanical prophylaxis, preferably with intermittent pneumatic compression. Inferior vena cava filter should not be used for primary prevention of VTE
Major trauma, high risk VTE	LMWH or low-dose unfractionated heparin and mechanical prophylaxis. Mechanical prophylaxis only, preferably with intermittent pneumatic compression, if high risk of bleeding. Add LMWH or unfractionated heparin when risk of bleeding diminishes

INR, international normalized ratio; LMWH, low molecular weight heparin. VTE, venous thromboembolism

Adapted from Guyatt GH *et al.* (2012). Antithrombotic therapy and prevention of thrombosis, 9th ed. American College of Chest Physicians Evidence-Based Clinical Practice Guidelines. *Chest* **141**(suppl), 7S–47S.

Table 16.1.6 Recommendations for prevention of venous thromboembolism in patients with medical conditions

Medical conditions in hospital	Recommendation
Acutely ill hospitalized medical patients, low risk VTE	No prophylaxis
Acutely ill hospitalized medical patients, increased risk VTE	Low-dose unfractionated heparin, LMWH or fondaparinux. Compression stockings *or* intermittent pneumatic compression if high risk of bleeding
Critically ill, critical care unit	Low-dose unfractionated heparin or LMWH
Critically ill, critical care unit, high risk bleeding	Compression stockings and/or intermittent pneumatic compression. Pharmacological prophylaxis when risk of bleeding decreases
Chronically immobilized, nursing home or at home	No thromboprophylaxis
Outpatients, solid tumours and additional risk factors for VTE	LMWH or low-dose unfractionated heparin
Outpatients, thrombophillia, no prior VTE	No thromboprophylaxis

LMWH, low molecular weight heparin; VTE, venous thromboembolism.

Adapted from Guyatt GH *et al.* (2012). Antithrombotic therapy and prevention of thrombosis, 9th ed. American College of Chest Physicians Evidence-Based Clinical Practice Guidelines. *Chest* **141**(suppl), 7S–47S.

the pulmonary component of the second sound was accentuated in 23% and 15% of cases. DVT was clinically apparent in 11% of patients with PE in PIOPED, but more frequently in PIOPED II (47%). A right ventricular lift, third heart sound, or pleural friction rub were uncommon, each occurring in 4% or less of patients with PE.

Most patients with PE who had rales (crepitations) had pulmonary parenchymal abnormalities, atelectasis, or a pleural effusion on the chest radiograph.

Among patients with PE and no other source of fever, temperature below 39.9 °C was present in 12% and fever of 39.9 °C or higher occurred in 2%. Fever in patients with pulmonary haemorrhage/infarction was not more frequent than among those with no pulmonary haemorrhage/infarction. Clinical evidence

Table 16.1.7 Recommendations for prevention of venous thromboembolism during long-distance air travel

Long-distance travel	Frequent ambulation, calf muscle exercise
Additional risk factors for VTE	Frequent ambulation, calf muscle exercise, *and* below-knee graduated compression stockings providing 15–30 mmHg of pressure at ankle. Recommend against aspirin or anticoagulants

LMWH, low molecular weight heparin; VTE, venous thromboembolism.

Adapted from Guyatt GH *et al.* (2012). Antithrombotic therapy and prevention of thrombosis, 9th ed. American College of Chest Physicians Evidence-Based Clinical Practice Guidelines. *Chest* **141**(suppl), 7S–47S.

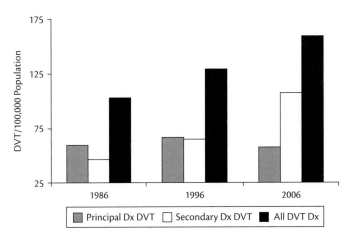

Fig. 16.1.1 Population-based prevalence of deep venous thrombosis (DVT) in the United States of America according to year. Incidence of principal diagnosis of DVT (admitting diagnosis) did not change from 1986 to 2006. Secondary diagnoses of DVT (occurring during hospitalization) increased. Total incidence of DVT increased in parallel. Grey bars, principal diagnosis DVT; white bars, secondary diagnosis DVT; black bars, all DVT diagnoses.
Data from Stein PD, Matta F, Dalen JE (2011). Is the campaign to prevent venous thromboembolism in hospitalized patients working? *Chest*, **139**, 1317–21.

of DVT was often present in patients with PE and otherwise unexplained fever.

Circulatory collapse (systolic blood pressure <80 mmHg or loss of consciousness) was an uncommon mode of presentation: 15% in PIOPED and in 8% in PIOPED II. However, patients with circulatory collapse may not be candidates for recruitment into trials of diagnostic investigations or therapies, and patients with circulatory collapse often die within the first few hours, hence it may be that the incidence of circulatory collapse as determined from published series is falsely low. Patients with pulmonary infarction have less severe PE than patients with isolated dyspnoea, and those with circulatory collapse probably have the most severe of all.

Combinations of symptoms and signs

Dyspnoea or tachypnoea (respiratory rate ≥20/min) was present in 90% and 84% of patients with acute PE and no pre-existing cardiac or pulmonary disease in PIOPED and PIOPED II. Dyspnoea or tachypnoea or pleuritic pain was present in 97% and 92% respectively. Dyspnoea or tachyponea or pleuritic pain or radiographic evidence of atelectasis or a parenchymal abnormality was present in 98%. The remaining patients usually had either DVT or an

Table 16.1.8 Recommendations for treatment of venous thromboembolism and/or pulmonary thromboembolism

Condition	Treatment
High clinical suspicion of DVT or PE or intermediate clinical suspicion if results of diagnostic tests delayed >4 h	Give anticoagulants while awaiting outcome of diagnostic tests
Confirmed proximal DVT or PE	Initial treatment with LMWH, intravenous or subcutaneous or fondaparinux for ≥5 days and until INR >2.0 for 24 h
	Suggest LMWH or fondaparinux over intravenous or subcutaneous unfractionated heparin and LMWH once daily rather than twice daily
	Start vitamin K antagonists with LMWH, unfractionated heparin or fondaparinux on first treatment day
	Continue vitamin K antagonist for 3 months, longer treatment for unprovoked PE, second unprovoked episode of DVT, or cancer, providing low to moderate risk of bleeding
	For long term treatment, prefer vitamin K antagonist over LMWH if no cancer, and LMWH over vitamin K antagonist if cancer. Either are preferred over dabigatran or rivaroxaban
	Suggest early ambulation and compression stockings
	Recommend *against* inferior vena cava filter unless contraindication to anticoagulants
Acute proximal DVT	Suggest anticoagulants alone over catheter directed or systemic thrombolysis or operative thrombectomy
Acute proximal DVT	Home treatment if circumstances adequate
Isolated distal DVT	Serial imaging for 2 weeks rather than anticoagulation unless severe symptoms or risk factors for proximal extension. Treat with anticoagulants if proximal extension
Distal superficial vein thrombosis, >5 cm	Prophylactic doses of fondaparinux of LMWH for 45 days
Low risk PE	Early discharge if adequate home circumstances
Massive PE, hypotension (systolic blood pressure <90 mmHg) or high risk of developing hypotension, no high bleeding risk	Systemic thrombolytic therapy, short infusion time preferred (2 h). Infuse through peripheral vein rather than pulmonary artery
Massive PE, highly compromised patients unable to receive thrombolytic therapy or whose critical status does not allow sufficient time to infuse thrombolytic therapy	Catheter extraction or fragmentation or pulmonary embolectomy. Pulmonary embolectomy if failed catheter-assisted embolectomy

LMWH, low molecular weight heparin.

Adapted from Guyatt GH *et al.* (2012). Antithrombotic therapy and prevention of thrombosis, 9th ed. American College of Chest Physicians Evidence-Based Clinical Practice Guidelines. *Chest* **141**(suppl), 7S–47S.

Table 16.1.9 Predisposing factors for pulmonary embolism in all patients irrespective of previous cardiac or pulmonary disease (n = 383)

Predisposing factor	Cases (%)
Immobilization	54
Surgery	42
Lung disease	27
Malignancy	18
Coronary heart disease	20
Thrombophlebitis—ever	19
Myocardial infarction	13
Trauma—lower extremities	12
Heart failure	12
Chronic obstructive pulmonary disease	10
Stroke	10
Asthma	7
Pneumonia—acute	7
Prior PE	6
Oestrogen	6
Collagen vascular disease	4
Postpartum—3 months or less	2
Interstitial lung disease	2

Unpublished data from PIOPED in Stein PD (2016). *Pulmonary embolism*, 3rd edn. Wiley Blackwell, Oxford.

Table 16.1.10 Symptoms of pulmonary embolism in patients without pre-existing cardiac or pulmonary disease

Symptoms	PE (%)	
	PIOPED I (n = 117)	PIOPED II (n = 127–133)
Dyspnoea		
Dyspnoea (rest or exertion)	73	73
Dyspnoea (at rest)		55
Dyspnoea (exertion only)		16
Orthopnoea (≥2 pillow)		28
Pleuritic pain	66	44
Chest pain (not pleuritic)	4	19
Cough	37	34
Haemoptysis	13	5 [a]
Purulent		5
Clear		5
Nonproductive		20
Wheezing	9	21
Palpitations	10	
Calf or thigh swelling		41
Calf swelling only	28	33
Calf and thigh swelling		7
Thigh swelling only		1
Calf or thigh pain		44
Calf pain only	26 [b]	23
Calf and thigh pain		17
Thigh pain only		3

[a] Haemoptysis, patients with PE: 2, slightly pinkish; 4, blood-streaked; 1, all blood (<1 teaspoonful).

[b] 'Leg pain'.

Data from Stein PD, *et al.* (1991). Clinical, laboratory, roentgenographic and electrocardiographic findings in patients with acute pulmonary embolism and no pre-existing cardiac or pulmonary disease. *Chest*, **100**, 598–603 and Stein PD, *et al.* (2007). Clinical characteristics of patient with acute pulmonary embolism: data from PIOPED II. *Am J Med*, **120**, 871–9.

unexplained low Pao_2. PE was rarely diagnosed in the absence of dyspnoea or tachypnoea or pleuritic pain.

Dyspnoea or tachypnoea occurred in 92% of all patients with PE (irrespective of pre-existing cardiopulmonary disease) in whom the pulmonary emboli were in main or lobar pulmonary arteries, but in only 65% of patients in whom the largest PE was in segmental pulmonary arteries. Dyspnoea or tachypnoea or pleuritic pain occurred in 97% of patients with proximal PE and 77% of patients with pulmonary emboli in only segmental pulmonary arteries.

Accuracy of clinical assessment

To emphasize the point that the diagnosis of PE is difficult to make, senior staff physicians and postgraduate fellows taking part in the PIOPED study were uncertain of the diagnosis in most patients. Using individual judgement without any specific predetermined criteria, senior staff were correct in the diagnosis in 88% of cases when their clinical assessment indicated a high probability of PE. When their clinical assessment indicated a low probability of PE, senior staff correctly excluded PE in 86%. Postgraduate fellows, on the basis of clinical assessment, were more accurate in excluding PE than they were in making the diagnosis. Objective scoring systems for the probability of acute PE give probability assessments similar to those of experienced physicians and do not require experience or clinical judgement. An example of a scoring system that is mostly objective is shown in Table 16.1.12.

Differential diagnosis

The commonest presentation of acute PE is with dyspnoea and/or pleuritic chest pain. There are several other possible causes of these symptoms, the commonest being musculoskeletal pain and pneumonia. Musculoskeletal chest pain can be very similar to that caused by pleurisy, and splinting of the chest can lead to a perception of breathlessness that may be exacerbated by anxiety. If there is an obvious history of local trauma to the chest, then the patient will rarely present to the physician, but it is worthwhile to ask specifically whether there has been any trauma or unaccustomed physical activity, whether the pain can be brought on by particular movements, and to examine carefully for local tenderness of the ribs, muscles, or costal margins. However, tenderness can sometimes be found in cases of pleurisy, and chest pain was reproduced by palpation in 20% of patients with PE. Appropriate history often supports a diagnosis of musculoskeletal pain.

Pneumonia complicated by pleurisy can cause dyspnoea and chest pain. Important features to look for in the history include preceding systemic upset (flu-like symptoms), high fever, and rigors, and on examination, high fever, 'toxic appearance', and chest

Table 16.1.11 Signs of pulmonary embolism in patients without pre-existing cardiac or pulmonary disease

Signs	PE (%)	
	PIOPED I (*n* = 117)	**PIOPED II** (*n* = 127–133)
General		
Tachypnea (≥20/min)	70	54
Tachycardia (>100/min)	30	24
Diaphoresis	11	2
Cyanosis	1	0
Temperature >38.5°C (>101.3°F)	7	1
Cardiac examination (any abnormality)		21
Increased P2	23	15
Third heart sound	3	
Fourth heart sound	24	
Right ventricular lift	4	4
Jugular venous distension		14
Lung examination (any abnormality)		29
Rales (crackles)	51	18
Wheezes	5	2
Rhonchi		2
Decreased breath sounds		17
Pleural friction rub	3	0
DVT		
Calf or thigh	11	47 [a]
Calf only		32
Calf and thigh		14
Thigh only		2
Homans' sign	4	

P2, pulmonary component of second sound.

[a] Number of patients with PE who had one or more signs of DVT: oedema, 55; erythema, 5; tenderness, 32; palpable cord, 2.

Data from Stein PD *et al*, (1991). Clinical, laboratory, roentgenographic and electrocardiographic findings in patients with acute pulmonary embolism and no pre-existing cardiac or pulmonary disease. *Chest* **100**, 598–603 and Stein PD, *et al*. (2007). Clinical characteristics of patient with acute pulmonary embolism: data from PIOPED II. *Am J Med*, **120**, 871–9.

signs of pneumonic consolidation. If a positive diagnosis of another cause of dyspnoea and/or pleuritic chest pain cannot be made, then the default position should be to assume that the patient has PE until proven otherwise.

Investigation

Detection of evidence of thrombus within the circulation: D-dimer

As when considering the diagnosis of DVT, a 'negative' D-dimer test is useful for excluding PE in patients who are clinically thought to be at low risk, but a 'positive' result does not establish the diagnosis. Hence, when used in the appropriate clinical context, D-dimer

Table 16.1.12 A model to determine the clinical probability of pulmonary embolism according to Wells and associates

Clinical feature	Score (points)
Clinical signs and symptoms of DVT (objectively measured leg swelling and pain with palpation in the deep vein system)	3.0
Heart rate>100/min	1.5
Immobilization ≥3 consecutive days (bed rest except to access bathroom) or surgery in previous 4 weeks	1.5
Previous objectively diagnosed PE or DVT	1.5
Haemoptysis	1.0
Malignancy (cancer patients receiving treatment within 6 months or receiving palliative treatment)	1.0
PE as likely or more likely than alternative diagnosis (based on history, physical examination, chest radiograph, ECG, and blood tests)	3.0

Score: <2.0, low probability; ≤4, unlikely probability; >4, likely probability; >6.0, high probability.

Data from Wells, PS et al (2000). Derivation of a simple clinical model to categorize patients probability of pulmonary embolism: increasing the models utility with the SimpliRED D-dimer. *Thromb Haemost*, **83**, 416–420 and from Wells PS, *et al*. (2001). Excluding PE at the bedside without diagnostic imaging: management of patients with suspected PE presenting to the emergency department by using a simple clinical model and D-dimer. *Ann Intern Med*, **135**, 98–107.

testing is useful in defining a group of patients with suspected PE who do not require further investigation.

In ranking the D-dimer assays according to their sensitivity values and likelihood of increasing certainty for ruling out PE, the ELISA and quantitative rapid ELISA assays are significantly superior to the semiquantitative latex and whole-blood agglutination assays. The quantitative rapid ELISA assay is more convenient than the conventional ELISA and provides a high level of certainty for a negative diagnosis of PE as well as DVT. A particle-enhanced immunoturbidometric assay (quantitative latex agglutination) gives results comparable to the rapid ELISA.

The 3-month risk of PE in untreated patients with a negative rapid ELISA D-dimer measurement and low or intermediate clinical probability Geneva score was 0% (0 of 220). With a negative D-dimer by rapid ELISA or quantitative latex agglutination assay and an unlikely (≤4) Wells score, PE occurred in 0.4% (4 of 1028), and with an unlikely (≤10) revised Geneva score in 1 of 320 (0.3%).

Detection of the physical presence of thrombus in the pulmonary circulation
Ventilation–perfusion lung scans

By 2001 in the United States of America the use of CT pulmonary angiography surpassed the use of ventilation–perfusion lung scans for the diagnosis of acute PE, the use of ventilation–perfusion lung scans having fallen into disfavour after the PIOPED trial because in most patients they led to an indeterminate result. Now, two decades since PIOPED was published, advances have been made in imaging equipment, improved methods of interpretation, and new radiopharmaceuticals. With such advances, and recognizing the risk of radiation with CT angiography, radionuclear imaging is receiving renewed interest.

Based on the results of PIOPED, a high-probability lung ventilation–perfusion scan (Fig. 16.1.2) indicates PE in 87% of

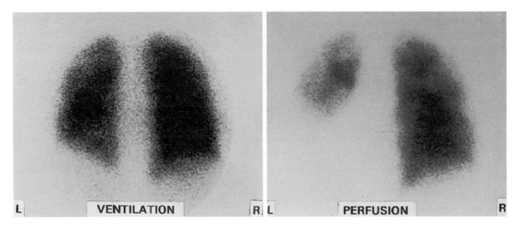

Fig. 16.1.2 Ventilation lung scan (left panel) and perfusion lung scan (right panel): posterior views with left (L) and right (R) indicated. The ventilation scan, equilibrium phase, shows nearly normal ventilation. The perfusion scan shows absent perfusion in the left lower lobe and mismatched perfusion defects in the left upper lobe. Perfusion defects (grey areas) are also shown in the right lung. This ventilation–perfusion lung scan was interpreted as showing high probability for PE.

patients (Table 16.1.13) and a normal scan excludes PE. In the absence of any other information an intermediate probability scan indicates a 30% chance of PE and a low-probability scan 14%. A low-probability ventilation–perfusion scan by the criteria used in PIOPED does not therefore exclude PE. Intermediate and low-probability interpretations may be grouped as 'nondiagnostic', which was frequently the case in PIOPED.

Prior clinical assessment in combination with interpretation of the ventilation–perfusion scan improves diagnostic validity (Table 16.1.13). If the ventilation–perfusion scan is interpreted as high probability for PE, and if the clinical impression is concordantly high, then the positive predictive value for PE is 96%. If the ventilation–perfusion scan is low probability and the clinical suspicion is concordantly low, then PE is excluded in 96% of patients.

The probability of PE can be determined based on the number of mismatched defects. Since PIOPED, criteria for the interpretation of very low probability lung scans (positive predictive value <10%) have been developed and tested. Fewer mismatched perfusion defects are required to diagnose PE among patients

with no prior cardiopulmonary disease. Adding clinical assessment to the stratification results in a more accurate evaluation. Outcome studies, as opposed to studies of accuracy as was PIOPED, showed that in patients with low probability, very low probability, or normal ventilation–perfusion lung scans there was no fatal PE and nonfatal PE in only 0.17% after 3–12 months without anticoagulants.

Using revised PIOPED criteria, some have shown that in patients with suspected acute PE and a normal chest radiograph the perfusion lung scan was diagnostic (high probability, normal or very low probability) in 89% of patients (Table 16.1.14). There were no nondiagnostic perfusion scans when interpreted by the PISAPED criteria (Table 16.1.15). After elimination of nondiagnostic scans, sensitivity with modified PIOPED criteria was 86% and specificity was 93%. With PISAPED criteria, sensitivity was 72% and specificity was 97%. It may be, therefore, that with updated techniques, perfusion scintigraphy in a patient with a normal chest radiograph can provide diagnostic accuracy similar to CT angiography at a lower cost and with a lower radiation dose.

Table 16.1.13 The probability of pulmonary embolism using clinical assessment in combination with ventilation–perfusion lung scans

Clinical science probability (%)	80–100		20–79		0–19		All probabilities	
Scan category	PE+/No of patients [a]	%	PE+/No of patients	%	PE+/No of patients	%	PE+/No of patients	%
High probability	28/29	96	70/80	88	5/9	56	103/118	87
Intermediate probability	27/41	66	66/236	28	11/68	16	104/345	30
Low probability	6/15	40	30/191	16	4/90	4	40/296	14
Near normal/normal	0/5	0	4/62	6	1/61	2	5/128	4
Total	61/90	68	170/569	30	21/228	9	252/887	28

[a] PE+ indicates angiogram reading that shows PE or determination of PE by the outcome classification committee on review. PE status is based on angiogram interpretation for 713 patients, on angiogram interpretation and outcome classification committee reassignment for 4 patients, and on clinical information alone (without definitive angiography) for 170 patients.

Reproduced from A National Investigation by the PIOPED Investigators (1990). Value of the ventilation/perfusion scan in acute pulmonary embolism—results of the Prospective Investigation of Pulmonary Embolism Diagnosis (PIOPED). Copyright 1990 American Medical Association.

Table 16.1.14 Modified PIOPED II scintigraphic criteria

Diagnosis	Criteria
PE present	High probability (≥2 segmental equivalents of perfusion scan-chest radiograph mismatch[a])
PE absent	Normal perfusion
Very low probability	Nonsegmental lesion, e.g. prominent hilum, cardiomegaly, elevated diaphragm, linear atelectasis, costophrenic angle effusion with no other perfusion defect in either lung
	Perfusion defect smaller than radiographic lesion
	1–3 small segmental defects
	A solitary chest radiographic–perfusion scan matched defect in the mid or upper lung zone confined to a single segment
	Stripe sign around perfusion defect (best tangential view)
	Pleural effusion ≥ 1/3 of the pleural cavity with no other perfusion defect in either lung
Not diagnostic	All other findings

[a] May be ≥2 large segmental mismatches, or 1 large and 2 moderate mismatches or 4 moderate segmental mismatches.

This research was originally published in *JNM*. Sostman H *et al.* Sensitivity and specificity of perfusion scintigraphy combined with chest radiography for acute pulmonary embolism in PIOPED II. *J Nucl Med.* 2008;49(11):1741–1748. Table 1. © by the Society of Nuclear Medicine and Molecular Imaging, Inc.

Although not routine practice in most centres, it can be useful to obtain a post-therapy baseline ventilation–perfusion lung scan for use in the event of suspected recurrent PE. This will assist in determining if abnormalities subsequently discovered on a ventilation–perfusion scan are new or residual. A residual abnormality of perfusion 1 year after PE is more frequent among patients with prior cardiopulmonary disease than among patients with none.

SPECT ventilation–perfusion lung scan imaging

Single-photon emission computed tomography (SPECT) ventilation–perfusion lung scan imaging may further improve the accuracy of pulmonary scintigraphy. SPECT offers the advantages of tomographic sections over traditional planar ventilation–perfusion imaging. The ability to obtain SPECT lung scans was still in its relatively

Table 16.1.15 PISAPED scintigraphic criteria

Diagnosis	Criteria
PE present	One or more wedge-shaped perfusion defects
PE absent	Normal or near normal perfusion
	Contour defect caused by enlarged heart, mediastinum, or diaphragm
	Perfusion defect, not wedge-shaped
Not diagnostic	Cannot classify as PE-positive or PE-negative

Modified from Sostman HD, *et al.* (2008). Sensitivity and specificity of perfusion scintigraphy combined with chest radiography for acute pulmonary embolism in PIOPED II. *J Nucl Med*, **49**, 1741–8.

early stages when the PIOPED investigation of planar lung scans was published. Dual- and triple-headed gamma cameras with ultra-high-resolution collimators have been developed, as have new radiopharmaceuticals for ventilatory studies, prominent among which is ^{99m}Tc-Technegas (Cyclomedica, Lucas Heights, Australia), which consists of ultrafine carbon particles that behave physiologically like a gas.

Many investigators have found SPECT ventilation–perfusion lung scan imaging to be better than planar imaging. Among its advantages are the avoidance of overlapping of small perfusion defects by normal tissue and a higher contrast resolution than planar scans. It can, therefore, detect abnormalities—particularly at the subsegmental level and in the lung bases—where the segments are tightly packed. Review showed that the sensitivity of SPECT was higher than planar lung scans in 4 of 5 investigations, and specificity was generally higher, equal, or only somewhat lower than planar ventilation–perfusion lung scans. Nondiagnostic SPECT lung scans were reported in ≤3% by most investigators.

Pulmonary angiography

Pulmonary angiography is no longer the diagnostic gold standard for PE (Fig. 16.1.3). It is associated with serious complications in about 1% of patients and has been replaced by contrast-enhanced CT.

Contrast-enhanced spiral CT

The sensitivity of multidetector (mostly 4-detector) CT angiography alone and in combination with CT venous-phase venography was investigated in PIOPED II. The CT angiogram among 824 patients was of insufficient quality for a conclusive interpretation in 6.2%. Among 773 patients with an adequate CT angiogram, the sensitivity of CT angiography was 83% and specificity was 96% (Fig. 16.1.4): positive predictive value was 86% and negative predictive value was 95%. Positive predictive values were 97% for PE in a main or lobar artery, 68% in those in whom the largest vessel with PE was a segmental pulmonary artery, and 25% among

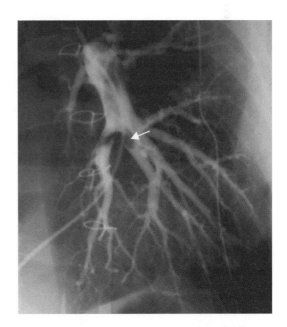

Fig. 16.1.3 Selective digital subtraction pulmonary angiogram of the left pulmonary artery showing multiple intraluminal filling defects indicative of pulmonary thromboemboli. One of these has been identified with an arrow.

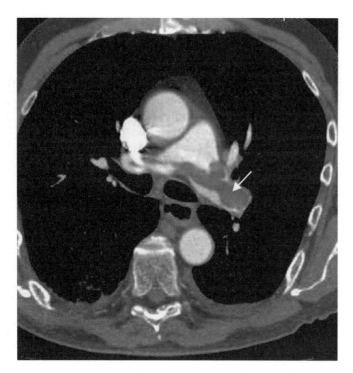

Fig. 16.1.4 Contrast-enhanced spiral CT showing a large intraluminal filling defect (arrow).

Table 16.1.16 Positive and negative predictive values of CT pulmonary angiography in relation to prior clinical assessment

	High clinical probability (Wells score >6) n/N (%)	Intermediate clinicalprobability (Wells score 2–6) n/N (%)	Low clinical probability[a] (Wells score <2) n/N (%)
CTA positive (positive predictive value)	22/23 (96)	93/101 (92)	22/38 (58)
CTA or CTV positive (positive predictive value)	27/28 (96)	100/111 (90)	24/42 (57)
CTA negative (negative predictive value)	9/15 (60)	121/136 (89)	158/164 (96) [a]
CTA and CTV negative (negative predictive value)	9/11 (82)	114/124 (92)	146/151 (97) [a]

CTA, CT pulmonary angiography; CTV, CT venous-phase imaging.

[a] To avoid bias for calculation of the negative predictive value in patients with a low-probability prior clinical assessment, only patients with a reference test diagnosis by V/Q scan or conventional pulmonary digital subtraction angiography were included.

Modified from Stein PD *et al.* (2006). PK for the PIOPED II Investigators. Multidetector computed tomography for acute pulmonary embolism. *N Engl J Med* **354**, 2317–27. With permission.

only a few patients in whom the largest PE was in a subsegmental branch.

The combination CT angiogram with venous-phase imaging of the pelvic and thigh veins (CT venogram) among 824 patients was of insufficient quality for a conclusive interpretation in 11%. Among the 737 patients with an adequate CT angiogram/CT venogram combination, the sensitivity was 90% and specificity was 95%, with positive predictive value 85% and negative predictive value 97%.

As with ventilation–perfusion scans, better prediction can be made if imaging results are interpreted in the light of clinical information (Table 16.1.16). Among patients with a high or intermediate probability prior clinical assessment based on the Wells score, a positive CT angiogram had a positive predictive value for PE of 96% and 92% respectively. In patients with a low or intermediate probability prior clinical assessment and a negative CT angiogram, the negative predictive values for exclusion of PE were 96% and 89% respectively. Positive and negative predictive values were considerably reduced when scan results were discordant with clinical probabilities.

MRI

Potential advantages of gadolinium-enhanced MR angiography are that it does not involve the use of iodinated contrast agents, it is minimally invasive, and patients are not exposed to ionizing radiation. In small studies it shows a sensitivity for PE in proximal or segmental branches that ranges from 77% to 100% and specificity that ranges from 95 to 98%, but sensitivity for subsegmental branches was not evaluated prior to PIOPED III. Gadolinium-enhanced venous-phase imaging of the veins of the pelvis and thighs in combination with imaging of the pulmonary arteries would permit a comprehensive study for thromboembolism comparable to the combination of contrast-enhanced spiral CT of the

pulmonary arteries in combination with venous-phase CT of the veins of the lower extremities.

The PIOPED III trial of the accuracy of gadolinium-enhanced MR pulmonary angiography showed that most centres had difficulty in obtaining adequate quality MR pulmonary angiograms (MRA). The investigators defined an adequate quality MRA as adequate opacification through subsegmental vessels. Among 371 patients, adequate quality images were obtained in the main or lobar pulmonary arteries in 91%, of the segmental pulmonary arteries in 87%, and of the subsegmental branches in 73%. Averaged across participating centres, MRAs were technically inadequate in 25%, but the figure at one centre was only 11%. Including patients with technically inadequate images, MRA identified 57% with PE. Technically adequate MRA had a sensitivity of 78% and specificity of 99%, and the sensitivity of MRA for detecting PE in a main or lobar pulmonary artery was 79%. Pulmonary embolism was rarely identified by MRA when the largest PE was in a segmental or subsegmental branch. Specificity was 98% to 100%, irrespective of the order of the vessel. The combination of a technically adequate MRA with MR venography (MRA/MRV) had a higher sensitivity than MRA alone, 92%, while maintaining a high specificity of 96%. However, either MRA or MRV was technically inadequate in 52% of patients. This led the investigators to conclude that MRA should only be considered at centres that routinely perform it well, and for patients who have contraindications to standard tests. Nephrogenic systemic fibrosis (also known as nephrogenic fibrosing dermopathy) has been reported in patients with moderate or severe renal failure and in patients on dialysis following MRA with gadolinium-containing contrast agents. Other diagnostic approaches are recommended in such patients.

Other tests

Electrocardiography

Electrocardiographic (ECG) abnormalities are common in acute PE (Table 16.1.17), with a normal ECG found in only 30% of patients. Acute ventricular dilatation is speculated to be the most likely cause of the ECG changes. Abnormalities of the ST segment and T wave are by far the most frequent observation, with nonspecific ST segment or T wave changes seen in about 50% of patients in whom the severity of PE ranged from mild to severe. Atrial flutter or atrial fibrillation in patients with acute PE is nearly always limited to individuals with prior heart disease. Electrocardiographic manifestations of acute cor pulmonale ($S_1Q_3T_3$, complete right bundle branch block, P pulmonale, or right axis deviation) are less common than ST segment or T wave changes and are not sensitive for right ventricular dilatation. One or more of these abnormalities occurred in 26% of patients with submassive or massive acute PE not associated with cardiac or pulmonary disease (32% of patients with massive PE). Left axis deviation occurs more frequently than right axis deviation.

The ECG may simulate an inferior infarction with Q waves and T wave inversion in leads II, III, and aVF, or anteroseptal infarction characterized by QS or QR waves in V1 and T wave inversion in the right precordial leads. The development of Q waves and extensive T wave inversion in the anterior and lateral leads has also been observed. However, a pseudoinfarction pattern is seen in only 3% of patients.

Table 16.1.17 Electrocardiographic manifestations of pulmonary embolisms in patients without prior cardiac or pulmonary disease ($n = 89$)

Patients with electrocardiographic findings [a]	(%)
Rhythm disturbances	
Atrial flutter	1
Atrial fibrillation	4
Atrial premature contractions	4
Ventricular premature contractions	4
P wave	
P pulmonale	2
QRS abnormalities	
Right axis deviation	2
Left axis deviation	13
Incomplete right bundle branch block	4
Complete right bundle branch block	6
Right ventricular hypertrophy	2
Pseudoinfarction	3
Low voltage (frontal plane)	3
ST segment and T wave	
Nonspecific ST segment or T wave abnormalities	49

[a] Some patients had more than one abnormality.

Data from Stein PD, *et al.* (1991). Clinical, laboratory, roentgenographic and electrocardiographic findings in patients with acute pulmonary embolism and no pre-existing cardiac or pulmonary disease. *Chest*, **100**, 598–603.

Inversion of the T waves is the most persistent ECG abnormality, disappearing in only 22% of patients 5 or 6 days after the PE was diagnosed, although resolving in 49% by 2 weeks. Depression of the ST segment tends to resolve somewhat faster, and abnormalities of depolarization resolve more quickly than abnormalities of repolarization. Well over half of the ECGs that showed pseudoinfarction, $S_1S_2S_3$, $S_1Q_3T_3$, right ventricular hypertrophy or right bundle branch block no longer show these abnormalities 5 or 6 days after the diagnosis is made.

Patients with ST segment abnormalities, T wave inversion, pseudoinfarction patterns, $S_1Q_3T_3$ patterns, incomplete right bundle branch block, right axis deviation, right ventricular hypertrophy, or ventricular premature beats have larger perfusion defects on the lung scan or larger defects on the pulmonary arteriogram than those with normal ECGs. Such patients have higher pulmonary arterial pressures and in general have a low partial pressure of oxygen in arterial blood.

The electrocardiographic abnormalities in patients with PE are not specific, although they may suggest the presence of PE. For example, patients with pneumonia often show QRS abnormalities or nonspecific ST-segment or T-wave changes comparable to those seen in PE.

Chest radiography

The findings on the plain chest radiograph—when used together with the history, physical examination, electrocardiogram and simple laboratory tests—assist in identifying PE. The chest radiograph, when normal in a patient who is dyspnoeic, hints that PE is a diagnostic possibility. Among patients with PE and no prior cardiopulmonary disease a normal chest radiograph is found in 16% (Table 16.1.18). Atelectasis or a pulmonary parenchymal abnormality are the most frequent abnormalities present (68%). Pleural effusions are found in about one-half of cases and are usually small, with most limited to blunting of the costophrenic angle. In some studies, an elevated hemidiaphragm is the most frequent abnormality. Westermark's sign (a prominent central pulmonary artery and decreased pulmonary vascularity) is identified by radiologists in only 7% of patients with PE.

In cases of PE, those with a normal plain chest radiograph have the lowest pulmonary artery mean pressures. The highest pulmonary artery mean pressures are in patients with a prominent central pulmonary artery or cardiomegaly.

Table 16.1.18 Chest radiograph findings in pulmonary embolism in patients with no previous cardiac or pulmonary disease ($n = 117$)

Patients with radiographic finding	(%)
Atelectasis or pulmonary parenchymal abnormality	68
Pleural effusion	48
Pleural based opacity	3
Elevated diaphragm hemidiaphragm	24
Decreased pulmonary vascularity	21
Prominent central pulmonary artery	15
Cardiomegaly	12
Westermark's sign [a]	7

[a] Prominent central pulmonary artery and decreased pulmonary vascularity.

Data modified from Stein PD *et al*, (1991). Clinical, laboratory, roentgenographic and electrocardiographic findings in patients with acute pulmonary embolism and no pre-existing cardiac or pulmonary disease. Chest 100, 598–603, with permission.

Echocardiography

Echocardiography may show right ventricular dilatation and evidence of pulmonary hypertension, which—in the proper clinical setting—may strengthen the clinical impression that PE has occurred. Transoesophageal echocardiography sometimes may show proximal pulmonary emboli, but it has limited value in this regard.

Arterial blood gases and alveolar–arterial oxygen difference

A low partial pressure of oxygen in arterial blood (Pao_2) is typical of acute PE and supports the diagnosis, but patients with acute PE can have a normal Pao_2. Among patients with acute PE and no prior cardiopulmonary disease who have measurements of the Pao_2 while breathing room air, 24% have a Pao_2 of 80 mmHg (10.5 kPa) or higher, and even among patients with submassive or massive acute PE, 12% have a Pao_2 of this level or higher. A normal alveolar–arterial oxygen difference (alveolar–arterial oxygen gradient) does not exclude acute PE. No value of the alveolar–arterial oxygen difference is diagnostic of PE, and no value can exclude the diagnosis.

Other routine blood tests

Among patients in whom a possible or definite cause for leucocytosis is eliminated, 80% of patients with PE have a normal white blood cell count, 6% a count of 10.1–11.9 × 10^9/litre, and 13% a count of higher than this. A white blood cell count of 20 × 10^9/litre or greater is rarely if ever seen. Leucocytosis is not more frequent in patients with the pulmonary haemorrhage/infarction syndrome than in other patients with acute PE.

Biomarkers

Cardiac troponin I (cTnI) and creatine kinase isoenzyme MB (CK-MB) are useful for assessment of prognosis in stable patients with acute PE who have right ventricular dilatation. Patients with a dilated right ventricle have a mortality from PE of 13% to 29% if cardiac biomarkers are elevated, compared with 4% if they are not. Elevated biomarkers are not prognostically significant if right ventricular size is normal. Only a few patients with PE had an abnormal CK-MB, which limits its value if used as the only indicator of prognosis.

Strategy for diagnosis

With increasing severity of PE, from pulmonary infarction to isolated dyspnoea to circulatory collapse, trends suggest that the prevalence of signs and symptoms increases, but generally recognized symptoms may be absent, even in patients with large pulmonary emboli. Clues that can assist the physician in assessing the possibility of PE, and avoiding inadvertent exclusion of the diagnosis are as follows:

- Dyspnoea—onset is usually, but not always, within minutes or hours, and may be present only on exertion. Frequent in patients with large pulmonary emboli, but often absent in those with small pulmonary emboli

- Orthopnea—often present in dyspnoeic patients with PE

- Circulatory collapse—may occur with PE in patients who do not have dyspnoea or tachypnoea or pleuritic pain

- Tachypnoea—frequent in patients with large pulmonary emboli, but often absent in those with small pulmonary emboli

- Crepitations (rales)—common among patients with pulmonary infarction, but less so in those with isolated dyspnoea or circulatory collapse; they occur in those with radiographic evidence of a parenchymal abnormality

- ECG—a normal ECG is frequent in patients with the pulmonary infarction syndrome, but uncommon in those with isolated dyspnoea; nonspecific ST segment and T wave changes are the most frequent abnormality

- Chest radiograph—abnormalities are more common among patients with pulmonary infarction but are often observed in those with isolated dyspnoea; patients with circulatory collapse may have a normal chest radiograph

- Ventilation–perfusion scan—a high-probability interpretation occurs in a minority of patients with the pulmonary infarction syndrome but in the majority of those with the isolated dyspnoea syndrome; a low-probability scan may occur in patients with PE and circulatory collapse

- Oxygenation—a Pao_2 higher than 80 mmHg (10.5 kPa) is not uncommon in patients with the pulmonary infarction syndrome, but such levels are uncommon in those with the isolated dyspnoea syndrome.

Subjecting all patients who might have a PE to complex, expensive, and/or invasive tests is best avoided. Management algorithms have been developed to identify those at very low risk, who can then be spared imaging tests. These algorithms typically use scoring systems to stratify the clinical probability that the particular patient has a PE, proceeding to D-dimer testing of those a clinical probability that is not high. Untreated patients with a low or intermediate clinical probability by Geneva score or 'unlikely' clinical probability by Wells score and negative D-dimer by rapid ELISA or quantitative latex agglutination test had a 3-month incidence of PE of 0% to 0.4%. There was no fatal PE on follow-up. Patients with such a clinical probability and D-dimer need not to be investigated further. Patients with a high clinical probability and patients with an elevated D-dimer proceed to tests for the presence of pulmonary emboli, typically by contrast-enhanced spiral CT. Recommendations for the approach to the diagnosis of acute PE based on use of a pretest scoring system (Table 16.1.12) and D-dimer followed by imaging are discussed below. Recommendations for the diagnostic approach to patients in whom PE is not excluded by clinical assessment in combination D-dimer test depend on clinical probability, age, gender, pregnancy, the complexity of associated lung disease as determined from the plain chest radiograph, and the severity of illness.

For patients with an elevated D-dimer and patients with a high-probability clinical assessment irrespective of the D-dimer, CT pulmonary angiography is recommended for most patients.

If CT angiography is negative and clinical probability is low or intermediate, treatment is unnecessary but a venous ultrasound is recommended if clinical assessment is intermediate or high probability. In those with a high-probability clinical assessment and negative CT angiogram, additional options include serial venous ultrasound examinations, pulmonary scintigraphy, and pulmonary digital subtraction angiography.

If CT angiography shows main or lobar pulmonary emboli, treatment is indicated irrespective of the clinical probability. With segmental or subsegmental pulmonary emboli the certainty of the CT diagnosis should be reassessed if clinical probability is low or intermediate, but treatment is indicated if the clinical probability is high. In those with segmental or subsegmental PE and a low or intermediate probability clinical assessment, pulmonary scintigraphy, a single venous ultrasound examination, or serial venous ultrasound examinations are optional. CT angiography should be repeated if image quality is poor.

Most believe that CT venography is unnecessary with CT pulmonary angiography because the risk from radiation outweighs the benefits of additional diagnoses. In patients with a high risk of lower-extremity DVT or elderly patients with low risk of radiation effects and limited cardiopulmonary reserve, CT venography is recommended by some. It appears safe to withhold treatment of isolated subsegmental PE provided that (1) pulmonary-respiratory reserve is good, (2) there is no evidence of DVT, (3) the major risk factor for PE was transient and no longer present, (4) there is no history of central venous catheterization or atrial fibrillation, and (5) the patient is willing and able to return for serial venous ultrasound examinations.

Other considerations
A venous ultrasound examination prior to imaging with CT angiography or prior to imaging with a ventilation–perfusion lung scan is optional and may guide treatment if positive. However, about 50% of patients with PE have negative noninvasive leg tests for DVT, even though DVT is the source of the PE.

Scintigraphy as the first imaging test
It may be that, with updated techniques, perfusion scintigraphy in a patient with a normal chest radiograph can provide diagnostic accuracy similar to CT angiography at a lower cost and with a lower radiation dose. Opinion is divided on whether perfusion lung scans or CT angiograms should be obtained as a first imaging test in patients with a nearly normal chest radiograph. Some opt for perfusion imaging only if the patient is pregnant or young or has a contraindication to CT angiography, as with chronic kidney disease. Patients with emphysema, chronic obstructive pulmonary disease, or poorly controlled asthma may require a ventilation scan in addition to a perfusion scan even if the chest radiograph appears nearly normal. Some suggest use of the PISAPED criteria for interpretation. Some now favour the use of SPECT scintigraphy over planar ventilation–perfusion lung scans.

Recommendations
For women of reproductive age
In women of reproductive age with a normal chest radiograph, if D-dimer is positive, most recommend either a perfusion lung scan as the first diagnostic test, or venous ultrasound to be followed by a perfusion lung scan. If the chest radiograph is abnormal, most recommend a CT pulmonary angiogram.

For patients who are pregnant
Most investigators recommend venous ultrasound before imaging tests with ionizing radiation in patients who are pregnant. The European Association for Nuclear Medicine recommends a perfusion scan without a ventilation scan, and a lower dose of radioisotope. Others believe that rapid diagnosis is crucial and radiation is a secondary issue. If a CT pulmonary angiogram is performed, imaging should be strictly limited to the thoracic cavity, and low kV_p, if applicable, should be utilized.

For haemodynamically stable young men
The effect of radiation on male reproduction is uncertain. In young men with a normal chest radiograph, opinions differ on which imaging test should be performed. In young men with an abnormal chest radiograph, most recommend CT pulmonary angiography as the first imaging test.

For haemodynamically stable older men and women
The risk of radiation-induced cancer is small with older men and women. Most recommend CT pulmonary angiography as the first imaging test in such patients, irrespective of whether the chest radiograph is normal. Opinion differs, however, and scintigraphy is recommended by many, particularly if the chest radiograph is normal.

For patients with allergy to iodinated contrast material
D-dimer with clinical assessment is recommended to exclude PE. Patients with mild iodine allergies may be treated with steroids prior to CT imaging. Venous ultrasound and pulmonary scintigraphy are recommended as alternative diagnostic tests in patients with severe iodine allergy. Serial venous ultrasound is an option, as is gadolinium-enhanced CT angiography.

For patients with impaired renal function
D-dimer with clinical assessment is recommended to exclude PE. If further investigation is warranted, venous ultrasound is recommended, followed by treatment if positive, and pulmonary scintigraphy if venous ultrasound is negative. Serial venous ultrasound is an option if scintigraphy is nondiagnostic. However, as always it is a matter of balancing benefits and risks, and if the index of suspicion is high, then many physicians will proceed with CT pulmonary angiography.

For patients in extremis
Bedside echocardiography in combination with bedside leg ultrasonography are generally recommended as rapidly obtainable bedside tests. In an appropriate clinical setting, either right ventricular enlargement or poor right ventricular function, or a positive venous ultrasound, can be interpreted as resulting from PE. Others recommend a portable perfusion scan or immediate transfer to an interventional catheterization laboratory, but in many instances neither of these will be available. A combination of a negative bedside echocardiogram and venous ultrasound suggests that the patient may be in extremis for some other reason than PE, but the diagnosis of PE can be pursued with CT angiography, if this is feasible, and such imaging may be appropriate if and when the patient stabilizes.

Serial noninvasive leg tests
Instead of imaging the lungs, an alternative strategy for the diagnosis of PE is to detect and treat DVT. Such a strategy can only be applied to patients with adequate cardiorespiratory reserve, because even a small recurrent PE might be dangerous if reserve is poor. In practice this means obtaining serial ultrasonography of the legs over a period of 2 weeks, and treating if DVT is shown. Among patients with suspected PE who had a nondiagnostic ventilation–perfusion lung scan, and negative noninvasive leg tests (one study required low or intermediate probability clinical assessment and another normal cardiorespiratory reserve), PE at 3 months follow-up occurred in only 0.4% to 0.6%. However, most now believe that with many safe and accurate imaging options available, management on the basis of serial noninvasive leg tests is rarely (if ever) indicated.

Treatment—general measures
All patients who are hypoxic should be given supplementary oxygen at high concentration (enough to restore normal Pao_2). In the early stages continuous monitoring of arterial oxygen tension by pulse oximetry is advised, with particularly careful clinical and

arterial blood gas monitoring of those with coincident chronic chest disease in case CO_2 retention is problematic.

Resuscitation

Patients with massive PE and circulatory collapse may look as though they are about to die, with cool peripheries, cyanosis, profound hypotension, and marked elevation of the jugular venous pulse. Features typical of long-standing pulmonary hypertension (palpable right ventricular heave, right ventricular gallop, loud P2, hepatomegaly, ascites, peripheral oedema) are unlikely to be present. This dramatic haemodynamic picture may not be simply due to the direct anatomical effects of occlusion of main pulmonary vessels (the same picture is not seen after pneumonectomy, when one pulmonary artery is tied off completely), but also secondary to pulmonary neurogenic reflexes and local release of vasoactive substances, including 5-hydroxytryptamine and thromboxane from activated platelets.

Every effort should be made to support the circulation until measures designed to deal with the embolus (usually thrombolysis—see below) can be applied and take effect.

Treatment—antithrombotic

It is common and sensible practice to begin anticoagulant treatment as soon as the diagnosis of PE is suspected, unless there are serious concerns about the potential side effects of anticoagulation or imaging is immediately available. The antithrombotic regimen is the same as for DVT: see Table 16.1.8 and Chapter 16.2.

Between 2012 and 2015 several novel oral anticoagulants—three direct oral factor Xa inhibitors (rivaroxaban, apixaban and edoxaban) and one oral direct thrombin inhibitor (dabigatran)—were approved by the United States Food and Drug Administration (FDA) for treatment of VTE. Some such drugs have also been approved for extended treatment (rivaroxaban, apixaban and dabigatran) or for prophylaxis (rivaroxaban and apixaban) following knee or hip replacement. None of these drugs requires monitoring of anticoagulant levels. They are as effective as conventional therapy with enoxaparin followed by a vitamin K antagonist in the treatment of DVT and PE, with extended treatment resulting in fewer recurrences of PE or DVT than with placebo.

All of the novel oral anticoagulants have comparable rates of bleeding or less bleeding than treatment with a low molecular–weight heparin/vitamin K antagonist. However, if bleeding occurs, there is not yet an antidote for the factor Xa inhibitors, although a specific antidote for dabigatran, namely the monoclonal antibody idarucizumab, was approved by the FDA on October 15, 2015. A factor Xa inhibitor antidote, the decoy receptor andexanet alfa, is being developed. It has received an FDA breakthrough therapy designation, which is intended to expedite its development and review.

Resolution rate with anticoagulants

Most patients (81%) treated with anticoagulants show complete CT angiographic resolution after 28 days, with emboli resolving at a faster rate in main or lobar pulmonary arteries than in segmental branches (Figure 16.1.5). Among patients with no prior cardiopulmonary disease who are treated with anticoagulants, resolution of 90% or more on perfusion lung scans is shown at 1 year in 91% of cases, compared with only 72% of those with prior cardiopulmonary disease.

Thrombolytic therapy

Thrombolytic therapy is not indicated for the routine treatment of PE. Hypotension, continuing hypoxemia while receiving high fractions of inspired oxygen (Fio_2), and requirement for

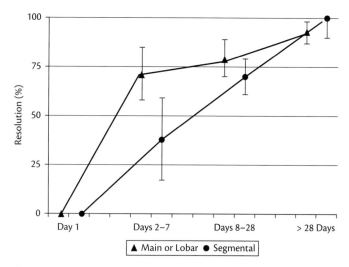

Fig. 16.1.5 Resolution of pulmonary emboli in main or lobar (▲) pulmonary arteries (PA) or segmental branches (●) according to number of days after initial CT angiogram. Bars = 95% confidence interval. Rate of resolution was slower in segmental branches.

Data from Stein PD, Yaekoub AY, Matta F, et al. (2010). Resolution of pulmonary embolism on CT pulmonary angiography. *AJR Am J Roentgenol*, **194**, 1263–8.

ventilatory support are indications for intervention. Analysis of data from 72 230 unstable (in shock or requiring ventilatory support) patients with PE throughout the United States of America from 1999 to 2008 showed that in-hospital mortality with thrombolytic therapy was 15% compared with 47% in those who did not receive thrombolytic therapy. Mortality was further reduced to 7.6% if a vena cava filter was used in addition to thrombolytic therapy compared with 33% mortality in those who received a vena cava filter, but no thrombolytic therapy. All-cause mortality in unstable patients was lower with thrombolytic therapy in every age group, including the elderly, irrespective of comorbid conditions.

Right ventricular dysfunction on the echocardiogram of normotensive patients with PE may indicate impending haemodynamic instability. For this group meta-analysis showed mortality was 1.4% with thrombolytics versus 2.9% with anticoagulants, but this benefit was offset by major bleeding in 7.7% with thrombolytics, versus 2.3% with anticoagulants.

A more rapid lysis of pulmonary thromboemboli occurs with thrombolytic agents than occurs spontaneously in patients treated only with anticoagulants, but pulmonary reperfusion as demonstrated on perfusion lung scans is similar after 2 weeks in patients treated with thrombolytic agents and patients treated with anticoagulants.

In 1973 the Urokinase Pulmonary Embolism Trial showed no improvement of mortality and no difference of the rate of recurrence of PE among stable patients treated with thrombolytic therapy and patients treated with anticoagulants. There have been no subsequent prospective randomized trials to contradict these results, although a trend suggesting a lower rate of recurrent PE has been shown among patients with right ventricular dysfunction who were treated with tissue plasminogen activator.

Thrombolysis has risks. Based on pooled data the frequency of major bleeding from tissue plasminogen activator among patients with PE in randomized trials was 14.7%. This occurred despite the fact that all studies excluded patients at a high risk of bleeding, such those with recent surgery, recent biopsy, peptic ulcer disease, blood dyscrasia, or severe hepatic or renal disease. The risk of intracranial haemorrhage with tissue plasminogen activator (2%) was higher among patients with PE than among patients who received tissue plasminogen activator for myocardial infarction. Even though there are risks of thrombolysis, mortality is lower in unstable patients (in shock or requiring ventilatory support) who receive thrombolysis than those who do not receive it.

Regimens of thrombolytic therapy

Regimens approved by the United States Food and Drug Administration for treatment of acute PE are:

◆ streptokinase 250 000 IU over 30 min followed by 100 000 IU/h for 24 h (no longer available in the United States)

◆ urokinase 4400 IU/kg over 10 min followed by 4400 IU/kg per h for 12 h

◆ tissue plasminogen activator (alteplase) 100 mg (50 million IU)/2 h. (In Europe, rt-PA is administrated using a 10-mg bolus, followed by a 90-mg continuous IV infusion with concomitant unfractionated heparin.)

In the United States, it is recommended that heparin be discontinued during thrombolytic therapy and reinstituted upon discontinuation of thrombolytic therapy.

Inferior vena cava occlusion

An inferior vena cava filter is recommended in a patient with proximal DVT or PE if anticoagulants are contraindicated, PE has recurred while on adequate anticoagulant therapy, or PE is severe (hypotension, right ventricular failure on physical examination) and any recurrent PE may be fatal. Insertion of an inferior vena cava filter is strongly recommended in patients following pulmonary embolectomy and pulmonary thromboendarterectomy.

Mortality is lower in unstable patients (in shock or on ventilatory support) who receive a vena cava filter (51% all-cause in-hospital mortality with no filter and no thrombolytic therapy versus 33% mortality with filter but no thrombolytic therapy; 18% mortality with thrombolytic therapy versus 7.6% mortality with thrombolytic therapy plus filter). Mortality is also lower in stable patients who require thrombolytic therapy for impending instability. Stable patients with PE who receive thrombolytic therapy because of a high risk of becoming unstable, and stable patients with PE who have solid malignant tumours or chronic obstructive pulmonary disease also appear to have a lower in-hospital all-cause case fatality rate if they receive a vena cava filter. These observations are based on administrative data from the Nationwide Inpatient Sample that includes thousands of hospitalized patients with PE in the United States of America.

The Prévention du Risque d'Embolie Pulmonaire par Interruption Cave (PREPIC) study, a randomized controlled trial of permanent filters plus anticoagulants (n=200) compared with anticoagulants alone (n=200) was performed in patients with proximal DVT, with or without symptomatic PE. Fewer patients in the filter group showed symptomatic PE at 1 year (1.1% versus 5.0%) and at 8 years 6.2% versus 15.1%) after recruitment. Recurrent DVT, however, was more frequent in the filter group and there was no difference in mortality.

Routine insertion of an inferior vena cava filter is not indicated solely on the basis of a continuing predisposition for DVT, although in special circumstances this may be the best approach, e.g. in high-risk patients with DVT, severe pulmonary hypertension, and minimal cardiopulmonary reserve.

Several vena cava filters have been designed for percutaneous insertion and many are retrievable. They differ in outer diameter of the delivery system, maximal caval diameter into which they can be inserted, hook design, retrievability, biocompatibility, and filtering efficiency. They may be effective alone in preventing PE, but anticoagulant therapy after insertion of a filter is recommended for the duration of treatment that would be required without a filter. Thereafter, anticoagulant therapy can be discontinued even though the filter remains in place. Complications of permanent vena cava filters include improper anatomical placement, filter deformation, filter fracture, insufficient opening of the filter, and filter migration; also perforation, thrombosis, and stenosis of the cava wall. Symptomatic occlusion of the inferior vena cava is the most frequent complication, occurring in about 9% of patients. Complications at the site of insertion of the catheter do not differ from complications observed locally with other catheter techniques. DVT at the puncture site generally has been reported in 8% to 25%. Retrievable vena cava filters typically are successfully removed after 1 to 3 months, but some have been successfully removed after 1 year.

PE after insertion of an inferior vena cava filter is uncommon (1%), and fatal embolism is rare. Possible mechanisms that can explain PE after filter insertion are (1) ineffective filtration, especially with tilting of the filter, (2) growth of trapped thrombi through the filter, (3) thrombosis on the proximal side of the filter, (4) filter migration, (5) filter retraction from the caval wall, (6) embolization through collaterals, (7) embolization from sites other than the inferior vena cava, and (8) incorrect position of the filter. Over the last two decades, the use of inferior vena cava filters in the United States of America has increased markedly in patients with PE, patients with DVT alone, and patients at risk who had neither PE nor DVT. The use for primary prevention in patients who do not have DVT or PE has accelerated. Extensive use of permanent and retrievable vena cava filters indicates a liberalization of indications, but despite the benefits of retrievability, retrieval has been attempted in only a minority of patients.

Catheter interventions

Catheter-tip devices for the extraction or the fragmentation of PE have the potential of producing immediate relief from massive PE. Such interventions may be particularly useful in patients in whom there is a contraindication to thrombolytic therapy. A suction-tip device for extraction of PE has been used in some patients, and thrombus fragmentation with a guide wire, angiographic catheter, balloon catheter, or specially designed devices has been reported in small case series or case reports. The release of fragmented thromboemboli into the distal pulmonary arterial branches is not a problem. A registry of management strategies used by hospitals throughout Germany showed use of catheter fragmentation in 1.3% to 6.8% of patients with PE, depending on severity.

Although originally it was thought that catheter embolectomy or fragmentation could substitute for thrombolytic therapy, it now appears to be an adjunct to thrombolysis, allowing a larger surface area of the fragmented emboli to be exposed to thrombolytic agent. Among patients who undergo fragmentation with standard angiographic catheters, the rate of successful clinical outcome with a local infusion of thrombolytic agents in combination with fragmentation is higher than with a systemic infusion.

Pulmonary embolectomy

Thrombolytic therapy is likely to give better results than embolectomy, although the latter may have life-saving potential in some instances. The average operative mortality in the United States of America among 620 unstable patients operated from 2004 to 2008 was 40%, and among 1550 stable patients mortality was 23%. These data reflect average results. Advanced centres with expertise might show a lower mortality. A candidate for pulmonary embolectomy should meet the following criteria: (1) massive PE, angiographically documented if possible; (2) haemodynamic instability (shock) despite heparin therapy and resuscitative efforts; and (3) failure of thrombolytic therapy or a contraindication to its use.

Chronic pulmonary thromboembolic hypertension

The vast majority of PE resolve because of natural thrombolytic processes. Residual emboli, if any, undergo fibrovascular organization causing chronic obstruction to pulmonary arterial blood flow. It is estimated that 2.8% of patients with PE develop chronic thromboembolic pulmonary hypertension, usually within 3 years after the acute PE. The predominant symptom of chronic thromboembolic pulmonary hypertension is unexplained dyspnoea on exertion, often following an asymptomatic period of several months or years after the acute PE. The reference standard for the diagnosis is combined right heart catheterization to quantify the haemodynamic impairment, and conventional pulmonary angiography to determine the extent and proximal location of the chronic thromboembolic obstruction. CT pulmonary angiography is essential to exclude rare conditions that may present with similar signs and symptoms such as fibrous mediastinitis, mediastinal carcinoma and pulmonary artery sarcoma.

Pulmonary thromboendarterectomy in an experienced centre is the treatment of choice in symptomatic patients with surgically accessible thromboemboli. Early diagnosis is important because the surgical mortality in patients who have progressed to dyspnoea at rest is substantially greater than among those with less severe symptoms. Neither anticoagulants nor vasodilators are effective, with the haemodynamic and symptomatic benefits of medical therapy being modest in comparison to those resulting from successful pulmonary thromboendarterectomy. See Chapter 15.2 for further discussion.

Further reading

Agnelli G, et al. (2013) AMPLIFY Investigators: Oral apixaban for the treatment of acute venous thromboembolism. N Engl J Med, 369, 799–808.
Agnelli G, Becattini C (2010). Acute pulmonary embolism. N Engl J Med, 363, 266–74.
Chatterjee S, et al. (2014). Thrombolysis for pulmonary embolism and risk of all-cause mortality, major bleeding, and intracranial hemorrhage: a meta-analysis. JAMA, 311, 2414–21.
Collaborative Study by the PIOPED Investigators (1990). Value of the ventilation/perfusion scan in acute pulmonary embolism—results of the Prospective Investigation of Pulmonary Embolism Diagnosis (PIOPED). JAMA, 263, 2753–59.
Fedullo P, et al. (2011). Chronic thromboembolic pulmonary hypertension. Am J Resp Crit Care Med, 183, 1605–13.
Guyatt GH, et al. (2012). Antithrombotic therapy and prevention of thrombosis, 9th ed: American College of Chest Physicians evidence-based clinical practice guidelines. Chest, 141(suppl), 7S–47S.
Mismetti P, et al. (2015). PREPIC2 Study Group. Effect of a retrievable inferior vena cava filter plus anticoagulation vs anticoagulation alone on risk of recurrent pulmonary embolism: a randomized clinical trial. JAMA, 313, 1627–35.
PREPIC Study Group (2005). Eight-year follow-up of patients with permanent vena cava filters in the prevention of pulmonary embolism: the PREPIC (Prevention du Risque d'Embolie Pulmonaire par Interruption Cave) randomized study. Circulation, 112, 416–22.
Schulman S, et al; RE-COVER II Trial Investigators (2014). Treatment of acute venous thromboembolism with dabigatran or warfarin and pooled analysis. Circulation, 18, 129, 764–72.
Sostman, HD et al. (2008). Sensitivity and specificity of perfusion scintigraphy combined with chest radiography for acute pulmonary embolism in PIOPED II. J Nucl Med, 49, 1741–8.
Stein PD (2016). Pulmonary embolism, 3rd edition. Wiley Blackwell, Oxford.
Stein PD, Matta F (2012). Thrombolytic therapy in unstable patients with acute pulmonary embolism: save lives but underused. Am J Med, 125, 465–70.
Stein PD, Matta F (2012). Pulmonary embolectomy for acute pulmonary embolism. Am J Med, 125, 471–7.
Stein PD, et al. (1991). Clinical, laboratory, roentgenographic and electrocardiographic findings in patients with acute pulmonary embolism and no pre-existing cardiac or pulmonary disease. Chest, 100, 598–603.
Stein PD, et al. (2004). D-dimer for the exclusion of deep venous thrombosis and acute pulmonary embolism: a systematic review. Ann Intern Med, 140, 589–602.
Stein PD, et al. (2006). Diagnostic pathways in acute pulmonary embolism: Recommendations of the PIOPED II investigators. Am J Med, 119, 1048–55.
Stein PD, et al. (2006). Multidetector computed tomography for acute pulmonary embolism. N Engl J Med, 354, 2317–27.
Stein PD, et al. (2007). Clinical characteristics of patient with acute pulmonary embolism: data from PIOPED II. Am J Med, 120, 871–9.
Stein PD, et al. (2010). Early discharge of patients with venous thromboembolism: implications regarding therapy. Clin Appl Thromb Hemost, 16, 141–5.
Stein PD, et al. (2010). Outcome in stable patients with acute pulmonary embolism who had right ventricular enlargement and/or elevated levels of troponin I. Am J Cardiol, 106, 558–63.
Stein PD, et al. (2010). Silent pulmonary embolism in patients with deep venous thrombosis: a systematic review. Am J Med, 123, 426–31.
Stein PD, et al. (2011). Elevated cardiac biomarkers with normal right ventricular size indicate an unlikely diagnosis of acute pulmonary embolism in stable patients. Clin Appl Thromb Hemost, 17, E153–7.
Stein PD, et al. (2011). Prognosis based on cardiac biomarkers and right ventricular size in stable patients with acute pulmonary embolism. Am J Cardiol, 107, 774–7.
Stein PD, et al. (2012). Diagnosis and management of isolated subsegmental pulmonary embolism: Review and assessment of the options. Clin Appl Thromb Hemost, 18, 20–6.
Stein PD, et al. (2012). Impact of vena cava filters on in-hospital case fatality rates from pulmonary embolism. Am J Med, 125, 478–84.
Stein PD, et al. (2012). Trends in case fatality rates in patients with pulmonary embolism according to stability and treatment. Thrombosis Research, 130, 841–46.
Stein PD, Matta F (2013). Treatment of unstable pulmonary embolism in elderly and those with comorbid conditions. Am J Med, 126, 304–10.
Stein PD, et al. (2014). A critical review of SPECT imaging in pulmonary embolism. Clin Transl Imaging, 2, 379–390.
Tapson VF (2008). Acute pulmonary embolism. N Engl J Med, 358, 1037–52.
van Belle A, et al. (2006). Effectiveness of managing suspected pulmonary embolism using an algorithm combining clinical probability, D-dimer testing, and computed tomography. JAMA, 295, 172–9.
Wells PS, et al. (1997). Value of assessment of pretest probability of deep-vein thrombosis in clinical management. Lancet, 350, 1795–8.
Wells PS, et al. (2000). Derivation of a simple clinical model to categorize patients probability of pulmonary embolism: increasing the models utility with the SimpliRED D-dimer. Thromb Haemost, 83, 416–20.
Wells PS, et al. (2001). Excluding PE at the bedside without diagnostic imaging: management of patients with suspected PE presenting to the emergency department by using a simple clinical model and D-dimer. Ann Intern Med, 135, 98–107.

CHAPTER 16.2

Therapeutic anticoagulation

David Keeling

Essentials

Low molecular weight heparins (LMWH) have largely replaced unfractionated heparin. Their much more predictable anticoagulant response combined with high bioavailability after subcutaneous injection means that the dose can be calculated by body weight and given subcutaneously without any monitoring or dose adjustment. Their widespread use resulted in most patients with deep vein thrombosis being managed as outpatients, and this is also increasingly the case for uncomplicated pulmonary embolism.

New oral direct inhibitors of anticoagulation that specifically target thrombin or factor Xa have been developed and are now an option for treating acute venous thromboembolism (VTE) and for stroke prevention in atrial fibrillation.

Particular issues—(1) in patients with cancer and VTE, giving LMWH for the first 6 months of long-term anticoagulant therapy has been shown to be superior to vitamin K antagonist; (2) high-dose loading regimens of warfarin are unnecessary and may increase the risk of overanticoagulation and bleeding; (3) warfarin for venous thromboembolism and atrial fibrillation should be given with a target INR of 2.5 (range 2.0–3.0); for patients with prosthetic heart valves the target INR is usually greater; (4) indefinite anticoagulation is required for patients with atrial fibrillation or a mechanical heart valve; for venous thromboembolism a careful clinical decision is required regarding duration of treatment; (5) for patients with atrial fibrillation anticoagulation is much more effective than aspirin in preventing stroke; (6) if warfarin needs to be stopped for surgery, full-dose heparin does not have to be given perioperatively unless the risk of thromboembolism is high, and warfarin can be continued in patients having dental extractions

Introduction

The main indications for therapeutic anticoagulation are venous thromboembolism (VTE)—deep vein thrombosis (DVT) and pulmonary embolism (PE) (see Chapter 16.1)—and the prevention of stroke in patients with atrial fibrillation or mechanical heart valves. Oral vitamin K antagonists (in the United Kingdom, mostly warfarin) have been the mainstay of treatment, but the new oral direct inhibitors of thrombin or factor Xa are being increasingly used to treat VTE and to prevent stroke in atrial fibrillation. When warfarin is used in acute venous thromboembolism, initial anticoagulation with heparin is required because warfarin takes time to become effective.

Therapeutic anticoagulation for venous thromboembolism

DVT and PE are aspects of the same disease—VTE. Forty per cent of patients with DVT without clinical evidence of PE have evidence of emboli on lung scanning. The principles of therapeutic anticoagulation are the same for both. In proximal DVT and PE, this has involved immediate anticoagulation with heparin followed by a period of anticoagulation with warfarin (or other oral vitamin K antagonist). Distal DVT can be managed in the same way, but an alternative strategy is to use serial noninvasive testing (e.g. ultrasonography), which only reliably detects proximal thrombosis, to ensure that suspected distal thrombosis does not extend above the knee, withholding treatment if it does not.

There is clear evidence that immediately acting anticoagulation is needed in the initial phase and that anticoagulation with oral vitamin K antagonists alone is inadequate. Warfarin can be commenced on the first day and heparin is continued for 5 days or until the international normalized ratio (INR) is greater than 2.0 for 2 consecutive days, whichever is the longer. Extending the period of heparinization from 5 to 10 days is not more effective and increases the risk of heparin-induced thrombocytopenia. The new oral direct inhibitors act immediately and rivaroxaban and apixaban have been used to treat acute VTE without initial heparin (see below). Dabigatran and edoxaban have also been used for acute VTE, but with initial heparin.

Heparin

Heparin, a glycosaminoglycan, is composed of alternating uronic acid and glucosamine saccharides that are sulfated to a varying degree. Its mode of action is to potentiate the activity of the serine protease inhibitor (serpin) antithrombin, whose main mode of action is to inhibit thrombin, but which also inhibits several other coagulant proteases such as factor Xa. A specific pentasaccharide sequence (see 'Fondaparinux', below) determined by the sulfation pattern along the heparin chain binds to antithrombin and causes a conformational change, giving it full activation against factor Xa but only partial activation against thrombin. Heparins of 18 saccharides (molecular weight (MW) 5400) or more can extend across the intermolecular gap and also bind to thrombin giving full antithrombin activity, which is lost if the chains are shorter. Unfractionated or standard heparins are a mixture of chains of different lengths (MW 5000–35 000, mean 13 000) and low molecular weight heparins (LMWH, MW 2000–8000, mean 5000) are derived from them by enzymatic or physicochemical cleavage. LMWH have, with good reason, largely replaced unfractionated heparin for the treatment of venous thromboembolism, but the use of the latter is discussed first.

Anticoagulation with unfractionated heparin

Unfractionated heparin has most often been given by continuous intravenous infusion, the rate of which has to be adjusted, usually by measuring the activated partial thromboplastin time (APTT). An inadequate APTT response in the first 24 h may increase the risk of recurrence of thromboembolism, although this does not seem to be critical if the starting infusion rate is at least 1250 IU/h. A validated regimen is to give a bolus dose of 80 IU/kg and to start the infusion at 18 IU/kg/h, performing the first APTT estimate after 6 h. The dose is then usually adjusted to maintain the APTT between 1.5 to 2.5 times the average laboratory control value. With older APTT reagents, this corresponded to a therapeutic heparin level of 0.3 to 0.7 IU/ml by anti-Xa assay. However, many current APTT reagents show an increased sensitivity to unfractionated heparin and, with these, higher ratios should be aimed for. The local laboratory should advise on the appropriate therapeutic range with its reagent. When the dose is therapeutic, the APTT should be checked daily.

An alternative is to give unfractionated heparin subcutaneously once every 12 h, and a meta-analysis suggested that this might be more effective and at least as safe as continuous intravenous infusion. A reasonable starting dose is 250 IU/kg, adjusting the dose according to the mid-interval APTT.

Anticoagulation with LMWH

Although much is made of the greater anti-Xa/antithrombin ratio of the LMWH, their key clinical property is that they produce a much more predictable anticoagulant response than unfractionated heparin. This, combined with the fact that they have very high bioavailability after subcutaneous injection, means that the dose can be calculated by body weight and be given subcutaneously without any monitoring or dose adjustment. The actual dosage used differs slightly with the different LMWH and the manufacturers' recommendations should be followed, but a typical dose is 200 IU/kg once a day. They are at least as effective and at least as safe as unfractionated heparin, even when given once a day. Their widespread use resulted in most patients with DVT being managed as outpatients, and this is also increasingly the case for low-risk PE. LMWH is renally excreted and so should be used with caution in patients with renal failure: it is possible to adjust the dose based on anti-Xa levels, but renal impairment is one of the few situations where unfractionated heparin, monitored by the APTT, may be preferred by some physicians.

In patients with cancer, giving LMWH for the first 6 months of long-term anticoagulant therapy has been shown to be superior to switching to a vitamin K antagonist.

Complications of heparin treatment

If a patient on intravenous unfractionated heparin is excessively anticoagulated, it is usually sufficient simply to stop the infusion, the half-life being 1 to 2 h. If bleeding is severe, the heparin can be neutralized with protamine sulfate, giving 1 mg for every 100 IU that has been infused over the previous hour. The reversal of LMWH is more problematic. Although protamine sulfate may not neutralize the smaller chains, it is often clinically effective, though estimating an appropriate dose is more difficult (the maximum dose is 50 mg, so this is often given if the subcutaneous injection was recent).

Heparin-induced thrombocytopenia is a feared complication, but much less common now that short courses of LMWH are used. It is due to the development of an antibody to the heparin–platelet factor 4 complex and can be associated with serious venous and arterial thrombosis. Heparin must be stopped if heparin-induced thrombocytopenia is likely and an alternative anticoagulant substituted in full dosage (e.g. danaparoid or argatroban).

Fondaparinux

The specific pentasaccharide sequence of heparin that binds to antithrombin has been chemically synthesized and is marketed as the drug fondaparinux. Like LMWH it is given by subcutaneous injection with no monitoring. It directs antithrombin's action against Xa, is equivalent to heparin in the treatment of venous thromboembolism, and is superior to heparin in the treatment of unstable angina and non-ST elevation myocardial infarction. It carries virtually no risk of heparin-induced thrombocytopenia.

Warfarin

The oral vitamin K antagonists have for decades been the mainstay of long-term anticoagulant therapy. Warfarin is the commonest vitamin K antagonist given; acenocoumarol (which has a shorter half-life) and phenindione (which has a higher incidence of skin rashes) are seldom used in the United Kingdom. The procoagulant factors II, VII, IX, and X (and the anticoagulants protein C and protein S) need vitamin K for the γ-carboxylation of the glutamic acid residues that form their gla domains. Without this post-translational modification they cannot bind calcium, and as a consequence cannot bind to anionic phospholipid surfaces such that assembly of the key coagulation complexes is disrupted.

Warfarin takes a number of days to become effective, so heparin is given initially if immediate anticoagulation is needed When warfarin is started, the vitamin K-dependent factors fall according to their half-lives. Factor VII and protein C have the shortest half-lives, so that despite a prolongation of the INR due to factor VII deficiency, warfarin may initially be procoagulant. This is the mechanism for the rare problem of warfarin-induced skin necrosis, most often described in those with protein C deficiency.

Initiation and monitoring of anticoagulation with warfarin

Monitoring of warfarin treatment is by the INR. This is a manipulation of the prothrombin time (PT) to allow for the different sensitivities of various laboratory reagents to the warfarin-induced coagulopathy. The INR equals $(PT/MNPT)^{ISI}$ where MNPT is the (mean normal) control PT and ISI is the international sensitivity index of the thromboplastin used in the assay. For the treatment of DVT and PE, the target INR should be 2.5 (target range 2.0–3.0).

If the initial coagulation tests are not prolonged, it has been customary to give 10 mg of warfarin on the first evening and check the INR the following morning, adjusting the dose according to the daily INR results until the patient is stable. With these regimens, most patients received 10 mg of warfarin on the first 2 days. There is, however, no evidence to suggest a 10 mg loading dose is superior to 5 mg, and regimens that start with 5 mg doses, or a single 10 mg dose followed by 5 mg doses, may be preferable to regimens that start with repeated 10 mg doses. This is the case in patients with an increased risk of bleeding, e.g. elderly people (>60 years old), and those with liver disease or cardiac failure. The dosing algorithm used in Oxford is shown in Table 16.2.1.

When patients are stable, they may go for up to 8 weeks between INR checks. If the INR is unstable, patients are seen more frequently, but it should be noted that with warfarin it takes approximately 1 week (5 times the half-life of 36 h) to reach a new steady state after dose adjustment, hence more frequent dosage alteration is inadvisable.

Table 16.2.1 A warfarin induction regimen

Days 1 and 2	Day 3		Day 4	
	INR	Dose (mg)	INR	Dose (mg)
Give 5 mg each evening if baseline INR < 1.4	<1.5	10	<1.6	10
	1.5–2.0	5	1.6–1.7	7
	2.1–2.5	3	1.8–1.9	6
	2.6–3.0	1	2.0–2.3	5
	>3.0*	0	2.4–2.7	4
			2.8–3.0	3
			3.1–3.5	2
			3.6–4.0	1
			>4.0*	0

*and seek advice on further management

Complications of warfarin treatment

The only major complication of warfarin treatment is bleeding. Risk factors for bleeding are increasing age, a history of stroke, a history of gastrointestinal bleeding, anaemia, renal impairment, diabetes, and recent myocardial infarction. A significant problem in control is the starting and stopping of other medication. Many drugs interact with warfarin (see Table 16.2.2 for those with the most evidence) such that patient (and doctor) education and constant vigilance are essential. Close monitoring of the INR is advised when concomitant medication is altered.

The approach taken to reverse over-anticoagulation with warfarin depends on the circumstances (see Box 16.2.1). Prothrombin

Table 16.2.2 Many drugs interact with warfarin; the evidence is strongest for those listed

Potentiation	Inhibition
Amiodarone	Barbiturates
Cimetidine	Carbamazepine
Clofibrate	Chlordiazepoxide
Cotrimoxazole	Colestyramine
Erythromycin	Griseofulvin
Fluconazole	Rifampicin
Isoniazid	Sucralfate
Metronidazole	
Miconazole	
Omeprazole	
Paracetamol	
Phenylbutazone	
Piroxicam	
Propafenone	
Propranolol	
Statins	
Sulfinpyrazone	

Box 16.2.1 Management of over-anticoagulation with warfarin

Major bleeding

◆ Stop warfarin

◆ Give prothrombin complex concentrate (PCC) 25–50 IU/kg (or fresh frozen plasma (FFP) 15 ml/kg if PCC not available)

◆ Give phytomenadione 5 mg intravenously

Minor bleeding

◆ Stop warfarin

◆ Give phytomenadione 1–3 mg intravenously

High INR without bleeding

◆ Stop warfarin until INR <5

◆ If INR >8 give phytomenadione 1–5 mg orally

---

complex concentrates, unlike fresh frozen plasma, reliably and rapidly correct the defect and should be used in life-threatening situations such as intracranial bleeding. Small doses of phytomenadione (vitamin K_1) can lower a high INR without making subsequent anticoagulation difficult, as is the case if high doses are given.

New oral direct inhibitors of anticoagulation

The ideal anticoagulant would be orally active, have a wide therapeutic index, predictable pharmacokinetics and dynamics (negating the need for monitoring), minimal interactions with other drugs and food, a rapid onset of action, an antidote, and minimal nonanticoagulant side effects. Heparin needs to be given parenterally. Warfarin has a slow onset of action, a narrow therapeutic index, unpredictable pharmacokinetics and dynamics, and significant drug and dietary interactions that make regular monitoring essential. New anticoagulants were therefore much sort after, and various parts of the coagulation cascade have been targeted by potential new drugs (Fig. 16.2.1). Oral direct thrombin inhibitors and the oral direct Xa inhibitors have now emerged into clinical practice: they directly inhibit their target coagulation factors and so do not require antithrombin for their action.

Oral direct thrombin (IIa) inhibitors

Dabigatran etexilate is orally absorbed and rapidly converted to dabigatran, which inhibits both free and clot-bound thrombin. Peak levels occur 2 h after a dose and the half-life is 12–17 h, the drug being 80% renally excreted. A fixed dose of 150 mg twice a day has been shown to be as effective as warfarin in the treatment of acute venous thromboembolism, though heparin was still given for the first 5 days. It has also been compared with warfarin for the prevention of stroke and systemic embolization in atrial fibrillation, with 110 mg twice a day showing similar efficacy with reduced major bleeding, and 150 mg twice a day showing improved efficacy with similar major bleeding.

A specific antidote for dabigatran, the monoclonal antibody idarucizumab, has recently been approved by the FDA.

Oral direct Xa inhibitors

Several oral direct Xa inhibitors have been developed (e.g. rivaroxaban, apixaban, edoxaban). All have a rapid onset of action and inhibit free Xa, also Xa bound in the prothrombinase complex.

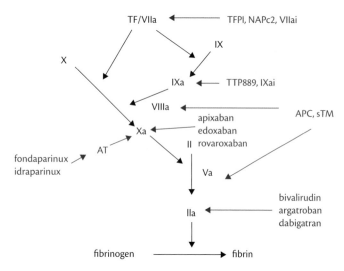

Fig. 16.2.1 New anticoagulants. Roman numerals represent the coagulation factors (a indicates the activated forms). APC, activated protein C; AT, antithrombin; NAPc2, nematode anticoagulant peptide; sTM, soluble thrombomodulin; TF, tissue factor; TFPI, tissue factor pathway inhibitor; TTP899, IXa inhibitor in development; VIIai and IXai, active site inhibited VIIa and IXa.

- *Rivaroxaban* has a half-life of 7–13 h and renal clearance is 33%. 15 mg twice a day for 3 weeks followed by 20 mg once a day is as effective as warfarin in the treatment of venous thromboembolism, with reduced major bleeding; 20 mg once a day is equivalent to warfarin for the prevention of stoke and systemic embolization in atrial fibrillation,

- *Apixaban* has a half-life of 10–14 h and renal clearance is 25%. 10 mg twice a day for 1 week followed by 5 mg twice a day is as effective as warfarin in the treatment of venous thromboembolism with reduced major bleeding; 5 mg twice a day is more effective than warfarin for the prevention of stoke and systemic embolization in atrial fibrillation with less major bleeding.

- *Edoxaban* has a half-life of 8–10 h and renal clearance is 50%. 60 mg once a day is as effective as warfarin in the treatment of venous thromboembolism but heparin was still used for the first 5 days. 60 mg once a day is as effective as warfarin for the prevention of stoke and systemic embolization in atrial fibrillation with less major bleeding; 30 mg once a day is used in those with renal impairment or low body weight.

At present there are no factor Xa inhibitor antidotes, but a decoy receptor–andexanet alfa–is in an advanced stage of development.

Selecting an anticoagulant

The oral direct inhibitors offer an alternative to vitamin K antagonists for the treatment and secondary prevention of VTE and for stroke prevention in atrial fibrillation. They cannot be used in patients with mechanical heart valves. Logistically they are much simpler to use as they do not require dose adjustment or monitoring. The lack of treatments to reverse the effects of oral direct inhibitors is a disadvantage compared to vitamin K antagonists, but they have short half-lives, seem to have a significantly reduced incidence of intracranial bleeding as compared to vitamin K antagonists, and antidotes should be available in the near future. They are not a good choice for the poorly compliant, and renal function should be assessed before they are prescribed.

Duration of anticoagulation after venous thromboembolism

After the acute event, 6 months of anticoagulation has been shown to be more effective than 6 weeks of anticoagulation, and 3 months has been shown to be equivalent to 6 months. The difficult clinical decision is to decide who should get long-term anticoagulation, which is a matter of balancing the risk of recurrence against the risk of bleeding on warfarin: 2–3% of people on warfarin have a major bleed each year and the case fatality is 10%, giving a fatality rate of 0.25% per year (mostly from intracranial haemorrhage). However, warfarin is highly (90–95%) effective at preventing recurrence. The risk of a recurrent venous thromboembolism (VTE) after a first VTE is approximately 5% per year, which with a case fatality rate of 5% also gives a fatality rate of 0.25% per year. Other factors that may either increase the risk of bleeding or increase the risk of recurrence need to be taken into account. The risk of recurrence is higher for proximal DVT and PE than for distal DVT, and it is lower if a transient risk factor was present (e.g. recent surgery, use of the contraceptive pill).

For patients with a first episode of distal DVT (whether provoked or unprovoked), or a first episode of proximal DVT or PE secondary to a transient (reversible) risk factor, treatment is recommended for 3 months. For patients with a first episode of unprovoked proximal DVT or PE, treatment is recommended for at least 3 months and consideration should be given to long-term treatment where there are no risk factors for bleeding and where anticoagulant control is good. Raised D-dimers after discontinuing anticoagulation increase the risk of recurrence. Factor V Leiden and the prothrombin mutation do not increase the risk of recurrence to a clinically significant extent. Whether deficiencies of antithrombin, protein C, or protein S increase the risk of recurrence is less clear, but testing for these is less helpful than paying attention to the history and considering a D-dimer test. Antiphospholipid antibodies are thought to increase the risk of recurrence, but the evidence is from poor quality studies. If the first event was a symptomatic PE subsequent events are more likely to be PE as compared to if the first event was a DVT. For patients with two or more episodes of objectively documented venous thromboembolism or those with a first event and an ongoing risk factor (such as cancer), indefinite treatment should be considered. Taking all this into account, a reasonable approach is indicated in Table 16.2.3.

Fibrinolysis for venous thromboembolism

Thrombolytic agents dissolve thrombi by directly or indirectly activating the zymogen plasminogen to plasmin. Plasmin then degrades fibrin to soluble peptides, but cannot distinguish fibrin in pathological thrombi from fibrin in haemostatic plugs.

Table 16.2.3 Duration of warfarin treatment

Event	Duration of treatment
1st calf DVT	3 months
1st proximal DVT or PE with TRF [a]	
1st unprovoked proximal DVT or PE	3 months or long term
1st proximal DVT or PE with ongoing risk factor	Long term
Recurrent VTE	

[a] TRF, transient risk factor (e.g. surgery, combined pill, pregnancy, plaster cast).

The use of thrombolytic agents for venous thromboembolism requires careful individual assessment. It is not often given in DVT, though its use should be considered in iliofemoral thrombosis. Thrombolysis in massive PE may be life-saving but for submassive PE, although thrombolysis achieves more rapid resolution than heparin alone, there is no clear evidence of lasting benefit (see Chapter 16.1).

Streptokinase (which forms a complex with plasminogen that then activates free plasminogen), urokinase, and tissue plasminogen activator (tPA) have all been used. For PE, streptokinase is recommended as a 250 000-IU loading dose followed by an infusion for 24 h at 100 000 IU/h. Urokinase is given as a 4400 IU/kg loading dose followed by 2200 IU/kg for 12 h. Following the success of rapid fibrinolytic regimens in myocardial infarction, tPA given as 100 mg over 2 h has been used for PE, and the use of more rapid regimens with the other two agents has also been suggested (see Chapter 16.1 for further discussion).

Anticoagulation in particular clinical circumstances

Treatment of venous thromboembolism in pregnancy

Heparin and LMWH do not cross the placenta and can be used in pregnancy. LMWH is more convenient, and the osteopenia sometimes seen with prolonged use of unfractionated heparin seems to be less of a problem with LMWH. Warfarin, which crosses the placenta, can cause an embryopathy if given between 6 and 12 weeks of gestation. At any time, it can cause fetal bleeding and has been associated with central nervous system abnormalities. The oral direct inhibitors cannot be used in pregnancy.

The usual treatment recommended for venous thromboembolism in pregnancy is to continue with full-dose subcutaneous LMWH until term. Warfarin can be used for the 6 weeks of the puerperium: women taking warfarin can breastfeed.

Therapeutic anticoagulation for atrial fibrillation

Atrial fibrillation affects 2 to 5% of people over the age of 60, and is associated with a stroke rate of 5% a year. In patients with atrial fibrillation, warfarin given to a target INR of 2.5 (target range 2.0–3.0) prevents two-thirds of fatal or disabling strokes, though it becomes less effective when the INR is less than 2.0. Aspirin reduces stroke in atrial fibrillation by only approximately 20%. Compared to warfarin the oral direct inhibitors are as or more effective with the same or reduced major bleeding (see above).

In patients with atrial fibrillation, the following increase the risk of stroke: congestive heart failure, hypertension, increasing age, diabetes, previous ischaemic stroke, or transient ischaemic attack, vascular disease, and female sex. One scheme used to assess patients (CHA_2DS_2-VASc) gives points for these risk factors. Patient with a score of zero do not usually receive anticoagulation, whereas those with a score of 2 or more are usually anticoagulated. Women with a score of 1 are not anticoagulated, but for men there has been a trend to recommend anticoagulation.

Warfarin or one of the oral direct inhibitors can be used. If warfarin is used rapid anticoagulation is not usually required and a slow-loading regimen (such as starting patients on 3 mg of warfarin daily for 1 week and determining subsequent doses by weekly INR measurement) is safe and achieves therapeutic anticoagulation in most patients within 3 to 4 weeks.

Table 16.2.4 Management of warfarin anticoagulation perioperatively, recommendations for bridging when warfarin is stopped 5 days before surgery

Risk	Preoperatively	Postoperatively until INR> 2
High risk e.g. VTE within 1 month; prosthetic mitral valve; AF and history of stroke	Treatment-dose heparin[a] (either IV UFH or SC LMWH)	Treatment-dose heparin[a] (either IV UFH or SC LMWH)
Low risk e.g. VTE >3 months ago, bi-leaflet aortic valve with no other risk factors, AF without previous stroke	Nil or prophylactic LMWH	Prophylactic LMWH

AF, atrial fibrillation; IV, intravenous; LMWH; low molecular weight heparin; SC, subcutaneous; UFH, unfractionated heparin; VTE, venous thromboembolism.

[a] Stop full-dose IV UFH 6 h before surgery and check APTT before operation begins, omit full-dose SC LMWH on day of surgery. Therapeutic dose heparin must not be given for at least 48 h after high bleeding risk surgery.

Therapeutic anticoagulation in patients with prosthetic heart valves

Vitamin K antagonists are recommended for all patients with mechanical prosthetic heart valves, the overall risk of embolic stroke if not anticoagulated being 8% per year. Emboli are more common from mitral prosthetic valves than aortic prosthetic valves, and caged-ball valves are more thrombogenic than bi-leaflet or tilting-disk valves.

Various national and international recommendations are made regarding the target INR in patients with prosthetic valves, with 3.5 traditionally being advised. This is still reasonable for caged-ball valves, but for tilting-disks and bi-leaflet valves the target INR can possibly be lower, e.g. 2.5 (range 2.0–3.0) for aortic valves and 3.0 (range 2.5–3.5) for mitral valves. When a new valve is inserted, it is recommended that unfractionated heparin or LMWH be given until the INR is stable and at a therapeutic level for 2 consecutive days.

Perioperative management of therapeutic anticoagulation

Warfarin does not need to be stopped for dentistry, nor for some minor surgery. For many operations, however, warfarin will need to be temporarily discontinued. It can generally be stopped 5 days before surgery and the INR be checked on the day of surgery (checking the day before obviates the risk of cancellation as a small dose of oral vitamin K can be given if necessary). The main clinical decision is whether to give bridging therapy with treatment-dose heparin perioperatively when the INR is less than 2.0. This depends on balancing the risk of bleeding with the risk of thromboembolism. For those at high risk of thromboembolism, such as patients with a prosthetic mitral valve, treatment-dose heparin is usually given (Table 16.2.4).

The new oral direct inhibitors of anticoagulation have short half-lives and so bridging is not required. They can normally be stopped 1 or 2 days preoperatively, although renal function needs to be taken into consideration, particularly for dabigatran. They must not be given for at least 48 h after high bleeding risk surgery.

Further reading

Ageno W, *et al.* (2012). Oral anticoagulant therapy: Antithrombotic therapy and prevention of thrombosis, 9th ed: American College of Chest Physicians Evidence-Based Clinical Practice Guidelines. *Chest*, **141**, e44–88S.

Connolly SJ, *et al.* (2009). Dabigatran versus warfarin in patients with atrial fibrillation. *N Engl J Med*, **361**, 1139–51.

Giugliano RP, *et al.*(2013). Edoxaban versus warfarin in patients with atrial fibrillation. *N Engl J Med*, **369**, 2093–104.

Granger CB, *et al.* (2011). Apixaban versus warfarin in patients with atrial fibrillation. *N Engl J Med*, **365**, 981–92.

Kearon C, *et al.* (2012). Antithrombotic therapy for VTE disease: Antithrombotic therapy and prevention of thrombosis, 9th ed: American College of Chest Physicians Evidence-Based Clinical Practice Guidelines. *Chest*, **141**, e419–94S.

Keeling D, *et al.* (2011). Guidelines on oral anticoagulation with warfarin—fourth edition. *Br J Haematol*, **154**, 311–24.

Patel MR, *et al.* (2011). Rivaroxaban versus warfarin in nonvalvular atrial fibrillation. *N Engl J Med*, **365**, 883–91.

Weitz JI, *et al.* (2012). New antithrombotic drugs: Antithrombotic therapy and prevention of thrombosis, 9th ed: American College of Chest Physicians Evidence-Based Clinical Practice Guidelines. *Chest*, **141**, e120–51S.

Hypertension

SECTION 17

Hypertension

CHAPTER 17.1

Essential hypertension: definition, epidemiology, and pathophysiology

Bryan Williams

Essentials

'Essential hypertension' is high blood pressure for which there is no clearly defined aetiology. From a practical perspective, it is best defined as that level of blood pressure at which treatment to lower blood pressure results in significant clinical benefit—a level which will vary from patient to patient depending on their absolute cardiovascular risk.

Historically, most guidelines define 'hypertension' as an office blood pressure greater than or equal to 140/90 mmHg, but some recent recommendations prefer home or ambulatory blood pressure (blood pressure) averages. When using 24 h ambulatory blood pressure or home blood pressure averages to define hypertension, the diagnostic thresholds are lower than those used with office measurement, with a value of 135/85 mmHg typically used for both daytime ambulatory blood pressure and home measurements.

Isolated diastolic hypertension (systolic blood pressure (SBP) <140 mmHg, diastolic blood pressure (DBP) >90 mmHg) is more common in younger people, and isolated systolic hypertension (SBP >140 mmHg, DBP <90 mmHg) is the most common form of hypertension in older people.

American guidelines include a category of 'prehypertension' (SBP 120–139 mmHg and/or DBP 80–89 mmHg), the reason for this being that blood pressure in this range is associated with both adverse cardiovascular outcome and a high rate of progression to hypertension.

Epidemiology

In 2000, it was estimated 25% of the world's adult population were hypertensive, and predicted that this would rise to 29% by 2025. By the age of 60, more than one-half of adults in most regions of the world will be hypertensive.

There is a continuous relationship between blood pressure and cardiovascular risk from blood pressure values as low as 115/75 mmHg. The relationship is steeper for stroke than it is for coronary heart disease, and is magnified by age. There is a doubling in risk of stroke and ischaemic heart disease mortality for every 20/10 mmHg increase in blood pressure.

Most people with hypertension are over the age of 50 years, and in these SBP is by far the most important contributor to the burden of cardiovascular disease attributable to hypertension.

Pathogenesis and pathophysiology

The pathogenesis of essential hypertension is a complex interplay between (1) genetic predisposition, (2) lifestyle and environmental influences, and (3) disturbances in vascular structure and neurohumoral control mechanisms.

Genetic predisposition—blood pressure runs in families, with a remarkably consistent level of correlation of around 0.2 between first-degree relatives found in many studies. This means that if the blood pressure of one member of the family deviates from the norm by +10 mmHg, the first-degree relative will deviate by +2 mmHg on average. Variants in a large number of genes, involving virtually all of the main physiological systems affecting blood pressure, have shown association with blood pressure in one or more studies, but the effect of any individual variant is likely to be modest.

Lifestyle and environmental influences—the exploding prevalence of hypertension in economically developing regions reflects lifestyle changes, so-called 'Westernization', more than anything else, with the most important influences on blood pressure being sodium intake, obesity, and alcohol intake.

Pathophysiology—a characteristic finding in essential hypertension is an inappropriate increase in peripheral vascular resistance relative to the cardiac output. This is due to remodelling of small arteries (arterioles), which is characterized by an increase in their media/lumen ratio, but it is not clear whether these changes are a consequence or a cause of raised blood pressure. The functional integrity of large conduit arteries, i.e. the aorta, which becomes stiffer, also influences the development of hypertension—especially systolic hypertension. Endothelial dysfunction and decreased nitric oxide production are found in hypertension, but are more likely a consequence than a cause of elevated blood pressure. The specific role of the renin–angiotensin–aldosterone system in the development of essential hypertension remains unclear, but therapeutic agents that inhibit this system have proved to be very effective treatments. The sympathetic nervous system is involved in the acute and chronic regulation of blood pressure, but whether disturbances in it play a major role in the initiation and maintenance of chronic essential hypertension remains unknown.

The hypertensive phenotype and target organ damage

Although blood pressure measurement is used to define hypertension, hypertension is more than just blood pressure. Essential hypertension is commonly associated with metabolic disturbances (the 'insulin resistance phenotype') and multisystem structural damage that conspire to enhance cardiovascular risk beyond that which can be attributed to blood pressure alone.

Left ventricular hypertrophy is a classic feature of untreated or inadequately treated long-standing hypertension, and is a very potent predictor of premature cardiovascular disease and death. Inhibition of the renin–angiotensin–aldosterone system is particularly effective at regressing left ventricular hypertrophy, which is associated with dramatically improved prognosis for people with hypertension.

Hypertension is the single most important risk factor for stroke, and is increasingly recognized as a major factor contributing to the rate of cognitive decline in later life. Patients with renal disease often have hypertension, people with hypertension can develop renal disease, and the age-related decline in GFR is more rapid in people with essential hypertension, but renal function is usually well preserved throughout life in patients with mild to moderate essential hypertension. Retinal changes caused by hypertension are discussed in Chapter 17.2.

Implications of the evolution of hypertensive injury

The process of hypertensive injury to target organs evolves silently over many years. Current treatment guidelines have been developed from an evidence base relating to changes in hard clinical endpoints derived from studies in very elderly patients at the end of the hypertensive disease process. Future treatment strategies must surely focus on preventing the evolution of the silent disease process, rather than simply battling with its consequences.

Definitions of hypertension

The commonest form of hypertension has been termed 'essential hypertension', i.e. hypertension for which there is no clearly defined aetiology. Blood pressure is normally distributed within populations and thus the definition of 'hypertension' is a moving target. From a practical perspective it is best defined as that level of blood pressure at which treatment to lower blood pressure results in significant clinical benefit, which will change as new evidence from clinical trials emerges. This statement also highlights the conundrum in definition of 'hypertension' because the risk associated with blood pressure is a continuum and the level of pressure at which treatment results in 'significant clinical benefit' for any individual will depend on their absolute cardiovascular risk.

There is substantial evidence that treating systolic pressure (SBP) above 160 mmHg and/or a diastolic pressure (DBP) above 100 mmHg is beneficial; there is also evidence that treating pressures above 140/90 mmHg is worthwhile, especially in higher-risk

Table 17.1.1 Classification of hypertension. Grades 1–3 replace the old terminology of 'mild', 'moderate', and 'severe'. The 'high normal' blood pressure range corresponds to 'prehypertension' in the United States guideline

Category	Systolic		Diastolic
Optimal	<120	and	<80
Normal	120–129	and/or	80–84
High normal	130–139	and/or	85–89
Grade 1 hypertension	140–159	and/or	90–99
Grade 2 hypertension	160–179	and/or	100–109
Grade 3 hypertension	>180	and/or	>110
Isolated systolic hypertension	>140	and	<90

Reproduced from Giuseppe Mancia, Guy De Backer, Anna Dominiczak, *et al.*, 2007 ESH-ESC Practice Guidelines for the Management of Arterial Hypertension: ESH-ESC Task Force on the Management of Arterial Hypertension, *Journal of Hypertension*, 2007;**25**:1751–1762, with permission from Wolters Kluwer Health.

patients. Historically, most guidelines have therefore defined 'hypertension' as an office blood pressure of 140/90 mmHg or more, with various grades of hypertension also specified (Table 17.1.1). The hypertension guidelines in the United States of America include a category of 'prehypertension' (SBP 120–139 mmHg and/or DBP 80–89 mmHg), which is discussed later in this chapter.

It is important to note that the diagnostic thresholds for hypertension vary according to the method of measurement. The aforementioned blood pressure thresholds for diagnosis have been defined according to seated blood pressure measurements, so-called 'office blood pressures'. However, the increasing use of automated blood pressure monitoring, either at home or with ambulatory devices, has shown that there can be marked discrepancies between clinic blood pressure measurements and those obtained at home or when ambulatory. This has led to much discussion as to whether conventional clinic blood pressure measurements are still the best way of establishing the diagnosis of hypertension. When using 24h ambulatory blood pressure or home blood pressure averages to define hypertension, the diagnostic thresholds are lower than these office blood pressures, typically quoted values being 135/85 mmHg for both daytime ambulatory blood pressure monitoring and home blood pressure measurements.

Subtypes of hypertension

Various categories of blood pressure can be identified in populations, with isolated diastolic hypertension (IDH) (SBP <140 mmHg, DBP >90 mmHg) being more common in younger people and isolated systolic hypertension (SBP >140 mmHg, DBP <90 mmHg) being the most common form of hypertension in older people, with systolic/diastolic hypertension (SDH) (SBP>140 mmHg and DBP >90 mmHg) bridging the two extremes of age (Fig. 17.1.1).

Although traditionally DBP was considered to carry the greatest prognostic significance, it is now clear that this is no longer the case. Most people with hypertension are over the age of 50 years, and in them SBP is by far the most important contributor to the burden of cardiovascular disease attributable to hypertension. The different patterns of blood pressure and the relative importance of DBP and SBP with regard to prognosis reflect progression of the underlying pathology. The pathogenesis of hypertension in younger people is characterized by an increased peripheral vascular resistance. This

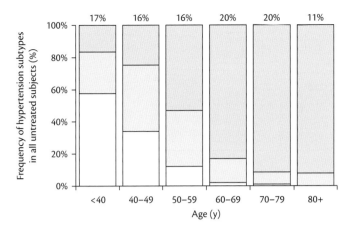

Fig. 17.1.1 Blood pressure subtypes in the United States of America according to age. The percentage values at the top of each column indicate the prevalence of hypertension in that age band.

Reproduced from Franklin SS *et al.*, Predominance of isolated systolic hypertension among middle-aged and elderly US hypertensives, *Hypertension* 2001;**37**:869–874 with permission of Wolters Kluwer Health.

results in an increased diastolic pressure, with any associated rise in systolic pressure 'cushioned' by a compliant aorta, hence the commonly observed IDH. With ageing there is progressive stiffening of the aorta, a consequent reduction in large-artery compliance, and a reduced capacity to sustain diastolic pressure and to cushion systolic pressure. The result is an age-related widening of pulse pressure as diastolic pressure falls alongside a progressive rise in SBP, hence the emergence of ISH (Fig. 17.1.2).

Epidemiology

Global prevalence

The global prevalence of hypertension when defined either as a blood pressure of ≥140/90 mmHg, or the use of antihypertensive medication, was estimated to be 972 million in the year 2000, representing about 25% of the world's adult population. The global prevalence of hypertension is expected to rise dramatically by about 60% by 2025, representing 29% of the world's adult population and affecting 1.6 billion people (Fig. 17.1.3). Most of this increase in the worldwide burden of hypertension is expected to result from an increase in the number of people with hypertension in economically developing regions, hence almost 75% of the world's hypertensive populations will be in economically developing regions by 2025.

The prevalence of hypertension in almost all regions of the world increases with age and more steeply in women. By the age of 60, more than one-half of adults in most regions of the world will be hypertensive. India and Asia have and will most likely continue to have the lowest rates of hypertension, whereas the highest rates are likely to remain in Latin America, the Caribbean, former Soviet republics, and sub-Saharan Africa. Consequently, hypertension is set to remain the single most important preventable cause of premature death worldwide over the next two decades, with the World Health Organization (WHO) estimating that about 7.1 million deaths per year may be attributable to hypertension, and that suboptimal blood pressure (SBP ≥115 mmHg by their definition) is responsible for 62% of cerebrovascular disease and 49% of ischaemic heart disease worldwide, with little variation by sex.

Lifetime risk

The prevalence of hypertension increases with age, affecting over one-half of those aged 60 to 69 years and over three-quarters of those aged over 70 years in the United States of America and most developed countries. As indicated above, almost all of the age-related rise in the prevalence of hypertension is due to a progressive rise in SBP. The lifetime probability of developing hypertension is about 90% for men and women who were not hypertensive at 55 or 65 years old and survived to age 80 to 85 (Fig. 17.1.4).

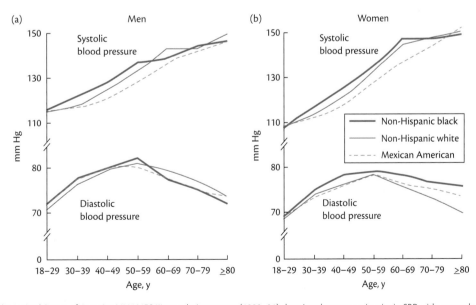

Fig. 17.1.2 Data from the United States of America NHANES III population survey (1988–91) showing the progressive rise in SBP with age and the rise in DBP up until age *c*.50 years, after which DBP falls and pulse pressure widens. This pattern is typical of Westernized countries and explains the high prevalence of isolated systolic hypertension in older people in these countries.

Reproduced from Burt VL *et al.*, Prevalence of hypertension in the US adult population, *Hypertension*, 1995;**23**:305–313 with permission of Wolters Kluwer Health.

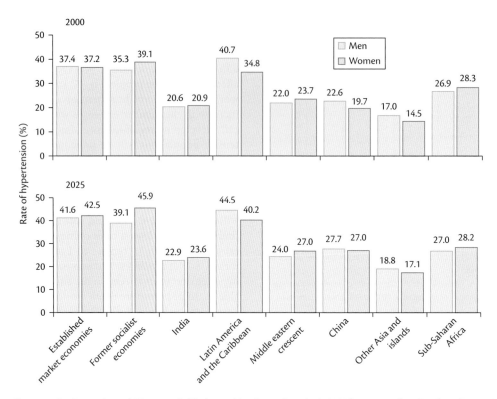

Fig. 17.1.3 Frequency of hypertension in people aged 20 years and older by world region and gender in 2000 (upper panel) and projected to 2025 (lower panel).
Reprinted from *The Lancet*, Vol. 365, Kearney PM, *et al.*, Global burden of hypertension: analysis of world-wide data, pp. 217–23. Copyright (2005), with permission from Elsevier.

Cardiovascular morbidity and mortality associated with hypertension

Elevated blood pressure increases the risk of cardiovascular morbidity and mortality. Data from observational studies of over 1 million people has indicated a continuous relationship between blood pressure and cardiovascular risk from blood pressure values as low as 115/75 mmHg (Fig. 17.1.5). The relationship is steeper for stroke than it is for coronary heart disease and is magnified by age. For every 20/10 mmHg increase in blood pressure, there is a doubling in risk of stroke and ischaemic heart disease mortality. Hypertension also increases the risk of congestive cardiac failure, endstage renal disease, and dementia. Moreover, data

from the Framingham Heart Study also indicates that there is a doubling of risk of cardiovascular complications in patients with blood pressure levels above normal but not yet classified as having overt hypertension (Fig. 17.1.6). This was the basis for the American guidelines introducing the term 'prehypertension' (SBP 120–139 mmHg and/or DBP 80–89 mmHg) to emphasize that this level of blood pressure (1) is not benign, (2) is associated with an elevated cardiovascular disease risk, and (3) predicts with a high degree of certainty that blood pressure is on an upward trajectory and that affected people are almost certain to develop more severe hypertension, unless there is intervention with effective in lifestyle changes and/or drug therapy.

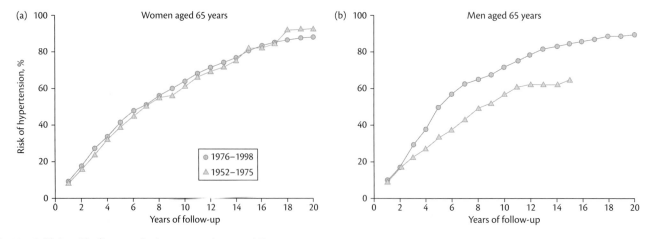

Fig. 17.1.4 Lifetime risk of hypertension in women and men aged 65 years.
Residual lifetime risk for developing hypertension in middle-aged women and men, the Framingham Heart Study, Ramachandran *et al. JAMA* 2002;**287**:1003–1010.

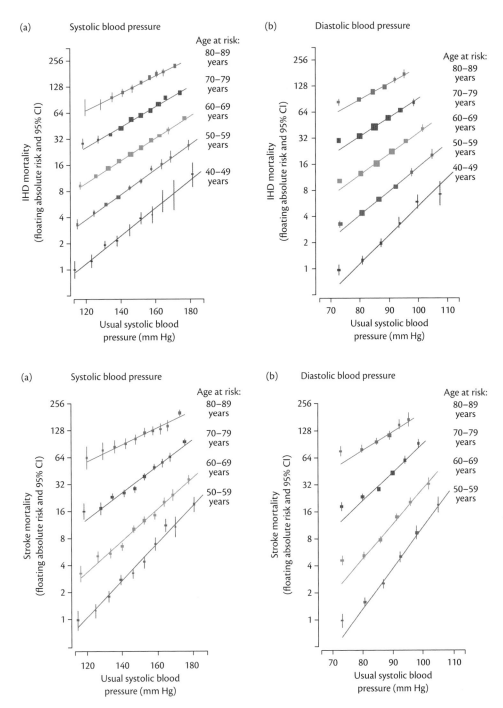

Fig. 17.1.5 Relationship between usual blood pressure at the start of a decade and the risk of ischaemic heart disease (IHD, top panel) and stroke (bottom panel) mortality rates in that decade, for each decade for each decade of life.

Reprinted from *The Lancet*, Vol. 360, Lewington *et al.*, Age-specific relevance of usual blood pressure to vascular mortality: a meta-analysis of individual data for one million adults in 61 prospective studies, pp. 1903–1913. Copyright (2002), with permission from Elsevier.

Systolic blood pressure as the main risk factor

For many years DBP was considered the main denominator for defining the threshold and treatment targets for hypertension. This is no longer the case. As indicated above, there is a progressive rise in DBP up to about the age of 50 years and thereafter it usually falls. By contrast, SBP begins to rise relentlessly from the age of around 40 years (Figs. 17.1.1 and 17.1.2). Thus, at the age of peak prevalence of hypertension (i.e. older than 60 years), SBP is the major

contributor to the diagnosis of the condition and its associated risk. Below the age of 50 years, DBP is also important. Figure 17.1.7 illustrates the shift in the major risk burden attributable to hypertension, from DBP to SBP, at about the age of 50 years. However, because most hypertension (>75%) occurs over the age of 50 years, SBP rather than DBP is by far the most important contributor to the huge global cardiovascular risk burden attributable to hypertension. SBP is also the most difficult to treat, which has led some

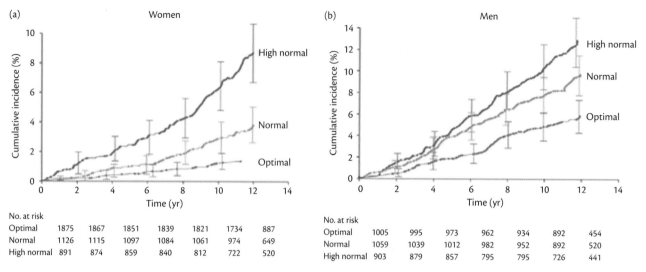

Fig. 17.1.6 High normal blood pressure and the risk of cardiovascular disease. Cumulative incidence of cardiovascular events in women (a) and men (b) without hypertension, according to blood pressure category at the baseline examination. For this analysis, optimal blood pressure was defined as SBP <120 mmHg and DBP <80 mmHg, normal blood pressure as SBP 120–129 mmHg and/or DBP 80–84 mmHg, and high normal blood pressure as SBP 130–139 mmHg and/or DBP 85–89 mm Hg. 95% confidence intervals are shown.
N Engl J Med 2001;**345**:1291–1297.

to argue that for patients over the age of 50 years the attention of doctors should be focused solely on the SBP.

What method of blood pressure measurement best predicts cardiovascular outcome?

A recent review of the literature looked at studies comparing ambulatory blood pressure monitoring (ABPM) vs clinic blood pressure monitoring (CBPM), home blood pressure monitoring (HBPM) vs CBPM, and studies that compared all three monitoring methods. Of nine studies comparing ABPM with CBPM, eight found ABPM to be superior, with one showing no difference. Of three studies comparing HBPM with CBPM, two found HBPM to be better, and one showed no difference. Of the two studies that compared all three methods, one showed HBPM similar to ABPM, with both superior to CBPM, and the other study showed no difference

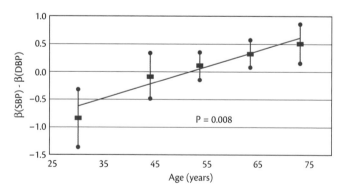

Fig. 17.1.7 The impact of DBP and SBP on the risk of coronary heart disease as a function of age. A β-coefficient level less than 0.0 indicates a stronger effect of DBP on coronary heart disease (CHD) risk, a β-coefficient level greater than 0.0 indicates a greater importance of SBP. The 'switch' from DBP to SBP occurs at around age 50 years.
Franklin SS, *et al.* Does the relation of blood pressure to coronary heart disease risk change with aging? *Circulation* 2001; **103**:1245. (http://circ.ahajournals.org/cgi/content/abstract/103/9/1245).

between the methods. These reviews are the basis of arguments that, in healthcare systems where they are readily available, ABPM or HBPM should be used as the basis for diagnosing (and therefore treating) hypertension.

Pathogenesis and pathophysiology of hypertension

The pathogenesis of essential hypertension has remained something of an enigma, in part reflecting the fact that the basis for the diagnosis, i.e. an elevated blood pressure, has so many potential causes. From a physiological perspective, the pressure in the circulation is the product of the cardiac output (CO) and impedance to flow, i.e. peripheral resistance (PR):

$$blood\ pressure = CO \times PR$$

Both cardiac output and peripheral resistance can be influenced by a number of control mechanisms, including activity of the renin–angiotensin–aldosterone system, activity of the sympathetic nervous system, and other factors influencing salt and water homeostasis. In addition, vascular structural changes associated with hypertension play a role in accentuating its severity and conferring resistance to treatment. These structural changes include small-artery remodelling that results in a reduced media/lumen ratio (which increases peripheral resistance) and large-artery stiffening (which changes pulse wave characteristics and reduces the compliance of the circulation). Recent reports suggest that a reduced diameter of the proximal aorta may also be a factor contributing to the development of hypertension. Whether structural changes precede and predispose to the onset of hypertension, or follow it, or both, remains a subject of considerable debate.

In some cases (probably <10%) a discrete cause for hypertension will be identified (see Chapter 17.3). In most other circumstances the pathogenesis of essential hypertension, i.e. hypertension that is not due to a recognized secondary cause, is a complex interplay between (1) genetic predisposition, (2) lifestyle and environmental influences, and (3) disturbances in structure and the aforementioned control mechanisms. These are in turn compounded by the effects of ageing on the cardiovascular and renal systems.

Genetic factors (this section written by Professor Nilesh J. Samani)

Historical perspective

The history of the genetics of hypertension is marked by a celebrated debate in the 1950s and 1960s between Platt and Pickering, two doyens of British medicine. On the basis of a finding of a bimodal distribution of blood pressures in some families of patients with hypertension, and evidence of hypertension transmitted over three generations in a few pedigrees, Platt argued that hypertension was a distinct genetic disorder with a likely autosomal dominant mode of inheritance. By contrast, Pickering and colleagues showed that in the general population there was no obvious discontinuity of blood pressure distribution and that the familial resemblance of blood pressure spanned the whole range of blood pressures, and was not different for those with hypertension. Thus, Pickering argued that blood pressure, like height and weight, was a quantitative trait, and that although there was a significant genetic contribution, this was polygenic and that hypertension represented one extreme of the trait but was not a distinct disorder, except perhaps for rare monogenetic forms embedded in the blood pressure distribution curve. Today, the overwhelming mass of evidence supports the Pickering concept, although several mendelian disorders that predispose to hypertension have been described (see Chapter 17.4).

Genetic epidemiology of blood pressure and hypertension

The extent of familial aggregation of blood pressure has been studied in diverse ethnic groups living in distinct places, ranging from Polynesians to Middle Americans. A remarkably consistent level of correlation of around 0.2 between first-degree relatives has been found, meaning that if the blood pressure of one member of the family deviates from the norm by +10 mmHg, the first-degree relative will deviate by +2 mmHg on average. Studies in children and infants suggest that the familial resemblance in blood pressure starts very early and is maintained throughout life.

Attempts to partition the familial resemblance of blood pressure between shared genes and shared environment have been made through studies of adoptees and twins. In the Montreal Adoption Study, correlations between natural siblings compared with adoptive siblings, and between parents and natural children compared with parents and adopted children, were at least twice as great. Similarly, several studies have documented much higher correlations in blood pressure between monozygotic twins (0.55–0.85) compared with dizygotic twins (0.25–0.50), although the results from twin studies have to be viewed with caution as there is substantial evidence of excess sharing of sociocultural environments by twin pairs, especially monozygotic.

However, taken altogether the epidemiological data suggest that genetic factors account for about 40 to 45% of the population variability of blood pressure, common household environment for about 10 to 15%, and nonfamilial factors for the remaining 40 to 45%.

Although determination of familial correlations of blood pressure provides an overall view of the impact of heredity in determining blood pressure, a more relevant measure of the importance of genetic factors in determining susceptibility to hypertension is

relative risk. This is the ratio of the risk of an individual developing the condition given its presence in a first-degree relative compared with the overall population risk. For relatively rare monogenetic conditions such as cystic fibrosis, relative risk is as high as 500. For common and complex polygenic disorders, relative risk tends to be much lower. For hypertension, relative risk estimates vary between 2 and 5 depending on the criteria used to define family history. Values are highest when both parents have hypertension before the age of 55 years.

Genes involved in 'essential hypertension'

Given the importance of hypertension as a risk factor for several cardiovascular diseases, a huge effort has been made in the last 20 years to identify genes where variants affect blood pressure and increase risk of hypertension or hypertension-related end-organ damage. Most of the studies have involved association analyses of so-called candidate genes whose products are known, or suspected to, be involved in regulation of blood pressure. A smaller number have used linkage analyses in collections of affected sib pairs to identify genetic loci in a systematic manner. Variants in a large number of genes, involving virtually all the main physiological systems affecting blood pressure, such as the renin–angiotensin–aldosterone system (Table 17.1.2) and the sympathetic system, have shown association with blood pressure in one or more studies. The findings to date suggest that the effect of any individual variant is likely to be modest. For example, a meta-analysis of 32 case–control studies (corresponding to 13 760 patients) of the methionine to threonine (M235T) polymorphism in the angiotensinogen gene, one of the most studied variants, found that the *TT* genotype conferred a 31% increased risk of hypertension compared with the *MM* genotype. There is evidence that variants may act in an additive or epistatic fashion. For example, one prospective study of 678 initially normotensive subjects found that combined carriage of the angiotensin converting enzyme *DD* genotype (at the insertion (I)/deletion (D) polymorphism in the gene), the tryptophan (*Trp*) allele at codon 460 in the α-adducin gene, and the *CC* genotype at the −344C/T promoter polymorphism in aldosterone synthase *CC* genotype, increased the risk of developing hypertension by 252% over a median follow-up of 9.1 years compared with other genotypes.

The *Trp* allele of α-adducin, part of a ubiquitous α/β heterodimeric cytoskeletal protein which affects sodium absorption in

Table 17.1.2 Some genes with evidence for common variants influencing blood pressure or risk of hypertension

Gene	Role
Angiotensinogen	Substrate for renin
Angiotensin converting enzyme	Converts angiotensin I to angiotensin II
Angiotensin receptor (type 1)	Main vascular receptor for angiotensin II
Aldosterone synthase	Promotes synthesis of aldosterone
α-Adducin	Cytoskeletal protein involved in sodium homeostasis
G protein β3 subunit	Involved in G-protein signalling

Reprinted from *The Lancet*, Vol 349, Cusi D *et al*. Polymorphisms of α-adducin and salt sensitivity in patients with essential hypertension. 349, 1353–7 (1997), with permission from Elsevier.

the kidney, has also been associated with greater blood-pressure-lowering response to thiazide diuretics, and in one study of hypertensive subjects diuretic therapy was associated with a lower risk of combined myocardial infarction or stroke than other antihypertensive therapies in carriers of this adducin variant. Such findings raise the prospect of better prediction and individually tailored treatment for hypertension. However, inconsistent findings between studies reflecting, at least in part, poorly understood gene–gene and gene–environment interactions, have hampered progress and significant clinical application so far.

While genetic dissection of essential hypertension has proved challenging, the genetic basis of several monogenic forms of hypertension has been elucidated during the same period. The findings have provided novel and illuminating insights into the molecular regulation of blood pressure and particularly the role of the kidney and sodium homeostasis. See Chapter 17.4 for further discussion.

Environmental and lifestyle influences on the development of hypertension

The prevalence of hypertension can be powerfully influenced by local lifestyles and customs. There are a number of lines of evidence that support this conclusion, including studies of migrant populations, comparisons between different communities, prospective population studies, and randomized trials of lifestyle interventions. There is little doubt that the exploding prevalence of hypertension in economically developing regions reflects lifestyle changes, so-called 'Westernization', more than anything else.

Migrant studies

Migration studies have provided powerful evidence to illustrate the importance of the local environment and lifestyle on the level of blood pressure and the prevalence of hypertension. Studies of migration from rural to urban areas of Africa and Australia typically report marked increases in migrant blood pressure, body weight, and sodium intake, coincident with the adoption of more sedentary lifestyles, usually within months of migration. This latter point is important because it helps discriminate between powerful lifestyle factors and genetics—i.e. the changes in blood pressure are more nurture than nature.

Population studies

Studies of specific populations are often very informative. Populations in specific regions of the world, e.g. primitive rural populations such as the Yanamamo Indians of Brazil, do not show much evidence of an age-related rise in blood pressure, suggesting that the progressive rise in SBP seen in urban populations is not inevitable. This could reflect genetic differences in vascular structure in discrete populations, but most likely reflects influence of the local environment, and customs. Evidence in support of this conclusion comes from a classic study which compared Italian nuns with a control group of women from the same town. In the control group, blood pressure typically rose with age, whereas the nuns, from a similar genetic background, showed no such rise in blood pressure over 20 years of follow-up. Thus, essential hypertension is undoubtedly a 'disease of urbanization', reflecting the impact of a number of specific lifestyle factors.

Specific lifestyle influences on blood pressure

The most important lifestyle/environmental influences on blood pressure are sodium intake, obesity, and alcohol intake. Early nutritional deficiency may be important, and recent evidence suggests that psychosocial factors are likely to play some role in the development of essential hypertension. A small socio-economic gradient of blood pressure has also been observed. Interestingly, this gradient is negative for developed countries and positive for developing countries, which probably reflects the higher prevalence of obesity and higher intakes of alcohol and salt among those of higher socio-economic status in developing countries, compared to the reverse in more economically developed regions of the world. With regard to dietary influences on blood pressure, recent evidence (discussed later) suggests that diets rich in fruit and vegetables with low total and saturated fats may protect against hypertension. Low calcium intake, although associated with hypertension in population studies, is now considered to play no part in pathogenesis.

Dietary salt intake

There has been vigorous debate about the role of dietary salt in the genesis of hypertension. It is clear that sodium balance is a key factor determining the blood pressure of an individual. Moreover, it is intriguing that the various monogenic forms of hypertension that have been characterized by genetic studies all involve disturbances to renal sodium handling (see Chapter 17.4). Review of the evidence from population-based studies and studies of dietary intervention support the hypothesis that dietary sodium intake has an important impact on blood pressure, and recent studies have also highlighted the importance of salt intake in the genesis of hypertension in children and the effectiveness of sodium restriction at reducing blood pressure. That said, there will clearly be some patients whose blood pressure will be more sensitive to dietary sodium intake than others. As indicated in Chapter 17.2, dietary sodium restriction forms part of the lifestyle interventions recommended by all guidelines as part of the treatment strategy for hypertension, and to delay the development of hypertension in people with prehypertension.

A related but different question is whether dietary sodium restriction could influence not only blood pressure, but also cardiovascular disease outcomes. Recent studies suggest that this is likely to be the case. People allocated to a sodium-restricted diet experienced a 30% lower incidence of cardiovascular events in the next 10–15 years, irrespective of sex, ethnic origin, age, body mass, and blood pressure. As the people randomized into these studies were not hypertensive (blood pressure c.125/85 mmHg) it is conceivable that the benefits, impressive as they are, might have been even greater in a hypertensive population. These findings support current guideline recommendations and underline the importance of education and national health policies to reduce dietary sodium intake.

Obesity and blood pressure

Fat people generally have higher blood pressures than lean people. Fat arms can lead to overestimation of blood pressure when small cuffs are used, but the relation between body weight and blood pressure persists after correcting for arm circumference. Although body mass index (BMI) is often used to define obesity, visceral adiposity seems to be more important in defining the relationship between blood pressure and obesity. Visceral obesity also increases the likelihood of coexisting 'metabolic syndrome' (see 'Hypertension and the metabolic syndrome' later in the chapter) in people with hypertension. In untreated hypertensive people, fat tends to preferentially accumulate intra-abdominally and intrathoracically, and the magnitude of the visceral adiposity is quantitatively related to the blood pressure. Importantly, the adiposity–blood pressure link is observable from early childhood and a key predictor of the likelihood of developing overt hypertension.

Recent analysis of longitudinal data from the Bogalusa Heart Study (Louisiana, USA) tracked the association between obesity in childhood and the risk of developing hypertension. Excess adiposity was present in one-fifth of those with normal blood pressure, one-third of those with prehypertension, and more than one-half of those with hypertension. Moreover, these associations were evident in people as young as 4 to 11 years, suggesting that the avoidance of obesity could markedly reduce the prevalence of hypertension in middle-aged adults. In support of the strength of the association between BMI and the risk of developing hypertension, in a study of 36 424 Israel Defense Forces employees (mean age *c.*35 years), BMI was the strongest predictor of prehypertension, with a 10 to 15% increase in risk for every 1 kg/m^2 increase in BMI. The strong cause–effect relationship between obesity and hypertension has been confirmed by intervention studies showing that weight reduction results in a fall in blood pressure.

Alcohol intake and blood pressure

Epidemiological data have consistently shown an association between alcohol intake and blood pressure, and intervention trials confirm that blood pressure falls when alcohol is withdrawn from heavy drinkers. Analysis of data from the National Health and Nutrition Examination Survey (NHANES, 1999–2000) showed that an alcohol intake of up to two drinks per day had no effect on blood pressure, which is consistent with previous reports that moderate drinking (2–3 units daily) does not appear to exert a pressor effect. Heavier alcohol intakes, patterns of alcohol consumption, and the types of alcohol consumed can also influence blood pressure. Binge drinking can exert a pressor effect, but the mechanism accounting for the pressor effects of alcohol remain undefined. However, whatever the mechanism, data from the WHO Global Burden of Disease survey in 2000 attributed 16% of all hypertensive disease to alcohol.

There has been controversy about whether moderate alcohol consumption might actually reduce cardiovascular disease risk. For example, in a prospective study of almost half a million men and women in the United States of America, the relative risk of death from cardiovascular disease in moderate drinkers compared with nondrinkers was 0.7 for men and 0.6 for women. However, it is important to emphasize that these kind of analyses run the risk of confounding by an unmeasured disease effect modifier that tracks with different patterns of alcohol consumption.

Sleep and blood pressure

Blood pressure characteristically falls during sleep. A recent longitudinal analysis of the first NHANES (*n* = 4810) examined the impact of sleep duration on the risk of developing hypertension. This risk was increased by about twofold in adults in middle age who sleep for less than 5 h each night. Even after adjusting for obesity and diabetes (the risk of which also increase with sleep deprivation), the risk remained around 1.6-fold. There are a number of mechanisms that might account for this relationship: it may simply reflect a longer duration of sympathetic nervous system activation as a consequence of less time asleep and hence a higher 24 h average blood pressure load, giving rise to a higher risk of longer-term cardiovascular structural damage and hence to sustained hypertension.

There is also a clear association between obstructive sleep apnoea and hypertension. An apnoea–hypopnoea index of 15 or more (i.e. breathing decreases or stops ≥15 times per hour of sleep) is associated with a threefold increase in the risk of developing hypertension. Moreover, in such patients continuous positive airway pressure can be effective in lowering both night-time and, to a lesser extent, daytime blood pressure. Doctors should therefore consider sleep deprivation and obstructive sleep apnoea in their assessment of people developing hypertension.

Psychosocial stress and blood pressure

Blood pressure elevation is a well-recognized acute stress response, and the act of taking the blood pressure can increase the SBP by up to 75 mmHg in some patients. However, the role of chronic stress in the pathogenesis of hypertension has been difficult to assess, (1) because of individual variability in the response to stress, (2) because it is difficult to objectively measure chronic stress, and (3) because stress can induce behavioural and lifestyle choices that could influence blood pressure independently of stress per se.

One measure of stress that appears to be robust in predicting blood pressure is an individual's perception of control in their employment. Using ABPM it has been shown that in men—but not in women—job strain is associated with an elevated blood pressure, both at work and also while at home and during sleep. Job strain in this context was defined as having a highly demanding job, but with the individual having little control over it. By contrast, people employed in equally demanding jobs, but where they have an element of control over their work, have less stress and less elevation of blood pressure. This effect of job strain on blood pressure is independent of other environmental and lifestyle influences, and is as strong as the impact of obesity.

Early origins of hypertension—impact of fetal and infant growth

An associated between low birth weight and risk of developing hypertension and premature cardiovascular disease has been recognized in many epidemiological studies. A large family-based study recently explored the mechanisms underlying the associations of birth weight and gestational age with SBP measured at 17 to 19 years of age. This suggested that the inverse associations of birth weight and gestational age with SBP are not explained by confounding resulting from a family's socio-economic status, or other factors that are shared by siblings. Variations in maternal metabolic or vascular health during pregnancy or placental implantation and function may explain these associations. Other studies have suggested that this relationship may relate to fetal programming of increased risk for hypertension via a reduction in nephron number, thereby increasing salt sensitivity.

Another hypothesis has suggested that increased nutritional support to promote 'catch-up growth' in the immediate postnatal period for babies who are small for gestational age could ameliorate the risk for developing hypertension. This hypothesis was tested in a cohort of small for gestational age babies who had been fed with either a standard or nutrient-enriched (28% more protein than standard) formula after birth. The enriched feed promoted faster postnatal weight gain and was associated with higher (not lower) blood pressure in later childhood, which does not support the promotion of faster weight gain in infants born small for gestational age.

Prehypertension predicts hypertension

The presence of mild elevation in blood pressure for age predicts the likelihood of developing hypertension. In a study of patients with prehypertension (SBP 120–139 mmHg and/or DBP 80–89 mmHg) the annual rate of progression to hypertension (≥140/90 mmHg) was greater than 15% per year despite lifestyle advice. In addition to an elevated blood pressure, people with prehypertension often also have the characteristic metabolic phenotype associated with hypertension (see below) and evidence of endothelial dysfunction and cardiovascular structural damage. This may explain why an analysis of data from the Women's Health Study in the United States of America, involving over 60 000 women followed for 7 years, showed that the presence of prehypertension was associated with an almost doubling in risk of any cardiovascular event—including death, myocardial infarction, stroke, or hospitalization for heart failure—when compared to those with normal blood pressure. Prehypertension was also more common in people with diabetes, when it was associated with an almost fourfold increase in risk of cardiovascular disease when compared to people without diabetes and normal blood pressure.

Kidney, vascular structure, and neurohumoral control systems and the development of hypertension

The maintenance of an adequate mean arterial pressure is fundamental to life, hence there are many homeostatic mechanisms designed to achieve this despite fluctuations in posture, volume status, exercise, and other metabolic demands. There is considerable redundancy within these control systems, such that inhibition of one system is compensated for by increased activity of another, which is important when considering the design of effective strategies to lower blood pressure.

Kidney

The kidney is important for blood pressure regulation via two key mechanisms: (1) the regulation of sodium and volume homeostasis, and (2) the regulation of the activity of the renin–angiotensin–aldosterone system. The transplantation of a kidney from a genetically hypertensive rat into a normotensive control rat results in the development of hypertension in the recipient, and the converse is also true. In humans, significant renal impairment is invariably associated with hypertension, which in large part relates to disturbances in sodium handling, and as stated previously almost all of the single-gene defects resulting in the development of hypertension involve disturbances in the renal tubular handling of sodium (see Chapter 17.4).

The kidney is also intimately involved with sensing and setting of blood pressure via the activity of the renin–angiotensin–aldosterone system. Reduced renal perfusion pressure (e.g. in renal artery stenosis) results in activation of the renin–angiotensin–aldosterone system, which in turn elevates blood pressure to try and restore renal perfusion pressure via a number of mechanisms (see 'Renin–angiotensin–aldosterone system' below).

Structure of small arteries

A characteristic finding in essential hypertension is an inappropriate increase in peripheral vascular resistance relative to the cardiac output. The main site of this resistance is small arteries (arterioles), which undergo inward eutrophic remodelling that is characterized by an increase in their media/lumen ratio. These changes result from vascular remodelling, i.e. rearrangement of existing material in the vascular media around a smaller lumen, and there is often also evidence of some hypertrophy and/or hyperplasia of the resident myocytes.

There has been much debate about whether these changes in small-artery structure antedate and thus contribute to the development of hypertension, and/or whether they are the consequence of an elevated blood pressure and the trophic effects of neurohumoral activation (i.e. sympathetic nervous system and the renin–angiotensin–aldosterone system) in people with hypertension. Whatever the mechanism, recent studies of small arteries isolated from biopsies in humans, or retinal vascular structural changes (especially narrowing), suggest that the magnitude of structural changes of the small arteries is strongly predictive of future cardiovascular events. It is also predictive of the likelihood and magnitude of structural changes elsewhere, i.e. left ventricular hypertrophy.

Structure of large arteries

The functional integrity of large conduit arteries such as the aorta also influences the development of hypertension, especially systolic hypertension. The pulsatile nature of blood flow exerts chronic cyclical stress on the walls of these arteries, and over time this results in deterioration in their elastic properties as a consequence of thinning, splitting, and fragmentation of the elastin fibres within the media. This process is accelerated in people with hypertension, resulting in progressive dilatation in aortic root diameter and arterial stiffening. In turn, this reduction in arterial compliance increases pulse wave velocity, increases systolic pressure and central aortic pulse pressure, and reduces diastolic pressure. This explains the very high prevalence of systolic hypertension with advancing age (see Fig. 17.1.2) and the progressive age-related disappearance of diastolic hypertension.

The process of age-related stiffening of the aorta is accelerated by post-translational modification of vascular wall proteins such as collagen by the formation of advanced glycation end products (AGEs). AGE formation is accelerated in people with diabetes, thereby explaining the earlier onset of isolated systolic hypertension in patients with this condition. It is conceivable that if aortic function and especially its elasticity were genetically determined, then accelerated degeneration of aortic elastic function could also be a factor in the development of systolic hypertension in younger people. Aside from aortic function, there is current debate about whether the diameter of the aortic root is causally related to the likelihood of developing hypertension. This has been prompted by recent observations that central aortic pulse pressure appears to be inversely related to aortic root diameter, prompting speculation that a smaller effective root diameter might also contribute to the development of hypertension.

Endothelium

The endothelium plays a key role in the regulation of vascular tone. Endothelial cells form nitric oxide (NO) from L-arginine via the activity of nitric oxide synthase (eNOS), which is tonically activated by shear stress and relaxes vascular tone. NO also inhibits platelet aggregation and inhibits vascular smooth muscle cell proliferation. Hypertension, even in its earliest stages, has been associated with 'endothelial dysfunction', usually by demonstrating a reduction in forearm blood flow in response to agents that promote NO release such as acetyl choline or its mimetics. NO production has also been shown to be decreased in people with hypertension.

It is not clear whether endothelial dysfunction and decreased NO production are a cause or consequence of an elevated blood pressure, but the latter seems most likely. Whatever the mechanism, a reduction in NO production would be expected to increase vascular tone and may also contribute to vascular proliferation and remodelling (see above). NO donors such as glyeryl trinitrate (GTN) are very effective at lowering blood pressure in the acute setting, and are especially effective at reducing central aortic pressure. However, the use of NO donors to lower blood pressure outside of the acute setting has been bedevilled by their short duration of action and the fact that tolerance to them develops rapidly. The actions of some commonly used antihypertensive drugs, angiotensin converting enzyme (ACE) inhibitors and angiotensin receptor blockers (ARBs), have in part been attributed to their local potentiation of NO.

The endothelium also produces a powerful vascoconstrictor, endothelin. This seems less important in the chronic regulation of blood pressure, even though inhibitors of endothelin have been shown to lower it. The biology and actions of NO and endothelin are discussed in greater detail elsewhere (Chapter 1.1).

Oxidative stress

Numerous studies in experimental animals and humans have indicated that hypertension is associated with markers of increased systemic oxidative stress, i.e. the increased production of oxygen free radicals such as superoxide and hydrogen peroxide. These are short-lived reactive species that have the potential to cause cellular damage via oxidation of proteins, lipids and DNA. They also react with and inactivate NO, thereby providing a mechanism for reduced NO levels and increased vascular tone. The mechanism for increased oxidative stress in hypertension is not known, but studies have suggested that this may in part relate to activation of NADH/NADPH oxidase within vascular cells. Of interest, this vascular oxidase is activated by angiotensin II, which provides a link between the renin–angiotensin–aldosterone system and endothelial dysfunction and may contribute to the pressor effect of angiotensin II.

Renin–angiotensin–aldosterone system

The renin–angiotensin–aldosterone system, whose main effector molecules are angiotensin II and aldosterone, plays an important role in the regulation of blood pressure via a number of mechanisms. Angiotensin II is produced by an enzymatic cascade (Fig. 17.1.8). Renin synthesis—the rate-limiting step for the production of angiotensin II—may take place in a number of tissues apart from the kidney, including the adrenal, heart, the blood vessel wall, and brain. In the kidney renin is produced by the juxtaglomerular apparatus in response to falls in renal perfusion pressure, sodium depletion, and increased sympathetic nerve activity. However, the renin–angiotensin–aldosterone system is active both in the circulation and locally within tissues.

The two principle angiotensin receptors are AT1 and AT2. The major actions of angiotensin II are via the AT1 receptor, which is the target for the ARB class of blood-pressure-lowering agents. The AT2 receptor is less ubiquitously expressed than the AT1 receptor, is markedly up-regulated during tissue repair, and its activation produces effects that appear to oppose those of AT1 activation, suggesting that the two receptors may operate a yin–yang relationship.

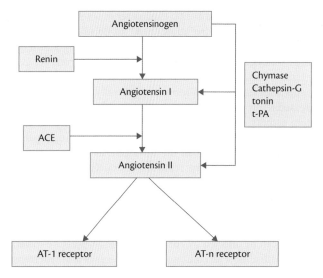

Fig. 17.1.8 The renin–angiotensin system. The enzyme renin cleaves its substrate angiotensinogen to generate the decapeptide angiotensin I, which is then cleaved by angiotensin converting enzyme (ACE) to generate angiotensin II, which binds to a family of specific angiotensin receptors. Its main effect on blood pressure regulation is via the AT-1 receptor, the functions of other angiotensin receptors (AT-n) being poorly defined. Angiotensin II can also be generated by other proteolytic enzyme systems such as chymases and tissue plasminogen activators (t-PA). These pathways may be important for local angiotensin II generation in disease.

Angiotensin II elevates blood pressure by a number of different mechanisms: (1) it is a direct pressor agent promoting vasoconstriction, and it also increases superoxide production by the endothelium, which reduces NO availability (see above); (2) it increases sodium reabsorption by the kidney via direct tubular effects and via simulation of aldosterone release from the adrenal cortex; (3) it can have trophic effects on vascular cell growth and has been implicated in the small-artery remodelling process that results in increased peripheral vascular resistance; (4) it acts centrally on AT1 receptors in the nucleus tractus solitarius (NTS) to desensitize the afferent component of the baroreceptor reflex.

In addition to these pressor actions, angiotensin II has also been implicated in the development of end-organ damage through (1) trophic effects on the myocardium, resulting in left ventricular hypertrophy; (2) the development of glomerular hypertension, albuminuria, and interstitial fibrosis, leading to chronic renal disease; (3) pro-oxidant effects, contributing to the development of atherosclerosis. Consequently, the renin–angiotensin–aldosterone system has become a popular target for drug therapy to lower blood pressure and limit its cardiovascular consequences.

Aldosterone is the other effector molecule of the renin–angiotensin–aldosterone system. It is produced by the adrenal cortex in response to many stimuli, including sodium and volume depletion, angiotensin II, excess potassium intake, trauma, and stress. It acts on the distal tubule of the kidney to promote sodium absorption in exchange for potassium. An inappropriate increase in production of aldosterone can lead to the development of hypertension (e.g. Conn's syndrome and adrenal hyperplasia), as discussed in Chapter 17.3.

The specific role of the renin–angiotensin–aldosterone system in the development of essential hypertension remains unclear, although therapeutic agents that inhibit this system have proved to be very effective treatments. Plasma renin levels vary widely in essential hypertension, from low (30%), to normal (50%), to high (20%): they are inversely related to sodium loading and tend to decline with ageing. Thus patients with low renin levels are generally older and have volume-dependent hypertension. Hypertensive patients with higher renin levels are generally younger, and their increased renin may reflect increased levels of sympathetic nervous system activity (see next section). Black people at any age have a high prevalence of low-renin hypertension, suggesting a primary role for sodium retention in the pathogenesis of their hypertension. Although the baseline renin level is rarely measured in routine clinical practice, age has been used as a surrogate in the recent hypertension guidelines in the United Kingdom for predicting the most effective initial therapy in people with essential hypertension. If plasma renin levels are measured, it is important to recognize that they can be affected by concomitant blood-pressure-lowering therapy, with almost all commonly used classes of antihypertensive drugs increasing plasma renin, the main exception being β-blockers which suppress plasma renin.

Sympathetic nervous system

The sympathetic nervous system is involved in the acute and chronic regulation of blood pressure. It is known to be involved in the regulation of arteriolar resistance, cardiac output and volume regulation, renin release by the kidney, and catecholamine and mineralocorticoid release by the adrenal gland. It is by necessity a complex system that involves (1) vasomotor control centres within the brain; (2) the peripheral nervous system providing efferent and afferent signals; and (3) the adrenal medulla. Several nuclei within the central nervous system are involved in the regulation of blood pressure, with control integrated in the rostral ventrolateral nucleus of the medulla oblongata—the vasomotor centre—that is particularly influenced by the NTS which receives its input from

peripheral afferents such as baroreceptor activation in the aortic arch, carotid sinus, and cardiac ventricles and atria. The NTS also receives excitatory and inhibitory inputs from other regions of the brain, e.g. the brain stem and cortex, and its outputs to the vasomotor centre tend to inhibit sympathetic outflow and thus buffer acute rises in blood pressure—the baroreceptor reflex arc. Another important influence on the rostral ventrolateral nucleus–NTS complex is the action of angiotensin II. The area postrema in the floor of the fourth ventricle does not have a blood–brain barrier, which allows circulating angiotensin II to blunt the inhibitory effect of the NTS on the rostral ventrolateral nucleus, thereby increasing central sympathetic outflow. The various inputs and outputs are summarized in Fig. 17.1.9.

Environmental and behavioural impacts on blood pressure are primarily coordinated via the hypothalamus. The posterolateral hypothalamus is responsible for the classical 'fight or flight' response, and lesions in this area reduce blood pressure. By contrast, lesions in the anterior hypothalamus can substantially increase blood pressure.

The peripheral vascular α-adrenergic system ($α_1$ receptors) is also important in maintaining enhanced vascular resistance in hypertension, with some studies suggesting that peripheral α-adrenergic responsiveness might be especially enhanced in black people with hypertension.

The importance of the sympathetic nervous system in the regulation of blood pressure is beyond question, but a key unanswered question is whether disturbances to the regulation of the sympathetic nervous system play a major role in the initiation and maintenance of chronic essential hypertension. Most surveys of younger people with prehypertension or stage 1 hypertension indicate the presence of an elevated heart rate, indicative of sympathetic nervous system activation. Other studies have reported elevated circulating catecholamine levels in young patients with

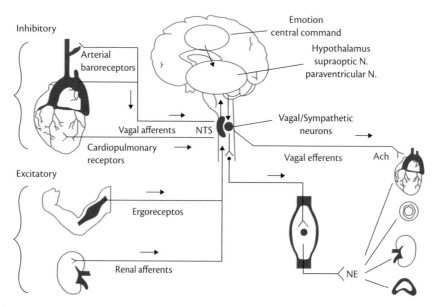

Fig. 17.1.9 Organization of the nervous system control of blood pressure. Peripheral inhibitory and excitatory inputs are integrated in the nucleus tractus solitarius (NTS), whose central inputs are integrated via the hypothalamus. The NTS regulates sympathetic outflow via the rostral centrolateral nuclei of the medulla oblongata. The balance of sympathetic and vagal outflow influences cardiac output, heart rate, vasoconstrictor tone, renin release, and renal blood flow, also catecholamine and mineralocorticoid release.

Adapted from Abboud FM (1982) The sympathetic system in hypertension. State-of-the-art review. *Hypertension*, 1982; **4**(Suppl II); 208–225.

prehypertension, and that such elevations predict the risk of developing hypertension. Further studies have used radiolabelled norepinephrine (noradrenaline) to demonstrate enhanced 'spillover' indicative of enhanced sympathetic nervous system activity, or microneurography to demonstrate increased sympathetic nervous system activity in young hypertensives. It must be emphasized, however, that simple demonstration of enhanced activity of a particular system at a single snapshot in time cannot be taken as evidence of a direct causal role: the critical question is whether the level of activity is appropriate or inappropriate in the context of the overall integrated physiological regulation of blood pressure. In this regard, a full understanding of the role of the sympathetic nervous system in the genesis of essential hypertension in humans has been hindered by the complexity of the system under study and the rather crude instruments used to evaluate the system *in vivo*. Some remain to be convinced of the importance of the sympathetic nervous system in the genesis of essential hypertension, while others argue that given the importance of the sympathetic nervous system in regulating blood pressure, then—even if essential hypertension has an unrelated aetiology—abnormal activity of the sympathetic nervous system must be permissive in maintaining blood pressure elevation.

Sympathetic nervous system, obesity, and the metabolic syndrome

Obesity is associated with increased muscle sympathetic nerve activity, and increased sympathetic nervous system activity has been implicated in the pathogenesis of obesity-related hypertension. Hypertension is often associated with features of a metabolic syndrome (see 'Hypertension and the metabolic syndrome' in the next section) characterized by insulin resistance, dyslipidaemia, and impaired glucose tolerance. Increased sympathetic nervous system activity has also been implicated in the development of this syndrome, and drugs therapies that reduce central sympathetic outflow or block α_1 adrenergic receptors improve insulin sensitivity and features of the metabolic syndrome.

Natriuretic peptides

The natriuretic peptide system—including atrial natriuretic peptide (ANP), brain natriuretic peptide (BNP), and C-type natriuretic peptide (CNP)—is an endocrine system that is involved in the regulation of salt and water homeostasis. ANP is secreted primarily by the right atrium in response to atrial wall stretch. BNP was initially identified in the brain, hence the name, but is predominantly produced in the ventricles in response to stretch. CNP is produced by vascular endothelial cells and in the kidney. These natriuretic peptides bind to specific cell membrane receptors on target tissues and induce natriuresis and diuresis; they also decrease renin secretion and aldosterone, and induce vasodilatation and a modest fall in blood pressure. These physiological actions suggested a potential role for reduced natriuretic peptide levels or action in the pathogenesis of hypertension, hence these have been measured in patients with essential hypertension. The results have been conflicting, with no clear pattern emerging. This in part reflects the fact that levels of natriuretic peptides, especially BNP, will be elevated in people with early or established left ventricular dysfunction and other hypertension-related complications, but it does not preclude a future role for drugs that augment the activity of natriuretic peptides in the clinical management of hypertension.

The hypertensive phenotype and target organ damage in hypertension

Although blood pressure measurement is used to define hypertension, hypertension is more than just blood pressure. Essential hypertension is commonly associated with metabolic disturbances and multisystem structural damage that conspire to enhance cardiovascular risk beyond that which can be attributed to blood pressure alone.

Hypertension and the metabolic syndrome

Few people with essential hypertension simply have an elevated blood pressure: many also have associated disturbances in metabolism which are typical of the 'insulin resistance phenotype', notably predisposition to impaired glucose tolerance, elevated triglyceride levels, reduced HDL-cholesterol values, and hyperuricaemia. These metabolic disturbances appear to precede and may even predict the likelihood of developing hypertension: in large prospective population studies in the United States of America and Europe the development of hypertension could be predicted by a person's initial metabolic profile. Even in those with optimal initial blood pressure levels (<120/80 mmHg), increasing obesity and the aforementioned abnormal lipid profile were major predictors of the development of hypertension.

With regard to obesity, the accumulation of visceral fat (i.e. abdominal obesity) is most strongly associated with hypertension and attendant metabolic disturbances. Indeed, the link between visceral fat content and indices of insulin resistance and metabolic syndrome is demonstrable even in lean patients when MRI is used to quantify visceral fat. Moreover, the link between visceral adiposity and blood pressure is present from early childhood and explains the approximately twofold increase in risk of developing type 2 diabetes in patients with essential hypertension.

The frequent coexistence of obesity with other features of metabolic syndrome in patients with hypertension underscores the need to view hypertension as more than just blood pressure in the context of cardiovascular disease risk management, and it points to the importance of early lifestyle interventions as the foundation for prevention and treatment.

Vascular structural changes and atherosclerosis

Aorta and large arteries

The arterial system is designed to convert the pulsatile flow generated by cardiac contraction into steady flow in the capillary bed. Thus the aorta is both a conduit and an elastic reservoir designed to buffer pulsatile blood flow. Over time, recurrent pulsatile stress produces uncoiling, disruption, and calcification of elastic fibres within the aortic wall. At the same time, relatively inelastic collagen is increased and made more rigid by post-translational modification by the accumulation of AGEs. Such age-related processes cause loss of the normal elastic reservoir function of the aorta and other large arteries. These changes are accelerated by the presence of high blood pressure and hence occur at an earlier age in hypertensive patients.

In addition to these structural changes, elevation in pressure itself contributes to a loss of large-artery compliance and buffering because, as pressure increases, the elastic fibres become fully stretched, thereby transferring load-bearing function to the relatively inelastic collagen fibres. As a result of these changes, the pressure wave generated by left ventricular contraction is no longer buffered by the aorta and proximal large arteries, but instead is transmitted into the arterial tree with greater amplitude. This is manifested clinically as increased brachial pulse pressure, with higher systolic and lower diastolic pressures. More importantly, the resulting increase in pulse wave velocity and changes in arterial haemodynamics contribute to an elevation in central aortic systolic and pulse pressures and an increase in ventricular loading conditions—changes that cannot always be appreciated by measurement of the brachial blood pressure alone.

Increased large-artery stiffening and reduced compliance also reduces the sensitivity of the carotid and aortic baroceptors to stretch, which blunts the normal rapid buffering of changes in blood pressure. As a result, blood pressure becomes more labile and the circulatory adaptation to acute postural changes may become impaired, producing symptoms of postural dizziness in older people.

Resistance vessels

The characteristic structural change in the smaller arteries and arterioles of hypertensive patients is an increase in wall/lumen ratio, the characteristics and pathogenesis of which have been discussed earlier. These changes have important functional consequences. The vessels can still dilate in response to stimuli such as warmth or drugs, but maximal vasodilatation is reduced. The converse is also true; responsiveness to pressor agents or stimuli becomes enhanced. These structural changes in resistance vessels also contribute to the characteristic increase in vascular resistance in hypertension, and they render vital organs more susceptible to ischaemic damage at the small-vessel level, e.g. small-vessel ischaemic brain damage.

Atheroma in hypertension

Hypertension is associated with an increased risk of generalized atherosclerotic disease. This is likely to result from an interplay of many factors, including pressure and haemodynamic stress, metabolic disturbances, inflammatory and oxidative stresses, endothelial disturbances, and neurohumoral activation.

The overwhelming importance of haemodynamic factors and pressure is illustrated by (1) the predilection for atheroma to develop at sites of increased haemodynamic stress within the circulation, e.g. arterial bifurcations; and (2) the fact that atheroma is rarely observed in a low-pressure circulation, e.g. the pulmonary circulation or venous system (unless pulmonary hypertension develops, or veins are grafted into the arterial circulation). Two recent studies have been important in establishing a direct link between pressure and the development and/or regression of atherosclerosis. Using a mouse genetically prone to develop atheroma, the placement of a suprarenal clip was used to generate aortic constriction (a high renin state) and hypertension. The atheromatous plaque area was greatly increased by the presence of hypertension and was not obviously ameliorated by administration of an ARB. This study therefore suggested that pressure and not activation of the renin–angiotensin–aldosterone system was the main cause of accelerated atheroma in this model. Further data from a human study that used intravascular ultrasonography to quantify changes in coronary atheroma suggested that the patients' in-trial blood pressure determined whether there was progression, stabilization, or regression of atheromatous plaque over a 2 year period. Thus, a large body of evidence supports the hypothesis that blood pressure plays a key role in the initiation and progression of atheroma in humans. It is also likely that haemodynamic stress plays an important role in the process of plaque rupture, as well as the plaque burden.

The heart in hypertension

Left ventricular hypertrophy is a classic feature of untreated, or inadequately treated, long-standing hypertension. In this regard it can be considered the hypertensive equivalent of the glycated Hb_{A1c} for patients with diabetes: it is an index of the prevailing blood pressure load. Left ventricular hypertrophy is demonstrable in about 50% of untreated hypertensive patients using echocardiography, but only 5 to 10% when using conventional ECG criteria (Sokolov–Lyon or Cornell duration product). Pressure load on the left ventricle is unquestionably the most important pathogenic factor, with ambulatory monitoring blood pressure measurements much better correlated with left ventricular hypertrophy than clinic measurements of pressure. Pressure load is compounded by stiffening of the aorta with ageing, but neurohumoral factors, including the activity of the sympathetic nervous system and renin–angiotensin–aldosterone system, also appear to be important.

Left ventricular hypertrophy is a very potent predictor of premature cardiovascular disease and death. Its presence on the ECG, especially when associated with a characteristic 'strain pattern' (see Chapter 3.1), is associated with a two- to threefold increase in risk of cardiovascular disease morbidity and mortality, including a marked increased risk of stroke and heart failure. Using echocardiography to characterize left ventricular hypertrophy, recent studies suggest that concentric hypertrophy carries a worse prognosis that eccentric hypertrophy (Fig. 17.1.10).

Pathological features

There are two pathological features of the cardiac changes in hypertension that culminate in the development of left ventricular

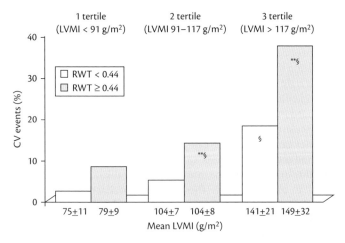

Fig. 17.1.10 Concentric vs eccentric left ventricular hypertrophy and cardiovascular risk in hypertensive patients. All patients had echocardiographic evidence of left ventricular hypertrophy (LVH). Concentric LVH was defined as a relative wall thickness (RWT) greater than or equal to 0.44. Cardiovascular events increased progressively per LVH tertile at follow-up, and were greater in each tertile of LVH in those with concentric LVH (shaded bars). CV, cardiovascular; LVMI, left ventricular mass index.

Data from Muiesan ML, et al., Hypertension 2004; **43**: 731–8.

hypertrophy: an increase in size of cardiomyocytes, which increases the muscular mass of the left ventricle, and an increase in extracellular matrix deposition within the ventricle, which contributes to an increase in wall stiffness. The increase in left ventricular mass and stiffness manifests initially as impaired relaxation during diastole, which is often detectable on echocardiography in hypertensive patients at diagnosis, even before the left ventricular mass is sufficiently increased to be classified as indicating hypertrophy. Over time, in untreated or poorly treated patients, cardiac changes will progress to impaired systolic function and ultimately overt heart failure.

Myocardial ischaemia

In addition to impaired cardiac diastolic and systolic function, the hypertensive heart is also predisposed to myocardial ischaemia because of (1) increased myocardial oxygen consumption due to increased cardiac afterload, (2) impaired endocardial blood flow due to the structural and functional changes in small arteries described above, (3) an increase in the systolic time interval and reduced diastolic filling time and pressures due to large-artery stiffening and impaired ventricular–vascular coupling, and (4) increased risk of coronary atheroma in people with hypertension.

Cardiac arrhythmias

The aforementioned structural and ischaemic changes also predispose to an increased prevalence of simple and complex ventricular arrhythmias in people with hypertensive left ventricular hypertrophy. In addition, it has recently been recognized that atrial fibrillation is much commoner in older people with hypertension. Moreover, in hypertensive patients with left ventricular hypertrophy the risk of developing atrial fibrillation is at least twofold greater, and increases further as a function of advancing age, increased systolic pressure, increased left ventricular mass, and increased left atrial diameter. The combination of these latter two cardiac features is a particularly potent predictor of the risk of developing atrial fibrillation in hypertensive patients.

Regression of left ventricular hypertrophy

Recent clinical studies suggest that inhibition of the renin–angiotensin–aldosterone system is particularly effective at regressing left ventricular hypertrophy. This is important, because there is now clear evidence that regression of the ECG manifestations of left ventricular hypertrophy is associated with dramatically improved prognosis for people with hypertension (50% reduction in risk of cardiovascular death over 5 years). Moreover, blockade of the renin–angiotensin–aldosterone system may be particularly effective at reducing the risk of developing atrial fibrillation in people with hypertensive left ventricular hypertrophy. Consensus in guidelines is that lowering blood pressure is of paramount importance for patients with left ventricular hypertrophy, but that effective renin–angiotensin–aldosterone system blockade should also be part of the treatment strategy.

The brain in hypertension

Hypertension is the single most important risk factor for stroke and is increasingly recognized as a major factor contributing to the rate of cognitive decline in later life. All categories of stroke—ischaemic (large and small vessel), haemorrhagic, and embolic—are increased in hypertensive patients.

Cerebral (atherothrombotic) infarction

Infarction accounts for about 80% of the strokes suffered by patients with hypertension. It is usually attributable to atheroma of one of the larger cerebral arteries (usually the middle cerebral artery), or to small-vessel (lacunar) infarction. Although poorly characterized, it is likely that embolic stroke is also more common in people with hypertension, especially those with left ventricular hypertrophy, because of the increased likelihood of paroxysmal or sustained atrial fibrillation on a background of increased left atrial size.

Intracerebral haemorrhage

This accounts for 10 to 15% of strokes in patients with hypertension and is usually the result of rupture of a small intracerebral degenerative microaneurysm (Charcot–Bouchard aneurysm). These lesions develop in the small (<200 μm diameter) perforating arteries in the region of the basal ganglia, thalamus, and internal capsule. Hyaline degeneration (lipohyalinosis) occurs in the aneurysmal wall, with a defect in the media at the neck of the aneurysm. The incidence of Charcot–Bouchard aneurysms is closely correlated with age and blood pressure, the two factors acting additively so that lesions are rarely if ever seen in younger normotensive people. The relationship between blood pressure and haemorrhagic stroke appears to be steeper in people of Chinese/East Asian origin.

The remaining strokes in hypertensive patients are due to subarachnoid haemorrhage. Transient ischaemic attacks due to disease of extracranial vessels are also more frequent in hypertensive subjects.

Hypertension and cognitive function

Hypertension is increasingly recognized as an important cause of dementia, with increased blood pressure in mid life associated with an increased risk of dementia in later life. Cognitive decline is related to diffuse small-vessel cerebrovascular disease in untreated hypertension and in older patients. Functional imaging studies have shown relative reductions in blood flow in parietal and forebrain areas in hypertensive patients during memory tasks and areas of cortical and subcortical hypometabolism. More advanced vascular disease gives rise to multiple, punctate, hyperintense white matter lesions on MRI scanning. These are due to focal ischaemia, either as a result of lipohyalinosis or microatheromatous disease, tortuosity, and narrowing of the perforating arteries. All degrees of impairment of cognitive performance may occur as a result of these lesions, ranging from effects only detectable with sensitive psychometric testing, to lacunar strokes and Binswanger's disease.

Hypertensive encephalopathy

The brain is protected from wide fluctuations in blood pressure by blood flow autoregulation, i.e. the intrinsic capacity of the cerebral vessels to constrict in the face of increased pressure and dilate in the face of decreased pressure to maintain a constant flow. Resistance vessel remodelling and hypertrophy may enhance protection against higher perfusion pressures, thereby extending the upper limits of the autoregulatory range in long-standing hypertension. However, such remodelling may also impair the autoregulation of blood flow when faced with decreased pressure because of impaired capacity of hypertrophied resistance vessels to dilate, thereby predisposing to small-vessel ischaemia. In severe hypertension focal areas of vasodilatation can develop if blood pressure rises above the autoregulatory range, resulting in localized perivascular oedema and fibrinoid necrosis. Focal haemorrhages, ischaemia, and infarction may result, giving rise to the clinical picture of encephalopathy (see Chapter 17.5).

The kidney in hypertension

Patients with renal disease often have hypertension, and people with hypertension can develop renal disease. The age-related decline in GFR is more rapid in people with essential hypertension. However, GFR is usually well preserved throughout life in patients with mild to moderate essential hypertension, hence the development of endstage renal disease in such patients is unusual in the absence of any other renal lesions. The decline in GFR, when it does occur, is due to progressive glomerulosclerosis, most likely driven by raised intraglomerular capillary pressures, which also explain the increased urinary albumin excretion rates in these patients. Increased urinary albumin excretion rate has in turn been linked to increased likelihood of more widespread endothelial/vascular dysfunction and an increased risk of premature cardiovascular disease and death, hence the kidney—and urinary albumin excretion rate in particular—has been proposed as the earliest clinical indicator of significant pressure mediated vascular injury.

Significant hypertension-induced glomerulosclerosis is much more likely in two settings (1) severe and accelerated hypertension, resulting in so-called hypertensive nephropathy; and (2) in the presence of intrinsic renal disease, i.e. due to diabetes or glomerulonephritis. Effective control of blood pressure is of substantial importance in retarding the progression of renal impairment in these settings.

Another important association between hypertension and renal disease is atheromatous renal vascular disease. In these patients, hypertension is usually moderate to severe, and the condition is characteristically associated with a progressive ischaemic nephropathy due either to proximal renal artery (often ostial) disease and/or smaller branch artery disease. It may be associated with small-vessel cholesterol embolization, the affected patients usually being older, with evidence of widespread atheromatous disease.

The eye in hypertension

The findings in the retina of patients with hypertension range from mild generalized retinal–arteriolar narrowing, through to the development of more significant changes of flame-shaped or blot-shaped haemorrhages, cottonwool spots, hard exudates, microaneurysms, or a combination of all of these factors. Swelling of the optic disc can also be seen. The classification of these changes and their pathophysiology and significance are discussed in Chapter 17.2.

The evolution of hypertensive injury—from physiology to philosophy

The process of hypertensive injury to target organs evolves silently over many years, the magnitude and rate of progression determined largely by the level of blood pressure, but also by individual susceptibility (Fig. 17.1.11). In the prehypertensive phase, patients may already have disturbances in blood pressure regulation, i.e. responses to pressor stimuli, visceral obesity, and subtle features of the metabolic syndrome. The injurious process and metabolic disturbances then progress though a silent phase, often lasting many years, during which there is subtle damage to many target organs as cited above, i.e. vascular wall, myocardium, brain, kidney, and eye. This subtle early damage is potentially preventable and/or reversible, but progresses if untreated to more sinister markers of

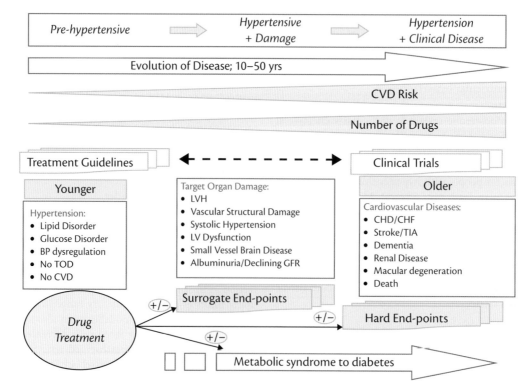

Fig. 17.1.11 The clinical progression of hypertension. blood pressure, blood pressure; CHD, coronary heart disease; CHF, congestive heart failure; CVD, cardiovascular disease; GFR, glomerular filtration rate; LV, left ventricular; TIA, transient ischaemic attack; TOD, target organ damage.

more advanced damage—the so-called intermediate or surrogate disease markers that can be detected in many cases by simple tests such as the ECG, or urinalysis for albumin or protein. Untreated or poorly treated, this progressive hypertension-mediated damage culminates in overt cardiovascular, renal, and cerebrovascular disease and clinical events—the so-called 'hard clinical endpoints' that form the evidence base for treatment guidelines. Alongside, the metabolic syndrome is evolving, increasing the risk of developing diabetes and magnifying the cardiovascular risk burden associated with the blood pressure elevation. Along the way, the conduit arteries are stiffening with damage and age, and the systolic pressure is rising and becoming more difficult to treat.

Current treatment guidelines have been developed from an evidence base relating to changes in hard clinical endpoints derived from studies in very elderly patients at the end of the hypertensive disease process. Somehow, we have to try to translate that evidence into strategies for treating younger patients at the start of the disease process when their risk of clinical events is low. Future treatment strategies must surely focus on preventing the evolution of the silent disease process, rather than simply battling with its consequences. To meet that challenge, we need more and better studies of younger patients with hypertension to better characterize the impact of treatments on the evolution of hypertensive disease, and to determine the robustness of the associated intermediate or surrogate disease markers at predicting treatment benefit.

Further reading

Epidemiology

Asia Pacific Cohort Studies Collaboration (APCSC) (2005). Joint effects of systolic blood pressure and serum cholesterol on cardiovascular disease in the Asia Pacific region. *Circulation*, **112**, 3384–90.

Chobanian AV (2007). Isolated systolic hypertension in the elderly. *N Engl J Med*, **357**, 789–96.

Ezzati M, *et al.* (2002). Selected major risk factors and global and regional burden of disease. *Lancet*, **360**, 1347–60.

Franklin SS, *et al.* (1997). Hemodynamic patterns of age-related changes in blood pressure: the Framingham Heart Study. *Circulation*, **96**, 308–15.

Lawes CMM, *et al.* (2006). Blood pressure and the global burden of disease 2000. Part I: estimates of blood pressure levels. *J Hypertens*, **24**, 413–22.

Lawes CMM, *et al.* (2008). Global burden of blood pressure related disease, 2001. *Lancet*, **371**, 1513–18.

Lewington S, *et al.* (2002). Age-specific relevance of usual blood pressure to vascular mortality: a meta-analysis of individual data for one million adults in 61 prospective studies. *Lancet*, **360**, 1903–13.

MacMahonS, Meal B, Rodgers A (2005). Hypertension—time to move on. *Lancet*, **365**, 1108–9.

National Clinical Guideline Centre (2011). *Hypertension—the clinical management of primary hypertension in adults.* Clinical Guideline 127. <http://www.nice.org.uk/guidance/cg127>.

Staessen JA, *et al.* (2003). Cardiovascular prevention and blood pressure reduction: a quantitative overview updated until 1st March 2003. *J Hypertens*, **21**, 1055–76.

Vasan RS, *et al.* (2001). Impact of high-normal blood pressure on the risk of cardiovascular disease. *New Engl J Med*, **345**, 1291–7.

Wang Y, Wang QJ (2004). The prevalence of prehypertension and hypertension among US adults according to the new joint national committee guidelines: new challenges of the old problem. *Arch Intern Med*, **164**, 2126–34.

William B, *et al.* (2008). Systolic pressure is all that matters. *Lancet*, **371**, 2219–21.

Yusuf S, *et al.* (2004). Effect of potentially modifiable risk factors associated with myocardial infarction in 52 countries (the INTERHEART study): case-control study. *Lancet*, **364**, 937–52.

Pathophysiology

Aksnesa TA, *et al.* (2007). Prevention of new-onset atrial fibrillation and its predictors with angiotensin II-receptor blockers in the treatment of hypertension and heart failure. *J Hypertens*, **25**, 15–23.

Cusi D, *et al.* (1997). Polymorphisms of α-adducin and salt sensitivity in patients with essential hypertension. *Lancet*, **349**, 1353–57.

Devereux RB, *et al.* (2004). Prognostic significance of left ventricular mass change during treatment of hypertension. *JAMA*, **292**, 2386–8.

Drukteinis J, *et al.* (2007). Cardiac and systemic hemodynamic characteristics of hypertension and prehypertension in adolescents and young adults. the Strong Heart Study. *Circulation*, **115**, 221–7.

Elliott WJ, Meyer PM (2007). Incident diabetes in clinical trials of antihypertensive drugs: a network meta-analysis. *Lancet*, **369**, 201–207.

Lip GYH, Blann AD (2000). Does hypertension confer a prothrombotic state? Virchow's triad revisited. *Circulation*, **101**, 218–20.

Mancia G, *et al.* (2007). The sympathetic nervous system and the metabolic syndrome. *J Hypertens*, **25**, 909–20.

Mancini JGB, *et al.* (2004). Surrogate markers for cardiovascular disease. *Circulation*, **109** Suppl, IV22–30.

Mason JM, *et al.* (2005). The diabetogenic potential of thiazide-type diuretic and beta-blocker combinations in patients with hypertension. *J Hypertens*, **23**, 1777–81.

Okin PM, *et al.* (2004). Electrocardiographic strain pattern and prediction of cardiovascular morbidity and mortality in hypertensive patients. *Hypertension*, **44**, 48–54.

Okin PM, *et al.* (2006). Electrocardiographic strain pattern and prediction of new-onset congestive heart failure in hypertensive patients: the Losartan Intervention for Endpoint Reduction in Hypertension (LIFE) study. *Circulation*, **113**, 67–73.

Pepine CJ, Cooper-DeHoff RM (2004). Cardiovascular therapies and risk of the development of diabetes. *J Am Coll Cardiol*, **44**, 609–12.

Psaty BM, *et al.* (2002). Diuretic therapy, the alpha-adducin gene variant, and the risk of myocardial infarction or stroke in persons with treated hypertension. *JAMA*, **287**, 1680–9.

Sironi AM, *et al.* (2004). Visceral fat in hypertension. *Hypertension*, **44**, 127–33.

Srinivasan SR, Myers L, Berenson GS (2006). Changes in metabolic syndrome variables since childhood in prehypertensive and hypertensive subjects: the Bogalusa Heart Study. *Hypertension*, **48**, 33–9.

Staessen JA, *et al.* (2001). Effects of three candidate genes on prevalence and incidence of hypertension in a Caucasian population. *J Hypertens*, **19**, 1349–58.

Stevens LA, *et al.* (2006). Assessing kidney function—measured and estimated glomerular filtration rate. *New Engl J Med*, **354**, 2473–83.

Swales JD (1985). *Platt versus Pickering: an episode in recent medical history.* London: Keynes Press.

Taddei S, *et al.* (2000). Endothelial dysfunction in hypertension. *J Nephrol*, **13**, 205–10.

Wang JG, *et al.* (2006). Carotid intima-media thickness and antihypertensive treatment: a meta-analysis of randomized controlled trials. *Stroke*, **37**, 1933–40.

Ward R (1990). Familial aggregation and genetic epidemiology of blood pressure. In: Laragh JH, Brenner BM (eds) *Hypertension: pathophysiology, diagnosis and management*, pp. 81–100. New York: Raven Press.

Weber MA, *et al.* (2014). Clinical practice guidelines for the management of hypertension in the community a statement by the American Society of Hypertension and the International Society of Hypertension. *J Hypertens*, **32**, 3–15.

Williams B (1994). Insulin resistance: the shape of things to come. *Lancet*, **344**, 521–4.

Wong T, Mitchell P (2007). The eye in hypertension. *Lancet*, **369**, 425–35.

CHAPTER 17.2

Essential hypertension: diagnosis, assessment, and treatment

Bryan Williams and John D. Firth

Essentials

Essential hypertension is almost invariably symptomless, and usually detected by routine screening or opportunistic measurement of blood pressure. Key questions to answer in the assessment of a person presenting with an elevated blood pressure are: (1) Do they have hypertension, i.e. is the blood pressure persistently elevated? (2) Are there any associated clinical features that might warrant further evaluation to exclude secondary causes of hypertension? (3) Are there factors that might be contributing to an elevated blood pressure, including lifestyle or dietary factors or concomitant medication? (4) Is there any associated target organ damage or comorbidity that influences the overall cardiovascular disease risk and subsequent treatment of the patient?

Diagnosis

It is normal to find large variations in blood pressure measured in a single individual, hence it should be measured as accurately as possible using the British Hypertension Society protocol. All adults should have their blood pressure measured routinely at least every 5 years. Automated home blood pressure measurements (HBPM) and ambulatory blood pressure measurement (ABPM) recordings provide much more information than standard office blood pressure measurements with regard to diagnosis and efficacy of treatment of hypertension, and some recent guidelines recommend that they should be used routinely for diagnosis.

The appropriate thresholds for diagnosis of hypertension depending on the method of blood pressure measurement are (1) office or clinic—systolic blood pressure (SBP) 140 mmHg, diastolic blood pressure (DBP) 90 mmHg; (2) ABPM 24 h—SBP 130 mmHg, DBP 80 mmHg; daytime—SBP 135 mmHg, DBP 85 mmHg; night-time—SBP 120 mmHg, DBP 70 mmHg; and (3) home measurements—SBP 135 mmHg, DBP 85 mmHg. The European Society of Hypertension classification of hypertension is described in Chapter 17.1.

Isolated office hypertension ('white coat' hypertension) should be diagnosed whenever office blood pressure is greater than or equal to 140/90 mmHg on at least three occasions, while 24 h mean and daytime blood pressures are within their normal range.

Clinical examination and investigation

Fundoscopy is the most convenient method of directly visualizing vascular pathology and provides important prognostic information.

Three grades are recognized: (1) mild—generalized and focal arteriolar narrowing, arteriolar wall opacification, and arteriovenous nipping; (2) moderate—as (1) plus flame-shaped blot haemorrhages and/or cotton wool spots and/or hard exudates and/or microaneurysms; and (3) severe—as (2) plus swelling of the optic disc.

Aside from measurement of blood pressure and fundal examination as detailed above, particular features to look for on examination are evidence of secondary effects of sustained hypertension on the heart, and features that might suggest the presence of a secondary cause of hypertension (coarctation—absent/delayed femoral pulses, cardiac murmur; and renovascular disease—renal bruit).

Patients with essential hypertension need only a limited number of routine investigations, namely (1) urine strip test for blood and urinary albumin:creatinine ratio (ACR) for proteinuria; (2) serum creatinine and electrolytes; (3) blood glucose—ideally fasted; (4) cholesterol and HDL-cholesterol—ideally fasted; and (5) 12-lead electrocardiogram (ECG).

Management

The treatment of hypertension is directed towards reducing risk rather than treating symptoms, and best advice and treatment is informed by formal estimation of a patient's overall cardiovascular risk.

There is international consensus that, for office blood pressure, an optimal treatment target should be less than 140/90 mmHg in patients under the age of 60 years. Recommendations differ for older patients: current American guidelines suggest treating to a goal of less than 150/90 mmHg for patients aged over 60 years, whereas the British Hypertension Society/NICE guideline recommends the same higher target for those over 80 years. Most international guidelines no longer recommend lower blood pressure targets for populations at higher cardiovascular rise, e.g. patients with diabetes, although the most recent European guideline suggests a target for DBP of below 85 mmHg in this group. Although early studies focused primarily on DBP as the treatment target, SBP is invariably more difficult to control and should be the main focus of treatment.

The most effective lifestyle interventions for reducing blood pressure are (1) modifications to diet to induce weight loss, (2) regular aerobic exercise, and (3) reduction of excessive alcohol and/or sodium intake; all smokers should be offered advice and help to quit to reduce cardiovascular (and other) risks. Many patients will require more than one drug to control blood pressure: monotherapy is rarely sufficient. The blood pressure response to an individual class of blood pressure lowering medication is heterogeneous, hence there is no 'perfect drug' for every patient, but some trials have indicated that certain comorbidities or target organ damage provide compelling indications for inclusion of specific classes of drug therapy in the treatment regimen.

There is wide variation in the international guidelines with regard to the preferred initial therapy for essential hypertension: (1) the (American) Joint National Committee (JNC) 8 guideline recommends initial drug treatment with an angiotensin converting enzyme inhibitor (ACE inhibitor), angiotensin receptor blocker (ARB), calcium channel blocker (CCB), or thiazide-type diuretic (TTD) in non-black hypertensive patients, with a CCB or TTD preferred in black patients; (2) the recent European guideline suggests that all five main classes of blood pressure lowering drugs (ACE inhibitor, ARB, β-blockers, CCB, and TTD) are all suitable as initial therapy; (3) the British Hypertension Society/NICE guideline suggests that the most appropriate initial blood pressure lowering agent for (a) people aged 55 years or over, and for black people of African or Caribbean family origin of any age, is a CCB, with a TTD preferred if a CCB is not suitable, and (b) for people under 55 years of age an ACE inhibitor or a low-cost ARB is preferred initial therapy.

All guidelines recognize that combinations of blood pressure lowering drugs are often required to achieve recommended blood pressure goals. European guidelines suggest various suitable combinations of treatments. American guidelines recommend selecting any two of the medications recommended as suitable for the particular patient as initial therapy. The British guideline provides explicit guidance on preferred combinations of treatment if one agent fails to achieve adequate control: step 2—a CCB combined with either an ACE inhibitor or ARB; step 3—add a TTD; step 4—add higher-dose TTD, spironolactone, an α-blocker or a β-blocker.

Patients with hypertension and deemed to be at high cardiovascular risk (>20% over 10 years) should receive advice to adjust their lifestyles and be considered for treatment with statin therapy and low-dose aspirin to optimize their risk reduction.

Indications for specialist referral include uncertainty about the decision to treat, investigations to exclude secondary hypertension, severe and complicated hypertension, and resistant hypertension.

Clinical presentation

Symptoms

Essential hypertension is invariably symptomless and usually detected by routine screening or opportunistic measurement of blood pressure. However, once a patient has been labelled as 'hypertensive' it is not uncommon for them to associate preceding symptoms to their elevated blood pressure. Some patients will claim that they can recognize when their blood pressure is elevated, usually on the basis of symptoms such as plethoric features, palpitations, dizziness, or a feeling of tension. Screening surveys have demonstrated that these symptoms occur no more commonly in untreated hypertensive patients than they do in the normotensive population. However, there are two important caveats to the symptomless nature of essential hypertension: (1) symptoms may develop as a

consequence of target organ damage, (2) headache may be a feature of severe hypertension.

Headache

Most headaches in hypertensive patients are tension headaches, not related to blood pressure at all, although they become more common when patients become aware of the diagnosis. The classic hypertensive headache is present on waking in the morning, situated in the occipital region, radiating to the frontal area, throbbing in quality, and wears off during the course of the day. It is generally associated with more severe hypertension. Effective treatment of hypertension reduces the incidence of such headaches. Morning headaches in obese hypertensive patients may be related to sleep apnoea.

Epistaxis

Epistaxis is not associated with mild hypertension but is more common in moderate to severe hypertension. However, the associated anxiety can elevate blood pressure when patients present with bleeding, hence it is particularly important that patients are not automatically labelled as hypertensive, with care taken to dissociate hypertension as a cause of epistaxis from a pressor response to the epistaxis itself.

Male impotence

Patients rarely volunteer information about impotence, but there is an increased prevalence of erectile dysfunction in untreated hypertensive men. This is related to two factors: remodelling of small arteries and increased risk of atheroma, both of which vascular changes can reduce penile blood flow despite the elevation in blood pressure. Furthermore, erectile dysfunction can develop or worsen as a consequence of treatment, for the most part related to the reduction in blood pressure before any concomitant change in vascular structure.

Nocturia

This is common in people with untreated hypertension as a consequence of a reduction in urine-concentrating capacity. The symptoms usually improve with treatment.

Symptoms associated with target organ damage

If patients develop cardiac, vascular, cerebrovascular, and/or renal complications as a consequence of long-standing untreated or poorly treated hypertension, then symptoms related to these complications may be present. Target organ damage and associated symptoms are discussed in Chapter 17.1.

Aims of assessment

There are several important issues that must be considered in the assessment of people presenting with an elevated blood pressure:

- Does the patient have hypertension, i.e. is the blood pressure persistently elevated?

- Are there any associated clinical features that might warrant further evaluation to exclude secondary causes of hypertension? (see below and Chapter 17.3)

- Are there factors that might be contributing to an elevated blood pressure, including lifestyle or dietary factors or concomitant medication?

- Is there any associated target organ damage or comorbidity that influences the overall cardiovascular disease risk and subsequent treatment of the patient?

These factors, along with the age and ethnicity of the patient, will inform the decision to treat, the urgency of the need to treat, the need for further investigation, and the choice of treatment.

Physical examination

Blood pressure measurement

Large variations in blood pressure measured in a single individual are normal, hence it should be measured as accurately as possible using the British Hypertension Society (BHS) protocol (Box 17.2.1). Blood pressure should initially be measured in both arms because there can be large inter-arm difference in blood pressure. The finding of a difference of greater than 20 mmHg may indicate the presence of underlying vascular disease, especially subclavian stenosis. When there is a significant inter-arm difference in blood pressure reading, the arm with the higher pressure should be used for all subsequent measurements.

All adults should have their blood pressure measured routinely at least every 5 years. Those with high-normal blood pressure (systolic blood pressure (SBP) 130–139 mmHg or diastolic blood pressure (DBP) 85–89 mmHg) and those who have had high blood pressure readings at any time previously should have their blood pressure re-measured annually. These measurements can be made in the clinic, in the home setting, or using ambulatory blood pressure monitoring (ABPM), as described later in the chapter.

Seated blood pressure recordings are generally sufficient, with the patient seated and rested for a few minutes beforehand. At least two measurements should be taken, and if the first measurement is more than 10 mmHg higher than the subsequent one, then it should be discarded and a further reading taken. Standing blood pressure (after at least 2 min standing) should be measured in elderly or diabetic patients to exclude significant orthostatic hypotension.

The timing of blood pressure measurement should take account of the timing of medication. Treatment decisions should not be based on single blood pressure readings: the average of two readings at each of at least three visits (depending on severity) should be used to guide the decision to treat. The time between visits will vary according to the severity of the hypertension, ranging from days or weeks to months. In patients with severe hypertension, especially when there is unequivocal evidence of target organ damage, the decision to treat may be made at the time of first presentation.

When measuring blood pressure, the upper arm should be supported at heart level during recordings, and it is important that an appropriate cuff size is used, with the bladder encircling at least 80% of the upper arm. Using too large a cuff results in an underestimation of blood pressure and too small a cuff will lead to overestimation. If the auscultatory method is used to measure blood pressure, then Korotkoff phase I (first appearance of sound) and phase V sounds (disappearance of sound) should be taken for SBP and DBP, respectively. If phase V goes to zero, then phase IV (muffling of sound) should be recorded.

The beat-to-beat variability associated with atrial fibrillation can make blood pressure measurement difficult and semiautomatic or automated devices can be very inaccurate in such circumstances, in which case multiple readings of auscultatory measurements are recommended.

Blood pressure monitors

The sphygmomanometer has been the mainstay of blood pressure measurement for over 100 years, but its use is likely to decline as a consequence of the decommissioning of mercury-based devices and the emergence of automated and semiautomated devices for routine blood pressure measurement in the office and home and for ABPM.

It is important to note that there are different diagnostic thresholds for the diagnosis of hypertension dependent on the method of measurement, i.e. when using multiple home or ambulatory blood pressure values to measure an average blood pressure, then the average value used to define hypertension is lower than the equivalent office blood pressure threshold of 140/90 mmHg (Table 17.2.1) and it should be noted—as stated above—that automated devices are inaccurate in patients with atrial fibrillation, in whom blood pressure should be measured manually. Detailed guidance on blood pressure measurement and a wide range of validated monitors is available from <http://www.bhsoc.org>.

Ambulatory blood pressure measurements (ABPM)

ABPM recordings provide much more information than standard office blood pressure measurements with regard to diagnosis and

---

Box 17.2.1 British Hypertension Society protocol for blood pressure measurement

- Use a properly maintained, calibrated, and validated device

- Measure sitting blood pressure routinely: standing blood pressure should be recorded at the initial estimation in elderly and diabetic patients

- Remove light clothing, support arm at heart level, ensure hand relaxed and avoid talking during the measurement procedure

- Use cuff of appropriate size, and rapidly inflate the cuff to 20 mmHg above the point where the brachial pulse disappears

- Lower cuff pressure slowly (2 mm/s)

- Read blood pressure to the nearest 2 mmHg

- Measure diastolic as disappearance of sounds (phase V)

- Take the mean of at least two readings: more recordings are needed if marked differences between initial measurements are found

- Do not treat on the basis of an isolated reading

Reprinted by permission from Macmillan Publishers Ltd: *Journal of Human Hypertension*, **18**, 139–185 (2004).

Table 17.2.1 Diagnostic thresholds for hypertension according to different methods of measurement

	SBP (mmHg)	DBP (mmHg)
Office or clinic	140	90
24 hour	125	80
Day	135	85
Night	120	70
Home	135	85

DBP, diastolic blood pressure; SBP, systolic blood pressure.

efficacy of treatment of hypertension. When compared to office blood pressure, there is a much steeper relationship between ABPM averages and target organ damage indices and cardiovascular events, no doubt reflecting that fact that more measurements are obtained and the 'white coat' or 'office' effect (see 'White coat' or isolated office hypertension, below) is eliminated. Generally, ABPM devices are programmed to record blood pressure at 20 min intervals during the day and 30 min intervals at night. A diary is provided to record activity and sleep patterns. In addition to the 24 h blood pressure average, ABPM also provides information on blood pressure profiles, e.g. daytime and night-time averages, the 'dipper status', i.e. the relationship between night-time and daytime blood pressure averages, blood pressure variability throughout the day, the morning surge in blood pressure, and—more recently—indices of aortic function via the ambulatory stiffness index. Each of these parameters adds value over and above the assessment of office blood pressure, hence such techniques are increasingly used for the assessment of people with hypertension. Clinical indications for the use of ABPM are shown in Box 17.2.2.

Home blood pressure measurements (HBPM)

It is increasingly common for patients to measure their own blood pressure at home using monitors that measure blood pressure on the upper arm, wrist, or finger. The average of frequent measurements may be more reproducible and reliable than clinic measures, and HBPM has been shown to be a better predictor of clinical outcomes. Validated devices should be used, with an average of duplicate morning and evening HBPM recorded daily for at least 4 days and ideally for 7 days. The measurements should be recorded seated after 5 min rest, with those taken on the first day discarded. Advocates of HBPM argue that it may reduce unnecessary treatment (by revealing the diagnosis of 'white coat' hypertension; see next section) and increase treatment compliance, against which must be balanced the fact that in some patients it can lead to inappropriate concern and anxiety.

'White coat' or isolated office hypertension

In some patients office blood pressure is persistently elevated although their 24 h blood pressure or home blood pressure averages are within the normal range. This has been termed white coat hypertension or isolated office hypertension. It is important to note that blood pressure will generally fall with repeated readings in all patients, hence it is the chronicity of the office blood pressure elevation that is important to establish the diagnosis.

Box 17.2.2 Possible indications for ambulatory blood pressure monitoring

- Unusual blood pressure variability
- Possible 'white coat' hypertension
- Informing equivocal treatment decisions
- Evaluation of nocturnal hypertension
- Evaluation of drug-resistant hypertension
- Determining the efficacy of drug treatment over 24 h
- Diagnosis and treatment of hypertension in pregnancy
- Evaluation of symptomatic hypotension

White coat or isolated office hypertension should be diagnosed whenever office blood pressure is 140/90 mmHg or more on at least three occasions, while 24 h mean and daytime blood pressures are within their normal range. The diagnosis can also be based on home blood pressure values, i.e. average home readings below 135/85 mmHg and office values 140/90 mmHg or more.

Surveys suggest that white coat or isolated office hypertension may be present in as many as 15% of the general population and approximately one-third of all hypertensives. There is considerable debate about its prognostic significance: some studies report association with evidence of hypertensive target organ damage, but others do not. However, overall it appears that white coat hypertension is not benign, with the associated risk probably sitting between those with hypertension confirmed by office readings and ABPM, and those with definitively normal pressures by all methods of measurement. When white coat hypertension is diagnosed, the best advice is to monitor blood pressure and target organ damage via ABPM or home blood pressure averages and not treat unless these pressures are persistently elevated.

Masked hypertension

Less attention has been paid to masked hypertension, i.e. patients with a normal office blood pressure but elevated ABPM or home blood pressure averages, than to those with white coat hypertension. Estimates of prevalence range from 10% to 30% of the population, hence a normal office blood pressure does not exclude hypertension. Moreover, as HBPM becomes more popular, the detection of masked hypertension will increase. These patients are more likely to have target organ damage and are at increased cardiovascular risk, perhaps more so than those with white coat hypertension. Masked hypertension should be considered in patients who have clinical evidence of hypertensive target organ damage, but in whom office blood pressure appears normal. Treatment should be offered to such patients, aimed at controlling the home blood pressure average.

Cost-effectiveness of different methods of diagnosing hypertension

A more expensive method of confirming a diagnosis of hypertension may be more cost-effective if, by increasing the accuracy of diagnosis, it avoids treatment costs in some patients. There are no studies that have compared clinic blood pressure monitoring with both ABPM and HBPM from a cost-effectiveness perspective, but the NICE analysis of 2011 concluded that ABPM was the most cost-effective option. However, this conclusion depends on a wide range of assumptions, including the costs of ABPM and HBPM, the frequency and cost of subsequent measurements of blood pressure in those deemed not to be hypertensive, and the costs of treatment of those declared to have hypertension.

Establishing the diagnosis of hypertension

In most healthcare systems hypertension will and should continue to be diagnosed on the basis of office blood pressure measurements. Within the United Kingdom, the most recent NICE recommendations (2011) are that unless severe hypertension (>180/110 mmHg) is found a clinic measurement in excess of 140/90 mmHg should be followed by ABPM, with at least two measurements taken per hour during the person's normal waking hours and an average value of at least 14 readings used to confirm the diagnosis (>135/85 mmHg). HBPM can be used if the patient cannot tolerate ABPM. The most

Table 17.2.2 Modern classification of hypertensive retinopathy

Mild hypertensive retinopathy	Retinal arteriolar signs, such as generalized and focal arteriolar narrowing, arteriolar wall opacification, and arteriovenous nipping
Moderate hypertensive retinopathy	The signs above plus flame-shaped or blot-shaped haemorrhages, cotton wool spots, hard exudates, microaneurysms, or a combination of all of these factors
Severe hypertensive retinopathy	The signs above plus swelling of the optic disc

recent American guidelines (JNC8) do not make new comment on diagnosis of hypertension, and the recent European guidelines (2013) continue to regard conventional office blood pressure measurements as the gold standard for screening, diagnosis, and management.

Fundal examination

Fundoscopy is the most convenient method of directly visualizing vascular pathology and provides important prognostic information. Signs of hypertensive retinopathy are frequently seen in adults 40 years and older, and are predictive of incident stroke, congestive heart failure, and cardiovascular mortality—independently of traditional risk factors.

The Keith Wagener classification of fundal appearances has been used for many years, but has serious shortcomings. This classification identified four grades of hypertensive retinopathy. Grade I and II changes, which result from arteriolar thickening, are often difficult to differentiate from each other, and the prognostic significance of the grade I and II subclassification is unclear. A more practical three-grade classification (i.e. mild, moderate, and severe) has been proposed (Table 17.2.2). The mild changes of generalized retinal–arteriolar narrowing and arteriovenous nipping are related to both the blood pressure at diagnosis and chronic exposure to an elevated blood pressure, hence they appear to be an index of the chronicity of blood pressure elevation (Fig. 17.2.1a). The changes of moderate hypertensive retinopathy are the changes of mild retinopathy plus flame-shaped or blot-shaped haemorrhages, cotton

wool spots, hard exudates, microaneurysms, or a combination of all of these factors. Severe retinopathy (malignant or accelerated hypertension) is characterized by all of the aforementioned changes plus swelling of the optic disc (Fig. 17.2.1b). These moderate and severe fundal changes are more closely related to more recent elevation of blood pressure, suggesting they are the consequence of more transient and severe blood pressure elevation.

The flame-shaped haemorrhages are superficial and shaped due to constraints imposed by nerve fibres. Dot and blot haemorrhages are deeper than the nerve fibres and thus are not so constrained. Haemorrhages usually disappear after a few weeks of effective blood pressure control. There are two types of exudates: hard or waxy exudates represent the end result of fluid leakage into the fibre layers of the retina from damaged vessels, with fluid reabsorption leaving a protein–lipid residue that is slowly removed by macrophages; soft exudates or cotton wool patches are usually larger than hard exudates and have a woolly, ill-defined edge, but they are not true exudates, rather nerve fibre infarcts caused by hypertensive vascular occlusion. Unlike hard exudates, these lesions disappear within a few weeks of establishing adequate antihypertensive therapy.

Severe fundal changes are characterized by disc swelling (i.e. papilloedema) resulting from raised pressure in the disc head secondary to severe vascular damage and increased permeability. Venous distension is followed by increased vascularity of the optic disc, which has a pink appearance with blurring of the disc margins and loss of the optic cup. Raising of the optic disc with anterior displacement of the vessels occurs later. The surrounding retina often shows oedema, small radial haemorrhages, and cotton wool exudates. Moderate or severe fundal changes represent malignant or accelerated hypertension and carry the same adverse prognosis and should be treated as a medical emergency (see Chapter 17.5).

Other fundal changes associated with hypertension

Hypertension also predisposes to the development of a number of sight-threatening complications that can be detected by fundoscopy.

Retinal vein occlusion

This is characterized by dilated and tortuous retinal veins and the presence of retinal haemorrhages, cotton wool spots, and oedema of the macula and optic disc. In the case of central retinal vein occlusion, all four fundal quadrants are involved (Fig. 17.2.2a); only

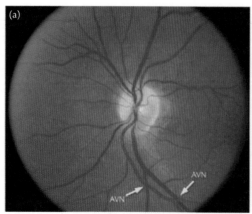
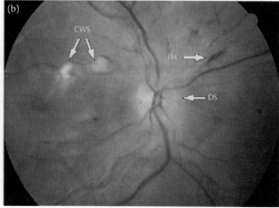

Fig. 17.2.1 (a) Signs of mild hypertensive retinopathy. (b) Signs of severe hypertensive retinopathy. AVN, arteriovenous nipping; CWS, cotton wool spots; DS, swelling of the optic disc; FH, flame-shaped retinal haemorrhage.

Reprinted from *The Lancet*, Vol. 369, Wong T, Mitchell P, The eye in hypertension, pp. 425–35. Copyright (2007), with permission from Elsevier.

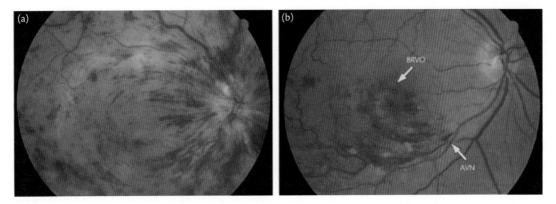

Fig. 17.2.2 (a) Central retinal vein occlusion involving all four fundal quadrants. (b) Branch retinal vein occlusion (BRVO) involving a single fundal quadrant, also showing a good example of arteriovenous nipping (AVN).

Reprinted from *The Lancet*, Vol. 369, Wong T, Mitchell P, *The eye in hypertension*, pp. 425–35. Copyright (2007), with permission from Elsevier.

one fundal quadrant is involved if there is a branch vein occlusion (Fig. 17.2.2b). Central retinal vein occlusion can either be ischaemic or nonischaemic, patients with an ischaemic central retinal vein occlusion typically having poor visual acuity and a relative afferent pupillary defect. Ophthalmic follow-up is needed to diagnose and prevent the two main complications of retinal vein occlusion, namely neovascularization and macular oedema.

Retinal arteriolar embolization

Due to cholesterol crystals, platelet/fibrin clot, or calcium, this is twice as common in people with hypertension compared to those who are normotensive, with the risk further accentuated in cigarette smokers and those with diabetes.

Retinal artery occlusion

Also more common in people with hypertension, central retinal artery occlusion typically presents with a sudden, painless, unilateral loss of vision, associated with a cherry red spot (Fig. 17.2.3a). Branch retinal artery occlusion (Fig. 17.2.3b) will present with a sudden, painless, visual field defect, and there may be only minimal impairment of central vision.

Retinal arterial macroaneurysms

These can be either fusiform or saccular. They are uncommon, but are usually only seen in patients with hypertension. When they

occur, about 20% are bilateral and 10% are multiple. They are usually discovered by routine fundoscopy in asymptomatic hypertensive patients, but can present acutely, with visual loss secondary to haemorrhage or exudation.

Nonarteritic ischaemic optic neuropathy

This is also more common in people with hypertension, occurring (in one series) with a yearly incidence of 1 in 10 000. It presents with sudden unilateral visual loss and optic disc oedema. There is no effective treatment and prospects for visual recovery are poor.

Other systems

All patients with hypertension should have a thorough physical examination (Box 17.2.3). Aside from measurement of blood pressure and fundal examination as detailed above, particular features to look for are evidence of secondary effects of sustained hypertension on the heart, features that might suggest the presence of a secondary cause of hypertension, and evidence of other vascular pathology (absent pulses, arterial bruits).

Cardiac examination may reveal a sustained apex beat, or features of cardiac failure that might be secondary to hypertension. It is sometimes said that the second component of the aortic sound is loud in moderate or severe hypertension, but this is not a reliable finding.

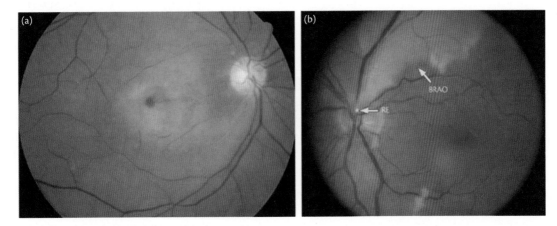

Fig. 17.2.3 (a) Central retinal artery occlusion with a characteristic cherry red spot. (b) Retinal–arteriolar emboli (RE) and retina branch artery occlusion (BRAO).

Reprinted from *The Lancet*, Vol. 369, Wong T, Mitchell P, The eye in hypertension, pp. 425–35. Copyright (2007), with permission from Elsevier.

Box 17.2.3 Initial assessment of the patient with hypertension

◆ Identifiable causes of hypertension:

- Drugs (NSAIDs, oral contraceptive, steroids, liquorice, sympathomimetics, i.e. some cold cures)

- Renal disease (present, past or family history, proteinuria and/or haematuria: palpable kidney(s)—polycystic)

- Renovascular disease (abdominal or loin bruit)

- Obstructive sleep apnoea (snoring, daytime somnolence)

- Coarctation (radiofemoral delay or weak femoral pulses)

- Phaeochromocytoma (paroxysmal symptoms)

- Conn's syndrome (tetany, muscle weakness, polyuria, hypokalaemia)

- Cushing's (classical clinical characteristics)

- Hypothyroidism or hyperthyroidism (classical clinical characteristics)

- Acromegaly (classical clinical characteristics)

◆ Contributory factors

- Overweight

- Excess alcohol (>3 units/day)

- Excess salt intake

- Lack of exercise

- Environmental stress

◆ Complications of hypertension/target organ damage

- Stroke, TIA, dementia, carotid bruits

- LVH and/or LV strain on ECG, heart failure

- Myocardial infarction, angina, CABG or angioplasty

- Peripheral vascular disease

- Fundal haemorrhages or exudates, papilloedema

- Proteinuria

- Renal impairment (raised serum creatinine)

◆ Cardiovascular disease risk factors

- Smoking

- Diabetes

- Total cholesterol:high-density lipoprotein-cholesterol ratio

- Family history

- Age

- Sex

◆ Drug contraindications

CABG, coronary artery bypass graft; LVH, left ventricular hypertrophy; NSAIDs, nonsteroidal anti-inflammatory drugs; TIA, transient ischaemic attack.

In coarctation of the aorta the femoral pulses will be absent or diminished and delayed, and there may be various murmurs (usually a systolic murmur at the sternal border and a continuous murmur at the back of the chest), also visible or palpable collateral arteries on the back of the chest or in the axillae. Blood pressure measured in the legs will be lower than that in the arms.

An abdominal bruit is reported in 4% to 20% of normal people, most commonly in those aged over 40 years, when it is typically systolic and audible only between the xiphisternum and the umbilicus. In patients with severe hypertension that is difficult to control, the finding of an abdominal bruit in both systole and diastole strongly supports the diagnosis of renovascular hypertension, but a bruit confined to systole is much less likely to be of significance.

Routine investigation

Patients with essential hypertension need only a limited number of routine investigations, which must include:

◆ urine strip test for haematuria

◆ urinary albumin:creatinine ratio (ACR) for proteinuria

◆ serum creatinine and electrolytes

◆ blood glucose—ideally fasted

◆ cholesterol and HDL-cholesterol —ideally fasted

◆ ECG

These routine investigations help inform the assessment of target organ damage and cardiovascular disease risk. With regard to renal function, it is now almost universal laboratory practice to report an 'estimated' GFR (eGFR) calculated using an algorithm based on the serum creatinine measurement and the patient's age. Testing for proteinuria should be by quantification on a spot urine sample of the urinary albumin/creatinine ratio (ACR). More sophisticated assessment tools are available, but the list above is sufficient for routine clinical practice. Note that only two of these routine investigations contribute to the detection of underlying causes of hypertension, namely urinalysis (renal causes) and serum creatinine and electrolytes (renal causes and mineralocorticoid excess), although the ECG may very rarely show U waves as a clue to one of the hypokalaemic syndromes. Indications for further investigation for causes of secondary hypertension are given in Chapter 17.3.

A chest radiograph and urine microscopy are not routinely required. Echocardiography is more sensitive at detecting left ventricular hypertrophy than an ECG, but is not required routinely, although it is valuable to confirm or refute the presence of left ventricular hypertrophy when the ECG shows voltage criteria suggestive of this.

Assessment of cardiovascular disease risk

The cardiovascular risk associated with hypertension is not eliminated by the treatment of blood pressure alone. This is because many patients have established cardiovascular damage which may not necessarily reverse with treatment of blood pressure, also lifestyle habits such as smoking and dietary factors that may not have changed since therapy was initiated. Other factors are also important: patients with high blood pressure often have associated disturbances in their metabolic profile (especially lipids and glucose tolerance) that contribute to their risk, which has led many international guidelines to recommend that cardiovascular risk should be formally assessed in all patients with hypertension to determine whether they are at low, medium, or high risk.

Risk calculations based on the Framingham cohort have been used in the United States of America and the United Kingdom, and European guidelines have used a risk score based on mortality data from European countries. Pragmatism in risk assessment is important, with the risk factors cited in the guidelines being conventional markers that can easily be documented in a basic clinical setting, i.e. SBP, age, gender, low-density lipoprotein (LDL) cholesterol, presence of diabetes, smoking history, and the presence or absence of structural damage, e.g. ECG evidence of left ventricular hypertrophy. Recent surveys suggest that more than 90% of population-attributable risk for cardiovascular disease can be explained by these risk factors. The use of more sophisticated risk assessment by adding any of the recently advocated biomarkers, such as C-reactive protein, adds little to the conventional methods of cardiovascular risk estimation.

Cardiovascular disease risk thresholds for intervention currently define 'high-risk' patients as having a 10-year Framingham-derived cardiovascular disease risk of 20% or more, and such patients should be offered antihypertensive drug treatment if their blood pressure is elevated. The typical hypertensive male aged 55 years or more has this level of cardiovascular disease risk, and it is likely that even lower thresholds would be cost-effective for intervention. Formal cardiovascular disease risk estimation is not necessary for patients with hypertension and established cardiovascular disease, diabetes, or overt end organ damage: they are already at sufficient cardiovascular disease risk to benefit from multifactorial risk factor intervention. Whether treatment to reduce blood pressure should be recommended for those with an estimated 10-year cardiovascular risk of less than 20% remains a contentious matter.

Patients with hypertension and deemed to be at high risk should receive strong advice to adjust their lifestyles and be considered for treatment with statin therapy and low-dose aspirin to optimize their risk reduction (see next section).

Clinical management

Initial considerations

Blood pressure is elevated sporadically in everybody. Key objectives in the assessment of essential hypertension are to establish whether blood pressure is persistently elevated; the level to which blood pressure is elevated, i.e. the severity of hypertension; and the presence or absence of hypertension-mediated target organ damage. The initial assessment is usually followed by a period of observation, the duration of which will be dependent on the severity of the hypertension and the associated cardiovascular disease risk and damage. Lifestyle advice should be provided during this observation period, with drug therapy initiated depending on the level of blood pressure and overall cardiovascular disease risk at the end of the observation period.

Establishing the diagnosis

Patients with essential hypertension usually present in one of three ways:

◆ as an asymptomatic individual whose blood pressure has been measured at routine examination for employment, insurance,

or as a result of screening or preoperatively—the most common presentation

◆ as a patient whose blood pressure has been measured opportunistically when presenting with an unrelated disorder; or

◆ as a result of symptoms produced by hypertension, or by the acute or chronic complications of hypertension—the least common presentation.

Repeated blood pressure measurements over a period of observation are usually necessary to establish the diagnosis. Exceptions to this are patients presenting with severe hypertension in whom fundal examination or other assessment of target organ damage (e.g. left ventricular hypertrophy or renal impairment) clearly reveals the presence of hypertension-mediated damage, indicative of the fact that the blood pressure needs treatment.

The period of observation required before initiating drug therapy is dependent on the severity of the hypertension and the presence or absence of cardiovascular disease, diabetes and/or target organ damage. Those with more severe hypertension and disease require emergency or urgent intervention with drug therapy to lower their blood pressure, whereas those with less severe hypertension and/or the absence of damage or disease can be monitored over a longer period—up to many months—before initiating drug therapy. This period of observation is important because it is used to repeat blood pressure measurements, confirm the presence of sustained hypertension, and get a more accurate appreciation of the associated risk, also to implement lifestyle interventions that may reduce blood pressure.

Diagnostic thresholds for therapeutic intervention, the observation period and treatment targets

The diagnostic thresholds and appropriate interventions for the levels of hypertension severity are shown in Fig. 17.2.4, and the recommended period of observation for different grades of hypertension are shown in Table 17.2.3. Although there is general consensus about the management of grade II (i.e. ≥160/100 mmHg) or more severe hypertension, the British guidelines have traditionally been more cautious than other guidelines with regard to drug therapy for uncomplicated grade I hypertension (140–159/90–99 mmHg) (Figure 17.2.4 and Table 17.2.3). Most other guidelines recommend treating all patients under the age of 60 years with a blood pressure sustained above 140/90 mmHg, whereas the British guidelines have recommended drug therapy for those with grade I hypertension only when there is associated cardiovascular disease or target organ damage, or a calculated risk of cardiovascular disease at least 20% over 10 years. There is genuine uncertainty about the cost-effectiveness of treating otherwise low-risk people with grade I hypertension, but this must be balanced by recognition that the greatest burden of blood pressure-attributable disease in populations is in those with grade I hypertension because it is so common. Moreover, blood pressure will invariably continue to rise in patients with grade I hypertension, and there is concern that the subtle vascular damage that is occurring while these patients remain untreated may not be reversible when treatment is eventually initiated at higher levels of pressure. Thus, while a prolonged period of observation and lifestyle intervention for uncomplicated, low-risk, grade I hypertension is considered acceptable, it is inevitable that most of these patients will eventually (if not immediately) require drug treatment. Further differences between guidelines relate to

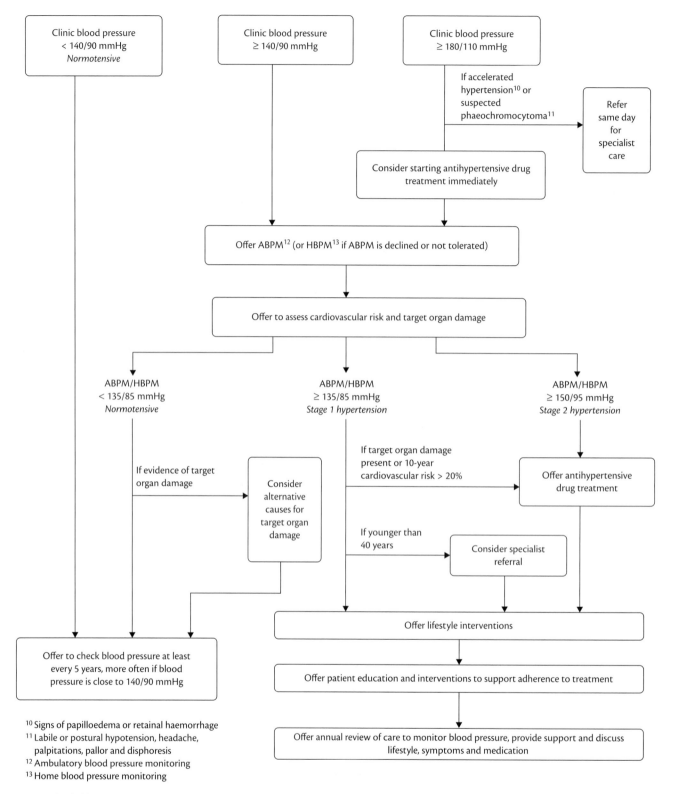

Fig. 17.2.4 Thresholds and appropriate inventions depending on blood pressure. Note: if ABPM or HBPM are not available, then proceed as advised in Table 17.2.3. From National Clinical Guideline Centre (2011). *Hypertension—the clinical management of primary hypertension in adults.* Clinical Guideline 127.

older patients: current American guidelines suggest treating to a goal of less than 150/90 mmHg for patients over 60 years of age, whereas the British guideline recommends the same higher target for those over 80 years of age, and the European guideline suggests a systolic target of 140–150 mmHg in patients over 80 years of age 'provided they are in good physical and mental conditions'.

Initial advice

The treatment of hypertension is directed towards reducing risk rather than treating symptoms. It is imperative, therefore, to explain the significance of high blood pressure at the earliest opportunity. Many patients find difficulty in grasping the concept of blood pressure variability and are often alarmed by the inevitable occasional

Table 17.2.3 Typical observation periods for different grades of hypertension and associated cardiovascular disease, diabetes, and/or target organ damage

Grade of hypertension	Typical observation period
Accelerated (malignant) hypertension (papilloedema and/or fundal haemorrhages and exudates, or with acute cardiovascular complications e.g. aortic dissection)	Immediate treatment—usually requiring acute hospital admission (see Chapter 17.5)
BP ≥220/120 mmHg	Treat immediately—hospital admission not usually required
Grade III hypertension BP >180–219/110–119 mmHg	Confirm by repeated measurements over 1–2 weeks, then treat
Grade II hypertension BP 160–179/100–109 mmHg	In the presence of cardiovascular disease, diabetes, or target organ damage: confirm over 3–4 weeks, then treat No cardiovascular disease, diabetes, or target organ damage: lifestyle measures, re-measure weekly initially, and treat if BP persists at these levels over 4–12 weeks
Grade I hypertension: BP 140–159/90–99 mmHg	Cardiovascular disease, diabetes, or target organ damage: either confirm or refute diagnosis by (a) ABPM) or HBPM, or (b) repeat clinic measurement within weeks, then treat if diagnosis confirmed No clinical cardiovascular disease, diabetes or target organ damage: lifestyle advice and either confirm or refute diagnosis by (a) ABPM or HBPM, or (b) re-measure clinic BP at monthly intervals for 3–6 months. If mild hypertension persists, estimate 10-year cardiovascular diseases risk and treat if this is ≥20% (if <20%, keep under annual review)

ABPM, ambulatory blood pressure measurement; BP, blood pressure; HBPM, home blood pressure measurement.

Modified and updated from Williams B, *et al.* (2004). *BMJ*, **328**, 364–40.

high reading. Discussion of the rationale for evaluation and treatment, together with an explanation of the nature of high blood pressure and its very high prevalence, reassures patients and may improve adherence to treatment. Further comprehensive advice for patients may be obtained from http://www.bpassoc.org.uk.

Lifestyle advice

Blood pressure is strongly influenced by lifestyle factors such as diet and exercise and their consequences such as on body weight. Effective lifestyle modification for patients with grade I hypertension may lower blood pressure as much as a single blood pressure lowering drug, and combinations of two or more lifestyle modifications may be even more effective. Lifestyle interventions may reduce the need for drug therapy for people with mild hypertension, can enhance the antihypertensive effects of blood pressure lowering medication, and can favourably influence overall cardiovascular disease risk.

The most effective lifestyle interventions for reducing blood pressure in clinical trials are modifications to diet to induce weight loss, regular aerobic exercise, and restrictions in alcohol and sodium intake. The expected reductions in blood pressure with these lifestyle manoeuvres are shown in Table 17.2.4, and recommended lifestyle interventions to reduce blood pressure and/or cardiovascular disease risk are shown in Box 17.2.4.

Patients are often enthusiastic to try lifestyle changes rather than take drug therapy. This is a reasonable initial option in patients with grade I hypertension who do not have associated target organ damage or high cardiovascular disease risk. In patients with more severe hypertension or those at high risk, lifestyle measures should be recommended alongside drug therapy. This is important because these measures may improve the effectiveness of drug therapy and also contribute to a reduction in overall cardiovascular risk. Note, however, that effective implementation of lifestyle measures requires enthusiasm, knowledge, patience, and considerable time spent with patients and other family members. It is best undertaken by well-trained health professionals, e.g. practice or clinic nurses, and should be supported by clear written information.

Weight reduction

Many patients with hypertension are overweight, and weight reduction by calorie restriction is an appropriate recommendation.

Table 17.2.4 Blood pressure reductions associated with lifestyle interventions for patients with hypertension

Intervention	Recommendation	Expected SBP reduction (range)
Weight reduction	Maintain ideal BMI (20–25 kg/m²)	5–10 mmHg per 10 kg weight loss
DASH eating plan	Consume diet rich in fruit, vegetables, low-fat dairy products with reduced content of saturated and total fat	8–14 mmHg
Dietary sodium restriction	Reduce dietary sodium intake to <100 mmol/day (<2.4 g sodium or <6 g sodium chloride)	2–8 mmHg
Physical activity	Engage in regular aerobic physical activity, e.g. brisk walking for at least 30 min most days	4–9 mmHg
Alcohol moderation	Men ≤21 units/week	2–4 mmHg
	Women ≤14 units/week	

BMI, body mass index; DASH, Dietary Approaches to Stop Hypertension; SBP, systolic blood pressure.

> **Box 17.2.4** Lifestyle measures that lower blood pressure and reduce cardiovascular disease risk
>
> **Measures to lower blood pressure**
> - Weight reduction
> - Reduced salt intake
> - Limitation of alcohol consumption
> - Increased physical activity
> - Increased fruit and vegetable consumption
> - Reduced total fat and saturated fat intake
>
> **Measures to reduce cardiovascular disease risk**
> - Cessation of smoking
> - Reduced total fat and saturated fat intake
> - Replacement of saturated fats with monounsaturated fats
> - Increased consumption of oily fish

The blood pressure lowering effect of weight reduction may be enhanced by increased regular aerobic physical exercise, by alcohol moderation in heavy drinkers, and by a reduction in sodium intake. On average, blood pressure may fall by as much as 1 mmHg per kg weight loss, although results vary in studies and the maximum overall effect of combined lifestyle interventions is an average of 10 mmHg fall in SBP. Body mass index (BMI) is frequently used as a measure of overweight, but other measures of obesity—particularly central obesity—are better markers of adverse cardiovascular outcomes in people with hypertension. In this regard, weight reduction also has beneficial effects on associated risk factors such as insulin resistance, risk of developing diabetes, and dyslipidaemia.

Dietary salt reduction

Sodium intake influences blood pressure and all international guidelines recommend dietary sodium restriction. Dietary salt reduction from an average of 10 to 5 g/day (5 g = 1 teaspoon) lowers blood pressure by about 5/2 mmHg, with larger blood pressure falls in elderly people, blacks, and those with higher initial blood pressure levels. About one-third of people will achieve a reduction of 5/5 mmHg or more. These effects are additive to the blood pressure lowering effect of a healthy diet, e.g. the Dietary Approaches to Stop Hypertension (DASH) diet (<http://www.nhlbi.nih.gov/health/public/heart/hbp/dash/>).

Many patients will already be aware of the relationship between salt and blood pressure and will have discontinued adding salt at the table and even when cooking, but few are aware of the large amount of salt in processed foods, such as bread (one slice contains 0.5 g salt), some breakfast cereals, ready-prepared meals, and flavour enhancers such as stock cubes or manufactured sauces. Patients, and those who cook for patients, should be provided with specific written advice, such as that from http://www.bpassoc.org.uk.

Increased fruit and vegetable consumption

Using the DASH diet, which increased vegetable consumption from two to seven portions per day, blood pressure was lowered by around 7/3 mmHg in hypertensive patients. Hypertensive patients should therefore be given clear advice to increase fruit and vegetable intake to at least five portions per day. When this is combined with an increased use of low-fat dairy products and reduction of total and saturated fat, then blood pressure falls averaging 11/6 mmHg are seen. The mechanism whereby fruit and vegetable consumption lowers blood pressure is uncertain, but it may be due to an associated increase in potassium intake, as suggested by some supplementation studies.

Physical activity

Regular physical activity, especially when combined with dietary measures, can be particularly effective at reducing blood pressure (Table 17.2.4). The activity should be regular, aerobic (e.g. brisk walking), and tailored to the individual. For example, three vigorous training sessions per week may be appropriate for fit younger patients, or brisk walking for 20 min/day in older patients. This activity will be expected to reduce SBP and DBP by about 2–3 mmHg, with the combination of exercise and diet reducing both by 5–6 mmHg. Heavy physical exercise should be discouraged in people with severe hypertension or those in whom hypertension is poorly controlled. Exercise can be recommended once drug therapy has been started and blood pressure is better controlled.

In addition to its effects on blood pressure, physical exercise appears to exert a strong protective effect against cardiovascular mortality and is associated with a lower risk of coronary heart disease in men and women. Protection is lost when exercise is discontinued. Any activity appears to be of benefit, but people who are more active appear to gain more protection. A reasonable strategy is regular aerobic exercise (e.g. brisk walking) for at least 30 min, ideally on most days, but at least 3 days per week.

Alcohol intake

An alcohol intake of above 21 units per week is associated with blood pressure elevation, and binge drinking is associated with an increased risk of stroke. Hypertensive patients should be advised to limit their alcohol intake to 21 units per week (men) and 14 units per week (women). On average, structured interventions to reduce alcohol consumption have a small effect on blood pressure, reducing SBP (and possibly DBP) by about 2–3 mmHg. Consumption of smaller amounts of alcohol, up to the recommended limit, may protect against cardiovascular disease and should not be discouraged.

Caffeine consumption

Following caffeine consumption there is a dose-related increase in SBP of 5–15 mmHg and of DBP of 5–10 mmHg that persists for several hours. A systematic review of studies of median duration 8 weeks showed that people drinking an average of five cups of caffeinated coffee a day had blood pressure 2.4 mmHg (systolic) and 1.2 mmHg (diastolic) higher than controls (no coffee, or decaffeinated coffee). There is no good data on the effect of withdrawing or limiting caffeine intake in patients with hypertension.

Sleep and blood pressure

Blood pressure characteristically falls during sleep, and sleep duration impacts on the risk of developing hypertension. The risk of developing hypertension in one survey was increased by about twofold in adults in middle age who sleep 5 h or less each night. This may simply reflect a higher 24 h average blood pressure load and longer duration of sympathetic nervous system activation as a consequence of less time asleep, which in turn would give rise to a higher risk of longer-term cardiovascular structural damage, leading to sustained hypertension. Whatever the mechanism, sleep deprivation should be considered in the assessment of people developing hypertension. Consistent with the association between sleep deprivation and hypertension, high blood pressure is more common in patients with obstructive sleep apnoea. Although this could be explained by the fact that both conditions are commoner in males and in obese individuals, a few studies indicate that continuous positive airways pressure can reduce blood pressure, particularly nocturnal pressures, implying a causal relationship.

Lifestyle strategies to reduce cardiovascular risk in hypertensive patients

Cigarette smoking

Patients with hypertension should be encouraged and given support to stop smoking. Nicotine replacement therapy and other strategies are safe and effective in people with hypertension and double the chance of quitting smoking. Those who fail on their first attempt to quit should be encouraged to continue trying: the chance of success increases with the number of quit attempts. Although smoking is not a major contributor to an elevated blood pressure, it does significantly amplify the cardiovascular risk associated with hypertension. Smoking is a major factor related to the persistent increase in coronary and stroke mortality in men with treated hypertension. Those who stop smoking experience a rapid decline in risk, by as much as 50% after 1 year, but up to 10 years may be needed to reach the risk level of those who have never smoked.

Reduced dietary saturated fat intake

Reducing dietary fat intake can reduce serum cholesterol values, which can reduce the risk of cardiovascular disease. All patients should be advised to keep total dietary intake of fat to less than one-third of their total energy intake, to keep the intake of saturated fats to less than one-third of their total fat intake, and to replace saturated fats by an increased intake of monounsaturated fats. These dietary changes can be very effective, but reduce serum cholesterol by only about 6% on average, in part because of difficulty in sustaining such dietary discipline. A regular intake of fish and other sources of n-3 fatty acids (at least two servings of fish per week) will further improve lipid profiles and has been shown to reduce blood pressure.

Lifestyle modifications that are ineffective at lowering blood pressure

Dietary supplements

The best available evidence does not support the use of calcium, magnesium, or potassium supplementation (i.e. tablets), individually or in combination, to achieve a worthwhile reduction in blood pressure. Inadequate information is available from randomized controlled trials to support the recommendation for garlic, herbal, or other complementary medicines.

Psychological stress reduction

Structured interventions to reduce stress, e.g. stress management programmes, meditation, yoga, cognitive therapies, breathing exercises, biofeedback, and acupuncture have been shown to modestly reduce blood pressure in some but not all studies. However, many of these interventions are time consuming and have been short term, and it is difficult to know whether they would be an effective intervention for adequate blood pressure control over the longer term.

Clinical management

Pharmacological treatments

The treatment of hypertension has been subjected to many large randomized controlled trials that have compared active treatments with placebo, and different treatment strategies with each other. Hypertension has the most impressive evidence base in medicine to guide treatment decisions, and analysis of this has provided important guiding principles with regard to treatment strategies:

◆ Effective blood pressure lowering is overwhelmingly important in reducing the risk of major cardiovascular events in people with hypertension, thus the first priority in treatment is to control blood pressure.

◆ Many patients will require more than one drug to control blood pressure; monotherapy is rarely sufficient.

◆ Although early studies focused primarily on DBP as the treatment target, SBP is invariably more difficult to control and should now be the main focus of treatment.

◆ The blood pressure response to an individual class of blood pressure lowering medication is heterogeneous, hence there is no 'perfect drug' for every patient.

◆ Some trials have indicated that certain comorbidities or target organ damage provide compelling indications for inclusion of specific classes of drug therapy in the treatment regimen.

◆ There is inadequate clinical outcome data for treatment studies of younger patients as most of the studies, especially the more recent ones, have been conducted in patients over the age of 55 years, and typically with a mean age over 65 years.

Blood pressure lowering therapy is effective at reducing the risk of stroke, myocardial infarction, heart failure, chronic renal disease, peripheral vascular disease, and death. It may also be effective at reducing the risk of vascular dementia. On average, lowering blood pressure by 20/10 mmHg will reduce the risk of major cardiovascular events by one-half, with the reduction in stroke risk appearing to follow the predicted reduction in risk based on the epidemiological association between stroke and blood pressure. There appears to be a shortfall in the reduction in risk of ischaemic heart disease with blood pressure lowering when compared to epidemiological predictions, which is best addressed by attention to concomitant risk factors. Importantly, the risk reduction associated with blood pressure lowering appears to be continuous across a wide range of blood pressures, thus the absolute benefit from treatment is greatest in those with the highest absolute cardiovascular disease risk. This provides the rational for advocating the use of complementary strategies to reduce cardiovascular disease risk, e.g. statins and antiplatelet therapy, in those with established vascular disease, target organ damage, or at high calculated cardiovascular disease risk, i.e. a calculated cardiovascular disease risk of 20% or more over 10 years.

The main classes of blood pressure lowering therapies are summarized in this section. The over-riding treatment priority is to control blood pressure, but there is general consensus among international guidelines about indications and contraindications for the use of specific classes of blood pressure lowering therapy in specific clinical situations, and these are detailed in Tables 17.2.5 and 17.2.6. It is important to note that these lists are not comprehensive and

Table 17.2.5 Indications favouring the use of specific classes of blood pressure lowering drugs

Thiazide diuretics	Isolated systolic hypertension (elderly)
	Heart failure
	Hypertension in blacks
ACE inhibitors	Heart failure
	LV dysfunction
	Postmyocardial infarction
	Diabetic nephropathy
	Nondiabetic nephropathy
	LV hypertrophy
	Carotid atherosclerosis
	Proteinuria/microalbuminuria
	Atrial fibrillation
	Metabolic syndrome
Angiotensin receptor blockers	Heart failure
	Post myocardial infarction
	Diabetic nephropathy
	Proteinuria/microalbuminuria
	LV hypertrophy
	Atrial fibrillation
	Metabolic syndrome
	ACEi-induced cough
β-Blockers	Angina pectoris
	Post myocardial infarction
	Heart failure
	Tachyarrhythmias
	Glaucoma
	Pregnancy
Calcium antagonists (dihydropyridines)	Isolated systolic hypertension (elderly)
	Angina pectoris
	LV hypertrophy
	Carotid/coronary atherosclerosis
	Pregnancy
	Hypertension in blacks
Diuretics (antialdosterone)	Heart failure
	Post myocardial infarction
Calcium antagonist (verapamil/diltiazem)	Angina pectoris
	Carotid atherosclerosis
	Supraventricular tachycardia
Loop diuretics	Stage 4 and 5 chronic kidney renal disease
	Heart failure

Table 17.2.6 Compelling and possible contraindications to specific classes of blood pressure lowering therapies

	Compelling	Possible
Thiazide diuretics	Gout	Metabolic syndrome
		Glucose intolerance
		Pregnancy
β-Blockers	Asthma	Peripheral artery disease
	AV block (grade 2 or 3)	Metabolic syndrome
		Glucose intolerance
		Athletes and physically active patients
		Chronic obstructive pulmonary disease
Calcium antagonists (dihydropiridines)		Tachyarrhythmias
		Heart failure
Calcium antagonists (verapamil, diltiazem)	AV block (grade 2 or 3)	
	Heart failure	
ACE inhibitors	Pregnancy	
	Angioneurotic oedema	
	Hyperkalaemia	
	Bilateral renal artery stenosis	
Angiotensin receptor antagonists	Pregnancy	
	Hyperkalaemia	
	Bilateral renal artery stenosis	
Diuretics (antialdosterone)	Renal failure	
	Hyperkalaemia	

ACE, angiotensin converting enzyme; AV, atrioventricular.

Data from Williams, *et al.* BHS Guidelines 2004. *Guidelines for management of hypertension: report of the fourth working party of the British Hypertension Society,* 2004—BHS IV.

hypertension. Commonly used examples include chlortalidone, hydrochlorthiazide, and bendroflumethiazide. TTDs lower blood pressure by a complex series of mechanisms. Urinary loss of sodium resulting from a blockade of renal tubular reabsorption of sodium is integral to the antihypertensive effect. The early changes in salt and water balance are often accompanied by counter-activation of several vasoconstrictor mechanisms, including the renin–angiotensin–aldosterone system, which may transiently raise peripheral vascular resistance and attenuate blood pressure lowering. There is subsequently a gradual reduction in peripheral vascular resistance and a new steady state of reduced total body sodium and blood pressure.

The sustained actions of thiazide/thiazide-like diuretics on the kidney make them preferable to loop diuretics for the control of blood pressure. This is because loop diuretics are shorter acting, and the short-term sodium and water loss is usually compensated for by sodium retention during the latter part of the dosing interval and reduced blood pressure lowering efficacy. There is really no place for loop diuretics in the routine management of essential hypertension, but TTDs become ineffective in patients with a glomerular

are subject to change as new evidence emerges, and the reader is directed towards the information sheets for each specific drug for more detailed prescribing information.

Diuretics
Thiazides
Thiazide-type diuretics (TTDs) were the first major class of drug used to treat hypertension on a large scale and they remain one of the main therapeutic options for the treatment of essential

filtration rate below 30 ml/min and in such patients loop diuretics are often required for effective blood pressure lowering, especially when there is clinical evidence of sodium and water retention.

The main adverse effects of TTDs are hypokalaemia, hyponatraemia (less commonly), impaired glucose tolerance, and small increments in blood levels of LDL cholesterol and triglycerides. TTDs elevate serum uric acid levels and should be avoided in patients predisposed to gout. They should also be avoided in those receiving lithium because of a high risk of lithium toxicity. An incidental advantage of thiazides may be reduction in osteoporosis as a result of calcium retention.

To minimize the adverse effects of TTDs, low doses of these drugs have been recommended by guidelines for the treatment of essential hypertension, and these are well tolerated. On the basis of some small studies it has been assumed that the dose response to TTDs is generally flat (unlike the adverse effect profile), and this has been used to further justify the low-dose strategy for TTDs, but it should be emphasized that some patients do respond to and tolerate higher doses. Moreover, when thiazides are combined with drugs that block the renin–angiotensin system, e.g. ACE inhibition, then the dose response is steeper and higher doses may be used in patients with more resistant hypertension (see below).

Potassium-retaining diuretics

Potassium-retaining diuretics, e.g. spironolactone or amiloride, are effective blood pressure lowering agents that are much less commonly used for the routine treatment of hypertension. They can be very effective in combination with TTDs, and are increasingly used as part of a multidrug strategy for the treatment of resistant hypertension (see below). They are used and effective in large doses in the treatment of primary aldosteronism. They have the advantage over TTDs in not causing hypokalaemia or hyperuricaemia and do not impair glucose tolerance, but spironolactone causes nipple tenderness and gynaecomastia in some patients, which is dose dependent and can limit its use. Moreover, if potassium-sparing diuretics are used in combination with drugs that block the activity of the renin–angiotensin system or in patients with renal impairment, then monitoring of serum potassium is required because of the increased risk of hyperkalaemia.

β-Adrenoceptor blocking drugs (β-blockers)

β-Blockers reduce blood pressure and cardiovascular events in patients with hypertension. Most β-blockers, with the exception of those with strong intrinsic sympathomimetic activity, reduce cardiac output due to their negative chronotropic and inotropic effects. As with diuretics, short-term haemodynamic responses can be offset by counter-activation of vasoconstrictor mechanisms, which may limit initial blood pressure lowering. Longer-term reduction in arterial pressure, which occurs over days, is due to restoration of vascular resistance to pretreatment levels. Partial blockade of renin release from the kidney may contribute to the later haemodynamic response.

β-Blockers differ in their duration of action, their selectivity for β_1-receptors, lipophilicity, and partial agonist activity. Side effects include lethargy, aches in the limbs on exercise, impaired concentration and memory, erectile dysfunction, vivid dreams, and exacerbation of symptoms of peripheral vascular disease and Raynaud's syndrome. They are contraindicated in asthma and can cause adverse metabolic effects, including impaired glucose tolerance and worsening of dyslipidaemia—notably reduced

HDL-cholesterol and raised triglycerides. There is accumulating evidence that β-blockers increase the likelihood of new-onset diabetes, particularly when combined with TTDs. Moreover, recent meta-analyses suggest that there is a shortfall in cardiovascular protection with β-blocker-based treatment for hypertension (especially in stroke reduction) when compared to treatment with other main drug classes. As a consequence, British and American guidelines do not recommend β-blockers as an initial therapy for uncomplicated hypertension, and they should only be used when there is a compelling indication other than blood pressure control, e.g. in patients with hypertension and angina or chronic heart failure. One exception is in younger women of childbearing potential, in whom β-blockers are often very effective at lowering blood pressure, perhaps due to higher renin levels of younger people, and safer than ACE inhibition or angiotensin receptor blockers (ARBs) in those anticipating pregnancy.

Calcium channel blockers

This class of drug has been extensively used in treating hypertension since the 1970s: they are very effective at reducing blood pressure and have an extensive evidence base supporting their use. In addition to their blood pressure lowering properties, they are also effective antianginal agents.

There are two main groups of calcium channel blocker (CCB), the dihydropyridines (e.g. amlodipine, nifedipine) and the nondihydropyridines (e.g. diltiazem, verapamil). The dihydropyridine CCBs act mainly by inducing relaxation of arterial smooth muscle by blocking L-type calcium channels, thereby inducing peripheral vascular relaxation with a fall in vascular resistance and arterial pressure. Nondihydropyridine CCBs also block calcium channels in cardiac muscle and reduce cardiac output. Verapamil has an additional antiarrhythmic action through its effects on the atrioventricular node.

The earlier formulations of some dihydropyridines, such as capsular nifedipine, had a rapid onset of action, unpredictable effects on blood pressure, and were accompanied by reflex sympathetic stimulation and tachycardia. With the availability of longer-acting formulations of dihydropyridine CCBs, these shorter-acting CCBs have no place in the management of hypertension, even (and especially) in the emergency setting (see Chapter 17.5).

Side effects of dihydropyridine CCBs include dose-dependent peripheral oedema, which is not due to fluid retention but results from transudation of fluid from the vascular compartments into the dependent tissues due to precapillary arteriolar dilatation. This oedema does not respond to diuretic therapy but is alleviated by limb elevation, and there is emerging evidence that it may be reduced by coadministration of an ACE inhibitor or ARB because of their effects on venous capacitance. Gum hypertrophy can occur with dihydropyridine CCBs, but is rarely seen with nondihydropyridine CCBs. Nondihydropyridine CCBs cause less peripheral oedema but are negatively inotropic and negatively chronotropic and should therefore be avoided in patients with compromised left ventricular function, and used with caution in combination with β-blockers. Verapamil use is commonly accompanied by constipation.

Blockade of the renin–angiotensin system

The renin–angiotensin system has become a very popular target for drug development to treat hypertension. Inhibition of the renin–angiotensin system is predictably effective at lowering blood pressure by inhibiting the various central and peripheral pressor effects of angiotensin II, and blockade may also lower blood pressure by other mechanisms involving improvements in endothelial function, vagal tone, and baroreceptor function, and via inhibition of the renal tubular reabsorption of sodium. In addition, inhibition of the renin–angiotensin system has been promoted by clinical trial evidence showing reduced morbidity and mortality with these treatments in patients with heart failure, delay in the progression of renal disease, and reduction in cardiovascular events in patients at high cardiovascular risk.

ACE inhibitors

The ACE inhibitors, which block the conversion of angiotensin I to angiotensin II, were the first effective strategy to inhibit the renin–angiotensin system and have been used to treat hypertension since the late 1970s. The resulting reduction in levels of angiotensin II leads to vasodilatation and a fall in blood pressure. Angiotensin II has many additional actions that are potentially harmful to the cardiovascular system and have been implicated in the pathogenesis of structural changes in the heart, blood vessels, and kidneys in hypertension.

Sharp falls in blood pressure following the introduction of ACE inhibitors may occur when the renin–angiotensin system is activated, e.g. in patients who are dehydrated, in heart failure, or have accelerated hypertension. This is rarely a problem when therapy is initiated in uncomplicated hypertensive patients. Side effects of ACE inhibitors include the development of a persistent dry cough in about 20% of users. This is more common in women and in people from Asia, and only disappears after discontinuation of the drug. Another rare but important complication is angio-oedema, which occurs in around 1% but is much more common in the black population (c.4%). ACE inhibitors should be avoided in women of childbearing potential because of the danger of fetal renal malformation. They should not be used in patients with bilateral renal artery disease because they may precipitate deterioration in renal function and renal failure. It should be routine practice to check the serum creatinine 10–14 days after initiation of ACE inhibition, and to stop the drug if this has risen by more than 25%: lesser elevations can be tolerated. Particularly careful monitoring of renal function and serum potassium is required in patients with more advanced renal impairment of any cause because of the risk of hyperkalaemia.

Angiotensin receptor blockers (ARBs)

In the 1990s, the ARBs, which are highly selective inhibitors of the angiotensin II type 1 receptor (AT-1), emerged as an alternative to ACE inhibition. In general they are as effective as ACE inhibitors at reducing blood pressure, but appear to have a longer duration of action, and in common with ACE inhibitors they inhibit the actions of angiotensin II on the cardiovascular system and kidney. They are very well tolerated by patients, with a placebo-like adverse effect profile. Cough and angio-oedema are much less likely to occur than with ACE inhibitors and most guidelines recommend switching patients to an ARB when an ACE-induced cough occurs. Cautions and contraindications are similar to those outlined for ACE inhibitors.

Direct renin inhibition

A third strategy to inhibit the renin–angiotensin system for the treatment of hypertension is direct renin inhibition, the first non-peptide, orally active, direct renin inhibitor being aliskiren. This has high specificity for renin and is a potent renin inhibitor with a long half-life (c.24 h). It inhibits the rate-limiting step in angiotensin production, notably the renin-dependent conversion of angiotensinogen to angiotensin I, and in initial studies appeared to have similar blood pressure lowering efficacy to other means of inhibiting the renin system, i.e. ACE inhibition or ARBs, but with less side effects than ACE inhibition. However, the combination of aliskiren with ACE inhibitor or ARBs was found to have serious adverse cardiovascular and renal outcomes in a large clinical trial (ALTITUDE) that was stopped following interim data analysis, as a result of which some regulatory authorities have stated that the combination of these drugs is contraindicated (in patients with diabetes) or not recommended (in other patients), and recommended that aliskiren should not be used in those with eGFR <30 ml/min (CKD4).

α-Adrenergic blocking drugs

The original members of this class (e.g. prazosin) were short acting drugs that blocked the activation of α_1 adrenoceptors in the vasculature, leading to vasodilatation. The dosages that were initially recommended were too high, and postural hypotension and syncope proved serious problems that retarded the acceptance of this class of drugs, although the use of lower doses and the development of longer-acting agents (e.g. doxazosin) has largely overcome this problem. Blockade of sphincteric receptors improves symptoms in patients with benign prostatic hypertrophy, and occasionally these same sphincteric effects can worsen symptoms of stress incontinence in women. Uniquely among antihypertensive drugs, the α_1-antagonists produce modest favourable changes in plasma lipids, with a reduction in total and LDL cholesterol and triglycerides, and an increase in high-density lipoprotein (HDL) cholesterol.

Centrally acting sympatholytic drugs

Some of the earliest drugs developed to treat hypertension targeted the activation of the sympathetic nervous system at various levels, including the cardiovascular regulatory nuclei in the brainstem, the peripheral autonomic ganglia, and the post ganglionic sympathetic neuron. With one or two exceptions, few of these agents have any residual role to play in the modern treatment of hypertension because side effects are common, often unpleasant, and potentially harmful.

Methyldopa

Methyldopa reduces sympathetic outflow from the brainstem. It was originally developed in the late 1950s and for many years it was one of the mainstays of antihypertensive therapy. However, it frequently causes sedation, impaired psychomotor performance, dry mouth, and erectile dysfunction. This unfavourable impact upon quality of life led to it being replaced by more effective drugs, although it is still used extensively in the management of hypertension of pregnancy, which is now its main indication.

Clonidine

Clonidine is now rarely used because of its short duration of action and risk of a withdrawal syndrome after discontinuing the drug: sudden discontinuation results in a rebound rise in catecholamines with features that may resemble phaeochromocytoma, such as severe hypertension, tachycardia, and sweating. This is exacerbated when patients are also receiving nonselective β-blockers such as propranolol. The syndrome is treated by readministering the drug and then gradually discontinuing it, or the intravenous infusion of labetalol in an emergency.

Moxonidine

Moxonidine is a newer centrally acting agent that is an imidazoline receptor agonist, acting to reduce sympathetic outflow and blood pressure. It has a lower incidence of side effects and is better tolerated than other centrally acting agents.

Direct vasodilators

Hydralazine

Hydralazine was previously extensively used as part of a stepped care regimen. However, its main disadvantages were sympathetic activation and the development of a lupus-like syndrome, particularly in patients with the slow acetylator genotype, which together with the need for multiple daily dosage have resulted in its replacement by other agents, except for occasional use in severe hypertension and hypertension associated with pregnancy. No end-point trials have been carried out.

Minoxidil

Minoxidil is a very potent vasodilator. Its use is confined to specialist centres for the treatment of severe and resistant hypertension because of its side effects, which include stimulation of body hair growth, tachycardia, and severe fluid retention. For this reason, combination with a potent loop diuretic and a β-blocker is almost always necessary.

Pharmacological treatment strategies

Initial drug therapy

After a suitable period of observation and after assessment of concomitant risk factors, comorbid disease and overall cardiovascular disease risk, a decision may be reached to treat the patient with drug therapy. However, even when this is contemplated it is important to continue to emphasize the importance of lifestyle changes to reduce cardiovascular risk and enhance the efficiency of blood pressure lowering medications, and it is also important to view the patient's blood pressure in the context of their overall cardiovascular risk burden and decide whether other therapies such as statins and antiplatelet therapy might also be appropriate.

Once a decision has been made to initiate drug therapy, it is usual to commence treatment with a single drug. Monotherapy will on average reduce systolic pressure by 7 to 13 mmHg and diastolic pressure by 4 to 8 mmHg. This will give some indication as to whether monotherapy is likely to be effective at achieving the recommended blood pressure goal, but there is marked heterogeneity in response among individuals to particular drugs. Treatment should normally commence with a low dose of the drug selected. If an adequate response is not obtained, the dose of the initial drug can be increased. However, if there has not been much response to the starting dose and the patient's blood pressure remains well short of the target blood pressure, then a more appropriate action would be to add a second drug, either separately or as a combination tablet, mindful of the fact that most people with hypertension require two or more drugs to adequately control their blood pressure. Alternatively, if the initial drug produced a weak response, or none at all, and the patient could conceivably get to their blood pressure goal on monotherapy, then the first drug could be discontinued and replaced with another class of antihypertensive agent.

Initial therapy with a two-drug combination

The heterogeneity of blood pressure responses to different classes of blood pressure lowering drugs and the likelihood that most people will be uncontrolled by monotherapy, has led to the suggestion that more people should be initiated on treatment with low-dose combination therapy. Low-dose two-drug combination therapy

has been recommended in European and American hypertension guidelines for the treatment of patients whose blood pressure is greater than 20/10 mmHg above their goal blood pressure and therefore unlikely to achieve their goal blood pressure with monotherapy (Figs. 17.2.5 and 17.2.6). The concept of initial therapy with a two-drug combination has in part been driven by concern that the up-titration of treatment in people at high risk may be too slow and leave them at risk for too long.

Choice of initial therapy

There is wide variation in the international guidelines with regard to the preferred initial therapy for essential hypertension. In the United States of America, the Joint National Committee 8 (JNC8) guideline recommends initial drug treatment with an ACE inhibitor, ARB, CCB, or TTD in nonblack hypertensive patients, with a CCB or TTD preferred in black patients (Fig. 17.2.6).

The recent European guideline suggests that all five main classes of blood pressure lowering drugs (ACE inhibitors, ARBs, β-blockers, CCBs, and diuretics) are suitable as initial therapy, and that choice would in part reflect physician preference and the concomitant conditions and specific indications and contraindications for different drug classes in an individual patient (Table 17.2.6).

The British Hypertension Society/NICE guideline adopts a different approach, suggesting that the most appropriate initial blood pressure lowering agent (1) for people 55 years or older, and for black people of African or Caribbean family origin of any age, is a CCB, with a thiazide-like diuretic preferred if a CCB is not suitable; and (b) for people aged under 55 years an ACE inhibitor or a low-cost ARB is preferred initial therapy (Fig. 17.2.7). The rationale for this recommendation was founded on the observation that plasma renin levels fall as people age and are lower in blacks at any age. Therefore drugs that target the renin system are more likely to be more effective initial therapy in higher-renin younger patients, whereas the converse in true with ageing. The argument against the use of β-blockers as a preferred initial therapy (especially for older patients), unless there are compelling other indications (Table 17.2.6), is because they appear less effective at reducing the risk of stroke than the alternatives, are associated with an increased risk of developing diabetes, and are the least cost-effective treatment option for essential hypertension.

Combination therapy for controlling blood pressure

All guidelines recognize that combinations of blood pressure lowering drugs are often required to achieve recommended blood pressure goals. The European guidelines provide a diagram to illustrate suitable combinations of treatment (Fig. 17.2.5). The American JNC8 guidelines (Fig. 17.2.6) recommend selecting any two of the medications recommended as suitable for the particular patient as initial therapy. Only the British guideline (Fig. 17.2.7) provides explicit guidance on preferred combinations of treatment:

* step 2—a CCB (C) combined with either an ACE inhibitor or ARB (A)

* step 3—add a thiazide-like diuretic (D)

* step 4—add higher-dose thiazide-like diuretic, spironolactone, an α-blocker or a β-blocker.

The preference for the combination of A + C at step 2 is based on data, e.g. the ACCOMPLISH study, suggesting that A + C may be more effective than A + D at preventing cardiovascular events, despite similarities in blood pressure control.

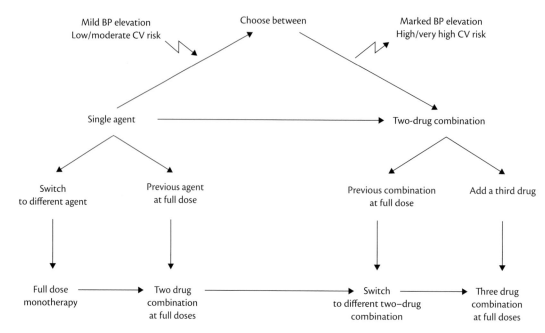

BP = blood pressure; CV = cardiovascular.

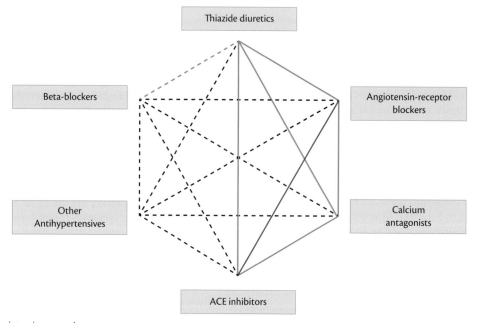

ACE - angiotensin-converting enzyme.

Fig. 17.2.5 European Society of Hypertension/European Society of Cardiology guideline recommendations: (a) Monotherapy vs combination treatment strategies to treat hypertension. Moving from a less intensive to more intensive treatment should be done whenever the blood pressure target is not achieved. (b) Possible combinations of classes of antihypertensive drugs. Green continuous lines, preferred combinations; green dashed line, useful combination (with some limitations); black dashed lines, possible but less well tested combinations; red continuous line, not recommended. Only dihydropyridine calcium channel blockers should normally be combined with a β-blocker.

From Mancia G, et al. (2013). 2013 ESH/ESC guidelines for the management of arterial hypertension: the task force for the management of arterial hypertension of the European Society of Hypertension (ESH) and of the European Society of Cardiology (ESC). *Eur Heart J*, **34**, 2159–219.

Resistant hypertension

Drug-resistant hypertension can be defined as blood pressure that is not controlled despite treatment with an appropriate combination of three drug therapies (e.g. A + C + D—see Fig. 17.2.7) prescribed at their maximum recommended and tolerated doses. In the absence of evidence of target organ damage, white coat hypertension should be excluded by 24 h ambulatory monitoring if this has not already been done. Other causes for resistant hypertension include (1) secondary hypertension (e.g. renovascular or endocrine); (2) ingestion of drugs that may raise blood pressure (e.g. nonsteroidal anti-inflammatory agents); (3) heavy alcohol intake; (4) sleep apnoea; (5) sodium and fluid retention as a result

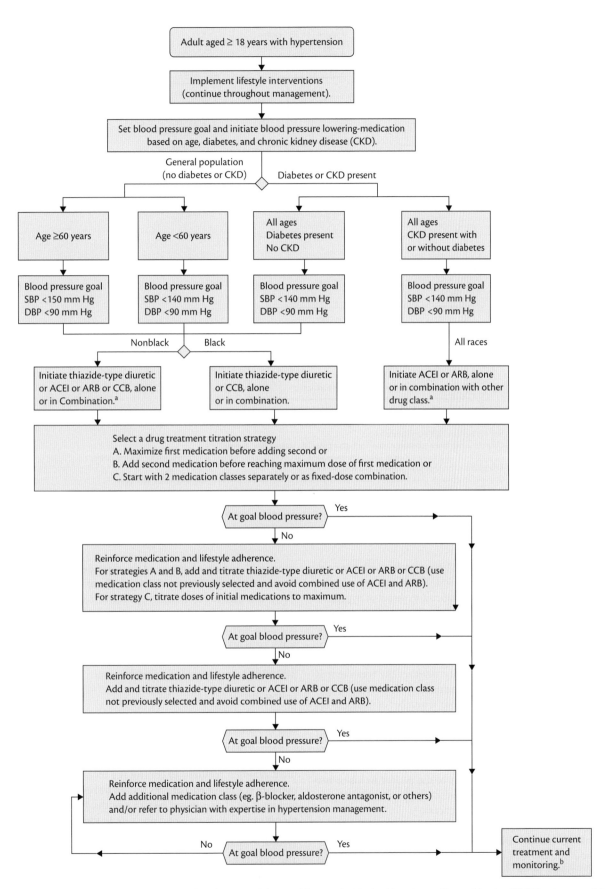

Fig. 17.2.6 JNC8 hypertension guideline management algorithm. Note: (a) ACE inhibitor and ARBs should not be used in combination; (b) if blood pressure fails to be maintained at goal, re-enter the algorithm where appropriate based on the current individual therapeutic plan.

From James PA, *et al*. (2014). 2014 Evidence-based guidelines for the management of high blood pressure in adults. Report from the panel members appointed to the Eighth Joint National Committee (JNC8). *JAMA*, **311**, 507–520.)

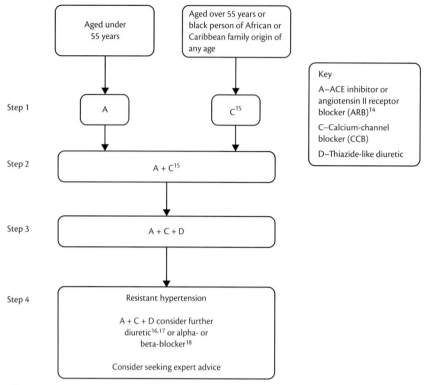

Fig. 17.2.7 British Hypertension Society/NICE treatment algorithm for the treatment of essential hypertension.
From National Institute for Health and Care Excellence (2011) CG 127 *Hypertension: management of hypertension in adults in primary care.* Available from <www.nice.org.uk/CG127>.

of inadequate diuretic therapy; and (6) poor patient adherence to treatment.

Poor adherence to therapy is often difficult to detect in hypertensive patients and can lead to expensive investigations for secondary causes. One way of detecting effectiveness of treatment is to use ABPM to monitor blood pressure after directly observed consumption of medication. Although this may not resolve the problem of adherence to treatment, it will identify whether the treatment is effective if adhered to, thus avoiding the need for further investigations. Where adherence is obviously poor, a number of manoeuvres can help to improve it. The treatment should be made as simple as possible, using once-daily drugs and combination tablets, and a carer needs to be involved in administering medication to those who are confused. Whenever possible, effective communication with full information and involvement of the patient in his or her treatment is essential. Nurses, pharmacists, and other health professionals can play a vital role in this process.

Most patients with truly drug-resistant hypertension (i.e. those who are taking their medications as prescribed) are likely to be retaining sodium and will respond to further diuretic therapy. A suppressed plasma renin despite treatment with A + C + D would be indicative of sodium retention because these treatments would be expected to elevate plasma renin, hence the preferred initial approach to treatment in this situation is further diuretic therapy,

either with increased dosage of the thiazide diuretic, or using low-dose spironolactone (e.g. 25 mg/day), or amiloride (10–20 mg/day), with careful monitoring of electrolytes. A recent randomized cross-over trial found the addition of spironolactone to be more effective than that of bisoprolol or doxazosin in this context. For some patients with very severe drug-resistant hypertension it may be necessary to use a combination of monoxidil, loop diuretic, and β-blocker to improve blood pressure control.

Follow-up

It is essential that patients are monitored regularly and it is important that this message is conveyed to the patient. In the early stages of treatment the frequency of monitoring will be determined by the response to therapy, comorbidities, and the complexity of the treatment regimen required to control the blood pressure. Once blood pressure is controlled, patients should be reviewed at least annually, and most will be reviewed every 6 months. Patients are increasingly monitoring their own blood pressure in the intervening period.

Withdrawal of therapy

The vast majority of patients with hypertension require lifelong therapy. Some with grade I hypertension who make substantial adjustments to their lifestyle may obtain sufficient fall in their blood pressure to warrant withdrawal of monotherapy. However, patients with target organ damage or those at high cardiovascular disease risk should not usually have their therapy withdrawn, unless there is a compelling clinical reason to do so. It is also important to note that in patients with previously severe hypertension that has subsequently been well controlled, treatment withdrawal may not always result in an immediate increase in blood pressure. This can sometimes convey the false impression that treatment may no longer be required because blood pressure can sometimes take many months to progressively rise back to dangerously high pretreatment values. Thus, any patient who discontinues therapy must remain under review with regular monitoring of their blood pressure, and all but a very few will require treatment again.

Other issues

Indications for specialist referral

There are circumstances when referral to a specialist centre is indicated for the management of hypertension. These include uncertainty about the decision to treat, investigations to exclude secondary hypertension, severe and complicated hypertension, and resistant hypertension, among others as detailed in Box 17.2.5.

Medication to reduce cardiovascular risk

Blood pressure should not be treated in isolation and should be considered as part of a comprehensive strategy to reduce cardiovascular disease risk. In this regard, patients at high risk, i.e. those with established cardiovascular disease, target organ damage, and/or diabetes, or those with a calculated cardiovascular disease risk which is elevated (e.g. ≥20% over 10 years), should be offered additional interventions to reduce risk. These include reinforcement of lifestyle advice, especially smoking cessation, and treatment with statin therapy to further reduce their risk of stroke and coronary disease. The routine use of statins to reduce total cholesterol values by 1 mmol/litre has been associated with a reduction in the risk of ischaemic heart disease events by about one-third and stroke by about one-fifth, over and above the benefit already accrued from blood pressure lowering. Moreover, the relative risk reduction associated with statin therapy in higher-risk hypertensive patients is not dependent on a high baseline cholesterol value.

Once blood pressure has been controlled, higher-risk hypertensive patients should also be considered for treatment with low-dose aspirin (75 mg/day). This has been shown to reduce the incidence of myocardial infarction in higher-risk patients over 50 years old and should be offered routinely to patients who come into this category and who do not have contraindications. In view of the increased incidence of haemorrhage, it is not indicated in lower-risk hypertensive patients.

Intercurrent illness

Patients who develop intercurrent illness that is likely to lead to volume depletion (e.g. diarrhoea, vomiting, high fever) should be told to stop taking their antihypertensive medications (particularly diuretics, ACEi and ARBs) until they are able to eat and drink normally. This is very important if they develop postural dizziness, which is a marker of significant intravascular volume depletion in this clinical context.

Other treatments for hypertension
Renal denervation

Initial uncontrolled and unblinded studies reported impressive reduction in blood pressure in patients with resistant hypertension, but a subsequent blinded randomized trial (SIMPLICITY HTN-3) failed to show benefit. A total of 531 patients were randomized in a 2:1 (active:sham) ratio: the mean reduction in SBP at 6 months in the denervation group was 14 mmHg, compared with 12 mmHg in the controls. Following these findings a larger ongoing trial (SIMPLICITY HTN-4) was stopped. This treatment should not be offered to patients with hypertension in routine clinical practice.

Electrical stimulation of carotid sinus baroreceptors

Non-randomized studies have suggested that baroreflex activation therapy, whereby an implantable device is used to stimulate the carotid sinus baroreflex system, can significantly reduce blood pressure in patients with resistant hypertension. These studies were followed by the Rheos Pivotal Trial in which 265 patients had a device implanted, and were randomized 1 month after implantation to receive baroreflex activation therapy immediately, or to have device activation delayed for 6 months. At 6 months, 42% of those whose device had been activated at 1 month had achieved SBP below 140 mmHg, compared to 24% of those whose device had not been switched on; by 12 months over 50% of both groups had achieved this blood pressure target. Follow-up over 22–53 months suggested that the effect on blood pressure was maintained. However, the place of baroreflex activation therapy in the management of hypertension is not yet clear, and it should only be offered in the context of clinical trials.

Box 17.2.5 Recommended and possible indications for specialist referral for patients with hypertension

- ◆ Urgent treatment needed:
  - • Accelerated hypertension (severe hypertension with grade III–IV retinopathy)
  - • Particularly severe hypertension (>220/120 mmHg)
  - • Impending complications (e.g. TIA, left ventricular failure)
- ◆ Possible underlying cause:
  - • Any clue in history or examination of a secondary cause, e.g. hypokalaemia with increased or high-normal plasma sodium (Conn's syndrome)
  - • Elevated serum creatinine
  - • Proteinuria or haematuria
  - • Sudden-onset or worsening of hypertension
  - • Resistance to multidrug regimen, i.e. ≥3 drugs
  - • Young age (any hypertension <20 years; needing treatment <30 years)
- ◆ Therapeutic problems:
  - • Multiple drug intolerance
  - • Multiple drug contraindications
  - • Persistent non-adherence or non-compliance
- ◆ Special situations:
  - • Unusual blood pressure variability
  - • Possible white coat hypertension
  - • Hypertension in pregnancy

Hypertension in specific groups of patients

People of black African origin

Hypertension is more prevalent in blacks, is associated with more target organ damage, and consequently carries a worse prognosis, with a particularly high risk of stroke. Black patients as a group tend to respond better to diuretics, CCBs, and dietary salt restriction than white patients. ACE inhibitors, ARBs, and β-blockers are generally less effective as initial therapy, but become more effective when combined with diuretics and/or CCBs.

Older people

Most people with hypertension are elderly. If a blood pressure of 140/90 mmHg or more is used to define hypertension, then over 70% of people over the age of 60 years will be hypertensive, with most of these having isolated systolic hypertension. Surveys suggest that doctors consistently underestimate the risks and undertreat hypertension in older people, which is somewhat paradoxical in that elderly people have much higher absolute risk than younger people with hypertension and therefore much to gain from blood pressure lowering. There are, however, some important considerations when treating older people:

- The arterial wall stiffening that gives rise to systolic hypertension and increased pulse pressure (isolated systolic hypertension) is also associated with impaired baroreflex sensitivity, with increased risk of orthostatic hypotension, hence it is important to record lying and standing blood pressure in elderly patients.

- eGFR declines with age and renal conservation of sodium and fluid in the face of depletion is impaired, thus elderly patients are more prone to dehydration as a result of diuretic therapy.

- Clearance of drugs and their active metabolites is decreased as a result of declining hepatic and renal function.

- Cardiac function and reserve are often reduced, such that patients are much more likely to develop cardiac failure. This explains why end-point trials of hypertension treatment have consistently shown reductions in morbidity and mortality from cardiac failure.

- Comorbidity is much more common.

- Communication and adherence with therapy may be more difficult with decline in cognitive function. Some evidence from clinical trials suggests that this decline may be retarded by antihypertensive treatment.

Despite these considerations, elderly people tolerate blood pressure lowering medications well, and the benefits of blood pressure reduction are impressive with regard to reductions in morbidity and mortality due to stroke, ischaemic heart disease, and heart failure. As a general rule, drug regimens should be as simple as possible and dosages increased more gradually, the greatest danger resulting from lowering pressure too much and too rapidly. Until recently there was uncertainty about the risks and benefits of treating hypertension in very elderly people (>80 years of age), but studies in this age group confirm that treatment can be well tolerated and associated with impressive reductions in the risk of stroke, heart failure, and mortality. However, it must be recognized that highly selected (very fit) elderly patients are recruited into trials, and physicians working in medical admission units will be all too familiar with the scenario of the elderly patient, taking a plethora of antihypertensives, who is admitted after a collapse. Biological rather than chronological age should be the deciding factor in initiating antihypertensive treatment, but there is never any substitute for clinical common sense—the elderly man with mild cognitive impairment, prone to falls, and with occasional dizziness on standing up, is not likely to be well served by the doctor who advocates medication to reduce marginally elevated blood pressure.

Children

Although secondary hypertension is more common in children than in adults, no specific cause is found for hypertension in most adolescents. The criteria for drug treatment, however, have to be modified because of the lower normal blood pressure range. The JNC guidelines recommend that blood pressures above the 95th percentile—taking into account age, height, and sex—should be considered elevated. In principle, treatment regimens are the same as those recommended for adults, with appropriate dose adjustment.

Further reading

Blood pressure measurement

Agabiti-Rosei E, *et al.* (2007). Central blood pressure measurements and antihypertensive therapy: A consensus document. *Hypertension,* **50**, 1–7.

European Society of Hypertension (2008). Guidelines for blood pressure monitoring at home: a summary report of the Second International Consensus Conference on Home Blood Pressure Monitoring. *J Hypertens,* **26**, 1505–26.

Kikuya M, *et al.* (2007). Diagnostic thresholds for ambulatory blood pressure monitoring based on 10-year cardiovascular risk. *Circulation,* **115**, 2145–52.

O'Brien E, *et al.* (2003). European Society of Hypertension recommendations for conventional, ambulatory and home blood pressure measurement. *J Hypertens,* **21**, 821–48.

Pickering TG, *et al.* (2008). Call to action on use and reimbursement for home blood pressure monitoring: a joint scientific statement from the American Heart Association, American Society of Hypertension, and Preventive Cardiovascular Nurses Association. *Hypertension,* **52**, 10–29.

Verdecchia P, *et al.* (2002). Properly defining white coat hypertension. *Eur Heart J,* **23**, 106–9.

Lifestyle interventions

Appel LJ, *et al.* (1997). A clinical trial of the effects of dietary patterns on blood pressure. *N Engl J Med,* **336**, 1117–24.

Beilin LJ, Puddey IB (2006). Alcohol and hypertension—an update. *Hypertension,* **47**, 1035–8.

Cook NR, *et al.* (2007). Long term effects of dietary sodium reduction on cardiovascular disease outcomes: observational follow-up of trials of hypertension prevention. *BMJ,* **334**, 885–92.

Dickinson HO, *et al.* (2006). Lifestyle interventions to reduce raised blood pressure: a systematic review of randomized controlled trials. *J Hypertens,* **24**, 215–33.

Gangwisch JE, *et al.* (2006). Short sleep duration as a risk factor for hypertension: analyses of the First National Health and Nutrition Examination Survey. *Hypertension,* **47**, 833–9.

He FJ, MacGregor GA (2006). Importance of salt in determining blood pressure in children meta-analysis of controlled trials. *Hypertension,* **48**, 861–9.

Clinical trials and pharmacological treatment

Blood Pressure Lowering Treatment Trialists' Collaboration (2003). Effects of different blood-pressure lowering regimens on major cardiovascular events: results of prospectively-designed overviews of randomised trials. *Lancet,* **362**, 1527–45.

Hanon O, *et al.* (2003). Effect of antihypertensive treatment on cognitive functions. *J Hypertens*, **24**, 2101–7.

Jamerson K, Weber MA, Bakris GL, *et al.* (2008). Benazepril plus amlodipine or hydrochlorothiazide for hypertension in high-risk patients. *N Engl J Med*, **359**, 2417–28.

Julius S, *et al.* (2006). for the Trial of Preventing Hypertension (TROPHY) Study Investigators. Feasibility of treating prehypertension with an angiotensin-receptor blocker. *N Engl J Med*, **354**, 1685–97.

Lawes CM, *et al.* (2004). Blood pressure and stroke: An overview of published trials. *Stroke*, **35**, 776–85.

Lindholm LH, Carlberg B, Samuelsson O (2005). Should β blockers remain first choice in the treatment of primary hypertension? A meta-analysis. *Lancet*, **366**, 1545–53.

Mancia G, Grassi G (2002). Systolic and diastolic blood pressure control in antihypertensive drug trials. *J Hypertens*, **20**, 1461–4.

Staessen JA, *et al.* (2003). Cardiovascular prevention and blood pressure reduction: a quantitative overview updated until 1st March 2003. *J Hypertens*, **21**, 1055–76.

Williams B (2004). Protection against stroke and dementia: an update on the latest clinical trial evidence. *Curr Hypertens Rep*, **6**, 307–13.

Williams B (2007). Beta-blockers and the treatment of hypertension. *J Hypertens*, **25**, 1351–3.

Williams B (2007). Hypertension in the young—preventing the evolution of disease versus prevention of clinical events. *J Am Coll Cardiol*, **50**, 840–2.

Williams B, *et al.* (2015). Spironolactone versus placebo, bisoprolol, and doxazosin to determine the optimal treatment for drug-resistant hypertension (PATHWAY-2): a randomised, double-blind, crossover trial. Lancet Published Online September 21, 2015 <http://dx.doi.org/10.1016/ S0140-6736(15)00257-3>.

Zhang H, Thijs L, Staessen JA (2006). Blood pressure lowering for primary and secondary prevention of stroke. *Hypertension*, **48**, 187–95.

Other treatments for hypertension

Bhatt DL, *et al.* (2014). A controlled trial of renal denervation for resistant hypertension. *N Engl J Med,* **370**, 1393–1401.

Bisognano JD, *et al.* (2011). Baroreflex activation therapy lowers blood pressure in patients with resistant hypertension: results from the double-blinded, randomized, placebo-controlled Rheos Pivotal Trial. *J Am Coll Cardiol,* **58,** 765–773.

Gassler JP, Bisognano JD (2014). Baroreflex activation therapy in hypertension. *J Hum Hypertens,* **28,** 469–474.

Other therapies to reduce cardiovascular risk in hypertensive patients

Emberson J, *et al.* (2004). Evaluating the impact of population and high-risk strategies for the primary prevention of CVD. *Eur Heart J,* **25,** 484–91.

Gaziano TA, Opie LH, Weinstein MC (2006). Cardiovascular disease prevention with a multidrug regimen in the developing world: a cost-effectiveness analysis. *Lancet*, **368**, 679–86.

Heart Protection Study Collaborative Group (2002). MRC/BHF Heart Protection Study of antioxidant vitamin supplementation in 20 536 high-risk individuals: a randomised placebo-controlled trial. *Lancet*, **360**, 23–33.

Patrono C, *et al.* (2005). Low-dose aspirin for the prevention of athero-thrombosis. *N Engl J Med*, **353**, 2373–83.

Sever PS, *et al.* (2003). Prevention of coronary and stroke events with atorvastatin in hypertensive patients who have average or lower-then-average cholesterol concentrations, in the Anglo Scandinavian Cardiac Outcomes Trial-Lipid Lowering Arm (ASCOT-LLA): A multicentre randomised controlled trial. *Lancet*, **361**, 1149–58.

Wald NJ, Law MR (2003). A strategy to reduce cardiovascular disease by more than 80%. *BMJ*, **326**, 1419–23.

Treatment guidelines

Adams, Jr, HP, *et al.* (2007). Guidelines for the early management of adults with ischemic stroke. *Circulation*, **115**, e478–534.

Broderick J, *et al.* (2007). Guidelines for the management of spontaneous intracerebral hemorrhage in adults: update. *Stroke*, **38**, 2001–2023.

Chobanian AV, *et al.* (2003). The seventh report of the Joint National Committee on Prevention, Detection, Evaluation and Treatment of High Blood Pressure: the JNC VII Report. *JAMA*, **289**, 2560–72.

Colhoun DA, *et al.* (2008). Resistant hypertension: Diagnosis evaluation and treatment. A scientific statement from the American heart association professional education committee of the council for high blood pressure research. *Hypertension*, **117**, e510–26.

Conroy RM, *et al.* (2003). Estimation of ten-year risk of fatal cardiovascular disease in Europe: the SCORE project. *Eur Heart J*, **24**, 987–1003.

Douglas JG, *et al.* (2003). The Hypertension in African Americans Working Group. Management of high blood pressure in African Americans. *Arch Intern Med*, **163**, 525–41.

James PA, *et al.* (2014). 2014 Evidence-Based guidelines for the management of high blood pressure in adults. Report from the panel members appointed to the Eighth Joint National Committee (JNC8). *JAMA,* **311,** 507–520.

Higgens B, *et al.* (2007). Pharmacological management of hypertension. *Clin Med*, 7, 612–16. [Key features of the UK BHS/NICE hypertension guideline update in 2006, with link to the full guideline resource: http://www.nice.org.uk/CG034guidance.]

Mancia G, *et al.* (2013). 2013 ESH/ESC guidelines for the management of arterial hypertension: the task force for the management of arterial hypertension of the European Society of Hypertension (ESH) and of the European Society of Cardiology (ESC). *Eur Heart J*, **34**, 2159–2219.

Mendis S, *et al.* (2007). World Health Organization (WHO) and International Society of Hypertension (ISH) risk prediction charts: assessment of cardiovascular risk for prevention and control of cardiovascular disease in low and middle-income countries. *J Hypertens*, **25**, 1578–82.

National Clinical Guideline Centre (2011). *Hypertension—the clinical management of primary hypertension in adults*. Clinical Guideline 127. <http://www.nice.org.uk/guidance/cg127>.

Task Force for the Management of Arterial Hypertension of the European Society of Hypertension (ESH) and of the European Society of Cardiology (ESC). (2007). Guidelines for the management of arterial hypertension. *J Hypertens*, **25**, 1105–87.

Williams B (2006). Evolution of hypertensive disease: a revolution in guidelines. *Lancet*, **368**, 6–8.

Williams B (2009). Resistant hypertension. *Lancet*, **374**, 1396–1398.

CHAPTER 17.3

Secondary hypertension

Morris J. Brown and Fraz A. Mir

Essentials

The term 'secondary hypertension' is used to describe patients whose blood pressure is elevated by a single, identifiable cause, with an important subdivision being into reversible and irreversible causes: clinically, it is important to exclude the former, but not necessarily to find the latter.

In the first two decades of life, the prevalence of secondary hypertension is greater than that of essential hypertension; thereafter, a patient is much more likely to have essential hypertension, but investigations for secondary hypertension should still be assiduous in the twenties and thirties because the alternative entails so many years of tablet-taking.

All patients with hypertension should have a minimum set of investigations (see Chapter 17.2). Common indications for further investigations are (1) any evidence of an underlying cause on history or examination; (2) proteinuria, haematuria, or elevated serum creatinine (eGFR<30; CKD 4/5); (3) hypokalaemia, even if caused by diuretics; (4) accelerated (malignant) hypertension; (5) documented recent onset or recent worsening of hypertension; (6) resistant hypertension (not controlled with three antihypertensive drugs); (7) young age—any hypertension at less than 20 years; any hypertension needing treatment at less than 35 years.

The minimum screen in younger patients should include serum electrolytes, plasma bicarbonate, renin, and metanephrines (or catecholamines) to exclude phaeochromocytoma; 24-h urinary sodium excretion should be measured either in all patients, or in those with abnormal renin levels.

Primary hyperaldosteronism (Conn's syndrome)

Recent studies suggest that aldosterone-producing adrenal adenomas are the single commonest known cause of hypertension. Primary hyperaldosteronism causes increased sodium retention through the epithelial sodium channel (ENaC) in the distal tubule and cortical collecting duct, which leads to hypertension. It can be caused by (1) Conn's adenoma—a small (0.5–3.5 cm) benign tumour of the adrenal gland; (2) bilateral adrenal hyperplasia—where there are macro- or micronodules in the adrenal cortex; (3) the very rare condition of glucocorticoid-remediable aldosteronism (see Chapter 17.4).

Diagnosis— this usually consists of three confirmatory features: suggestive clinical biochemistry; radiological imaging showing an adenoma; lateralization on selective adrenal sampling. A good blood pressure response to aldosterone antagonism with spironolactone can provide further reassurance but is not an essential, or always present, part of the diagnosis. The classic clinical picture is hypertension with plasma electrolytes showing low K^+, elevated bicarbonate, and Na^+ typically at the upper end of the normal range, together with suppressed plasma renin and elevated aldosterone. However, none of these findings is invariable, and a high index of suspicion is warranted in patients with hypertension resistant to conventional therapy. A suppressed plasma renin, despite treatment with 'A+C+D' drugs which normally elevate renin, is the most useful clue, whereas plasma aldosterone itself is often within the normal range but inappropriately high for the level of renin.

The imaging, like the biochemistry, is straightforward in classical patients, since the adrenals are easily imaged in most patients by either CT or MRI. However, patients with little intra-abdominal fat remain challenging, and it is important also to recognize that adrenals reported as 'bulky' often hide a small (<1 cm) adenoma. The key objective, once an adenoma is seen or suspected, is proving functional lateralization. This can be difficult, but is essential for predicting that removal of one adrenal will have a substantial benefit, as well as indicating which adrenal to remove. The most reliable technique in most specialist centres is adrenal vein sampling: all samples need to be assayed for aldosterone and cortisol, with the ratio compared between the two sides.

Management—medical treatment is preferred for bilateral adrenal hyperplasia, control of hypertension and hypokalaemia before surgery for adenoma, older patients with adenoma who are well controlled, or where there is any doubt about diagnosis or lateralization. Spironolactone is the treatment of choice but causes gynaecomastia in men. Eplerenone or amiloride are less effective alternatives, and amiloride can be used cautiously in combination with either of the other two drugs. Elective surgery is indicated for younger patients with adenomas, and older patients intolerant of—or uncontrolled by—medical treatment.

Renovascular hypertension

This is most commonly due to intrinsic disease of the intima (acquired, atherosclerosis, etc.) or media (congenital, fibromuscular dysplasia (FMD), etc.). FMD accounts for only 10–20% of all cases, but is the commonest cause under the age of 40.

Most cases of renovascular hypertension are probably not diagnosed because of the absence of sensitive clinical or biochemical markers. The main clinical clue is the finding in 50% of cases of a bruit anteriorly or posteriorly over a renal area, but it is important to remember that such a bruit is never diagnostic. In centres where it is routinely measured in younger patients, an elevated plasma renin is the commonest trigger to investigation for FMD. The diagnosis is made radiologically, most commonly by CT or MR angiography.

In FMD, angioplasty is usually curative, with about three-quarters of patients able to discontinue antihypertensive treatment. In atheromatous disease, angioplasty is much less likely to be successful. Complete cure of hypertension is rare, and recent studies suggest no benefit in prevention of decline of renal function in most cases.

Coarctation of the aorta

Coarctation causes less than 1% of all cases of hypertension. The classical clinical finding is radio–femoral pulse delay or weak lower limb pulses. Diagnosis is confirmed by two-dimensional echocardiography, or by CT or MR angiography. Treatment is by surgery, balloon dilatation, or stenting.

Phaeochromocytoma

Phaeochromocytomas are rare tumours of chromaffin tissue that account for 0.1 to 1% of cases of hypertension: 90% are benign and 90% are located in the adrenal gland (4% of adrenal incidentalomas are phaeochromocytomas). Most are sporadic, but some are associated with genetic syndromes, including von Hippel–Lindau and multiple endocrine neoplasia (MEN) type 2.

Hypertension, usually in association with one or more symptoms of headache, sweating, anxiety, and palpitations, is the most common presentation. Other rarer presentations include unexplained heart failure or paroxysmal arrhythmia.

Diagnosis—this is usually not difficult once the possibility of phaeochromocytoma has been entertained; more difficult is excluding the diagnosis in patients who have clinical and/or biochemical features of physiological catecholamine excess. Investigation must first determine whether the patient has a phaeochromocytoma, and then where the tumour is. The best screening test is to measure plasma normetanephrine (normetadrenaline) and metanephrine (metadrenaline) levels or, if unavailable, 24-h urine metanephrines: both assays in a reliable laboratory are more sensitive and specific than measurement of catecholamines or vanillylmandelic acid (VMA). Detection of elevated metadrenaline is a useful clue to the usual adrenal location of the phaeochromocytoma. A pharmacological suppression test can be performed where doubt about the diagnosis remains: physiological elevations of noradrenaline release are temporarily suppressed by administration of the ganglion-blocking drug pentolinium, or the centrally acting α_2-agonist clonidine, but these drugs do not suppress autonomous secretion by tumour. CT or MRI scanning usually provides excellent imaging of the adrenal. Radioisotope scanning with the iodinated analogue of noradrenaline, m-iodobenzylguanidine (mIBG), is usually helpful in localizing extra-adrenal tumours. Selective venous sampling is occasionally required.

Management—surgery is the definitive treatment that cures hypertension in most patients; the task for the physician is to make it safe. This should be done by α-blockade with phenoxybenzamine, with a low dose of a β_1-selective blocker used to prevent reflex tachycardia.

Introduction

The term 'secondary hypertension' is used to describe patients whose blood pressure is elevated by a single, identifiable cause. Until recently, there has been an optimistic view that description of new causes of hypertension would mean that those regarded as having 'essential hypertension' would be an ever-diminishing group. However, as discussed in Chapter 17.1, genome-wide investigation into the genetic bases of hypertension have shown that there are no common inherited susceptibility alleles that can explain more than 1 to 2 mmHg of a person's blood pressure. Hence it is now almost certain that essential hypertension differs from secondary hypertension not only in being unexplained, but in being, within each patient, due to a multiplicity of inherited and acquired characteristics.

An important subdivision of secondary hypertension is into reversible and irreversible causes: clinically it is important to exclude the former, but not necessarily to find the latter. Their elucidation may lead to improved medical therapy, e.g. by predicting the best diuretic in the monogenic causes of low-renin hypertension, or help assess prognosis, as in the patient with proteinuria. However, the resource implications of finding causes, which can be considerable, need to be balanced against achievable gains. These in turn are influenced by the patient's age, usually meaning that a search for secondary causes is easier to justify in young patients in whom small benefits are multiplied over many years.

Age-related prevalence of secondary hypertension

Whereas essential hypertension is clearly an age-related phenomenon, the same is less true of secondary hypertension, although different causes predominate at different ages. The net likelihood of a given patient with hypertension having a secondary cause is higher at a young age (Fig. 17.3.1). In the first two decades, essential hypertension is so uncommon that even the absolute prevalence of secondary hypertension is greater than that of essential hypertension. Thereafter, a patient is much more likely to have essential hypertension, but investigations for secondary hypertension should still be aggressive in patients in their twenties and thirties because the alternative entails so many years of tablet-taking.

In the first decade of life the main causes of secondary hypertension are (1) the monogenic syndromes causing low-renin (Na^+-dependent) hypertension and (2) congenital causes (e.g. coarctation). However, the rarity of blood pressure measurement or of complications in the first decade means diagnosis is often later, hence these are also the main causes of hypertension diagnosed in the second decade. Additional causes by this time are some acquired renal diseases, and the familial phaeochromocytoma syndromes. Conn's syndrome becomes the commonest cause for the next two to three decades; primary hyperaldosteronism as a whole is becoming increasingly recognized as a secondary cause in adults. From the fifth decade onwards, atheromatous renal artery stenosis is also an important cause of hypertension.

The clinical approach to secondary hypertension

All patients with hypertension should have a minimum set of investigations, as described in Chapter 17.2. Common indications for further investigations are shown in Box 17.3.1.

If possible, patients with blood pressure requiring treatment in their twenties or thirties should be investigated before initiation of treatment because this is rarely pressing at a young age, and some of the tests are easier to interpret off treatment.

The minimum screen in younger patients should include serum electrolytes, plasma bicarbonate, plasma renin, and metanephrines

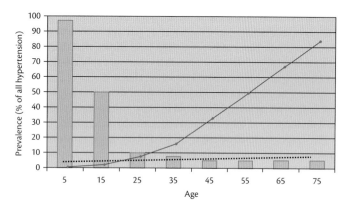

Fig. 17.3.1 The age-related prevalence of secondary hypertension. The red line shows the prevalence of essential hypertension by age (years), the dotted line the prevalence of secondary hypertension by age, and the bars show the percentage of all hypertensives with a secondary cause.

to exclude a phaeochromocytoma; 24-h electrolyte excretion should be measured either in all patients, or in those with abnormal renin levels. Sodium intake is most readily estimated at steady state (i.e. no recent change in diet or drugs) by measuring sodium excretion: intakes between 100 and 200 mmol (c.6–12 g)/day have little effect upon plasma renin, whereas outside this range there is a steep inverse relationship.

Further investigations pursuing specific diagnoses that might be considered in particular cases (Table 17.3.1) are described in the following sections.

Primary hyperaldosteronism (Conn's syndrome)

History

In 1955, with the words 'to our surprise and delight, a cortical adenoma was observed to be arising from the right adrenal gland', Jerome Conn reported the first observation of the benign aldosterone-secreting tumour that now bears his name. The patient had presented with severe hypertension and hypokalaemia, shortly after the discovery of aldosterone ('electrocortin') in London by the Taits in 1953. On detecting a high level of aldosterone in the

---

Box 17.3.1 Indications for investigation for secondary causes of hypertension

- Any evidence of an underlying cause in the history or examination (Table 17.3.1)
- Proteinuria, haematuria, or elevated serum creatinine (eGFR<30; CKD 4/5)
- Hypokalaemia even if caused by diuretics
- Accelerated (malignant) hypertension
- Documented recent onset or recent worsening of hypertension
- Resistant hypertension (not controlled with three antihypertensive drugs)
- Young age—any hypertension <20 years; any hypertension needing treatment <35 years

---

patient's urine, Conn decided not to remove both adrenals. There is an historical irony in this entirely correct decision: not so much because the patient retained her left adrenal, but because the finding of unilateral disease in this patient has largely pre-empted the same decision being made in patients with truly bilateral disease.

Conn's report led to a flurry of similar diagnoses and optimism that as much as 20% of hypertension might be due to his tumour. However, it soon became apparent that no adenoma could be found in perhaps 50% of patients with the clinical and biochemical features of primary hyperaldosteronism, some being diagnosed instead as having bilateral nodular hyperplasia. With waning enthusiasm for finding a curable cause of hypertension, estimated prevalence fell to less than 1% of hypertension, but the picture again reversed with the recognition that not all patients with primary hyperaldosteronism have an elevated plasma aldosterone concentration; indeed, it is now estimated that 5–10% of hypertensive patients have a potentially curable cause. Whereas previously low-renin hypertension was often considered a separate diagnosis, increasingly it is felt that even in such patients aldosterone drives the suppression of renin and that smaller adenomas are found when newer radiotracer imaging modalities are employed.

Aetiology and pathology

Conn's adenoma is a small (0.5–3.5 cm) benign tumour. Although aldosterone is normally secreted selectively by the (outer) zona glomerulosa of the adrenal, classical Conn's adenomas arise from the cortisol-secreting zona fasciculata, and secrete more cortisol than aldosterone; occasionally, the extra cortisol may be sufficient to cause suppression of the contralateral adrenal. In recent years, it has become apparent that aldosterone-producing adenomas of the zona glomerulosa are also common, but are commonly missed because of their smaller size. Adenomas arising in the two zones are characterized by somatic mutations in different genes (*KCNJ5*, a K$^+$ channel, in zona fasciculata tumours; Cav1.3 (*ATP2B3*), an L-type Ca^{2+} channel, and Na$^+$,K$^+$-ATPase (*ATP1A1*) in zona glomerulosa tumours). Presentation in pregnancy and after the menopause of aldosterone-producing adrenal adenomas harbouring activating mutations of CTNNB1, encoding β-catenin in the Wnt cell-differentiation pathway, has also been described.

Bilateral adrenal hyperplasia is a distinct condition in which either radiologically or histologically there are macro- or micronodules in the adrenal cortex where the monolayered arcades of the normal zona glomerulosa are replaced by bi- or multicellular layered arcades. In the one type of primary hyperaldosteronism of known cause—glucocorticoid-remediable aldosteronism (see Chapter 17.4)—there is no anatomical lesion in the adrenals other than expansion of the zona glomerulosa.

It remains unknown whether some patients develop single adenomas on the background of nodular hyperplasia, with suppression of all but the dominant nodule, or whether unilateral adenomas are usually a different condition from hyperplasia. In favour of the latter are a number of biochemical and pharmacological differences, and the fact that patients with glucocorticoid-remediable hyperaldosteronism never develop a superadded adenoma. Patients with classical Conn's adenomas show an exaggerated diurnal rhythm in aldosterone secretion, consistent with an enhanced ACTH-dependent cAMP pathway. By contrast, patients with hyperplasia, and those with the small zona glomerulosa tumours, show exaggerated aldosterone response to stimulation by angiotensin II and therefore have higher erect than supine aldosterone levels.

Table 17.3.1 Evidence in history, examination, or routine investigations suggesting a secondary cause for hypertension

Clinical	Evidence	Condition to consider
History	Paroxysmal features—palpitations, sweating, pallor, panic, headache or chest pain, cool peripheries	Phaeochromocytoma
	Flushing, labile blood pressure	Carcinoid syndrome
	Personal or family history of renal disease	Renal hypertension
	Pregnancy	Pre-eclampsia, HELLP syndrome
	Drug history—oestrogen-containing oral contraceptives; corticosteroids; non-steroidal anti-inflammatory drugs; sympathomimetics (amphetmaines, cocaine, cold cures, nasal decongestants); corticosteroids; ciclosporin; leflunomide; liquorice; caffeine; carbenoxalone; sodium bicarbonate (often found in excessive amounts in effervescent medictions, antacids); ergotamine; triptans; monoamine oxidase inhibitors (with tyramine-containing foods); erythropoietin; chronic arsenic exposure; long-term alcohol use; smoking cessation therapies; tramadol (enhances serotonergic and adrenergic transmission)	Drug-induced hypertension
	Tetany, muscle weakness, fatigue	Conn's syndrome
Examination	General appearance	Cushing's syndrome, acromegaly, thyroid disorders, obstructive sleep apnoea
	Palpable kidney(s)	Adult polycystic kidney disease, tuberous sclerosis
	Abdominal or loin bruits	Renovascular disease
	Delayed or weak femoral pulses	Coarctation of the aorta
Investigations	Proteinuria, haematuria, or elevated serum creatinine (eGFR<30; CKD 4/5)	Renal or renovascular disease
	Hypokalaemia, metabolic alkalosis	Conn's syndrome
	Hypercalcaemia	Hyperparathyroidsim
	Hyperglycaemia	Phaeochromocytoma

Primary hyperaldosteronism causes increased sodium retention through the epithelial sodium channel (ENaC) in the distal tubule and cortical collecting duct. The chronic sodium retention leads to hypertension, which is an essential feature of Conn's syndrome. Electroneutrality in the tubular cell is retained by secreting K^+ and/or H^+ ions in exchange for the Na^+ with consequent hypokalaemic alkalosis.

Epidemiology

Adenomas are slightly commoner in women, bilateral hyperplasia commoner in men. Conn's syndrome is not a cause of childhood hypertension, except for the rare monogenic syndrome of glucocorticoid-remediable hyperaldosteronism. Hyperplasia is said to be commoner among older patients with hypertension. However, it is difficult clinically to distinguish hyperplasia from small zona glomerulosa adenomas. Since it is likely that the latter have been present for many years or decades before presenting with often resistant hypertension, the best and easiest time to look for them is in younger patients, where hyperplasia is less likely and surgical treatment is most rewarding. Another condition which needs distinguishing from aldosterone-producing adenomas in older patients is nonfunctioning adrenal adenomas ('incidentalomas'), which are present in at least 4% of people over 50.

Overall prevalence remains contentious because of the detailed investigations required to establish presence or absence of functioning adenomas. In younger patients, where nonfunctioning adenomas and low-renin hypertension are both uncommon, and response to surgery is more clear cut, a conservative estimate would be 2% of those with hypertension, but the discovery of the smaller zona glomerulosa tumours may double this number. The prevalence among older patients with hypertension is probably similar. At present, a higher proportion of the older age group are likely to be investigated, having presented with either resistant hypertension or an adrenal incidentaloma, but in reality a smaller proportion are likely to benefit from surgery. Whether investigations reduce or increase in coming years may depend on the success of less invasive modalities than in current use for both investigation and treatment of adenomas, and extension of the latter into bilateral disease.

Clinical features

Patients with primary hyperaldosteronism 'escape' from the effects of aldosterone before sufficient Na^+ is retained to cause overt oedema, hence the clues and confirmation of the diagnosis are largely biochemical. The classic picture in Conn's syndrome is hypertension in which the plasma electrolytes show a low K^+, elevated bicarbonate, and a Na^+ typically at the upper end of the normal range, but sometimes above this. The hypertension is often resistant to treatment with conventional treatment for the patient's age group—e.g. angiotensin converting enzyme (ACE) inhibition in a younger patient, or to multiple drugs including a thiazide diuretic in the older age groups. It is important to mention, however, that the classical hallmark—hypokalaemia—is not always present, and yet the consequences of K^+ depletion—weakness, tiredness, U wave on ECG—might still be manifest. The severity of hypokalaemia varies steeply with the Na^+ load presented to the ENaC, this depending partly on dietary Na^+ intake and partly on drugs—principally thiazide diuretics—which affect the proportion of the filtered Na$^+$ load reaching the distal tubule. The commonest reason for the biochemical features of Conn's to be masked is concurrent treatment with a calcium channel blocker. Hence, when considering the possibility of Conn's in a patient with hypertension apparently resistant to conventional treatment, it is important to look not just at the current plasma electrolytes but at an historical set of results for any finding of hypokalaemia or alkalosis, and also to reflect that hypokalaemia on a low dose of thiazide is a reason for pursuing (rather than dismissing) the diagnosis of primary hyperaldosteronism.

Differential diagnosis

The hypokalaemic hypertensive is an interesting diagnostic challenge that can usually be solved by a series of logical moves. The finding of a Conn's adenoma is the most satisfying outcome because surgical excision is most likely to lead to long-term cure. The other curable cause is liquorice consumption which, taken in excess, inhibits the enzyme 11β-hydroxysteroid dehydrogenase (11HSD) and permits cortisol access to the mineralocorticoid receptor (see 'Apparent mineralocorticoid excess' in Chapter 17.4). Excess production of cortisol in Cushing's syndrome can also mimic Conn's. This is most likely to happen when there is ectopic ACTH production or with a malignant adrenocortical tumour, resulting in gross excess of cortisol and consequent saturation of the 11HSD enzyme (Fig. 17.3.2). Cosecreting, or coexisting, aldosterone- and cortisol-producing adenomas should also be considered, although generally the clinical picture is predominantly of one or the other.

Clinical investigation

Electrolytes

The critical tests in the investigation of hypokalaemic hypertension are plasma and urine electrolytes, and plasma renin and aldosterone. If the recommendations described above for screening tests in young patients with hypertension have been observed, all but the plasma aldosterone should already have been performed. The urine K$^+$ (which can be performed on a spot sample) is usually in excess of 40 mmol/litre if hypokalaemia is due to increased urinary loss, but this test is valuable only when performed when plasma K$^+$ is low. Because transient hypokalaemia is common, and hypokalaemia commonly transient even in Conn's syndrome, it is important not to postpone urine K$^+$ estimation and risk missing a one-off opportunity for sparing a patient the further investigations required for renal K$^+$ loss.

Renin

Of the triad of hypokalaemia, suppressed plasma renin, and elevated aldosterone, the renin is of most importance in the diagnosis of Conn's—although renin suppression is not invariable, even in untreated patients. The diagnosis should be entertained in the absence of an elevated aldosterone, especially in patients where a suppressed renin is unexpected: the younger patient (aged <45 years), particularly if already on an ACE inhibitor or angiotensin receptor blocker (ARB); and the older patient with resistant hypertension, receiving multiple drugs which normally elevate renin.

The main confounders in interpretation of the plasma renin level are drugs. A low renin in the presence of β-blockade is of no significance, and a β-blocker (which is unlikely to help with blood pressure control in Conn's anyway) should be discontinued or substituted by an ACE inhibitor or ARB 2 weeks before renin measurement. Conversely, spironolactone or amiloride will 'desuppress' renin in most patients, and this should be borne in mind if the patient was already receiving one of these drugs prior to investigation.

Renin itself is very stable in blood, providing this is not chilled (which cryoactivates the renin precursor, prorenin). Although changes in posture and activity cause two- to threefold changes in renin, the range of renin between high- and low-renin patients is some 1000-fold, hence it is simple to interpret results taken in routine outpatient clinics or surgeries, providing the blood sample (taken into an EDTA tube) reaches the laboratory for plasma separation on the same day as the blood is taken.

Aldosterone

Plasma aldosterone is often elevated above the normal range (100–400 pmol/litre), and is generally higher in patients with macroadenomas (>1 cm) than in those with microadenomas or hyperplasia.

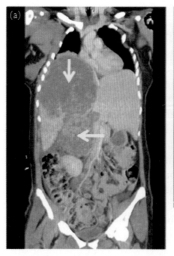
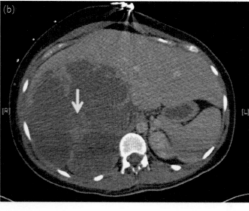

Fig. 17.3.2 Coronal (panel A) and axial (panel B) CT scan images of a large right-sided malignant adrenocortical tumour (horizontal arrow) that is invading the liver (vertical arrows).

In patients with adenomas there is an exaggerated influence of ACTH leading to pronounced diurnal variation in aldosterone levels, which are more likely to be normal when sampled in the afternoon. By contrast, patients with hyperplasia have an exaggerated response to angiotensin II, so that levels may actually rise during the day in response to activity and be normalized by drugs blocking the renin system, particularly angiotensin receptor blockade. However, the most profound influences are serum K^+ and the use of calcium channel blocker treatment, which (as already stated) is probably now the commonest reason for the diagnosis of Conn's syndrome to be missed.

Aldosterone/renin ratio

The recognition that aldosterone is often normal—even, sometimes, after correction of hypokalaemia and withdrawal of calcium channel blocker—led to the concept of the aldosterone/renin ratio. However, in practice, because renin is log-normally distributed and aldosterone distribution is normal, the aldosterone/renin ratio is always high in low-renin patients (except in the rare low-renin, low-aldosterone differential diagnoses considered above for hypokalaemic hypertension) and the vast majority of those with an elevated aldosterone/renin ratio do not have primary hyperaldosteronism, hence the key question is how to avoid unnecessary investigations in these cases. The empirical answer is that in the absence of other clues—hypokalaemia, high/high-normal plasma Na^+, alkalosis—investigation be undertaken only in patients with resistant hypertension.

Saline (fludrocortisone) suppression

A possible dynamic test before proceeding to radiological investigations is the saline (or salt + fludrocortisone) suppression test, which in principle is equivalent to the outpatient dexamethasone test for Cushing's syndrome. In practice the classical test prescribes sodium and potassium loading during the 3 days of suppression by fludrocortisone 400 micrograms daily, and the consequent risk of severe hypertension necessitates close observation. Simplified protocols using either fludrocortisone or saline suppression alone are also sometimes followed. However, many investigators regard suppression as unreliable and unnecessary: perhaps its role in diagnosis can best be reserved for a late stage in the diagnostic algorithm, in patients where the case for surgery is borderline, and when extra certainty about diagnosis is required.

Genetic testing

This is rarely required, but if there is a family history of early-onset hypertension, and particularly of strokes at a young age, the patient should be screened for glucocorticoid-remediable aldosteronism (see Chapter 17.4), of which there are only a few known families in the United Kingdom. Interestingly, research is increasingly providing fascinating insights into the genetics of aldosterone-producing adenomas, which in turn may lead to improved diagnosis in future, without the need for adrenal venous sampling. Further discussion can be found in the 'Aetiology and pathology' section of this chapter.

Scanning

The adrenals are easily imaged by either CT or MRI, except when there is a dearth of intra-abdominal fat (Fig. 17.3.3). Under such circumstances, where the patient is very slim, skilled ultrasonography may be superior to CT or MRI. There is no proven advantage of one of these two modalities over the other. MRI may be preferred in younger patients, to spare radiation, and the fat-suppression sequence is useful for differentiating adenomas both from other adrenal masses, and sometimes the adjacent normal adrenal. Resolution may be higher with CT, but the limit for both modalities is not so much inherent resolution as the existence of 0.3–0.6-cm adenomas that do not create a discrete bulge within an adrenal limb, and even 1-cm adenomas at the bifurcation of the two limbs can be difficult to distinguish from a normal gland. It is valuable to request coronal reconstructions, which may show or confirm adenomas less evident on the axial views. Neither MRI nor CT can differentiate functional from incidental adenomas.

Functional lateralization

This is the key but most difficult stage of diagnosis. Lateralization is essential in predicting that removal of one adrenal will have a

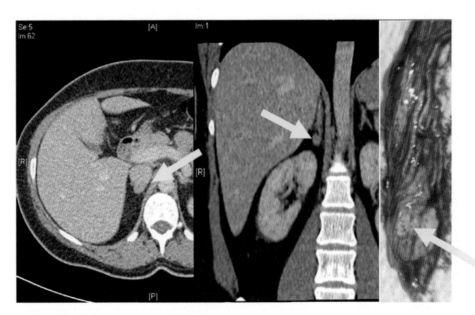

Fig. 17.3.3 Conn's adenoma (arrow): CT transverse view (left), coronal view (middle), surgical specimen (right).

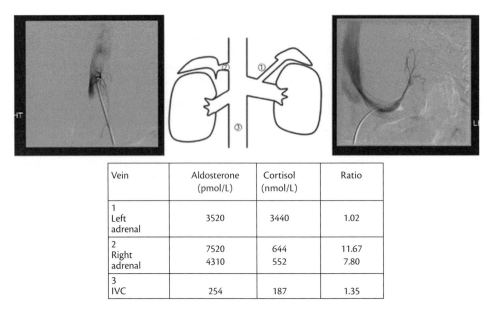

Vein	Aldosterone (pmol/L)	Cortisol (nmol/L)	Ratio
1 Left adrenal	3520	3440	1.02
2 Right adrenal	7520 4310	644 552	11.67 7.80
3 IVC	254	187	1.35

Fig. 17.3.4 Adrenal vein sampling for a right adrenal adenoma.

substantial benefit, as well as indicating which adrenal to remove, although it might occasionally be omitted in younger patients (aged <35 years) with macroadenomas, or where the tumour is more than 3.5 cm in diameter and needs to be removed to exclude a mixed adrenal carcinoma.

At present, the only reliable form of lateralization available at most specialist centres is adrenal vein sampling. This is technically demanding and should be undertaken only by experienced radiologists (Fig. 17.3.4). On the left side, the adrenal vein is the only vein to enter the renal vein superiorly, and cannulation is relatively straightforward. On the right, however, the adrenal vein is one of several small veins (<1 mm diameter) entering the inferior vena cava posteriorly. A fish-hooked 'Cobra' catheter with side-holes maximizes the chances of success at 80%, providing several veins are sampled, with reference samples also taken in the inferior vena cava above and below the adrenal veins.

All samples need to be assayed for aldosterone and cortisol, with the ratio compared between the two sides: a ratio above 4 is usually diagnostic, and above 10 is definitive. Ratios of two- to fourfold can be compatible with lateralization, but are best confirmed on repeat sampling. In such cases accuracy might be enhanced by simultaneous sampling from both veins, or—if aldosterone levels were low on the first occasion—by prior ACTH stimulation. Some centres advocate these additional procedures as a routine, but they increase both the cost and duration of adrenal vein sampling at a time when the increased recognition of Conn's syndrome requires increased access to tests for lateralization. When the right adrenal vein cannot be cannulated—revealed by a cortisol concentration less than 20% above that in the inferior vena cava—it is very risky to draw conclusions from the left sample alone: concentrations of aldosterone can be very high, even in a normal vein, because adrenal vein blood flow is so low.

Isotope scans can also be used for lateralization. ^{131}I-cholesterol (or ^{75}Se-methyl-19-norcholesterol) can be bought or generated for scanning in any nuclear medicine department, but ^{11}C-metomidate (Fig. 17.3.5) must be synthesized on site in centres with a cyclotron and positron emission tomography (PET) scanner. The cholesterol scans rely on its role as precursor of steroid synthesis, and the scan is performed 1 week after isotope administration to permit cholesterol turnover and elimination from non-adrenal sites. However, the technique has a generally unreliable record, possibly because the dexamethasone taken during the week of investigation has variable influence on zona glomerulosa as well as zona fasciculata uptake. Metomidate binds to synthetic enzymes in both the aldosterone and cortisol pathway, but appears relatively selective for those expressed in aldosterone-producing adenomas.

Treatment

Medical

Medical treatment is preferred for bilateral adrenal hyperplasia, before surgery for adenoma, in older patients with adenoma who are well controlled, or where there is any doubt about diagnosis or lateralization.

Chronic medical treatment is by K^+-sparing diuretic, preferably spironolactone or amiloride. Spironolactone is a competitive antagonist of aldosterone, hence patients with very high aldosterone levels may require higher doses than used in resistant hypertension. While this is possible for preoperative use, long-term administration causes gynaecomastia. High-dose amiloride (20–40 mg daily) is better tolerated but less effective. Eplerenone also avoids the gynaecomastia of spironolactone, but again is less effective and currently much more expensive. A possible strategy is to combine eplerenone or a low dose of spironolactone (≤25 mg daily) with amiloride, but vigilant monitoring of plasma electrolytes is required.

It may not be possible to control blood pressure entirely by diuresis, especially in older patients, where calcium channel blockers or α-blockers can usefully be added. In patients who are difficult to control, the maximum useful dose of diuretic can be found by titrating dose against plasma renin: once this is de-suppressed it becomes logical to add ACE inhibition or an ARB. In patients with bilateral hyperplasia, one of these classes is often required, even when renin is suppressed. This may reflect either the resistant nature of hypertension that often ensues with long-standing hyperaldosteronism, or the increased sensitivity to angiotensin in salt-loaded patients.

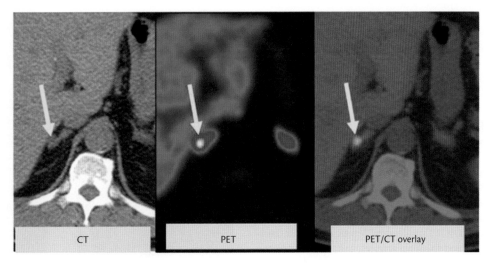

| CT | PET | PET/CT overlay |

Fig. 17.3.5 ^{11}C-metomidate PET/CT scan of a right adrenal aldosteronoma. Uptake correctly differentiated hot and cold nodules, as confirmed by presence and absence of aldosterone secretion from the nodules when cultured postoperatively.

Surgical

Elective surgery is indicated for younger patients with adenomas, and older patients intolerant of medical treatment, or uncontrolled by it. A good blood pressure response to spironolactone augurs well for cure by surgery, but the opposite is not necessarily true: a poor response does not exclude benefit from surgery. It is best not to promise any patient complete cure, but rather a substantial reduction in number of medicines required to control blood pressure. A bonus in many patients is alleviation of chronic fatigue, presumably attributable to total body K$^+$ depletion.

Surgery should be undertaken by a surgeon experienced in laparoscopic adrenalectomy, but patients warned that anatomical anomalies, or perioperative eventualities such as tear of the inferior vena cava, may necessitate conversion to open adrenalectomy in about 1/40 procedures. No special preoperative care is required, although it is sensible to undertake assessment to exclude hypercortisolism in those patients with large adenomas. Diuretics should be withdrawn from the time of surgery, but any additional antihypertensive treatment continued until any change in blood pressure becomes clear over the following weeks. In the future, alcohol ablation of adenomas is looking a viable option, preserving the adjacent normal adrenal gland. Left-side adenomas, sitting close to the stomach, are accessible for both diagnostic fine-needle aspiration, and therapeutic ablation, delivered using endoscopic ultrasound. This development should lower the bar at which intervention for a benign tumour is considered. Ablation also opens up the possibility of cure for the increasing number of patients found to have bilateral aldosterone-producing adenomas but in whom bilateral adrenalectomy would never be considered an option.

Prognosis

Most (70–80%) younger patients with adenomas are cured of hypertension and hypokalaemia. Older patients are less likely to come off all antihypertensive treatment, but hypokalaemia is rarely persistent if they have been well selected for surgery, and the average number of medicines is more than halved, with improved blood pressure control in the remainder. The lesser success of surgery in older patients is due to a mixture of longer duration of hypertension, associated essential hypertension, and lingering suspicion that the smaller adenomas are part of the bilateral hyperplasia spectrum, with residual disease in the contralateral adrenal. Residual hypertension can be exquisitely sensitive to low doses of an ARB, and there may be a role for routine prophylactic treatment of older patients to prevent hyperplasia of the remaining adrenal.

Renal hypertension

The principal curable cause is renovascular hypertension. This is usually due to a stenosis in one or both renal arteries, but can be due to a suprarenal aortic stenosis. Other curable causes include renal tumours (hypernephroma and, the rarest of all secondary causes, a juxtaglomerular renin-secreting tumour); a unilateral, poorly functioning scarred or hydronephrotic kidney which hypersecretes renin, and can be removed without unacceptable loss of renal function (so-called Page kidneys; Fig. 17.3.6); and various

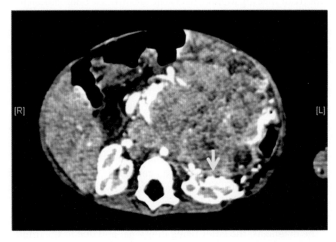

Fig. 17.3.6 A Page kidney. CT scan image showing a left-sided neuroblastoma compressing the kidney (arrow). The compression impedes renal blood flow, resulting in excess secretion of the hormone renin and consequently hypertension. Named after Irvine Page (1901–89) who demonstrated that wrapping cellophane tightly around an animal's kidney caused arterial blood pressure to rise. The patient's hypertension was cured after surgery to remove the tumour.

causes of acute/subacute glomerulonephritis, some associated with systemic disorders whose treatment by immunosuppression cures the hypertension and underlying disorder. Interestingly, aortic dissection, often itself a complication of arterial hypertension, may extend into the renal arteries and thereby exacerbate hypertension by causing increased secretion of renin.

Renovascular hypertension

This is most commonly due to intrinsic disease of the intima (acquired—atherosclerosis) or media (congenital—fibromuscular dysplasia). Extrinsic narrowing can be caused by ligamentous bands or by tumours (e.g. neurofibromas).

Fibromuscular dysplasia (FMD) accounts for only 10 to 20% of all patients with renovascular hypertension, but is the commonest cause under the age of 40. It is a nonatherosclerotic and noninflammatory disease of small and medium arteries, usually affecting the media, less commonly the adventitia (<25%), and rarely the intima. The classical 'string of beads' appearance seen at arteriography results from proliferation of the extracellular matrix and disruption of the internal elastic lamina, causing multiple stenoses and post-stenotic saccular aneurysms. The condition affects women more often than men, and there is usually no family history of hypertension. FMD involves extrarenal arteries in about one-quarter of patients, with cerebral infarction recorded due to relative hypotension and hypoperfusion of FMD-affected carotid arteries following successful renal angioplasty.

The typical medial form of FMD does not affect the proximal part of the renal arteries and is bilateral in about one-third of cases. Other vascular beds, e.g. the cerebral arteries, can be affected. Complications (other than renal ischaemia) are rare, whereas dissection or thrombosis can ensue in the rarer intimal or adventitial form of FMD. Rupture of renal artery aneurysms is rare.

Atheromatous renal artery stenosis has the same risk factors as atheromatous disease of other arteries, which often coexists. It is thus commoner in older men, and whereas FMD rarely causes renal impairment, atheromatous disease is often discovered in the context of investigation of hypertension with chronic kidney disease. Apart from the obvious difference in biology of FMD and atheromatous renovascular hypertension, there is a difference in location of the stenosis, which is more likely to be proximal in atheromatous disease (Fig. 17.3.8).

Mechanism of hypertension

Unilateral renal artery stenosis gives rise to an endocrine disorder, because reduced pressure in the afferent arteriole causes juxtaglomerular hyperplasia and increased renin secretion. The consequent increase in angiotensin II formation causes hypertension, partly by vasoconstriction and partly through increased aldosterone secretion. Although secondary hyperaldosteronism is not usually a marked feature of renal artery stenosis, the combination of hypokalaemia and hyponatraemia should raise suspicion of the diagnosis, the latter being dilutional and due to the inhibition by angiotensin II of free water clearance. The effect on renin secretion is less predictable when renal artery stenosis affects both renal arteries: sometimes it is high, but sometimes bilateral reduction in GFR leads to sufficient sodium retention that renin is suppressed.

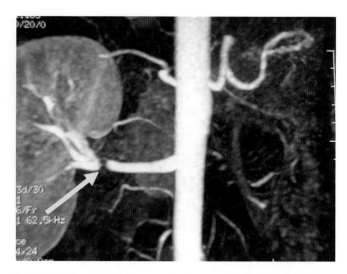

Fig. 17.3.7 MR angiogram demonstrating fibromuscular dysplasia of the right renal artery causing stenosis (arrow).

Diagnosis

Most cases of renovascular hypertension are probably not diagnosed because of the absence of sensitive clinical or biochemical markers. Lack of a family history of hypertension in younger patients, or recent onset (or exacerbation) of hypertension in older patients is more likely than in essential hypertension. Acute shortness of breath, due to flash pulmonary oedema, can be the presenting feature of bilateral renal artery stenosis. However, the main clinical clue is the finding, in about one-half of the patients, of a bruit anteriorly or posteriorly over a renal area. It is important to remember, however, that such a bruit is never diagnostic: normal abdominal arteries can give rise to innocent flow murmurs in younger patients and in older patients a bruit could arise from any of a number of arteries within the abdomen. The response to antihypertensive drugs can also give clues: in particular poor response to β-blockade in younger patients, or rapid worsening of renal function in older patients.

The diagnosis of renal artery stenosis is made radiologically. The cheapest investigation is a nuclear medicine scan using technetium-labelled MAG3, both the uptake and elimination of this being delayed on the ischaemic side, with the difference in excretion rate between sides greatly increased following a single dose of captopril (25 mg) because of dilatation of the efferent arterioles in glomeruli and consequent reduction in filtration fraction. For this reason the scan is best performed initially with captopril; if abnormal, it is repeated on a subsequent visit without captopril, with partial or complete normalization being evidence that the previous abnormality was due to vascular rather than renal parenchymal disease. However, the MAG3 scan is not always positive, with chronic use of ACE inhibitors being a cause of some false negatives, and it may also miss bilateral renal artery stenoses that do not cause significant asymmetry between the kidneys.

Partly for these reasons, nuclear imaging is not performed for suspected renal artery stenosis in most centres, with investigation proceeding to direct imaging of the renal arteries by CT or MR angiography (Fig. 17.3.7 and Fig. 17.3.8). In patients under 20 years of age some form of angiography should always be undertaken, except in those with low-renin syndromes, because of the high likelihood of a secondary cause being present, and that this will be a vascular abnormality. As well as providing an accurate estimate in

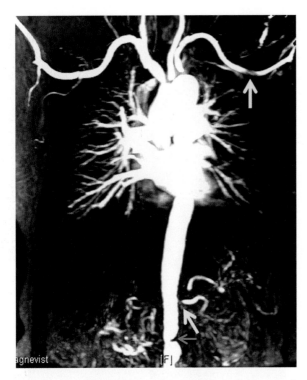

Fig. 17.3.8 MRI scan image showing a concomitant left renal artery stenosis (yellow arrow at bottom of image), and left subclavian artery stenosis (yellow arrow at top of image). There is also an infrarenal aortic stenosis (blue arrow). This patient presented with a subclavian steal syndrome and lower blood pressure readings in the left arm.

most patients of the severity of any stenosis, angiography will also detect suprarenal aortic stenoses. False-positive and false-negative diagnoses still occur; e.g. the poststenotic dilatations of FMD can—if they expand proximally around the artery—be a cause of stenoses being missed. However, the risk of diagnostic error can be reduced by careful review of images taken in more than one projection, and it is useful to remember that stenoses are not usually isolated lesions in both FMD and atheromatous disease (Fig. 17.3.8).

Some centres use Doppler flow measurements for diagnosis, but these are more user-dependent than angiography, which is still required subsequently for anatomical diagnosis. On the other hand, there are some patients in whom an anatomical diagnosis is made first, but the severity is in question. Here it can be useful to perform Doppler or MAG3 scan as the second investigation before proceeding to treatment. Another investigation that is sometimes helpful at this stage is renal vein sampling for renin determination, the main use for which is before removing a kidney thought responsible for causing hypertension through elevated renin secretion. The contralateral—anatomically normal—kidney has often sustained microvascular damage as a consequence of prolonged hypertension and renin excess, and is found to secrete as much renin as (or more than) the diseased kidney. Nephrectomy should not normally be contemplated where significant renal function remains, but in any circumstance there would rarely be an indication for removing a kidney showing less than 25% excess renin secretion compared to the contralateral side.

Treatment

There are several options, one of which is simply to continue optimal drug treatment if for any reason the risks of other intervention appear excessive. Among interventions, the options are as for any other arterial stenosis, namely angioplasty, stenting or surgery. For FMD, angioplasty is usually curative, and about three-quarters can discontinue antihypertensive treatment. In atheromatous disease, angioplasty is much less likely to be successful, especially for lesions at the origin of the artery, and restenosis can occur. It is reasonable to recommend stenting as a backup procedure when angioplasty has failed. Complete cure of hypertension is very much less likely than in FMD. In the past, the purpose of intervention was often to try to protect or improve renal function. The ASTRAL and CORAL trials have largely rebutted this objective, although some argue that patients were excluded from participation where clinicians were certain of benefit from intervention. Few nephrologists now pursue renal revascularization with the same vigour that was common five or ten years ago.

Sometimes angioplasty is unsuccessful because balloon inflation fails to dent the stenosis. Surgery is required in this situation, or when failure can be predicted because stenosis is due to external compression or there is complete occlusion. As renovascular surgery is not common today outside the transplant arena, a favoured surgical procedure is autotransplantation to the pelvis.

Coarctation of the aorta

Coarctation of the aorta, a congenital cause of hypertension, was described pathologically in the 1700s and recognized clinically in the early 1900s. The term describes a constriction of the aorta at the point where the fetal arterial duct originates, and the condition should ideally be diagnosed in early childhood, with most cases treated before hypertension develops. Coarctation represents 5 to 8% of all causes of congenital heart disease, but less than 1% of all cases of hypertension. However, sometimes diagnosis is delayed until the patient presents in adulthood with hypertension, and high blood pressure can sometimes develop even after surgical cure of the coarctation. Coarctation may also develop at a much lower level in the aorta secondary to long-standing aortitis. The mechanism of hypertension is predominantly the relative renal ischaemia consequent on low perfusion pressure in the aorta beyond the coarctation.

The classical clinical finding in coarctation is radiofemoral pulse delay or weak lower limb pulses, confirmed by measurement of reduced blood pressure in the legs. Of greater sensitivity and specificity in the clinic is a bruit—systolic or continuous—over the front and back of the praecordium, which arises in the intercostal collaterals.

The diagnosis should be confirmed by two-dimensional (2D) echocardiography (suprasternal view) or by CT or MR angiography (Figs 17.3.9 and 17.3.10). Treatment is by surgery, balloon dilatation, or stenting. Surgery or balloon dilation are the preferred approaches in childhood, balloon dilation and stent implantation in adolescents and adults. Although upper limb hypertension is usually cured, recurrence has been attributed to a variety of unproven factors, including a systemic vasculopathy.

Phaeochromocytoma

Aetiology and pathology

Catecholamine biochemistry

Catecholamine biochemistry is summarized in Fig. 17.3.11. The final step in the biosynthetic pathway is the *N*-methylation of

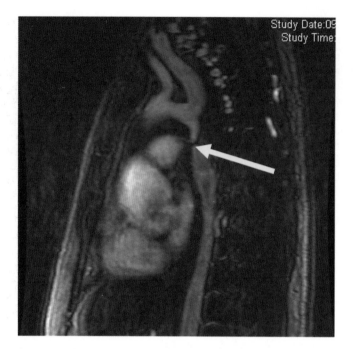

Fig. 17.3.9 MR angiogram showing coarctation of the aorta (arrow).

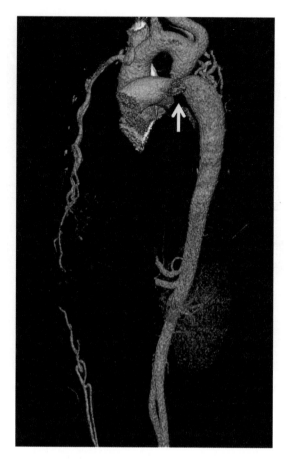

Fig. 17.3.10 3D CT reconstruction of coarctation of the aorta (arrow).

noradrenaline (norepinephrine) to adrenaline (epinephrine), which outside the brain occurs only in the adrenal medulla because the enzyme phenylethanolamine *N*-methyltransferase in the adrenal is dependent for induction on glucocorticoids, secreted at high concentration into the adrenal portocapillary circulation. The clinical importance of this is that extra-adrenal phaeochromocytomas rarely produce adrenaline.

The metabolism of catecholamines is different from normal in phaeochromocytoma in that adrenaline and noradrenaline are liberated directly into the bloodstream, rather than mainly into the synaptic gap around sympathetic nerve endings. Noradrenaline released from these is largely recaptured by neuronal and extraneuronal uptake, and metabolized before any free amine escapes into the bloodstream. Consequently, the proportion of parent amine (noradrenaline) to metabolite (adrenaline) is usually higher in blood and urine in the presence of a phaeochromocytoma than in any other cause of elevated catecholamine production.

Pathology

Phaeochromocytomas arise in chromaffin tissue and their anatomical distribution closely parallels the sites where this tissue is present at the time of birth. The term phaeochromocytoma reflects the dusky colour of the cut surface of the tumour, whereas the term chromaffin refers to the brownish colour caused by contact with dichromate salts, which oxidize the catecholamines.

Most phaeochromocytomas are benign, but the pathologist can rarely provide a clear distinction between those that are benign and those that are malignant: benign tumours can appear to be invading the capsule of the tumour, which is often ill-defined, while malignant tumours may show no mitoses because of their slow rate of division. Yearly surveillance, or earlier if indicated clinically, with measurement of plasma metanephrine levels is recommended.

Genetics

Several mutations cause syndromes that include phaeochromocytoma (Table 17.3.2), the clinical and biochemical features of

which are variable. Only tumours associated with mutations of succinate dehydrogenase (SDH, subunits B or D) commonly occur outside the adrenal, where they are sometimes referred to as paragangliomas rather than extra-adrenal phaeochromocytomas, and paragangliomas in the head or neck are restricted to *SDHD* (or rarely *SDHC*) mutations. *VHL* and *RET* mutations may cause multiple tumour types, the site of these being determined by the site of mutation in the gene: e.g. VHL type 2c missense mutations cause only phaeochromocytoma, while the gene deletions of type 1 cause renal cell carcinoma but not phaeochromocytoma. The main value of genotyping has become prediction of multiple (but usually benign) extra-adrenal phaeochromocytomas in patients with *SDHD* mutations, while patients with *SDHB* mutations have a high incidence of malignancy.

Some of the mutations in *VHL* or *SDH* also occur in sporadic tumours. This observation, together with the biochemical connection between VHL and SDH, has suggested that one underlying cause of phaeochromocytoma is failure to suppress hypoxia-induced cell proliferation. Oxygen detection by prolyl hydroxylases normally leads to degradation of hypoxia-inducible factors in a process that requires the VHL protein: if VHL is defective, or prolyl hydroxylases are inhibited by accumulation of succinate, then the degradation of hypoxia-inducible factors is altered and cell proliferation is stimulated.

Epidemiology

Phaeochromocytoma is a rare tumour, responsible for probably 0.1 to 1% of hypertensives, although it is possible that some of

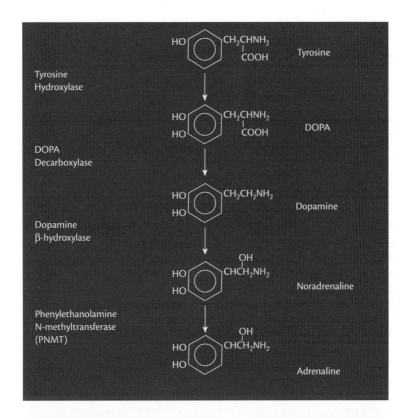

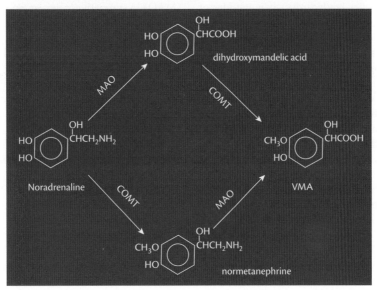

Fig. 17.3.11 The biosynthetic pathway for epinephrine and norepinephrine (upper panel), and for metabolism of norepinephrine (lower panel). COMT, catechol-O-methyltransferase; DOPA, dihydroxyphenylalanine; MAO, monoamine oxidase; VMA, vanillylmandelic acid.

its non-blood-pressure presentations are overlooked and that we selectively detect patients in whom pressure natriuresis no longer compensates for the effect of vasoconstriction upon blood pressure. However, despite its rarity, phaeochromocytoma justifies the disproportionate interest that it commands among physicians, combining the potential for being lethal if not diagnosed and treated, and for cure in most patients if diagnosed. The need for maintaining a high awareness of the condition is emphasized by the small number of deaths each year due to undiagnosed phaeochromocytoma in both anaesthetic and obstetric practice.

Clinical features

Hypertension is the most common presentation of phaeochromocytoma in clinical practice, but other rare presentations include unexplained heart failure or paroxysmal arrhythmias. Patients with large tumours occasionally remain asymptomatic, and this is the norm for small phaeochromocytomas detected through regular screening of patients with a genetic diagnosis.

In hypertensive patients a spontaneous history or direct enquiry will usually reveal at least one of a group of characteristic symptoms.

Table 17.3.2 Genes associated with familial forms of phaeochromocytoma

Gene	Chromosome	Exons	Protein	Frequency of germ-line mutations in apparent sporadic phaeochromocytoma (%)	Frequency of malignant disease (%)
VHL	3p25–26	3	pVHL19 and pVHL30	2–1	5
RET	10qll.2	21	Tyrosine kinase receptor	<5	3
NF1	17qll.2	59	Neurofibromin	Unknown	11
SDHB	1P36.13	8	Catalytic iron-sulphur protein	3–10	50
SDHD	Hq23	4	CybS (membrane-spanning subunit)	4–7	<3

VHL, von Hippel–Lindau syndrome; RET, a proto-oncogene encoding a receptor tyrosine kinase; NF1, neurofibromatosis type 1; SDHB, succinate dehydrogenase B; SDHD, succinate dehydrogenase D.

The classical triad comprises headache, sweating, and palpitations; less frequent are episodes of pallor, a feeling of 'impending doom', and paraesthesiae. Spontaneous haemorrhage and infarction in the tumour can be associated with local pain and (on occasion) systemic features of tissue necrosis, and rarely the patient can present with the features of full-blown retroperitoneal haemorrhage, coupled to a pathognomonic swinging blood pressure.

Most of the symptoms of phaeochromocytoma can be readily ascribed to the expected effects of catecholamine excess, and disappear rapidly on initiation of appropriate treatment. Because large tumours principally secrete noradrenaline, even when arising within the adrenal gland, tachycardia is usually only modest, and can be replaced altogether by reflex bradycardia when episodes of hypertension are triggered by release of noradrenaline alone. The bradycardia can be severe enough—if the hypertension is high enough—to be misdiagnosed as asystolic cardiac arrest, and the correct treatment is not atropine but phentolamine to reduce the blood pressure. Severe bradycardia is also recorded in response to the paradoxical rise in blood pressure when patients with phaeochromocytoma are inadvertently given a nonselective β-blocker such as propranolol. Often, however, the clinical features are less impressive than might be expected, possibly because the adrenoceptors have been down-regulated by years of exposure before the diagnosis is first entertained.

Examination may reveal a bruit over the tumour. A Raynaud's type of discolouration over the extremities and the larger joints in the limbs can be caused by ischaemia.

Clinical investigation

The diagnosis of phaeochromocytoma is usually not difficult once the possibility has been entertained; often more difficult is excluding the diagnosis in patients who have clinical and/or biochemical features of physiological catecholamine excess. There are two distinct questions to ask in order. 'Does the patient have a phaeochromocytoma?', and 'Where is it?'. It is unwise to use radiological tests to answer the first question because of the risk of false positives and false negatives.

Biochemical analyses of catecholamines and their metabolites

Twenty-four-hour urine samples measure integrated catecholamine release and provide a useful screening test, with catecholamine metabolites less temperamental to assay than the more unstable catecholamines themselves. Vanillylmandelic acid (VMA) measured by high-performance liquid chromatography (HPLC) is least prone to interference, L-DOPA and paracetamol being the main concerns, and although now regarded as less sensitive than some alternatives it is still the exception for VMA to be entirely normal in a patient with hypertension due to a phaeochromocytoma. Metanephrines (sometimes called metadrenalines) measured by radioimmunoassay or gas chromatography–mass spectrometry (GCMS) are more sensitive and more specific than VMA, with the assay of 'fractionated metanephrines' permitting separate evaluation of noradrenaline and adrenaline secretion. The ability to differentiate physiological release of noradrenaline from sympathetic nerve endings from pathological secretion from a phaeochromocytoma arises because of the presence of two different enzymes in the two locations: monoamine oxidase (MAO) in sympathetic nerves, and catechol-O-methyltransferase (COMT) in the adrenal medulla and phaeochromocytoma (see Fig. 17.3.11).

The measurement of free catecholamines in plasma (which have a very short half-life) by HPLC with electrochemical detection allows short bursts of secretion during a possible phaeochromocytoma crisis to be detected. However, the technique is susceptible to interference, especially in the adrenaline peak, and the finding of an adrenaline concentration that is higher than that of noradrenaline should be regarded as suspect. Dopamine levels are usually undetectable in plasma, whereas it is the major catecholamine in urine as a product of renal decarboxylation of plasma dihydroxyphenylalanine. Only several-fold increases in urinary dopamine are of diagnostic value, and are more likely to indicate neuroblastoma (in a child) or melanoma (which secretes dopamine as a by-product of melanin synthesis) than phaeochromocytoma.

Most adrenal phaeochromocytomas secrete adrenaline (and therefore metadrenaline), the exceptions being patients with very large tumours, which completely disrupt the portocapillary supply of cortisol required to induce phenylethanolamine N-methyltransferase, and patients with von Hippel–Lindau syndrome, who often have normal adrenaline levels even when their tumour is small. By contrast, in patients with multiple endocrine neoplasia (MEN) an elevated plasma adrenaline concentration is the first biochemical abnormality. Usually the normal adrenal predominance of adrenaline over noradrenaline is reversed as the tumour enlarges. Occasionally even large tumours secrete mainly adrenaline if either the tumour's centre is infarcted, leaving a rim still exposed to cortical cortisol supply, or the tumour itself is secreting ACTH or corticotrophin releasing factor (CRF). This secretion may be triggered by α-blocker therapy, and typical Cushing's features are then absent (as with any ectopic ACTH tumour).

Phaeochromocytomas often secrete one or more neuropeptides: somatostatin may exaggerate the episodic nature of catecholamine discharge by inhibiting catecholamine release as soon as a discharge starts, and it may also contribute to a reversible form of diabetes in phaeochromocytoma.

Suppression tests

The use of plasma or urine metanephrine measurements, in a reliable laboratory, has reduced the number of patients with ambiguous results. In deciding which of the 'grey zone' patients need further investigations, it is also helpful to remember that modest increases in noradrenaline secretion are usually insufficient to cause severe hypertension. This is partly because of receptor (and postreceptor) desensitization, and partly volume depletion consequent on pressure natriuresis. Where doubt about the diagnosis remains, a pharmacological suppression test can be performed prior to imaging. Whereas physiological elevations of noradrenaline release are temporarily suppressed by administration of the ganglion-blocking drug pentolinium, or the centrally acting α_2-agonist clonidine, these drugs do not suppress autonomous secretion by tumour.

Pentolinium should not be used in patients with an eGFR less than 60 ml/min. After the patient has rested supine for 30 min, plasma catecholamines are measured in two baseline samples taken 5 min apart from an intravenous cannula, and in two further samples taken 10 and 20 min after an intravenous bolus of pentolinium 2.5 mg. Patients should remain supine for a further 60 min, and their erect arterial pressure checked before they are allowed to leave the clinic. A normal response to pentolinium is a fall of both plasma noradrenaline and adrenaline concentrations into the normal range, or by 50% from baseline. However, there may be little fall in plasma catecholamine values when the basal levels are already within the normal range.

In the clonidine test, blood is taken hourly for 3 h before and after oral administration of clonidine 300 μg. Plasma noradrenaline or normetanephrine should fall by 50%, but adrenaline is little affected. Clonidine is more useful than pentolinium for patients with normal basal levels of noradrenaline or normetanephrine.

Localization of phaeochromocytomas

A substantial clue to localization is provided by measurement of plasma adrenaline (or metadrenaline) or fractionated urinary metanephrines (as stated previously, extra-adrenal tumours rarely produce adrenaline). CT or MRI scanning provides excellent imaging of the adrenal, where 90% of phaeochromocytomas are found (Fig. 17.3.12). They are usually much larger than Conn's tumours, and may appear heterogeneous.

It is best to withhold CT/MRI scanning for extra-adrenal phaeochromocytomas until the radiologist can be given some clue as to where to concentrate. This can be achieved by radioisotope scanning with the iodinated analogue of noradrenaline, m-iodobenzylguanidine (mIBG), in about 85% of patients. This may carry either an [123I] or [131I] label, the former being more sensitive but also more expensive, and may be misinterpreted if users are unaware that normal adrenal glands also accumulate mIBG. There is a case for undertaking mIBG scanning in addition to CT, even for patients found to have an adrenal phaeochromocytoma, to identify extra-adrenal secondary deposits when tumours are malignant, and because there may be coexisting adrenal and extra-adrenal phaeochromocytomas. PET scans have been used and may be positive when mIBG is unhelpful. ^{18}F-DOPA appears to be the most accurate of these, but available only when there is a centre doing neurological research for which a routine supply of this radiotracer is required. ^{68}Ga-DOTANOC, a somatostatin receptor analogue, is acquiring a reputation for higher sensitivity than mIBG, with good specificity.

Selective venous sampling remains of occasional value when diagnostic problems persist. About 25 samples of blood are collected under fluoroscopic guidance from various sites, with an arterial sample invaluable for interpreting the results because it enables sites with a positive venoarterial difference to be readily detected. Because of the short half-life of catecholamines in the circulation (c.1 min), the concentration at the tumour site is usually several-fold greater than elsewhere. This procedure should not usually be used for adrenal phaeochromocytomas, an exception being patients with von Hippel–Lindau syndrome with small adrenal masses, in whom all other biochemical tests may be normal, and the diagnosis of phaeochromocytoma is suggested by a reversal of the normal excess of adrenaline to noradrenaline in the adrenal vein.

Because phaeochromocytomas are vascular tumours, they provide a good tumour blush, and occasionally angiography is required

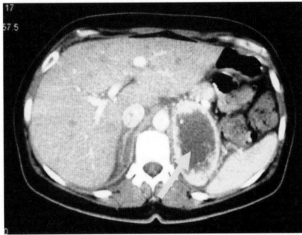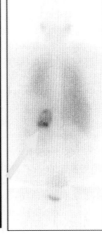

Fig. 17.3.12) CT (left) and m-iodobenzylguanidine (mIBG) scan (right) of a patient with a left adrenal phaeochromocytoma. Both scans illustrate typical nonhomogeneous appearance due to large area of haemorrhage/infarction at the centre of the tumour.

to resolve equivocal scans. Patients must be fully α-blocked and preferably also β-blocked prior to angiography.

Other investigations

It is important to check blood glucose in every patient as there may be α-mediated inhibition of insulin release prior to effective treatment, and all patients should be screened for an associated medullary carcinoma of the thyroid. Routine slit lamp examination of the fundi has resulted in more frequent diagnosis of von Hippel–Lindau syndrome, sometimes as a *de novo* occurrence.

Treatment

Medical management before surgery

The definitive treatment for phaeochromocytoma is surgical, with laparoscopic surgery possible for most adrenal tumours. Even the small number of phaeochromocytomas that are recognized to be malignant preoperatively (e.g. by the presence of bone or liver metastases) may still benefit from resection of the primary tumour. The task for the physician is to make surgery safe, for which the mainstay of medical treatment is α-blockade, but not all patients—especially those without elevated plasma adrenaline levels—require β-blockade. The objective of treatment is not solely control of blood pressure, but also the expansion of blood volume, which is invariably reduced. Indeed, phaeochromocytoma represents the pure vasoconstriction end of the vasoconstriction-volume spectrum, and the hypertensive patient is best seen as the exception where pressure natriuresis has failed to compensate adequately for vasoconstriction. Normotension is an indication, not contraindication, for the use of α-blockade to restore volume preoperatively.

The α-blocker of choice is phenoxybenzamine, which is an irreversible blocker that actually destroys the α-receptor by alkylation. More modern α-blockers, such as doxazosin, and the mixed α- and β-blocker labetalol (a much stronger β-blocker than it is α-blocker), cause competitive blockade, which can be overcome by a surge of noradrenaline release from the tumour. An additional advantage of phenoxybenzamine is that it will block both α_1- and α_2-receptors, with blockade of the latter possibly advantageous because extrasynaptic α_2-receptors mediate some of the direct vasoconstriction caused by circulating (non-neuronal) catecholamines. The diabetogenic effect of catecholamines is also an α_2-mediated response. The starting dose of phenoxybenzamine is 10 mg once or twice daily, with increases titrated against blood pressure up to a maximum of 90 mg daily. The effect of irreversible antagonists is cumulative, with the effect of the drug—and each subsequent dose increment—taking several days to reach maximum.

There is rarely any urgency for surgery, which should not normally be considered in less than 1 month after initiation of treatment in patients with symptomatic phaeochromocytomas. Indeed, the more severe the initial clinical picture, the greater the need for prolonged α-blockade to expand intravascular volume. In most patients there is a low filling pressure at presentation, evident clinically as a jugular venous pressure visible only when the patient lies flat, and any postural hypotension should be assumed to reflect continuing hypovolaemia, not excessive α-blockade, until the venous pressure is normalized. Usually volume expansion will occur spontaneously with phenoxybenzamine treatment, but expansion should be achieved with intravenous saline if there is persistent hypovolaemia when patients are admitted a few

days before surgery. During the preoperative admission the dose of phenoxybenzamine should be increased until there is at least a 10 mmHg postural fall in blood pressure.

The need for β-blockade is indicated by tachycardia, which may become apparent only after treatment with phenoxybenzamine, and the dose of β-blocking drug necessary is generally lower than that used in the treatment of hypertension. It is usually better to use a β_1-selective agent so that the peripheral vasodilatation mediated by β_2-receptors is not affected. Occasionally, pronounced β_2-receptor mediated effects, including tachycardia or tremor, can oblige use of a nonselective β-blocker, although blood pressure control may then be more difficult and require addition of a calcium blocker. The reason for using as low a dose of β-blocker as possible is that there may be a period of hypotension immediately upon removal of the phaeochromocytoma, despite the preoperative preparation that has been outlined. This hypotension should normally be offset by the ability to mount a tachycardia. The correct treatment is by volume replacement, supplemented if necessary by β-agonists, most vasoconstrictor drugs being ineffective because of the slow washout of phenoxybenzamine.

Malignant phaeochromocytomas

The treatment of malignant phaeochromocytomas remains uncertain and unsatisfactory. The rate of growth is usually slow, but the prognosis for affected individuals can vary between the extremes of local recurrence at intervals of many years, and rapid demise sometimes precipitated by surgery. The tumours are not particularly sensitive either to chemotherapy or to radiotherapy, although the variability of response may still make them worth trying. There has been interest in the use of therapeutic doses of mIBG as a means of targeting high doses of radioactivity to the tumour: some patients show considerable regression after such treatment, but long-term results are less certain.

It is rare for the pharmacological effects of the tumour to be the principal problem if the primary tumour has been removed or debulked. High doses of phenoxybenzamine are preferable to α-methyltyrosine, used as an inhibitor of noradrenaline synthesis. There is anecdotal evidence that therapy with high doses of an ARB might slow progression through reflex activation of renin and hence AT_2-receptor mediated apoptosis.

Prognosis and genetic screening

Most (90%) phaeochromocytomas are benign, and the proportion is probably even higher for adrenal tumours, whereas those that are extra-adrenal have a greater than 10% likelihood of proving malignant. The latter should be screened for mutations in the *SDHB* gene, which carry greater than 50% risk of malignancy. Other genetic screening will be influenced by a mixture of clinical features and cost considerations. A history (or family history) of other relevant tumours will lead to a search for von Hippel–Lindau syndrome or MEN type 2. There is some consensus that all patients presenting under the age of 45 years should have structured genetic counselling and screening, and this is particularly important in much younger patients. All patients should be followed indefinitely with at least an annual measurement of arterial pressure and analysis of one of the indices of catecholamine secretion, as mentioned previously. The removal of a phaeochromocytoma cures hypertension in most patients, especially those that are young.

Other endocrine causes of hypertension

Conn's syndrome and phaeochromocytoma have been singled out for attention in this chapter as the two endocrine conditions most likely to present as hypertension. However, hypertension is a feature of several other endocrinopathies: Cushing's syndrome, acromegaly, hyperparathyroidism, and is a common complication of type 2 diabetes. The hypertension of Cushing's syndrome is usually modest, except in ectopic ACTH where there is saturation by high cortisol levels of 11β-hydroxysteroid dehydrogenase 2 (which normally converts cortisol to the inactive cortisone). The cause of the hypertension in other syndromes is less clear cut and often not corrected by surgical cure of the primary problem.

Further reading

Primary hyperaldosteronism

Brown MJ, Hopper RV (1999). Calcium-channel blockade can mask the diagnosis of Conn's syndrome. *Postgrad Med J*, **75**, 235–6.

Choi M, et al. (2011). K+ channel mutations in adrenal aldosterone-producing adenomas and hereditary hypertension. *Science*, **331**(6018), 768–72.

Dluhy RG, Lifton RP (1999). Glucocorticoid-remediable aldosteronism. *J Clin Endocrinol Metab*, **84**, 4341–4.

Ganguly A (1998). Primary aldosteronism. *N Engl J Med*, **339**, 1828–34.

Gordon RD, et al. (1994). High incidence of primary aldosteronism in 199 patients referred with hypertension. *Clin Exp Pharmacol Physiol*, **21**, 315–18.

Hood SJ, et al. (2007). The Spironolactone, Amiloride, Losartan, and Thiazide (SALT) double-blind crossover trial in patients with low-renin hypertension and elevated aldosterone-renin ratio. *Circulation*, **116**, 268–75.

Kaplan NM (2004). The current epidemic of primary aldosteronism: causes and consequences. *J Hypertens*, **22**, 863–9.

Mir FA, Brown MJ, Appleton DS (2007). Lessons in the diagnosis and management of Conn's syndrome. *Clin Med*, **7**, 530–2.

Mulatero P, et al. (2006). Comparison of confirmatory tests for the diagnosis of primary aldosteronism. *J Clin Endocrinol Metab*, **91**, 2618–23.

Rossi GP, et al. (2006). A prospective study of the prevalence of primary aldosteronism in 1,125 hypertensive patients. *J Am Coll Cardiol*, **48**, 2293–300.

Stewart PM (1999). Mineralocorticoid hypertension. *Lancet*, **353**, 1341–7.

Stowasser M, et al. (2003). High rate of detection of primary aldosteronism, including surgically treatable forms, after 'non-selective' screening of hypertensive patients. *J Hypertens*, **21**, 2149–57.

Young WF Jr (2007). The incidentally discovered adrenal mass. *N Engl J Med*, **356**, 601–10.

Renovascular hypertension and coarctation

Caliezi C, Reber P (2006). Images in clinical medicine. Fibromuscular dysplasia of the renal artery. *N Engl J Med*, **355**, 2131.

Rosenthal E (2005). Coarctation of the aorta from fetus to adult: curable condition or lifelong disease process? *Heart*, **91**, 1495–502.

Safian RD, Textor SC (2001). Renal-artery stenosis. *N Engl J Med*, **344**, 431–42.

White CJ (2006). Catheter-based therapy for atherosclerotic renal artery stenosis. *Circulation*, **113**, 1464–73.

Phaeochromocytoma

Allison DJ, et al. (1983). Role of venous sampling in locating a phaeochromocytoma. *BMJ*, **286**, 1122–4.

Brown MJ, et al. (1981). Increased sensitivity and accuracy of phaeochromocytoma diagnosis achieved by use of plasma epinephrine estimations and a pentolinium suppression test. *Lancet*, **i**, 174–7.

Brown MJ, et al. (2009). Phaeochromocytoma. *Horm Metab Res*, **41**, 655–7.

Col V, et al. (1999). Laparoscopic adrenalectomy for phaeochromocytoma: endocrinological and surgical aspects of a new therapeutic approach. *Clin Endocrinol (Oxf)*, **50**, 121–5.

Manger WM (1997). Pheochromocytoma. Springer Verlag, Berlin.

Richards FM, et al. (1998). Molecular genetic analysis of von Hippel-Lindau disease. *J Intern Med*, **243**, 527–33.

Sisson JC, Shulkin BL (1999). Nuclear medicine imaging of pheochromocytoma and neuroblastoma. *Q J Nucl Med*, **43**, 217–23.

CHAPTER 17.4

Mendelian disorders causing hypertension

Nilesh J. Samani and Maciej Tomaszewski

Essentials

Several mendelian disorders with hypertension as the predominant manifestation have been characterized at the molecular level. Features that may suggest one of these very rare conditions include a young age of onset, moderate to severe hypertension, strong family history, consanguinity (for the autosomal recessive disorders), and electrolyte abnormalities, particularly of potassium (although this is not invariable).

Glucocorticoid-remediable aldosteronism—an autosomal dominant condition caused by a chimeric gene where the regulatory elements of the 11β-hydroxylase gene become attached to the coding region of aldosterone synthase. Hypertension responds to a low daily dose of exogenous glucocorticoid.

Apparent mineralocorticoid excess—an autosomal recessive disorder caused by mutations causing loss of function in the type 2 11β-hydroxysteroid dehydrogenase gene that normally inactivates cortisol in the kidney and prevents it binding to the mineralocorticoid receptor. Hypertension responds to spironolactone.

Liddle's syndrome—an autosomal dominant condition caused by activating mutations in genes encoding the β- or γ-subunits of the trimeric epithelial sodium channel. Hypertension responds to direct inhibitors triamterene or amiloride.

Pseudohypoaldosteronism type 2 (PHA2, Gordon's syndrome)—an autosomal dominant condition, caused by mutations in the *WNK1* or *WNK4* serine-threonine kinases genes, the Kelch-like 3 (*KLHL3*) gene or the cullin 3 (*CUL3*) gene. These genes regulate salt reabsorption by the Na-Cl cotransporter (SLC12A3) and the linked process of potassium secretion by the renal outer medullary potassium channel (ROMK). The hypertension and physiological abnormalities are corrected by thiazide diuretics.

Introduction

Several rare mendelian disorders where hypertension is the predominant manifestation have been characterized at the molecular level (Box 17.4.1). These include glucocorticoid-remediable aldosteronism, the syndrome of apparent mineralocorticoid excess, Liddle's syndrome, and Gordon's syndrome. Hypertension and hypokalaemia are features of 11β-hydroxylase and 17β-hydroxylase deficiency—two rare recessive gene disorders of adrenal steroid-synthesizing enzymes that, among others, cause congenital adrenal hyperplasia. 11β-Hydroxylase deficiency usually presents in infancy or early childhood with virilization of both sexes, while presentation of 17β-hydroxylase deficiency may be delayed until adolescence or adulthood. Hypertension due to a phaeochromocytoma may be a feature of multiple endocrine neoplasia type 2 (MEN2, Sipple's syndrome), which when familial is inherited in an autosomal dominant pattern, or rarely to be a feature of neurofibromatosis (von Recklinghausen's disease).

Glucocorticoid-remediable aldosteronism

Glucocorticoid-remediable aldosteronism (GRA, OMIM 103900) is a form of mineralocorticoid hypertension that is inherited in an autosomal dominant fashion. The hypertension is accompanied by hypokalaemia (not invariably), a tendency to metabolic alkalosis, an elevated plasma aldosterone level and a suppressed renin level. Patients are usually suspected of having primary aldosteronism (Conn's syndrome, see Chapter 17.3), although the age of onset,

---

Box 17.4.1 Mendelian forms of blood pressure variation

Hypertension

- Glucocorticoid-remediable aldosteronism (GRA)
- Syndrome of apparent mineralocorticoid excess (AME)
- Liddle's syndrome
- Gordon's syndrome (pseudohypoaldosteronism type II, PHA-II)
- Hypertension exacerbated by pregnancy
- 11β-Hydroxylase deficiency
- 17β-Hydroxylase deficiency
- Multiple endocrine neoplasia type 2 with phaeochromocytoma

Hypotension

- Pseudohypoaldosteronism type 1
- Gitleman's syndrome
- Bartter syndrome
- 11β-hydroxylase deficiency
- Aldosterone synthase deficiency

usually in the first two decades of life, is younger than typical of primary aldosteronism. Intracranial aneurysms are common and the first manifestation may be a presentation with intracranial haemorrhage.

The two hallmark features of GRA are the presence of large amounts of two abnormal steroids—18-hydroxycortisol and 18-oxocortisol—in the urine, and the paradoxical response of the hypertension, with return of plasma aldosterone to a normal level and disappearance of the abnormal steroids, following treatment over a few days with a low daily dose of exogenous glucocorticoid, e.g. 0.5 to 1.0 mg of dexamethasone (hence the name).

Patients with GRA have a chimeric gene due to an unequal crossing-over event at meiosis between two adjacent and highly homologous genes involved in adrenocorticosteroid synthesis—aldosterone synthase (*CYP11B2*) (normally expressed only in the zona glomerulosa, involved in aldosterone synthesis and regulated by angiotensin II) and 11β-hydroxylase (*CYP11B1*) (expressed in the zona fasciculata, involved in glucocorticoid synthesis and regulated by ACTH). In the chimeric gene, the regulatory elements of *CYP11B1* have become attached to the aldosterone synthase coding region of *CYP11B2* (Fig. 17.4.1a). This leads to ACTH-driven production of aldosterone (and the other abnormal hormones) in the zona fasciculata, hence the clinical syndrome and its suppression by glucocorticoids.

The mainstay of treatment for GRA is glucocorticoids, with physiological doses (or only slightly higher, e.g. 0.125 mg of dexamethasone or 2.5 mg of prednisolone daily) sufficing. Response can be monitored by measuring the suppression of aldosterone production. Selective mineralocorticoid receptor blockers, such as spironolactone, can provide useful adjunctive treatment.

Syndrome of apparent mineralocorticoid excess

The syndrome of apparent mineralocorticoid excess (AME, OMIM 218030) is an autosomal recessive disorder that usually presents in childhood with hypertension, hypokalaemia, and low renin activity. Despite the clinical features of mineralocorticoid excess, levels of all known mineralocorticoid hormones are low, yet the hypertension responds to spironolactone or amiloride. Patients with the disorder cannot metabolize cortisol to its inactive metabolite cortisone normally, resulting in a prolonged half-life of cortisol and a characteristic increase in urinary cortisol (compound F) compared with cortisone (compound E) ratio.

Elucidating the defect causing AME first required the solution of another paradox—why cortisol, which circulates at a level several-fold greater than aldosterone, does not overwhelmingly activate the renal mineralocorticoid receptor *in vivo* despite the two having equal affinity *in vitro*. The reason relates to the enzyme 11β-hydroxysteroid dehydrogenase (11β-HSD), which has two isoforms. Type 1 11β-HSD is located in the liver, adipose tissue, muscle, pancreatic islets, and gonad and converts cortisone to cortisol. Type 2 11β-HSD is expressed in the mineralocorticoid target tissues—kidney, colon, and salivary gland—and inactivates cortisol to cortisone. In the kidney the enzyme plays the crucial role of protecting the mineralcorticoid receptor on the distal tubule from activation by cortisol. In subjects with AME a variety of loss-of-function mutations in the type 2 11β-HSD gene cause a deficiency of the enzyme, allowing cortisol access to the mineralocorticoid receptor (Fig. 17.4.1b).

The severe form of AME, due to disabling mutations in type 2 11β-HSD, usually presents in childhood. Recently a milder form, termed AME type II, has been described, which is characterized by a later age of presentation (>30 years), a more variable degree of hypertension, and less impact on biochemical parameters. These patients have alterations in 11β-HSD2 that produce a partial rather than absolute decrease in enzymatic activity, hence classification into distinct subcategories may be inappropriate, with AME best regarded as a spectrum of mineralocorticoid hypertension with severity reflecting the underlying genetic defect. The mainstay of treatment of AME is spironolactone. A low-salt diet is also important.

AME resembles the syndrome observed in subjects ingesting large amounts of liquorice or taking the now redundant antiulcer drug carbenoxolone, both of which contain glycyrrhetinic acid, an inhibitor of type 2 11β-HSD, thus explaining the hypertension and hypokalaemia observed with these compounds. Spillover access of cortisol to the mineralocorticoid receptor may also, at least partly, explain the hypertension accompanying some forms of Cushing's syndrome and glucocorticoid resistance.

Liddle's syndrome

Liddle described a family in which the siblings were affected by early-onset hypertension and hypokalaemia, but with low renin and aldosterone levels (OMIM 177200). The clue to the nature of the molecular defect underlying this autosomal dominant disorder came from the observation that the hypertension does not respond to spironolactone, the mineralocorticoid receptor antagonist, but does respond to direct inhibitors (such as triamterene or amiloride) of the trimeric epithelial sodium channel—a key channel responsible for sodium reabsorption in the distal nephron. Subsequent work revealed activating mutations in genes (*SCNN1B*, *SCNN1G*) encoding the β- or γ-subunits of the channel (Fig. 17.4.1c), All mutations so far identified cause an alteration or deletion of a proline-rich (PY) motif in the C-terminal cytoplasmic tails of the subunits that is necessary for regulatory proteins such as Nedd4 to bind and internalize the channel. When this mechanism is impaired, the number of channels located in the apical membrane is increased, leading to over-reabsorption of sodium and water.

Pseudohypoaldosteronism type 2 (Gordon's syndrome)

Pseudohypoaldosteronism type 2 (PHA2, OMIM 145260), also known as Gordon's syndrome, is an autosomal dominant disorder that causes elevated blood pressure accompanied by hyperkalaemia, despite normal renal glomerular filtration. Mild hyperchloraemia, metabolic acidosis, and suppressed plasma renin activity are common associated findings. Hypercalciuria can also be a feature, leading to osteopenia, osteoporosis, and kidney stone disease. The hypertension and biochemical abnormalities are corrected by thiazide diuretics.

Mutations in at least four genes are recognized causes of PHA2. Initially some cases of PHA2 were linked to mutations in two genes, *WNK1* and *WNK4*, members of the WNK family of serine-threonine kinases. The genetic defects in both *WNK1* and *WNK4*,

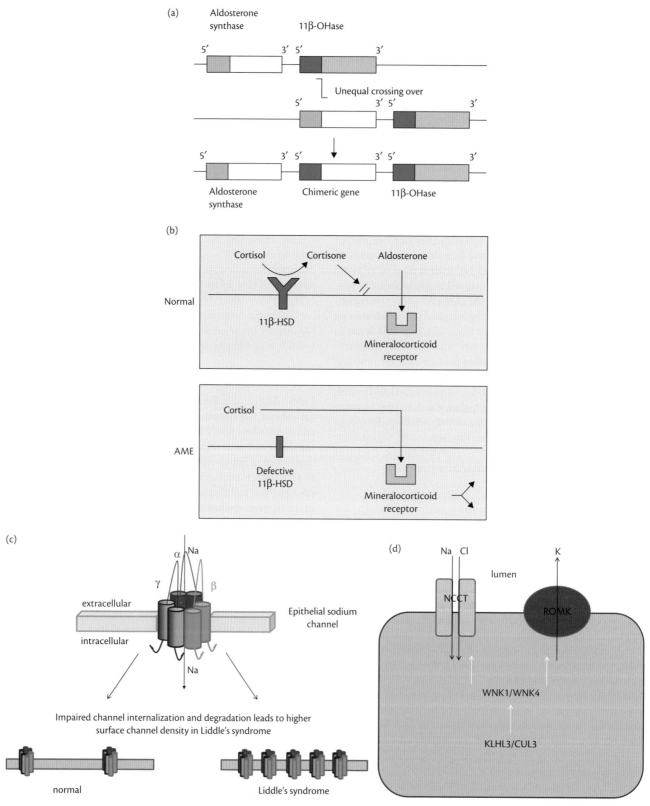

Fig. 17.4.1 Mechanisms underlying four forms of monogenetic hypertension. (a) Glucocorticoid-remediable aldosteronism (GRA). In GRA an unequal crossing event leads to a chimaeric gene where the coding region of aldosterone synthase becomes attached to the regulatory region for 11β-hydroxylase. The chimaeric gene produces excess amounts of aldosterone under the regulation of ACTH. (b) Syndrome of apparent mineralocorticoid excess (AME). The mineralocorticoid receptor in the distal renal tubule is normally protected from stimulation by cortisol by the activity of the 11β-hydroxysteroid dehydrogenase enzyme. In AME, mutations in the enzyme allow cortisol to gain access to the receptor. (c) Liddle's syndrome. The trimeric epithelial sodium channel mediates sodium reuptake in the distal renal tubule. In Liddle's syndrome, mutations in the β and γ subunits of the channel impair its intracellular biodegradation and lead to excessive channel density and activity on the surface of distal renal tubular epithelium. (d) Gordon's syndrome. WNK1 and WNK4 regulate thiazide-sensitive sodium-chloride cotransporter (NCCT) and potassium secretion via ROMK in the distal nephron. Mutations in WNK1/WNK4 or genes responsible for their intracellular degradation (KLHL3 and CUL3) lead to increased sodium reabsorption via overactive NCCT and impaired potassium secretion through ROMK.

by increasing their expression/activity in the distal nephron, lead to enhanced phosphorylation of two other enzymes, STE20/SPS1-related proline-alanine-rich protein kinase (SPAK) and oxidative stress-responsive kinase-1 (OSR1). Both SPAK and OSR1 are key regulators of the Na-Cl cotransporter, NCCT (encoded by the *SLC12A3* gene), which is responsible for sodium reabsorption in the distal convoluted tubule and the linked process of potassium secretion by the renal outer medullary potassium channel (ROMK). Na-Cl cotransporter overactivity is the chief biochemical abnormality of the syndrome and the primary driver of enhanced sodium reabsorption, volume expansion, inhibition of renin secretion, and hypertension.

Decreased potassium excretion leading to hyperkalaemia in PHA2 results from two processes. Firstly, increased Na-Cl cotransporter activity, by increasing sodium reabsorption in the distal convoluted tubule, leads to reduced sodium delivery to the connecting tubule, which results in a drop in electrochemical gradient necessary to maintain activity of ROMK channels that transfer K⁺ from blood to urine across the distal tubule epithelium. Secondly, enhanced internalization of ROMK channels in PHA2 leads to their decreased expression/activity on the surface of tubular epithelium.

More recently, mutations in two novel genes, *Kelch-like 3* (*KLHL3*) and *Cullin 3* (*CUL3*), were reported to account for a majority (≈80%) of causal genetic defects in patients with PHA2. The mutations are inherited in either autosomal dominant (*KLHL3* and *CUL3*) or recessive (*KLHL3*) manner. The products of both genes are a part of ubiquitin ligase complex responsible for intracellular degradation of more than 50 proteins, including WNKs. The most likely molecular mechanism by which genetic defects in these genes lead to PHA2 is disruption of WNKs intracellular degradation and accumulation of WNK4/WNK1 and subsequent changes in the activity of Na-Cl cotransporter /ROMK channel.

The Na-Cl transporter is the target for thiazide diuretics, which explains the specific clinical response of PHA2 to this class of drugs. Defects in the Na-Cl cotransporter lead to the salt-losing Gitelman's syndrome, which as described below is the mirror image of PHA2.

Other monogenetic forms of hypertension

A missense mutation in the ligand-binding domain of the mineralocorticoid receptor has been found to cause an autosomal dominant form of hypertension that is markedly accelerated in pregnancy. The mutation, *MR S810L*, causes partial, aldosterone-independent activation of the receptor, causing carriers to develop hypertension before age 20. Compounds such as progesterone that normally bind to but do not activate the mineralocorticoid receptor are all potent agonists of the mutant receptor, hence *MR S810L* carriers have dramatic acceleration of hypertension during pregnancy stimulated by the 100-fold rise in progesterone. Although the *MR S810L* mutation is extremely rare, the finding does raise the question of whether related mechanisms may underlie other forms of hypertension in pregnancy.

Genetic defects causing hypotension

A number of mendelian syndromes where hypotension is a feature have recently been characterized at the molecular level (Table 17.4.1). Many are mirror images of the genetic abnormalities causing the mendelian forms of hypertension described above.

Table 17.4.1 Biochemical and therapeutic characteristics of glucocorticoid-remediable aldosteronism (GRA), syndrome of apparent mineralocorticoid excess (AME), Liddle's syndrome, and Gordon's syndrome

	GRA	AME	Liddle's	Gordon's
Plasma electrolytes	↑Na ↓K	↑Na ↓K	↑Na ↓K	↑Na ↑K
Plasma aldosterone	↑	↓	↓	↑↓
Plasma renin	↓	↓	↓	↓
Specific treatment	Dexamethasone	Spironolactone	Amiloride	Thiazide

Note that while the biochemical changes are characteristic, they are not invariably present.

Pseudohypoaldosteronism type 1 (PHA1) occurs in two forms, autosomal recessive and autosomal dominant. Both are characterized by life-threatening dehydration in the neonatal period, hypotension, salt wasting, hyperkalaemia, metabolic acidosis, and marked elevation of renin and aldosterone. The autosomal recessive form (OMIM 264350) is due to inactivating mutations (compare with Liddle's syndrome) in one of the genes *SCNN1A*, *SCCN1B*, or *SCNN1G*, encoding (respectively) the α, β, and γ subunits of the epithelial sodium channel, while the autosomal dominant form (OMIM 177735) is due to loss-of-function mutations in the gene *NR3C2*, encoding the mineralocorticoid receptor.

Gitelman's syndrome (OMIM 263800) is an autosomal recessive disorder characterized by hypotension, neuromuscular abnormalities, hypokalaemia, hypomagnesaemia, hypocalciuria, metabolic alkalosis, and an activated renin–angiotensin system. It arises due to inactivating mutations in the gene encoding the renal thiazide-sensitive Na-Cl cotransporter (*SLC12A3*), and typically presents in adolescence or early adulthood with neuromuscular signs and symptoms.

Bartter's syndrome is caused by mutations in one or more of the genes that encode regulators of chloride transport within the thick ascending limb of nephron. There are several types of Bartter's syndrome. The gene defects responsible are in genes encoding bumetanide-sensitive sodium-(potassium)-chloride cotransporter 2 (*SLC12A1*) (type 1, OMIM 601678), ATP-regulated potassium channel ROMK (*KCNJ1*) (type 2, OMIM 241200), chloride channel Kb (*CLCNKB*) (type 3, OMIM 607364), barttin (*BSDN*) (type 4a, OMIM 602522), and both *CLCNKA* and *CLCNKB* genes (type 4b, OMIM 613090).

The manifestation of these autosomal recessive disorders is heterogeneous, but the most typical clinical presentations include early onset (infancy or childhood), hypovolaemia and polyuria, low or normal blood pressure, elevated prostaglandin levels and nephrocalcinosis. The recently identified Bartter-like syndrome occurring in subjects with mutations in the *CASR* gene (which encodes extracellular basolateral calcium sensing receptor) manifests as hypocalcemic hypercalciuria.

Does my patient have a recognized form of monogenetic hypertension?

Identification that a patient has GRA, AME, Liddle's syndrome, or Gordon's syndrome has important consequences for treatment

(Table 17.4.1) and family screening. Phenotypic expression is highly variable, but all of the syndromes are extremely rare and suspicion will usually go unrewarded. Features that may suggest a diagnosis of mendelian hypertension include a young age of onset, moderate to severe hypertension, strong family history, consanguinity (for the autosomal recessive disorders), and electrolyte abnormalities, particularly of potassium (although this is not invariable). A good starting point, as described in Chapter 17.3, is the measurement of plasma renin activity and plasma aldosterone. If the aldosterone is significantly elevated then the differential diagnosis lies between the various forms of Conn's syndrome and GRA. Diagnosis of GRA would be supported by the finding of elevated 18-hydroxycortisol and 18-oxocortisol in the urine, and a positive dexamethasone suppression test, suppression of plasma aldosterone levels to less than 4 ng/dl with 0.75 to 2.0 mg/day for at least 2 days being reported to have a greater than 90% specificity and sensitivity for the diagnosis, and GRA can now also be relatively easily confirmed by finding a chimeric gene fragment with DNA testing.

If the aldosterone level is suppressed, then finding an increased ratio of cortisol/cortisone metabolites in the urine would support a diagnosis of AME. The presence of hyperkalaemia, hyperchloraemia, and metabolic acidosis would suggest a diagnosis of Gordon's syndrome. No biochemical abnormalities specifically support a diagnosis of Liddle's syndrome, but it typically presents with hyporeninaemic hypoaldosteronism. Ultimately, diagnosis of AME, Liddle's syndrome, and Gordon's syndrome also requires DNA confirmation, but this is not as straightforward as it is with GRA since several different mutations can give rise to each syndrome.

Further reading

Boyden LM, *et al.* (2012). Mutations in kelch-like 3 and cullin 3 cause hypertension and electrolyte abnormalities. *Nature*, **482**(7383), 98–102.

Geller DS, *et al.* (2000). Activating mineralocorticoid receptor mutation in hypertension exacerbated by pregnancy. *Science*, **289**, 119–23.

Lifton RP, *et al.* (1992). A chimaeric 11β-hydroxylase/aldosterone synthase gene causes glucocorticoid-remediable aldosteronism and human hypertension. *Nature*, **355**, 262–65.

Lifton RP, *et al.* (2001). Molecular mechanisms of human hypertension. *Cell*, **104**, 545–56.

Mune T, *et al.* (1995). Human hypertension caused by mutations in the kidney isozyme of 11β-hydroxysteroid dehydrogenase. *Nat Genet*, **10**, 394–9.

Shimkets RA, *et al.* (1994). Liddle's syndrome: Heritable human hypertension caused by mutations in the β subunit of the epithelial sodium channel. *Cell*, **79**, 407–14.

Wilson FH, *et al.* (2001). Human hypertension caused by mutations in WNK kinases. *Science*, **293**, 1107–12.

CHAPTER 17.5

Hypertensive urgencies and emergencies

Gregory Y. H. Lip and D. Gareth Beevers

Essentials

Hypertensive urgencies and emergencies occur most commonly in patients with previous hypertension, especially if inadequately managed. About 40% of cases have an underlying cause, most commonly renovascular disease, primary renal diseases, phaeochromocytoma, and connective tissue disorders. Hypertensive emergencies occur when severely elevated or sudden marked increase in blood pressure is associated with acute end-organ damage.

The key pathophysiological process is intense peripheral vasoconstriction, resulting in a rapid rise in blood pressure and a vicious circle of events, including ischaemia of the brain and peripheral organs.

Hypertensive urgencies

Malignant phase hypertension is a rare condition (1–3 per 100 000 per year, more common in black people) characterized by very high blood pressure, with bilateral retinal haemorrhages and/or exudates or cotton wool spots, with or without papilloedema.

Presentation is typically with visual disturbance, with or without headaches. Urinalysis may demonstrate proteinuria and haematuria, even in the absence of primary renal disease. Some patients with mild renal impairment at first presentation may improve, or even regain normal renal function, but this is unlikely to occur in those with more severe renal impairment at presentation.

Patients with severe hypertension who are asymptomatic require controlled reduction in blood pressure with oral antihypertensive agents. Over-rapid blood pressure reduction may be hazardous, leading on occasion to ischaemic complications such as stroke, myocardial infarction, or blindness. The maximum initial fall in blood pressure should not exceed 25% of the presenting value, with the initial aim of treatment being to lower the diastolic pressure to about 100 to 105 mmHg over a period of 2 to 3 days. The first-line oral antihypertensive agent is either a short-acting calcium antagonist (such as nifedipine, 10–20 mg of the tablet formulation: sublingual or capsular preparations should never be used) or a β-blocker (such as atenolol, 25 mg initial dose).

Hypertensive emergencies

Patients who are symptomatic with acute life-threatening complications of severe hypertension, such as hypertensive encephalopathy, hypertensive left ventricular failure, or aortic dissection, require parenteral antihypertensive therapy to promptly reduce the blood pressure in a carefully controlled manner. Blood pressure should be reduced by 25% over several hours, depending on the clinical situation, usually with a target diastolic blood pressure of less than 100 to 110 mmHg. The first-line treatment for most hypertensive emergencies is either intravenous sodium nitroprusside or intravenous labetalol, with β-blockade essential in patients with aortic dissection.

Hypertensive emergencies and urgencies carry a poor short- and long-term prognosis unless adequately managed. Initial over-rapid reduction of blood pressure to a normal value is dangerous, but—in the long term—blood pressure should eventually be reduced to accepted blood pressure targets.

Introduction

Hypertensive emergencies occur when severe hypertension is associated with acute end-organ damage. These can take a variety of forms and can occur at any age. They may be acute life-threatening medical conditions, and are associated with either severe hypertension or sudden marked increases in blood pressure (Box 17.5.1). Symptomatic patients with complications such as aortic dissection and hypertensive encephalopathy require parenteral antihypertensive therapy to reduce the blood pressure promptly, but in a controlled manner and with careful monitoring because over-rapid treatment may in itself be hazardous, leading, on occasions, to ischaemic complications such as stroke, myocardial infarction, or blindness. Thus, in patients who have severe hypertension but are asymptomatic, slower, controlled, reduction in blood pressure should be achieved with oral antihypertensive agents, making such situations hypertensive 'urgencies' rather than 'emergencies'.

In general, there has been a decline in the incidence of hypertensive emergencies over the past 20 years in the Western world, which may possibly be the result of the more effective detection, diagnosis, and treatment of mild to moderate hypertension.

If patients with hypertensive emergencies are not recognized or treated appropriately, the mortality and morbidity can be very high, with the 1-year mortality being 70 to 90%, and the 5-year mortality 100%. With adequate blood pressure control, the 1-year and 5-year mortality rates decrease to 25 and 50%, respectively.

Hypertensive emergencies occur most commonly in patients with previous hypertension, especially if inadequately managed. Nevertheless, some patients can present with hypertensive emergencies de novo, without any previous history of hypertension.

Box 17.5.1 Hypertensive emergencies and urgencies

Hypertensive emergencies

- Hypertensive encephalopathy
- Hypertensive left ventricular failure
- Hypertension with myocardial infarction or unstable angina
- Hypertension with aortic dissection
- Severe hypertension with subarachnoid haemorrhage or stroke
- Phaeochromocytoma crisis
- Recreational drugs—amphetamines, LSD, cocaine, MDMA (ecstasy), etc.
- Perioperative hypertension
- Severe pre-eclampsia or eclampsia

Hypertensive urgencies

- Malignant hypertension
- Chronic renal failure
- Pre-eclampsia
- Severe nonmalignant hypertension

LSD, lysergic acid diethylamide; MDMA, 3,4-methylenedioxymethamphetamine.

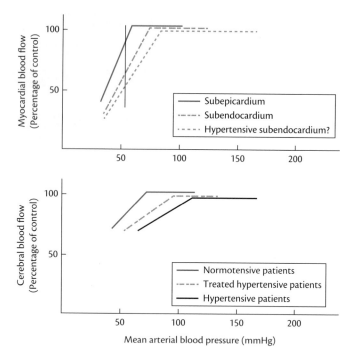

Fig. 17.5.1 Autoregulation of myocardial and cerebral blood flow in normotensive and hypertensive patients.
Reprinted from *The Lancet*, Vol. **330**, Strandgaard S and Haunsø S, Why does antihypertensive treatment prevent stroke but not myocardial infarction?, pp. 658–60. Copyright (1987), with permission from Elsevier.

Very severe and malignant hypertension are more likely to be associated with underlying causes such as renovascular disease, primary renal diseases, phaeochromocytoma, and connective tissue disorders, but malignant hypertension complicating primary hyperaldosteronism (Conn's syndrome) is very rare. About 40% of patients with malignant hypertension have an underlying cause.

Pathophysiology

The common denominator in hypertensive emergencies is intense peripheral vasoconstriction, resulting in a rapid rise in blood pressure and a vicious circle of events, including ischaemia of the brain and peripheral organs. This ischaemia stimulates neurohormone and cytokine release, exacerbating vasoconstriction and ischaemia, further increasing blood pressure, and resulting in target organ damage. In addition, myointimal proliferation in the vasculature may exacerbate the situation, as can disseminated intravascular coagulation. Also, renal ischaemia leads to activation of the renin–angiotensin system, causing further rise in blood pressure and microvascular damage.

With mild to moderate elevation of blood pressure, the initial response of the vasculature is arterial and arteriolar vasoconstriction—such autoregulation maintaining tissue perfusion at a relatively constant level and preventing the raised blood pressure from damaging smaller, more distal blood vessels. Later, arteriolar hypertrophy also minimizes the transmission of pressure to the capillary circulation. In normotensive subjects, the upper limit of autoregulation can be a mean arterial pressure of 120 mmHg (equivalent to 160/100 mmHg), but in chronic hypertension, where the vessels are hypertrophied by long-standing hypertension, the lower limit of autoregulation of cerebral blood flow is shifted towards higher blood pressures (Fig. 17.5.1), with impairment of the tolerance to acute hypotension. However, the

process of autoregulation fails with rapid and severe rises in blood pressure, leading to a rise in pressure in the arterioles and capillaries, causing vascular damage. Disruption of the endothelium allows plasma constituents (including fibrinoid material) to enter the vessel wall, narrowing or obliterating the lumen in many tissue beds, the level at which fibrinoid necrosis occurs depending upon the baseline blood pressure. In the cerebral circulation, this can lead to the development of cerebral oedema and the clinical picture of hypertensive encephalopathy.

In addition to protecting the tissues against the effects of hypertension, autoregulation maintains perfusion during the treatment of hypertension via arterial and arteriolar vasodilatation. However, falls in blood pressure below the autoregulatory range can lead to organ ischaemia, and the arteriolar hypertrophy induced by chronic hypertension means that target organ ischaemia will occur at a higher pressure than in previously normotensive subjects.

Malignant hypertension, a hypertensive 'urgency'

The malignant phase of hypertension is a rare condition characterized by very high blood pressure, with bilateral retinal haemorrhages and/or exudates or cotton wool spots, with or without papilloedema (Fig. 17.5.2). Its pathophysiological definition is based on the histological hallmark of fibrinoid necrosis of arterioles in many tissues, particularly the kidney—changes which are broadly similar to those seen in the haemolytic–uraemic syndrome or scleroderma. Mucoid intimal proliferation in renal interlobular arteries and ischaemic collapse of the glomerular tufts may also be seen. Myointimal hyperplasia is a common finding in black patients, with the consequent intrarenal vascular disease leading to ischaemia of the juxtaglomerular apparatus and activation of the

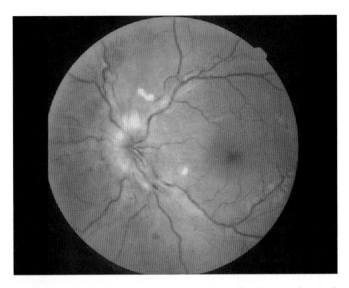

Fig. 17.5.2 Ocular fundus in hypertension, showing papilloedema, exudates, and a few haemorrhages.

renin–angiotensin system with further vasoconstriction and wall damage, as well as exacerbation of hypertension.

Epidemiology

Malignant hypertension may be becoming rarer in some countries, particularly among white populations, but it still remains a common problem in developing countries and in other populations with health and social deprivation, where it is an important cause of endstage renal failure. In west Birmingham in the United Kingdom, the incidence of malignant hypertension is around 1 to 2 per 100 000 population per year, with no clear reduction between 1970 and 2006 in the number of new cases seen, the mean duration of known hypertension before presentation, presenting blood pressures, or the number of antihypertensive drugs that were being used. These data are reinforced by an analysis from Amsterdam of 122 patients with malignant hypertension in a multiethnic population, where the incidence rate was approximately 2.6 per 100 000 per year, and was higher among blacks.

Although essential hypertension is usually the most common underlying cause of malignant hypertension in adults, secondary causes (especially renal disease) are more prevalent among younger patients, being identified in up to 40% of white and 10% of black subjects. In children (aged <16 years) with malignant hypertension, parenchymal renal disease is the commonest cause (63%), with 33% having renovascular hypertension (aortoarteritis and fibromuscular dysplasia), and only 5% with essential hypertension.

There is an association between cigarette smoking and malignant hypertension that remains unexplained. Very rarely, the oral contraceptive pill may be implicated, consistent with the well-recognized increase in blood pressure in some women taking the combined oestrogen/progesterone oral contraceptive pill. It is uncertain whether oral contraceptives cause hypertension directly, or whether they simply exaggerate a tendency in women who already have a propensity to raised blood pressure.

Malignant hypertension can occur in older people, and is more common in Afro-Caribbean than in white and Indo-Asian populations. Possible reasons for this include the relative resistance of black patients to some antihypertensive therapies and, perhaps, poorer drug compliance. In many series, black individuals had higher systolic blood pressures and more renal dysfunction than whites.

One reason for the failure of malignant hypertension to decline in some centres may be inadequate medical screening facilities among poorly educated people with a limited understanding of the nature of the disease and the need to comply with antihypertensive therapy. Any reduction in the incidence of malignant hypertension may be because increasing use of drug therapy in milder grades of hypertension prevents progression to the malignant phase. Nevertheless, it is possible that there has been no real decline in malignant hypertension, but merely a failure to recognize this life-threatening condition.

Note that the diagnosis of malignant hypertension is usually based on the association of severely elevated blood pressure with a Keith and Wagener stage III or IV retinopathy.

More recently, there is a proposal to consider that malignant hypertension with retinopathy is only one of a number of possible presentation(s) of acute hypertension with multiorgan damage, that is, hypertension multiorgan damage (MOD). Indeed, we recognise that these hypertensive emergencies, when retinopathy is lacking, is associated acute elevation of BP associated with impairment of at least three different target organs.

Clinical features

The predominant presenting symptom is visual disturbance with or without headaches, but some patients with malignant hypertension remain asymptomatic, and others present at a late stage of their disease, this proportion ranging from 10% to 75% in one series from Nigeria.

In the west Birmingham series, the presenting mean systolic and diastolic blood pressures have remained surprisingly similar over the 30 years surveyed (average blood pressure 229/142 mmHg), despite improvements in antihypertensive therapy. Heart failure, angina, or myocardial infarction are complicating features in approximately 20% of patients, and the ECG shows that many patients have cardiomegaly and left ventricular hypertrophy. Nevertheless, some patients do have normal chest radiographs, ECGs, or echocardiograms despite very high blood pressure, suggesting that hypertension may have been of recent onset.

Investigation

All patients with malignant hypertension need a detailed clinical history and examination, and investigation with blood tests (full blood count, serum biochemistry including electrolytes and renal function), 12-lead ECG, chest radiography, and urinalysis. Fundoscopy and retinal photography are mandatory. Urinalysis may demonstrate proteinuria and haematuria, even in the absence of primary renal disease, but the presence of proteinuria is a poor prognostic sign. The kidneys should be imaged by abdominal ultrasonography to assess renal size and appearance, with a low threshold for proceeding to renal angiography to look for renal artery stenosis if the kidneys are asymmetric. A 24-h urine collection is necessary for catecholamines (see Chapter 17.3) and so is protein excretion assessment in all patients (or the latter can be estimated by albumin/creatinine ratio, ACR). These initial screening tests serve to identify patients in whom additional investigations may be appropriate to detect an underlying cause of hypertension.

The full blood count and film may reveal the anaemia of chronic renal failure or occasionally a microangiopathic haemolytic anaemia—with red cell fragmentation and intravascular haemolysis—possibly related to the degree of arteriolar fibrinoid necrosis. Serum urea and creatinine should initially be measured daily: renal impairment may have significant prognostic implications.

Mild hypokalaemia due to secondary hyperaldosteronism may be present, which usually resolves after control of the hypertension. Only very rarely does hypokalaemia indicate primary hyperaldosteronism (Conn's syndrome), but if it is extreme or persists despite good blood pressure control, then the characteristic findings of low renin levels, but high aldosterone concentrations, may be present. More commonly, both plasma renin and aldosterone levels are high in malignant hypertension, usually attributed to juxtaglomerular ischaemia. The inflammatory markers erythrocyte sedimentation rate (ESR) and C-reactive protein (CRP) are often modestly elevated in malignant hypertension, but measurement of autoantibodies (antinuclear antibodies and antineutrophil cytoplasmic antibodies) can be used to discern uncommon cases due to vasculitis. Renal biopsy is required to make a specific diagnosis in some instances, but should not be performed until blood pressure is controlled.

The chest radiograph may show cardiomegaly and the presence of pulmonary oedema. In a recent series of patients with malignant hypertension undergoing echocardiography, cardiac hypertrophy was common and associated with systolic dysfunction and a dilated left atrium, irrespective of the duration of known hypertension. These structural/functional abnormalities may predispose patients to cardiovascular complications including heart failure and cardiac arrhythmias, such as atrial fibrillation.

Hypertension and atrial fibrillation commonly coexist, and both are additive to the risk of stroke. In particular, the presence of uncontrolled hypertension increases the risk of stroke and thromboembolism associated with this common arrhythmia.

Complications

Retinopathy

As described above and in Chapter 17.2, the most widely used classification of hypertensive changes in the fundus is that of Keith, Wagener, and Barker—the strength of this being the correlation in the original description between clinical findings and prognosis (Table 17.5.1). However, this classification has now been made obsolete by advances in the understanding of the pathophysiology of arterial hypertension and the availability of effective antihypertensive therapy. Ophthalmoscopic grading of the retinal changes in hypertension has been simplified into mild, moderate, and severe levels (see Chapter 17.2), and can be further reduced into two groups: grade A (nonmalignant)—arteriolar narrowing and focal constriction, which also correlate with age and general cardiovascular status as well as blood pressure; and grade B (malignant)—linear flame-shaped haemorrhages, and/or exudates, and/or cotton wool spots, with or without disc swelling. Papilloedema is an unreliable physical sign, and its presence or absence in the context of other grade-B changes does not indicate a worse prognosis.

Grades 1 and 2 are broadly similar and are related to age and general cardiovascular status as well as blood pressure. Grades 3 and 4 are much more alike and both are now considered to be 'malignant'. See Chapter 17.2 for further discussion.

Similar retinal appearances with haemorrhages and papilloedema can occur in severe anaemia, connective tissue disease, and infective endocarditis. Idiopathic intracranial hypertension with bilateral papilloedema is itself associated with hypertension and obesity but this is not indicative of hypertension entering its malignant phase. Nevertheless, severe hypertension and lone bilateral papilloedema may be a variant of malignant hypertension, with similar clinical features and prognosis. The retinal features of malignant hypertension regress over a period of 2 to 3 months, if good blood pressure control is achieved.

Renal involvement

Renal involvement in malignant hypertension has been referred to as malignant nephrosclerosis, manifest as haematuria, proteinuria, and (sometimes) acute renal failure. Renal failure is the commonest cause of death, with presenting urea and creatinine levels independent predictors of survival.

When antihypertensive therapy is initiated and blood pressure control achieved, the effect on renal function is variable. In the short term, renal function stabilizes in 10% of cases, deteriorates progressively in 30%, and deteriorates transiently before improving over a matter of weeks in the remainder. Renal failure is more frequent (two- to threefold) in black, than in white, individuals (Fig. 17.5.3), but mainly because of higher serum creatinine levels at presentation.

Isles and coworkers have suggested that the renal outcome of patients with malignant hypertension can be considered in three groups, each with a different renal prognosis: (1) patients whose serum creatinine is less than 300 μmol/litre at presentation, who do well with effective antihypertensive therapy; (2) patients with chronic renal failure (serum creatinine >300 μmol/litre) who do not require renal dialysis immediately, but are unlikely to maintain or

Table 17.5.1 The Keith, Wagener, and Barker classification of hypertensive retinopathy

	Grade 1	Grade 2	Grade 3	Grade 4
Retinal findings	Mild narrowing or sclerosis of the retinal arterioles	Moderate to marked sclerosis of the retinal arterioles	Retinal oedema, cotton wool spots and haemorrhages	All the above and optic disc oedema
		Exaggerated arterial light reflex	Sclerosis and spastic lesions of retinal arterioles	
		Venous compression at arteriovenous crossings ('nipping')	Macular star	
Percentage surviving in original series				
1 year	90	88	65	21
3 years	70	62	22	6
5 years	70	54	20	1

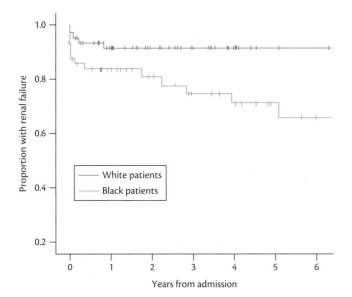

Fig. 17.5.3 Proportion with renal failure after presentation with malignant hypertension, stratified for ethnicity.
From Van den Born BJ et al. (2006). Ethnic disparities in the incidence, presentation and complications of malignant hypertension. *J Hypertens*, **24**, 2299–304 .

recover renal function, except possibly in the short term, and commonly progress to endstage renal failure; and (3) a small group with acute renal failure. It is possible that some of these patients may have poststreptococcal acute nephritic syndrome, characterized by retinopathy, fluid retention, and usually complete renal recovery.

In the west Birmingham series, Lip *et al.* did not find such a clear distinction based on serum creatinine and found that renal function continued to deteriorate among many patients with malignant hypertension, despite good blood pressure control at follow-up. About half of the patients with severe renal impairment at presentation demonstrated either static or improved renal function, and there was no evidence that those cases where renal function remained static were those with less renal impairment at presentation. The severity of malignant hypertension at presentation did not predict outcome, but the quality of control of systolic blood pressure at follow-up and the height of the serum creatinine at presentation did, suggesting that careful monitoring of renal function and aggressive treatment of blood pressure is mandatory in patients with this condition.

High serum urate levels are associated with greater renal impairment at baseline, as well as higher diastolic blood pressures, but are not predictive of deterioration in renal function or overall survival in patients with malignant hypertension.

There are varying reports of the frequency of renovascular disease in malignant hypertension, which may be due to the frequency with which renal angiography is performed. In older patients, renal artery stenosis is likely to be due to atheromatous disease, which itself may be a consequence of chronic hypertension and chronic hyperlipidaemia, as well as cigarette smoking. In younger patients, and particularly in women, renal artery stenosis may be due to fibromuscular dysplasia of the renal arteries, with the characteristic 'string of beads' appearance on renal angiography. The value of surgical or angioplastic correction of atheromatous disease is debatable, possibly producing no better results than effective blood pressure control with antihypertensive drugs. In patients with fibromuscular dysplasia, however, renal angioplasty with stenting is worthwhile and will often lead to a normal blood pressure level.

Management

All patients with malignant hypertension require assessment, investigation, and commencement of therapy under supervision, preferably as an in-patient. Blood pressure should be measured 4-hourly, with the initial aim of treatment being to lower the diastolic pressure near about 100 to 105 mmHg over a period of 2 to 3 days, with oral therapy and dose escalation at daily intervals, if necessary. The maximum initial fall in blood pressure should not exceed 25% of the presenting value, gradual reduction allowing adaptation of disordered tissue autoregulation and avoidance of target organ ischaemia. More aggressive antihypertensive therapy is both unnecessary and dangerous, as it may reduce the blood pressure to below the autoregulatory range, leading to ischaemic events such as strokes, heart attack, or renal failure.

The first-line oral antihypertensive agent is either a short-acting calcium antagonist (such as nifedipine) or a β-blocker (such as atenolol). An appropriate dose of nifedipine is 10 to 20 mg of the tablet formulation, which can be repeated or increased, as necessary, to bring about gradual reduction in blood pressure. Nifedipine is not absorbed from the oral mucosa, and there have been reports of complications including visual loss, cerebral infarction, and myocardial infarction with nifedipine therapy using the short-acting sublingual capsules, which produce unpredictable falls in blood pressure and should never be used. β-Blockers are useful alternatives, but should be avoided in patients with asthma or where there is a high suspicion of an underlying phaeochromocytoma. It is sensible to start with small doses, such as 25 mg of atenolol, increasing dose as necessary. The combination of oral atenolol and nifedipine is often a well-tolerated and effective regime.

Diuretics should be restricted to those with evidence of fluid overload. Some patients are volume depleted, presumably secondary to a pressure-related diuresis and activation of the renin–angiotensin system. Captopril and the other angiotensin converting enzyme (ACE) inhibitors can produce rapid and dangerous falls in blood pressure, particularly in patients with hypokalaemic secondary hyperaldosteronism and hyponatraemia secondary to juxtaglomerular ischaemia or renovascular disease, which may be unrecognized in the acute situation.

Over a period of about 1 to 2 weeks, further antihypertensive drugs should be added in to achieve a gradual reduction of blood pressure to less than 140/85 mmHg. Triple or quadruple drug regimens are invariably necessary in the long term.

Drugs for the treatment of hypertensive emergencies and urgencies are summarized in Tables 17.5.2 and 17.5.3.

Prognosis

If malignant hypertension is left untreated, around 80% of patients die within 2 years, hence the name. In west Birmingham, between 1965 and 2006, after a median follow-up of 103 months (range 1–539 months), 40% were alive and not requiring renal replacement therapy, 3.2% were on long-term haemodialysis, and 40% were dead, with the remainder lost to follow-up. The commonest causes of death were renal failure (39.7%), stroke (23.8%), myocardial infarction (11.1%), and heart failure (10.3%).

Table 17.5.2 Oral drugs for hypertensive emergencies and urgencies

Category	Example	Comment
β-Blockers	Atenolol (25–50 mg)	Safe unless contraindicated
Calcium channel blockers	Nifedipine capsules	Dangerous
	Nifedipine tablets (10–20 mg)	Safe
	Amlodipine	Onset of action is slow (c.5 days)
	Verapamil	Useful if tachycardia or associated supraventricular arrhythmia
	Nicardipine	Not better than nifedipine by mouth
α-Blockers	Prazosin	Little experience
	Doxazosin	Little experience
	Phenoxybenzamine	Phaeochromocytoma
Diuretics	Thiazides	Slow onset
	Loop diuretics	Only if heart failure
ACE inhibitors	Captopril (6.25–50 mg, 3 times a day)	If patient on diuretic, or if renal artery stenosis is undiagnosed, may cause rapid falls in blood pressure and acute renal failure

The advent of effective and tolerable antihypertensive drug therapy has improved prognosis. For example, in the west Birmingham series, 5-year survival rates improved from 31.4% prior to 1967 to 91.9% for the years 1997 to 2006 (Fig. 17.5.4). The series by Scarpelli and coworkers reported a 12-year survival rate of about 69%, although patients with malignant hypertension diagnosed after 1980 had a 100% survival rate. More contemporaneous data from the Amsterdam series, describing patient incidents between 1993 and 2005, showed that 10% had died and 19% needed renal replacement therapy after a mean follow-up of 4 years. Hence, whatever the cause of malignant hypertension, progressive renal impairment is still a common complicating factor, with many patients needing dialysis in the long term.

The importance of early diagnosis is emphasized as patients tend to develop clinical symptoms only at a late stage of their disease. Black men with malignant hypertension have a poor prognosis when compared with other ethnic groups or women; they also present with more severe hypertension and greater renal damage, which are independent predictors of outcome and explain the poorer prognosis.

Hypertensive emergencies

Hypertensive left ventricular failure

Hypertension causes heart failure by a number of mechanisms: these include pressure overload on the heart due to the raised peripheral vascular resistance, reduced left ventricular compliance (e.g. in left ventricular hypertrophy), an increased risk for coronary artery disease and the precipitation of cardiac arrhythmias (such as atrial fibrillation). Severe hypertension results in a significant increase in afterload and may result in decompensation of the failing heart.

In very severe hypertension with marked pulmonary oedema, intravenous sodium nitroprusside may be necessary to reduce preload and afterload in addition to conventional management with opioids and loop diuretics. However, metabolism of nitroprusside to cyanide, possibly leading to the development of cyanide or (rarely) thiocyanate toxicity, may be a limitation. This manifests with altered mental status and lactic acidosis, and can be fatal. The risk of toxicity is increased in children, also with prolonged treatment (>24–48 h), underlying renal insufficiency, and requirement for high doses (>2 µg/kg per min). An infusion of sodium thiosulfate can be used in affected patients to provide a sulfur donor to detoxify cyanide into thiocyanate.

Nitrates may also be used to treat hypertensive left ventricular failure, but they are less potent than sodium nitroprusside. ACE inhibitors should be considered only after the patient's condition is stabilized, when they are well established to be life-saving in those with left ventricular systolic impairment, lead to long-term regression of left ventricular hypertrophy, and may also improve heart failure secondary to diastolic dysfunction.

Hypertensive encephalopathy

Hypertensive encephalopathy refers to the presence of signs of cerebral oedema caused by breakthrough hyperperfusion following severe and sudden rises in blood pressure. There is failure of autoregulatory vasoconstriction with focal or generalized dilatation of small arteries and arterioles. This leads to high cerebral blood flow, dysfunction of the blood–brain barrier, and the formation of brain oedema, which is thought to cause the clinical symptoms. The condition is now very rare, and it is essential to perform a CT or an MRI scan to ensure that this hypertensive emergency is distinguished from other neurological syndromes associated with high blood pressure, including intracerebral or subarachnoid haemorrhage, ischaemic stroke, or lacunar infarction.

Hypertensive encephalopathy is usually associated with a history of hypertension that has been inadequately treated, or where previous treatment has been discontinued. It is characterized by the insidious onset of headache, nausea, and vomiting, followed by visual disturbances and fluctuating, nonlocalizing neurological symptoms such as restlessness, confusion, and—if the hypertension is not treated—seizures and coma. Severe retinopathy is frequently, but not always, present.

CT or MRI may demonstrate white matter oedema, and one of these tests is mandatory to exclude cerebral haemorrhage or infarction. Indeed, the increased use of CT scanning has demonstrated that almost all patients who appear to have hypertensive encephalopathy have cerebral infarction or haemorrhage with surrounding oedema and space-occupying cerebral symptoms. Lumbar puncture is not indicated in the management of patients with malignant hypertension; but if obtained (perhaps in ignorance of the diagnosis) the cerebrospinal fluid is usually normal, although at an increased pressure. The ECG may show variable transient, focal, or bilateral abnormalities.

Sodium nitroprusside is the drug of choice for genuine hypertensive encephalopathy, but is not usually given if there is a cerebral infarct or haemorrhage. Parenteral labetalol and nitrates have also been used successfully. Rarely, diazoxide and hydralazine have been given, but they can cause precipitate and life-threatening acute falls in blood pressure, and they require concurrent β-blocker administration to minimize reflex sympathetic stimulation. Sublingual

Table 17.5.3 Parenteral drugs for the treatment of hypertensive emergencies

	Action	Administration	Use and adverse effects	Comment
Sodium nitroprusside	Dilates both arterioles and veins via generation of cGMP which then activates calcium-sensitive potassium channels in the cell membrane	IV infusion; rapid onset and offset of action, minimizing the risk of hypotension Recommended starting dose is 0.25–0.5 µg/kg per min, increased as necessary to a maximum dose of 8–10 µg/kg per min, for up to 10 min Nitroprusside should not be given to pregnant women	Can cause intrapulmonary shunting and coronary 'steal' Thiocynate and cyanide toxicity manifest by clinical deterioration, muscle twitching, altered mental status, and lactic acidosis, and can be fatal	The most effective parenteral drug for most hypertensive emergencies Easy to control on a minute-to-minute basis
Glyceryl trinitrate (nitroglycerine)	Similar action to nitroprusside, but greater venodilatation	IV infusion, 5–100 µg/min Onset of action is 2–5 min, duration of action 5–10 min	Headache (due to direct vasodilatation) and tachycardia (reflex sympathetic activation) Vomiting Methaemoglobinaemia	Most useful in patients with symptomatic coronary disease and in those with hypertension following surgery
Labetalol	Combined β- and α-blocker	Rapid onset of action (5 min or less) Bolus of 20 mg initially, followed by 20–80 mg every 10 min to a total dose of 300 mg The infusion rate is 0.5–2 mg/min	Avoid in patients with contraindications to β-blockers	Safe in patients with active coronary disease since it does not increase the heart rate Also useful in the perioperative care of patients with severe hypertension
Esmolol	β-Blocker	Rapid onset and offset of action IV infusion, titrated to heart rate and blood pressure response	Reduces myocardial ischaemia Avoid in patients with contraindications to β-blockers	Useful in tachycardias, hyperdynamic heart, arrhythmias (e.g. atrial fibrillation), perioperative hypertension, aortic dissection
Nicardipine	Dihydropyridine calcium channel blocker	IV infusion at 5–15 mg/h	Headache and flushing Tachycardia	Becoming more popular Useful for most hypertensive emergencies, except acute heart failure
Diazoxide	Arteriolar vasodilator that has little effect on the venous circulation	IV bolus 50–150 mg or infusion 2–10 mg/h Peak effect seen within 15 min, lasts for 4–24 h	Do not use in patients with angina pectoris, myocardial infarction, pulmonary oedema, or a dissecting aortic aneurysm Can cause marked fluid retention and a diuretic may be needed	Give β-blocker to block reflex activation of the sympathetic nervous system Rarely used nowadays as may cause excessive blood pressure reduction which is difficult to reverse
Hydralazine	Direct arteriolar vasodilator	IV bolus Initial dose is 10–20 mg Fall in blood pressure begins within 10–30 min and lasts 2–4 h	Tachycardia, flushing, headache, vomiting Aggravation of angina Hypotensive response to hydralazine is less predictable	Used in pregnant women
Phentolamine	α-Adrenergic blocker	IV bolus, 5–10 mg every 5–15 min as necessary	Severe hypertension due to phaeochromocytoma and other syndromes of increased catecholamine activity, such as drug abuse, MAO-induced hypertension, etc.	Tachyphylaxis means that doses need to be escalated

IV, intravenous; MAO, monoamine oxidase.

nifedipine capsules should never be used (see 'Management' above). Phentolamine is used only in patients with severe hypertension due to increased catecholamine activity, such as that seen in phaeochromocytoma, or after tyramine ingestion in a patient being treated with a monoamine oxidase inhibitor. ACE inhibitors are best avoided in the early stage as they may, even in a very low dose, cause precipitate falls in blood pressure and life-threatening reduction in cerebral perfusion, particularly when patients are fluid depleted due to diuretic therapy or in the presence of renal artery stenosis.

Severe pre-eclampsia and eclampsia are discussed in detail elsewhere (see Chapter 14.4). They may present with clinical features

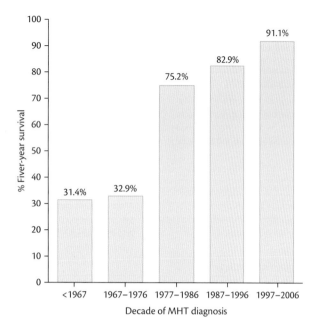

Fig. 17.5.4 Five-year survival by decade of diagnosis. MHT, malignant phase hypertension.

American Journal of Hypertension, Lane DA, Lip GYH, Beevers DG, Improving survival of malignant hypertension patients over 40 years. **22**: 1199–204, copyright (2009). Oxford University Press.

similar to hypertensive encephalopathy, and treatment is broadly similar, with labetalol infusions, magnesium sulfate, and early delivery of the fetus.

Hypertension with unstable angina or acute myocardial infarction

In a patient presenting with an acute coronary syndrome (unstable angina or acute myocardial infarction) and severe hypertension, a 'true' hypertensive emergency, such as aortic dissection, must first be ruled out. The risk of bleeding and stroke is significantly increased if anticoagulation with heparin, antiplatelet therapies (such as glycoprotein IIb/IIIa inhibitors), or thrombolytic therapy is administered.

The appropriate initial treatment of patients with severe hypertension (>180/110 mmHg) and an acute coronary syndrome should include the initiation of intravenous nitrates, with intravenous labetalol, sodium nitroprusside, or nicardipine as alternatives. The reduction of blood pressure should not be too abrupt: as with malignant hypertension, a gradual reduction is recommended in an endeavour to avoid further myocardial or brain ischaemia. As stated previously, sublingual nifedipine—once considered as a first-line drug—should not be used in view of its negligible oral absorption and the unpredictable hypotensive effects from later gastric absorption.

Anticoagulation or thrombolytic therapy can be administered when the blood pressure is adequately controlled (<180/110 mmHg). In many centres, revascularization with primary percutaneous coronary angioplasty is increasingly the initial management option for acute ST segment elevation myocardial infarction (STEMI).

Hypertension with acute stroke and after a stroke

It is common to find modestly elevated blood pressure in patients admitted to hospital following an acute stroke. Cerebral autoregulation is commonly impaired in this context, with flow becoming pressure dependent. Thus, excessive antihypertensive treatment may serve to worsen the cerebral damage resulting from intracerebral infarction or haemorrhage, and stroke physicians are very wary about lowering the blood pressure. There are few randomized controlled trials to inform the management of this common problem. Current consensus only recommends acute blood pressure lowering where there is associated acute end-organ damage—e.g. cardiac (acute myocardial infarction, severe left ventricular failure) or vascular urgencies (aortic dissection), hypertensive encephalopathy, acute renal failure, concurrent coagulant therapy (thrombolysis, intravenous heparin, etc.), or persistent blood pressure elevation with a threshold greater than 200/120 mmHg for ischaemic stroke and greater than 180/105 mmHg for haemorrhagic stroke. In these cases, oral therapy with small doses of nifedipine or atenolol may be required. Parenteral treatment or sublingual nifedipine is always contraindicated. The calcium antagonist nimodipine has beneficial effects on cerebral vasospasm following subarachnoid haemorrhage, but these effects are not related to the small fall in blood pressure with this drug.

Severe hypertension after a stroke is a risk factor for further stokes, and long-term treatment is worthwhile. It is unclear whether the immediate treatment of mild hypertension is of benefit. The role of antihypertensive medication before, during, and after a stroke can, therefore, be summarized as follows:

- *Before a stroke*, it is of benefit to have blood pressure reduced to below 140/85 mmHg, as stroke prevention can be achieved.

- *During a stroke*, it is detrimental to have hypertension treated aggressively, in view of the disordered cerebral autoregulation.

- *After a stroke*, the epidemiological associations of hypertension with recurrent stroke have not been entirely consistent, with some studies showing no association or a J-shaped relationship.

In recent years many studies have reported on the effects of antihypertensive drugs—predominantly ACE inhibitors or angiotensin receptor blockers—in the early poststroke setting. The Heart Outcomes Prevention Evaluation (HOPE) study reported a subset of 1013 subjects with a previous history of stroke or transient ischaemic attack (TIA), where there was a nonsignificant 15% reduction in total stroke recurrence with ramipril. In the PROGRESS trial, 6105 normotensive and hypertensive patients with a history of ischaemic or haemorrhagic stroke or TIA were randomized to perindopril (± indapamide), which reduced recurrent stroke by 28% and major vascular events by 26% during 4 years of follow-up.

The Morbidity and Mortality after Stroke Eprosartan Study (MOSES) compared eprosartan (an angiotensin receptor blocker) to nitrendipine (a dihydropyridine calcium channel blocker) in hypertensive-stroke survivors and found a 21% risk reduction in the primary endpoint of all cardiovascular and cerebrovascular events and a 25% reduction in recurrent cerebrovascular events in the eprosartan-treated patients.

In the CATIS Randomized Clinical Trial, patients with acute ischaemic stroke (*n* = 2038) were randomly assigned to receive antihypertensive treatment (aimed at lowering systolic blood pressure by 10% to 25% within the first 24 h after randomization, achieving blood pressure less than 140/90 mmHg within 7 days, and maintaining this level during hospitalization) or to discontinue all antihypertensive medications (control) during hospitalization (*n* = 2033). In this trial, blood pressure reduction with antihypertensive medications, compared with the absence of hypertensive medication, did not reduce the likelihood of death and major disability at 14 days or hospital discharge.

Management of blood pressure in a patient with aortic dissection

The detailed presentation, diagnosis, and treatment of aortic dissection is discussed in Chapter 14.1. On suspicion of the diagnosis, whether or not surgery is indicated, all patients should be treated pharmacologically to reduce the systolic blood pressure to around 110 mmHg and the heart rate to 60 to 70 beats/min, thus reducing the force of systolic ejection to reduce aortic shear stress and limit the size of the dissection. Labetalol is an effective agent, or alternatively, sodium nitroprusside in conjunction with a β-blocker may be used. Patients should ideally have haemodynamic monitoring with an arterial line in position. Diagnostic tests are then performed on an urgent basis to confirm the dissection, identifying whether the ascending aorta is involved, and defining any vascular abnormalities resulting from the dissection.

Further reading

Bloxham CA, Beevers DG, Walker JM (1979). Malignant hypertension and cigarette smoking. *Br Med J*, **i**, 581–3.

Cremer A, *et al.* (2015). From malignant hypertension to hypertension-MOD: a modern definition for an old but still dangerous emergency. *J Hum Hypertens*. 2015 Nov 19. doi:10.1038/jhh.2015.112.

Gudbrandsson T, *et al.* (1979). Malignant hypertension. Improving prognosis in a rare disease. *Acta Med Scand*, **206**, 495–9.

Harvey JM, *et al.* (1992). Renal biopsy findings in hypertensive patients with proteinuria. *Lancet*, **340**, 1435–6.

He J, *et al.* (2014). Effects of immediate blood pressure reduction on death and major disability in patients with acute ischemic stroke: the CATIS randomized clinical trial. *JAMA*, **311**, 479–89.

Isles CG, McLay A, Boulton Jones JM (1984). Recovery in malignant hypertension presenting as acute renal failure. *Q J Med*, **212**, 439–52.

Jhetam D, *et al.* (1982). The malignant phase of essential hypertension in Johannesburg blacks. *S Afr Med J*, **61**, 899–902.

Kadiri S, Olutade BO (1991). The clinical presentation of malignant hypertension in Nigerians. *J Hum Hypertens*, **5**, 339–43.

Keith NM, Wagener HP, Barker NW (1939). Some different types of essential hypertension: their course and prognosis. *Am J Med Sci*, **196**, 332–43.

Kumar P, *et al.* (1996). Malignant hypertension in children in India. *Nephrol Dial Trans*, **11**, 1261–6.

Lane DA, Lip GYH, Beevas DG (2009). Improving survival of malignant hypertension patients over 40 years, *Am J Hypertens*, **22**, 1199–204.

Leishman AWD (1959). Hypertension—treated and untreated: a study of 400 cases. *Br Med J*, **i**, 1361–3.

Lim KG, *et al.* (1987). Malignant hypertension in women of childbearing age and its relation to the contraceptive pill. *BMJ*, **294**, 1057–9.

Lip GYH *et al.* (1995). Severe hypertension and lone bilateral papilloedema: a variant of malignant phase hypertension. *Blood Press*, **4**, 339–42.

Lip GYH, *et al.* (1995). Malignant hypertension in the elderly. *Q J Med*, **88**, 641–7.

Lip GYH, Beevers M, Beevers DG (1997). Does renal function improve following diagnosis of malignant phase hypertension? *J Hypertens*, **15**, 1309–15.

Lip GYH, Beevers M, Beevers DG (2000). Serum urate is associated with baseline renal dysfunction but not survival or deterioration in renal function in malignant phase hypertension. *J Hypertens*, **18**, 97–101.

Lip GY, et al. (2010). Refining clinical risk stratification for predicting stroke and thromboembolism in atrial fibrillation using a novel risk factor-based approach: the euro heart survey on atrial fibrillation. *Chest*, 137, 263–72.

Mamdani BH, *et al.* (1974). Recovery from prolonged renal failure in patients with accelerated hypertension. *N Engl J Med*, **291**, 1343–4.

Pitcock JA, *et al.* (1976). Malignant hypertension in blacks. Malignant intrarenal arterial disease as observed by light and electron microscopy. *Hum Pathol*, 7, 333–46.

Scarpelli PT, *et al.* (1997). Accelerated (malignant) hypertension: a study of 121 cases between 1974 and 1996. *Nephrology*, **10**, 207–15.

Schrader J, *et al.* (2005). Morbidity and mortality after stroke, eprosartan compared with nitrendipine for secondary prevention: principal results of a prospective randomized controlled study (MOSES). *Stroke*, **36**, 1218–26.

Strandgaard S, Paulson OB (1996). Antihypertensive drugs and cerebral circulation. *Eur J Clin Invest*, **26**, 625–30.

Van den Born BJ, *et al.* (2006). Ethnic disparities in the incidence, presentation and complications of malignant hypertension. *J Hypertens*, **24**, 2299–304.

Veriava Y, *et al.* (1990). Hypertension as a cause of end-stage renal failure in South Africa. *J Hum Hypertens*, **4**, 379–83.

Webster J, *et al.* (1993). Accelerated hypertension—patterns of mortality and clinical factors affecting outcome in treated patients. *Q J Med*, **86**, 485–93.

Zampaglione P, *et al.* (1996). Hypertensive urgencies and emergencies. Prevalence and clinical presentation. *Hypertension*, **27**, 144–7.

Heart disease in pregnancy

CHAPTER 18.1

Heart disease in pregnancy

Catherine E. G. Head

Essentials

Pregnancy is a vasodilator state in which plasma volume and cardiac output increase such that many symptoms and signs of cardiac disease can occur physiologically. Disproportionate symptoms or abnormal signs such as a diastolic murmur require investigation as usual; necessary radiological investigations should not be withheld as the risks to the fetus are generally low.

Prepregnancy risk assessment—this is ideally based on data related to the specific cardiac abnormality, with prepregnancy functional status an important predictor of outcome. Issues of particular note are (1) pregnancy is high risk in pulmonary hypertension or severe left ventricular dysfunction—effective contraception and termination should be offered; (2) women at risk of aortic dissection are at increased risk during pregnancy—prepregnancy elective replacement of the aortic root should be considered if its diameter at its widest point is greater than 4.5–5.0 cm, depending on the underlying aetiology; β-blockers and regular echo monitoring should continue through pregnancy.

Delivery of the baby—vaginal delivery is recommended, other than in the presence of a dilated aortic root, aneurysm, or dissection, or if the fetal INR is elevated. Low-dose infusions of epidural anaesthesia and oxytoxic drugs are safe.

Heart conditions arising in pregnancy

Peripartum cardiomyopathy—this should be considered in any woman presenting peripartum with dyspnoea or tachycardia.

Myocardial infarction—when occurring in pregnancy this may be due to coronary dissection: immediate angiography with percutaneous coronary intervention is the management of choice, but thrombolysis is not contraindicated.

Pregnancy in women with known cardiac disorders

Valve diseases and cardiomyopathies—(1) Symptomatic mitral stenosis—may be managed medically with diuretics, β-blockade, and maintenance of sinus rhythm; failing this, balloon valvuloplasty is usually successful. (2) Aortic stenosis—women with satisfactory prepregnancy haemodynamics are at low risk of problems in pregnancy. (3) Hypertrophic cardiomyopathy—patients generally tolerate pregnancy well.

Congenital cardiac lesions—low-risk conditions include atrial septal defect, restrictive ventricular septal defect, and corrected tetralogy of Fallot in the absence of severe pulmonary regurgitation or aortic

root dilatation. All cases other than those at low risk should be managed by a multidisciplinary team in a specialist centre.

Anticoagulation—the optimal anticoagulation management of a pregnant patient with a mechanical prosthetic valve is not known. Continued warfarin therapy carries the risk of warfarin embryopathy for the fetus, but switching to heparin increases the maternal risk of thromboembolism, although newer regimens using low molecular weight heparin with monitoring of anti-Xa levels almost certainly perform better than historical regimens using unfractionated heparin.

Introduction

Cardiac disease is the commonest cause of maternal death in the United Kingdom. Historically most of these women had rheumatic mitral stenosis, but in the developed world today the leading causes are sudden adult death syndrome (SADS), cardiomyopathy, aortic dissection, and myocardial infarction, followed by congenital heart disease and pulmonary hypertension. Maternal death is fortunately rare, but the proportion of pregnant women who have cardiac disease is increasing, reflecting both the improved survival of adults with congenital heart disease and changes in pregnancy demographics.

Cardiovascular changes in pregnancy

Early in gestation the up-regulation of nitric oxide synthesis by oestradiol causes arterial vasodilatation and a reduction in both systemic and pulmonary vascular resistance. Simultaneously the normal fall in heart rate at the end of the menstrual cycle fails to occur, and the heart rate increases by 10 to 20 beats/min for the duration of the pregnancy. The reduction in afterload and blood pressure stimulates an increase in plasma volume and hence preload by activation of the renin–angiotensin–aldosterone system. End diastolic volume, stroke volume and contractility increase such that cardiac output reaches about 140% of prepregnancy level by mid gestation. These changes combined with the development of the low-resistance uteroplacental circulation cause blood pressure (systolic and diastolic) to decline by around 10 mmHg to a nadir at about 20 weeks, before returning to prepregnancy levels by term. Although central venous pressure and pulmonary capillary wedge pressure remain unchanged, serum colloid osmotic pressure is reduced by plasma expansion and the pregnant woman is therefore at increased risk of pulmonary oedema. The 50% increase in plasma volume combined with the 25% increase in red cell mass accounts for a haemoglobin level of around 11 g/dl—the physiological anaemia of pregnancy.

Labour, particularly the second stage, is associated with a further increase in cardiac output as pain increases heart rate via the sympathetic response and stroke volume is augmented by autotransfusion during contractions and postpartum. This means that the later stages of labour are a period of high risk for pulmonary oedema.

Structural changes to the heart and great vessels occur. Orifice areas of all four valves increase, causing a higher incidence of valvular regurgitation. Changes in the extracellular matrix of the aortic media increase compliance but also, in combination with the increased cardiac output, the risk of dissection.

Cardiac clinical features of normal pregnancy

Fatigue, dizziness, palpitation, oedema, dyspnoea, and reduced exercise tolerance may occur in a normal pregnancy. Pressure of the uterus on the inferior vena cava when supine can significantly reduce preload and therefore cardiac output, causing presyncope. Symptoms are rapidly relieved by turning on one side. The increased cardiac output of pregnancy, together with the relative sinus tachycardia and the increased tendency to ectopy, may be experienced as palpitation, often particularly when at rest lying down. Physiological hyperventilation of pregnancy is perceived as breathlessness, particularly when speaking, by most women at some point during a normal pregnancy.

Normal cardiovascular examination findings in pregnancy are

* increased volume 'bounding' peripheral pulses
* third heart sound
* soft ejection systolic murmur at the left sternal edge
* peripheral oedema

Abnormal findings that require further assessment include:

* fourth heart sound
* diastolic murmur

Cardiovascular investigation in pregnancy

Electrocardiogram

The rotated position of the heart causes left axis deviation. Common findings also include the presence of a Q wave and T wave inversion in lead III, and inverted T waves in V1 and V2. Changes in autonomic control and ion channel expression result in an increase in corrected QT interval and QT dispersion.

Exercise testing

Maximal exercise testing is safe for both mother and fetus in a normal pregnancy, with maximal oxygen uptake the same as that of nonpregnant matched controls in non-weight-bearing (static cycle) protocols. European Society of Cardiology guidelines recommend submaximal testing to 80% of target heart rate in asymptomatic pregnant patients with suspected cardiovascular disease. Semi-recumbent cycle ergometry is usually the most comfortable modality. There is no specific data on the use of exercise testing to diagnose ischaemic heart disease during pregnancy and so sensible extrapolation from the nonpregnant data should be used, remembering that nonspecific 'T' wave changes can be normal in pregnancy. Prepregnancy testing is useful in risk stratification.

Chest radiograph/CT

The fetal absorbed dose of ionizing radiation is less than 0.01 mGy from a chest radiograph and less than 1 mGy from a chest CT. Maximum recommended total occupational exposure during pregnancy is 1 mGy, the mean annual dose received from background radiation. The threshold dose for fetal malformation is 50–100 mGy, and while there is no threshold associated with an increased rate of later malignancy, the relative risk is modest at × 1.4 for a dose of over 10 mGy. Thus a chest radiograph or CT necessary to make a diagnosis should not be withheld from a pregnant woman.

Echocardiogram

Echocardiography is safe and useful. Views are standard other than for the absence of a subcostal view in later pregnancy. Normal findings include a small increase in the size of all cardiac chambers, mild regurgitation of all four valves, and the presence of a small pericardial effusion.

Cardiac catheterization

Diagnostic cardiac catheterization is rarely indicated in pregnancy, but percutaneous intervention may be required for valvular or coronary disease. Most interventional cardiac procedures are associated with a total maternal exposure of less than 50 mGy (usually 1–10 mGy), of which c.20% reaches the fetus. External shielding of the pelvis and abdomen is of limited protective value as most fetal exposure is caused by internally scattered radiation. However, fetal doses can be reduced by use of adjunctive imaging modalities such as transoesophageal echo, use of the transradial route for coronary intervention, and imaging of the woman in the first trimester with an empty bladder. A wedge should be placed under one hip during the procedure to prevent aortocaval compression.

MRI

MRI avoids ionizing radiation and yields very high-quality diagnostic information but is associated with theoretical fetal risk from heat, noise, and electromagnetic fields. If MRI is necessary in pregnancy, often for imaging of the aorta, the first trimester and gadolinium contrast are avoided.

Prepregnancy assessment and risk stratification

In all but the most straightforward cases a planned pregnancy is preferable to one that is unplanned. Prior to pregnancy a full clinical assessment should be made, including measurement of oxygen saturation, ECG, chest radiography, and echocardiogram. Prepregnancy functional capacity is an important predictor of a woman's ability to tolerate pregnancy, with those in New York Heart Association (NYHA) classes I and II generally having a good outcome. Treadmill exercise testing can be useful to define this: achievement of a level of above 7 METS (multiples of resting oxygen consumption) being used empirically by some centres to predict a good outcome. Invasive investigation may also be necessary. An estimate of maternal and fetal risk can then be given, together with recommendations for any medical, interventional, or surgical treatment before conception (Tables 18.1.1 and Box 18.1.1). Although it is a difficult issue to discuss, it is also important that the prospective mother is fully aware of her expected lifespan and capacity.

Table 18.1.1 Classification of maternal risk of pregnancy

Risk class	Risk of pregnancy by medical conditions
I	No detectable increased risk of maternal mortality and no/mild increase in morbidity
II	Small increased risk of maternal mortality or moderate increase in morbidity
III	Significantly increased risk of maternal mortality or severe morbidity. Expert counselling required. If pregnancy is decided upon, intensive specialist cardiac and obstetric monitoring needed throughout pregnancy, childbirth, and the puerperium
IV	Extremely high risk of maternal mortality or severe morbidity; pregnancy contraindicated. If pregnancy occurs termination should be discussed. If pregnancy continues, care as for class III

Maternal

In parallel with the known lesion-specific risks, generic scoring systems can be used to predict the risk of an adverse maternal event, but these are highly population dependent. The best overall maternal risk predictor is probably the modified World Health Organization (WHO) risk classification, which integrates all known maternal cardiovascular risk factors, both lesion-specific and generic.

Fetal

Maternal baseline NYHA III or IV, cyanosis, left heart obstruction, smoking, anticoagulation, and multiple pregnancy are adverse

Box 18.1.1 Maternal risk of pregnancy for women with various cardiac conditions

Conditions in which pregnancy risk is WHO I

- Uncomplicated, small or mild
  - pulmonary stenosis
  - patent ductus arteriosus
  - mitral valve prolapse
- Successfully repaired simple lesions (atrial or ventricular septal defect, patent ductus arteriosus, anomalous pulmonary venous drainage)
- Atrial or ventricular ectopic beats, isolated

Conditions in which pregnancy risk is WHO II or III

WHO II (if otherwise well and uncomplicated)

- Unoperated atrial or ventricular septal defect
- Repaired tetralogy of Fallot
- Most arrhythmias

WHO II–III (depending on individual)

- Mild left ventricular impairment
- Hypertrophic cardiomyopathy
- Native or tissue valvular heart disease not considered WHO I or IV
- Marfan syndrome without aortic dilatation

- Aorta <45 mm in aortic disease associated with bicuspid aortic valve
- Repaired coarctation

WHO III

- Mechanical valve
- Systemic right ventricle
- Fontan circulation
- Cyanotic heart disease (unrepaired)
- Other complex congenital heart disease
- Aortic dilatation 40–45 mm in Marfan syndrome
- Aortic dilatation 45–50 mm in aortic disease associated with bicuspid aortic valve

Conditions in which pregnancy risk is WHO IV (pregnancy contraindicated)

- Pulmonary arterial hypertension of any cause
- Severe systemic ventricular dysfunction (LVEF <30%, NYHA III–IV)
- Previous peripartum cardiomyopathy with any residual impairment of left ventricular function
- Severe mitral stenosis, severe symptomatic aortic stenosis
- Marfan syndrome with aorta dilated >45 mm
- Aortic dilatation >50 mm in aortic disease associated with bicuspid aortic valve
- Native severe coarctation

predictors of fetal and neonatal outcome, especially prematurity and low birth weight. Recurrence risk of any nonmonogenic congenital heart disease is 3 to 6%, which is up to a tenfold increase over the general population. Affected women should be offered fetal echocardiography and families with multiple cases of congenital heart disease should be offered referral to a clinical geneticist.

Management—general principles

Antenatal care

Women in WHO class I can generally be managed locally, but in all other cases antenatal care should be multidisciplinary either in, or shared with, a specialist centre. Many cardiac drugs are relatively or absolutely contraindicated in pregnancy, and therapy should be reviewed before conception. In general warfarin should be changed to subcutaneous low molecular weight heparin (LMWH), with anti-Xa level monitoring, for the duration of pregnancy, except in the case of mechanical valve replacements discussed below.

Cardiac surgery during pregnancy

Maternal mortality rates are similar to those reported for emergency procedures in nonpregnant patients, but rates of fetal loss associated with cardiopulmonary bypass are high (15–33%). Modifications to standard cardiopulmonary bypass may improve fetal outcome, but consideration should also be given to early delivery, balancing the risk of fetal loss against those of prematurity.

Labour and delivery

In women in risk classes WHO III and IV, delivery should occur at the tertiary centre with a written management plan in place. Awaiting spontaneous onset of labour is the norm, with induction indicated for the standard obstetric reasons, maternal cardiac decompensation, or for practical reasons, for example when the mother lives far from the intended site of delivery. In the United Kingdom current NICE guidelines do not recommend antibiotic prophylaxis for delivery.

Vaginal delivery is generally recommended. There is not complete consensus on cardiac indications for caesarean section, but these are generally agreed to be:

* aortopathy with aortic root >4.5 cm or rapidly dilating

* aortic dissection

* warfarin therapy within the preceding 2 weeks (although the maternal INR may be normal, the fetus clears warfarin more slowly and may still be at risk of cerebral haemorrhage)

Low-dose epidural anaesthesia does not cause excessive vasodilatation, and with adequate volume expansion is the analgesia of choice. Invasive blood pressure monitoring is advisable in women with obstructive lesions (e.g. aortic stenosis), in whom large fluid shifts may be poorly tolerated. Observation and monitoring on a high-dependency unit may be required for up to 1 week postpartum.

Specific cardiac conditions in pregnancy

Cardiomyopathy

Peripartum cardiomyopathy

This is defined as the development of left ventricular (LV) systolic dysfunction that occurs between the last month of pregnancy and 5 months postpartum in the absence of an identifiable cause or previous cardiac disease. Incidence in Western countries is 1 in 4000. Risk factors include multiple pregnancy, multiparity, hypertension, increased maternal age, and black ethnicity. There is evidence for infective, inflammatory, and autoimmune mechanisms, with the final common pathway oxidative stress leading to proteolytic cleavage of prolactin into a potent angiostatic factor and proapoptotic fragments. Clinical features are those of LV failure; the diagnosis should be suspected in any peripartum woman with dyspnoea, orthopnoea, paroxysmal nocturnal dyspnoea, or tachycardia. Echocardiography is key in the diagnosis, both to establish LV systolic dysfunction and to exclude other cardiac causes (Fig. 18.1.1). Management is as standard for LV failure, with oxygen, diuretics, vasodilators (angiotensin converting enzyme (ACE) inhibitors postpartum only), β-blockers, and occasionally digoxin. There is a high risk of thromboembolism, necessitating the addition of a prophylactic or, in high-risk cases, treatment dose of LMWH. There is some preliminary evidence to support the use of bromocriptine, an inhibitor of prolactin secretion, and larger trials are in progress.

Mortality is 9 to 15%, usually occurring within 3 months and predicted by poor NYHA class at presentation, larger LV dimensions, lower ejection fraction (LVEF), and lack of contractile reserve on dobutamine stress echocardiography. Cases refractory to standard medical therapy may require intensive care with inotropic support and consideration of a ventricular assist device or cardiac transplantation.

Up to 60% of patients recover normal resting LV function, which is crucial to the outcome of a future pregnancy (Fig. 18.1.2). We counsel against subsequent pregnancy in women whose LV function has not recovered and offer termination of unplanned pregnancy. In those who are NYHA I with a normal resting echocardiogram we attempt to refine their risk by exercise stress echocardiography, judging empirically that women with a normal contractile reserve are less likely to deteriorate during a pregnancy. This, however, will not predict cases of recurrence of the original pathological process and thus a further pregnancy will always involve a degree of risk.

Dilated cardiomyopathy

As in peripartum cardiomyopathy the diagnosis depends on the identification of LV dilatation and dysfunction in the absence of an identifiable cause. Women may present with a pre-existing diagnosis or *de novo* in pregnancy. An LVEF less than 40% is a predictor of adverse events in pregnancy, and less than 30% or NYHA III/IV clinical status is a contraindication. Management is largely as discussed for peripartum cardiomyopathy, with the important addition of consideration of termination of pregnancy for women with worsening symptoms or ventricular function prior to fetal viability.

Hypertrophic cardiomyopathy

Women with hypertrophic cardiomyopathy generally tolerate pregnancy well, with outcome predicted by prepregnancy functional status. An asymptomatic woman has a better than 90% chance of remaining so throughout her pregnancy. Reported mortality rates are 0 to 1%, with the two deaths in a recent series both being high-risk cases who had been advised against pregnancy. Prepregnancy assessment should include exercise testing, echocardiography, and standard assessment of sudden cardiac death risk. Women with a high outflow tract gradient are at increased risk and those with severe systolic or diastolic dysfunction should be advised against pregnancy. Women with moderate diastolic dysfunction may require diuretic treatment if they do not cope with volume expansion. β-Blockers should be continued and atrial fibrillation cardioverted if it occurs. An implantable cardioverter-defibrillator is no bar to pregnancy. During labour cardiac filling pressures should be maintained by fluid infusion, especially in the event of postpartum haemorrhage, and any epidural analgesia/anaesthesia should be low dose to avoid vasodilatation.

Ischaemic heart disease

In the 10 years from 1994 a small decrease in the female prevalence of hypertension and smoking, combined with an increase in diabetes and obesity, resulted in an unchanged prevalence of cardiovascular disease in women. However, the proportion of live births occurring to women in their thirties or older has more than doubled over the last 30 years, such that the prevalence of coronary atheroma in pregnant women is increasing.

Known ischaemic heart disease prepregnancy is rare and should be assessed as if risk-stratifying for noncardiac surgery. Previous percutaneous coronary intervention (PCI) or coronary artery bypass grafting (CABG) is no bar to pregnancy if functional status is good and ventricular function normal. Angina presenting in pregnancy should be managed with standard medical therapy, other than a statin as these are teratogenic. PCI is feasible, as described above. Drug-eluting stents should be avoided as their safety is unknown in pregnancy and their use would require prolonged dual

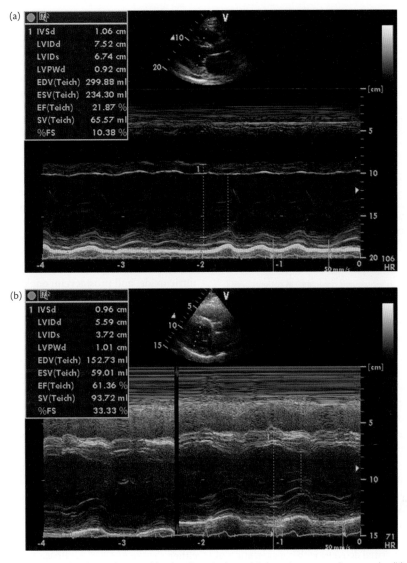

Fig. 18.1.1 Left ventricular dimensions on M-mode echocardiogram. (a) Dilated impaired ventricle in peripartum cardiomyopathy; (b) normal ventricle.

antiplatelet therapy. Troponin I is unaffected by normal pregnancy and delivery.

In the United States of America myocardial infarction occurs in 3 to 6 in 100 000 deliveries, with mortality 5 to 7%. Most cases occur in the third trimester, largely peripartum. Risk factors include thrombophilia, infection, and transfusion in addition to standard coronary risk factors. Coronary atheroma is present in less than half of cases (43%), with the remainder caused by spontaneous dissection, thrombosis, or embolus. In 29% of cases angiography is entirely normal and coronary spasm the presumed diagnosis; this has been reported following administration of the vasoconstrictor ergometrine to prevent postpartum haemorrhage (transfusion, listed above as a risk factor, may be a surrogate marker for this). Immediate angiography is the management of choice as it allows percutaneous intervention and appropriate targeting of secondary coronary prevention. Thrombolysis is not contraindicated, but best avoided 2 weeks peripartum because of the risk of postpartum haemorrhage. Aspirin is safe, but there is only case report evidence about other antiplatelet drugs.

Aortopathy

Dilated aortic root

Aortic root dilatation secondary to cystic medial necrosis occurs in association with Marfan's syndrome and related disorders, Turner's syndrome, familial thoracic aneurysm, bicuspid aortic valve, and repaired tetralogy of Fallot, but has also been reported in healthy pregnant women. Together with hypertension, atherosclerosis, and infection it confers a risk of type A dissection, most commonly in the third trimester or peripartum—the time of greatest haemodynamic shear stress to the aortic wall. Most of the literature concerns Marfan's syndrome, with an overall pregnancy mortality of 1%. It is important to note that although prepregnancy aortic root dimensions less than 4 cm tend to remain stable during pregnancy, dissection can occur in a nondilated root, especially if there is a family history. Although the number of reported cases is small, the risk in Marfan's syndrome appears to increase significantly if the aortic root diameter is greater than 4.5 cm, in which case elective aortic root replacement before conception should be considered. The risk of dissection is lower in other conditions, such as bicuspid

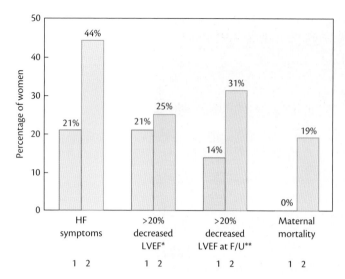

Fig. 18.1.2 Maternal complications in subsequent pregnancy in patients with previous peripartum cardiomyopathy. Group 1, LVEF >50% prior to subsequent pregnancy; group 2, LVEF <50%. HF, heart failure. *During subsequent pregnancy or early postpartum period, **at average of 6 years after subsequent pregnancy. From Elkayam U. (2002). Pregnant again after peripartum cardiomyopathy: to be or not to be? *Eur Heart J*, **23**, 753–6, with permission.

aortic valve and tetralogy of Fallot, and a prepregnancy threshold of 5 cm is used for prophylactic surgery. In small women an indexed measurement of 2.7 cm/m² body surface are (BSA) is more useful. The aorta should be screened by echocardiography and MRI/CT before conception and by echocardiogram every 4 to 12 weeks during pregnancy and the puerperium (Fig. 18.1.3). It is recommended that, regardless of root diameter, all higher-risk women are fully β-blocked throughout pregnancy. If despite these measures the root dilates rapidly or dissects, the management of choice is caesarean delivery of a viable fetus followed by root replacement. If the fetus is nonviable, surgery should proceed, accepting the risk of fetal loss. Low-risk cases should have a normal delivery with consideration of an assisted second stage, but caesarean section should be considered when maximum aortic dimension exceeds 4.5 cm. Obstetric complications of Marfan's syndrome include recurrent miscarriage, preterm rupture of membranes, and postpartum haemorrhage. Ehlers–Danlos type IV (associated with aortic involvement) confers a significant risk of uterine rupture and is therefore a contraindication to pregnancy.

Coarctation of the aorta

Pregnancy is low risk in repaired coarctation as long as there is no aneurysm at the site of repair: MRI or CT should be performed before conception to exclude this. Two recent series reported a single death, by type A dissection, in 104 women (20 unrepaired) undergoing 244 pregnancies. The incidence of hypertension is fourfold higher than in the general pregnant population, particularly in those women with a residual or native gradient higher than 20 mmHg. This should ideally be corrected prior to pregnancy. In the presence of a significant gradient the concerns are dual: maternal hypertension, with risk of aortic dissection and stroke, and hypotension of the fetoplacental unit. Blood pressure should therefore be measured in the right arm and either leg, using β-blockers as the first-line antihypertensive agent to achieve systolic pressures of less than 140 mmHg in the arm and more than 70 mmHg

in the leg. Delivery should usually be vaginal, with consideration of assisted second stage in the presence of a significant gradient or hypertension, unless an aneurysm is present. Angioplasty and stenting of coarctation during pregnancy and the puerperium is not recommended because of the increased predisposition to dissection during this period, although there are no series from which to estimate risk.

Pulmonary hypertension

Pulmonary hypertension (mPAP >25 mmHg at rest or 30 mmHg on exercise) of any cause is high risk for pregnancy, with maternal mortality around 30%. Effective contraception or termination should be advised. Women who elect to continue should be monitored closely in a specialist centre and advised strongly to reconsider termination should they deteriorate in the first or second trimester.

Suggested treatments include bed rest, oxygen, anticoagulation, and targeted pulmonary vascular therapies such as sildenafil, nitric oxide, and prostacyclin analogues, but the evidence is scant. Bosentan is not recommended as it has been associated with animal teratogenesis. One small series reported an improved maternal mortality with a regimen of oxygen, heparin before delivery, and warfarin after 48 h; 60% of infants were liveborn, with most premature. Early reports of the use of nebulized iloprost, intravenous epoprostenol, and oral sildenafil are optimistic, but numbers are small and deaths still occur.

In the presence of a right-to-left shunt (Eisenmenger's syndrome), systemic vasodilatation should be avoided, as this increases shunting and therefore cyanosis, and thromboembolic prophylaxis should be considered.

Admission for bed rest and timing of delivery are determined by the clinical status of the woman. There is no evidence to support the choice of either vaginal or caesarean delivery for cardiac reasons: vaginal delivery is associated with a lower average blood loss but also increased maternal effort. In practice early caesarean delivery is often required because of intrauterine growth retardation. In either case regional anaesthesia is preferable to general anaesthesia, as positive pressure ventilation reduces preload. Invasive blood pressure monitoring is required, and oxytocic drugs should be given as a low-dose infusion, rather than a bolus dose. Monitoring should continue for at least a week after delivery because the risk of sudden death postpartum is high.

Valvular lesions
Mitral stenosis

This is generally rheumatic in aetiology, occurring predominantly in those born outside the developed world. The volume expansion and tachycardia of pregnancy can unmask a previously clinically silent lesion. Death rates are low but pulmonary oedema or arrhythmia occur in one-third, particularly those with valve area less than 1.5 cm² or a history of cardiac events. Medical therapy includes β-blockade to increase time for diastolic filling, diuretics, and consideration of anticoagulation, as left atrial thrombus has been reported in pregnancy even in sinus rhythm. New atrial fibrillation should be cardioverted promptly. If NYHA III/IV symptoms develop despite medical therapy, and the valve is morphologically suitable, balloon mitral valvuloplasty is the treatment of choice, being clinically successful in more than 95% with significantly lower rates of fetal loss than surgery.

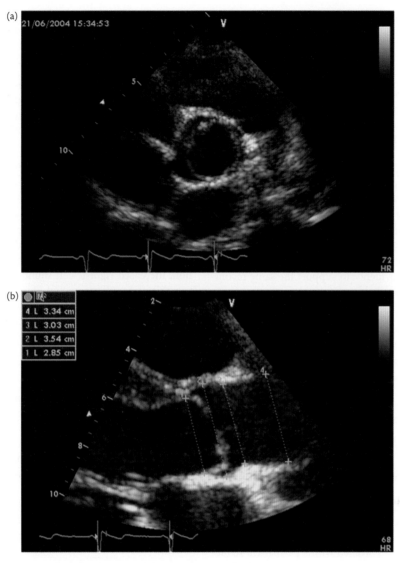

Fig. 18.1.3 Bicuspid aortic valve: (a) in short axis, (b) showing the aortic root measurements used in monitoring.

Aortic stenosis and bicuspid aortic valve

Bicuspid aortic valve (Fig. 18.1.3) in the absence of any stenosis or aortic dilatation can be managed as a normal pregnancy.

Aortic stenosis is well tolerated if before pregnancy the patient is asymptomatic, has a normal resting ECG, echocardiography shows normal LV function with peak aortic valve gradient less than 80 mmHg and mean less than 50 mmHg, and a treadmill exercise test to target heart rate (220 minus age) reveals no ST segment change or arrhythmia and a normal haemodynamic response. Otherwise aortic stenosis should be relieved before conception using balloon dilatation or a tissue valve if feasible, to avoid mechanical valve replacement. A recent series reported a 10% complication rate in pregnant women with peak gradient more than 64 mmHg or valve area less than 1 cm^2 and no complications in those with less severe stenosis. The valve gradient will increase as pregnancy progresses and failure to do so is a warning sign of ventricular dysfunction. There is benefit in bed rest and β-blockade if a pregnant woman presents or becomes severely symptomatic with dyspnoea, angina or syncope, but balloon valvuloplasty may need to be considered. Valve replacement during pregnancy carries a maternal mortality of 1.5 to 6% and fetal mortality of 30%. Delivery should generally be vaginal, avoiding vasodilatation and fluid shifts, with consideration of caesarean delivery under general anaesthetic in severe symptomatic cases only. It is unknown whether pregnancy accelerates the progression of congenital aortic stenosis.

Pulmonary stenosis

This is generally well tolerated, although in severe cases may precipitate right heart failure, tricuspid regurgitation, or atrial arrhythmia. Women with a prepregnancy peak echo gradient of more than 64 mmHg or symptoms should be considered for balloon valvuloplasty or surgery before conception. Balloon valvuloplasty is also possible during pregnancy if symptoms develop. It has been suggested that women with pulmonary stenosis are at increased risk of hypertensive disorders and preterm delivery, but this requires confirmation.

Mitral and aortic regurgitation

Left-sided valve regurgitation is generally very well tolerated in pregnancy if ventricular function is normal. The offloading of the left ventricle caused by systemic vasodilatation is beneficial, but diuretics and vasodilators such as nitrates may be necessary in addition. ACE inhibitors are contraindicated in pregnancy.

Small left-to-right shunts

Atrial septal defect

In the presence of a normal pulmonary vascular resistance an unrepaired atrial septal defect should be well tolerated. The pre-existing tendency to atrial arrhythmia may increase with the increase in cardiac output. The potential to shunt right to left in combination with the hypercoagulable state of pregnancy increases the risk of paradoxical embolism, especially with increases in intrathoracic pressure during labour. There should therefore be a low threshold for the use of compression stockings and prophylactic heparin in the presence of immobility or additional risk factors for venous thrombosis. This also applies to patients known to have a patent foramen ovale. Surgical or device closure of the atrial septal defect removes this risk and if planned should therefore be carried out before pregnancy, although there is no evidence to support the same recommendation for patent foramen ovale.

Ventricular septal defect or patent ductus arteriosus

A small defect with normal right-sided pressures confers no added risk in pregnancy. Because of the large pressure gradient across the defect, paradoxical embolism is extremely unlikely. Large defects causing pulmonary vascular disease (Eisenmenger's syndrome) are high risk as discussed earlier.

Complex congenital heart disease

For full descriptions of these lesions and their sequelae see Chapter 12.

Transposition of the great arteries—post Mustard or Senning atrial repair

Successful tolerance of pregnancy depends largely on good function of the systemic right ventricle and its atrioventricular valve. In a total of 195 pregnancies reported in 104 women there were 2 deaths, 1 heart transplant, and 7 women with a permanent reduction in ventricular function or functional class. Atrial arrhythmia occurs in 10 to 20%, those with a previous history being at higher risk. There is an increased incidence of miscarriage, prematurity, and low birth weight. More recently, repair has been by the arterial switch operation, following which pregnancy appears to be well tolerated, but the number reported remains small.

Congenitally corrected transposition of the great arteries

Outcome of this rare condition (where the circulation is physiologically 'corrected', with blood passing from the pulmonary veins to the left atrium, to the right ventricle, to the aorta) depends on systemic right ventricular function and the presence of associated lesions such as complete heart block, ventricular septal defect, or pulmonary stenosis.

Fontan operation for univentricular circulation

These patients have two separate circulations in series and are therefore usually not cyanosed, but they experience a chronic low-output state and are at risk of ventricular failure, atrial arrhythmia, and thrombosis. They are generally anticoagulated with warfarin, which should be converted to full-dose LMWH for the duration of pregnancy. Maternal outcome again depends on functional capacity and ventricular function. If these are satisfactory and the woman

accepts the two- to threefold increase in the rate of first trimester fetal loss, then there is no reason to advise against pregnancy, as any deterioration appears to be reversible.

Surgically corrected tetralogy of Fallot

Women with good functional capacity and no significant haemodynamic abnormality tolerate pregnancy well, although the presence of severe pulmonary regurgitation confers a 20 to 30% risk of symptomatic heart failure. If the mother carries del22q11 the recurrence risk is 50%.

Cyanotic heart disease without pulmonary hypertension

Cyanosis is associated with a poorer outcome for both mother and fetus. The risk of paradoxical embolism should be reduced by appropriate hydration, mobilization, use of compression stockings, and consideration of thromboprophylaxis. Because cyanosis also confers an increased bleeding tendency, full-dose anticoagulants are not used routinely, but only if there is an additional indication. Increased right-to-left shunting can occur with the systemic vasodilatation of pregnancy, causing worsening cyanosis. Fetal outcome is dependent on maternal saturation: the chance of a live birth decreases from 92% with prepregnancy maternal saturation over 90%, to 12% if maternal saturation is less than 85%, and many of these infants are premature or of low birth weight.

Prosthetic valves

Bioprosthetic valves do not confer increased risk if haemodynamics are normal, and they do not degenerate more rapidly in pregnancy as previously feared. The management of a mechanical prosthesis is far less straightforward and represents a conflict of interest between the mother and fetus. Complication rates associated with the alternative anticoagulation regimens are shown in Table 18.1.2. The increased rate of fetal loss associated with all effective anticoagulation may reflect retroplacental haemorrhage.

A relatively safe option for the mother is to remain on warfarin for the duration of the pregnancy, changing to dose-adjusted unfractionated or LMWH at 36 weeks (to allow the fetus to clear the warfarin) if vaginal delivery is planned, or at 38 weeks for elective caesarean delivery. This strategy is associated with a risk of warfarin embryopathy, which is significantly reduced if the dose required to achieve target INR is less than 6 mg daily.

Heparin does not cross the placenta, hence a strategy of substituting heparin for warfarin during the period of organogenesis (6–12 weeks) abolishes the risk of warfarin embryopathy, but it doubles the maternal thromboembolism rate. Heparin throughout pregnancy has historically been associated with a high risk of thromboembolism, but has not always been appropriately dose-adjusted. With twice-daily dosing of LMWH and anti-Xa levels monitored fortnightly, achieving a level of 1 to 1.2 IU/ml 4 to 6 h post dose, the thromboembolism rate in a recent meta-analysis was only 2%.

Arrhythmia

Ectopy occurs in most pregnancies, but sustained arrhythmia in less than 1%. A pre-existing tachyarrhythmia confers a 50% chance of a recurrence of supraventricular tachycardia and 25% of ventricular tachycardia. The principles of diagnosis and management are the same as in the nonpregnant state—only recurrent symptomatic or life-threatening arrhythmia should be treated and underlying

Table 18.1.2 Complication rates (%) of anticoagulation regimens in pregnant women with mechanical heart valves

Regimen	Maternal thromboembolism	Maternal death	Fetal abnormality	Fetal loss[a]	Source
Warfarin to 38/40, then heparin	4	2	6	34	Chan et al. (2000)
Heparin 6–12/40, warfarin otherwise	9	4	0[b]	16	Chan et al. (2000)
Heparin throughout	25	7	0	44	Chan et al. (2000)
Heparin anti-Xa adjusted throughout	2	0	0	12[c]	Oran et al. (2004)

[a] Refers to abortion, stillbirth, or neonatal death.

[b] If heparin instituted at or before 6/40.

[c] Abortion and stillbirth only.

causes such as thyroid disease should be sought and corrected. Vagal manoeuvres are useful as a first line to diagnose or terminate a narrow complex tachycardia. Adenosine is safe in pregnancy, as is DC cardioversion with fetal monitoring. The risk/benefit ratio of all drugs should be assessed: no drug is absolutely contraindicated, as maternal haemodynamic instability may result in worse fetal outcome. Bradyarrhythmia is rare; the presence of a permanent pacemaker or implantable cardioverter-defibrillator is no problem, but the permanent pacemaker may need to be reprogrammed for delivery. Equipment for temporary pacing during labour is recommended, though not usually needed, for nonpaced women with complete heart block.

Contraception

Barrier methods

These are safe for all cardiac patients and have the added benefit of protection against sexually transmitted diseases, but reported failure rates are 2 to 26 per 100 woman years.

Hormonal methods

The oestrogen component of the combined oral contraceptive, whether oral or transdermal, confers an increased risk of thrombosis that is not completely abolished by warfarin. These preparations are therefore contraindicated in women who already have a high thrombotic risk, i.e. pulmonary hypertension, the Fontan circulation, older mechanical valves, dilated cardiac chambers with the risk of atrial fibrillation, or in cyanosed patients in whom paradoxical embolism may occur. The standard progesterone-only 'minipill' is safe, but is less reliable than the combined oral contraceptive pill and therefore not the method of choice for women in whom avoidance of pregnancy is critical. Recommended progesterone-only preparations, more reliable as they act by suppression of ovulation, include daily oral desogestrel, 3 monthly depot medroxyprogesterone, and a subcutaneous etonogestrel implant, which is the method of choice for complex congenital heart disease. Women concurrently taking the endothelin antagonist bosentan require additional protection.

Intrauterine devices

These are not contraindicated, but insertion of the device can be associated with bacteraemia and also a vasovagal response, which can be life-threatening in a haemodynamically unstable patient such as those with a Fontan circulation or Eisenmenger's syndrome.

Sterilization

Sterilization by tubal ligation may be appropriate for women in whom pregnancy would be high risk. However, failure may result in ectopic pregnancy and the surgery is not trivial, especially in women at risk of paradoxical embolism, as it includes a head-down tilt and distension of the abdomen with CO_2. Sterilization of the male partner is not generally advised if he has a much longer potential lifespan than his partner and may therefore wish to father children in a subsequent relationship.

Further reading

Bates SM, et al. (2008). Venous thromboembolism, thrombophilia, antithrombotic therapy, and pregnancy. ACCP Clinical Practice Guideline. Chest, **133**, 844S–66S.

Beauchesne LM, et al. (2001). Coarctation of the aorta: outcome of pregnancy. J Am Coll Cardiol, **38**, 1728–33.

Chan WS, Anand S, Ginsberg JS (2000). Anticoagulation of pregnant women with mechanical heart valves: a systematic review of the literature. Arch Intern Med, **160**, 191–6.

Gowda RM, et al. (2003). Cardiac arrhythmias in pregnancy: clinical and therapeutic considerations. Int J Cardiol, **88**, 129–33.

James AH, et al. (2006). Acute myocardial infarction in pregnancy: a United States population-based study. Circulation, **113**, 1564–71.

Meijboom LJ, et al. (2005). Pregnancy and aortic root growth in the Marfan syndrome: a prospective study. Eur Heart J, **26**, 914–20.

Oran B, Lee-Parritz A, Ansell J (2004). Low molecular weight heparin for the prophylaxis of thromboembolism in women with prosthetic mechanical heart valves during pregnancy. Thromb Haemost, **92**, 747–51.

Presbitero P, et al. (1994). Pregnancy in cyanotic congenital heart disease. Outcome of mother and fetus. Circulation, **89**, 2673–6.

Silversides CK, et al. (2003). Cardiac risk in pregnant women with rheumatic mitral stenosis. Am J Cardiol, **91**, 1382–5.

Silversides CK, et al. (2003). Early and intermediate-term outcomes of pregnancy with congenital aortic stenosis. Am J Cardiol, **91**, 1386–9.

Siu SC, et al. (2001). Prospective multicenter study of pregnancy outcomes in women with heart disease. Circulation, **104**, 515–21.

Sliwa K, et al. (2010). Current state of knowledge on aetiology, diagnosis, management and therapy of peripartum cardiomyopathy: a position statement from the Heart Failure Association of the European Society of Cardiology Working Group on peripartum cardiomyopathy. Eur J Heart Fail, **12**, 767–78.

Steer PJ, Gatzoulis MA, Baker P (ed.) (2006). Heart disease and pregnancy, London: RCOG Press.

Task Force on the Management of Cardiovascular Diseases During Pregnancy of the European Society of Cardiology (2011). ESC Guidelines on the management of cardiovascular diseases during pregnancy. Eur Heart J, **32**, 3147–97.

Thaman R, *et al.* (2003). Pregnancy associated complications in women with hypertrophic cardiomyopathy. *Heart*, **89**, 752–6.

Thorne S, MacGregor A, Nelson-Piercy C (2006). Risks of contraception and pregnancy in heart disease. *Heart*, **92**, 1520–5.

Thorne SA, *et al.* (2006). Pregnancy and contraception in heart disease and pulmonary arterial hypertension. *J Fam Plann Reprod Health Care*, **32**, 75–81.

Veldtman GR, *et al.* (2004). Outcomes of pregnancy in women with tetralogy of Fallot. *J Am Coll Cardiol*, **44**, 174–80.

Vitale N, *et al.* (1999). Dose-dependent fetal complications of warfarin in pregnant women with mechanical heart valves. *J Am Coll Cardiol*, **33**, 1637–41.

Vriend JWJ, *et al.* (2005). Outcome of pregnancy in patients after repair of aortic coarctation. *Eur Heart J*, **26**, 2173–8.

Walker F (2007). Pregnancy and the various forms of the Fontan circulation. *Heart*, **93**, 152–4.

Weiss BM, Hess OM. (2000). Pulmonary vascular disease and pregnancy: current controversies, management strategies, and perspectives. *Eur Heart J*, **21**, 104–15.

SECTION 19

Chronic peripheral oedema and lymphoedema

CHAPTER 19.1

Chronic peripheral oedema and lymphoedema

Peter S. Mortimer

Essentials

Lymph transport, not venous reabsorption, is the main process responsible for interstitial fluid drainage. All peripheral oedema is either absolute or relative lymph drainage failure. Oedema develops when the microvascular filtration rate exceeds lymph drainage for a sufficient period, either because the filtration rate is high or because lymph flow is low, or a combination of the two. Lymphoedema is strictly peripheral oedema due solely to a failure of lymph drainage. Most peripheral oedema arises from microvascular fluid filtration overwhelming lymph drainage, e.g. heart failure, but lymphoedema supervenes as lymph function declines if high filtration is sustained.

Causes of lymphoedema

Lymph drainage may fail either because of a defect intrinsic to the lymph conducting pathways (primary lymphoedema), or because of irreversible damage from some factor(s) originating from outside the lymphatic system (secondary lymphoedema).

Primary lymphoedema is caused by genetic faults in lymphatic development. These faults may be chromosomal abnormalities as seen in Turner's syndrome, germline mutations such as in the vascular endothelial growth factor receptor-3 gene which causes Milroy's disease, or as a somatic mutation as in congenital lymphatic malformations, but for most forms of lymphoedema the genetic cause is unknown.

For secondary lymphoedema filariasis is by far the most common cause of lymphoedema worldwide. In the developed world most cases are secondary to cancer treatment and poor mobility.

Clinical features and management

Lymphoedema causes persistent swelling which is often associated with recurrent cellulitis. Response to diuretics is poor. The oedema does pit, but prolonged pressure may be required as the skin becomes thickened and warty. The investigation of choice for confirming lymphoedema is lymphoscintigraphy.

No drug or surgical therapy is known to improve lymph drainage. Current best practice aims to (1) improve lymph drainage through physiological principles known to stimulate lymph flow, and (2) control any excessive microvascular fluid filtration. Exercise and movement combined with compression form the basis of stimulating lymph flow. This generates a high interstitial pressure during muscle contractions to drive lymph drainage. Low pressures during

skeletal muscle relaxation permit lymphatic vessel refilling before further muscle contraction repeats the cycle.

Cellulitis, often recurrent, occurs in up to 50% of lymphoedema cases. The mechanism is presumed to be disturbed immune cell trafficking. Each attack can cause further decline in lymph drainage and worse swelling. Prevention and prompt treatment of cellulitis is crucial to the control of lymphoedema.

Introduction

The primary function of the lymphatic vessels is to drain the plasma filtrate within body tissues and return it to the blood circulation. Lymphatic vessels also have an important immune surveillance function, as they are the main drainage route from the tissues for immune active cells such as dendritic cells, lymphocytes and macrophages. Intestinal lymphatics are responsible for fat absorption. Defects in lymphatic function can lead to lymph accumulation in tissues and swelling (lymphoedema), dampened immune responses (infection), and disturbed fat homeostasis. Lymphatic vessels are also the preferential route for cancer spread.

Oedema

Oedema is an excess of interstitial fluid and is an important sign of ill health in clinical medicine. The usual clinical approach to peripheral oedema is to consider a single diagnosis such as heart failure, nephrotic syndrome, venous obstruction, or lymphoedema. This viewpoint fails to appreciate the many dynamic physiological forces contributing to oedema development and in particular the central role of the lymphatic drainage system in tissue fluid (and consequently plasma volume) homeostasis. Hence the clinician's approach to peripheral oedema is often misguided and the necessary medical intervention inappropriate (e.g. empirical use of diuretics). Management of peripheral oedema is better based on physiological principles that can then guide treatment.

Pathophysiology

Lymph transport, not venous reabsorption, is the main process responsible for interstitial fluid drainage. Oedema develops when the microvascular (from capillaries and venules) filtration rate exceeds lymph drainage for a sufficient period, either because the filtration rate is high or because lymph flow is low, or a combination

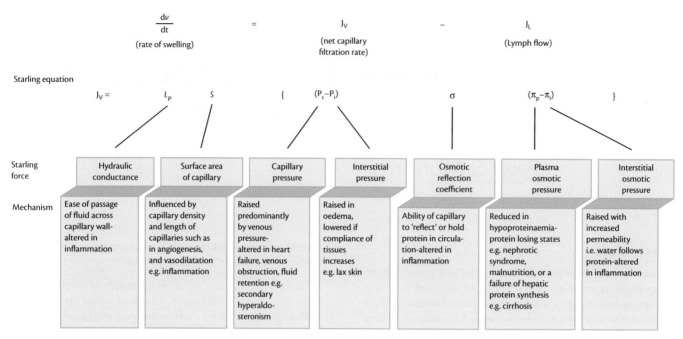

Fig. 19.1.1 Physiology of oedema.

of the two. Filtration rate is governed by the Starling principle of fluid exchange, which is described succinctly and quantitatively by the Starling equation for flow across a semipermeable membrane (Fig. 19.1.1).

In simple terms, filtration of fluid from capillary into interstitium is driven by the hydraulic (water) pressure gradient across the wall $(P_c - P_i)$ and is opposed by the osmotic pressure gradient $(\pi_p - \pi_i)$, which is the 'suction' force keeping fluid in the circulation.

The Starling equation provides a logical approach for classifying oedema that is due to increased filtration (Box 19.1.1)

Traditionally it has been taught that the arterial end of capillaries filters fluid while the venous end reabsorbs the bulk of fluid filtered. This view is not supported by modern evidence, which demonstrates that in most vascular beds there is a net but dwindling filtration along the entire length of well-perfused capillaries. The sum of all Starling forces is not an absorptive force in venous capillaries but a slight filtration force (except e.g. following haemorrhage, when capillary pressure drops sufficiently for transient absorption to occur). Even under such circumstances Starling forces soon re-equilibrate and slight filtration is restored. Sustained reabsorption of fluid is a normal feature of some microcirculatory beds, namely intestinal mucosa, renal peritubular, and lymph node capillaries, but not peripheral tissues. Since the old concept of sustained fluid absorption by venous capillaries is no longer tenable, the major responsibility for drainage of interstitial fluid is through the lymphatic system.

Restraining factors against oedema include (1) elevation of interstitial fluid pressure, (2) fall in interstitial colloid osmotic pressure (COP), and (3) increased lymph flow. Stiffness in tissues resists swelling. A small increase in interstitial fluid in a stiff tissue (low compliance) will cause a relatively large increase in interstitial pressure (P_i), which then opposes filtration. Placing a bandage or rigid stocking around a leg will reduce compliance and resist stretch. Consequently P_i will increase more steeply for a given interstitial volume increase and the increased P_i will oppose filtration. Relating

to interstitial COP, an increase in filtration rate will dilute the interstitial protein concentration and consequently reduce the osmotic pressure (π immediately outside the semipermeable membrane).

Box 19.1.1 Starling forces in the classification of oedema

1 Raised capillary pressure

Capillary pressure is more susceptible to changes in venous pressure than systemic (arterial) blood pressure because postcapillary resistance is much lower than precapillary resistance. Peripheral venous pressure is raised in:

- right ventricular failure
- salt and water overload (e.g. overtransfusion)
- venous obstruction
- venous reflux (chronic venous disease) e.g. following deep vein thrombosis, primary varicose veins
- dependency (the effect of gravity)

2 Reduced plasma osmotic pressure (COP)

This essentially means hypoalbuminaemia, which can arise from:

- malnutrition
- intestinal disease (malabsorption or protein loss)
- nephrotic syndrome
- hepatic failure to synthesize albumin—due to liver disease or chronic inflammatory states

3 Increased capillary permeability

Inflammation can cause a breakdown in the endothelial barrier, facilitating the passage of both plasma proteins and water across the capillary wall. In addition, vasodilatation causes a rise in capillary pressure (and blood flow).

The resulting increase in the osmotic pressure gradient will raise the suction force keeping fluid within the blood compartment.

Increases in interstitial fluid pressure and volume stimulate lymph flow. Lymph drainage is a complex process involving absorption of protein and fluid (as well as other macromolecules, microorganisms, immune cells, and cancer cells) from the interstitium into initial lymphatic vessels (also known as lymphatics) and then downstream through vessels of ever-enlarging diameter until reaching the main collecting lymphatics that pump lymph to the sentinel lymph nodes. Valves ensure unidirectional flow. Transport of interstitial fluid into and along initial lymphatics is largely a passive process dependent upon changes in tissue (interstitial) pressure from movement (active and passive exercise), massage, and local arterial pulsation and—in more central tissues—breathing. The larger collecting lymphatics contract and are mainly responsible for pumping lymph against gravity. Successive segments of collecting lymphatics behave like 'mini hearts' in series, and their contractile cycle bears striking similarities to the cardiac cycle. Sympathetic input influences the pumping rate, while the diastolic filling (preload or supply from upstream lymphatics) controls the force of contraction. Flow in collecting lymphatics is only as good as the supply from initial (noncontractile) lymphatics. Influx of calcium ions is important for smooth muscle contraction in the walls of the collecting lymphatics, hence calcium channel antagonists may cause oedema by paralysing lymphatic pumping.

The lymph vessels return the capillary filtrate back to the bloodstream via the lymph nodes and eventually the thoracic duct. This completes the extravascular circulation of fluid and protein and maintains tissue volume homeostasis. Lymph flow should respond to increases in capillary filtration and so prevent oedema. By failing to compensate for increased capillary filtration and so permit swelling, the lymphatic is to some extent failing in its duty to preventing all types of oedema. Differences in lymph drainage capacity could be the explanation for differing levels of leg oedema seen in patients with right-sided heart failure despite no difference in ejection fraction. Similarly, peripheral oedema that persists after heart failure has been successfully treated is likely to be lymphatic in origin.

True lymphoedema is strictly oedema arising from reduced lymph transport that is unable to cope with normal levels of capillary filtration. Most oedema arises from increased capillary filtration overwhelming lymph transport capacity for a sustained period of time. Once high lymph flow cannot be sustained and transport capacity fails, 'true' lymphoedema ensues. This pathophysiology is comparable with that occurring in high-output cardiac failure.

Aetiology

Lymph drainage may fail either because of a defect intrinsic to the lymph conducting pathways (primary lymphoedema, Figs. 19.1.2a and 19.1.2b) or because of irreversible damage from some factor(s) originating from outside the lymphatic system (secondary lymphoedema, Fig. 19.1.2c).

Physiologically there are only a limited number of ways that lymphatics can fail. They may be reduced in number (aplasia/hypoplasia), obliterated or damaged without repair (failed lymphangiogenesis), or obstructed; they may lose contractility (pump failure), or become incompetent (valvular reflux). A lack of sensitive methods for investigation makes it difficult to distinguish between these mechanisms.

Primary lymphoedema

A defining moment in lymphatic research came with the discovery of the receptor vascular endothelial growth factor receptor-3 (VEGFR-3) and its ligands VEGF-C and VEGF-D as the main signalling mechanism for lymphangiogenesis. Lymphatic endothelial cells differentiate from blood endothelial cells in the cardinal vein early in embryonal development, after the onset of circulation. SOX18 and PROX1 genes commit to a lymphatic lineage. VEGF-C and CCBE1 drive lymphatic capillary sprouting and migration. Mutations in SOX18 and CCBE1 are causal for primary lymphoedema in humans. In mice, deletion of Flt4 (= VEGFR-3) leads to defects in blood as well as lymphatic vessels and embryonic death, indicating an early role in both cardio- and lymphovascular function for this gene. Heterozygous missense point mutations leading to tyrosine kinase inactivation have been found in VEGFR3 in patients with congenital familial lymphoedema (Milroy's disease, OMIM 153100). The phenotype manifests with inheritable lymphoedema at or soon after birth, with swelling confined to one or both feet and ankles due to impaired function of initial lymphatics. A phenotype similar to Milroy's is microcephaly lymphoedema syndrome for which the mutation is in KIF11, hence it is important to measure head circumference in congenital lymphoedema confined to the feet and legs.

The forkhead transcription factor FOXC2 is involved in the specification of the lymphatic capillary vs collecting lymphatic vessel phenotype. It is also important for the development and maintenance of lymphatic (and venous) valves. Heterozygous loss-of-function mutations in FOXC2 cause lymphoedema–distichiasis (OMIM 153400), a dominantly inherited late-onset (postpubertal) lymphoedema associated with a double row of (ingrowing) eyelashes (distichiasis). Unlike Milroy's disease the lymphatic vasculature is well formed or even hyperplastic, but a defect in lymphatic valves results in lymph reflux. Swelling may not manifest until the fifth decade, indicating how genetic abnormalities can cause late-onset lymphoedema. The phenotype can also cause congenital heart disease, emphasizing the close relationship between cardiovascular and lymphatic development.

Primary lymphoedema may be sporadic and involve several limbs, genitalia, or even the face (multisegmental). A failure in lymphatic development may also manifest with internal lymphatic abnormalities such as pleural/pericardial effusions, and pulmonary or intestinal lymphangiectasia. Intestinal lymphangiectasia or disturbances in mesenteric lymph drainage may result in chylous reflux, with chyle rerouting to various parts of the body, e.g. chylous effusion or ascites. The fat as well as protein content of such fluids should be measured for diagnosis. Mutations in CCBE1 cause generalized lymphatic dysplasia with widespread lymphatic abnormalities, both peripheral and internal. To date, nine mutations have been discovered which are causal for primary lymphoedema. Emberger's syndrome (OMIM 614038), caused by mutations in the transcription factor GATA2, manifests with myelodysplasia which predisposes to acute myeloid leukaemia. Systemic immunodeficiency is an associated feature, indicating the close relationship between the lymphatic system and immune competence.

Primary lymphoedema may occur in isolation or as part of a syndrome, e.g. Turner's, Noonan's (OMIM 163950) or Proteus (OMIM 176920). For most forms of primary lymphoedema the genetic cause remains unknown. Swelling usually presents at or after puberty, particularly in females, and affects the distal leg. Familial

Causes of Primary Lymphoedema

(a)

SYNDROMIC (Lymphoedema not the dominant feature)		SYSTEMIC / VISCERAL INVOLVEMENT		MALFORMATION		LYMPHOEDEMA (Dominant feature)		PROLIFERATIVE
CHROMOSOMAL	SINGLE GENE DISORDER	GENERALISED LYMPHATIC DYSPLASIA	MULTISEGMENT* ASYMMETRICAL LYMPHOEDEMA WITH SYSTEMIC INVOLVEMENT+	TISSUE OVERGROWTH / VASCULAR ANOMALIES	LYMPHATIC MALFORMATION	CONGENITAL	LATE ONSET > 1 YEAR	
Turner (45, XO) Prader-Willi	Noonan / Cardio-facio-cutaneous (RAS-MAPKinase pathway)	Hennekam syndrome (CCBE1, FAT4) PIEZO1 related lymphatic disorder (PIEZO1)	Multisegment Asymmetrical Lymphoedema with systemic involvement	Klippel-Trenaunay syndrome Parkes-Weber (RASA1)	Truncular Lymphatic malformation**	Milroy (VEGFR3 or VEGFC)	Lymphoedema distichiasis (FOXC2)	Lymphangiomatosis Gorham-Stout disease Generalized lymphatic anomaly
Phelan McDermid Syndrome (22q terminal deletion/ Ring chromosome 22) Velocardiofacial syndrome (22q11 mircodeletion) Down Syndrome Trisomy 21	Charge syndrome (CDH7) Aagenes syndrome Choanal Atresia-Lymphoedema (PTPN14) Ectodermal Dysplasia, Anhidrotic, Immunodeficiency; Osteopetrosis and Lymphoedema[OL-EDA-ID syndrome] (IKBKG (NEMO)) Fabry disease (GLA) Hypotrichosis-Lymphoedema-Telangiectasia (SOX18) Microcephaly with or without Chorioretinopathy, Lymphoedema or Mental Retardation [MCLMR] (KIF11)			Proteus / CLOVE / Fibroadipose hyperplasia /Macrocephaly Capillary Malformation (AKT/PIK3CA Related Overgrowth Spectrum (PROS))	Atruncular Lymphatic malformation*** (Lymphangioma) Mixed vascular malformation	Congenital Unisegmental Congenital Multisegmental (i.e. more than one segment)	Meige disease 4 Limb lymphoedema (GJC2) Emberger syndrome (GATA 2) Unisegmental Lymphoedema Multisegmental Lymphoedema Yellow Nail syndrome	Lymphangioleio myomatosis (TSC1 / TSC2)

With Chromosome or Genetic cause in red

*Multisegment = more than one body part (e.g. upper or lower limbs, genitalia, head/neck/trunk but not including bilateral lower limbs)

+Systemic/Visceral involvement includes hydrops fetalis, pleural or pericardial effusions, pulmonary or intestinal lymphangiectasia, chylous reflux

**Truncular = communicating with main lymphatic channels

*** Atruncular = isolated, aberrant system not communicating with main lymph channels

Fig. 19.1.2 (a) Causes of primary lymphoedema. (b) Classification and diagnostic algorithm for primary lymphatic dysplasia (c) Causes of secondary lymphoedema.
Part (b) is adapted from Connell F et al. (2013). The classification and diagnostic algorithm for primary lymphatic dysplasia: an update from 2010 to include molecular findings. *Clin Genet*, **84**, 3031–4.

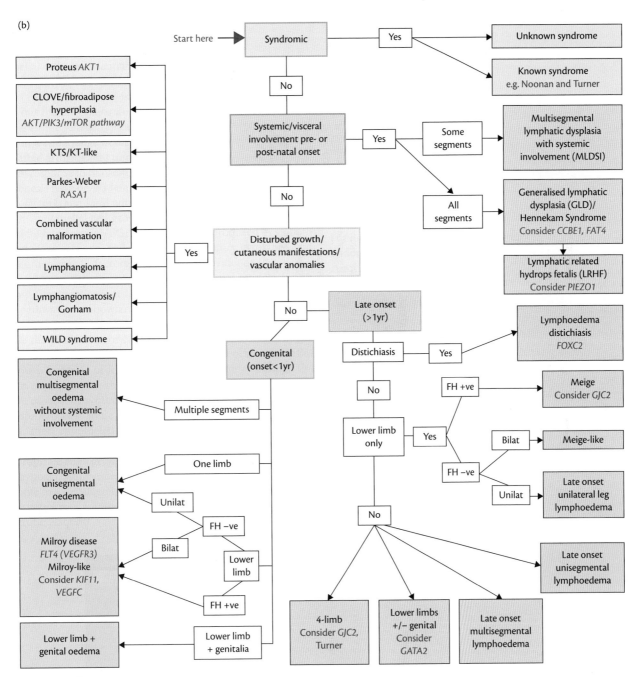

Fig. 19.1.2 Continued

Causes of Secondary Lymphoedema

CANCER		INFECTION		INFLAMMATION		VASCULAR	TRAUMA			DRUGS
TREATMENT	TUMOUR	FILARIASIS	LYMPHANGITIS CELLULITIS ERYSIPELAS	LYMPHATIC OCCLUSION	GRANULOMATOUS DISEAS	VENOUS DISEASE	SURGERY	ACCIDENT	FACTITIOUS	
Sentinel lymphnode biopsy or lymphadenectomy	Inflammatory cancer			Podoconiosis	Crohn's	Post Thrombotic Syndrome	Lymphatic vessel and node removal	Extensive soft tissue injury	Tourniquet application (Secretan's syndrome)	Calcium channel antagonists
Radiotherapy	Kaposi sarcoma			Pretibial myxoedema	Oro-facial granulomatosis	Venous leg ulcers	Vein harvesting	Burns		Rapamycin inhibitors e.g. sirolimus
Taxanes	Lymphangiosarcoma			Dermatitis / Eczema	Ano-genital granulomatosis	Intravenous drug abuse	Chronic regional pain syndrome (Type II)			
	Relapsed tumour			Rheumatoid arthritis	Mycobacterial disease	IVC Obstruction				
				Psoriasis	Rosacea	Retro-peritoneal fibrosis				
				Hidradenitis suppurativa		Left iliac vein compression (May-Thurner Syndrome)				

Fig. 19.1.2 Continued

(c)

forms in which lymphangiograms demonstrate a reduction in size and number of superficial lymphatic collecting vessels but no other phenotypic features are called Meige's disease (OMIM 153200). Lymphoedema of the proximal obstructive type with unilateral whole-limb swelling is sporadic in type. Lymphangiograms of this form of lymphoedema demonstrate obstruction at the inguinal nodes, so called ilio-inguinal nodal sclerosis, but no cause can be found. In cases of proximal obstruction it is of the utmost importance to exclude tumour or iliac vein thrombosis.

It is not unusual for lymphoedema to associate with hypertrophy of other tissues giving rise to increased limb girth or length. Those cases of unilateral limb swelling associated with overgrowth and vascular abnormalities such as port wine stain and/or varicose veins are likely to be a form of Klippel–Trenaunay syndrome.

The yellow nail syndrome, although given an OMIM number (153300), rarely has a family history and is of unknown cause.

Secondary lymphoedema

Filariasis is by far the most common cause of lymphoedema worldwide (filarial elephantiasis). It is endemic in eastern Asia, the Indian subcontinent, west and east Africa, Brazil, and the Caribbean. Microfilaria introduced into the skin by mosquitoes migrate towards and enter initial lymphatics. Adult worms develop within the main collector vessels close to the nodes, resulting in lymphatic dilatation and lymphadenitis.

In developed countries surgical removal or irradiation (or both) of lymph nodes for cancer treatment results in lymphoedema. In breast-cancer-related lymphoedema (BCRL) the exact mechanisms for development are unclear, but a simple 'stopcock' obstruction in the axilla from scarring seems unlikely. Lymphoedema can develop in some patients after one (sentinel) node removal, but not in others who have had a complete axillary clearance. The incidence of arm lymphoedema remains stubbornly high at over 1 in 5 despite developments such as breast-conserving surgery and sentinel lymph node biopsy. Obesity is a strong risk factor for BCRL and weight loss has been shown to improve existing lymphoedema significantly.

Cancer rarely presents with lymphoedema, except in advanced disease, but relapsed tumour frequently results in lymphoedema due to obstruction or infiltration of collateral lymphatic routes that have hitherto permitted escape of lymph. Kaposi's sarcoma is thought to arise from human herpesvirus-8-induced reprogramming of lymphatic endothelial cells. Vascular plaques in skin and lymphoedema characterize Kaposi's sarcoma. Lymphangiosarcoma is a highly malignant tumour of endothelial cells which usually arises in long-standing lymphoedema.

Lymphangitis or cellulitis probably only causes lymphoedema when the lymphatics are perilously vulnerable. Any patient suffering recurrent lymphangitis/cellulitis in the same region is likely to have pre-existing impaired lymphatic function. Recurrent attacks of cellulitis frequently lead to a stepwise deterioration in swelling.

Podoconiosis (endemic elephantiasis) is a form of endemic nonfilarial lymphoedema caused by microparticles of silica that penetrate the feet during barefoot walking in soil containing silica and aluminosilicates in tropical west and east Africa, certain volcanic islands, and Central America (see Chapter 9.5.8).

Functional lymphoedema may develop as a result of immobility and dependency due to infirmity following stroke, severe arthritis, or respiratory disease, with long periods spent in a chair. It is probably the lack of exercise as much as increased weight that causes lymphoedema to develop with obesity and sleep apnoea syndrome.

Lymphoedema is a common consequence of post-thrombotic syndrome (following deep vein thrombosis) and severe longstanding venous reflux due to varicose veins. High filtration rates from the ambulatory venous hypertension slowly exhaust lymph drainage in a manner equivalent to high-output cardiac failure. Irreversibly impaired lymph drainage eventually results. Lymphoedema can also result from long-term inflammatory states such as rheumatoid arthritis and chronic hand or foot dermatitis (with or without infection).

Epidemiology

An estimated 15 million people suffer from leg lymphoedema in filariasis-endemic areas of the world. Other lymphatic manifestations such as genital lymphoedema and hydrocoele are equally common. The prevalence of lymphoedema due to podoconiosis is estimated at 3.4% in Ethiopia rising to 5.6% in western Ethiopia.

In the United Kingdom secondary forms of lymphoedema, particularly cancer-related lymphoedema, are generally considered more frequent than primary forms. A study investigating lymphoedema in south-west London ascertained a prevalence of 1.33 per 1000 population, rising to 1 in 200 over 65 years of age, and with three noncancer patients for every cancer patient identified. 29% of the cases had experienced cellulitis in the preceding year, with one-quarter of them requiring admission. Time off work was attributed to the lymphoedema in 80% of cases, with employment status affected in 9%. Quality of life suffered with clear deficits in many domains of the well-validated SF-36 questionnaire.

More than one in five women who survive breast cancer will develop arm lymphoedema. Other cancers such as cervix, uterus, vulva, prostate, penis, head and neck, melanoma, and sarcoma have smaller numbers presenting with lymphoedema as a result of treatment or through progressive disease

Prevention

Identification of patients at risk of lymphoedema relies on awareness of its causes. In breast cancer the strongest risk factors are obesity, stage of cancer, extent of surgery and postoperative infection. In filariasis and podoconiosis prevention of infection through good skin and foot care seems the most important.

Clinical features

Lymphoedema is rarely considered at presentation and consequently diagnosis is usually delayed while other possible causes of swelling are investigated and excluded. Any chronic oedema, irrespective of cause, will mean lymphatic failure either absolute (lymphatic insufficiency with normal lymph load i.e. microvascular fluid filtration not increased) or relative (high lymph load from increased microvascular fluid filtration overwhelming lymph drainage capacity).

Lymphoedema most commonly affects the extremities, particularly the leg, although midline swelling affecting head and neck or genitalia can be an isolated finding. Truncal oedema is often observed in the adjoining quadrant of the trunk to an affected limb because of the shared lymph routes within the same lymph drainage basin. Oedema that is symmetrical (equal between right and left legs) is more likely to have systemic origins, e.g. right-sided heart failure or hypoproteinaemia. Oedema that is asymmetrical (more in one leg than the other) implies a local cause, e.g. impaired venous or lymph drainage, but both systemic and local causes can coexist. In a patient with advanced cancer leg oedema may result from a combination of hypoproteinaemia (liver metastases), impaired lymph drainage (original lymphadenectomy and/or lymphatic infiltration by tumour), venous obstruction (deep vein thrombosis or vein compression by tumour), immobility, and dependency.

History

Swelling frequently develops rapidly—within a day—but may be mild and intermittent at first. Pain may feature initially, prompting diagnoses such as deep vein thrombosis, soft tissue injury, or infection (although cellulitis often triggers lymphoedema). With time, oedema becomes more permanent and painless, although discomfort, aching, and heaviness are common symptoms. Functional impairment is slight until swelling becomes more severe (Fig. 19.1.3).

Lymphoedema does not respond much to elevation or diuretics, except in the early stages or when it is compounded by increased capillary filtration. Chronic oedema that does not reduce significantly overnight is likely to be lymphatic in origin.

Clinical signs

It is often said that lymphoedema does not pit, but this is not true unless the advanced stages of fibrosis (elephantiasis) have been established. To demonstrate pitting in lymphoedema sustained pressure for some 20 s may be necessary, owing to the firmer (and thicker) nature of the skin and subcutaneous tissues. The skin may double in thickness in lymphoedema, particularly at the base of the second toe, where it may become impossible to pinch up a fold of skin. An inability to pinch and lift a fold of skin at the base

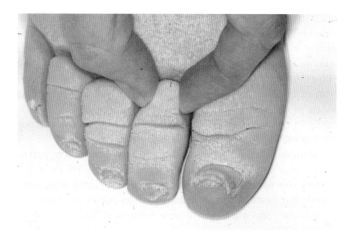

Fig. 19.1.4 Kaposi–Stemmer sign: the inability to pinch and pick up a fold of skin at the base of the second toe (due to thickened skin).

of the second toe is referred to as the (Kaposi–)Stemmer sign and is pathognomonic of lymphoedema (Fig. 19.1.4, Table 19.1.1). As the skin thickens so creases become enhanced and a warty texture (hyperkeratosis) develops.

Accumulation of lymph under pressure in dermal lymphatics can result in lymph blisters that bulge on the surface (lymphangiectasia) and weep lymph. When associated with dermal fibrosis the surface bulges are firmer and resemble cobblestones (papillomatosis). The resemblance of the skin texture to elephant hide explains the term elephantiasis. Intestinal lymph that is rerouted or refluxes into more dependent regions of the body will appear milky (chyle) due to its high fat content. Chyle may reflux into the lower limbs, genitalia, peritoneal cavity, urinary and genital tracts, pleural cavity, and other cavities such as synovial joints and pericardium. Chyle will only appear if the lymphatic incompetence extends up to the preaortic lymphatics and cisterna chyli.

Cellulitis (erysipelas)

In addition to swelling, impaired lymph drainage also predisposes to infection because of the role the lymphatic system plays in immunosurveillance. Acute inflammatory episodes identical to cellulitis can often be recurrent and frequent. Such events occur irrespective of the cause of the lymphoedema. In filarial lymphoedema secondary bacterial infections appear to be important for the progression of the elephantiasis. 'Acute attacks' manifest with increased oedema, pain, fever, or flu-like symptoms and can be

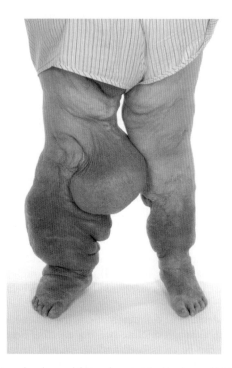

Fig. 19.1.3 Lymphoedema exhibiting characteristic skin changes (thickened skin with warty surface change and in more advanced cases 'cobblestone' papillomatosis) together with loss of shape and folds developing around the ankles.

Table 19.1.1 Criteria for diagnosis of lymphoedema

Symptoms	Persistent swelling (can be intermittent at first)
	Oedema does not resolve with overnight elevation
	Poor response to diuretics
	Associated with cellulitis
Signs	Pitting oedema (but difficult to pit)
	Thickened, warty skin
	Kaposi–Stemmer sign
Investigation	Abnormal lymph drainage routes or impaired transport on lymphoscintigraphy

prevented with long-term penicillin and improvements in skin hygiene. In primary and cancer-related lymphoedema recurrent cellulitis can be as common as in filariasis, suggesting that disturbed immune cell trafficking associated with the lymphoedema is the fundamental cause.

Differential diagnosis of the swollen limb

Both excessive capillary filtration and compromised lymph drainage frequently coexist (Fig. 19.1.5).

'Venous' oedema

Most cases of chronic venous disease giving rise to venous hypertension do not manifest with oedema because of increased lymph flow in response to increased capillary filtration. This suggests that the development of oedema in post-thrombotic syndrome and venous ulceration is as much a failure of lymph drainage as it is due solely to overwhelming microvascular fluid filtration. Correction of the superficial vein incompetence by surgery may not resolve the oedema because of co-existent and permanent lymphatic insufficiency.

Lipodermatosclerosis

Chronic 'congestion' in the lower leg resulting from both increased capillary filtration and impaired lymph drainage will often result in lipodermatosclerosis. This manifests with skin redness, induration of underlying subcutaneous tissues, and oedema. It is usually seen just above the medial malleolus or anterior gaiter region (Fig. 19.1.6). Lipodermatosclerosis is reported to occur with venous disease but it can frequently be seen with lymphoedema in the absence of venous disease. It is frequently mistaken for cellulitis but antibiotics have little effect. Only 'decongestion' through compression or elevation improves the condition.

'Armchair' legs (dependency syndrome)

This syndrome refers to those patients who sit in a chair day and night with their legs dependent. Immobility results in minimal lymph drainage and 'functional lymphoedema' ensues, i.e. there is no stimulation of lymph drainage from movement. The associated increased capillary filtration from gravitational forces leads to profound lower limb oedema. Patients predisposed are those suffering cardiac or respiratory failure who cannot lie flat, those paralysed from stroke or spinal damage including spina bifida, and those with crippling arthritis, particularly rheumatoid. Becoming more common with this scenario are excessively obese individuals with or without obstructive sleep apnoea.

Lipoedema (lipodystrophy, lipohypertrophy, lipidosis)

Frequently misdiagnosed as lymphoedema, lipoedema is almost exclusive to females with onset at or after puberty. Lipoedema (lip = fat, oedema = swelling) results in excessive fat deposition below the waist (and sometimes upper arms), but not affecting the feet. This gives rise to a disproportionate, large, pear-shaped lower half with thick, heavy, chunky legs (Fig. 19.1.7). The skin is soft, tender, and bruises easily. Pain may be a striking feature. Distinction from a gynoid-distributed obesity may be difficult, but lipoedema is not influenced by dieting and is therefore distinct from morbid obesity. Lipedema is a genetic condition with either X-linked

dominant inheritance or, more likely, autosomal dominant inheritance with sex limitation.

Clinical investigation

The investigation of choice for confirming that oedema is primarily of lymphatic origin is lymphoscintigraphy (isotope lymphography). Traditional direct-contrast radiographic lymphography is now rarely undertaken to investigate lymphoedema. MRI or CT is of value in identifying a cause for lymphatic obstruction, e.g. cancer.

Indocyanine Green lymphography has recently been developed to facilitate imaging of superficial lymphatic collecting vessels prior to lymphatico-venous anastomosis surgery. It can visualize lymphatic pumping.

Lymphoscintigraphy

A radiolabelled protein or colloid is administered via a subcutaneous or intradermal injection, and its absorption and transport through lymphatic vessels to lymph nodes is imaged by gamma camera. Theoretically lymphoscintigraphy permits examination of lymph drainage from any site to which radiolabelled tracer can be administered, as has happened with sentinel node mapping for melanoma, breast, and genital cancer management. For the investigation of a swollen limb tracer is administered bilaterally into feet or hands. Lymph drainage routes can be crudely imaged and abnormalities identified (Fig. 19.1.8). Offline calculation of time–activity curves over regions of interest permit quantitative analysis of lymph drainage. Lymphoscintigraphy is very specific, i.e. there are few false positives, but it is only 90% sensitive and may miss lymphoedema.

MRI

MRI (or CT) demonstrates a thicker skin and a 'honeycomb' pattern in the swollen subcutaneous compartment of lymphoedema. Following deep vein thrombosis of the leg the subfascial muscle compartment is enlarged, but not so in lymphoedema. MRI and CT are more objective than ultrasonography for identifying enlarged lymph nodes or pathology responsible for lymphatic obstruction such as pelvic tumour. MRI can be helpful to differentiate fat from fluid in cases of lipoedema/lipodystrophy and where there is tissue overgrowth of fat or muscle (e.g. Proteus syndrome).

Colour Doppler duplex ultrasound

Venous disease (primary varicose veins or post-thrombotic syndrome) may cause or contribute to lower limb swelling. Venous duplex ultrasonography is helpful for identifying venous reflux. Iliac vein thrombosis or compression can be a cause of whole-leg swelling.

Gene testing

Gene testing is now the definitive means of diagnosing Milroy's disease (mutations in *VEGFR3*) and lymphoedema distichiasis syndrome (OMIM 153400, mutations in *FOXC2*). Gene testing should become available for Emberger's syndrome (*GATA2*) and microcephaly lymphoedema syndrome (OMIM 152950, mutation in *KIF11*).

Treatment

Physical therapy

No drug or surgical therapy is known to improve lymph drainage. The treatment of lymphoedema relies on improving lymph

CONGENITAL			ACQUIRED				
VASCULAR	LYMPHATIC	OTHER	VASCULAR	LYMPHATIC	INFLAMMATORY	MUSCULO-SKELETAL	TUMOURS
Vascular malformation	Lymphoedema	Tissue overgrowth/ Hemihypertrophy	DVT	Lymphoedema	Cellulitis / Erysipelas	Ruptured Baker's cyst	Metastatic cancer
Diffuse phlebectasia	Lymphatic malformation	Plexiform neurofibroma	Post-Thrombotic syndrome	Armchair legs/dependency syndrome	Eczema	Haematoma or ruptured muscle	Sarcoma
Klippel Trenaunay syndrome	Lymphangioma	Proteus syndrome	Chronic venous reflux	Lipodermatosclerosis	Psoriasis	Pathological fracture	Kaposi sarcoma
Parkes-Weber syndrome		Hamartoma	Venous obstruction	Surgical trauma	Recurrent Herpes simplex	Achilles tendonitis	Lymphangiosarcoma
Maffucci's		Gigantism	Vein obliteration (IV drug abuse, chemotherapy)	Accidental trauma	Rheumatoid arthritis	Myositis ossificans	
				Vein harvesting			
				Facctitial (Tourniquet)			
				Pre-Tibial myxoedema			
				Chronic regional pain syndrome			

Fig. 19.1.5 Causes of a Chronically Swollen Limb

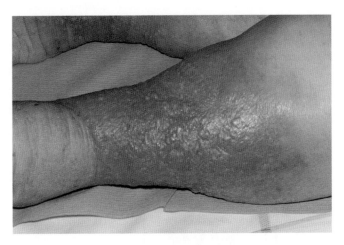

Fig. 19.1.6 Lipodermatosclerosis, a consequence of chronic congestion, manifests with fixed plum-red discolouration of skin, subcutaneous induration, and oedema—and is often mistaken for cellulitis.

drainage through the application of simple physiological principles known to stimulate lymph flow, while at the same time restoring any excessive capillary filtration to as near normal as possible. The principles of treatment are generic, but obviously vary according to individual circumstances dependent on site, e.g. facial vs leg lymphoedema, and cause, e.g. genetic lymphoedema in a child vs lymphoedema in advanced cancer.

Unlike blood flow, which is predominantly driven by the heart, lymph flow falls to low levels unless stimulated by movement and in

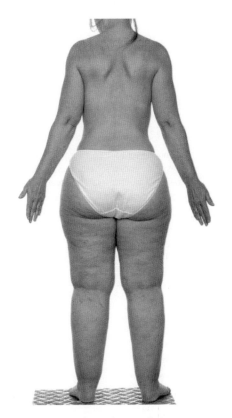

Fig. 19.1.7 Lipoedema—a condition almost exclusive to women resulting in excess subcutaneous fat on hips, buttocks, thighs, or legs giving rise to disproportionately large lower limbs and often mistaken for lymphoedema.

particular exercise. Alternating changes in interstitial fluid pressure (by active or passive exercise or massage) increase initial lymphatic filling and flow within initial lymphatics. Increases in lymph load to collecting lymphatics will stimulate greater contractility within these main pumping vessels. Patients with leg lymphoedema often notice that walking reduces swelling. The addition of a bandage or stocking will enhance the effect of movement. The idea of compression is not to squeeze fluid out of the limb with force like squeezing toothpaste out of a tube, but to create an outer collar to the leg that resists expansion of the calf muscle during contraction. This generates a high interstitial pressure during muscle contractions to drive lymph drainage. Low pressures during skeletal muscle relaxation permit lymphatic vessel refilling before further muscle contraction repeats the cycle. Compression without movement (active or passive exercises) does not improve lymph drainage. Isotonic muscle exercise and compression will be particularly helpful in circumstances where lymphatic collector contractility is impaired (normally once lymph has entered a lymphatic collecting vessel smooth muscle contractions drive lymph forwards and valves ensure unidirectional flow). Compression has the added benefit of lowering venous pressure in the leg, so reducing fluid filtration and lymph load.

Manual lymphatic drainage therapy (MLD), a specific form of lymphatic massage, operates on the same principle of stimulating alternating rises and falls in interstitial pressure and is used to decongest more proximal regions of the body, e.g. the adjoining quadrant of the trunk to a swollen limb, through which lymph from the limb needs to pass before being directed to a normally functioning lymphatic basin. In right-arm lymphoedema MLD would serve to direct collateral lymph drainage to normally draining lymph routes in the contralateral left axilla and so complement the effect of any compression and exercise to the right arm.

In moderate to severe lymphoedema treatment with an intensive course of MLD, multilayer lymphoedema bandaging, and exercise (decongestive lymphatic therapy/combined decongestive therapy) can reverse more or less all the comorbidity from swelling, including 'elephantiasis' skin changes. Once swelling has been reduced and limb shape improved, control is maintained through exercise while wearing appropriately fitted compression garments. In elderly and infirm individuals the application and removal of hosiery can be problematic, but if good technique is taught and aids to application provided then most patients will manage. Velcro wraps (e.g. Farrow wraps) provide easily applied graduated support.

Elevation of the legs is often wrongly chosen over exercise as treatment. Elevation helps oedema by lowering venous pressure and consequently reducing capillary pressure, not by improving lymph drainage. While exercise is preferred to elevation as treatment, elevation is recommended during periods of rest.

Intermittent pneumatic compression pumps probably displace fluid as much as improve lymph flow. Nevertheless, they may prove helpful for patients spending considerable time in chairs and in cases of oedema associated with high filtration.

Drug therapy

Too often diuretics are prescribed for oedema on an empirical basis without due thought for the underlying pathophysiology. Diuretics have very little effect in established lymphoedema because their main action is to reduce capillary filtration. They should only be prescribed in circumstances of salt and water retention, whereupon

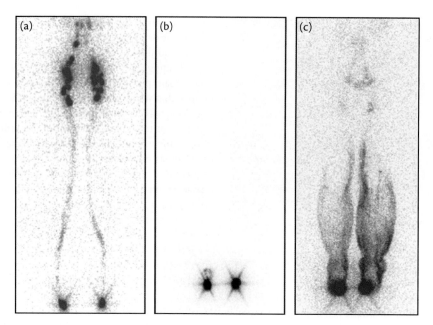

Fig. 19.1.8 Lymphoscintigraphy is the investigation of choice for determining if limb swelling is due to lymphoedema. Following a web space injection (hand or foot) of a radiolabelled colloid ($^{99\,m}$Tc–antimony sulfide colloid) the transport of radioactivity is imaged by gamma camera. Image abnormalities or a quantitative reduction in radioactivity in a region of interest within draining lymph nodes indicates lymphoedema. (a) Normal lymphoscintigraphy. (b) A patient with Milroy's disease and identified mutation in the *VEGFR3* gene giving rise to dysfunctional initial (absorbing) lymphatics in the feet. (c) A patient with lymphoedema–distichiasis due to mutation in the *FOXC2* gene that results in lymph reflux due to lymphatic valve failure.

Table 19.1.2 Antibacterials for cellulitis[a, b]

Situation	First-line antibacterials	If allergic to penicillin	Second-line antibacterials	Comments
Acute cellulitis + septicaemia (inpatient admission)	Flucloxacillin 1–2g IV q6h[c,6] _or_ amoxicillin 2g IV q8h[c] (see main text)	Clindamycin 600mg IV q6h[13]	Clindamycin 600mg IV q6h (if poor or no response by 48h)	Switch to PO flucloxacillin 500mg q.d.s. _or_ amoxicillin 500mg t.d.s. _or_ clindamycin 300mg q.d.s. when: no fever for 48h _and_ inflammation much resolved _and_ falling CRP. Then continue as below.
Acute cellulitis (home care) or emergency back-up supply of antibacterials	Flucloxacillin 500mg q.d.s. _or_ amoxicillin 500mg t.d.s.[d]	Erythromycin[e] 500mg q.d.s. _or_ clarithromycin[e] 500mg b.d.	Clindamycin 300mg q.d.s. If fails to resolve, convert to first-line IV regimen above	Give for a minimum of 2 weeks. Continue antibacterials until the acute inflammation has completely resolved; in severe cases this may take 1–2 months. (Note: residual 'staining' may persist beyond this.)
Prophylaxis if 2+ episodes of cellulitis per year	Phenoxymethylpenicillin 250mg b.d.(500mg b.d. if BMI ≥33)[14]	Erythromycin[e] 250mg once daily _or_ clarithromycin[e] 250mg once daily	Clindamycin 150mg once daily _or_ doxycycline 50mg once daily[f]	Continue for 2 years, after 1 year, halve the dose of phenoxymethylpenicillin; if acute cellulitis develops after dose reduction/discontinuation, treat the acute cellulitis and then commence _life-long_ prophylaxis

a but follow local guidelines, particularly for IV antibacterials

b PO unless stated otherwise

c add gentamicin 5mg/kg IV daily for 1 week if anogenital region involved, adjust dose according to renal function and gentamicin plasma concentration

d if *Staph. aureus* infection suspected (folliculitis, pus formation, crusted dermatitis), flucloxacillin 500mg q.d.s. should definitely be used

e for patients taking astemizole, tolterodine or statins, do *not* prescribe macrolide antibacterials (clarithromycin, erythromycin); doxycycline

f in these circumstances, review by local specialist lymphoedema services and advice from a microbiologist is recommended. There is a need to balance the use of certain antibiotics (e.g. clindamycin, cefalexin) as prophylaxis against the risk of predisposing to *C. difficile* infection.

spironolactone may be preferred. Rutoside (a glycoside) has been advocated, but clinical effect is minimal.

Calcium channel antagonists should be avoided in lymphoedema because they encourage oedema. The mechanism is unclear, but lymphatic pumping is paralysed in animal studies.

Skin care and prevention of infection

The main risk factors for cellulitis (erysipelas) are lymphatic insufficiency and loss of skin integrity (wounds, interdigital skin breaks, and leg ulcers). Good skin care is the first consideration when treating lymphoedema. This has been well demonstrated in elephantiasis and podoconiosis. Avoidance of skin damage (including sterile needle puncture), good hygiene, regular emollients, treatment of any dermatitis or fungal infection, and antisepsis following minor wounds are important. Consensus recommendations for the treatment of cellulitis with lymphoedema are found in Table 19.1.2 and at <http://www.thebls.com/cellulitis>.

Recurrent cellulitis can be a particular problem. Prophylactic phenoxymethylpenicillin 250 mg twice daily for 12 months halves rates of infection compared to placebo. Obesity, multiple previous attacks, and lymphoedema are associated with increased failure of prophylaxis.

Surgery

Surgery can involve removal of excess tissue (reducing/debulking operations or liposuction) or bypassing of local lymphatic defects. The availability of centres offering microsurgical lymphovenous and lymphatic–lymphatic anastomoses remains limited. Surgery rarely if ever obviates the need for long-term compression hosiery.

Genital lymphoedema

Genital lymphoedema may arise from a genetic fault in lymphatic development, in which case internal lymph problems, e.g. intestinal lymphangiectasia, may coexist. Acquired forms may result from filariasis, cancer treatment, infection (cellulitis), anogenital granulomatosis/Crohn's disease, and hidradenitis suppurativa. Control of any inflammation is essential for control of oedema.

Facial lymphoedema

Impaired lymph drainage within skin and subcutaneous local lymphatics is likely to be a factor in cases of facial swelling, particularly periorbital oedema associated with rosacea, dermatomyositis, and thyroid disease. Head and neck lymphoedema has become a greater burden with the increased incidence of head and neck cancer treatment.

Further reading

Alitalo K (2011). The lymphatic vasculature in disease. *Nat Med*, **17**, 13718–0.

British Lymphology Society (2005). *Consensus document on the management of cellulitis in lymphoedema.* <http://www.thebls.com/concensus.php> (updated 2013)

Brorson H (2000). Liposuction gives complete reduction of chronic large arm lymphoedema after breast cancer. *Acta Oncol*, **39**, 407–20.

Browse NL, Burnand KG, Mortimer PS (2003). *Diseases of the lymphatics.* Arnold, London.

Burnand KG, et al. (2002). Value of isotope lymphography in the diagnosis of lymphoedema of the leg. *Br J Surg*, **89**, 74–8.

Child AH, et al. (2010). Lipedema: an inherited condition. *Am J Med Genet A*, **152A**, 970–6.

Connell FC, et al. (2013). The classification and diagnostic algorithm for primary lymphatic dysplasia: an update from 2010 to include molecular findings. *Clin Genet*, **84**, 3031–4.

DiSipio T, Rye S, Newman B, Hayes S (2013). Incidence of unilateral arm lymphoedema after breast cancer: a systematic review and meta-analysis. *Lancet Oncol*, **14**, 5001–5.

Foldi M, Foldi E, Kubik S (2003). *Textbook of lymphology for physicians and lymphoedema therapists.* Urban & Fischer, San Francisco, CA.

International Society of Lymphology (2013). The diagnosis and treatment of peripheral lymphedema: 2013 Consensus Document of the International Society of Lymphology. *Lymphology*, **46**, 1–11.

Lee BB, et al. (2013) Diagnosis and treatment of primary lymphedema. Consensus document of the International Union of Phlebology (IUP)-2013. *Int Angiol*, **32**, 541–74.

Levick JR (2009). *An introduction to cardiovascular physiology*, 5th edition. CRC Press, London.

Levick JR, Michel CC (2010). Microvascular fluid exchange and the revised Starling principle. *Cardiovasc Res*, **87**, 1982–10.

Lymphoedema Framework Project (2006). *Best practice for the management of lymphoedema, international consensus.* Medical Education Partnership, London. <http://www.lympho.org/mod_turbolead/upload/file/Lympho/Best_practice_20_July.pdf>.

Mihara M, et al. (2014). High-accuracy diagnosis and regional classification of lymphedema using indocyanine green fluorescent lymphography after gynecologic cancer treatment. *Ann Plast Surg*, **72**, 204–8.

Moffatt C, et al. (2003). Lymphoedema: an underestimated health problem. *Q J Med*, **96**, 731–8.

Mortimer PS, Levick JR (2004). Chronic peripheral oedema: the critical role of the lymphatic system. *Clin Med*, **4**, 4448–53.

Nutman TB (ed.) (2000). *Lymphatic filariasis.* Imperial College Press, London.

Thomas KS, et al.; UK Dermatology Clinical Trials Network's PATCH I Trial Team (2013). Penicillin to prevent recurrent leg cellulitis. *N Engl J Med*, **368**, 1695–703.

Twycross RG, Wilcock A (2011). *Palliative care formulary*, 4th edition. <http://www.palliativedrugs.com>.

Zuther JE, Norton S (2013). *Lymphedema management*, 3rd edition. Thieme, New York.

Idiopathic oedema of women

Idiopathic oedema of women

John D. Firth

Essentials

Idiopathic oedema is an unsatisfactory label that is applied to women who complain of swelling, typically variable, with diagnosis requiring exclusion of known causes of oedema and (most authors would agree) demonstration of weight gain, from morning to evening, of more than 1.4 kg.

The cause of idiopathic oedema is (by definition) unknown: hypotheses include abnormal capillary permeability/leakage, re-feeding oedema, and diuretic-induced oedema. There is no clear relationship to the menstrual cycle. Even if not a primary cause, the use and abuse of diuretics can complicate and exacerbate the problem.

Management is difficult, but patients can be helped by a sympathetic approach from the physician and (1) encouragement to lose weight if they are obese; (2) avoidance of excess dietary salt; and (3) weaning from consumption of high doses of diuretics that can cause or exacerbate the tiredness, lethargy, weakness, and dizziness that are suffered by many.

Definition and diagnosis

In some women fluid retention occurs in the absence of any clear explanation and is termed idiopathic oedema. Since the condition typically fluctuates in severity from one time to another it is sometimes called cyclical or periodic oedema, but these terms mislead; first, because there is rarely any recognizable periodicity, and second, because the condition is not related to menstrual periods. Most women retain fluid just before the menses and lose this fluid immediately afterwards. Idiopathic oedema occurs most commonly in women aged 20 to 40 years, but has no clear relationship with the menstrual cycle and can persist after the menopause or oophorectomy.

The diagnosis of idiopathic oedema depends on the exclusion of other causes of oedema, including cardiac, hepatic, renal, allergic, or hypoproteinaemic disease, venous or lymphatic obstruction, and use of some medications. The role of diuretics, causally or in treatment, is contentious, as discussed below. However, it is always unsatisfactory when a diagnosis is made by exclusion of other conditions rather than on the basis of 'positive' criteria. Such criteria for the diagnosis of idiopathic oedema have not been universally agreed, although both Thorn and McKendry (see Kay *et al.* for discussion) have made proposals that (1) require evidence of substantial weight gain during the course of the day from morning to evening, with a figure of more than 1.4 kg often quoted, although this does not provide a clear-cut separation from normal, and (2) demand the presence of (loosely specified) emotional or psychological factors. Many authors comment on the aggravation of swelling by prolonged sitting or standing, but this does not feature in the diagnostic criteria mentioned.

Clinical features

The patient's complaint is of swelling, which usually waxes and wanes but can be constant. In the morning the face and eyelids feel swollen and heavy. By the end of the day the areas worst affected are the hands, breasts, trunk, abdomen, thighs, ankles, and feet. Rings no longer fit the swollen fingers, and undergarments and clothes can feel so uncomfortably tight that they have to be removed or replaced with something larger. The feet and ankles may be relatively spared, hence the disposition of oedema tends to be different from that in most other oedematous states, where it begins distally in the feet and ankles and progresses proximally.

Episodes or exacerbations of fluid retention often occur unpredictably, but obesity, emotional stress, and consumption of high-carbohydrate food are thought to be triggers in some. Sufferers are often mentally and physically lethargic during periods of fluid retention, frequently expressing the view that they feel bloated and ugly, even though this may not be apparent to the observer. Many appear to be emotionally labile or anxious and some are depressed, invariably (and perhaps correctly) claiming that this is secondary to the fluid retention. Other common symptoms include carpal tunnel syndrome, nonarticular rheumatism, palpitations, nonulcer dyspepsia, and headaches, and idiopathic oedema may be a factor in women troubled by severe cellulite.

Women with idiopathic oedema are often very concerned about their weight. One study showed an association between symptoms of this condition and abnormal attitudes to eating. Some patients will report that they episodically severely reduce their food intake, perhaps making them susceptible to the phenomenon of re-feeding oedema when they start eating again.

Aside from oedema, which may or may not be present at the time of medical assessment, examination is unremarkable, as are routine investigations for the cause of oedema. Those patients that have used diuretics may have a hypokalaemic hypochloraemic metabolic alkalosis.

Idiopathic oedema has been reported to be associated with a range of conditions including obesity, diabetes and psychiatric disorders. Apart from depression, the latter may include purging behaviours (self-induced vomiting, laxative abuse, diuretic abuse). Making the diagnosis of an additional 'idiopathic' condition in such circumstances is fraught with difficulties.

Pathophysiology

The cause of idiopathic oedema is not known (by definition). Because of pooling of extracellular fluid in the legs when standing, normal weight gain during the day is typically around 1 kg, and diurnal weight fluctuation of more than 1.4 kg is required for diagnosis, but weight may fluctuate from day to day by up to 4 or 5 kg. During periods of weight gain the patient may be oliguric, passing low volumes of urine in which there is little sodium (<20 mmol/litre). There are three main pathophysiological hypotheses.

Abnormal capillary permeability

The blood vessels of women with idiopathic oedema are more permeable to albumin, the fractional catabolic rate of albumin is increased, both intravascular and total body albumin pools are smaller, and the plasma volume decreases by more on standing than in normal controls. Activation of the sympathetic nervous system, renin–angiotensin–aldosterone system, and high levels of antidiuretic hormone (ADH) in the plasma that are consistent with intravascular volume depletion have all been reported, and these changes provide a plausible explanation for why the kidney retains salt and water in idiopathic oedema. They also form the background to postural water-loading or sodium-loading tests that have been advocated as diagnostic tools, although these are not used routinely in clinical practice. After similar loading on two separate occasions, patients with idiopathic oedema who remain upright throughout the test excrete less water or sodium than they do if they remain supine. However, the prime mover remains uncertain: decreased release of dopamine has been reported, as has generalized impairment of hypothalamic function.

Re-feeding oedema

If women concerned about their weight engage in 'crash dieting' followed by binge eating, then they may induce re-feeding oedema. This has led some authors to the conclusion that idiopathic oedema may be a presentation of eating disorder. Why re-feeding should precipitate oedema is not clear, but in a study of malnourished patients with anorexia nervosa, those re-fed with a low-sodium diet were less susceptible to oedema than those re-fed with a normal-sodium diet.

Diuretic-induced oedema

Many patients seen in hospital practice will already be taking diuretics or have taken them in the past, and some will be consuming large doses of loop agents every day. One influential study reported 10 such patients who started to take diuretics because of concern about swelling or their body weight and who continued to take them because cessation provoked rapid weight gain, facial bloating, and abdominal distension. When prevailed upon to stop diuretics they each gained weight (up to 5 kg), reaching a maximum in 4 to 10 days, but by 20 days 7 of the 10 had fallen to below their previous weight, and 9 of the 10 remained free of oedema over a long period of follow-up without taking diuretics. This led the authors to suggest that diuretic abuse might be the cause of all cases of idiopathic oedema. This view is not held by most with experience in the field, but rebound oedema on diuretic withdrawal can undoubtedly be an exacerbating feature, and it is appropriate to look for evidence of diuretic abuse if the patient denies taking such drugs and yet routine biochemical testing of blood and urine suggests the possibility.

Management

Women with idiopathic oedema frequently complain that doctors have not taken their condition seriously, and there is no doubt that it is a frustrating disorder for both patients and their physicians. Sympathetic explanation of the nature of the problem helps management.

A patient who is obese should be given advice as to how to lose weight, and—independent of any effect on weight—some find that reducing dietary sodium and carbohydrate intake helps. They should be advised to avoid long periods of standing or sitting and to wear loose-fitting clothing, although most will have discovered these things for themselves. Avoidance of an excessive dietary intake of sodium is a sensible recommendation. On theoretical grounds the use of elastic stockings would also seem appropriate, since these might reduce the postural reduction in plasma volume seen in idiopathic oedema. However, few find that the benefits of elastic stockings outweigh their disadvantages and it is difficult to get most patients to persist with them for long enough to see whether or not they really would be of help.

Diuretics are a real problem. It seems intuitively obvious to most patients and to many doctors that someone who is retaining fluid would benefit from a diuretic, hence many patients with idiopathic oedema end up on very large doses of loop agents, often combined with amiloride or spironolactone. Rather than helping, these may worsen symptoms of tiredness, lethargy, weakness, and dizziness by exacerbating intravascular volume depletion, and attempts to stop typically lead to rebound oedema. Long-term use of high doses of furosemide can also cause medullary nephrocalcinosis and variable degrees of renal insufficiency. Explanation is the key here, in that if patients recognize rebound oedema for what it is and relieve oedema with supine rest rather than renewed consumption of high doses of diuretics, then there is a reasonable chance that they can be weaned off diuretics with benefit.

A range of agents including levodopa, carbidopa, bromocriptine, captopril, and ephedrine have been tried in idiopathic oedema. None is of widely proven benefit. There is a single report that aminaphtone (aminophenazone) produced improvement in 70% of cases in a small series, but this drug (formerly used as an antipyretic and analgesic, but which can cause leucocytopenia) is not widely available. A recent controlled study suggested that nonsurgical periodontal therapy led to improvement in idiopathic oedema and hypothesized that this might be by reducing a source of systemic inflammation. However, the duration of follow-up was very short (4 weeks), and further studies of adequate duration are needed to know whether or not such treatment should be recommended for this chronic condition.

Further reading

Bihun JA, McSherry J, Marciano D. (1993). Idiopathic oedema and eating disorders: evidence for an association. *Int J Eat Disord*, **14**, 197–201.

Dunningan MG, *et al.* (2004). Unexplained swelling symptoms in women (idiopathic oedema) comprise one component of a common polysymptomatic syndrome. *QJM*, **97**, 755–64.

Joseph R, *et al.* (2011). Non-surgical periodontal therapy improves serum levels of C-reactive protein and edematous states in female patients with idiopathic oedema. *J Periodontol*, **82**, 201–9.

Kay A, Davis CL (1999). Idiopathic edema. *Am J Kidney Dis*, **34**, 405–23.

MacGregor GA, *et al.* (1979). Is 'idiopathic' oedema idiopathic? *Lancet*, **i**, 397–400.

Marks AD (1983). Intermittent fluid retention in women. Is it idiopathic edema? *Postgrad Med*, **73**, 75–83.

Pereira de Godoy JM (2008). Aminaphtone in idiopathic cyclic oedema syndrome. *Phlebology*, **23**, 118–19.

Sabatini S (2001). Hormonal insights into the pathogenesis of cyclic idiopathic edema. *Semin Nephrol*, **21**, 244–50.

Streeten DH (1995). Idiopathic edema. Pathogenesis, clinical features, and treatment. *Endocrinol Metabol Clin North Am*, **24**, 531–47.

Index

Notes: Abbreviations used in the index can be found on pages xv–xvii
vs. indicates a comparison or differential diagnosis
Page numbers suffixed with *f* refer to material in figures, *t* tables and *b* boxes